瓣膜性心脏病
Braunwald心脏病学姊妹篇

Valvular Heart Disease: A Companion to
Braunwald's Heart Disease

第5版 | Fifth Edition

中文精要·英文影印版

◎ 主编

[美] 凯瑟琳·M. 奥托（Catherine M. Otto）

[美] 罗伯特·O. 博诺（Robert O. Bonow）

◎ 编译

吴永健　编译委员会主任委员
许海燕

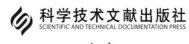

科学技术文献出版社
SCIENTIFIC AND TECHNICAL DOCUMENTATION PRESS
·北京·

图书在版编目（CIP）数据

瓣膜性心脏病：Braunwald心脏病学姊妹篇：第5版 /（美）凯瑟琳·M. 奥托（Catherine M. Otto），（美）罗伯特·O. 博诺（Robert O. Bonow）主编；吴永健，许海燕编译. —北京：科学技术文献出版社，2023.4

书名原文：Valvular Heart Disease: A Companion to Braunwald's Heart Disease（Fifth Edition）

ISBN 978-7-5189-9603-2

Ⅰ . ①瓣…　Ⅱ . ①凯…　②罗…　③吴…　④许…　Ⅲ . ①心脏瓣膜疾病—诊疗　Ⅳ . ① R542.5

中国版本图书馆 CIP 数据核字（2022）第 177300 号

著作权合同登记号 图字：01-2022-5275

中文简体字版权专有权归科学技术文献出版社所有

Elsevier (Singapore) Pte Ltd.
3 Killiney Road,
#08-01 Winsland House I,
Singapore 239519
Tel: (65) 6349-0200; Fax: (65) 6733-1817

瓣膜性心脏病：Braunwald心脏病学姊妹篇（第5版）

策划编辑：张　蓉　　　　　　责任编辑：张　蓉　赵　楠　　　　　　责任校对：张永霞　　　　　　责任出版：张志平

出　版　者　科学技术文献出版社
地　　　址　北京市复兴路15号　　邮编　100038
编　务　部　（010）58882938，58882087（传真）
发　行　部　（010）58882868，58882870（传真）
邮　购　部　（010）58882873
官 方 网 址　www.stdp.com.cn
发　行　者　科学技术文献出版社发行　全国各地新华书店经销
印　刷　者　北京地大彩印有限公司
版　　　次　2023 年 4 月第 1 版　2023 年 4 月第 1 次印刷
开　　　本　889×1194　1/16
字　　　数　1069千
印　　　张　42
书　　　号　ISBN 978-7-5189-9603-2
定　　　价　598.00元

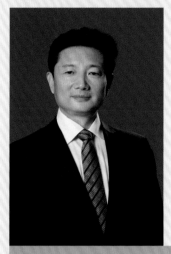

吴永健

主任医师，教授，博士研究生导师
中国医学科学院阜外医院冠心病中心主任、结构性
心脏病中心副主任

【社会任职】

现任中华医学会心血管病学分会委员、中国医师协会心血管内科医师分会常务委员、中国医师协会心脏重症专业委员会副主任委员、世界中医药学会联合会心脏康复专业委员会主任委员、海峡两岸医药卫生交流协会心脏重症专家委员会副主任委员等；担任《中国循环杂志》《中国介入心脏病学杂志》编委，《中华心血管病杂志》、英国*HEART*杂志通讯编委等。

【专业特长】

主要从事冠心病和老年瓣膜性心脏病介入治疗及其相关研究，是我国最早开展不用开胸经导管进行主动脉瓣膜置换的专家之一，从零开始探索我国经导管主动脉瓣膜置换术体系，打造国内首个经导管主动脉瓣膜置换术影像学核心实验室；已完成经导管主动脉瓣膜置换术1000余例；推广标准化经导管主动脉瓣膜置换术体系在全国100多家医院应用。

【学术成果】

承担国家和省部级科研课题12项，横向课题10项；参与研发多款其他瓣膜，并获得专利30余项；参与制定我国首个《经导管主动脉瓣置换术中国专家共识》；在国际上首次提出CT"多平面评估体系"。

编译主任委员简介

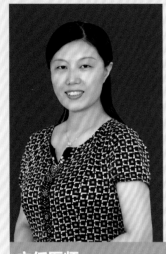

许海燕

主任医师
中国医学科学院阜外医院心内科

【社会任职】

现任中国医师协会心血管医师分会临床研究工作组委员、中国中西医结合学会心血管病专业委员会委员。

【专业特长】

擅长冠心病和瓣膜性心脏病的临床诊治、风险评估、预防康复和长期管理；最早开展了经导管主动脉瓣置换术的术前老年综合评估和围手术期序贯综合康复治疗。

【学术成果】

负责完成中国成人心脏瓣膜病队列研究；构建了我国老年心脏瓣膜疾病多功能大数据平台和多维度综合评估技术标准。

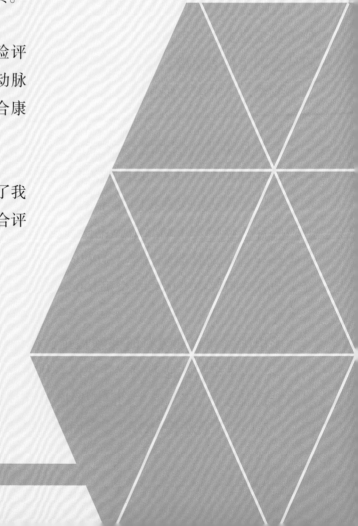

Thomas Michael Bashore, MD
Professor of Medicine
Duke University Medical Center
Durham, North Carolina

Robert O. Bonow, MD, MS
Goldberg Distinguished Professor
  of Cardiology
Department of Medicine
Northwestern University Feinberg School
  of Medicine
Chicago, Illinois

Alan C. Braverman, MD
Alumni Endowed Professor in
  Cardiovascular Diseases
Department of Medicine
Washington University School of Medicine
Saint Louis, Missouri

John D. Carroll, MD
Director, Interventional Cardiology
Division of Cardiology
University of Colorado Denver
Aurora, Colorado

Javier G. Castillo, MD
Director, Hispanic Heart Center
Cardiovascular Surgery
The Mount Sinai Hospital
New York, New York

João L. Cavalcante, MD
Director, Cardiac MRI, Structural CT,
  and Cardiovascular Imaging Research Center & Core Lab
Minneapolis Heart Institute
Abbott Northwestern Hospital
Minneapolis, Minnesota

John B. Chambers, MD
Professor of Clinical Cardiology
Cardiothoracic Department
Guy's and St Thomas' Hospitals
London, United Kingdom

Andrew Cheng, MD
Assistant Professor
Department of Medicine
University of Washington/VA Puget Sound Health Care System
Seattle, Washington

Milind Desai, MD
Haslam Family Endowed Chair in CV
  Medicine
Director, Clinical Operations
Cardiovascular Medicine
Heart and Vascular Institute
Professor of Medicine
Cleveland Clinic Lerner College of Medicine
Cleveland Clinic
Cleveland, Ohio

Danny Dvir, MD
Cardiology
Shaarei Tzedek Medical Centre
Hebrew University
Jerusalem, Israel
Affiliate Assistant Professor of Medicine
University of Washington School of Medicine
Seattle, Washington

Marc R. Dweck, MD, PhD
BHF Senior Lecturer and Consultant
  Cardiologist
Center for Cardiovascular Science
University of Edinburgh
Edinburgh, United Kingdom

Maurice Enriquez-Sarano, MD
Division of Cardiovascular Diseases
  and Internal Medicine
Mayo Clinic
Rochester, Minnesota

John P. Erwin III, MD
Chair, Department of Internal Medicine
NorthShore University HealthSystem
Chicago, Illinois

Arturo Evangelista, MD
Department of Cardiology
Hospital Universitari Vall d´Hebron
Corazón-Quironsalud-Teknon Institute
Barcelona, Spain

Russell J. Everett, MD, PhD
Specialty Trainee in Cardiology
Center for Cardiovascular Sciences
University of Edinburgh
Edinburgh, United Kingdom

Benjamin H. Freed, MD
Assistant Professor of Medicine
Division of Cardiology
Department of Medicine

Northwestern University Feinberg School
of Medicine
Chicago, Illinois

Paul Grayburn, MD
Director, Cardiology Research
Internal Medicine
Baylor University Medical Center
Dallas, Texas

Rebecca T. Hahn, MD
Director of Interventional Echocardiography
Center for Interventional and Vascular
Therapy
Department of Medicine
Irving Medical Center
New York, New York

Mohanad Hamandi, MD
Postdoctoral Fellow
Cardiovascular Research
The Heart Hospital Baylor Plano
Plano, Texas

Howard C. Hermann, MD
John W. Bryfogle Jr. Professor of
Cardiovascular Medicine
Cardiovascular Division
Perelman School of Medicine of the
University of Pennsylvania
Philadelphia, Pennsylvania

Bernard Iung, MD
Cardiologist
Department of Cardiology
Bichat Hospital
Professor of Cardiology
Université de Paris
Paris, France

Yuli Y. Kim, MD
Medical Director
Philadelphia Adult Congenital Heart Center
Hospital of the University of Pennsylvania and The Children's
Hospital of Philadelphia
Philadelphia, Pennsylvania

Susheel Kodali, MD
Assistant Professor of Medicine
Center for Interventional Vascular Therapy
Columbia University Irving Medical Center
New York, New York

Eric V. Krieger, MD
Associate Professor
Division of Cardiology
Department of Internal Medicine
University of Washington School
of Medicine
Seattle, Washington

Roberto M. Lang, MD
Professor of Medicine and Radiology
Director, Noninvasive Cardiac Imaging
Laboratories
Section of Cardiology
Heart and Vascular Center
University of Chicago Medicine
Chicago, Illinois

James Lee, MD
Associate Director of Echocardiography
Advanced Cardiovascular Imaging
Division of Cardiology
Henry Ford Heart and Vascular Institute
Detroit, Michigan

Grace Lin, MD
Associate Professor
Cardiovascular Diseases
Mayo Clinic
Rochester, Minnesota

Brian R. Lindman, MD, MSc
Associate Professor of Medicine
Medical Director, Structural Heart and Valve Center
Cardiovascular Division
Vanderbilt University Medical Center
Nashville, Tennessee

Jason P. Linefsky, MD
Associate Professor of Medicine
Department of Medicine
Emory University School of Medicine
Decatur, Georgia

Michael J. Mack, MD
Medical Director, Cardiovascular Service Line
Cardiovascular Services
Baylor Scott & White Health
Dallas, Texas

S. Chris Malaisrie, MD
Attending Cardiac Surgeon
Professor of Surgery
Bluhm Cardiovascular Institute
Northwestern Medicine
Department of Surgery
Division of Cardiac Surgery
Northwestern University Feinberg School
of Medicine
Chicago, Illinois

Patrick M. McCarthy, MD
Executive Director
Bluhm Cardiovascular Institute
Vice President, Northwestern Medical Group
Chief, Cardiac Surgery
Heller-Sacks Professor of Surgery
Department of Surgery
Division of Cardiac Surgery
Northwestern University/Northwestern
Memorial Hospital
Chicago, Illinois

David Messika-Zeitoun, MD, PhD
Professor of Cardiology
Department of Cardiology
University of Ottawa Heart Institute
Ottawa, Ontario, Canada

Akhil Narang, MD
Assistant Professor of Medicine
Northwestern University Feinberg School
  of Medicine
Chicago, Illinois

David E. Newby, MD, PhD
BHF John Wheatley Chair of Cardiology
Center for Cardiovascular Sciences
University of Edinburgh
Edinburgh, United Kingdom

Patrick T. O'Gara, MD
Senior Physician
Division of Cardiovascular Medicine
Watkins Family Distinguished Chair in
  Cardiology
Brigham and Women's Hospital
Professor of Medicine
Harvard Medical School
Boston, Massachusetts

Catherine M. Otto, MD
Professor of Medicine
J. Ward Kennedy-Hamilton Endowed Chair in Cardiology
Department of Medicine
Division of Cardiology
University of Washington School of Medicine
Seattle, Washington

Donald C. Oxorn, MD
Professor of Anesthesiology
Adjunct Professor of Medicine (Cardiology)
University of Washington School of Medicine
Seattle, Washington

Amisha Patel, MD
Assistant Professor of Medicine
Center for Interventional Vascular Therapy
Columbia University Irving Medical Center
New York, New York

Philippe Pibarot, DVM, PhD
Professor of Medicine
Department of Medicine
Laval University
Québec Heart & Lung Institute
Québec City, Québec, Canada

Jyothy Puthumana, MD
Associate Professor of Cardiology
Northwestern University Feinberg School
  of Medicine
Chicago, Illinois

Robert A. Quaife, MD
Professor of Medicine and Radiology
University of Colorado School of Medicine
Director, Advanced Cardiac Imaging
University of Colorado Hospital
Anschutz Medical Campus
Aurora, Colorado

Ernesto E. Salcedo, MD
Professor of Medicine
Medicine/Cardiology
University of Colorado Denver
Denver, Colorado

Paul Schoenhagen, MD
Professor
Department of Radiology
Cleveland Clinic Lerner College of Medicine
Cleveland, Ohio

Karen K. Stout, MD
Associate Chief
Division of Cardiology
Professor of Medicine
University of Washington School
  of Medicine
Seattle, Washington

George Thanassoulis, MD, MSc
Associate Professor of Medicine
McGill University Health Center
Montreal, Québec, Canada

James Thomas, MD
Professor of Medicine
Northwestern University Feinberg School
  of Medicine
Chicago, Illinois

Pilar Tornos, MD
Department of Cardiology
Hospital Quirónsalud
Barcelona, Spain

Wendy Tsang, MD, MSc
Assistant Professor
Division of Cardiology
Toronto General Hospital
University of Toronto
Toronto, Ontario, Canada

Alec Vahanian, MD
Professor of Cardiology
Université de Paris
Paris, France

Andrew Wang, MD
Professor of Medicine
Vice Chief for Clinical Servcies
Duke University Medical Center
Durham, North Carolina

编译委员会名单

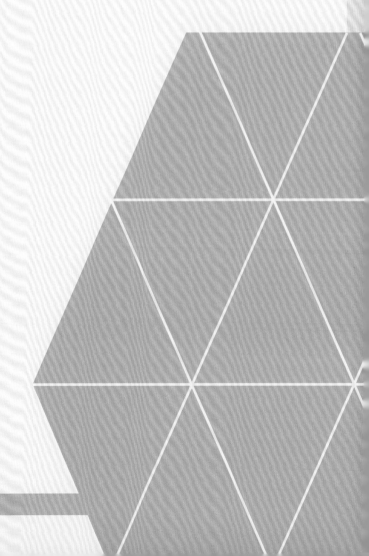

目前，瓣膜性心脏病仍然是一个重要的临床问题。据估计，全世界有1700万人受到该疾病的影响，仅在美国，该病每年会造成约2万人死亡，近10万人住院。近年来，在瓣膜性心脏病的流行病学、评估和疾病管理方面取得了许多重要进展。尽管风湿热在高收入国家已基本消失，但在这些地区由于人口老龄化，瓣膜病的发病率在逐年增加。而在低收入国家，由于风湿性心脏病的发病率尚未下降，同时老年人的数量和高龄相关的瓣膜疾病却在增加，所以瓣膜性心脏病的发病率也在上升。

在对瓣膜性心脏病患者进行评估时，临床病史仍然是最重要且不能轻易忽视的信息，因为对活动能力的评估和对疾病进展的估计对于决定是否采取有创干预措施具有至关重要的意义。以三维超声心动图、心脏MRI和CT为代表的无创成像技术的出现为瓣膜性心脏病的诊治提供了丰富解剖学和功能信息。基于导管的瓣膜介入技术已成为瓣膜病治疗领域的最重要进展。正是因为瓣膜介入技术的出现，结构性心脏病作为一个新兴的亚专业才能取得如此繁荣的发展。尽管如此，开胸手术在瓣膜性心脏病患者的治疗方面仍发挥着重要作用。因而在瓣膜性心脏病患者治疗决策的制定中，应更多采取"心脏团队"模式，即包括一名心脏病专家、一名在多模态影像评估方面有经验的医师、一名介入心脏病专家和一名心脏外科医师。

Valvular Heart Disease: A Companion to Braunwald's Heart Disease（*Fifth Edition*）的主编Catherine M. Otto和Robert O. Bonow是瓣膜性心脏病领域的世界级专家。本书系统而深入地介绍了瓣膜性心脏病的发病机制、病理生理学、临床表现、影像学、疾病自然史和治疗方案，并详细阐述了瓣膜置换治疗方面的难点。

Valvular Heart Disease: A Companion to Braunwald's Heart Disease（*Fifth Edition*）吸取了前几版内容的精华，所有章节都经过了彻底的修订，并增加了4个新的章节。该系列教材已成为瓣膜病领域最先进的教科书。在本书编辑过程中，有18位新作者参与其中，每一位都是其所编写领域的权威。感谢编辑和

作者的重要贡献，并欢迎这本杰出的新教材加入日益壮大的Braunwald心脏病学系列书籍的大家庭。

Eugene Braunwald, MD

Peter Libby, MD

Douglas L. Mann, MD

Gordon F. Tomaselli, MD

Deepak Bhatt, MD, MPH

Scott Solomon, MD

瓣膜性心脏病（瓣膜病）的基础科研、临床评估和治疗技术正在以惊人的速度发展。在瓣膜病知识迅速扩增的背景下，我们很高兴推出 *Valvular Heart Disease: A Companion to Braunwald's Heart Disease*（*Fifth Edition*）。相信这本书将成为心脏病学及外科医师、在职医师和各级学生的宝贵、权威的学习资源。

与 *Valvular Heart Disease: A Companion to Braunwald's Heart Disease* 的前几版相同，第五版广泛涵盖瓣膜性心脏病领域最重要的内容，不仅提供了瓣膜性心脏病诊断和治疗的基础知识，并且阐述了令人兴奋的新进展及其改变心脏瓣膜病患者临床预后的可能性。在来自美国、加拿大和欧洲等国际知名学者的帮助下，我们对该版本进行了彻底的修订，以保持内容的推陈出新和即时性。在28个章节的编写过程中，约50%的新作者加入，他们均在各自的学科领域具有非常高的成就并得到认可。各章节经过了重新编排，尤其是将主动脉瓣和二尖瓣疾病的影像学和介入治疗紧密联系起来。

本书从了解瓣膜性心脏病的基础开始，包括流行病学、三维解剖学、疾病的分子生物学机制、遗传和临床风险因素、医学治疗基本原则，以及患者个体化手术风险的评估方法。在主动脉瓣疾病相关章节中，分别讨论了主动脉瓣狭窄、主动脉瓣反流和二叶式主动脉瓣疾病，并详细介绍了经导管主动脉瓣置换术和外科主动脉瓣置换术的患者选择和手术操作问题。接下来的8章涉及二尖瓣疾病的不同方面，包括风湿性二尖瓣狭窄、原发性二尖瓣反流、继发性二尖瓣反流、经导管介入治疗和二尖瓣外科手术。重点章节讨论了影像学在经导管介入治疗围手术期所发挥的重要作用。本书最后一部分讨论了三尖瓣疾病、肺动脉瓣疾病、心内膜炎、人工瓣膜、人工瓣膜狭窄的经导管介入，以及妊娠期瓣膜性心脏病的治疗管理。

本书涉及的热门话题和关键治疗技术包括经导管主动脉瓣置换术、经导管二尖瓣球囊成形术、原发性和继发性二尖瓣反流的经导管修复术、外科二尖瓣修复和置换、三尖瓣反流的干预措施、经导管肺动脉瓣植入术和瓣中瓣经导管主动脉瓣置换术的时机与方法，以及人工瓣膜患者的管理、主动脉瓣和二尖瓣的影像学、妊娠期女性瓣膜病的管理和心内膜炎诊断与治疗的进展。

Valvular Heart Disease: A Companion to Braunwald's Heart Disease（*Fifth Edition*）还包括750多幅更新的解剖与生理学、方法学、流程图和临床实例插图，并且在线版本中还提供了更多的数字和视频内容。各章还包括美国心脏学会（American College of Cardiology，ACC）/美国心脏协会（American Heart Association，AHA）和欧洲心脏病学会（European Society of Cardiology，ECS）/欧洲心胸外科协会（European Association of Cardio-Thoracic Surgery，EACTS）的指南推荐，每章的相关推荐均已用表格总结出。

感谢所有作者，他们投入了大量时间和精力，确保了*Valvular Heart Disease: A Companion to Braunwald's Heart Disease*（*Fifth Edition*）的高质量和权威性。同时很高兴本书成为*Braunwald*心脏病学系列书籍中的全新成员。本书可在配套网站上在线阅读，且电子版包括比印刷版更多的图表。这些图表还可直接从网站下载，用于电子幻灯片演示。此外，还有大量视频内容，对许多章节的印刷版内容进行了补充。

尽管在诊断和治疗（包括手术和介入治疗）方面取得了进展，瓣膜性心脏病仍然是全世界发病和死亡的主要原因。风湿性心脏病仍然是世界上许多发展中国家所共同面临的公共健康问题，先天性的主动脉瓣和二尖瓣疾病是造成发达国家和发展中国家中青年主动脉瓣狭窄、主动脉瓣反流和二尖瓣反流的主要原因。随着世界范围人口老龄化进程加快，越来越多的老年患者患有退行性主动脉瓣狭窄和二尖瓣反流，并经常出现与年龄相关的医疗并发症，给医疗决策的制定带来挑战。现阶段，大多数其他形式心血管疾病的治疗决策可由多个大规模随机对照临床试验所建立的证据基础来指导，而瓣膜疾病的证据基础却因临床试验缺乏而受到限制。在瓣膜病领域，专家的临床判断和经验是合理决策和优化患者管理的基石，该点比任何其他领域都重要。*Valvular Heart Disease: A Companion to Braunwald's Heart Disease*（*Fifth Edition*）一书汇集了笔者的理论知识、工作经验和专业性临床判断，相信其将成为瓣膜性心脏病领域一线工作人员的宝贵资源。

Robert O. Bonow, MD, MS

Catherine M. Otto, MD

衷心地感谢许多帮助这本书最终成为现实的朋友们，特别是向杰出的各章节作者为本书付出时间和努力表达深深的谢意，同时感谢Elsevier出版社工作人员的指导和密切合作。最后，最重要的是感谢家人们的理解、鼓励和支持。

随着人口老龄化的不断加剧及经导管瓣膜介入技术的飞速发展，瓣膜性心脏病已逐渐由外科治疗的方式向介入治疗方式过渡。老年瓣膜性心脏病的病因、病理改变和临床表现与过去相比均发生了很大变化。近些年，无论基础研究还是临床研究均取得了显著成绩。经导管的器械研发和治疗技术日新月异，而其无论从技术路线、诊疗思路、手术操作和结果评价均存在明显不同。可以说，在心血管疾病的所有亚专业中，瓣膜性心脏病是发展最快的。因此，对于广大从业者而言，迫切需要一部专业著作进行学习。

由Catherine M. Otto和Robert O. Bonow主编的*Valvular Heart Disease: A Companion to Braunwald's Heart Disease*（*Fifth Edition*）已问世，其作为*Braunwald*心脏病学的系列丛书，是目前瓣膜性心脏病领域广受欢迎的专业著作。与既往该领域的其他专著不同，该图书更加重视瓣膜性心脏病经导管治疗。因此，该图书不仅适用于心脏外科医师，同样适用于心脏内科医师，尤其是介入心脏病学医师。图书中对如何进行临床和影像学评估、手术操作的讲解均非常具体，体现了编写人员直接的临床经验和感受。很多部分的表述让从事该技术的专业人员有一种"感同身受"的体会。为了让读者更加系统地掌握瓣膜性心脏病的相关知识和技术，该图书亦对瓣膜性心脏病的基础知识（如病因、病理学和病理生理学）均进行了深入浅出的讲解。书中配有大量的解剖图谱和表格，让读者非常容易地学习和理解。其对于从事瓣膜性心脏病基础和临床研究的专业人员而言的确是一本好的学习用书和工作参考书。

为尽快将该图书介绍给中国读者，玲珑医学经努力获得了该图书在中国的Elsevier出版授权，并与科学技术文献出版社联合出版这部影印版的*Valvular Heart Disease: A Companion to Braunwald's Heart Disease*（*Fifth Edition*）。所谓影印版即编译者对每一章节重点内容进行提炼，以此读者既可快速了解该章节的主要内容，也可对所感兴趣的章节详细阅读英文原文。这是在图书进口和翻译工作中的一次大胆尝试，主要考虑到我国读者的英文阅读能力普遍提高，且临床工作比较繁忙，阅读成为一种奢侈，而本书可满足读者不同的需求。参与本图书的编译者大多为来自中国医学科学院阜外医院瓣膜性心脏病团队的一线人员，他们参与到本书的编译既是一种学习，也是一种责任和荣誉。衷心地希望编译者的学习和劳动能够为广大的读者朋友所认同。当然，因是首次尝试编译工作，个中问题和不足在所难免，还望读者朋友提出批评和指正。期待这本影印版的瓣膜性心脏病专著能够给读者朋友带来帮助。

吴永健　许海燕

2022年12月

中文目录

Braunwald的心脏病书籍系列

BRAUNWALD'S HEART DISEASE COMPANIONS

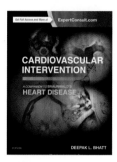

BHATT
Cardiovascular Intervention

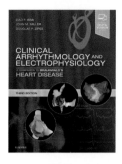

ISSA, MILLER, AND ZIPES
Clinical Arrhythmology and Electrophysiology

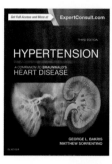

BAKRIS AND SORRENTINO
Hypertension

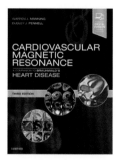

MANNING AND PENNELL
Cardiovascular Magnetic Resonance

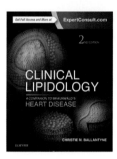

BALLANTYNE
Clinical Lipidology

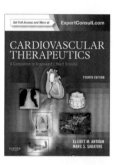

ANTMAN AND SABATINE
Cardiovascular Therapeutics

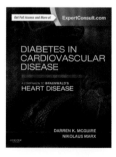

MCGUIRE AND MARX
Diabetes in Cardiovascular Disease

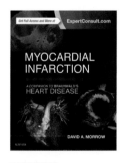

MORROW
Myocardial Infarction

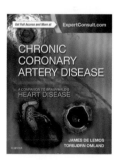

DE LEMOS AND OMLAND
Chronic Coronary Artery Disease

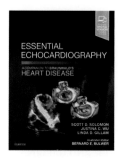

SOLOMON, WU, AND GILLAM
Essential Echocardiography

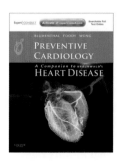

BLUMENTHAL, FOODY, AND WONG
Preventive Cardiology

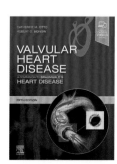

OTTO AND BONOW
Valvular Heart Disease

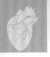

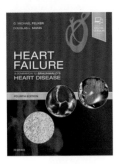

FELKER AND MANN
Heart Failure

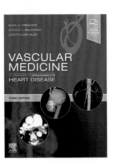

CREAGER
Vascular Medicine

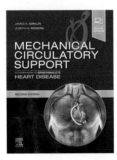

KIRKLIN AND ROGERS
Mechanical Circulatory Support

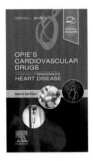

BHATT
Opie's Cardiovascular Drugs

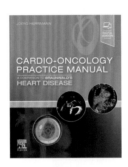

HERRMANN
Cardio-Oncology Practice Manual

BRAUNWALD'S HEART DISEASE REVIEW AND ASSESSMENT

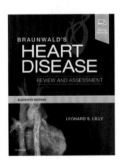

LILLY
Braunwald's Heart Disease Review and Assessment

BRAUNWALD'S HEART DISEASE IMAGING COMPANIONS

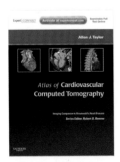

TAYLOR
Atlas of Cardiovascular Computed Tomography

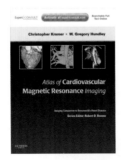

KRAMER AND HUNDLEY
Atlas of Cardiovascular Magnetic Resonance Imaging

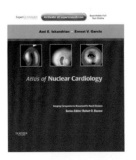

ISKANDRIAN AND GARCIA
Atlas of Nuclear Cardiology

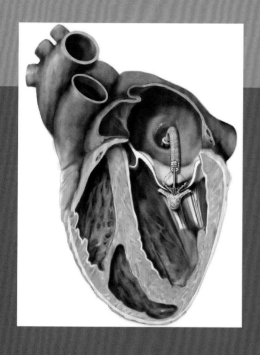

第1章
瓣膜性心脏病的流行病学

　　瓣膜性心脏病是一组常见疾病，先天或后天、遗传或环境因素导致瓣膜解剖或功能异常。目前关于瓣膜性心脏病的流行病学数据并不完善，各国调查研究均有不同局限性，总体瓣膜病的检出率仍较低，粗略估计全球有2.5%的人群患病。不同人口和地域国家的瓣膜性心脏病疾病谱和病因均有明显不同，在发展中国家，风湿热和慢性风湿性心脏病是最常见病因，全球每年新发急性风湿热患者为47.1万，2016年估计慢性风湿性心脏病患者为3000万，心内膜心肌纤维化在非洲赤道地区是瓣膜性心脏病的第二病因；而在发达国家，20世纪后半叶，随着经济发展，风湿热的发病逐渐减少，钙化性退行性变和继发性二尖瓣反流在老年人中更多见，年轻患者多为二尖瓣脱垂和二叶式主动脉瓣畸形。在美国，瓣膜病在老年人中最常见，其在75岁以上老年人中占13%。近年来，药物引起的瓣膜病也有所增加，感染性心内膜炎多与体内植入性器械和静脉用药相关，生物人工瓣膜衰败在各国家和地区也均成为主要问题。各国医疗资源参差不齐，全球主要挑战是预防慢性风湿性心脏病，其需要社会、政府和医疗系统共同合作。本章详细介绍了瓣膜性心脏病的发病率、病因和分类。

许海燕

Epidemiology of Valvular Heart Disease

John B. Chambers

CHAPTER OUTLINE

KEY POINTS

- Valve disease is globally common, affecting approximately 2.5% of the population.
- In industrially underdeveloped countries, rheumatic disease (RhD) is the most common cause. Endomyocardial fibrosis is an underresearched disease common in equatorial Africa.
- In industrially developed regions, diseases of old age predominate, particularly calcific aortic stenosis and secondary mitral regurgitation.
- In the United States, valve disease is most common among the elderly, with a prevalence of 13% among those older than 75 years.

- Drug-induced valve disease is increasing as a result of 5-HT2B receptor agonists.
- Infective endocarditis is increasingly related to medical devices and intravenous drug use.
- Failure of biological replacement valves is a major burden in all regions of the world.
- Substantial variation in access to health care exists in all countries, including those that are industrially developed.
- The main global challenge is to prevent chronic RhD, which will require collaborations among social, political, and medical programs.

Heart valve disease is the term for any deviation from normal valve anatomy or function. This includes a wide spectrum of severity, from mild mitral prolapse to a flail mitral leaflet or aortic sclerosis to critical aortic stenosis. The term does not describe a unitary diagnosis but instead a set of conditions affecting one or more of the four heart valves caused by genetic, environmental, or acquired pathologic processes that vary with geography and demography.

Our knowledge of the epidemiology of valve disease is incomplete. The global disease survey[1,2] used 56,356 unique sources of data from 195 countries to estimate incidence, prevalence, mortality, and disability rates arising from 328 diseases and injuries. Rheumatic disease (RhD) and infective endocarditis (IE) were the only valve diseases recorded.

National or large-scale screening programs for RhD exist in some countries (e.g., Australia, Cambodia, Fiji, India, Laos, Mali, Mozambique, New Caledonia, New Zealand, Nicaragua, Pakistan, Samoa, South Africa, Tonga, Yemen),[3] but most surveys of RhD are of children and young adults and are restricted geographically and by time. Countrywide estimates are usually extrapolated from these small studies to people of all ages and socioeconomic classes and therefore remain uncertain. In the industrially developed world, there have been population surveys of all types of valve disease in the United States[4] and Norway[5] and studies of the elderly in the United Kingdom.[6] Otherwise, work has focused on aortic stenosis,[7,8] mitral prolapse,[9] or bicuspid aortic valve.[10,11]

There are other limitations to our knowledge. Estimates of the prevalence of valve disease vary with the method of diagnosis, which for RhD was originally clinical but more recently includes echocardiography, which is approximately 10 times more sensitive than auscultation.[12] The prevalence and types of valve disease differ whether

TABLE 1.1   Principal Causes of Valve Disease with Prevalence or Incidence When Known.

	Prevalence in Economically Poorer Countries	Prevalence in Economically Richer Countries	References
Causes			
Chronic rheumatic heart disease	0.9%–4.0%	0.3%	17–22
Endomyocardial fibrosis	20%[a]		23
Calcific aortic stenosis		0.4%[b]	3
Bicuspid aortic valve		0.5%–0.8%[b]	9,10
Mitral regurgitation		1.7%	3
Mitral prolapse		2%–3%	8,23
Prolapse and mitral regurgitation		0.2%–0.3%	20,21
Secondary mitral regurgitation		1.4%[c]	
Failing biological replacement valves			
Aortic dilation			
Inflammatory conditions (e.g., SLE, rheumatoid arthritis)			
Drugs, carcinoid, radiation			
Incidence per 100,000 Population per Annum			
Acute rheumatic fever, all attacks	10–374	30	17–19
Acute rheumatic fever, first attack	8–51	≤10	17–19,22
New rheumatic heart disease	20		24
Infective endocarditis	3.4	1.4–6.2	25,26

[a]Coastal Mozambique.
[b]The world population is 7,000,000,000. The proportion older than 60 years is about 10%, or 700,000,000. Assuming a prevalence of aortic stenosis of 1.74% in this age group[3] gives a world prevalence of aortic stenosis of 12 million. The prevalence of bicuspid valve is 35 million based on a population prevalence of 0.5%.[10] In a study of patients with bicuspid aortic valves with a mean age of 32 years at baseline and followed for 20 years, 28 (13%) of 212 needed aortic valve replacement for severe aortic stenosis.[27] This suggests that about 4.5 million in the world could have severe aortic stenosis as a result of a bicuspid aortic valve and that the total as a result of nonrheumatic disease (calcific stenosis in those older than 65 years and bicuspid aortic valve in those younger than 65) could be 16.5 million.
[c]Estimated as U.S. population prevalence of mitral regurgitation minus prevalence of mitral regurgitation caused by mitral prolapse.
SLE, Systemic lupus erythematosus.

assessment occurs by community screening,[4,6,8] open access echocardiography,[13,14] or hospital services.[15] For example, the frequency of bicuspid aortic valves is 0.5% to 0.8% in community surveys,[10,11] 2% in a postmortem study,[16] and approximately 67% among patients in their 40s who have aortic valve replacement.[17]

The limitations make it difficult to talk about the epidemiology of valve disease in general, but there are two broad patterns (Table 1.1).[3,8–10,17–26] The first occurs in economically disadvantaged areas of the world characterized by poor housing, sanitation, and nutrition and with inadequate access to medical care. These areas include parts of Africa, the Indian subcontinent, the Middle East, and South America.

Valve disease is predominantly caused by rheumatic fever (RhF) and chronic RhD. Patients are typically young, and the morbidity and mortality rates are high. Acute RhF occurs mainly between the ages of 5 and 15 years, and heart failure, usually as a result of acute rheumatic mitral regurgitation, occurs most commonly within a year of the acute episode.[18,19] In Ethiopia, 20% with RhD die before the age of 5 years and 80% before 25 years.[20] Endocarditis, stroke, and heart failure are common sequelae. Mitral prolapse occurs within the differential diagnosis of chronic RhD diagnosed by echocardiography. There are also a number of geographically localized diseases. Endomyocardial fibrosis (EMF) is second in incidence to RhD in Equatorial Africa. Subvalvar

aneurysms are the third most common cause of mitral regurgitation after RhD and mitral prolapse in sub-Saharan Africa.

The second pattern occurs in economically richer areas, where the epidemiology of valve disease changed (Box 1.1)[27] in the second half of the 20th century, with a decrease in the incidence of rheumatic fever as a result of better housing to reduce overcrowding, better nutrition,[21] and better health care. There also was a change in streptococcal serotypes. Rheumatogenic serotypes were found in 50% of children with pharyngitis in Chicago between 1961 and 1968, compared with 11% between 2000 and 2004.[22] Calcific degeneration, secondary mitral regurgitation, and aortic dilation leading to aortic regurgitation predominantly affect older people; mitral prolapse and bicuspid aortic valve are found in younger people.

New types of valve disease are increasing in frequency as a result of drugs or radiation exposure. IE has a different pattern from that in the developing world. With older populations, more *Staphylococcus aureus* and more cases as a result of health care, mainly hemodialysis and implanted electrical devices.[28] Tricuspid regurgitation as a result of endocardial pacing systems and defibrillators is also increasingly seen.[23]

These two patterns are usually taken to apply broadly to the industrially underdeveloped and developed regions of the world. However, this is an oversimplification because pockets of poverty exist in the

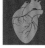

> ### BOX 1.1 Changing Epidemiology of Valve Disease in Industrialized Countries
>
> - Reasons for reduced rheumatic disease with a decrease in acute rheumatic fever cases:
>   Better housing and reduced overcrowding
>   Better nutrition
>   Better health care (e.g., treatment of throat infections, better secondary prophylaxis)
>   Fall in rheumatogenic serotypes[a]
> - Increasing age expectancy, leading to more degenerative disease
> - New types of valve disease requiring treatment (e.g., radiation, drugs)
> - More health care–related endocarditis
> - Biological replacement valves used in younger patients resulting in more reoperations, including valve-in-valve transcatheter procedures
> - More mild disease as a result of increased use of echocardiography

[a]There were rheumatogenic serotypes in 50% of children with pharyngitis in Chicago between 1961 and 1968, compared with 11% between 2000 and 2004.[27]

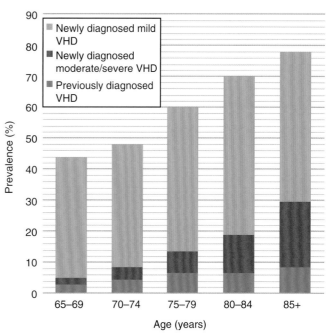

Fig. 1.1 Newly Detected and Previously Known Valvular Heart Disease *(VHD)* **by Age From the OxVALVE Study.** Subjects 65 years of age or older without known valve disease and who were registered with one of five primary care medical centers were invited to participate. For the first 2500 enrolled participants, the mean age (SD) was 73 (6) years, 51.5% were female, and 99% were white. The plot illustrates that a substantial burden of valve disease was not previously detected. (From d'Arcy JL, Coffey S, Loudon MA, et al. Large-scale community echocardiographic screening reveals a major burden of undiagnosed valvular heart disease in older people: the OxVALVE Population Cohort Study. Eur Heart J 2016;37:3515-3522.)

industrially developed world (e.g., indigenous populations of Australia and New Zealand). Conversely, richer people in the disadvantaged areas of the world are more likely to reflect patterns of valve disease usually seen in the industrially developed areas. Many countries, such as India and China, are in the process of rapid development and have a falling incidence of RhF while retaining a higher prevalence of chronic rheumatic heart disease among the more elderly population than seen in the United States or Western Europe.[18]

INCIDENCE AND PREVALENCE OF VALVE DISEASE

Valve disease remains underdetected[6,12] (Fig. 1.1) in developed and developing countries. In the developing world, the detection rate is approximately 10% using clinical examination alone without systematic echocardiographic screening.[12,24] In the United States,[4] the prevalence of moderate or severe valve disease is 1.8% when estimated from echocardiograms performed as clinically indicated compared with an age-corrected population prevalence of 2.5%. In the U.K. Oxford Valve (OxVALVE) study,[6] the prevalence of previously undiagnosed moderate or severe valve disease was 6.4% for people aged 65 years of age or older and was already identified in another 4.9% (see Fig. 1.1).

A survey of open access studies found that significant valve disease was suspected from a murmur in 127 patients but was unsuspected in 177 cases.[14] Postmortem examinations show that only about 50% of aortic stenosis cases may be diagnosed before death,[25] and undetected or underinvestigated aortic stenosis is an important cause of perioperative and maternal deaths.[26] Detection rates may increase in the future with improved access to point-of-care echocardiography,[29,30] perhaps aided by improved analysis of murmurs using artificial intelligence linked with mobile phone technology.

Access to valve surgery is restricted. In India and Africa, valve operations are performed at a rate of 1.8 per 100,000 people each year.[31] This compares with 28 operations per 100,000 people in the Netherlands[32] and 122 operations per 100,000 people in the United States. In Brazil, only 11,000 operations are performed each year, and 80% of those needing surgery remain on a waiting list.[27] There is also variation in access to surgery in industrially developed countries. A comparison of rates of aortic valve replacement in the United Kingdom against estimated need found a variance between observed and expected ranging between −356 and +230.[33] The causes of this variance have not been explored but may partly reflect the activity of community

physicians. The elderly are particularly disadvantaged, and about one third with aortic stenosis are denied surgery inappropriately.[34] Developing a transcatheter program leads to an increase in conventional surgical rates[35] because clinically inappropriate perceptual barriers to referral are lifted.

Valve Disease in Industrially Underdeveloped Areas

The global burden of RhD was assessed in a World Health Organization (WHO) report in 2005,[36] two reports in 2011,[18,37] and the global burden of disease study most recently updated in 2017.[1,2] All but the first of these used echocardiographic diagnosis, but the criteria for echocardiographic diagnosis have changed.

Incidence of Rheumatic Fever and Chronic Rheumatic Disease

The annual incidence of all first or subsequent attacks of acute RhF worldwide is estimated at 471,000 cases[38] based on a meta-analysis of regional reports. The median annual incidence ranges from 10 to 374 cases per 100,000 people.[38,39] The incidence is decreasing in all WHO regions for which data exist, except in the Americas, where the incidence is increasing slightly (Fig. 1.2).[18,19,39] It is higher in surveys with active surveillance (8 to 51 cases per 100,000) than in surveys using passive surveillance (5 to 35 per 100,000).[40] Estimates of the incidence of first attack are based on few data but annual incidences are 23 per 100,000 people per annum (p.a.) in Kuwait, 35 per 100,000 in Iran, 51 per 100,000 in India, 80 per 100,000 in a Maori population in New Zealand,[40] and 194 per 100,000 in an indigenous population in the Northern Territories of Australia.[41]

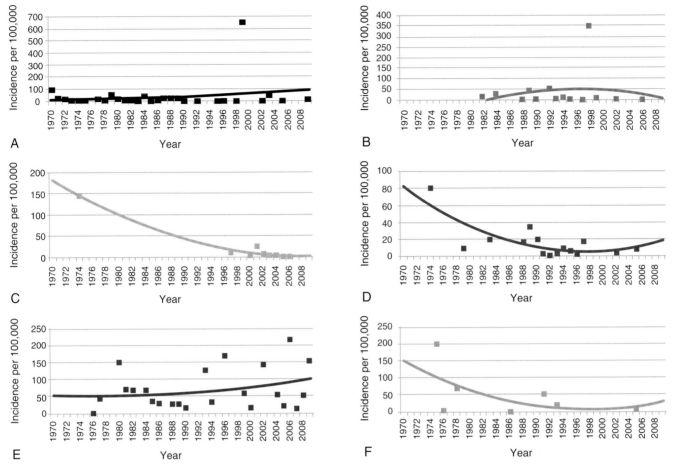

Fig. 1.2 Patterns of Change in Incidence of Acute Rheumatic Fever in World Health Organization (WHO) Regions. Incidence was approximately stable in every WHO region other than the Americas, where there is a slight increase. (A) The Americas. (B) Europe. (C) Africa. (D) Eastern Mediterranean. (E) Western Pacific. (F) Southeast Asia. Acute rheumatic fever continues to occur sporadically in industrially developed areas, such as in Utah,[39] and the annual incidence is 30 cases per 100,000 people[37] for all attacks but less than 10 cases per 100,000 people p.a. for first attacks.[19] (From Seckeler MD, Hoke TR. The worldwide epidemiology of acute rheumatic fever and rheumatic heart disease. Clin Epidemiol 2011;3:67-84.)

Males and females were equally affected by first attacks in one study,[40] and females more frequently affected in another.[41] The incidence peaks at age 5 to 14 at 150 per 100,000 men, falling to approximately 55 per 100,000 at 15 to 24 years of age and to 25 per 100,000 at 25 to 34 years of age.[41] The recurrence rate is 4.5% during the first year and 12.5% at 5 years.[41] There are no data on the incidence of first attack from Africa.

The incidence of new RhD is 27% to 35% at 1 year, 44% to 51% by 5 years, and 52% to 61% at 10 years.[42,43] Allowing that 60% of people with acute RhF develop chronic RhD, the annual incidence of new cases of RhD globally has been estimated at 282,000.[38] However, there are major geographic differences, with a mean of 160 cases per 100,000 people (95% CI: 80–230) based on a meta-analysis of 37 population surveys.[43] The estimated incidence is 23.5 cases per 100,000 people in Soweto,[44] but with a J-shaped age-dependence curve and with 30 cases per 100,000 for those 15 to 19 years of age, 15 cases per 100,000 for those 19 years of age, and 53 cases per 100,000 for those older than 60 years.

Prevalence of Rheumatic Disease

The global disease survey[1] estimated a worldwide prevalence of chronic RhD of at just under 30 million in 2016, an increase of 3.4% compared with 2006. The prevalence is increasing in all WHO regions other than

Europe (Fig. 1.3).[18,22,40–43] RhD is estimated to cause 4.3 million cases of heart failure, which is 6.9% of the total number of cases, and to produce an age-standardized mortality rate of 4.7 deaths per 100,000 people p.a.[2]

In surveys concentrating on RhD, prevalence estimates have changed in recent years with the use of echocardiography and with the evolution of echocardiographic criteria for diagnosis. A seminal study in 2007 in Cambodia and Mozambique[12] found a prevalence of 230 cases per 100,000 children as estimated by clinical examination but 2810 cases per 100,000 using echocardiography. The WHO 2006 criteria[42] used a combination of clinical examination and echocardiography to give a prevalence of 2110 cases per 100,000 (95% CI: 1410–3140),[43] compared with only 270 cases per 100,000 (95% CI: 160–440) based on clinical diagnosis.[43]

There were concerns about the limitations of clinical examination and the specificity and variability of echocardiographic criteria. A retrospective re-evaluation of results gave a range in prevalence for the same population of 510 to 3040 cases per 100,000, depending on the echocardiographic criteria used.[45] These concerns led to a World Heart Federation consensus[46] statement in 2012 that categorized RhD as definite or borderline using a combination of regurgitation, gradient, and morphology (Fig. 1.4 and Box 1.2),[45] Using these criteria, the

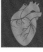

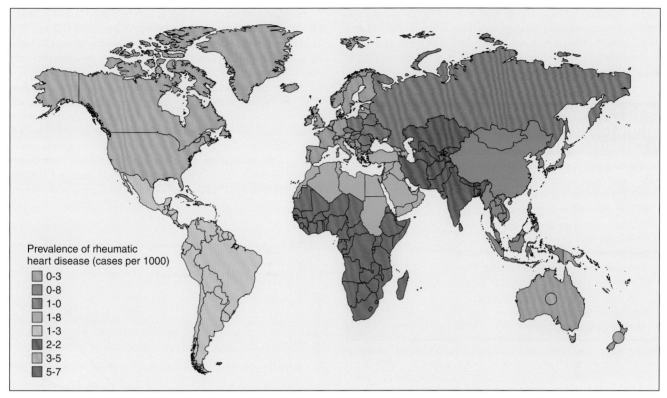

Fig. 1.3 Worldwide Prevalence of Chronic Rheumatic Disease. These prevalence estimates are based on the World Health Organization (WHO) 2006 criteria,[40] which used a combination of clinical examination and echocardiography. The prevalence of 2110 cases per 100,000 people (95% CI: 1410–3140)[22] compared with only 270 cases (95% CI: 160–440) per 100,000 people based on clinical diagnosis.[22] However, there were concerns about the limitations of clinical examination and the specificity and variability of echocardiographic criteria. A retrospective re-evaluation of results gave a large range in prevalence in the same population of 510 to 3040 cases per 100,000, depending on the echocardiographic criteria used.[41] Prevalence increases with age from 470 per 100,000 at age 5, about 1500 per 100,000 at age 10, and 2100 per 100,000 at age 16 to 35 years.[42] Prevalence is inversely related to income. In a lower-income area of Cape Town, the prevalence was 2700 cases per 100,000 school children in a lower-income area compared with only 1250 cases per 100,000 in a higher-income area.[43] In the same study, the average prevalence was 2000 cases per 100,000 in South Africa compared with 3000 cases per 100,000 in Ethiopia, which had a poorer more rural population. Similarly in Addis Ababa,[44] the prevalence of rheumatic disease was seven times higher among low- than high-socioeconomic-class school children. (From Carapetis JR. Rheumatic heart disease in developing countries. New Engl J Med 2007;357:439.)

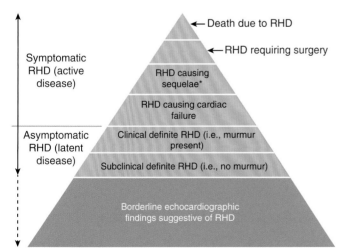

Fig. 1.4 Classification of Chronic Rheumatic Disease. Disease stage is based on echocardiographic imaging, physical examination, clinical symptoms, complications, and adverse outcomes. *RHD,* Rheumatic heart disease. (From Zühlke LJ, Steer AC. Estimates of the global burden of rheumatic heart disease. Global Heart 2013;8:189-195.)

prevalence of borderline or definite RhD ranges from 910 to 4020 cases per 100,000 people in different populations[47–54] (Fig. 1.5).

The echocardiographic criteria are relatively labor intensive to apply, and for the sake of screening children to give secondary prophylaxis, there is a move to handheld devices, nonphysician operators, and much simplified criteria, typically a 2-cm or larger mitral regurgitant jet or any aortic regurgitation.[54,55] This allows screening of 200 to 250 cases per day by one sonographer spending 2 minutes per patient.[56] This approach has high sensitivity but reduced specificity, and a more expert review is required to confirm a diagnosis.

There is uncertainty about the clinical significance of echocardiographic borderline RhD. Small studies with a follow-up at a maximum of 24 months suggest that two thirds of mild lesions remain unchanged, one third improve or resolve completely,[57,58] and one third become worse, particularly if there is regurgitation plus a morphologic abnormality.[59,60] A large, prospective, multicenter registry, the Global Rheumatic Heart Disease Registry (REMEDY),[25] aims to determine the natural history of borderline disease more accurately and whether secondary prophylaxis is beneficial. New Zealand does not give secondary antibiotic prophylaxis to borderline RhD but uses active surveillance with intervention only if the echocardiographic appearance changes. Resource-scarce countries may have to weigh the cost of screening programs against the need to combat tuberculosis (TB) and human immunodeficiency virus (HIV) infections, but they may choose to prescreen with auscultation. Sadiq et al.[61] screened 24,980 Pakistani children in this way.

BOX 1.2   World Heart Federation Criteria for the Diagnosis of Rheumatic Heart Disease in Patients 20 Years of Age or Younger

Definite diagnosis, one or more of the following criteria:
- Pathologic mitral regurgitation[a] and at least 2 morphologic features of rheumatic mitral valve disease[b]
- Mitral stenosis with mean gradient ≥4 mmHg
- Pathologic aortic regurgitation[a] and at least two morphologic features of rheumatic aortic valve disease[c]
- Borderline disease of the aortic and mitral valves

Borderline diagnosis, any of the following criteria:
- At least two morphologic features of rheumatic mitral valve disease[b] (in the absence of stenosis or regurgitation)
- Pathologic mitral regurgitation[a]
- Pathologic aortic regurgitation[a]

[a]The pathologic regurgitation diagnosis must include all of the following: (1) seen in two views, (2) jet length in at least one view of ≥ 2 cm (for mitral) or ≥ 1 cm (for aorta, (3) peak velocity ≥ 3 m/s, and (4) pan systolic (mitral) or pandiastolic (aortic) in at least one signal.
[b]Morphologic features of the mitral valve: anterior leaflet thickening ≥ 3 mm, chordal thickening, restricted leaflet motion, and excessive leaflet tip motion in systole.
[c]Morphologic features of the aortic valve: irregular or focal thickening, coaptation defect, restricted leaflet motion, and prolapse.
From Marijon E, Celermajer DS, Tafflet M, et al. Rheumatic heart disease screening by echocardiography. The inadequacy of World Health Organization criteria for optimizing the diagnosis of subclinical disease. Circulation 2009;120:663-668.

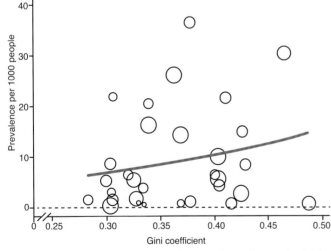

Fig. 1.5 Prevalence of Rheumatic Disease According to Social Inequality. The prevalence of rheumatic disease is plotted against the Gini coefficient, which is a measure of income inequality. The higher the coefficient, the greater the inequality. This relationship applies only in endemic areas. The Gini income distribution indices are 0.40 to 0.45 for the United States and 0.35 to 0.40 for the United Kingdom. (From Rothenbühler M, O'Sullivan CJ, Stortecky S, et al. Active surveillance for rheumatic heart disease in endemic regions: a systematic review and meta-analysis of prevalence among children and adolescents. Lancet Global Health 2014;2:e717-e726.)

Prevalence increases with age in endemic areas from 470 cases per 100,000 children at age 5, about 1500 cases per 100,000 at age 10, and 2100 cases per 100,000 at age 16.[62] Among Nicaraguan adults between the ages of 20 and 35 years, the prevalence based on echocardiography was 2200 cases per 100,000.[62] The prevalence of RhD is higher in rural than urban populations and higher in low-income populations (Fig, 1.6) because these factors affect living conditions and access to medical care, including secondary prophylaxis. In a lower-income area of Cape Town, the prevalence was 2700 cases per 100,000 school children compared with only 1250 cases per 100,000 in a higher-income area.[63] In the same study, the average prevalence was 2000 cases per 100,000 in South Africa compared with 3000 cases per 100,000 in Ethiopia, where there is a poorer and more rural population. Similarly,

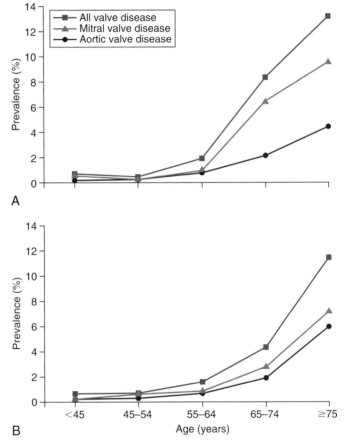

Fig. 1.6 Effect of Age on Prevalence of Valve Disease in Three Pooled Population-Based Studies. The study pooled echocardiographic data available from the National Heart, Lung, and Blood Institute (NHLBI) database for three population-based studies: the Coronary Artery Risk Development in Young Adults (CARDIA) study, the Atherosclerosis Risk in Communities (ARIC) study, and the Cardiovascular Health Study (CHS). In total, there were 11,911 subjects with echocardiograms (40% black and 59% white). These data were compared with those from the Olmsted County echocardiography register, for which the echocardiograms were performed for clinical reasons (data not shown). The population-based prevalence of all moderate or severe valve disease was 5.2%, which when corrected for the age and sex distribution of the U.S. population at the time of the data collection in 2000, was 2.5% (95% CI: 2.2%–2.7%). The prevalence rose for those older than age 64 and was 13.2% for those older than age 74. *Blue line* indicates all valve disease, *green line* indicates mitral valve disease, and *red line* indicates aortic valve disease. (Modified from Nkomo VT, Gardin JM, Skelton TN, et al. Burden of valvular heart diseases: a population-based study. Lancet 2006;368: 1005-1011.)

in Addis Ababa[64] the prevalence of RhD was seven times higher among low- than high-socioeconomic-class school children.

Throughout the industrially underdeveloped world, 10% to 35% of all cardiac admissions are a result of acute or chronic RhD.[65] RhD is the dominant cause of heart failure, with 4.3 million cases worldwide, representing 6.9% of the total cases.[1] In a study from the Northern Territories of Australia, the 10-year cumulative incidence of heart failure was 18.6% after acute RhF, 3.4% for atrial fibrillation, 4% for IE, and 3.6% for stroke, and the death rate was 10.3%.[42]

RhD, particularly mitral stenosis, is a major cause of mortality and morbidity in pregnancy. The prevalence among pregnant women is 230 cases per 100,000 in Fiji and South Africa.[66] The maternal mortality rate for RhD was 34% in a study from Senegal[67] and as high as 54% in the setting of severe mitral stenosis.

Valve Disease in Industrially Developed Areas

Few incidence figures exist, but it was estimated using hospital registries for the whole Swedish population between 2003 and 2010 as 63.9 cases per 100,000 patient-years.[65] The incidence rose with age, with 69% of all valve disease diagnosed in people 65 years of age or older. The most commonly occurring lesions were aortic stenosis, mitral regurgitation, and aortic regurgitation.

The population prevalence of valve disease was estimated at 2.5% in the United States[4] (Table 1.2) and 3.3% of those older than 25 years in Tromsø, Norway.[5] The prevalence was age dependent, beginning to rise at age 55 and becoming steeper after age 65. After age 75, the prevalence was 13.2% in the United States[4] but higher (18.7%) in the U.K. OxVALVE population (Fig. 1.7 and Table 1.3).[6] It is possible that patients volunteered for the U.K. OxVALVE study because of a known murmur or a cardiac symptom. The most common valve lesions were mitral regurgitation and aortic stenosis, and a similar prevalence of aortic stenosis was identified in Scandinavia.[7,68]

As expected, mild valve disease was more common, occurring in 44% of the OxVALVE population of 2500 community people[5] (see Fig. 1.1). In the U.S. population-based studies, there were no gender differences for mitral valve disease or aortic regurgitation, but there was a trend ($P = 0.06$) toward a higher prevalence of aortic stenosis among men, which became statistically significant ($P = 0.04$) after adjustment for age (odds ratio = 1.52). This may be explained by bicuspid aortic valves being more common in men. The factors associated with valve disease included age, low socioeconomic class,

and atrial fibrillation (Fig. 1.7).[6,69] Atrial fibrillation was also associated with valve disease in a survey of open access echocardiograms.[14]

Reports of selected patient groups inevitably record different results. In a study of 1797 men and women older than 60 years in long-term health care in the United States,[70] there were 22 (1.2%) with mitral stenosis, 591 (33%) with mitral regurgitation, 301 (17%) with aortic stenosis, and 526 (29%) with aortic regurgitation. The EuroHeart Surveys I and II[15,71] recorded the causes of moderate and severe disease occurring mainly in Western and Eastern Europe in inpatients or in medical or surgical outpatient clinics. The mean age was 65 years (SD = 14 years),[15] and age-related valve diseases were the most common causes[71] (Table 1.4). They included aortic stenosis (41% of the total), multiple valve disease (25%), and mitral regurgitation (21%) (see Table 1.4). Valve disease was reported for 29% of patients in the EuroHeart Failure survey.[72]

In the West, the frequency of chronic RhD fell after the 1950s. The proportion of aortic regurgitation of rheumatic origin was 62% in the period from 1932 to 1967, but it fell to 29% during the 1970–1974 period and 20% during the 1985–1989 period.[73–75] Chronic RhD is still reported in residents of care homes in Russia and China,[36] and the prevalence of RhD in nine urban and semi-urban provinces in China during the 2001–2002 period among middle-aged or older people using echocardiography was 186 cases in 100,000 people (Fig. 1.8).[76] Acute RhF continues to occur sporadically, such as in Utah,[77] and the annual incidence is 30 cases per 100,000 p.a.[36] for all attacks but 10 or fewer cases per 100,000 p.a. for first attacks.[40]

The rational for detecting mild RhD is to give secondary antibiotic prophylaxis. However, there is no recognized treatment to reduce the rate of progression of mild nonrheumatic valve disease, which is increasingly detected when echocardiography is used for relatively nonspecific indications such as dizziness or palpitation or noncardiac chest pain. In a survey of open access echocardiography,[14] mild valve disease of no hemodynamic significance was found in 8% of 1637 with no murmur. The natural history of mild disease is not as well known as that for moderate or severe disease, and there is a tendency for using surveillance, which carries the risk of causing health anxiety.[78]

CAUSES OF VALVE DISEASE

Rheumatic Fever

RhF occurs in children between the ages of 5 and 15 years. It usually results from the immune response to group A β-hemolytic streptococcal pharyngitis. The response occurs after 1 to 5 weeks and is caused by molecular mimicry of streptococcal M protein and human myosin and between the group A carbohydrate in the streptococci and valve tissue.

Genetically determined immune markers affect susceptibility to the initial infection and help determine the risk of developing chronic RhD.[79,80] HLA-DR7 has been the most frequently identified association. There is some evidence for a disordered signaling mechanisms and reactivation of the embryologic pathways.[81] Some streptococcal serotypes (emm-encoded types 3, 5, 6, 14, 18, 1 9, and 29) may be more likely than others to cause RhF.[79] These host and bacterial factors vary geographically. There is evidence from native Australians that pyoderma (rather than pharyngitis) and group C and group G streptococci may have an important role.[58]

RhF is uncommon after one episode of pharyngitis, but it occurs in up to 75% of people after recurrent episodes. Cardiac involvement occurs in 10% to 40% after the first attack of RhF[82] and more frequently after multiple attacks.[83]

A proliferative exudative inflammation of the collagen of the valve and annulus is characterized by modified histiocytes called Aschoff

TABLE 1.2 Prevalence of Valve Disease in Three Pooled Population-Based Studies.

	DATA BY AGE GROUP				
	18–44	45–54	55–64	65–74	≥75
Total participants	4351	696	1240	3879	1745
Mitral regurgitation	23 (0.5%)[a]	1 (0.1%)	12 (1.0%)	250 (6.4%)	163 (9.3%)
Mitral stenosis	0	1 (0.1%)	3 (0.2%)	7 (0.2%)	4 (0.2%)
Aortic regurgitation	10 (0.2%)	1 (0.1%)	8 (0.7%)	37 (1.0%)	34 (2%)
Aortic stenosis	1 (0.02%)	1 (0.1%)	2 (0.2%)	50 (1.3%)	48 (2.8%)

[a]Prevalence values are given as the number of cases (% of total participants in the age group).
Modified from Iung B, Baron G, Butchart EG, et al. A prospective study of patients with valvular heart disease in Europe: the Euro Heart Survey on Valvular Heart Disease. Eur Heart J 2003;24:1231-1243.

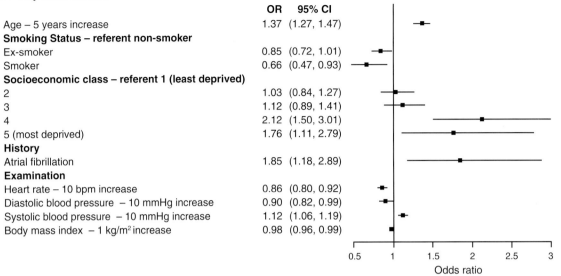

A Any valve disease

	OR	95% CI
Age – 5 years increase	1.37	(1.27, 1.47)
Smoking Status – referent non-smoker		
Ex-smoker	0.85	(0.72, 1.01)
Smoker	0.66	(0.47, 0.93)
Socioeconomic class – referent 1 (least deprived)		
2	1.03	(0.84, 1.27)
3	1.12	(0.89, 1.41)
4	2.12	(1.50, 3.01)
5 (most deprived)	1.76	(1.11, 2.79)
History		
Atrial fibrillation	1.85	(1.18, 2.89)
Examination		
Heart rate – 10 bpm increase	0.86	(0.80, 0.92)
Diastolic blood pressure – 10 mmHg increase	0.90	(0.82, 0.99)
Systolic blood pressure – 10 mmHg increase	1.12	(1.06, 1.19)
Body mass index – 1 kg/m² increase	0.98	(0.96, 0.99)

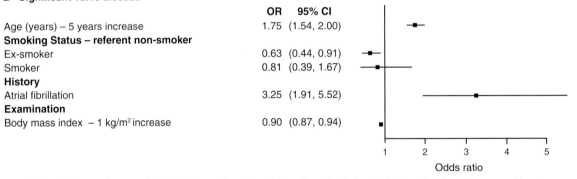

B Significant valve disease

	OR	95% CI
Age (years) – 5 years increase	1.75	(1.54, 2.00)
Smoking Status – referent non-smoker		
Ex-smoker	0.63	(0.44, 0.91)
Smoker	0.81	(0.39, 1.67)
History		
Atrial fibrillation	3.25	(1.91, 5.52)
Examination		
Body mass index – 1 kg/m² increase	0.90	(0.87, 0.94)

Fig. 1.7 Determinants of Valve Disease in a Population-Based Study. Subjects older than 65 years without known valve disease and who were registered with one of five primary care medical centers were invited to participate. For the first 2500 enrolled participants, the mean age (SD) was 73 (6) years; 51.5% were female, and 99% were white. This plot illustrates that a substantial burden of valve disease was not previously detected. This is a forest plot of odds ratios from multiple regression analysis of clinical associations with any valvular heart disease (A) and significant (moderate or severe) valvular heart disease (B). Only statistically significant variables are shown. *Dots* represent the odds ratio *(OR)*, and *whiskers* represent the 95% confidence interval *(CI)*. Socioeconomic class is determined according to national quintile. *bpm,* Beats per minute. (From d'Arcy JL, Coffey S, Loudon MA, et al. Large-scale community echocardiographic screening reveals a major burden of undiagnosed valvular heart disease in older people: the OxVALVE Population Cohort Study. Eur Heart J 2016;37:3515-3522.)

TABLE 1.3 Prevalence of Previously Undetected Valve Lesions in the OxVALVE UK Community Survey.

Valve Lesion	Mild	Moderate/Severe
Mitral regurgitation	494 (19.8%)	58 (2.3%)
Mitral stenosis	7 (0.3%)	2 (0.1%)
Aortic regurgitation	341 (13.6%)	41 (1.6%)
Aortic stenosis	866 (34.6%)	17 (0.7%)
Tricuspid regurgitation		67 (2.7%)
Pulmonary regurgitation		7 (0.3%)

Form Lindekleiv H, Løchen ML, Mathiesen EB, et al. Echocardiographic screening of the general population and long-term survival. A randomized clinical study. JAMA Int Med 2013;173:1592-1598.

bodies. The valve, annulus, and chordae are edematous and inflamed, leading to annular dilation and chordal elongation[83] and sometimes leading to mitral prolapse but otherwise to leaflet thickening and nodularity. These changes cause severe mitral regurgitation, which is the hallmark of acute RhF in the young. Much less is known about the mechanisms of aortic regurgitation, but there may be stretching of the cusps as a result of inflammation and subsequent prolapse.

The development of chronic RhD depends on the age at the time of the acute episodes, their severity and frequency,[83] and the magnitude of the immunologic response. It is more likely with multiple valve involvement, failure to obtain medical help and lack of secondary prophylaxis (Fig. 1.9).[83–90] The mitral valve is affected in more than 90% of cases.[56] Single valve involvement and mitral stenosis are more likely in older individuals with less active carditis.[82,83] Development of complications (e.g., atrial fibrillation, heart failure, stroke) occurs most commonly in the first year after an initial attack of RhF and more

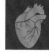

TABLE 1.4 Causes of Single Left-Sided Valve Disease in the EuroHeart Survey.

Cause	AS[a] (n = 1197)	AR (n = 369)	MS (n = 336)	MR (n = 877)
Degenerative (%)[b]	81.9	50.3	12.5	61.3
Rheumatic (%)	11.2	15.2	85.4	14.2
Endocarditis (%)	0.8	7.5	0.6	3.5
Inflammatory (%)	0.1	4.1	0	0.8
Congenital (%)	5.4	15.2	0.6	4.8
Ischemic (%)	0	0	0	7.3
Other (%)[c]	0.6	7.7	0.9	8.1

[a]Aortic stenosis was defined by Vmax > 2.5 m/s, mitral stenosis by an orifice area < 2.0 cm², and mitral or aortic regurgitation by the presence of ≥ 2/4 regurgitation.
[b]Defined as calcific aortic valve disease, mitral annulus calcification, and mitral prolapse. Subjects were recruited as inpatients or from medical or surgical outpatient clinics between April 1 and July 31, 2001, at participating hospitals, mainly located in western and eastern Europe. The mean age was 65 (SD = 14), and 16.8% were younger than 50, 50% were between 50 and 70, 30% were between 70 and 80, and 8.3% were older than 80 years.
[c]The overall frequency of right-sided disease was 42 (1.2%) and multiple valve disease was 713 (20%).
AR, Aortic regurgitation; AS, aortic stenosis; MR, mitral regurgitation; MS, mitral stenosis.
From Iung B, Baron G, Butchart EG, et al. A prospective study of patients with valvular heart disease in Europe: the Euro Heart Survey on Valvular Heart Disease. Eur Heart J 2003;24:1231-1243.

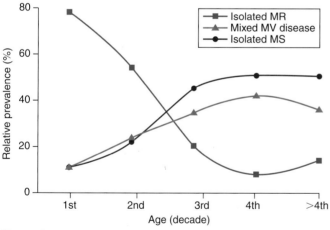

Fig. 1.8 Relationship Between Age and Type of Mitral Valve Disease. Time-course analysis (by decades) of the relative prevalence of isolated mitral regurgitation (MR), mixed (stenosis and regurgitation) mitral valve (MV) disease, and isolated mitral stenosis (MS). (Modified from Marcus RH, Sareli P, Pocock WA, et al. The spectrum of severe rheumatic mitral valve disease in a developing country. Correlations among clinical presentation, surgical pathological findings, and hemodynamic sequaelae. Ann Intern Med 1994;120:177-183.)

rapidly than after a second attack of RhF. This underlines the need for prevention. Complications and survival are also linked with comorbidities (e.g., alcohol use).

Endomyocardial Fibrosis

EMF is, after RhD, the second most frequent cause of acquired heart disease in Africa.[94] It was originally described in the equatorial region of Africa, Uganda, Nigeria, and Ivory Coast, but with the use of echocardiography, it was identified more widely, including in Egypt and South Africa. EMF occurs predominantly in children and adolescents. It affects males and females in similar proportion, although there is a second peak in women of reproductive age.[95] Echocardiography of a sample of 1063 people of all ages in coastal Mozambique found a prevalence of 20% (95% CI: 17.4%-22.2%).[96]

EMF begins as a febrile illness that is followed by a latent phase of 2 to 10 years. Symptoms then reappear as left ventricular (LV) and right ventricular (RV) thrombi and fibrosis develop, leading to RV, LV, or biventricular restrictive cardiomyopathy and enmeshment of the posterior mitral leaflet or nonseptal tricuspid valve leaflets.

The pathology of EMF remains uncertain. There is evidence for the reactivation of embryologic pathways[81] and postulated etiologic factors,[96] which are not mutually exclusive and include the following:

- Hypereosinophilia: Features are similar to hypereosinophilic syndromes, and the eosinophil count is transiently high in up to 30% of patients with EMF.
- Infection: EMF may be associated with helminth infection, schistosomiasis, filariasis, and *Mycoplasma* pneumonia.
- Autoimmunity: Immunoglobulin G (IgG) reactivity occurs to myocardial proteins.
- Genetic predisposition: The incidence is high among some ethnic groups.
- Diet: Eating uncooked cassava causes an EMF-like response in African green monkeys and may be relevant in humans, especially those eating protein-deficient diets.
- Geochemistry: Increased levels of cerium are found in the hearts of some patients with EMF living near the coast of Mozambique.

The incidence of EMF in southern Nigeria has decreased. This is thought to result from improved health care delivery and better living conditions.

Calcific Aortic Stenosis

The incidence and severity of aortic stenosis increase with age by a process of active lipid deposition, inflammation, neoangiogenesis, and calcification (see Chapter 3). Aortic stenosis shares a number of risk factors with other atherosclerotic processes. Psoriasis has been shown to be an independent risk for coronary disease and aortic stenosis,[97] possibly through inflammatory mechanisms.

Aortic valve sclerosis is defined by valve thickening and a peak transaortic velocity on echocardiography of less than 2.5 m/s. Approximately 20% of patients with sclerosis progress to stenosis within 10 years.[98,99] Aortic valve sclerosis is also associated with vascular disease and is a marker for a higher risk of myocardial infarction,[100] particularly in patients with no established coronary disease or those with low conventional risk profiles, such as women or patients younger than 55 years[101] (see Chapter 4).

Age-related calcification can affect the mitral annulus but rarely causes sufficient obstruction to require surgery, except occasionally in patients with chronic renal failure.[102] If calcification is found at the aortic valve and mitral annulus and in the aorta, there is a significant likelihood of associated three-vessel coronary disease.[103]

Aortic sclerosis is very common, with a population prevalence of 45% for those 65 years or older in Barcelona[8] and 34% of those in Oxford.[6] Prevalence is 73.5% among those older than 85 years.[8] The population prevalence of moderate or severe aortic stenosis was 0.4% among those older than 18 years in the United States[4] but 1.3% for those between the ages of 65 and 74 years and 2.4% for those older than 75 years. The Tromso[68] study showed a higher prevalence of 1.3% for those between the ages of 60 and 69 years, 3.9% for those between 70 and 79 years, and 9.8% for those between 80 and 89 years of age.

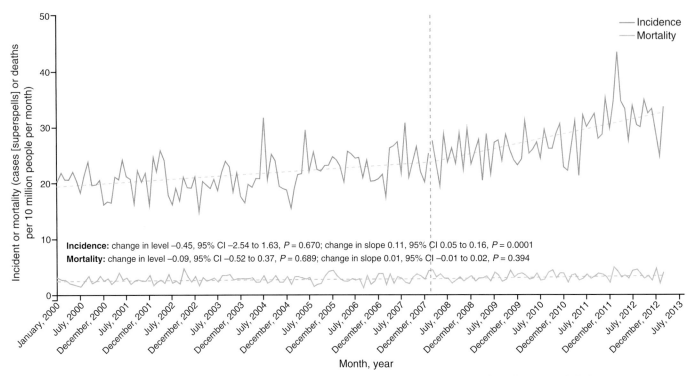

Fig. 1.9 Incidence of Infective Endocarditis and Infective Endocarditis–Related Mortality. Prophylaxis is no longer recommended for people at moderate risk for infective endocarditis (IE) before invasive dental procedures. However, prophylaxis is still recommended in the setting of replacement valves, prior endocarditis, or congenital lesions corrected by valves according to European, U.S., and Australian guidelines,[84–86] with the addition of rheumatic disease in indigenous Australians in the 2008 Australian guidelines[91] and valve disease in transplanted hearts in the United States.[92] There has been a gradual increase in the incidence of IE over the past 10 years,[93] with an estimated 35 more cases per month than would have been expected before the change. The figure shows the number of cases of IE (superspells) recorded each month *(solid blue line)* and associated in-patient mortality rate *(solid red line)*. Data are corrected for the change in the size of the English population. The vertical *dashed line* indicates March 2008, the month in which cessation of antibiotic prophylaxis for IE was recommended by the National Institute for Health and Care Excellence (NICE). The trend lines for IE incidence *(dashed blue line)* and associated in-patient mortality rates *(dashed red line)* before and after introduction of the NICE guidelines are shown. With the outlier value for incidence of IE in March 2012 removed the change in the incidence trend line remains significant (change in level of −0.28, 95% CI: −2.27 to 1.70, $P = 0.78$; change in slope of 0.09, 95% CI: 0.04 to 0.14, $P = 0.0001$). (From Dayer MJ, Jones S, Prendergast B, et al. Incidence of infective endocarditis in England, 2000-13: a secular trend, interrupted time-series analysis. Lancet 2015;385(9974):1219-1228.)

Two other studies[7,104] showed a prevalence rate between those in the Tromso[68] and US[4] studies. As expected from the age of the patients, aortic stenosis was identified in 8% of those admitted with a fractured hip.[105]

The incidence is changing. In Sweden[106] between 1989 and 2009, the crude incidence based on hospital coding remained approximately constant at between 19 and 26 cases per 100,000 people, but the age-adjusted incidence decreased from 15.0 to 11.4 cases per 100,000 men and 9.8 to 7.1 cases per 100,000 women. In contrast, an analysis[69] of hospital coding over a 10-year period in Scotland showed an increased rate of admission, rising from 24.6 cases per 100,000 people in 1997 to 36.5 cases in 2005. These disparities may reflect differences in risk factor management.

Mitral Prolapse

Mitral prolapse is defined by abnormal systolic displacement into the left atrium of the whole or part of one or both leaflets. It is associated with myxomatous infiltration or fibroelastic deficiency of the leaflets. These histopathologic changes may coexist,[107,108] and although fibroelastic deficiency is more common in the elderly,[107] it is not clear whether the two processes are genetically related or distinct.

Myxomatous degeneration causes leaflet thickening, annulus dilation, and abnormal chordae. The chordae are prone to stretching and rupture and may be deficient, particularly at the commissures or at the middle scallop of the posterior leaflet. Fibroelastic deficiency produces thin, smooth leaflets that are deficient in collagen, elastin, and proteoglycans and relatively mild annulus dilation and chordal lengthening.

Mitral prolapse may be sporadic or familial (i.e., syndromic and nonsyndromic). Genetic studies are based on small pedigrees that are subject to selection bias. Abnormalities of the gene encoding filamin A *(FLNA)* causes an X-linked mitral prolapse,[109] but the genes responsible for the more common nonsyndromic autosomal dominant inheritance pattern are not known, although they are located on chromosomes 16, 11, and 13.[108] Syndromic mitral prolapse is associated with Marfan syndrome and Ehlers-Danlos syndrome type IV, osteogenesis imperfecta, Loeys-Dietz syndrome, pseudoxanthoma elasticum, and aneurysms-osteoarthritis syndrome. It can be associated with mutations in several genes, including *FBN1, TGFBR1* or *TGFBR2*, and *MADH3*.[108]

Methods of defining prolapse have been refined with advances in echocardiography and particularly with the realization that the mitral

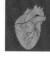

annulus is saddle shaped. Mitral prolapse is uncommon in children and young adults, but after the age of 30, the prevalence of prolapse using modern definitions is 2% to 3%[9,110] in unselected community populations, although the rate is higher in hospital series or for patients with syndromes associated with mitral valve prolapse or those with symptoms. Mitral prolapse is associated with tricuspid prolapse in 10% of cases[111] or, rarely, with aortic valve prolapse.

Mitral regurgitation occurs in 6% to 9% of all patients with prolapse,[42,112] but 25% in the setting of leaflet thickening as a result of myxomatous degeneration.[111] The grade of regurgitation depends on the degree of leaflet thickening and prolapse, and it is worse when ruptured chordae lead to flail or partially flail leaflet segments. In these cases, the mean 10-year survival rate without heart failure is only 37%.[113] However, there is a low risk of progression if the prolapse is mild with no more than mild mitral regurgitation and a normal left atrial size in sinus rhythm, and for these patients, follow-up may not be required.[114]

Secondary Mitral Regurgitation

Use of the terms *ischemic* and *secondary* is not fully standardized. *Ischemic regurgitation* typically is used for acute ischemic mitral regurgitation as a result of papillary muscle rupture. This requires emergency surgery (see Chapter 17). *Secondary mitral regurgitation* is a chronic condition that primarily results from LV dysfunction, which causes altered stresses on the mitral valve apparatus and restriction of the leaflets. Dilation of the annulus may also occur. Leaflet restriction may be asymmetric when it affects predominantly the posterior leaflet. This is most commonly associated with an inferoposterior myocardial infarction. It may also be symmetric, which results from more generalized LV dysfunction.

LV dysfunction leading to functional mitral regurgitation results from the causes of heart failure, which vary geographically. Important causes are ischemic disease, hypertension, and alcohol. In the West, probably 20% of patients with chronic left ventricular systolic dysfunction have severe secondary mitral regurgitation,[115] and 29% of patients in the EuroHeart Failure survey[72] had valve disease with secondary mitral regurgitation as the most likely cause. Chagas disease and HIV are important in endemic areas. Chagas disease caused 383,900 cases of heart failure in 2013,[1] which accounted for 0.6% of the global total and 11.4% in Brazil.

Secondary Aortic Regurgitation Resulting From Aortic Dilation

Functional aortic regurgitation results from dilation of the aortic root. Associated organic regurgitation often occurs as a result of a bicuspid aortic valve or arteriosclerosis. The risk factors for aortic dilation are age, weakness of the aortic wall, and the arteriosclerotic risk factors of hypertension, dyslipidemia, smoking, and diabetes. Weakness of the aortic wall as a result of medial necrosis occurs in Marfan syndrome and Ehlers-Danlos syndrome type IV.

Bicuspid aortic valve should be regarded as a general thoracic aortopathy, and it is associated with significant dilation of the aorta (to >40 mm) as a result of medial necrosis[116] in about 20% of cases.[117] Approximately one half affect the root, and the others affect the ascending aorta. Aortic dilation is more likely to be associated with coarctation,[118] but dissection is relatively uncommon and has a relatively high operative success, probably because of the youth and underlying good health of the patient. Prophylactic surgery is necessary in about 5% of cases during a 20-year follow-up[16] (see Chapter 11).

Vasculitides, especially giant cell arteritis and Takayasu arteritis, may weaken the arterial wall. Other causes of aortic dilation are trauma, cocaine, and amphetamines. In contradistinction to the usual symmetric fusiform dilation of a segment of aorta, a less common saccular aneurysm consisting of an outpouching of the aorta can result from inflammation from syphilis.

Secondary Tricuspid Regurgitation

Tricuspid regurgitation is associated with rheumatic mitral disease or mitral prolapse. It may sometimes result from organic involvement of the valve or annulus, but more often, it is a result of RV dilation due to pulmonary hypertension. If not corrected, it progresses after left-sided surgery, recurring in 75% 3 years after repair for mitral prolapse.[84] The 8-year mortality rate is 16% with tricuspid regurgitation, but it is only 5% without,[84] and the effect of tricuspid regurgitation on survival is independent of LV systolic function.[85] Secondary tricuspid regurgitation should therefore be repaired at the time of left-sided surgery, which provides freedom from severe tricuspid regurgitation for at least 10 years.[86]

Tricuspid regurgitation induced by endocardially implanted electrical devices is a growing phenomenon as the use of pacemaker and defibrillator systems increases. New or worsening tricuspid regurgitation in the absence of infection of the system occurs in 20% to 32% of cases[87,88] and occurs more commonly with implantable defibrillators than pacemakers.

Significant, grade 2 or higher tricuspid regurgitation is associated with progressive enlargement of the right heart and a poorer outcome for patients over 1 to 1.5 years than for those with no or grade 1 tricuspid regurgitation.[88] Tricuspid regurgitation does not resolve by changing the mode and does not depend on whether the RV lead is positioned at the apex or RV outflow tract. In a series of 41 patients[23] requiring surgery for severe tricuspid regurgitation 6 years after pacemaker or defibrillator placement, tricuspid regurgitation was caused by lead impingement in 16, adherence in 14, perforation (usually of the septal leaflet) in 7, and entanglement in 4. Tricuspid replacement was required in 22, and annuloplasty was needed in 19. Fibrosis and adherence can occur as early as 17 days after implantation. Tricuspid regurgitation can also develop as a result of percutaneous removal of endocardial electrodes; a flail tricuspid leaflet occurred in 19 (9.1%) of 208 patients.[89] Dense scarring causing tricuspid stenosis also occurs but is uncommon.

Infective Endocarditis

The estimated world incidence of IE in 2016 was 1,172,000 cases (95% CI: 1,068,000–1,280,000).[1] The incidence is probably similar in poor and rich countries at 3.4 cases per 100,000 people.[90] The estimated incidence in the West is 1.4 to 6.2 cases per 100,000.[24] This increases to 14.5 episodes per 100,000 patients-years in those older than 70 to 80 years.[93,119] However, the epidemiology is different.

In the industrially underdeveloped regions, patients with endocarditis are young, and about one half to three fourths have rheumatic heart disease; the others have prosthetic valves. The risk is 1% at 1 year after diagnosis of RhD, 2% at 5 years, and 4% at 10 years.[65] Health care–related IE is much less common than in the West.[90,120]

In the West, the epidemiology is different from that in the underdeveloped world, and it has changed in the past 20 years. Patients are older and are more likely to have diabetes and immune suppression.[121] There has been a reduction in the number with acquired heart disease and an increase in cases associated with health care, especially replacement heart valves, pacemakers,[122–124] or hemodialysis.[123] In the West, IE affects prosthetic valve in 20% to 30% of total cases,[125] and the incidence of prosthetic valve endocarditis is 464 cases per 100,000 people in the United Kingdom (relative risk of 70, compared with the general population) and 600 cases per 100,000 people in Holland.[126]

The major geographic variations depend largely on the frequency of medical devices used and on intravenous drug use.[28]

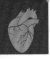

Hemodialysis-related IE is more common in the United States than in Europe (21% vs. 4%), with a lower use of native arteriovenous fistulas compared with Europe.[22,28] There is a male-to-female preponderance of 1.2 to 2.7:1, which is possibly related to bicuspid aortic valve being more common in men.

Oral streptococci are still the main infecting organisms[127] in underdeveloped areas, but *S. aureus* is becoming more common.[120] In the West, *S. aureus* was the predominant organism found in series reported from referral centers, which is likely related to a rise in health care–related IE and intravenous drug use. However, these series are biased to reporting severely ill patients, and population-based surveys of incidence report a gradual and statistically nonsignificant upward trend in the incidence of *S. aureus*–related IE[128] from 0.52 in 1991 to 0.82 per 100,000 p.a. in 2008. At the same time, the incidence of oral streptococcal IE fell from 0.81 to 0.65 per 100,000 p.a. Some organisms have a regional focus. *Brucella* is rare outside the Mediterranean and Middle East. *Bartonella* occurs in 1% to 4.4% cases in France, Canada, and Brazil and in up to 7% of cases in India. Non-HACEK (*Haemophilus*, *Aggregatibacter*, *Cardiobacterium*, *Eikenella*, and *Kingella*), gram-negative bacilli are rare causes of IE globally but occur in 9% to 15% of cases in South Africa, India, and Pakistan.[120]

A prospective cohort study[129] of patients admitted to 58 hospitals in 25 countries allows comparison of the West and developing countries. Of 2781 adults with definite IE, most were from the United States (*n* = 597 [21.5%]) or Europe (*n* = 1213 43.6%), but there were 254 (9.1%) from South America and other countries (*n* = 717 [25.8%]). The median age was 58, and 72.1% had native valve IE. Most patients (77.0%) presented within 30 days of disease onset and had few of the classic clinical hallmarks of IE. *S. aureus* was the most common pathogen (31.2%) overall but occurred in 43% of cases in the United States, compared with 17% in South America. Oral streptococcal infection occurred in 26% in South America and in only 9% in the United States.

In the same study, RhD occurred in less than 5%. Health care associated–IE occurred in 25% overall but 38% in the United States and only 20% in South America.[129] The in-hospital mortality rate in the United States was 17.7%, similar to that in the underdeveloped world, and stroke occurred in 17% of patients and heart failure in 32%. Surgery was performed in 48% of patients, a similar rate to that in the underdeveloped world.[130]

During recent years, use of antibiotic prophylaxis has diminished, with antibiotic prophylaxis before invasive dental procedures administered only in the setting of high-risk cardiac conditions such as replacement valves, prior endocarditis, or corrected adult congenital heart disease using valve conduits. These indications comply with the European Society of Cardiology (ESC), American Heart Association (AHA), and Australian guidelines,[91,131,132] with the addition of RhD in indigenous Australians in the 2008 Australian guidelines[91] and valve disease in transplanted hearts in the United States.[132]

Although there has been a gradual increase in the incidence of IE,[192] changes in the ESC and AHA guidelines have not affected this,[121,133] but two studies in the United States[134] and Germany[135] show an increase in incidence since guidelines changes about antibiotic prophylaxis were made. The U.S. study[134] suggested an increase in the incidence of streptococcal IE, but the study did not ascertain whether these cases were oral. In the United Kingdom, the 2008 National Institute for Health and Care Excellence (NICE) guidelines[136] recommended the withdrawal of all antibiotic prophylaxis in all groups for all procedures. There is evidence of a rise in the incidence of IE beginning with the change in the guidelines,[92] with an estimated 35 additional cases per month than would have been expected before the change in guidelines (Fig. 1.9).[16,133–139] NICE has subsequently softened its recommendations and now advises that antibiotic prophylaxis

can be given at the discretion of the physician, effectively bringing it in line with ESC and U.S. guidelines.

Replacement Heart Valves

Replacement valves are a treatment for valve disease but introduce a risk of structural valve deterioration, nonstructural deterioration, thrombosis or thromboembolic events, infection, or bleeding. The pattern of use of replacement valves is different in developed and underdeveloped regions, and 85% of valves are used for 11% of the world population.[137] In the underdeveloped world, safe anticoagulation may not be feasible. Repair is therefore performed even in patients with RhD in preference to the implantation of a replacement mechanical valve. Results may be good,[138] with a 90% survival rate at 10 and 14 years, compared with a 79% survival rate at 10 years and only a 44% survival rate at 14 years for valve replacement using mainly mechanical valves.

Poor international normalized ratio (INR) control was thought to explain the 2.17 times increased risk of dying with a mechanical than a biological valve and the 8.45 times higher risk for a Maori or 6.54 times higher risk for a Pacific Islander compared with white patients in New Zealand.[139] A biological valve may be used in a young person to avoid anticoagulation despite the known increased risk of early structural degeneration compared with use in older people. Reoperation for structural degeneration of biological replacement valves is a more common reason for surgery than in industrially developed areas, occurring in 41% of operations in Sao Paolo.[27]

However, there is a strong trend toward using biological valves in younger patients in the United States[140] and United Kingdom.[141] Despite guideline recommendations to implant mainly mechanical replacement aortic valves in patients younger than 60 years (see Chapter 14), the proportion of isolated aortic valve replacements using biological valve in people between 56 and 60 years of age increased from 25% in 2004 to 40% in 2008.[33,141] This discrepancy partly reflects the perceived longer durability of third-generation biological valves coupled with the possibility of a valve-in-valve transcatheter procedure to treat primary failure.[140]

In the United States, 31% of adult-sized children suitable for a mechanical valve between 2009 and 2013 elected to have a biological valve.[142] However, durability is limited in younger patients, particularly those younger than 40 years.[143,144] In a series from Ottawa, the rate of 10-year freedom from reoperation for aortic replacements was 50.9% for patients younger than 40 years at implantation, compared with 99.7% for those older than 60 years.[144] As a result, the need for redo procedures is increasing. In the United Kingdom, 7% of aortic valve operations are redo procedures.[33] Defining valve deterioration echocardiographically rather than by the need for a redo procedure suggests that failure in some designs of valve is more common than previously thought.[145]

Congenital Conditions

Congenital lesions account for approximately 5% of valve operations throughout the world. Bicuspid aortic valve is the most common abnormality and affects up to 2.0% of the population based on autopsy series[16] and 0.5% to 0.8% in larger population-based studies.[10,11] There is evidence of geographic clustering of cases,[146] which is likely a result of genetic factors[147,148] because the risk of a bicuspid aortic valve or aortic disease is about 10% among first-degree relatives of probands.[149,150] The male-to-female ratio is approximately 2:1. The valve is anatomically or truly bicuspid in one third of cases and functionally bicuspid in two thirds as a result of incomplete separation of two cusps in utero. In 80% of cases, the pattern is failure of right-left separation, which is more likely to be associated with aortic dilation.[151] Failure of separation of right and noncoronary cusps is more likely to be associated with mitral prolapse.[151]

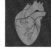

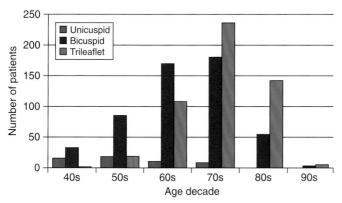

Fig. 1.10 Numbers of Cusps by Decade of Age for Patients Having Aortic Valve Surgery for Aortic Stenosis. Because the young are more likely to have surgery, the frequency of bicuspid disease is about one third of unselected surgical cases.[133] However, in detailed pathologic examinations of 932 surgically excised valves, the proportion of bicuspid valves in patients with aortic stenosis having surgery[16,134–139] was 67% for patients in their 40s, 57% for those in their 50s, 59% for those in their 60s, 42% for those in their 70s, 28% for those in their 80s, and 33% for those in their 90s.

During a 20-year follow-up, 24% of patients with a bicuspid aortic valve developed severe stenosis or regurgitation requiring surgery.[152,153] Events are far more common in those with even mild valve thickening at baseline, with surgical rates of 75% at 12 years in the setting of thickening, compared with only 8% for those without valve thickening.[152] Because the young are more likely to have surgery, the frequency of bicuspid disease is about one third of unselected surgical cases.[154] However, detailed pathologic examinations of surgically excised valves reported that among patients with bicuspid valves and aortic stenosis having surgery, 67% were in their 40s[17] and 28% were octogenarians[155–160] (Fig. 1.10).

Congenital mitral disease is uncommon. Congenital malformations[161,162] that affect the valve are double orifice, isolated cleft (without atrioventricular septal defect), dysplastic (associated with hypoplastic left heart), and Ebstein anomaly of the mitral valve. Those affecting the chordae are arcade mitral valve caused by unusually short chordae, and straddling mitral valve with chordae attached to both ventricles. In parachute mitral valves, the chordae tendineae are attached to only a single papillary muscle origin.

Submitral aneurysms occur in sub-Saharan African populations and are thought to be caused by a congenital weakness of the mitral annulus. The aneurysms arise in the posterior annulus and are often loculated and serpiginous, and they bulge in an extracardiac direction or into the left atrium.[58] They occasionally occur under the aortic valve, and some may be tuberculous in origin.[130]

Systemic Inflammatory Conditions

Endocardial involvement is relatively common in systemic lupus erythematosus (SLE), particularly in patients with antiphospholipid antibodies.[163,164] However, it is usually subclinical. Symptomatic, significant valve disease occurs after recurrent valvulitis. Subendothelial deposition of immunoglobulins and complement cause proliferation of blood vessels, inflammation, thrombosis, and fibrosis.

Fusion of the mitral valve commissures may lead to stenosis, but more commonly, there is generalized thickening of the leaflets (30% to 70%) with regurgitation (30% to 50%).[163,165,166] Libman-Sacks vegetations are usually less than 10 mm in diameter, sessile, of mixed echogenicity, and usually rounded. They may occur anywhere, but they most commonly occur at the leaflet edges on the atrial surface of the mitral valve and, less frequently, occur on the ventricular side of the aortic valve. The right-sided valves are rarely affected. Active

vegetations have central fibrinoid degeneration with fibrosis and inflammatory infiltrate, whereas healed vegetations have central fibrosis with little or no inflammation.

Valve lesions may occur in the absence of features of SLE in the antiphospholipid syndrome.[165] Antiphospholipid antibodies cause the following:[166]

- Activation of endothelial cells
- Increased uptake of oxidized low-density lipoprotein (LDL), leading to macrophage activation
- Interference with regulatory functions of prothrombin and decreased production of protein C and S

Rheumatoid arthritis[166] causes an immune-complex valvulitis with infiltration of plasma cells, histiocytes, lymphocytes, and eosinophils that leads to fibrosis and retraction. Nodules consist of central fibrinoid necrosis surrounded by mononuclear cells, histiocytes, Langhans giant cells, and a border of fibrous tissue. The nodules are 4 to 12 mm in diameter and develop at the base of the mitral or aortic valves. Occasionally, there may be more generalized valvulitis. Healed valvulitis leads to leaflet fibrosis and retraction, causing regurgitation.

Ankylosing spondylitis is associated with HLA-B27–mediated chronic inflammation and proliferative endarteritis of the aortic root and left-sided valves. This commonly causes the following:[166]

- Aortitis of the aortic root leads to thickening, dilation, and functional aortic regurgitation.
- Aortic valvulitis occurs with thickening of the leaflets and cusp retraction.
- Downward displacement of the aortic root leads to a subaortic bulge at the base of the anterior mitral leaflet. This causes retraction of the anterior mitral leaflet with reduced coaptation.

The frequency of valve disease is uncertain because reported series are small and tend to be biased toward those with severe disease. Aortic valve thickening has been reported in 40%, mitral valve thickening in 34%, and significant aortic dilation in 25%.[166]

Carcinoid, Drugs, and Radiation
Carcinoid
Carcinoid tumors arise from neural crest gastrointestinal enterochromaffin cells. They are rare, occurring in 1 of 75,000 people.[167] The carcinoid syndrome develops in about one half of patients as a result of hepatic spread, and carcinoid heart disease develops in 40% of this group.[168,169] The cardiac lesions are caused by the paraneoplastic effects of vasoactive substances, notably 5-hydroxytryptophan (5-HT). The drugs known to cause valve disease (Table 1.5) are agonists themselves or have metabolites that are agonists at 5-HT2B receptors. Drugs with an affinity for 5-HT2A and 5-HT2C receptors do not cause valve disease.

Drugs
Drug-induced lesions are similar to those found in carcinoid disease. However, in carcinoid, right-sided lesions predominate[167,168] because the vasoactive substances are inactivated in the lungs. Left-sided valves may be affected in the 5% of cases[167,168] with lung metastases or a patent foramen ovale. In contrast, drug-induced disease affects mainly the left-sided valves. Leaflet retraction is more extreme in carcinoid than in drug-induced valve disease.

Interaction with the 5-HT2B receptor stimulates cardiac fibroblast proliferation, leading to fibrous plaques with a pearly white appearance on valves and chordae. On echocardiography,[169] this produces the following:

- Valve thickening
- Chordal thickening and shortening
- Restriction of movement
- Failure of coaptation
- Regurgitation

TABLE 1.5 Drugs That Cause Valvopathy.

Agent	Valve Lesion	Prevalence
Anorexic Agents		
Fenfluramine	AR, MR, TR	20% women, 12% men
Benfluorex	AR	Case reports
Parkinson Disease Drugs		
Pergolide	AR, MR, TR	22%
Cabergoline	AR, MR, TR	34%
Migraine Drugs		
Ergotamine	AR, MR, TR	Case reports
Methysergide	AR, MR	Case reports
Other Agents		
MDMA	AR, MR	28%

AR, Aortic regurgitation; *MDMA*, methyl amphetamine; *MR*, mitral regurgitation; *TR*, tricuspid regurgitation.

The earliest sign of valve involvement is an increase in the tenting height of the mitral valve, which is the distance between the point of apposition and the plane of the annulus.[169] The incidence of valve involvement has been difficult to determine exactly because of methodologic problems:

- Lack of blinding
- Lack of controls
- Expectation of the reporting echocardiographer
- Linkage to compensation claims (anorexic drugs)
- Small population sizes
- Failure to recognize the specific features of drug-induced valve disease
- Effect of dose and duration of therapy
- Co-determinants of valve disease, including age and hypertension

The U.S. Food and Drug Administration (FDA) approved the use of fenfluramine in 1973 as an anorexic agent for short-term use (<3 months). Fenfluramine is metabolized to norfenfluramine, which has 5-HT2B activity.[170] In 1997, a report[171] suggested that a combination of fenfluramine with the noradrenergic agonist phentermine, taken for a mean of 11 months, induced mitral regurgitation in 92% of cases and aortic regurgitation in 79%. Fenfluramine and its D-isomer dexfenfluramine were withdrawn that year. A large observational study[172] showed a lower but still clinically significant prevalence of aortic or mitral valve regurgitation in 20% of women and 12% of men.

Benfluorex, an anorectic and hypolipidemic agent that is structurally related to fenfluramine, has been used to treat obesity in diabetes with metabolic syndrome since 1976. It is metabolized to norfenfluramine and causes valve lesions[173] similar to those found with fenfluramine. The exact incidence is uncertain because only case reports and small case-matched studies exist. It was withdrawn from use in Europe in 2009. Phentermine on its own has not been shown to cause valve lesions.

Bromocriptine has only weak 5-HT2B effects, but pergolide and cabergoline have much stronger effects and cause valve disease when used in the relatively large doses necessary for Parkinson disease.[174] The mean cumulative dose of cabergoline or peroxide associated with moderate or severe valve thickening in one study[175] was 4015 mg (SD = 3208 mg). By comparison, the dose was only 2820 mg (SD = 2523 mg) if there was no or only mild thickening.

There is controversy about whether valve disease can occur with the smaller doses of cabergoline used for microprolactinoma, typically with cumulative doses of 200 to 414 mg.[176] Studies of cabergoline have differed in dose, duration, and design, and there is evidence that the expectation of the echocardiographer affects the prevalence of abnormalities reported.[177] Valvopathy appears to be rare,[176] but it has been described in isolated case reports after relatively large doses used for periods in excess of 10 years.[177] Guidance in draft form suggests that regular surveillance echocardiography is not needed for patients taking doses of cabergoline of less than 2 mg per week.

The ergot alkaloids ergotamine, dihydroergotamine, and methysergide and their metabolite methylergonovine may cause endocardial fibrosis, but reports have been anecdotal,[178] and accurate estimates of incidence do not exist. 3,4-Methylenedioxy methamphetamine (MDMA) used recreationally has caused a high incidence of valve lesions.[179]

Radiation

Exposure to radiation may cause heavy thickening of the aortic valve and mitral annular calcification. It often occurs after high-dose, high-volume mediastinal irradiation given typically for Hodgkin disease and, less commonly, for breast cancer. Minor thickening is seen in 80% of cases, and this may progress to asymptomatic dysfunction in 11 years and to symptoms after another 4 years,[180] although the rate of progression varies. One study suggested that the effect of radiation may be potentiated by chemotherapy,[180] but this is uncertain. Valve changes are more likely to affect the left-sided valves, probably because of higher mechanical stresses, but the tricuspid and, less commonly, the pulmonary valve may also be involved.[181] The aortic and mitral valves are affected equally. The aortic valve typically shows the following:

- Generalized calcification and immobility similar to age-related calcific disease
- Posterior mitral annular calcification
- Thickening extending from the mitral-aortic fibrosa over the base of the anterior mitral leaflet

DISEASE BY VALVE TYPE

Aortic Stenosis and Regurgitation

In industrially underdeveloped regions, RhD remains the most common cause of aortic valve disease. In the industrially developed regions and among the elderly throughout the world, aortic valve disease is predominantly a result of calcific disease (Boxes 1.3 and 1.4). About 25% to 35% of people older than 65 years have aortic valve thickening,[6,7] and 2.8% of those 75 years of age or older have moderate or severe stenosis.[4] The most common cause of aortic stenosis or regurgitation in patients younger than 65 years is bicuspid aortic valve disease (see Fig. 1.6). The prevalence of aortic stenosis in the adult population older than 18[4] or older than 25 years[4] is 0.4% to 0.9%.[4,5]

In the U.S. population-based series, there was a trend ($P = 0.06$) toward a higher prevalence of aortic stenosis among men, and this became statistically significant ($P = 0.04$) after adjustment for age (odds ratio = 1.52). Rare or uncommon causes of aortic stenosis (see Box 1.4) include radiation exposure, ochronosis, familial hypercholesterolemia, and Paget disease of the bone. Ochronosis is an inherited absence of homogentisic acid oxidase. Homogentisic acid accumulates in connective tissue, including the endocardium, usually causing no hemodynamic impairment. However, deposits occasionally cause significant aortic stenosis requiring surgery.[158,159]

In the Helsinki Ageing Study,[7] echocardiograms were performed for 552 participants between 55 and 86 years of age. The prevalence of any aortic regurgitation was 29%, and the prevalence of moderate or severe regurgitation was 13%. The frequency of regurgitation increases with age, and in the United States, the prevalence of moderate or severe aortic regurgitation was 2% for those 75 years of age or older

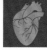

BOX 1.3   Causes of Aortic Regurgitation

Common
Rheumatic disease
Calcific disease
Aortic dilation
    Arteriosclerosis, Marfan syndrome, bicuspid, syphilis
Bicuspid valve
Endocarditis

Uncommon
Aortic dilation
    Dissection, Ehlers-Danlos syndrome, sinus of Valsalva aneurysm
Prolapse
Radiation
Drugs
Antiphospholipid syndrome

Rare
Carcinoid
Trauma: deceleration injury, instrumentation
Aortic dilation
    Reactive arthritis
    Giant cell arteritis
    Takayasu arteritis
    Wegener granulomatosis
    Sarcoidosis
    Behçet syndrome
Relapsing polychondritis
Pseudoxanthoma elasticum
Mucopolysaccharidoses, types I and IV

BOX 1.4   Causes of Aortic Stenosis

Common
Rheumatic disease
Calcific disease
Bicuspid valve

Uncommon
Radiation
Drugs
Congenital conditions (e.g., subaortic membrane)

Rare
Ochronosis[a]
Hypercholesterolemia in children
Paget disease
Other congenital conditions
Unicuspid or quadricuspid valve
Supravalvar stenosis

[a]Ochronosis is an inherited absence of homogentisic oxydase. Homogentisic acid accumulates in connective tissue, including the endocardium, and usually causes no hemodynamic impairment. However, deposits occasionally cause significant aortic stenosis requiring surgery.[164,165]

BOX 1.5   Causes of Mitral Stenosis

Common
Rheumatic disease
Calcific disease

Uncommon
Radiation
Systemic lupus erythematosus
Endomyocardial fibrosis
Carcinoid

Rare
Congenital conditions[140,141]
    Dysplastic valve (i.e., leaflet margins thickened and rolled, chordae shortened and thickened and matted together with fibrous tissue, underdeveloped papillary muscles, and reduced interpapillary muscle distance)
    Parachute mitral valve (single papillary muscle)
    Hypoplastic valve associated with hypoplastic left heart
    Supramitral ring
Whipple disease[168]
Fabry disease
Mucopolysaccharidoses, type I and IV[169]

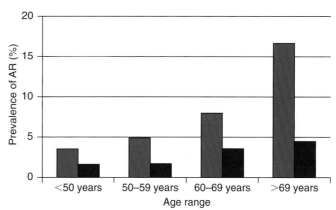

Fig. 1.11 Effect of Age on Prevalence of Aortic Regurgitation *(AR)*. Mild regurgitation (1+) *(blue bars)* was found in 97 (7.4%) of 1316 men and 160 (7.3%) of 2185 women. Moderate and severe regurgitation (≥2+) *(red bars)* was found in 38 (3.0%) of men and 55 (2.5%) of women. The range in prevalence for mild regurgitation was 4.5% to 16.4% by age ($P < 0.001$), and for moderate or severe regurgitation, it was 1.6% to 4.55% ($P < 0.002$). (From Lebowitz NE, Bella JN, Roman MJ, et al. Prevalence and correlates of aortic regurgitation in American Indians: the Strong Heart Study. J Am Coll Cardiol 2000;36:461-467.)

as a result of syphilitic aortic dilation occurred in 11% of 258 autopsies between 1932 and 1967.[73] However, the importance of syphilis declined after 1955. Rare causes of aortic regurgitation are given in Box 1.3.

Acute aortic regurgitation can occur as a result of endocarditis, dissection, or trauma. Over the past 30 years, IE has increased in frequency as a cause of aortic regurgitation from about 9% of surgical cases to 25%.[161,162]

Mitral Stenosis

RhD is the overwhelming cause of mitral stenosis worldwide (Box 1.5). It causes isolated mitral stenosis in 40% of cases. However, the population prevalence of mitral stenosis in industrially developed countries is only 0.1% to 0.2%[4,3] and accounts for only 10% of cases in European hospital-based series.[15] Although still predominantly rheumatic, it was

(Fig. 1.11). The prevalence of aortic regurgitation also depends on the diameter of the aortic root and ascending aorta,[160] indicating that it may be functional or may result from a combination of organic involvement and aortic dilation. The most common causes of aortic dilation are arteriosclerosis and medial necrosis. Aortic regurgitation

BOX 1.6   Causes of Mitral Regurgitation

Common
Secondary
Coronary disease
Hypertension
Alcohol
Chagas disease (South America)
Human immunodeficiency virus (HIV) infection

Primary or Organic
Rheumatic disease
Prolapse (myxomatous disease)
Endocarditis

Uncommon
Secondary
Idiopathic dilated myopathy
Chemotherapy
Systolic anterior motion: hypertrophic cardiomyopathy, Friedreich ataxia, amyloid

Primary or Organic
Radiation
Drugs
Systemic diseases: systemic lupus erythematosus, antiphospholipid syndrome, ankylosing spondylitis, rheumatoid arthritis
Traumatic: deceleration injury, instrumentation
Endomyocardial fibrosis

Rare
Secondary
African subvalvar aneurysm
Hemochromatosis
Fabry disease
Systemic sclerosis
Pseudoxanthoma elasticum

Primary or Organic
Congenital conditions: Ebstein mitral valve, double orifice, isolated cleft, dysplastic valve (associated with hypoplastic left heart), arcade mitral valve (short chordae), parachute mitral valve (single papillary muscle)

BOX 1.7   Causes of Tricuspid Valve Disease

Tricuspid Stenosis
Rheumatic disease
Pacemaker
Congenital conditions (e.g., tricuspid atresia, Ebstein anomaly)
Carcinoid

Tricuspid Regurgitation
Secondary
Pulmonary hypertension
RV dysfunction (e.g., cardiomyopathy, infarction)

Primary or Organic
Rheumatic disease
Myxomatous degeneration
Drugs interacting with 5-HT2B receptors
Carcinoid
Endocarditis
Trauma
Congenital conditions (e.g., Ebstein anomaly)
Pacemaker
Endomyocardial fibrosis

---

degenerative in approximately 10% of cases in the European survey.[15,71] Elderly patients, particularly those with renal failure, can develop heavy annular calcification, which may extend along the leaflets and cause moderate obstruction, although it is rarely severe enough to require valve surgery. The severity may be overestimated by the difficulty in imaging the leaflet tips and by a large atrial wave augmenting the estimated mean transmitral gradient.

Rare congenital causes include dysplastic valve (i.e., leaflet margins thickened and rolled, chordae shortened, thickened, and matted together with fibrous tissue, underdeveloped papillary muscles, and reduced interpapillary muscle distance). Other rare causes are SLE, Whipple disease, Fabry disease, and amyloid.[163–165]

Mitral Regurgitation

In industrially underdeveloped regions, RhD remains the most common cause, with EMF (see Endomyocardial Fibrosis) contributing in equatorial Africa or submitral aneurysms (see Congenital Conditions) contributing in South Africa. In the industrialized countries or among the elderly elsewhere, mitral regurgitation predominantly results from LV dysfunction (see Secondary Mitral Regurgitation), followed in frequency by mitral prolapse (see Mitral Prolapse).

The population prevalence of moderate or severe mitral regurgitation is 1.6% to 1.7%,[4,5] rising to 9.3% among those who are 75 years of age or older in the United States.[4] In a hospital-based European survey,[15] 32% of patients had mitral regurgitation. Uncommon or rare causes are given in Box 1.6.

Right-Sided Valve Disease

Right-sided disease is uncommon, occurring in 1.2% of patients in the EuroHeart Survey.[15] It was not mentioned in U.S. population-based studies,[4] and mild disease was found in only 3% of a population survey in the United Kingdom.[6]

Tricuspid Valve Disease

Tricuspid stenosis (Box 1.7) is almost always rheumatic and associated with rheumatic mitral disease, although it may also be congenital and is rarely associated with fibrosis caused by SLE or pacemakers. Abnormal tricuspid regurgitation is 90% due to left-sided disease, usually as a result of RV dilation due to pulmonary hypertension. It also results from any cause of RV disease, including cardiomyopathy and infarction. Tricuspid regurgitation associated with pacemaker electrodes is increasingly seen (see Secondary Tricuspid Regurgitation). Other causes of tricuspid regurgitation are given in Box 1.7.

Pulmonary Valve Disease

Pulmonary regurgitation commonly results from pulmonary hypertension (Box 1.8). Stenosis or regurgitation accounts for approximately 14% of all congenital cardiac lesions. The pulmonary valve is commonly affected by carcinoid. *S. aureus* endocarditis, whether community acquired or a result of intravenous drug use, can involve the valve.

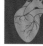

BOX 1.8 Causes of Pulmonary Valve Disease

Secondary Regurgitation
Pulmonary hypertension
Pulmonary artery aneurysm

Organic Causes
Congenital conditions
Carcinoid
Endocarditis

BOX 1.9 Causes of Multiple Valve Involvement

Rheumatic disease
Myxomatous disease
Endocarditis
Drugs
Carcinoid
Radiation

BOX 1.10 Steps To Eradicate Rheumatic Disease

- Improve living conditions.
- Educate about treatment.
- Treat streptococcal sore throats, even with a single dose of penicillin.
- Develop a vaccine.
- Identify valve involvement by population screening with echocardiography to give secondary prevention.
- Study developmental biology to modify progression to chronic lesions.
- Reclassify rheumatic disease as a notifiable condition to enable funding from organizations.

Multiple Valve Disease

Multiple valve involvement (Box 1.9) is common, occurring in 20% to 25% of participants in the EuroHeart survey[15,71] and 38.5% of people 65 years of age or older who were surveyed in Oxford.[6] In cases of RhD, isolated mitral stenosis is the most common disease, but combined aortic and mitral involvement is also frequently identified; aortic regurgitation is more likely to occur than stenosis. Tricuspid involvement is probably more common than thought because right-sided lesions may be difficult to detect by echocardiography because significant thickening does not occur.

CONCLUSIONS

Valve disease is common globally. It is underdetected, which adversely affects outcomes. Guidelines are based mainly on consensus opinions, and because there are almost no randomized, controlled trials, the need for more research is widely acknowledged.[25,182] Research and care-delivery initiatives aim to improve detection rates,[183] the delivery of secondary prophylaxis to patients with RHD (Box 1.10), and referral to specialist services for those with significant valve disease.[184] The challenge remains to deliver timely surgery for all valve disease and to maximize appropriate mitral repair rates for mitral prolapse.

REFERENCES

1. GBD 2016 Disease and Injury Incidence and Prevalence Collaborators. Global, regional and national incidence, prevalence, and years lived with disability for 328 diseases and injuries for 195 countries, 1990-2016: a systematic analysis for the Global Burden of Disease Study 2016. Lancet 2017;390:1211-1259.
2. GBD 2016 Causes of Death Collaborators. Global, regional and national age-sex specific mortality for 264 causes of death, 1980-2016: a systematic analysis for the Global Burden of Diseases Study 2016. Lancet 2017;390:1151-1210.
3. Nascimento BR, Nunes MCP, Lopes ELV, et al. Rheumatic heart disease echocardiographic screening: approaching practical and affordable solutions. Heart 2016. doi:10.1136/heartjnl-2015-308635.
4. Nkomo VT, Gardin JM, Skelton TN, et al. Burden of valvular heart diseases: a population-based study. Lancet 2006;368:1005-1011.
5. Lindekleiv H, Løchen M-L, Mathiesen EB, et al. Echocardiographic screening of the general population and long-term survival. A randomized clinical study. JAMA Intern Med 2013;173:1592-1598.
6. d'Arcy JL, Coffey S, Loudon MA, et al. Large-scale community echocardiographic screening reveals a major burden of undiagnosed valvular heart disease in older people: the OxVALVE Population Cohort Study. Eur Heart J 2016. doi:10.1093/eurheartj/ehw229.
7. Lindroos M, Kupari M, Heikkala J, Tilvis R. Prevalence of aortic valve abnormalities in the elderly: an echocardiographic study of a random population sample. J Am Coll Cardiol 1993;21:1220-1225.
8. Ferreira-Gonzalez I, Pinar-Sopena J, Ribera A, et al. Prevalence of calcific aortic valve disease in the elderly and associated risk factors: a population-based study in a Mediterranean area. Eur J Preventive Cardiol 2013;20:1022-1030.
9. Freed LA, Levy D, Levine RA, et al. Prevalence and clinical outcome of mitral-valve prolapse. N Engl J Med 1999;341:1-7.
10. Nistri S, Basso C, Marzari C, et al. Frequency of bicuspid aortic valve in conscripts by echocardiogram. Am J Cardiol 2005;96:718-721.
11. Movahed MR, Hepner AD, Ahmadi-Kashani M. Echocardiographic prevalence of bicuspid aortic valve in the population. Heart Lung Circ 2006;15:297-299.
12. Marijon E, Ou P, Celermajer S, et al. Prevalence of rheumatic heart disease detected by echocardiographic screening. N Engl J Med 2007;357:470-476.
13. van Heur LMSG, Baur LHB, Tent M, et al. Evaluation of an open access echocardiography service in the Netherlands: a mixed methods study of indications, outcomes, patient management and trends. BMC Health Serv Res 2010;10:37.
14. Chambers JB, Kabir S, Cajeat E. The detection of heart disease by open access echocardiography: a retrospective analysis. Br J Gen Pract 2014;64:86-87.
15. Iung B, Baron G, Butchart EG, et al. A prospective study of patients with valvular heart disease in Europe: the Euro Heart Survey on Valvular Heart Disease. Eur Heart J 2003;24:1231-1243.
16. Roberts WC. The congenitally bicuspid aortic valve. A study of 85 autopsy cases. Am J Cardiol 1970;26:72-83.
17. Roberts WC, Ko JM, Filardo G, et al. Valve structure and survival in quadragenarians having aortic valve replacement for aortic stenosis (±aortic regurgitation) with versus without coronary artery bypass grafting at a single US medical center (1993 to 2005). Am J Cardiol 2007;100:1683-1690.
18. Seckeler MD, Hoke TR. The worldwide epidemiology of acute rheumatic fever and rheumatic heart disease. Clin Epidemiol 2011;3:67-84.
19. Sliwa K, Zilla P. Rheumatic heart disease. The tip of the iceberg. Circulation 2012;125:3060-3062.
20. Oli K, Asmera J. Rheumatic heart disease in Ethiopia: could it be more malignant? Ethiop Med J 2004;42:1-8.
21. Gordis L. The virtual disappearance of rheumatic fever in the United States: lessons in the rise and fall of disease. Circulation 1985;72:1155-1162.
22. Shulman ST, Stollerman G, Beall B, et al. Temporal changes in streptoccal M protein types and the near disappearance of acute rheumatic fever in the United States. Clin Infect Dis 2006;42:441-447.

23. Lin G, Nishimura RA, Connolly HM, et al. Severe symptomatic tricuspid valve regurgitation due to permanent pacemaker or implantable cardioverter-defibrillator leads. J Am Coll Cardiol 2005;45:1672-1675.

24. Zühlke L, Engel ME, Karthikeyan G, et al. Characteristics, complications, and gaps in evidence-based interventions in rheumatic heart disease: the Global Rheumatic Heart Disease Registry (the REMEDY study). Eur Heart J 2015;36:1115-1122.

25. Andersen JA, Hansen BF, Lyndborg K. Isolated valvular aortic stenosis. Clinico-pathological findings in an autopsy material of elderly patients. Acta Med Scand 1975;197:61-64.

26. Anon 2001 Report of the National Confidential Enquiry into Perioperative Deaths. London: NECPOD; 2001:66-69.

27. Bocchi EA, Guimaraes G, Tarasoutshi F, et al. Cardiomyopathy, adult valve disease and heart failure in South America. Heart 2009;95:181-189.

28. Tleyjeh IM, Abdel-Latif A, Rahbi H, et al. A systematic review of population-based studies of infective endocarditis. Chest 2007;132:1025-1035.

29. Draper J, Subbiah S, Bailey R, Chambers JB. Murmur clinic: validation of a new model for detecting heart valve disease. Heart 2018. doi:10.1136/heartjnl-2018-313393.

30. Fabich N, Harrar H, Chambers J. 'Quick scan' cardiac ultrasound in a high-risk general practice population. Br J Cardiol 2016;23:27-29.

31. Pezzella A. Global aspects of cardiovascular surgery with focus on developing countries. Asian Cardiovasc Thorac Ann 2010;18:299-310.

32. Takkenberg JJM, Rajamannan NM, Rosenhek R, et al. The need for a global perspective on heart valve disease epidemiology. The SHVD working group on epidemiology of heart valve disease founding statement. J Heart Valve Dis 2008;17:135-139.

33. Bridgewater B, Kinsman R, Walton P, et al. Demonstrating quality: the sixth National Adult Cardiac Surgery database report. Henley on Thomas UK: Dendrite Clinical Systems Ltd; 2009.

34. Iung B. Management of the elderly patient with aortic stenosis. Heart 2008;94:519-524.

35. Grant SW, Devbhandari MP, Grayson AD, et al. What is the impact of providing a Transcatheter Aortic Valve Implantation (TAVI) service on conventional aortic valve surgical activity, patient risk factors and outcomes in the first two years? Heart 2012;96:1633-1637.

36. Carapetis JR, Steer AC, Mulholland EK, Weber M. The global burden of group A streptococcal diseases. Lancet Infect Dis 2005;5:685-694.

37. Jackson SJ, Steer AC, Campbell H. Systematic review: estimation of global burden of non-suppurative sequelae of upper respiratory tract infection: rheumatic fever and post streptococcal glomerulonephritis. Trop Med Int Health 2011;94:1534-1540.

38. Carapetis JR. Rheumatic heart disease in developing countries. N Engl J Med 2007;357:439.

39. Zülke LJ, Steer AC. Estimates of the global burden of rheumatic disease. Glob Heart 2013;8:189-195.

40. Tibazarwa KB, Volmink JA, Mayosi BM. Incidence of acute rheumatic fever in the world: a systematic review of population-based studies. Heart 2008;94:1534-1540.

41. Lawrence JG, Carapetis JR, Griffiths K, et al. Acute rheumatic fever and rheumatic heart disease. Incidence and progression in the Northern Territory of Australia 1997 to 2010. Circulation 2013;128:492-501.

42. He VYF, Ralph AP, Zhao Y, et al. Long-term outcomes from rheumatic fever and rheumatic heart disease. Circulation 2016;134:222-232.

43. Rothenbühler M, O'Sullivan CJ, Stortecky S, et al. Active surveillance for rheumatic heart disease in endemic regions: a systematic review and meta-analysis of prevalence among children and adolescents. Lancet Glob Health 2014;2:e717-e726.

44. Sliwa K, Carrington M, Mayosi BM, et al. Incidence and characterisation of newly diagnosed rheumatic heart disease in urban African adults: insights from the Heart of Soweto Study. Eur Heart J 2010;31:719-727.

45. Marijon E, Celermajer DS, Tafflet M, et al. Rheumatic heart disease screening by echocardiography. The inadequacy of World Health Organization criteria for optimizing the diagnosis of subclinical disease. Circulation 2009;120:663-668.

46. Remenyi B, Wilson N, Steer A, et al. World Heart Federation criteria for echocardiographic diagnosis of rheumatic heart disease—an evidence-based guideline. Nat Rev Cardiol 2012;9:297-309.

47. Roberts KV, Brown AD, Maguire GP, et al. Utility of auscultatory screening for detecting rheumatic heart disease in high-risk children in Australia's Northern Territory. Med J Aust 2013;199:196-199.

48. Beaton A, Okello E, Aliku T, et al. Latent rheumatic heart disease: outcomes 2 years after echocardiographic detection. Pediatr Cardiol 2014;35:1259-1267.

49. Roberts K, Maguire G, Brown A, et al. Echocardiographic screening for rheumatic heart disease in high and low risk Australian children. Circulation 2014;129:1953-1961.

50. Colquhoun SM, Kado JH, Remenyi B, et al. Echocardiographic screening in a resource poor setting: borderline rheumatic heart disease could be a normal variant. Int J Cardiol 2014;173:284-289.

51. Engel ME, Haileamlak A, Zuhlke L, et al. Prevalence of rheumatic heart disease in 4720 asymptomatic scholars from South Africa and Ethiopia. Heart 2015;101:1389-1394.

52. Mirabel M, Fauchier T, Bacquelin R, et al. Echocardiography screening to detect rheumatic heart disease: a cohort study of schoolchildren in French Pacific Islands. Int J Cardiol 2015;188:89-95.

53. Beaton A, Lu JC, Aliku T, et al. The utility of handheld echocardiography for early rheumatic heart disease diagnosis: a field study. Eur Heart J Cardiovasc Imaging 2015;16:475-482.

54. Mirabel M, Bacquelin R, Tafflet M, et al. Screening for rheumatic heart disease: evaluation of a focused cardiac ultrasound approach. Circ Cardiovasc Imaging 2015;8;e002324.

55. Mirabel M, Celermajer DS, Ferreira B, et al. Screening for rheumatic heart disease: evaluation of a simplified echocardiography-based approach. Eur Heart J Cardiovasc Imaging 2012;13:1024-1029.

56. Beaton A, Okello E, Lwabi P, et al. Echocardiography screening for rheumatic heart disease in Ugandan schoolchildren. Circulation 2012;125:3127-3132.

57. Saxena A, Zühlke L, Wilson N. Echocardiographic screening for rheumatic heart disease. Issues for the cardiology community. Global Heart 2013; 8:197-202.

58. Essop MR, Peters F. Contemporary issues in rheumatic fever and chronic rheumatic heart disease. Circulation 2014;130:2181-2188.

59. Tubridy-Clark M, Carapetis JR. Subclinical carditis in rheumatic fever: a systematic review. Int J Cardiol 2007;119:54-58.

60. Kane A, Mirabel M, Toure K, et al. Echocardiographic screening for rheumatic heart disease: age matters. Int J Cardiol 2013;168:888-891.

61. Sadiq M, Islam K, Abid R, et al. Prevalence of rheumatic heart disease in schoolchildren of urban Lahore. Heart 2009;95:353-357.

62. Paar JA, Berrios NM, Rose JD, et al. Prevalence of rheumatic heart disease in children and young adults in Nicaragua. Am J Cardiol 2010;105:1809-1814.

63. Engel ME, Haileamlak A, Zuhlke L, et al. Prevalence of rheumatic heart disease in 4720 asymptomatic scholars from South Africa and Ethiopia. Heart 2015;101:1389-1394. doi:10.1136/heartjnl-2015-307444.

64. Oli K, Porteous J. Prevalence of rheumatic heart disease among school children in Addis Ababa. East Afr Med J 1999;76:601-605.

65. Soler-Soler J, Galve E. Worldwide perspective of valve disease. Heart 2000;83:721-725.

66. Steer AC, Kado J, Jenney AW, et al. Acute rheumatic fever and rheumatic heart disease in Fiji: prospective surveillance, 2005-2007. Med J Aust 2009;190:133-135.

67. Diao M, Kane A, Ndiaye MB, et al. Pregnancy in women with heart disease in sub-Saharan Africa. Arch Cardiovasc Dis 2011;104:370-374.

68. Eveborn GW, Schirmer H, Heggelund G, et al. The evolving epidemiology of valvular aortic stenosis. The Tromsø Study. Heart 2013;99:396-400.

69. Berry C, Lloyd SM, Wang Y, et al. The changing course of aortic valve disease in Scotland: temporal trends in hospitalizations and mortality and prognostic importance of aortic stenosis. Eur Heart J 2013;34:1538-1547. http://dx.doi.org/10.1093/eurheartj/ehs339.

70. Aranow WS, Ahn C, Kronzon I. Prevalence of echocardiographic findings in 554 men and in 1,243 women aged >60 years in a long-term health care facility. Am J Cardiol 1997;79:379-380.

71. Iung B, Delgado V, Rosenhek R, et al. Contemporary presentation and management of valvular heart disease: The EURObservational Research Programme Valvular Heart Disease II Survey. Circulation. 2019 Sep 12. doi: 10.1161/CIRCULATIONAHA.119.041080. [Epub ahead of print]

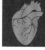

72. Cleland JGF, Swedberg K, Follath F, et al. The EuroHeart Failure survey programme—a survey on the quality of care among patients with heart failure in Europe. Part 1: patient characteristics and diagnosis. Eur Heart J 2003;24:442-463.

73. Barondess JA, Sande M. Some changing aspects of aortic regurgitation. Arch Intern Med 1969;124:600-605.

74. Acar J, Michel PL, Dorent R, et al. Evolution des etiologies des valvulopathies operees en France sur un periode de 20 ans. Arch Mal du Coeur 1992;85:411-415.

75. Olson LJ, Subramanian R, Edwards WD. Surgical pathology of pure aortic insufficiency: a study of 225 cases. Mayo Clin Proc 1984;59:835-841.

76. Zhimin W, Yubao Z, Lei S, et al. Prevalence of chronic rheumatic heart disease in Chinese adults. Int J Cardiol 2006;107:356-359.

77. Veasy LG, Wiedmeier SE, Orsmond GS, et al. Resurgence of acute rheumatic fever in the intermountain area of the United States. N Engl J Med 1987;316:421-427.

78. Stoate HG. Can health screening damage your health? J R Coll Gen Pract 1989;39:193-195.

79. Mishra TK. Acute rheumatic fever and rheumatic heart disease: current scenario. J Indian Acad Clin Med 2007;8:324-330.

80. Ramaswamy R, Spina GS, Fae KC, et al. Association of mannose-binding lectin gene polymorphism but not of mannose-binding serine protease 2 with chronic severe aortic regurgitation of rheumatic etiology. Clin Vaccine Immunol 2008;15:932-936.

81. Farrar EJ, Butcher JT. Valvular heart diseases in the developing world: developmental biology takes central stage. J Heart Valve Dis 2012;21:234-234.

82. Feinstein AR, Stern EK. Clinical effects of recurrent attacks of acute rheumatic fever: a prospective epidemiologic study of 105 episodes. J Chronic Dis 1967;20:13-27.

83. Marcus RH, Sareli P, Pocock WA, et al. The spectrum of severe rheumatic mitral valve disease in a developing country. Correlations among clinical presentation, surgical pathological findings, and hemodynamic sequelae. Ann Intern Med 1994;120:177-183.

84. Song H, Kim M-J, Chung CH, et al. Valvular heart disease: factors associated with development of late significant tricuspid regurgitation after successful left-sided valve surgery. Heart 2009;95:931-936

85. Nath J, Foster E, Heidenreich PA. Impact of tricuspid regurgitation on long-term survival. J Am Coll Cardiol. 2004;43:405-409. doi:10.1016/j.jacc.2003.09.036.

86. Kim JB, Yoo DG, Kim GC, et al. Mild-to-moderate functional tricuspid regurgitation in patients undergoing valve replacement for rheumatic mitral disease: the influence of tricuspid valve repair on clinical and echocardiographic outcomes. Heart 2012;98:24-30.

87. Kim JB, Spevack DM, Tunick PA, et al. The effect of transvenous pacemaker and implantable cardioverter defibrillator lead placement on tricuspid valve function: an observational study. J Am Soc Echocardiogr 2008;21:284-287.

88. Höke U, Auger D, Thijssen J, et al. Significant lead-induced tricuspid regurgitation is associated with poor prognosis at long-term follow-up. Heart 2014;100:960-968.

89. Franceschi F, Thuny F, Giorgi R, et al. Incidence, risk factors, and outcome of traumatic tricuspid regurgitation after percutaneous ventricular lead removal. J Am Coll Cardiol 2009;53:2168-2174.

90. Mirabel M, Andre R, Mikhail PB, Jouven X. Infective endocarditis in the Pacific: clinical characteristics, treatment and long-term outcomes. Open Heart 2014. doi:10.1136/openhrt-2014-000183.

91. Infective Endocarditis Prophylaxis Expert Group. Prevention of endocarditis. 2008 update from Therapeutic guidelines: antibiotic version 13, and Therapeutic guidelines: oral and dental version 1. Melbourne: Therapeutic Guidelines Limited; 2008.

92. Dayer MJ, Jones S, Prendergast B, et al. Incidence of infective endocarditis in England, 2000-13: a secular trend, interrupted time-series analysis. Lancet 2015;385(9974):1219-1228. PubMed PMID: 25467569.

93. Habib G, Hoen B, Tornon P, et al. Guidelines on the prevention, diagnosis, and treatment of infective endocarditis. Eur Heart J 2009;30:2369-2413.

94. Mayosi BM. Contemporary trends in the epidemiology and management of cardiomyopathy and pericarditis in sub-Saharan Africa. Heart 2007;93:1176-1183.

95. Mocumbi AOH, Falase AO. Recent advances in the epidemiology, diagnosis and treatment of endomyocardial fibrosis in Africa. Heart 2013;99:1481-1487.

96. Mocumbi AO, Yacoub S, Yacoub MH. Neglected tropical cardiomyopathies: II endomyocardial fibrosis: myocardial disease. Heart 2008;94:384-390.

97. Khalid U, Ahlehoff O, Gislason GH, et al. Increased risk of aortic valve stenosis in patients with psoriasis: a nationwide cohort study. Eur Heart J 2015;36:2177-2183.

98. Coffey S, Cox B, Williams MJA. The prevalence, incidence, progression, and risks of aortic valve sclerosis. J Am Coll Cardiol 2014;63:2852-2861.

99. Cosmi JE, Tunick PA, Rosenzweig BP, et al. The risk of development of aortic stenosis in patients with 'benign' aortic valve thickening. Arch Intern Med 2002;162:2345-2347.

100. Otto CM, Lind BK, Klitzman DW, et al. Association of aortic valve sclerosis with cardiovascular mortality and morbidity in the elderly. N Engl J Med 1999;341:142-147.

101. Hsu S-Y, Hsieh I-C, Chang S-H, et al. Aortic valve sclerosis is an echocardiographic indicator of significant coronary disease in patients undergoing diagnostic coronary angiography. Int J Clin Pract 2004;59:72-77.

102. Strauman E, Meyer B, Mistell M, et al. Aortic and mitral valve disease in patients with end stage renal failure on long-term haemodialysis. Br Heart J 1992;67:236-239.

103. Jeon D, Atar S, Brasch A, et al. Association of mitral valve annulus calcification, aortic valve sclerosis and aortic root calcification with abnormal myocardial single photon emission tomography in subjects age < 65 years old. J Am Coll Cardiol 2001;38:1988-1993.

104. Stewart BF, Siscovick D, Lind BK, et al. Clinical factors associated with calcific aortic valve disease: Cardiovascular Health Study. J Am Coll Cardiol 1997;29:630-634.

105. Loxdale SJ, Sneyd JR, Donovan A, et al. The role of routine pre-operative bedside echocardiography in detecting aortic stenosis in patients with a hip fracture. Anaesthesia 2012;67:51-54. doi:10.1111/j.1365-2044.2011.06942.x.

106. Martinsson A, Li X, Andersson C, et al. Temporal trends in the incidence and prognosis of aortic stenosis. A nationwide study of the Swedish population. Circulation 2015;131:988-994.

107. Pellerin D, Brecker S, Veyrat C. Degenerative mitral valve disease with emphasis on mitral valve prolapse. Heart 2002;88(Suppl IV):iv20-iv28.

108. Delling FN, Vasan RS. Epidemiology and pathophysiology of mitral valve prolapse. New insights into disease progression, genetics and molecular basis. Circulation 2014;129:2158-2170.

109. Kyndt F, Gueffet JP, Probst V, et al. Mutations in the gene incoding filamin A as a cause for familial cardiac valve dystrophy. Circulation 2007;115:40-49.

110. Devereux RB, Jones EC, Roman MJ, et al. Prevalence and correlates of mitral valve prolapse in a population-based sample of American Indians: the Strong Heart Study. Am J Med 2001;111:679-685.

111. Marks AR, Choong CY, Sanfilippo AJ, et al. Identification of high-risk and low-risk subgroups of patients with mitral-valve prolapse. N Engl J Med 1989;320:1031-1036.

112. Levy D, Savage D. Prevalence and clinical features of mitral valve prolapse. Am Heart J 1987;113:1281-1290.

113. Ling LH, Enriquez-Sarano M, Seward JB, et al. Clinical outcome of mitral regurgitation due to flail leaflet. N Engl J Med 1996;335:1417-1423.

114. Avierinos J-F, Gersh BJ, Melton LJ, et al. Natural history of asymptomatic mitral valve prolapse in the community. Circulation 2002;106:1355-1361.

115. Iung B, Vahanian A. Epidemiology of acquired valvular heart disease. Can J Cardiol 2014;30:962-970.

116. Tadros TM, Klein MD, Shapira OM. Ascending aortic dilatation associated with bicuspid aortic valve. Pathophysiology, molecular biology, and clinical implications. Circulation 2009;119:880-890.

117. Tzemos N, Therrien J, Yip J, et al. Outcomes in adults with bicuspid aortic valves. JAMA 2008;300:1317-1325.

118. Oliver JM, Alonso-Gonzalez R, Gonzalez AE, et al. Risk of aortic root or ascending aorta complications in patients with and without coarctation of the aorta. Am J Cardiol 2009;104:1001-1006.

119. Cabell CH Jr, Jollis JG, Peterson GE, et al Changing patient characteristics and the effect on mortality in endocarditis. Arch Intern Med 2002;162:90-94.

120. Yew HS, Murdoch DR. Global trends in infective endocarditis epidemiology. Curr Infect Dis Rep 2012;14:367-372.

121. Chirouze C, Hoen B, Duval X. Infective endocarditis epidemiology and consequences of prophylaxis guideline modifications: the dialectical evolution. Curr Infect Dis Rep 2014;16:440.

122. Friedman ND, Kaye KS, Stout JE, et al. Healthcare-associated bloodstream infections in adults: a reason to change the accepted definition of community-acquired infections. Ann Intern Med 2002;137:791-797.

123. Hill EE, Herigers P, Claus P, et al. Infective endocarditis: changing epidemiology and predictors of 6-month mortality: a prospective cohort study. Eur Heart J 2007;28:196-203.

124. Klug D, Lacroix D, Savoye C, et al. Systemic infection related to endocarditis on pacemaker leads: clinical presentation and management. Circulation 1997;95:2098-2107.

125. Selton-Suty C, Celard M, Moing V, et al. Preeminence of Staphylococcus aureus in infective endocarditis: a 1-year population-based study. Clin Infect Dis 2012;54:1230-1239.

126. Ostergaard L, Valour N, Ihlemann N, et al. Incidence of infective endocarditis among patients considered at high risk. Europe Heart J 2018; 39:623-629

127. Koegelenberg CF, Doubell AF, Orth H, et al. Infective endocarditis in the Western Cape Province of South Africa: a three year prospective study. Quart J Med 2003;96:217-225.

128. Duval X, Delahaye F, Alla F, et al. Temporal trends in infective endocarditis in the context of prophylaxis guideline modifications. Three successive population-based surveys. J Am Coll Cardiol 2012;59: 1968-1976.

129. Murdoch DR, Corey GR, Hoen B, et al. Clinical presentation, etiology, and outcome of infective endocarditis in the 21st century: the International Collaboration on Endocarditis–Prospective Cohort Study. Arch Intern Med 2009;169:463-473.

130. Nkomo VT. Epidemiology and prevention of valvular heart diseases and infective endocarditis in Africa. Heart 2007;93:1510-1519.

131. Habib G, Lancellotti P, Antunes MJ, et al. 2015 ESC guidelines for the management of infective endocarditis: the Task Force for the Management of Infective Endocarditis of the European Society of Cardiology (ESC) endorsed by: European Association for Cardio-Thoracic Surgery (EACTS), the European Association of Nuclear Medicine (EANM). Eur Heart J 2015;36:3075-3128. PubMed PMID: 26320109.

132. Nishimura RA, Carabello BA, Faxon DP, et al. ACC/AHA guideline update on valvular heart disease: focused update on infective endocarditis. Circulation 2008;118:887-896.

133. Cahill TJ, Harrison JL, Jewell JP, et al. Antibiotic prophylaxis for infective endocarditis: a systematic review and meta-analysis. Heart 2017; 103:937-944.

134. Pant S, Patel NL, Deshmukh A, et al. Trends in infective endocarditis incidence, microbiology, and valve replacement in the United States from 2000 to 2011. J Am Coll Cardiol 2015;65:2070-2076.

135. Keller K, von Bardeleben RS, Ostad MA, et al. Temporal trends in the prevalence if infective enodcarditis in Germany between 2005 and 2014. Am J Cardiol 2017;119(2):317-322

136. National Institute for Health and Care Excellence (NICE). Prophylaxis against infective endocarditis 2015 [NICE Clinical Guideline No 64]. Available from: http://www.nice.org.uk/guidance/cg64/chapter/Recommendations.

137. Zilla P, Brink J, Human P, Bezuidenhout D. Prosthetic heart valves: catering for the few. Biomaterials 2008;29:385-406.

138. Remenyi B, Webb R, Gentles T, et al. Improved long-term survival for rheumatic mitral valve repair compared to replacement in the young. World J Pediatr Congenit Heart Surg 2012;4:155-164.

139. North RA, Sadler L, Stewart AW, et al. Long-term survival and valve-related complications in young women with cardiac valve replacements. Circulation 1999;99:2669-2676.

140. Brown JM, O'Brien SM, Wu C, et al. Isolated aortic valve replacement in North America comprising 108,687 patients in 10 years: changes in risks, valve types, and outcomes in the Society of Thoracic Surgeons National Database. J Thorac Cardiovasc Surg 2009;137:82-90.

141. Dunning J, Gao H, Chambers J, et al. Aortic valve surgery—marked increases in volume and significant decreases in mechanical valve use; an analysis of 41,227 patients over 5 years from the Society for Cardiothoracic Surgery of Great Britain and Ireland National database. J Thorac Cardiovasc Surg 2011;142:776-782.

142. Saleeb SF, Newburger JW, Geva T, et al. Accelerated degeneration of a bovine pericardial bioprosthetic aortic valve in children and young adults. Circulation 2014;130:51-60.

143. Grunkemeier GL, Li H-H, Naftel DC, et al. Long-term performance of heart valve prostheses. Curr Probl Cardiol 2000;25:73-156.

144. Chan V, Malas T, Lapierre H, et al. Reoperation of left heart valve bioprostheses according to age at implantation. Circulation 2011;124 (Suppl 1):S75-S80.

145. Salaun E, Mahjoub H, Girerd N, et al. Rate, timing, correlates, and outcomes of hemodynamic valve deterioration after bioprosthetic surgical aortic valve replacement. Circulation 2018;138:971-985.

146. Le Gal G, Bertault V, Bezon E, et al. Heterogeneous geographic distribution of patients with aortic valve stenosis: arguments for new aetiological hypothesis. Heart 2005;91:247-249.

147. Garg V, Muth AN, Ransom MK, et al. Mutations in NOTCH1 cause aortic valve disease. Nature 2005;437:270-274.

148. McBride KL, Garg V. Heredity of bicuspid aortic valve: is family screening indicated? Heart 2011;97:1193-1195.

149. Huntington K, Hunter AGW, Chan K-L. A prospective study to assess the frequency of familial clustering of congenital bicuspid aortic valve. J Am Coll Cardiol 1997;30:1809-1812.

150. Cripe L, Andelfinger G, Martin LJ, et al. Bicuspid aortic valve is heritable. J Am Coll Cardiol 2004;44:138-143.

151. Schaefer BM, Lewin MB, Stout KK, et al. The bicuspid aortic valve: an integrated phenotypic classification of leaflet morphology and aortic root shape. Heart 2008;94:1634-1638.

152. Michelena HI, Desjardins VA, Avierinos J-F, et al. Natural history of asymptomatic patients with normally functioning or minimally dysfunctional bicuspid aortic valve in the community. Circulation 2008;117:2776-2784.

153. Masri A, Svensson LG, Griffin BP, Desai MY. Contemporary natural history of bicuspid aortic valve disease: a systematic review. Heart 2017; 103:1323-1330.

154. Dare AJ, Veinot JP, Edwards WD, et al. New observations on the etiology of aortic valve disease: a surgical pathologic study of 236 cases from 1990. Hum Pathol 1993;24:1330-1338.

155. Roberts WC, Ko JM, Filardo G, et al. Valve structure and survival in quinquagenarians having aortic valve replacement for aortic stenosis (±aortic regurgitation) with versus without coronary artery bypass grafting at a single US medical center 1993-2005. Am J Cardiol 2007;100:1584-1591.

156. Roberts WC, Ko JM, Filardo G, et al. Valve structure and survival in sexagenarians having aortic valve replacement for aortic stenosis (±aortic regurgitation) with versus without coronary artery bypass grafting at a single US medical center (1993 to 2005). Am J Cardiol 2007;100:1286-1292.

157. Roberts WC, Ko JM, Filardo G, et al. Valve structure and survival in septuagenarians having aortic valve replacement for aortic stenosis (±aortic regurgitation) with versus without coronary artery bypass grafting at a single US medical center (1993 to 2005). Am J Cardiol 2007;100:1157-1165.

158. Roberts WC, Ko JM, Garner WL, et al. Valve structure and survival in octogenarians having aortic valve replacement for aortic stenosis (±aortic regurgitation) with versus without coronary artery bypass grafting at a single US medical center 1993-2005. Am J Cardiol 2007;100:489-495.

159. Roberts WC, Ko JM, Matter GJ. Aortic valve replacement for aortic stenosis in nonagenarians. Am J Cardiol 2006;989:1251-1253.

160. Roberts WC, Ko JM. Frequency by decades of unicuspid, bicuspid, and tricuspid aortic valves in adults having isolated aortic valve replacement for aortic stenosis with or without associated aortic regurgitation. Circulation 2005;111:920-925.

161. Ruckman RN, Van Praagh R. Anatomic types of congenital mitral stenosis: report of 49 autopsy cases with consideration of diagnosis and surgical implications. Am J Cardiol 1978;42:592-601.

162. Seguela P-E, Houyel L, Acar P. Congenital malformations of the mitral valve. Arch Cardiovasc Dis 2011;104:465-479.

163. Roldan CA, Shively BK, Lau CC, et al. Systemic lupus erythematosus valve disease by transesophageal echocardiography and the role of antiphospholipid antibodies. J Am Coll Cardiol 1992;20:1127-1134.

164. Zuily S, Regnault V, Selton-Suty C, et al. Increased risk for heart valve disease associated with antiphospholipid antibodies in patients with systemic lupus erythematosis. Meta-analysis of echocardiographic studies. Circulation 2011;124:215-224.

165. Asherson RA, Cervera R. Antiphospholipid antibodies and the heart. Lessons and pitfalls for the cardiologist. Circulation 1991;84:920-923.

166. Roldan CA. Valvular and coronary heart disease in systemic inflammatory diseases. Heart 2008;94:1089-1101.

167. Fox DJ, Khattar RS. Carcinoid heart disease: presentation, diagnosis, and management. Heart 2004;90:1224-1228

168. Gustaffson BI, Hauso O, Drozdov I, et al. Carcinoid heart disease. Int J Cardiol 2008;129:318-324.

169. Lancellotti P, Livadariu E, Markov M, et al. Cabergoline and the risk of valvular lesions in endocrine disease. Eur J Endocrinol 2008;159:1-5.

170. Khan MA, Herzog CA, St Peter JV, et al. The prevalence of cardiac valvular insufficiency assessed by transthoracic echocardiography in obese patients treated with appetite-suppressant drugs. N Engl J Med 1998;339:713-718.

171. Connolly HM, Crary JL, McGoon MD, et al. Valvular heart disease associated with fenfluramine-phentermine. N Engl J Med 1997;337:581-588.

172. Dahl CF, Allen MR, Urie PM, et al. Valvular regurgitation and surgery associated with fenfluramine use: an analysis of 5743 individuals. BMC Med 2008;6:34.

173. Le Ven F, Tribouilloy C, Habib G, et al. Valvular heart disease associated with benfluorex therapy: results from the French multicentre registry. Eur J Echocardiogr 2011;12:265-271.

174. Antonini A, Poewe W. Fibrotic heart-valve reactions to dopamine-agonist treatment in Parkinson's disease. Lancet Neurol 2007;6:826-829.

175. Zanettini R, Antonini A, Gatto G, et al. Valvular heart disease and the use of dopamine agonists for Parkinson's disease. N Engl J Med 2007;356:39-46.

176. Sherlock M, Toogood AA, Steeds R. Dopamine agonist therapy for hyperprolactinaemia and cardiac valve dysfunction; a lot done but much more to do. Heart 2009;95:522-523.

177. Gu H, Luck S, Carroll P, et al. Cardiac valve disease and low-dose dopamine agonist therapy: an artefact of reporting bias? Clin Endocrinol 2011;74:608-610.

178. Redfield MM, Nicholson WJ, Edwards WD, et al. Valve disease associated with ergot alkaloid use. Echocardiographic and pathologic correlations. Ann Intern Med 1992;117:50-52.

179. Droogmans S, Cosyns B, D'Haenen H, et al. Possible association between 3,4-methylenedioxymethamphetamine abuse and valvular heart disease. Am J Cardiol 2007;100:1442-1445.

180. Carlson RG, Mayfield WR, Normann S, Alexander JA. Radiation-associated valvular disease. Chest 1991;99:538-545.

181. Veinot JP, Edwards WD. Pathology of radiation-induced heart disease: a surgical and autopsy study of 27 cases. Hum Pathol 1996;27:766-773.

182. Chambers JB, Shah BN, Prendergast B, et al. Valvular heart disease: a call for global collaborative research initiatives. Heart 2013;99:1797-1799. doi:10.1136/heartjnl-2013-303964.

183. Arden C, Chambers J, Ray S, et al. Can we improve the detection of heart valve disease? Heart 2014;100:271-273. E published 30 May 2013. doi:10.1136/heartjnl-2013-304223.

184. Lancellotti P, Rosenhek R, Pibarot P, et al. Heart valve clinics: organisation, structure and experiences. Eur Heart J 2013;34:1597-1606.

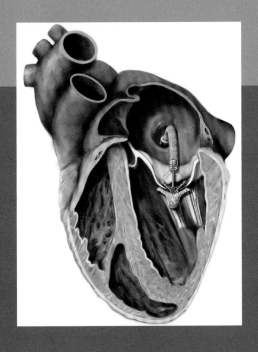

第2章
主动脉瓣及二尖瓣三维解剖

　　本章主要为读者介绍主动脉瓣与二尖瓣的解剖结构及三维超声检查在评估主动脉瓣及二尖瓣疾病中的应用。主动脉瓣与二尖瓣在解剖上由纤维结构相连，二者在功能上也是相互依赖关系。二尖瓣包含瓣环、瓣叶、瓣叶交界、腱索、乳头肌等解剖结构，这些解剖结构的协同作用确保了二尖瓣的正常功能。任何部分结构或功能的改变均可能导致二尖瓣功能失调，常见的包括退行性改变（如Barlow综合征或弹性纤维缺乏导致的瓣叶脱垂）和继发性改变（如缺血性心脏病导致的乳头肌移位），均可导致二尖瓣关闭不全。主动脉瓣的解剖结构要考虑到主动脉根部的整体结构。主动脉根部包括自左心室流出道水平至窦管交界水平的多种解剖结构，包含瓣环、瓣叶、瓣叶交界及主动脉窦。在主动脉疾病及二尖瓣疾病的评估方面，由于二者均是复杂的三维结构，相比二维超声检查的平面显像，三维超声检查可提供实时、详细的空间影像，对二尖瓣及主动脉瓣的结构、运动及功能的评估更为准确，不仅能更加准确区分其功能失调的机制，更可为手术治疗策略的制定（如修复治疗等）提供重要信息。同时，在经导管瓣膜介入治疗技术飞速发展的当下，三维超声检查在其中亦扮演着重要角色。

丰德京

Three-Dimensional Anatomy of the Aortic and Mitral Valves

Wendy Tsang, Benjamin H. Freed, Roberto M. Lang

CHAPTER OUTLINE

KEY POINTS

Mitral Valve

- Three-dimensional echocardiography (3DE) provides real-time, detailed, nonplanar images of the complex mitral valve (MV) apparatus, including the annulus, leaflets, chordae, and papillary muscles.
- Quantitative analysis of MV anatomy, function, and motion using 3DE is significantly more accurate and reproducible than two-dimensional echocardiographic (2DE) planar imaging.
- Assessment of degenerative MV disease with 3DE helps guide the optimal surgical strategy and improve postoperative outcome.
- 3DE provides mechanistic insight into the pathophysiology of ischemic mitral regurgitation (MR) and potential roles for surgical and transcatheter repair.
- Multiplanar imaging provides significantly more accurate measurements of the severity of MR compared with 2DE.
- 3DE plays an important role before, during, and after multiple catheter-based interventions, including valvuloplasty for mitral stenosis, edge-to-edge repair for MR, and closure of perivalvular leaks.

Aortic Valve

- The 3DE *en face* view improves the assessment of aortic root structures such as aortic valve leaflet number, aortic annular shape, and left ventricular outflow tract (LVOT) dimensions.
- Assessment of aortic stenosis severity is improved by substituting the 3DE planimetered area of the LVOT area into the continuity equation, by replacing the numerator of the continuity equation by 3DE-derived stroke volume, or by direct aortic valve area planimetry.
- Assessment of aortic regurgitation severity is improved with the use of 3DE planimetered vena contracta area.
- With 3DE, good visualization of prosthetic aortic valve rings from the LVOT perspective and the aorta is possible; however, reliable visualization of prosthetic aortic valve leaflets remains challenging.
- 3DE improves characterization of valve masses.
- 3DE plays an important role before, during, and after percutaneous procedures such as transcatheter aortic valve replacement and closure of paravalvular regurgitation.

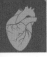

Advances in 3DE technology have ushered its use into mainstream clinical practice. It provides realistic images of the mitral and aortic valves and their spatial relationships with adjacent structures. It offers unique anatomic and functional insights that have furthered our understanding of the pathophysiology of valvular heart disease. In this chapter, we discuss the value of 3DE for the mitral and aortic valves in evaluating valve anatomy, volumetric quantification, presurgical planning, intraprocedural guidance, and postprocedural assessment.

MITRAL VALVE

Mitral Valve Anatomy

The MV is a complicated 3D structure involving multiple, distinct anatomic components. Optimal interaction of the elements comprising the annulus, commissures, leaflets, chordae tendineae, papillary muscles, and left ventricle (LV) is crucial for its functional integrity.

Mitral Valve Annulus

The mitral annulus is a fibromuscular ring to which the anterior and posterior MV leaflets attach. The normal MV annulus has a 3D saddle shape with its lowest points at the level of the anterolateral and posteromedial commissures. This enables proper leaflet apposition during systole and minimizes leaflet stress.[1] The annulus can be divided into the anterior and posterior annulus based on the insertion of the corresponding leaflets.

Mitral Valve Leaflets

The MV has an anterior and posterior leaflet. The atrial, or smooth, surface is free of attachments, whereas the LV, or rough, surface connects to the papillary muscles by the chordae tendineae. The posterior leaflet, which has a quadrangular shape, is attached to approximately three-fifths of the annular circumference. The semicircular anterior leaflet is attached to approximately two-fifths of the annular circumference.[2]

Although the posterior leaflet attaches to a larger portion of the annular circumference, the leaflet is shorter than the anterior one.

The leaflet segmentation proposed by Carpentier is the most widely classification used.[3] This schema takes advantage that the posterior leaflet has two well-defined indentations dividing it into three separate sections or *scallops*. The anterolateral scallop is defined as P1, the middle scallop is defined as P2, and the posteromedial scallop is defined as P3. The anterior leaflet typically has a smoother surface and is devoid of indentations. The segment of the anterior leaflet opposing P1 is designated A1 (anterior segment), the segment opposite to P2 is A2 (middle segment), and the segment opposite to P3 is A3 (posterior segment) (Fig. 2.1).

Mitral Valve Commissures

The commissures define a distinct area where the anterior and posterior leaflets appose each other during systole. Carpentier divides them into anterolateral and posteromedial commissures.[3] The amount of tissue in the commissures varies from several millimeters of leaflet tissue to distinct leaflet segments.

Mitral Valve Chordae

The chordae tendineae are responsible for determining the position and tension on the anterior and posterior leaflets at LV end-systole. The chordae are fibrous extensions originating from the heads of the papillary muscles and infrequently from the inferolateral LV wall. They are named according to their insertion site on the mitral leaflets. Marginal or primary chordae insert on the free margin of the mitral leaflets and help prevent marginal prolapse. Intermediate or secondary strut chordae insert on the LV surface of the leaflets, preventing billowing while reducing tension on the leaflet tissues.[4,5] These chords may also play a role in determining dynamic LV shape and function due to their contribution to LV-valve continuity.[6,7] Basal or tertiary chordae insert on the posterior leaflet base and mitral annulus. Their specific function is unclear.

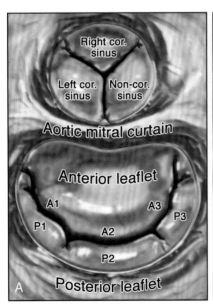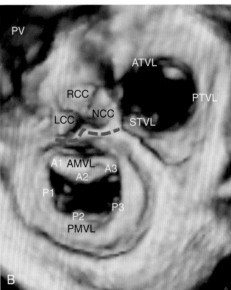

Fig. 2.1 Schematic diagram (A) and *en face* 3DE zoom mode image (B) of the mitral valve from the LA or surgeon's perspective depicts typical anatomic relationships. In this view, the aortic valve occupies the 12-o'clock position. The aortic-mitral curtain separates the anterior leaflet from the aortic valve. The Carpentier system divides the posterior leaflet into three scallops *(P1, P2, P3)* based on leaflet indentation. The anterior leaflet is then divided and classified as three segments based on their relationship to the posterior leaflet *(A1, A2, A3)*. *AMVL*, Anterior mitral valve leaflet; *ATVL*, anterior tricuspid valve leaflet; *LCC*, left coronary cusp; *NCC*, noncoronary cusp; *PMVL*, posterior mitral valve leaflet; *PTVL*, posterior tricuspid valve leaflet; *PV*, pulmonary valve; *RCC*, right coronary cusp; *STVL*, septal tricuspid valve leaflet.

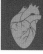

Papillary Muscles

There are two papillary muscles—the anterolateral and the posteromedial—that originate from the area between the apical and middle thirds of the LV free wall. The anterolateral papillary muscle is composed of an anterior and posterior head, and the posteromedial papillary muscle is usually composed of anterior, intermediate, and posterior heads.[8] Because the papillary muscles connect directly to the LV, any geometric change in LV shape can change the axial relationship of the chordae and leaflets, resulting in poor leaflet coaptation.

3DE and Mitral Valve Apparatus

With the advent of 3DE imaging, new parameters quantifying annular, coaptation, leaflet, and subvalvular geometry were easily obtained.[2,9] These measurements provided insights into MV mechanics and have been instrumental in guiding MV repair because 3DE allowed classification of MV dysfunction (Table 2.1). One study found a strong correlation ($r = 0.93$, $P < 0.0001$) between chordal length assessed preoperatively by 3DE and intraoperative measurements, emphasizing its important role in preprocedural surgical planning (Fig. 2.2).[10] Fig. 2.3 shows the most commonly used parameters.[2]

3DE Imaging
Image Acquisition

The main views used to acquire 3D transthoracic echocardiographic (TTE) images of the MV are the parasternal long-axis and apical four-chamber views (Table 2.2). Although the 2D TTE parasternal short-axis

view provides an *en face* view of the MV, it displays only the MV leaflets *en face* from the LV perspective.

When using 3D transesophageal echocardiography (TEE) for imaging, the 60-degree MV bi-commissural and 120-degree long-axis mid-esophageal views are best for visualizing the entire MV structure and its associated components.[11] The transgastric long-axis view of the MV is best used with multiplanar mode to assess subvalvular and valvular structures. 3D TEE provides significantly better anatomic detail compared with TTE due to its higher spatial resolution.

Image Display

After the 3D data set is acquired, plane cropping and rotation of the pyramidal volume can be performed to present a dynamic *en face* 3D rendering of the MV. 3DE facilitates communication between the imager and the cardiovascular surgeon because it can display the MV in a manner similar to the way the surgeon visualizes the valve in the operating room when approaching the valve from the left atrium (LA). This surgical view is obtained by viewing the MV from the LA and rotating the valve such that the aorta is directly above it at the 12-o'clock position (Fig. 2.4).

3DE Mechanisms of Mitral Valve Dysfunction
Degenerative Mitral Valve Disease

MV prolapse is the most common cause of MR in developed countries.[12] 3DE technology has considerably improved the ability of physicians to diagnose and surgically treat MV prolapse,[13] which primarily

Characteristic	Type 1	Type 2	Type IIIA	Type IIIB
Motion of leaflet margin	Normal	Prolapse or flail	Restricted leaflet opening	Restricted leaflet closure
Associated disease processes	Chronic atrial fibrillation Bacterial endocarditis	Degenerative disease (Barlow disease, fibroelastic deficiency)	Rheumatic disease	Myocardial infarction Dilated cardiomyopathy
Associated lesions	Annular dilation Leaflet perforation	Leaflet thickening Leaflet billowing Leaflet elongation Chordal thickening Chordal rupture	Commissure fusion Leaflet thickening Chordae thickening	Papillary displacement Chordae tethering Annular dilation

TABLE 2.1   **Carpentier Functional Classification for Mitral Valve Dysfunction.**

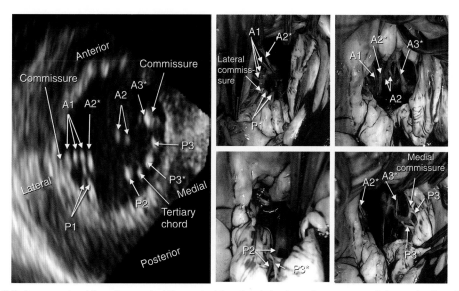

Fig. 2.2 An example of the alignment of the root of the chords is shown in an extracted short-axis plane from the 3D data set (*left*). The corresponding anatomy is demonstrated intraoperatively (*right*).

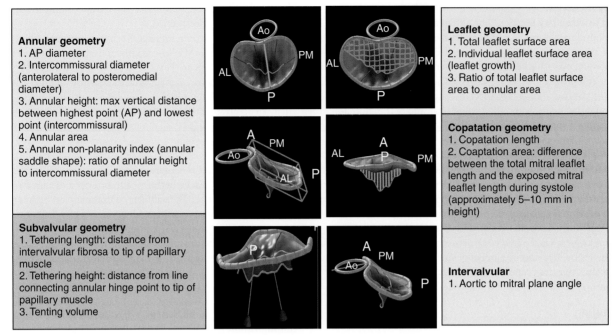

Annular geometry
1. AP diameter
2. Intercommissural diameter (anterolateral to posteromedial diameter)
3. Annular height: max vertical distance between highest point (AP) and lowest point (intercommissural)
4. Annular area
5. Annular non-planarity index (annular saddle shape): ratio of annular height to intercommissural diameter

Subvalvular geometry
1. Tethering length: distance from intervalvular fibrosa to tip of papillary muscle
2. Tethering height: distance from line connecting annular hinge point to tip of papillary muscle
3. Tenting volume

Leaflet geometry
1. Total leaflet surface area
2. Individual leaflet surface area (leaflet growth)
3. Ratio of total leaflet surface area to annular area

Copatation geometry
1. Copatation length
2. Coaptation area: difference between the total mitral leaflet length and the exposed mitral leaflet length during systole (approximately 5–10 mm in height)

Intervalvular
1. Aortic to mitral plane angle

Fig. 2.3 Volumetric reconstruction of the mitral valve with 3DE-based software allows measurements of mitral annulus, leaflet, coaptation line, intervalvular relationships, and subvalvular geometry. *A*, Anterior; *Ao*, aortic valve; *P*, posterior.

TABLE 2.2	3D Echocardiographic Acquisition and Display.		
Imaging	View	Mitral Valve	Aortic Valve
Acquisition	Transthoracic	Parasternal long-axis view Apical 4-chamber view	Parasternal long-axis view Parasternal short-axis view Apical 3-chamber view
	Transesophageal	Mid-esophageal ≈0° 4-chamber view Mid-esophageal ≈120° long-axis view	Mid-esophageal ≈60° aortic valve short-axis view Mid-esophageal ≈120° long-axis view
Display		Orient the aortic valve at the 12-o'clock position whether the valve is viewed from the LA or the LV	Orient the right coronary cusp at the 6-o'clock position whether viewed from the aorta or the LVOT

results from two distinctive types of degenerative diseases: Barlow disease and fibroelastic deficiency (Table 2.3). Barlow disease results from an excess of myxomatous tissue, which is an abnormal accumulation of mucopolysaccharides in one or both of the leaflets and many or only a few of the chordae.[14] In contrast, fibroelastic deficiency results from acute loss of mechanical integrity due to abnormalities of connective tissue structure and/or function.[14] It usually results in a localized or unisegmental prolapse due to elongated chordae or flail leaflet due to ruptured chordae (Fig. 2.5).

Many studies have shown that 3DE is superior to 2DE in accurately diagnosing the location of degenerative disease.[15–17] 3DE is less operator-dependent, and more reproducible than 2DE at any level of expertise. The diagnostic accuracy of 3D and 2D TEE was compared for a large number of patients undergoing MV repair due to prolapse, and echocardiographic findings were compared with surgical ones.[18] 3D TEE correctly identified the prolapsing scallop in 92% of patients versus 78% of patients using 2D TEE. The use of parametric maps, which are 3D images of the MV transformed into color-encoded topographic displays of MV anatomy in which the color gradations indicate the distance of the leaflet from the mitral annular plane toward the LA, have also improved diagnostic accuracy for novice readers (Fig. 2.6).[16]

One study found that 3D color-coded parametric maps of the MV allowed easy differentiation of MV prolapse versus MV billowing without the need to inspect multiple planes as needed with 2DE.[19]

In addition to its superior accuracy in diagnosing degenerative disease, 3DE also has the ability to differentiate Barlow disease from fibroelastic deficiency. When 3D quantitative parameters are used to differentiate patients with or without degenerative MV disease, billowing height and volume were the strongest predictors of degenerative MV disease.[15] 3D billowing height with a cutoff value of 1.0 mm differentiated normal from degenerative disease without overlap, whereas 3D billowing volume with a cutoff value of 1.15 mL differentiated Barlow disease from fibroelastic deficiency. These measurements were found to be highly reproducible.

3DE studies have increased our understanding of the pathophysiologic differences between fibroelastic deficiency and Barlow disease. These two entities have different alterations in annular dynamics and leaflet tissues.[20,21] In addition to significant leaflet prolapse, patients with Barlow disease have blunted annular dynamics during the cardiac cycle that exceed the extent of LV and atrial remodeling.[20] This suggests that there may be a primary abnormality of the mitral annulus that contributes to MR severity. These annular changes may also

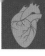

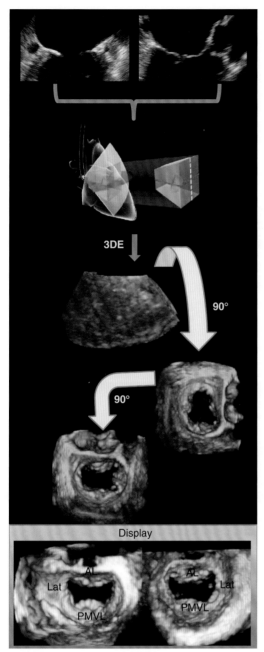

Fig. 2.4 3D TEE Acquisition and Presentation of the Mitral Valve. *Top,* Two orthogonal views of the mitral valve are optimized with biplane mode before 3D TEE acquisition. Once acquired, the 3DE pyramid should be rotated 90 degrees along the x-axis to obtain an *en face* view of the mitral valve. The 3DE pyramid should be rotated so that the aortic valve is located at the 12-o'clock position. The mitral valve should be displayed with the aortic valve at the 12-o'clock position regardless of whether the valve is viewed from the LA or LV perspective. *AL,* Anterolateral mitral valve leaflet, *Lat,* lateral, *PMVL,* posterior mitral valve leaflet.

TABLE 2.3   Key Differences Between Barlow Disease and Fibroelastic Deficiency.

Differentiating Characteristics	Barlow Disease	Fibroelastic Deficiency
Pathology	Excess of myxomatous tissue	Impaired production of connective tissue
Typical age of diagnosis	Younger (<40 years)	Older (>60 years)
Duration of disease	Years to decades	Days to months
Physical examination	Mid-systolic click and late systolic murmur	Holosystolic murmur
Leaflet involvement	Multisegmental	Unisegmental
Leaflet lesions	Leaflet billowing and thickening	Thin leaflets with thickened involved segment
Chordae lesions	Chordal thickening and elongation	Chordal elongation and chordal rupture
Carpentier classification	Type II	Type II
Type of dysfunction	Bileaflet prolapse	Prolapse and/or flail
Complexity of valve repair	More complex	Less complex

preserved annular function but little tissue reserve with reduced systolic leaflet area changes. They develop severe MR with fewer morphologic changes. Overall, these differences suggest that different surgical approaches may be required for repair.

With 3DE *en face* visualization of the MV, there has been greater recognition of the presence of deep cleft-like indentations in patients with degenerative valve disease (Fig. 2.7) and the importance of differentiating them from true clefts due to atrioventricular septal defects with or without an intact septum.[23] Understanding the role of these clefts in contributing to the MR is needed to determine feasibility for transcatheter edge-to-edge repair procedures and as a possible source of residual MR after device placement.

Ischemic Mitral Regurgitation

Ischemic MR is a pathophysiologic outcome of LV remodeling arising from ischemic heart disease. Classically, it was thought to primarily result from posteromedial papillary muscle dysfunction due to this muscle's dependence on a single blood supply. In the past decade, however, multiple 3DE studies have shown that papillary muscle dysfunction is not responsible for ischemic MR. A wide spectrum of geometric distortions that result from LV remodeling cause this type of valve dysfunction. The observations provided by 3DE have helped reshape our understanding of ischemic MR.

The MV is dynamic and changes from a saddle shape (i.e., hyperbolic paraboloid) during systole to a flatter configuration during diastole. During systole, competing forces act on the MV leaflets. Increased LV pressure acts to push the leaflets toward the LA, and tethering forces from the chordae act to pull the leaflets in the direction of the LV. The saddle-shape morphology is thought to balance these forces by optimizing leaflet curvature and minimizing mitral leaflet stress.[1] In the setting of a myocardial infarction and resultant LV remodeling, an outward and apical displacement of the posteromedial papillary muscle occurs, which tethers the MV leaflets into the LV, restricting their ability to coapt effectively at the level of the mitral annulus.[24] The mitral annulus also dilates, making leaflet coaptation even more difficult.[25]

explain the development of mitral annular disjunction that leads to a functional decoupling between the ventricle and the mitral annulus.[22] Despite greater prolapse severity and annular enlargement, patients with Barlow disease can have quantitatively similar MR severity compared with patients with fibroelastic deficiency due to compensation by increased mitral tissue reserve/distensibility during mid-to-late systole.[20] In contrast, patients with fibroelastic deficiency have relatively

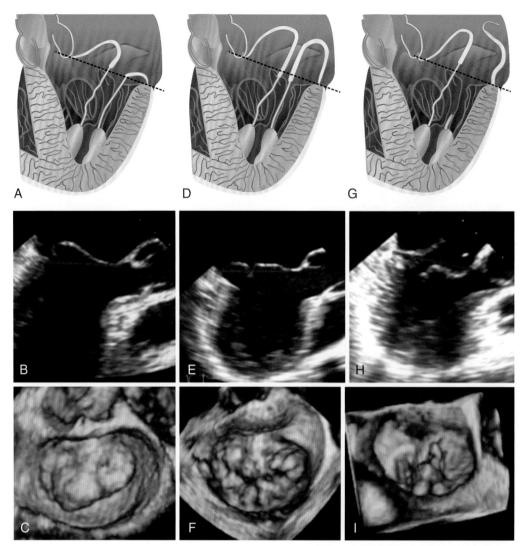

Fig. 2.5 Myxomatous Disease With Mitral Valve Prolapse. Schematic (A) demonstrates anterior leaflet prolapse with imaging from 2D TEE (B) and 3D TEE (C) as viewed *en face* from the LA. Leaflet prolapse is diagnosed when the free edge of the leaflet overrides the plane of the mitral annulus during systole. Schematic (D) demonstrates bileaflet billowing of the mitral valve due to chordae elongation with imaging from 2D TEE (E) and 3D TEE (F) as viewed *en face* from the LA. Leaflet billowing is diagnosed when there is systolic excursion of the leaflet body into the LA due to excess leaflet tissue, with the leaflet free edge remaining below the plane of the mitral annulus. Schematic (G) demonstrates anterior mitral leaflet prolapse and posterior mitral leaflet flail due to chordal rupture with a 2D TEE (H) example of P2 flail segment and corresponding 3D TEE (I) *en face* image as viewed from the LA.

Although some have used the terms *ischemic MR* and *functional MR* interchangeably, they have different meanings. Unlike ischemic MR, in which displacement of the posteromedial papillary muscle predominates, functional MR is a result of bilateral papillary muscle displacement (i.e., symmetric tethering) typically caused by dilated cardiomyopathy. The direction of the MR jet can help differentiate the two types of valvular dysfunction. The ischemic MR jet is usually eccentric and directed toward the posterior "restricted" leaflet, whereas the functional MR jet is commonly centrally directed toward the roof of the LA (Fig. 2.8).

3DE has provided insights into the pathophysiology of functional and ischemic MR. For example, several investigators using 3DE showed that increased sphericity of the LV, rather than contractile dysfunction, contributes significantly to bilateral papillary displacement, resulting in functional MR.[26,27] 3DE showed that anterior-apical myocardial

infarctions that extend to the inferior apex can also cause ischemic MR.[28] This suggests that inferior myocardial infarctions are not solely responsible for ischemic MR but that this entity can develop even when the myocardium immediately underlying the posteromedial papillary muscle is not directly involved.

Mitral leaflet tethering in ischemic mitral regurgitation. Mitral leaflet tethering is a major factor contributing to development of ischemic MR. 2DE has been extensively used to calculate MV tenting area and tenting length, but studies have shown that the asymmetry of these single-plane measurements is commonly inaccurate compared with intraoperative findings.[29] 3DE overcomes this limitation by providing more accurate and reproducible measurements. In one of the first studies to examine leaflet tethering with 3DE, patients with severe MR were shown to have significantly larger tenting lengths and volumes compared with control patients.[30]

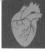

P2
flail

Medial
commissure

Barlows
prolapse

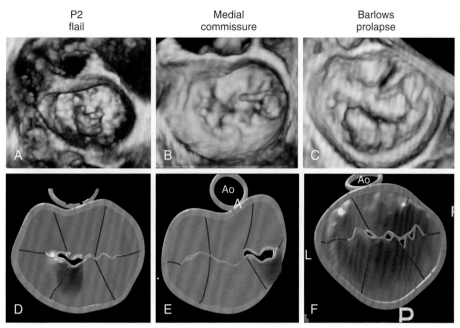

Fig. 2.6 *En face* 3D TEE images of the mitral valve as viewed from the LA demonstrate flail P2 segment (A) due to fibroelastic deficiency, flail medial commissure segment (B); and bileaflet prolapse (C) in a patient with Barlow disease. The corresponding parametric maps are for P2 flail (D), medial commissure flail (E), and Barlow disease (F), in which the color gradations toward orange indicate the distance of the leaflet from the mitral annular plane toward the LA. *A,* Anterior; *AL,* anterolateral; *Ao,* aortic valve; *P,* posterior.

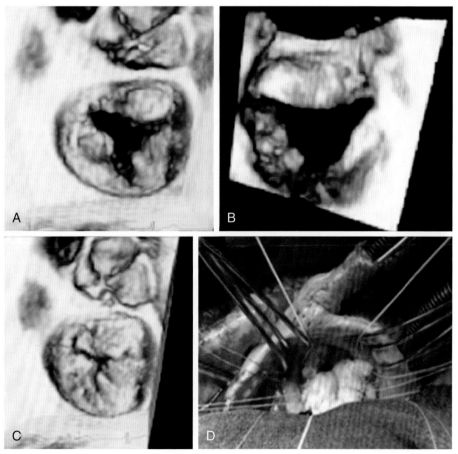

Fig. 2.7 (A) *En face* transesophageal image of the mitral valve as viewed from the LA during diastole demonstrates a pseudo-cleft in the posterior leaflet. (B) Image of the valve as seen from the left ventricle. (C) The image demonstrates the appearance of the valve during systole with the prolapsing segments. (D) Corresponding operative image of the valve demonstrates the significant prolapse with a deep fold.

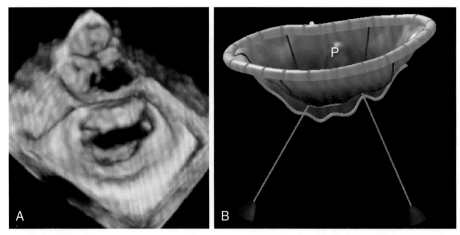

Fig. 2.8 (A) *En face* 3D TEE image of a mitral valve as viewed from the LA demonstrates symmetric bileaflet tethering due to dilated cardiomyopathy. (B) Corresponding parametric map depicts apical displacement of the chordae and subsequent tethering of both leaflets. *P*, Posterior.

This study found that the leaflet site where peak tenting occurred was different in each individual, suggesting that different chordae are involved in the disease process. Although MR severity is affected by the degree of tenting, tenting asymmetry is associated with greater degrees of regurgitation.

Mitral valve annulus in ischemic mitral regurgitation. Conformational changes of the MV annulus contributes to the development of ischemic MR. Multiple studies have shown that the annulus dilates and flattens, becoming essentially adynamic throughout the cardiac cycle.[24,30] 3DE imaging has revealed more subtle anatomic changes such as greater dilation in the anteroposterior dimension and greater overall dilation and flattening in anterior compared with inferior infarcts.[30,31] 3DE has been used to evaluate the dynamic changes in MV annular surface area and annular longitudinal displacement throughout the cardiac cycle.[32] It has been demonstrated that the mitral annular surface area is larger and the annular pulsatility and displacement lower in patients with ischemic MR. As the mitral annulus enlarges, it loses its motility, becoming progressively unable to modify its shape throughout the cardiac cycle.

Leaflet growth in ischemic mitral regurgitation. One of the most intriguing findings of 3DE is that while leaflet tethering and annular geometric changes drive the development of ischemic MR, leaflet growth occurs in an attempt to compensate for the decrease in leaflet coaptation.[33] In one of the earliest studies to examine this phenomenon, Chaput et al found that leaflet area increased by 35% in patients with LV dysfunction.[34] Two months after a myocardial infarction, tethered leaflet area and thickness were shown to be significantly increased compared with nontethered leaflets.[35] Studies using molecular histopathology showed that this leaflet growth was due to an increase in smooth muscle α-actin in tethered leaflets, indicating endothelial-mesenchymal transdifferentiation.

A 3DE study examined the interactions among leaflet tethering, annular dilation and flattening, and leaflet elongation.[36] The study authors measured multiple variables, including tenting length and volume, total leaflet area, total annular area, and coaptation length and area. They demonstrated that mitral leaflet coaptation decreases proportionally with the increased displacement of the papillary muscles, despite the presence of compensatory increased total leaflet area. The ratio of total leaflet area to total annular area required to ensure proper coaptation in mid-systole was decreased in patients with severe MR compared with patients with only mild MR. Coaptation area was the strongest determinant of MR severity. The reason why some patients

develop sufficient compensatory leaflet growth while others do not remains unknown.[37]

Treatment of ischemic mitral regurgitation. Multiple studies using 3DE after MV ring annuloplasty have shown that while this procedure reduces mitral annular size, it also reduces pulsatility and motion of the entire valve due to its inherent rigid structure.[32,38] Because of this insight, newer annuloplasty rings are being developed that better conform to the natural 3D dynamics of the MV annulus.[39] Quantification of the MV annular height and intercommissural diameter by 3DE is helpful in assessing the suitability of different customized prosthesis and repair strategies aimed at restoring or maintaining the saddle-shape of the annulus.[38] Despite this, annuloplasty rings in general do not address the tethering component and may be insufficient in decreasing MR. Patients with significant tethering on 3DE involving the posterior commissure (i.e., segments P2 and A3-P3) are at higher risk of recurrent MR after surgery. 3DE may play a role in selecting which ischemic MR patients should receive valve repair over replacement.

3DE Quantification of Mitral Regurgitation

Determining the severity of MR by quantitative analysis is an important step in the management of MV disease. Due to the complex geometry of the mitral apparatus, 3DE is uniquely suited for the assessment of MR. Delineation of the effective regurgitant orifice area by vena contracta area, proximal isovelocity surface area, and anatomical regurgitant surface area are some of the major strengths of 3DE (Table 2.4).[40]

3D Vena Contracta Area

Direct assessment of the vena contracta by 3DE reveals significant asymmetry of the vena contracta area in MR underscoring the poor estimation of the effective regurgitant orifice area by single-plane vena contracta width measurements.[41] This is particularly true of ischemic MR in which the MR jet is typically eccentric. 3DE vena contracta area provides a single, directly visualized, and reliable measurement of effective regurgitant orifice area, which classifies MR severity, similar to the current clinical practice of using the American Society of Echocardiography–recommended 2D integrative method (Fig. 2.9).[42]

Many studies have compared vena contracta area measurement by 3DE with various 2D quantitative parameters and have consistently found that the accuracy and reproducibility for MR severity is far superior when 3D vena contracta is used.[43–45] In a study comparing 2D

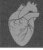

TABLE 2.4 3DE Quantitative Assessment of Mitral Regurgitation.

	Vena Contracta	Proximal Isovelocity Surface Area	Anatomic Regurgitant Orifice Area	Stroke Volumes
Benefits	TTE and TEE *En face* view of vena contracta Multplanar width assessment More accurate and reproducible	TTE and TEE Convergence is flattened proximal to orifice and elongated distal to orifice More accurate assessment of radius without geometric assumptions	Direct *en face* visualization of the mitral valve Can be calculated in real time	Integration of flow velocities throughout the entire cardiac cycle More accurate and reproducible
Limitations	3DE color Doppler limitations Requires proper selection of the systolic frame	Requires significant off-line processing 3DE color Doppler limitations	Limited TTE data Requires proper selection of the systolic frame	Limited TEE data Not valid with concomitant valvular disease or intracardiac shunting

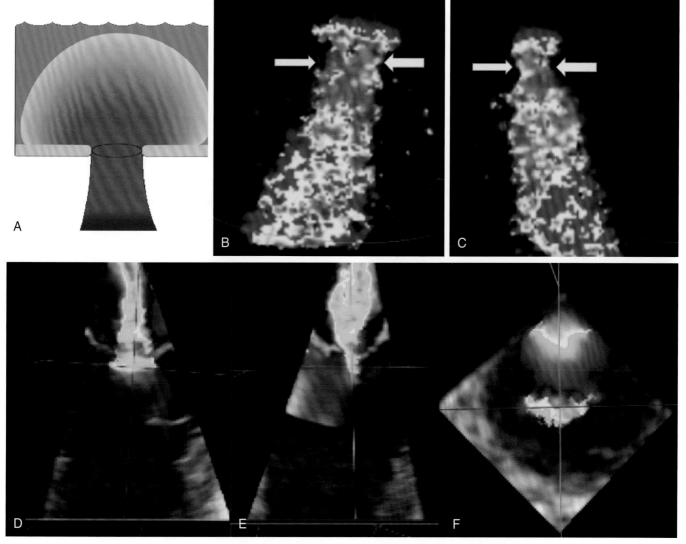

Fig. 2.9 (A) Illustration depicts the classic way of using the proximal isovelocity surface area (PISA) by visualizing the proximal surface area as a hemisphere (rather than a hemi-elliptical model). (B and C) Direct assessment of the mitral regurgitation (MR) jet by 3DE demonstrates that the vena contracta area is more oval than circular. (D–F) 3DE volumetric assessment of the MR jet reveals an ellipsoid effective regurgitant orifice area. These corrections allow more accurate measurements of the degree of MR and better guidance of therapy.

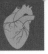

quantification of regurgitant orifice area by proximal isovelocity surface area method with 3D measured vena contracta area, the study authors found that a 3D vena contracta area cutoff of 0.41 cm^2 was 82% sensitive and 97% specific in differentiating moderate from severe MR.[43]

3D Proximal Isovelocity Surface Area

Two-dimensional methods of effective regurgitant orifice quantification assume that the proximal flow convergence region is hemispherical and that the regurgitant orifice is circular. 3D computational fluid dynamics models have demonstrated that, as the regurgitant orifice gets larger, the convergence region becomes spheroidal (flattened) near the orifice and ellipsoidal (elongated) far from the orifice.[46] Studies have shown that hemi-ellipsoidal models, rather than hemispherical models, result in a much more accurate estimation of the effective regurgitant orifice area in in vitro and clinical studies.[47,48]

3D Anatomic Regurgitant Orifice Area

Because 2D planimetry of the effective regurgitant orifice area in patients with MR is inaccurate due to the complex, nonplanar 3D geometry of the orifice, 3D anatomic regurgitant orifice area measurement may provide a reasonable alternative to determine the severity of MR.[49] Measurement of the anatomic regurgitant orifice area is accomplished by direct visualization of the MV *en face*.

There are several methods for determining the anatomic regurgitant orifice area. One method requires manual tracing of the leaflet edges in a 3D data set. This method demonstrates good correlation with 2D proximal isovelocity surface area–derived effective regurgitant orifice area but with better reproducibility.[49] Anatomic regurgitant orifice area can also be easily measured with the use of real-time 3D zoom mode of the MV acquired with TEE.[50]

3D Mitral Inflow and Left Ventricular Outflow Tract Stroke Volume

One of the great strengths of 3DE compared with 2DE is that it allows stroke volume quantification without geometric assumptions, flow profile assumptions, or reliance on single plane measurements. This technique uses 3D color Doppler data for a region of interest to calculate stroke volume. Several studies have demonstrated the accuracy of 3D-derived LV outflow and mitral inflow stroke volume measurements.[51,52]

A newer method for quantifying MV regurgitant volume involves using a single 3D TTE volume data set to obtain 3D-derived LV outflow and MV inflow stroke volumes. Thavendiranathan et al used this method for 44 patients without valvular disease and compared the results with standard 2D pulse wave Doppler measurements with cardiac magnetic resonance (CMR) velocity-encoded imaging as a reference.[53] The study authors demonstrated that LV outflow and MV inflow stroke volume measurements using real-time 3DE were significantly more accurate and reproducible than those obtained with 2DE. This technique was also highly feasible, with postprocessing data requiring less than 1 minute.

Limitations of 3D-Derived Quantitative Measurements for Mitral Regurgitation

Despite the improved accuracy and reproducibility in assessment of MR with 3DE, there are still many limitations with each technique. 3D-derived vena contracta area is subject to color Doppler limitations and depends on the proper selection of the systolic frame because it can significantly affect accurate and reproducible measurements.[54] Proximal isovelocity surface area still requires significant off-line processing and is not practical in a busy clinical setting. Although 3D

proximal velocity flow convergence is independent of the angle, the lower temporal resolution of 3D color Doppler may affect proper selection of the largest flow convergence region. Anatomic regurgitant orifice area requires proper selection of the systolic frame and is limited by the relatively poor temporal resolution of 3DE. 3D mitral inflow and LVOT stroke volume holds great promise, but this method requires further validation in patients with MR.

Mitral Stenosis

Although the prevalence of rheumatic MV disease has significantly diminished in the United States, it remains a major cause of mitral stenosis (MS) and MR worldwide.[55] Percutaneous mitral valvuloplasty is the preferred treatment for selected patients with MS.[12] Echocardiography plays an important role by confirming the diagnosis, evaluating the MV apparatus and its associated structures, and assessing the severity of MS.

3DE has many advantages over 2DE in examining the MV anatomy.[56] The echocardiographic Wilkins score, which includes leaflet thickening, valve calcification, and involvement of the subvalvular apparatus, was developed to predict which patients would benefit most from percutaneous mitral valvuloplasty. With 3DE and its ability to visualize the MV from the LA and LV perspective, the morphologic assessment of the MV becomes more accurate. The interobserver and intraobserver variability of the 3DE Wilkins score has been shown to be far superior to the 2DE assessment.[57] 3DE is better able than 2DE to identify commissural splitting and leaflet tears immediately after valvuloplasty in the catheterization laboratory.

There are several ways to quantitatively measure the severity of MS. Planimetry is the best method because it provides a direct method for measuring the MV area independent of loading conditions and associated cardiac conditions.[58] The major limitation of 2D-derived planimetry in MS is that there is no assurance that the selected plane used for planimetry is the smallest and most perpendicular (*en face*) view of the MV orifice.

Planimetry by 3DE is preferred to 2DE because it provides the narrowest orifice cross section of the MV funnel orifice, thereby providing a much more accurate assessment of the MV area. Many studies have shown the superiority of 3DE in the examination of patients with rheumatic MS.[57,59,60] The accuracy of 3DE planimetry has been proved to be superior to the accuracy of the invasive Gorlin method for measuring MV area.[59] 3DE planimetry also provides a more accurate assessment of the MV area before and after valvuloplasty compared with 2DE planimetry, 2DE pressure half-time, and the Gorlin method (Fig. 2.10).[60]

3DE is potentially useful for predicting embolic stroke in patients with MS. LA remodeling due to elevated LA pressure increases the risk of thrombus formation and subsequent embolic stroke. In some studies, the risk of systemic embolization approaches 10% to 20%.[61] In a study of 212 patients with MS, 3DE was used to assess LA volume, emptying fraction, and cross-sectional area.[62] The authors found that a more spherical LA shape was independently associated with an increased risk for embolic stroke independent of age and LA function.

AORTIC VALVE

Aortic Valve Anatomy
Aortic Valve Cusps

The aortic valve (AV) is composed of three cusps that are attached in a semilunar fashion along the entire length of the aortic root, with the highest point of attachment at the level of the sinotubular junction and the lowest in the LV myocardium below the anatomic ventricular-arterial

Pre   Valvuloplasty   Post

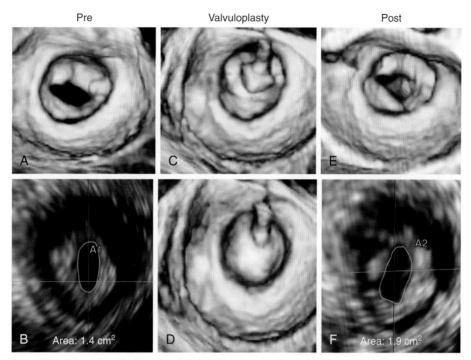

Fig. 2.10 TEE of the Mitral Valve. (A) 3D TEE LA view of a rheumatic mitral valve with thickened leaflets during diastole. (B) 3D TEE zoomed pre-valvuloplasty view of the mitral valve with an anatomic orifice area of 1.4 cm². (C and D) 3D TEE of mitral balloon valvuloplasty. (E and F) 3D TEE view of the mitral valve after valvuloplasty reveals an increase in the anatomic orifice area to 1.9 cm².

junction. The free edge of each cusp curves up from the commissures and is slightly thickened at the tip or midpoint, which is also known as the node of Arantius. Each cusp is identified by its relationship to the coronary arteries. The right and left coronary cusps lie below the off-take of the right and left coronary arteries, respectively, and the noncoronary cusp is adjacent to the interatrial septum.

Marked variation exists for all aspects of the cusps, including height, width, and surface area. The AV area is the area between the cusps during LV systole, and the shape of this area can be stellate, circular, triangular, or an intermediate form of these variants.[63]

Aortic Valve Annulus

Various definitions for the AV annulus exist because it is based on the AV cusp insertion points, which are not located in a single plane but along the length of the aortic root. Due to this anatomy, the surgical definition of aortic annulus refers to a semilunar crownlike structure demarcated by the hinges of the AV cusps, whereas the imaging definition refers to the virtual or projected ring that connects the three most basal insertion points of the cusps. 3D studies have revealed that the aortic annulus, when defined using the imaging definition, is not circular but elliptical.[64] Normal reported adult aortic annular area measurements by planimetry using 3DE images is 4.0 ± 0.8 cm.[265,66] 3DE studies have also found that the projected aortic annular area is largest in the first third of systole and smallest during isovolumic relaxation.[67]

Aortic Root Complex

The AV, the sinuses of Valsalva, and the fibrous intercusp triangles together form the aortic root complex.[68–70] The sinuses of Valsalva are areas of aortic root wall expansion defined by the insertion sites of the AV cusps, with the inferior margin located at the basal cusp insertion points and the superior margin at the sinotubular junction. Each sinus is separated from the others at its base by the intercusp triangle.[71] Absence of any of these intercusp triangles results in a loss of the coronet

shape of the cusp insertion points to a more ringlike shape, which is associated with valvular stenosis.[71]

The start of the aortic root from the LV is delineated by the basal attachments of the AV cusps, and the sinotubular ridge separates the aortic root from the ascending aorta. Along the anterior margin of the aortic root lie the subpulmonary infundibulum and, posteriorly, the orifice of the MV and the muscular interventricular septum. Overall, approximately two-thirds of the circumference of the lower part of the aortic root is connected to the septum, and the remaining one-third is connected by a fibrous continuity known as the aortic-mitral curtain to the MV (see Fig. 2.1).

Aortic Valve Physiology

During LV systole, the aortic cusps move toward the sinuses of Valsalva, and during diastole, they coapt at the level of the aortic annulus. When the aortic cusps are open, they do not strike the aortic wall due to the formation of vortices created by blood directed from the ridge at the sinotubular junction into the space between the cusps and the sinuses of Valsalva.[72] The coronary artery orifices are not occluded when the valve is open.[70] These vortices also promote valve closure. Due to the importance of these eddy flows in the sinuses, the curvature of the sinuses of Valsalva is central to determining the distribution of stress on the valve cusps.[73] Although blood flow contributes to the opening and closing of the AV, the actual motion of the aortic cusps does not completely parallel the blood flow pattern as the cusps open before any forward blood flow into the aorta and close before cessation of forward blood flow.[63,74–77]

3DE Imaging

3DE imaging of the AV can be challenging in patients with thin cusps and in those with heavily calcified valves because of significant cusp body dropout. This is caused by the orientation of the valve with respect to the echo probe and the artifacts caused by calcification of the valve.

Image Acquisition

The main views used to acquire 3D TTE images are the parasternal long-axis and short-axis views and the apical three-chamber view (see Table 2.2). The apical approach results in lower spatial resolution compared with the parasternal views, but this does not affect accurate assessment of AV morphology or LVOT assessment.

The main views used to acquire 3D TEE datasets include the mid-esophageal, the approximately 60-degree aortic valve short-axis view, and the approximately 120-degree long-axis view (Fig. 2.11).

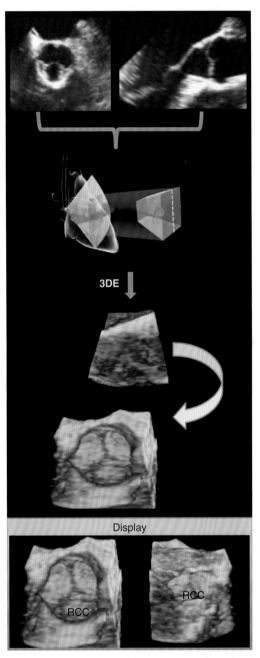

Fig. 2.11 3D TEE Acquisition and Presentation of the Aortic Valve. *Top*, Two orthogonal views (short and long axis) of the aortic valve are optimized with biplane mode before 3D TEE acquisition. Once acquired, the 3DE pyramid should be rotated 90 degrees along the y-axis so that an *en face* view of the aortic valve is presented. The aortic valve should be displayed with the right coronary cusp *(RCC)* located at the 6-o'clock position whether the valve is presented from the LV or aortic perspective.

Image Display

The AV should be imaged with the right coronary cusp located inferiorly, regardless whether the perspective is from the aorta or the LVOT.[11] The aortic perspective of the valve is best suited for assessing valve morphology, and the LV perspective may best delineate aortic tumors/vegetations or subvalvular obstructions (see Table 2.2).

Roles for 3DE
Aortic Valve Anatomy
Native valves. With 2DE, through-plane motion of the AV during the cardiac cycle often hampers adequate visualization of AV morphology. With 3DE, regardless of the actual spatial orientation of the aortic root, the true *en face* view of the AV is contained in the 3D data set. Although there are limitations to 3DE AV cusp body imaging, cusp edges often can be visualized.[13,78] 3DE, when compared with 2DE, has been shown to accurately identify abnormal aortic leaflet morphology, especially in bicuspid and quadricuspid aortic valves (Fig. 2.12).[79–83] 3DE has been useful for the assessment of cusp masses such as Lambl excrescences and AV papillary fibroelastomas.[84–86] The spatial relationship of the AV with surrounding structures such as the LVOT and mitral annulus also can be assessed.

Prosthetic valves. The strength of 3DE in the assessment of aortic mechanical and bioprosthetic valves is its ability to visualize the prosthetic valve ring *en face* regardless whether it is viewed from the LVOT or the aortic perspective.[87] This ability increases visualization and assessment of paravalvular regurgitation, allowing localization and severity quantification.[87,88] In contrast, the prosthetic leaflets are poorly visualized regardless of perspective because the AV lies far from the transducer and its location is oblique with respect to the angle of incidence of the ultrasound beam. This also explains why image quality of the native AV leaflets is relatively poor.

Endocarditis. 3DE is valuable in addressing native and prosthetic AV endocarditis because the *en face* view improves identification and localization of valve perforations compared with 2DE. For prosthetic valves, it allows accurate assessment of complications such as valve dehiscence with their associated regurgitation jets.[88–92] The ability to display valve images in a surgical perspective also enables better communication with surgeons. In prosthetic valve endocarditis, 3DE correlates well with surgical and 2D TEE findings, and it identifies additional vegetations not seen on 2D TEE.[88] 3DE can assist in differentiating vegetation from loose suture material, and the rocking motion of a partially dehisced valve is frequently better appreciated on 3D imaging. However, due to frame rate limitations on 3DE, 2DE remains superior for the identification of small mobile vegetations. The strength of 3DE lies in its ability to characterize the mass in more detail than just noting its presence or absence.

Aortic Stenosis Assessment

3DE has improved the accuracy and reproducibility of the aortic stenosis (AS) severity quantification through accurate LVOT area measurements, the use of direct volumetric measurement of stroke volume, and by direct planimetry of the AV area (Table 2.5).[93–97]

Left ventricular outflow tract. 3DE has shown that the LVOT cross-sectional area is not circular but is instead elliptical (Fig. 2.13). This difference is crucial because the calculation of AV area using the continuity equation uses a 2DE measured LVOT diameter that is substituted into a formula that assumes that the LVOT is circular, which results in an underestimation of AV area. Substitution with 3DE planimetered LVOT area into the continuity equation improves the accuracy of AV area calculations.[11,98–101]

3DE studies have demonstrated that the LVOT is less distensible in AS patients and that this reduced distensibility mainly affects the

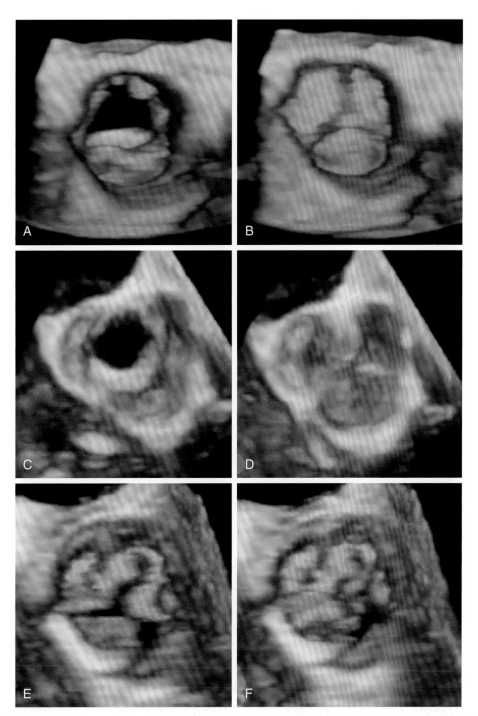

Fig. 2.12 3D TEE views of the aortic valve from the aorta perspective demonstrate a normal aortic valve during systole (A) and diastole (B), a unicuspid valve during systole (C) and diastole (D), and a sclerocalcific aortic valve during systole (E) and diastole (F).

minor axis. This minor axis corresponds to the anterior-posterior LVOT diameter measured by 2D TEE, which may cause an underestimation of LVOT area that results in a smaller stroke volume and an underestimation of AV area.[102]

Stroke volume quantification. There are two 3DE methods for improving stroke volume quantification. The first is to use 3DE-derived end-systolic and end-diastolic volumes to determine stroke volume, and the second is to use a direct volumetric measurement of stroke volume (Figs. 2.14 and 2.15).[103–106] AV area is calculated by dividing 3DE-derived stroke volume by AV continuous-wave Doppler time-velocity integral. Using these methods, 3DE has been shown to have superior accuracy compared with using 2D stroke volume calculations. This method is particularly useful for patients with distorted LVOT shapes because AV area determined by 3DE-determined stroke volume was significantly more accurate than 2DE-derived areas.[103]

Aortic valve planimetry. An alternative method for assessing AV area is direct planimetry of the AV area from 3DE data sets (Fig. 2.16).[107–110] Many studies have demonstrated that planimetered AV area is clinically feasible and relatively accurate compared

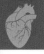

Quantification of Aortic Stenosis	3DE Contribution
Continuity equation	LVOT area: 3DE improves measurement of this elliptical structure
	Stroke volume derived from 3DE LV volumes: avoids LVOT measurement errors
	Direct volumetric quantification of stroke volume: avoids LVOT measurement errors
Direct planimetry	Direct tracing of the stenotic orifice area: recognizes the nonplanar nature of the stenotic orifice

TABLE 2.5   3DE Assessment of Aortic Stenosis.

with invasive measures and equivalent if not superior to 2D planimetry.[108,109,111] This improvement in accuracy results from the ability to trace the 3D shape of the stenotic orifice on 3DE, which is typically smaller than the planar orifice that can be traced from 2DE.

Transcatheter Aortic Valve Replacement

Transcatheter aortic valve replacement (TAVR) is a minimally invasive treatment option for patients with severe AS who are inoperable or have intermediate to high surgical risk. Insertion and placement of the valve results in compression of the native valve cusps between the prosthetic valve struts and the arterial wall. Different imaging modalities are used before, during, and after the procedure, and their use varies according to center expertise. When available, 3DE plays an important role in all of these stages.

Preprocedure: aortic root assessment. Accurate measurement of the aortic annulus is required to determine TAVR valve size. An undersized device may result in paravalvular insufficiency or valve detachment and embolization, whereas an oversized device may result in aortic dissection or rupture of the aortic annulus. Accurate

measurements of distances from the aortic annulus to the coronary ostium are important to avoid obstruction of the coronary ostium after valve implantation. Although many centers use computed tomography to obtain these measurements, there is a significant proportion of patients who are unable to undergo this test. For these patients, echocardiography with 3D use is superior to 2DE alone.

Quantitative 3DE measurements of the AV and root throughout the cardiac cycle can be obtained from manual measurements using multiplanar analysis or from semi-automated or fully automated analysis software.[112] With the use of 3DE multiplanar analysis, accurate cross-sectional planimetry and dimensions at all levels of the aortic root and the aortic cusp dimensions and distance from the projected aortic annulus to the coronary artery ostia can be obtained (Fig. 2.17).[65,113] Multiplanar analysis allows exact alignment of the cut planes to the structure in question, which is sometimes impossible to obtain in the 2D short-axis view and in hearts in a horizontal position or with aortic root pathology. With the use of multiplanar analysis, planar sagittal measurements of the aortic annulus have improved. The plane should be aligned between the left and noncoronary cusp commissure and through the middle of the right coronary cusp. It has also led to the realization that the coronal diameter, not this dimension, is the largest diameter of the aortic annulus (Fig. 2.18). Multiplanar analysis allows assessment of supravalvular and subvalvular anatomy within the 3D volume to evaluate for serial aortic outflow tract stenosis.

Overall, aortic root measurements obtained from 3DE demonstrate good correlation with measurements obtained by multislice computed tomography (MSCT) and/or CMR.[64,65,114–120] However, 3DE measurements are usually larger than those acquired with 2DE but smaller than those obtained with MSCT and CMR.[64,65,114–120] When comparing the accuracy of these imaging modalities using an in vitro gold standard, CMR was found to be the most accurate imaging modality, although 3DE and MSCT were reasonably accurate.[121] The amount of calcium decreased accuracy and interobserver reproducibility compared with 3DE and MSCT.[121]

Investigators have examined the impact of using aortic annular measurements obtained with different imaging modalities on the

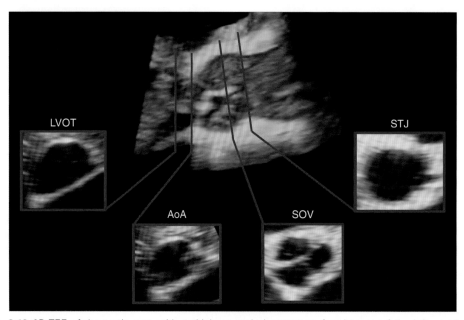

Fig. 2.13 3D TEE of the aortic root, with multiplanar analysis exact *en face* images of the left ventricular outflow tract *(LVOT)*, the aortic annulus *(AoA)*, the sinus of Valsalva *(SOV)*, and the sinotubular junction *(STJ)* can be obtained.

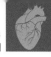

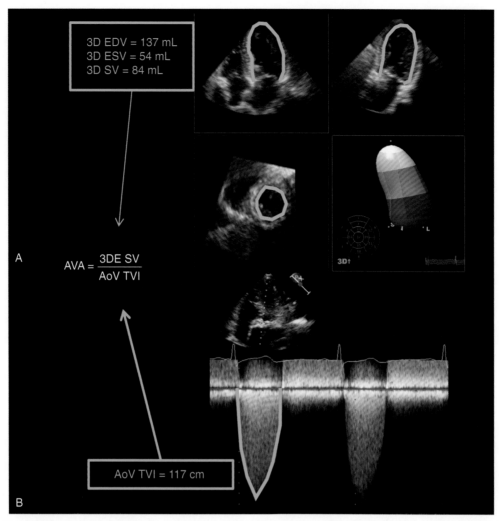

Fig. 2.14 Aortic valve area *(AVA)* assessment is improved by using 3D TTE-derived end-systolic *(ESV)* and end-diastolic volumes *(EDV)* (A) to determine stroke volume *(SV)* and dividing it by 2DE-derived aortic valve continuous-wave Doppler time-velocity integral *(TVI)* (B). The 3D TTE is obtained from a wide-angle, multibeat acquisition of the left ventricle.

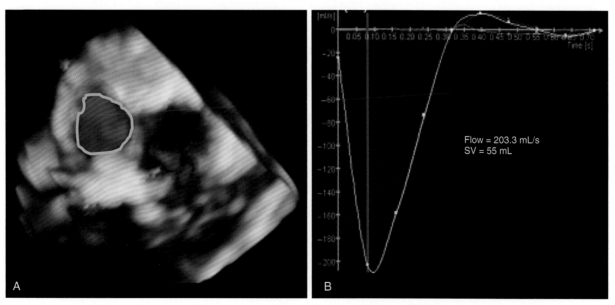

Fig. 2.15 **Direct Volumetric Measurement of Stroke Volume** *(SV)* **From 3D TEE.** (A) *En-face* view of blood flow through the aortic annulus from a single-beat, color Doppler, 3DE acquisition. From the region of interest *(green outline)*, 3DE software can calculate stroke volume through the valve. (B) Graph depicts blood flow through the valve obtained from the 3DE-based software.

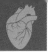

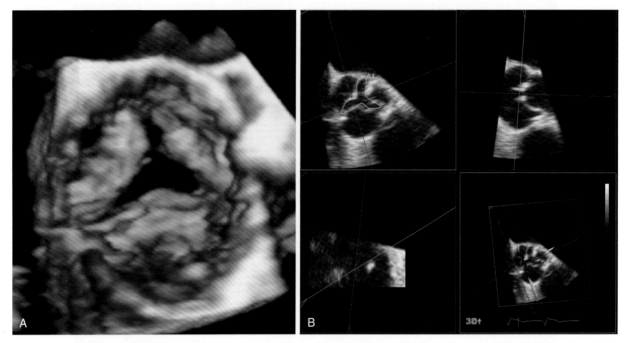

Fig. 2.16 (A) 3D TEE zoomed image of a stenotic aortic valve during maximal opening in systole. (B) Using multiplanar analysis, the aortic valve area can be measured.

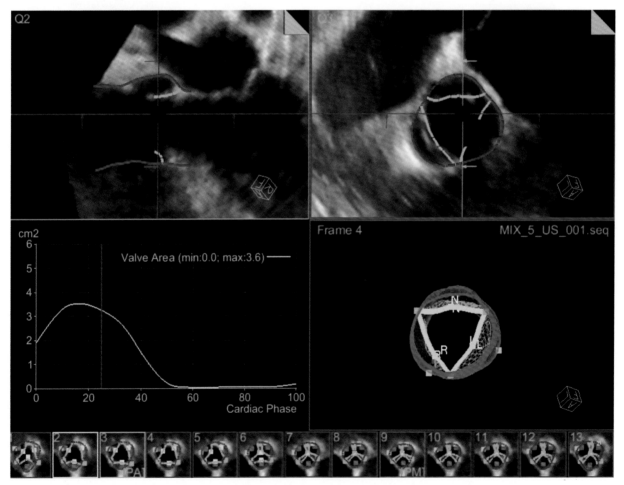

Fig. 2.17 Using specialized software from a 3D TEE data set, the aortic valve complex can be tracked throughout the cardiac cycle. Although almost any aortic root measurement can be obtained, in this example, the generated 3D model is tracking the aortic valve area.

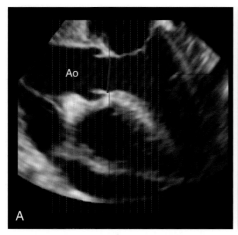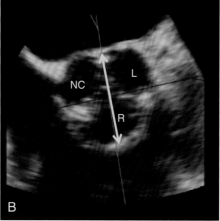

Fig. 2.18 To correctly measure the aortic *(Ao)* annulus anteroposterior (sagittal) diameter using a 3D dataset (A) at the level of the mid-sinuses of Valsalva (B), the plane should pass from between the non- and left commissures and through the middle of the right coronary sinus *(yellow line).*

choice of implanted percutaneous valve size. They found that the size of the implanted valve would have changed, from that chosen by 2DE in 40% to 42% of patients.[64] However, when these investigators studied the outcomes from prosthesis size determined from 2D TEE measurements, only a small number of patients had poor outcomes due to complications arising from the size of the implanted valve.[64] Even with the underestimation of echocardiographic measurements, there is no difference in outcomes because most guidelines for determining the size of aortic devices were developed using echocardiographic measurements.[115]

Periprocedure. TTE is playing an increasing role during TAVR procedures as conscious sedation protocols are being implemented, resulting in lower TEE use. However, TEE is still being used in a subset of patients and centers. When available, 3D TEE can help guide the catheter and the prosthetic valve into an optimal position. Advancing the device too far into the aorta may result in occlusion of the coronary ostia, whereas retraction toward the LVOT may interfere with the motion of the anterior mitral leaflet, resulting in MR.[122]

Postprocedure. 3D TEE is useful in evaluating results and identifying potential complications, including paravalvular and transvalvular regurgitation, new wall motion abnormalities, MR, damage to the aortic ring, aortic dissection, pericardial effusion, and

cardiac tamponade. In addition to localizing and quantifying paravalvular regurgitation, 3DE can direct percutaneous device closure of leaks.[123]

Aortic Regurgitation Assessment

3DE studies on aortic regurgitation (AR) have provided novel mechanistic insights. For example, for AR associated with aortic root dilatation, 3DE has found that there is remodeling of the cusps in response to the root dilatation but that it is insufficient in cases of central AR or excessive in eccentric AR.[124] Practically, 3DE improves AR assessment through superior assessments of AR mechanism and severity quantification.

Classification. Describing the mechanism of AR is important in determining surgical AV reparability. This can be achieved through the use of classification schemes that require assessment of cusp mobility, aortic root pathology, and cusp perforation (Table 2.6).[125–127] Use of these classification systems can guide repairs and reduce recurrence of AR.[128] The use of 3DE helps AR classification by improving assessment of leaflet mobility and quantifying changes in cusp size and shape throughout the cardiac cycle.[65,67]

Vena contracta. The vena contracta cross-sectional area, a surrogate for effective regurgitant orifice area, is a good predictor of

TABLE 2.6	**Functional Classification of Aortic Regurgitation and Repair Strategies.**	
Type of Aortic Regurgitation	**Mechanism of Aortic Regurgitation**	**Type of Aortic Valve Repair**
1A	Dilated sinotubular junction Normal cusp mobility	Sinotubular junction remodeling • Subcommissural annuloplasty
1B	Dilated sinuses of Valsalva Normal cusp mobility	Valve-sparing aortic root replacement
1C	Dilated ventriculo-aortic junction Normal cusp mobility	Subcommissural annuloplasty • Sinotubular junction annuloplasty
1D	Aortic cusp perforation Normal cusp mobility	Aortic cusp repair • Autologous or bovine pericardium
II	Aortic cusp prolapse Excessive cusp mobility	Cusp prolapse repair with subcommissural annuloplasty • Focal prolapse: plication, triangular resection • Generalized prolapse: free margin resuspension
III	Restricted cusp mobility Thickening, fibrosis, calcification	Cusp repair with subcommissural annuloplasty • Shaving, decalcification, patch

AR severity. However, quantification of the vena contracta with diameters from 2D color Doppler images can be inaccurate because the shape of regurgitant orifices can be asymmetric. 3DE multiplanar reconstruction of the vena contracta allows measurement of the cross-sectional area, which has been shown to be more accurate than 2D methods.[129–131] 3DE allows multiple jets of different directions to be measured. However, it may result in underestimation or overestimation when the vena contracta shape changes significantly throughout diastole. 3DE methods to directly measure the proximal isovelocity surface area are currently being studied.[132]

Stroke volume. 3DE can improve quantification of AR severity determined by comparing aortic stroke volume with mitral or pulmonic stroke volume. 3DE improves LV stroke volume measurements, which are similar to stroke volume at the LVOT in isolated AR. Another 3DE method involves computing the beat-to-beat difference between 3DE-determined left and right ventricular stroke volumes or LV outflow and mitral inflow.[133–135]

AORTIC-MITRAL VALVE INTERACTIONS

The MV and AV are anatomically linked through a shared fibrous border called the aortic-mitral curtain, and AV and MV functions are interdependent (see Fig. 2.1).[136] This relationship was fully appreciated with the development of 3DE.[67] It found that during the cardiac cycle when aortic annular area is at its maximum, mitral annular area is at its minimum, and vice versa. The angle between the AV and MV is smallest during LV ejection. Overall, the aortic-mitral fibrous continuity acts as an anchor affecting the function of both valves, and its effect likely plays a role in the efficiency of the heart as a pump.

This interaction also suggests that diseases or surgical processes that affect one valve may have unanticipated effects on the dynamics of the other valve. 3DE quantification of this coupling has been used to examine it in patients with degenerative MV disease before and after mitral annuloplasty repair.[137] In patients with degenerative MV disease, the AV appears unaffected. After MV repair, the AV annulus has reduced pulsatility and motion throughout the cardiac cycle due to the rigid structure of the mitral annuloplasty ring.

In patients with isolated AS, 3DE has found that the MV is affected with smaller mitral annular areas and reduced mitral annular function. These changes persist even with surgical or percutaneous treatment of the AV.[138,139] Clinically, this valvular coupling is observed by noting decreased MR severity after AV replacement.[140,141] Overall, diseases affecting the AV or MV and interventions to treat these diseases should include assessment of the impact on both valves.

CONCLUSIONS

3DE is an invaluable addition to the diagnosis and management of MV and AV disease. It has improved the anatomic assessment of these valves and offered mechanistic insights into diseased states. The use of 3DE has led to greater accuracy in quantification of stenosis and regurgitation and guided interventions with these abnormalities. Overall, the use of 3DE in evaluating the mitral and aortic valves is increasing and improving patient care.

REFERENCES

1. Salgo IS, Gorman JH, 3rd, Gorman RC, et al. Effect of annular shape on leaflet curvature in reducing mitral leaflet stress. Circulation 2002;106:711-717.
2. O'Gara P, Sugeng L, Lang R, et al. The role of imaging in chronic degenerative mitral regurgitation. JACC Cardiovasc Imaging 2008;1:221-237.
3. Carpentier A. Cardiac valve surgery—the "French correction". J Thorac Cardiovasc Surg 1983;86:323-337.
4. Timek TA, Nielsen SL, Green GR, et al. Influence of anterior mitral leaflet second-order chordae on leaflet dynamics and valve competence. Anna Thorac Surg 2001;72:535-540; discussion 541.
5. Messas E, Bel A, Szymanski C, et al. Relief of mitral leaflet tethering following chronic myocardial infarction by chordal cutting diminishes left ventricular remodeling. Circ Cardiovasc Imaging 2010;3:679-686.
6. Rodriguez F, Langer F, Harrington KB, et al. Effect of cutting second-order chordae on in-vivo anterior mitral leaflet compound curvature. J Heart Valve Dis 2005;14:592-601; discussion 601-602.
7. Rodriguez F, Langer F, Harrington KB, et al. Importance of mitral valve second-order chordae for left ventricular geometry, wall thickening mechanics, and global systolic function. Circulation 2004;110:II115-II122.
8. Dreyfus GD, Bahrami T, Alayle N, et al. Repair of anterior leaflet prolapse by papillary muscle repositioning: a new surgical option. Ann Thorac Surg 2001;71:1464-1470.
9. Berdajs D, Zund G, Camenisch C, et al. Annulus fibrosus of the mitral valve: reality or myth. J Card Surg 2007;22:406-409.
10. Obase K, Weinert L, Hollatz A, et al. Leaflet-chordal relations in patients with primary and secondary mitral regurgitation. J Am Soc Echocardiogr 2015;28:1302-1308.
11. Lang RM, Badano LP, Tsang W, et al. EAE/ASE recommendations for image acquisition and display using three-dimensional echocardiography. J Am Soc Echocardiogr 2012;25:3-46.
12. Nishimura RA, Otto CM, Bonow RO, et al. 2014 AHA/ACC Guideline for the management of patients with valvular heart disease: a report of the American College of Cardiology/American Heart Association Task Force on Practice Guidelines. Circulation 2014;129:e521-e643.
13. Sugeng L, Shernan SK, Salgo IS, et al. Live 3-dimensional transesophageal echocardiography initial experience using the fully-sampled matrix array probe. J Am Coll Cardiol 2008;52:446-449.
14. Anyanwu AC, Adams DH. Etiologic classification of degenerative mitral valve disease: Barlow's disease and fibroelastic deficiency. Semin Thorac Cardiovasc Surg 2007;19:90-96.
15. Chandra S, Salgo IS, Sugeng L, et al. Characterization of degenerative mitral valve disease using morphologic analysis of real-time three-dimensional echocardiographic images: objective insight into complexity and planning of mitral valve repair. Circ Cardiovasc Imaging 2011;4:24-32.
16. Tsang W, Weinert L, Sugeng L, et al. The value of three-dimensional echocardiography derived mitral valve parametric maps and the role of experience in the diagnosis of pathology. J Am Soc Echocardiogr. 2011;24(8):860-867.
17. Adams DH, Anyanwu AC, Sugeng L, Lang RM. Degenerative mitral valve regurgitation: surgical echocardiography. Curr Cardiol Rep 2008;10:226-232.
18. La Canna G, Arendar I, Maisano F, et al. Real-time three-dimensional transesophageal echocardiography for assessment of mitral valve functional anatomy in patients with prolapse-related regurgitation. Am J Cardiol 2011;107:1365-1374.
19. Addetia K, Mor-Avi V, Weinert L, et al. A new definition for an old entity: improved definition of mitral valve prolapse using three-dimensional echocardiography and color-coded parametric models. J Am Soc Echocardiogr 2014;27:8-16.
20. Clavel MA, Mantovani F, Malouf J, et al. Dynamic phenotypes of degenerative myxomatous mitral valve disease: quantitative 3-dimensional echocardiographic study. Circ Cardiovasc Imaging 2015;8.
21. Antoine C, Mantovani F, Benfari G, et al. Pathophysiology of degenerative mitral regurgitation: new 3-dimensional imaging insights. Circ Cardiovasc Imaging 2018;11:e005971.
22. Lee AP, Jin CN, Fan Y, et al. Functional implication of mitral annular disjunction in mitral valve prolapse: a quantitative dynamic 3D echocardiographic study. JACC Cardiovasc Imaging 2017;10:1424-1433.
23. Chui J, Anderson RH, Lang RM, Tsang W. The trileaflet mitral valve.. Am J Cardiol 2018;121:513-519.
24. Otsuji Y, Levine RA, Takeuchi M, et al. Mechanism of ischemic mitral regurgitation. J Cardiol 2008;51:145-156.

25. Grewal J, Suri R, Mankad S, et al. Mitral annular dynamics in myxomatous valve disease: new insights with real-time 3-dimensional echocardiography. Circulation 2010;121:1423-1431.

26. Dent JM, Spotnitz WD, Nolan SP, et al. Mechanism of mitral leaflet excursion. Am J Physiol 1995;269:H2100-H2108.

27. Otsuji Y, Handschumacher MD, Schwammenthal E, et al. Insights from three-dimensional echocardiography into the mechanism of functional mitral regurgitation: direct in vivo demonstration of altered leaflet tethering geometry. Circulation 1997;96:1999-2008.

28. Yosefy C, Beeri R, Guerrero JL, et al. Mitral regurgitation after anteroapical myocardial infarction: new mechanistic insights. Circulation 2011;123:1529-1536.

29. Daimon M, Shiota T, Gillinov AM, et al. Percutaneous mitral valve repair for chronic ischemic mitral regurgitation: a real-time three-dimensional echocardiographic study in an ovine model. Circulation 2005;111:2183-2189.

30. Watanabe N, Ogasawara Y, Yamaura Y, et al. Mitral annulus flattens in ischemic mitral regurgitation: geometric differences between inferior and anterior myocardial infarction: a real-time 3-dimensional echocardiographic study. Circulation 2005;112:I458-1462.

31. Vergnat M, Jassar AS, Jackson BM, et al. Ischemic mitral regurgitation: a quantitative three-dimensional echocardiographic analysis. Ann Thorac Surg 2011;91:157-164.

32. Veronesi F, Corsi C, Sugeng L, et al. Quantification of mitral apparatus dynamics in functional and ischemic mitral regurgitation using real-time 3-dimensional echocardiography. J Am Soc Echocardiogr 2008;21:347-354.

33. Lang RM, Tsang W, Weinert L, et al. Valvular heart disease. The value of 3-dimensional echocardiography. J Am Coll Cardiol 2011;58:1933-1944.

34. Chaput M, Handschumacher MD, Tournoux F, et al. Mitral leaflet adaptation to ventricular remodeling: occurrence and adequacy in patients with functional mitral regurgitation. Circulation 2008;118:845-852.

35. Dal-Bianco JP, Aikawa E, Bischoff J, et al. Active adaptation of the tethered mitral valve: insights into a compensatory mechanism for functional mitral regurgitation. Circulation 2009;120:334-342.

36. Saito K, Okura H, Watanabe N, et al. Influence of chronic tethering of the mitral valve on mitral leaflet size and coaptation in functional mitral regurgitation. JACC Cardiovasc Imaging 2012;5:337-345.

37. Lang RM, Adams DH. 3D echocardiographic quantification in functional mitral regurgitation. JACC Cardiovasc Imaging 2012;5:346-347.

38. Maffessanti F, Marsan NA, Tamborini G, et al. Quantitative analysis of mitral valve apparatus in mitral valve prolapse before and after annuloplasty: a three-dimensional intraoperative transesophageal study. J Am Soc Echocardiogr 2011;24:405-413.

39. Jensen MO, Jensen H, Levine RA, et al. Saddle-shaped mitral valve annuloplasty rings improve leaflet coaptation geometry. J Thorac Cardiovasc Surg 2011;142:697-703.

40. Bhave NM, Lang RM. Quantitative echocardiographic assessment of native mitral regurgitation: two- and three-dimensional techniques. J Heart Valve Dis 2011;20:483-492.

41. Kahlert P, Plicht B, Schenk IM, et al. Direct assessment of size and shape of noncircular vena contracta area in functional versus organic mitral regurgitation using real-time three-dimensional echocardiography. J Am Soc Echocardiogr 2008;21:912-921.

42. Little SH, Pirat B, Kumar R, et al. Three-dimensional color Doppler echocardiography for direct measurement of vena contracta area in mitral regurgitation: in vitro validation and clinical experience. JACC Cardiovasc Imaging 2008;1:695-704.

43. Zeng X, Levine RA, Hua L, et al. Diagnostic value of vena contracta area in the quantification of mitral regurgitation severity by color Doppler 3D echocardiography. Circ Cardiovasc Imaging 2011;4:506-513.

44. Marsan NA, Westenberg JJ, Ypenburg C, et al. Quantification of functional mitral regurgitation by real-time 3D echocardiography: comparison with 3D velocity-encoded cardiac magnetic resonance. JACC Cardiovasc Imaging 2009;2:1245-1252.

45. Yosefy C, Hung J, Chua S, et al. Direct measurement of vena contracta area by real-time 3-dimensional echocardiography for assessing severity of mitral regurgitation. Am J Cardiol 2009;104:978-983.

46. Shiota T, Jones M, Delabays A, et al. Direct measurement of three-dimensionally reconstructed flow convergence surface area and regurgitant flow in aortic regurgitation: in vitro and chronic animal model studies. Circulation 1997;96:3687-3695.

47. Matsumura Y, Saracino G, Sugioka K, et al. Determination of regurgitant orifice area with the use of a new three-dimensional flow convergence geometric assumption in functional mitral regurgitation. J Am Soc Echocardiogr 2008;21:1251-1256.

48. Shiota T, Sinclair B, Ishii M, et al. Three-dimensional reconstruction of color Doppler flow convergence regions and regurgitant jets: an in vitro quantitative study. J Am Coll Cardiol 1996;27:1511-1518.

49. Chandra S, Salgo IS, Sugeng L, et al. A three-dimensional insight into the complexity of flow convergence in mitral regurgitation: adjunctive benefit of anatomic regurgitant orifice area. Am J Physiol Heart Circ Physiol. 2011;301(3):H1015-H1024.

50. Altiok E, Hamada S, van Hall S, et al. Comparison of direct planimetry of mitral valve regurgitation orifice area by three-dimensional transesophageal echocardiography to effective regurgitant orifice area obtained by proximal flow convergence method and vena contracta area determined by color Doppler echocardiography. Am J Cardiol 2011;107:452-458.

51. Lodato JA, Weinert L, Baumann R, et al. Use of 3-dimensional color Doppler echocardiography to measure stroke volume in human beings: comparison with thermodilution. J Am Soc Echocardiogr 2007;20:103-112.

52. Pemberton J, Jerosch-Herold M, Li X, et al. Accuracy of real-time, three-dimensional Doppler echocardiography for stroke volume estimation compared with phase-encoded MRI: an in vivo study. Heart 2008;94:1212-1213.

53. Thavendiranathan P, Liu S, Datta S, et al. Automated quantification of mitral inflow and aortic outflow stroke volumes by three-dimensional real-time volume color-flow Doppler transthoracic echocardiography: comparison with pulsed-wave Doppler and cardiac magnetic resonance imaging. J Am Soc Echocardiogr 2012;25:56-65.

54. Buck T, Plicht B, Kahlert P, et al. Effect of dynamic flow rate and orifice area on mitral regurgitant stroke volume quantification using the proximal isovelocity surface area method. J Am Coll Cardiol 2008;52:767-778.

55. Steer AC, Carapetis JR. Prevention and treatment of rheumatic heart disease in the developing world. Nat Rev Cardiol 2009;6:689-698.

56. Mannaerts HF, Kamp O, Visser CA. Should mitral valve area assessment in patients with mitral stenosis be based on anatomical or on functional evaluation? A plea for 3D echocardiography as the new clinical standard. Eur Heart J 2004;25:2073-2074.

57. Zamorano J, Cordeiro P, Sugeng L, et al. Real-time three-dimensional echocardiography for rheumatic mitral valve stenosis evaluation: an accurate and novel approach. J Am Coll Cardiol 2004;43:2091-2096.

58. Baumgartner H, Hung J, Bermejo J, et al. Echocardiographic assessment of valve stenosis: EAE/ASE recommendations for clinical practice. J Am Soc Echocardiogr 2009;22:1-23; quiz 101-102.

59. Perez de Isla L, Casanova C, Almeria C, et al. Which method should be the reference method to evaluate the severity of rheumatic mitral stenosis? Gorlin's method versus 3D-echo. Eur J Echocardiogr 2007;8:470-473.

60. Zamorano J, Perez de Isla L, Sugeng L, et al. Non-invasive assessment of mitral valve area during percutaneous balloon mitral valvuloplasty: role of real-time 3D echocardiography. Eur Heart J 2004;25:2086-2091.

61. Selzer A, Cohn KE. Natural history of mitral stenosis: a review. Circulation 1972;45:878-890.

62. Nunes MC, Handschumacher MD, Levine RA, et al. Role of LA shape in predicting embolic cerebrovascular events in mitral stenosis: mechanistic insights from 3D echocardiography. JACC Cardiovasc Imaging 2014;7:453-461.

63. Handke M, Heinrichs G, Beyersdorf F, et al. In vivo analysis of aortic valve dynamics by transesophageal 3-dimensional echocardiography with high temporal resolution. J Thorac Cardiovasc Surg 2003;125:1412-1419.

64. Messika-Zeitoun D, Serfaty JM, Brochet E, et al. Multimodal assessment of the aortic annulus diameter: implications for transcatheter aortic valve implantation. J Am Coll Cardiol 2010;55:186-194.

65. Otani K, Takeuchi M, Kaku K, et al. Assessment of the aortic root using real-time 3D transesophageal echocardiography. Circ J 2010;74:2649-2657.

66. Kasprzak JD, Nosir YF, Dall'Agata A, et al. Quantification of the aortic valve area in three-dimensional echocardiographic data sets: analysis of orifice overestimation resulting from suboptimal cut-plane selection. Am Heart J 1998;135:995-1003.

67. Veronesi F, Corsi C, Sugeng L, et al. A study of functional anatomy of aortic-mitral valve coupling using 3D matrix transesophageal echocardiography. Circ Cardiovasc Imaging 2009;2:24-31.

68. Piazza N, de Jaegere P, Schultz C, et al. Anatomy of the aortic valvar complex and its implications for transcatheter implantation of the aortic valve. Circ Cardiovasc Interv 2008;1:74-81.

69. Anderson RH. Clinical anatomy of the aortic root. Heart 2000;84:670-673.

70. Underwood MJ, El Khoury G, Deronck D, et al. The aortic root: structure, function, and surgical reconstruction. Heart 2000;83:376-380.

71. Sutton JP, 3rd, Ho SY, Anderson RH. The forgotten interleaflet triangles: a review of the surgical anatomy of the aortic valve. Ann Thorac Surg 1995;59:419-427.

72. Thubrikar M, Nolan SP, Bosher LP, Deck JD. The cyclic changes and structure of the base of the aortic valve. Am Heart J 1980;99:217-224.

73. Thubrikar MJ, Nolan SP, Aouad J, Deck JD. Stress sharing between the sinus and leaflets of canine aortic valve. Ann Thorac Surg 1986;42:434-440.

74. Thubrikar M, Bosher LP, Nolan SP. The mechanism of opening of the aortic valve. J Thorac Cardiovasc Surg 1979;77:863-870.

75. Van Steenhoven AA, Verlaan CW, Veenstra PC, Reneman RS. In vivo cinematographic analysis of behavior of the aortic valve. Am J Physiol 1981;240:H286-H292.

76. Higashidate M, Tamiya K, Beppu T, Imai Y. Regulation of the aortic valve opening. In vivo dynamic measurement of aortic valve orifice area. J Thorac Cardiovasc Surg 1995;110:496-503.

77. Handke M, Jahnke C, Heinrichs G, et al. New three-dimensional echocardiographic system using digital radiofrequency data—visualization and quantitative analysis of aortic valve dynamics with high resolution: methods, feasibility, and initial clinical experience. Circulation 2003;107:2876-2879.

78. Kasprzak JD, Salustri A, Roelandt JR, Ten Cate FJ. Three-dimensional echocardiography of the aortic valve: feasibility, clinical potential, and limitations. Echocardiography 1998;15:127-138.

79. Armen TA, Vandse R, Bickle K, Nathan N. Three-dimensional echocardiographic evaluation of an incidental quadricuspid aortic valve. Eur J Echocardiogr 2008;9:318-320.

80. Burri MV, Nanda NC, Singh A, Panwar SR. Live/real time three-dimensional transthoracic echocardiographic identification of quadricuspid aortic valve. Echocardiography 2007;24:653-655.

81. Singh P, Dutta R, Nanda NC. Live/real time three-dimensional transthoracic echocardiographic assessment of bicuspid aortic valve morphology. Echocardiography 2009;26:478-480.

82. Unsworth B, Malik I, Mikhail GW. Recognising bicuspid aortic stenosis in patients referred for transcatheter aortic valve implantation: routine screening with three-dimensional transoesophageal echocardiography. Heart 2010;96:645.

83. Xiao Z, Meng W, Zhang E. Quadricuspid aortic valve by using intraoperative transesophageal echocardiography. Cardiovasc Ultrasound 2010;8:36.

84. Dichtl W, Muller LC, Pachinger O, et al. Images in cardiovascular medicine. Improved preoperative assessment of papillary fibroelastoma by dynamic three-dimensional echocardiography. Circulation 2002;106:1300.

85. Kelpis TG, Ninios VN, Economopoulos VA, Pitsis AA. Aortic valve papillary fibroelastoma: a three-dimensional transesophageal echocardiographic appearance. Ann Thorac Surg 2010;89:2043.

86. Samal AK, Nanda N, Thakur AC, et al. Three-dimensional echocardiographic assessment of Lambl's excrescences on the aortic valve. Echocardiography 1999;16:437-441.

87. Sugeng L, Shernan SK, Weinert L, et al. Real-time three-dimensional transesophageal echocardiography in valve disease: comparison with surgical findings and evaluation of prosthetic valves. J Am Soc Echocardiogr 2008;21:1347-1354.

88. Kort S. Real-time 3-dimensional echocardiography for prosthetic valve endocarditis: initial experience. J Am Soc Echocardiogr 2006;19:130-139.

89. Thompson KA, Shiota T, Tolstrup K, et al. Utility of three-dimensional transesophageal echocardiography in the diagnosis of valvular perforations. Am J Cardiol 2011;107:100-102.

90. Schwalm SA, Sugeng L, Raman J, et al. Assessment of mitral valve leaflet perforation as a result of infective endocarditis by 3-dimensional real-time echocardiography. J Am Soc Echocardiogr 2004;17:919-922.

91. Lang RM, Mor-Avi V, Sugeng L, et al. Three-dimensional echocardiography: the benefits of the additional dimension. J Am Coll Cardiol 2006;48:2053-2069.

92. Walker N, Bhan A, Desai J, Monaghan MJ. Myocardial abscess: a rare complication of valvular endocarditis demonstrated by 3D contrast echocardiography. Eur J Echocardiogr 2010;11:E37.

93. Marechaux S, Juthier F, Banfi C, et al. Illustration of the echocardiographic diagnosis of subaortic membrane stenosis in adults: surgical and live three-dimensional transoesophageal findings. Eur J Echocardiogr 2011;12:E2.

94. Bandarupalli N, Faulkner M, Nanda NC, Pothineni KR. Erroneous diagnosis of significant obstruction by Doppler in a patient with discrete subaortic membrane: correct diagnosis by 3D-transthoracic echocardiography. Echocardiography 2008;25:1004-1006.

95. Kelpis TG, Ninios VN, Dardas PS, Pitsis AA. Subaortic stenosis in an adult caused by two discrete membranes: a three-dimensional transesophageal echocardiographic visualization. Ann Thorac Surg 2009;88:1703.

96. Ge S, Warner JG, Jr., Fowle KM, et al. Morphology and dynamic change of discrete subaortic stenosis can be imaged and quantified with three-dimensional transesophageal echocardiography. J Am Soc Echocardiogr 1997;10:713-716.

97. Bharucha T, Ho SY, Vettukattil JJ. Multiplanar review analysis of three-dimensional echocardiographic datasets gives new insights into the morphology of subaortic stenosis. Eur J Echocardiogr 2008;9:614-620.

98. Perez de Isla L, Zamorano J, Perez de la Yglesia R, et al. [Quantification of aortic valve area using three-dimensional echocardiography]. Rev Esp Cardiol 2008;61:494-500.

99. Doddamani S, Bello R, Friedman MA, et al. Demonstration of left ventricular outflow tract eccentricity by real time 3D echocardiography: implications for the determination of aortic valve area. Echocardiography 2007;24:860-866.

100. Menzel T, Mohr-Kahaly S, Wagner S, et al. Calculation of left ventricular outflow tract area using three-dimensional echocardiography. Influence on quantification of aortic valve stenosis. Int J Card Imaging 1998;14:373-379.

101. Khaw AV, von Bardeleben RS, Strasser C, et al. Direct measurement of left ventricular outflow tract by transthoracic real-time 3D-echocardiography increases accuracy in assessment of aortic valve stenosis. Int J Cardiol 2009;136:64-71.

102. Mehrotra P, Jansen K, Flynn AW, et al. Differential left ventricular remodelling and longitudinal function distinguishes low flow from normal-flow preserved ejection fraction low-gradient severe aortic stenosis. Eur Heart J 2013;34:1906-1914.

103. Poh KK, Levine RA, Solis J, et al. Assessing aortic valve area in aortic stenosis by continuity equation: a novel approach using real-time three-dimensional echocardiography. Eur Heart J 2008;29:2526-2535.

104. Gutierrez-Chico JL, Zamorano JL, Prieto-Moriche E, et al. Real-time three-dimensional echocardiography in aortic stenosis: a novel, simple, and reliable method to improve accuracy in area calculation. Eur Heart J 2008;29:1296-1306.

105. Nakai H, Takeuchi M, Yoshitani H, et al. Pitfalls of anatomical aortic valve area measurements using two-dimensional transoesophageal echocardiography and the potential of three-dimensional transoesophageal echocardiography. Eur J Echocardiogr 2010;11:369-376.

106. Alunni G, Giorgi M, Sartori C, et al. Real time triplane echocardiography in aortic valve stenosis: validation, reliability, and feasibility of a new method for valve area quantification. Echocardiography 2010;27:644-650.

107. Blot-Souletie N, Hebrard A, Acar P, et al. Comparison of accuracy of aortic valve area assessment in aortic stenosis by real time three-dimensional echocardiography in biplane mode versus two-dimensional transthoracic and transesophageal echocardiography. Echocardiography 2007;24:1065-1072.

108. Ge S, Warner JG, Jr., Abraham TP, et al. Three-dimensional surface area of the aortic valve orifice by three-dimensional echocardiography: clinical validation of a novel index for assessment of aortic stenosis. Am Heart J 1998;136:1042-1050.

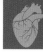

109. Goland S, Trento A, Iida K, et al. Assessment of aortic stenosis by three-dimensional echocardiography: an accurate and novel approach. Heart 2007;93:801-807.

110. Suradi H, Byers S, Green-Hess D, et al. Feasibility of using real time "Live 3D" echocardiography to visualize the stenotic aortic valve. Echocardiography 2010;27(8):1011-1020.

111. Machida T, Izumo M, Suzuki K, et al. Value of anatomical aortic valve area using real-time three-dimensional transoesophageal echocardiography in patients with aortic stenosis: a comparison between tricuspid and bicuspid aortic valves. Eur Heart J Cardiovasc Imaging 2015;16:1120-1128.

112. Calleja A, Thavendiranathan P, Ionasec RI, et al. Automated quantitative 3-dimensional modeling of the aortic valve and root by 3-dimensional transesophageal echocardiography in normals, aortic regurgitation, and aortic stenosis: comparison to computed tomography in normals and clinical implications. Circ Cardiovasc Imaging 2013;6:99-108.

113. Shibayama K, Harada K, Berdejo J, et al. Effect of transcatheter aortic valve replacement on the mitral valve apparatus and mitral regurgitation: real-time three-dimensional transesophageal echocardiography study. Circ Cardiovasc Imaging 2014;7:344-351.

114. Tops LF, Wood DA, Delgado V, et al. Noninvasive evaluation of the aortic root with multislice computed tomography implications for transcatheter aortic valve replacement. JACC Cardiovasc Imaging 2008;1:321-330.

115. Tuzcu EM, Kapadia SR, Schoenhagen P. Multimodality quantitative imaging of aortic root for transcatheter aortic valve implantation: more complex than it appears. J Am Coll Cardiol 2010;55:195-197.

116. Schoenhagen P, Tuzcu EM, Kapadia SR, et al. Three-dimensional imaging of the aortic valve and aortic root with computed tomography: new standards in an era of transcatheter valve repair/implantation. Eur Heart J 2009;30:2079-2086.

117. Ng AC, Delgado V, van der Kley F, et al. Comparison of aortic root dimensions and geometries before and after transcatheter aortic valve implantation by 2- and 3-dimensional transesophageal echocardiography and multislice computed tomography. Circulation Cardiovasc Imaging 2010;3:94-102.

118. Kurra V, Kapadia SR, Tuzcu EM, et al. Pre-procedural imaging of aortic root orientation and dimensions: comparison between X-ray angiographic planar imaging and 3-dimensional multidetector row computed tomography. JACC Cardiovasc Interv 2010;3:105-113.

119. Burman ED, Keegan J, Kilner PJ. Aortic root measurement by cardiovascular magnetic resonance: specification of planes and lines of measurement and corresponding normal values. Circ Cardiovasc Imaging 2008;1:104-113.

120. Paelinck BP, Van Herck PL, Rodrigus I, et al. Comparison of magnetic resonance imaging of aortic valve stenosis and aortic root to multimodality imaging for selection of transcatheter aortic valve implantation candidates. Am J Cardiol 2011;108(1):92-98

121. Tsang W, Bateman MG, Weinert L, et al. Accuracy of aortic annuli measurements obtained from three-dimensional echocardiography, computed tomography, and magnetic resonance imaging using an in vitro model.. J Am Coll Cardiol 2012;59:E2144.

122. Johnson MA, Munt B, Moss RR. Transcutaneous aortic valve implantation—a first line treatment for aortic valve disease? J Am Soc Echocardiogr 2010;23:377-379.

123. Altiok E, Frick M, Meyer CG, et al. Comparison of two- and three-dimensional transthoracic echocardiography to cardiac magnetic resonance imaging for assessment of paravalvular regurgitation after transcatheter aortic valve implantation. Am J Cardiol 2014;113:1859-1866.

124. Regeer MV, Kamperidis V, Versteegh MI, et al. Three-dimensional transoesophageal echocardiography of the aortic valve and root: changes in aortic root dilation and aortic regurgitation. Eur Heart J Cardiovasc Imaging 2016.

125. Haydar HS, He GW, Hovaguimian H, et al. Valve repair for aortic insufficiency: surgical classification and techniques. Eur J Cardiothorac Surg 1997;11:258-265.

126. Augoustides JG, Szeto WY, Bavaria JE. Advances in aortic valve repair: focus on functional approach, clinical outcomes, and central role of echocardiography. J Cardiothorac Vasc Anesth 2010;24:1016-1020.

127. El Khoury G, Glineur D, Rubay J, et al. Functional classification of aortic root/valve abnormalities and their correlation with etiologies and surgical procedures. Curr Opin Cardiol 2005;20:115-121.

128. Boodhwani M, de Kerchove L, Glineur D, et al. Repair-oriented classification of aortic insufficiency: impact on surgical techniques and clinical outcomes. J Thorac Cardiovasc Surg 2009;137:286-294.

129. Mori Y, Shiota T, Jones M, et al. Three-dimensional reconstruction of the color Doppler-imaged vena contracta for quantifying aortic regurgitation: studies in a chronic animal model. Circulation 1999;99:1611-1617.

130. Fang L, Hsiung MC, Miller AP, et al. Assessment of aortic regurgitation by live three-dimensional transthoracic echocardiographic measurements of vena contracta area: usefulness and validation. Echocardiography 2005;22:775-781.

131. Chin CH, Chen CH, Lo HS. The correlation between three-dimensional vena contracta area and aortic regurgitation index in patients with aortic regurgitation. Echocardiography 2010;27:161-166.

132. Pirat B, Little SH, Igo SR, et al. Direct measurement of proximal isovelocity surface area by real-time three-dimensional color Doppler for quantitation of aortic regurgitant volume: an in vitro validation. J Am Soc Echocardiogr 2009;22:306-313.

133. Li X, Jones M, Irvine T et al. Real-time 3-dimensional echocardiography for quantification of the difference in left ventricular versus right ventricular stroke volume in a chronic animal model study: improved results using C-scans for quantifying aortic regurgitation. J Am Soc Echocardiogr 2004;17:870-875.

134. Irvine T, Stetten GD, Sachdev V, et al. Quantification of aortic regurgitation by real-time 3-dimensional echocardiography in a chronic animal model: computation of aortic regurgitant volume as the difference between left and right ventricular stroke volumes. J Am Soc Echocardiogr 2001;14:1112-1118.

135. Choi J, Hong GR, Kim M, et al. Automatic quantification of aortic regurgitation using 3D full volume color doppler echocardiography: a validation study with cardiac magnetic resonance imaging. Int J Cardiovasc Imaging 2015;31:1379-1389.

136. Lansac E, Lim KH, Shomura Y, et al. Dynamic balance of the aortomitral junction. J Thorac Cardiovasc Surg 2002;123:911-918.

137. Veronesi F, Caiani EG, Sugeng L, et al. Effect of mitral valve repair on mitral-aortic coupling: a real-time three-dimensional transesophageal echocardiography study. J Am Soc Echocardiogr 2012;25(5):524-531.

138. Tsang W, Meineri M, Hahn RT, et al. A three-dimensional echocardiographic study on aortic-mitral coupling in transcatheter aortic valve replacement. Eur Heart J Cardiovasc Imaging 2013;14:950-956.

139. Tsang W, Veronesi F, Sugeng L, et al. Mitral valve dynamics in severe aortic stenosis before and after aortic valve replacement. J Am Soc Echocardiogr 2013;26:606-614.

140. Vanden Eynden F, Bouchard D, El-Hamamsy I, et al. Effect of aortic valve replacement for aortic stenosis on severity of mitral regurgitation. Ann Thorac Surg 2007;83:1279-1284.

141. Ruel M, Kapila V, Price J, et al. Natural history and predictors of outcome in patients with concomitant functional mitral regurgitation at the time of aortic valve replacement. Circulation 2006;114:I541-1546.

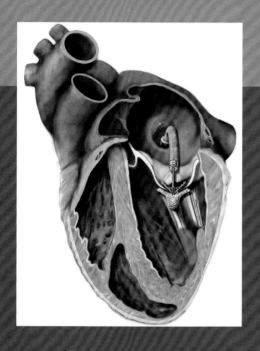

第3章
钙化性主动脉瓣疾病的分子机制

主动脉瓣狭窄以进行性瓣膜狭窄和压力超负荷引起的病理性左心室心肌肥厚为主要特征。本章主要阐释这两个受到高度调控的疾病过程的分子机制。

主动脉瓣的病理改变可分为两个阶段。起始阶段类似于动脉粥样硬化过程，内皮受损、炎症细胞浸润和脂质氧化起主导作用。增殖阶段由涉及成骨样细胞的多种信号通路驱动。成骨样细胞最可能来源于活化的瓣膜间质细胞，导致病理性细胞外基质重塑和瓣膜纤维化。被动的钙蓄积进一步强化瓣膜组织钙化。随着时间进展，增殖阶段最终形成钙化和血管损伤的自循环。

进行性瓣膜狭窄伴有左心室代偿性肥厚，以维持室壁压力和左心室功能，但流出道阻塞导致压力持续超负荷，最终使左心室发生病理性肥厚，其与生理性肥厚的分子机制有较大区别。病理性肥厚导致心肌纤维化、心内膜下缺血和细胞死亡，这是发生左心室功能失调、患者出现症状和不良事件的重要原因。

钙化性主动脉瓣疾病是一个复杂且受到高度调控的过程，尚无改变疾病自然史的治疗药物，但是几项有前景的临床试验正在进行。我们需要进一步探索其分子机制，以确定潜在的治疗靶点。

王　璨

Molecular Mechanisms of Calcific Aortic Valve Disease

Russell J. Everett, David E. Newby, Marc R. Dweck

CHAPTER OUTLINE

KEY POINTS

- Calcific aortic valve disease is an active, highly regulated process.
- The initiation phase has several similarities to atherosclerosis, including endothelial injury, inflammatory cell infiltration, and lipid oxidation.
- Valve interstitial cell activation leads to pathologic extracellular matrix remodeling and valvular fibrosis.
- Procalcific processes occur in the valve under the control of highly regulated osteoblast-like signaling (osteogenic) or passive calcium deposition and accumulation (dystrophic).

- The propagation phase eventually supersedes with a self-perpetuating cycle of mineralization, vascular injury, and disease progression.
- Sustained pressure overload leads to a pathologic hypertrophic response in the left ventricle that is characterized by myocardial fibrosis, subendocardial ischemia, and cell death, ultimately resulting in left ventricular decompensation.

BACKGROUND

Aortic valve disease represents a significant global health challenge. The prevalence of aortic stenosis increases exponentially with age and is the most common valve disease requiring surgery in the Western world.[1] Severe disease is estimated to affect 3.4% of people older than 75 years of age.[2]

Aortic stenosis is characterized by progressive narrowing of the valve and by the way in which the left ventricle (LV) adapts to the increased afterload imposed on it. Symptoms and adverse events are related to processes occurring in the myocardium and the valve. This chapter focuses on the molecular mechanisms underlying progressive narrowing of the valve and on the hypertrophic response of the LV. It also highlights potential therapeutic targets for this common clinical condition.

The Normal Aortic Valve

The normal aortic valve consists of three cusps attached at the base to the fibrous aortic root annulus and that coapt along their free edges during ventricular diastole to prevent retrograde flow into the LV. The cusps are usually less than 1 mm thick and consist of three layers: fibrosa, spongiosa, and ventricularis (Fig. 3.1).

The fibrosa layer faces the aorta, consists of collagen types I and III arranged circumferentially, and acts as the main load-bearing layer. The spongiosa connects the outer fibrosa and ventricularis layers, helping to lubricate their relative motion as they deform during the cardiac cycle. This layer predominantly comprises proteoglycans with a smaller percentage of collagen fibers and fibronectin and laminin as adhesive proteins. The ventricularis layer faces the LV and contains

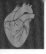

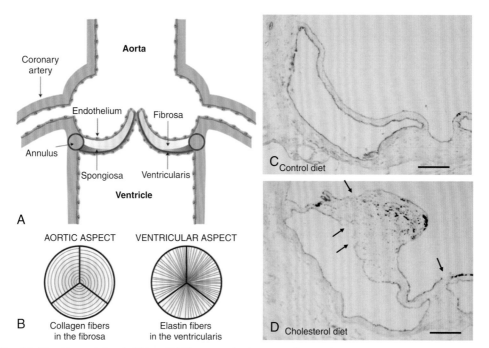

Fig. 3.1 The Normal Aortic Valve. (A) The normal valve comprises a three-layer structure. The fibrosa is found on the aortic aspect of the valve and contains mostly fibroblasts and collagen fibers. The spongiosa consists of glycosaminoglycans that lubricate relative motion of the two outermost layers and resist external compressive forces. The ventricularis faces the LV and contains radially orientated elastin fibers. An endothelial monolayer covers both aspects of the valve in continuity with surrounding tissues. (B) Short axis view of the aortic valve shows the circumferential orientation of collagen fibers in the fibrosa and radial orientation of elastin in the ventricularis. (C and D) Micrographs depict disruption of the aortic valve endothelium *(arrows)* in mice fed a control or Western-type diet for 16 weeks (immunohistochemical staining using anti–endothelial nitric oxide synthase antibody). (A and B from Dweck MR, Boon NA, Newby DE. Calcific aortic stenosis: a disease of the valve and myocardium. J Am Coll Cardiol 2012;60:1854-1863. C and D from Matsumoto Y, Adams V, Jacob S, et al. Regular exercise training prevents aortic valve disease in low-density lipoprotein-receptor-deficient mice. Circulation 2010;121:759-767.)

TABLE 3.1   Classification of Aortic Valve Cell Origins and Phenotypes.

Cell Type	Origin	Function
Endothelium	Endothelial endocardial cushion	Paracrine regulation of VIC function Maintenance of VIC population through ECM
	Circulating endothelial progenitors	Repair in response to injury Maintenance of VIC population through ECM
Quiescent, resident interstitial cells	Endothelial endocardial cushion (by ECM) or neural crest	Maintenance of valve structure/connective tissue production Secretion of antiangiogenic factors Potential osteogenic precursor
Interstitial cells of extravalvular origin	Bone marrow/circulating progenitor cells	Repair in response to injury Potential osteogenic precursor
Activated interstitial cells (α-SMA⁺)	Resident or circulating immune complex cells	Repair in response to injury (migration, proliferation) Angiogenic factor secretion with cusp thickening Robust ECM production/matrix remodeling enzyme expression Potential osteogenic precursor

ECM, Extracellular matrix; *SMA,* smooth muscle actin; *VIC,* valve interstitial cell.

radially orientated elastin fibers in addition to collagen. The elastin helps to mitigate radial strain when the valve is fully open and increases recoil to aid valve closure (Table 3.1).

General Concepts

Calcific aortic valve disease was long dismissed as a degenerative condition in which progressive "wear and tear" resulted in passive accumulation of calcium in the valve cusps. However, emerging evidence indicates that aortic valve disease instead develops as part of a highly complex and tightly regulated series of processes, each of which is potentially amenable to medical intervention.[3]

Contemporary thinking is that the pathophysiology of aortic stenosis can be subdivided into two distinct phases: an early *initiation phase* with many similarities to atherosclerosis, in which endothelial

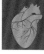

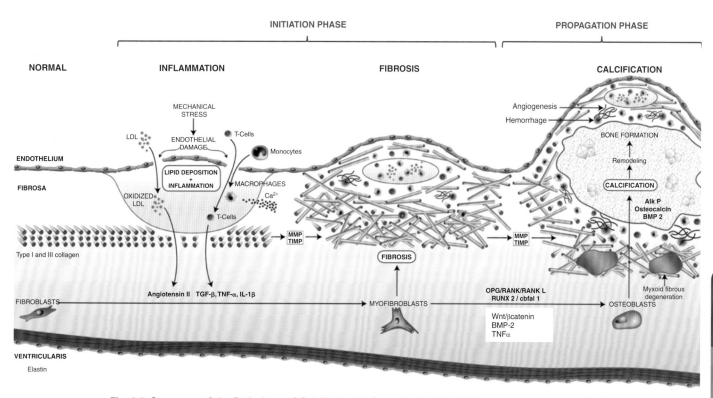

Fig. 3.2 Summary of the Pathology of Calcific Aortic Stenosis. Endothelial damage occurs as a result of increased mechanical stress and reduced sheer stress. This leads to infiltration of oxidized lipids and inflammatory cells. Inflammatory cytokines and other factors such as angiotensin II lead to activation of fibroblasts into myofibroblasts that secrete collagen. Increased collagen synthesis and the action of matrix metalloproteinases *(MMPs)* lead to extracellular matrix remodeling and valvular fibrosis. Valvular calcification begins with matrix vesicle secretion from macrophages but is accelerated under the control of valvular interstitial cells that differentiate into an osteoblast-like phenotype. This process is driven by a variety of osteogenic factors, such as WNT/β-catenin, RANKL/RANK signaling, and the CBFA/RUNX2 transcription factor. Osteoblast-like cells then coordinate further calcification in a process similar to skeletal bone formation that involves bone morphogenetic protein *(BMP)*, osteocalcin, and alkaline phosphatase signaling. This process is supported by angiogenesis, and valvular hemorrhage can be observed, which may accelerate disease progression. The propagation phase leads to progressive calcification and remodeling so that features of lamellar bone, microfractures, and hemopoietic tissue can be observed in end-stage calcific valve disease. *BMP,* Bone morphogenetic protein; *IL-1β,* interleukin-1β; *LDL,* low-density lipoprotein; *RANK,* receptor activator of nuclear κ-B; *RANKL,* receptor activator of nuclear κ-B ligand; *RAS,* renin-angiotensin system; *TGF,* transforming growth factor; *VIC,* valve interstitial cell. (Modified from Dweck MR, Boon NA, Newby DE. Calcific aortic stenosis: a disease of the valve and myocardium. J Am Coll Cardiol 2012;60:1854-1863.)

injury, valvular lipid deposition, and inflammation dominate, and a later *propagation phase*, in which osteogenic and procalcific mechanisms dominate and drive progressive valve narrowing (Fig. 3.2).[4,5]

Experimental Models

Although the description of cellular and molecular changes in human tissue is a critical component in research, empirical testing in animal models can provide important insights about whether a change is a pathophysiologic driver of calcific aortic valve disease or merely an epiphenomenon. When evaluating experimental data or deciding which model is useful for a particular study design, several important questions must be addressed (Table 3.2).

- Does the model require genetically altered animals, and do the mutations relate to the specific question at hand?
- What is the underlying stimulus driving calcification (e.g., hyperlipidemia, hypertension)?
- Are the histopathologic changes relevant to human disease (e.g., fibrosis, calcification)?

- Do the animals develop hemodynamically relevant aortic valve dysfunction and stenosis or only aortic valve sclerosis?

One criticism of preclinical animal models is that they have largely failed to accurately reflect human aortic stenosis, which has delayed development of effective medical therapies. Because of the difference between the human condition and that induced in animal models, data from the latter must always be interpreted with a degree of caution.

INITIATION PHASE

The initiating event in aortic stenosis is thought to be endothelial injury related to increased mechanical stress and reduced sheer stress. The aortic aspect of the valve cusps experience reduced shear stress compared with the ventricular aspect, with the noncoronary cusp experiencing even lower shear stress due to the absence of associated coronary blood flow. This may explain why valvular lesions appear to favor the aortic aspect of the valve and the noncoronary

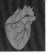

TABLE 3.2 Echocardiographic and Hemodynamic Changes in Animal Models of Aortic Valve Sclerosis and Stenosis.

Species/Strain	Diet	Histopathologic Changes in Aortic Valve	Hemodynamically Significant Stenosis
Mice			
C57BL/6	HF	Lipid deposition Modest calcification	No
ApoE$^{-/-}$	Chow	Lipid deposition Calcification Monocyte/inflammatory cell infiltration	<2%
	HF/HC	Lipid deposition Fibrosis Calcification Monocyte/inflammatory cell infiltration	<2%
Ldlr$^{-/-}$	HF/HC	Lipid deposition Calcification Monocyte/inflammatory cell infiltration	No
Ldlr$^{-/-}$/apoB$^{100/100}$	Chow	Lipid deposition Calcification Monocyte/inflammatory cell infiltration Myofibroblast activation	Yes, ≈30% of mice
	HF/HC	Lipid deposition Calcification Fibrosis Monocyte/inflammatory cell infiltration Myofibroblast activation	Yes, >50% of mice
EGFR$^{Wa2/Wa2}$	Chow	Fibrosis Calcification Inflammatory cell infiltration	Yes, but background strain dependent
eNOS$^{-/-}$	Chow	Bicuspid aortic valves in ≈40% of mice	No
Tricuspid offspring	HF/HC	Calcification Fibrosis	No
Bicuspid offspring	HF/HC	Calcification Fibrosis	Yes
Notch1$^{+/-}$	HF/HC	Calcification	No
Periostin$^{-/-}$	Chow	Calcification Fibrosis	Not known
	HF/HC	Reduced valve thickening and fibrosis	No
MGP$^{-/-}$	Chow	Calcification	Not known
Klotho$^{-/-}$	Chow	Calcification	No
Col1a2$^{Oim/Oim}$	Chow	Fibrosis/extracellular matrix disruption	No
Twist1$^{Tg/0}$	Chow	Hypercellular, thickened valves	No
Sox9$^{Fl/+}$/Col2a1^{Cre}	Chow	Calcification Fibrosis	No
Chm1$^{-/-}$	Chow	Neoangiogenesis Lipid deposition Calcification	Not known
Rabbits			
New Zealand White	HF/HC	Lipid deposition Calcification Inflammatory cell infiltration	<10% Mostly moderate sclerosis
	Chow + hypertension	Fibrosis Inflammation	<10%
Watanabe	HF/HC	Lipid deposition Fibrosis Calcification Inflammatory cell infiltration	No
Pigs			
Yorkshire Landrace	HF/HC	Lipid deposition	No

Apo, Apolipoprotein; *EGFR,* epidermal growth factor receptor; *eNOS,* endothelial nitric oxide synthetase; *HC,* high cholesterol; *HF,* high fat; *Ldlr,* low-density lipoprotein receptor; *MGP,* matrix Gla protein.

cusp in particular.[6] This is illustrated using the model of bicuspid aortic valve disease. Two rather than three valve cusps result in less efficient dissipation of mechanical stress, and as a result, patients with bicuspid valve disease almost universally develop aortic stenosis with more rapid disease progression, and on average, they require aortic valve replacement 5 to 10 years earlier.[7,8]

This early initiation phase of the disease is somewhat similar to atherosclerosis, with endothelial injury, lipid infiltration, and inflammation predominating. This may explain why the incidence of aortic stenosis is related to risk factors that are similar to those of atherosclerosis, with large longitudinal studies consistently demonstrating an association with factors such as age, smoking, hypertension, and hypercholesterolemia (Table 3.3).[9–11] Later in the initiation phase, angiogenesis can be observed alongside matrix remodeling and the earliest stage of valvular calcium formation.

Lipid Deposition

Similar to atherosclerosis, endothelial injury in aortic stenosis is followed by valvular lipid infiltration, predominantly lipoprotein(a) and low-density lipoprotein (LDL) cholesterol. Observational studies have shown that total cholesterol,[10,11] LDL,[9] and lipoprotein(a)[9,12] are independent risk factors for the development of aortic stenosis; high-density lipoprotein appears to be protective.[11]

Aortic valve calcification was linked to a single nucleotide polymorphism in the lipoprotein(a) locus in a large genome-wide linkage study.[12] This association led to hope that statin therapy might modify the progression of aortic stenosis and was supported by preclinical data (using the hypercholesterolemic mouse model of aortic stenosis). However, three randomized, controlled trials demonstrated that statins did not modify the natural history of this disease, suggesting that although lipid deposition and inflammation are involved in disease initiation, they are less important in driving disease progression.

The pathologic processes implicated in the propagation phase of aortic stenosis appear to be different from those in early initiation, but there has been renewed interest in lipid-lowering agents to modify disease progression since the development of the proprotein convertase subtilisin/kexin type 9 (PCSK9) inhibitors. PCSK9 is a hepatic convertase that internalizes LDL receptors, and PCSK9 inhibition can lead to dramatic reductions in circulating levels of LDL and

TABLE 3.3 Risk Factors for Calcific Aortic Valve Disease and Potential Molecular Mediators.

Risk Factor	Potential Molecular Mediators
Hypertension	Angiotensin II Force/shear-initiated signaling pathways Reactive oxygen species
Diabetes	Hyperglycemia Receptor for advanced glycation end products (RAGE) activation Angiotensin II Reactive oxygen species
Hyperlipidemia	Low-density lipoprotein Lipoprotein-related receptor protein 5/6 activation Local angiotensin II generation Reactive oxygen species
Smoking	Reactive oxygen species
Aging	Epigenetics Reactive oxygen species

lipoprotein(a).[13] The PCSK9 R46L loss-of-function mutation was associated with a lower risk of developing aortic stenosis in a large Danish observational study,[14] and in a small cross-sectional study, PSCK9 levels correlated with the presence but not the severity of aortic valve disease.[15] A randomized trial (NCT03051360) comparing the effect of PCSK9 inhibitor therapy with placebo on disease progression in patients with aortic stenosis is underway.

Inflammation

Similar to atherosclerosis, lipid deposition and oxidation in the valve induces a proinflammatory response. It is characterized by chemotaxis and infiltration of macrophages, T lymphocytes, and mast cells.[16] Inflammation in the valve may also be observed in the later stages of the disease related to recurrent valve injury, reactive oxygen species, cell death, and increased mechanical stress in the valve.

Consistent with this finding, elaboration of proinflammatory cytokines (e.g., tumor necrosis factor-α [TNF-α], interleukins IL-6 and IL-1) is also dramatically increased in humans and animals with calcific aortic valve disease.[17–21] Although few studies have examined the role of proinflammatory cytokines in the progression of calcific aortic valve disease in humans, three lines of evidence from nonclinical work suggest that they may play a role in initiation and progression of the disease.

First, aortic valves from IL-1 receptor antagonist (IL-1ra)–deficient mice are thickened, accumulate calcium, and develop mild aortic valve dysfunction (peak transvalvular velocity 2 m/s). This phenotype is abolished in IL-1ra/TNF-α double-knockout mice, suggesting that TNF-α is the major downstream mediator of IL-1–induced inflammation at least in this murine model.[17]

Second, a growing body of work suggests that activation of receptors for advanced glycosylation end products (RAGEs) is likely to accelerate cardiovascular calcification. Specifically, overexpression of S100A12 accelerates vascular calcification in hypercholesterolemic mice by what appears to be a nicotinamide adenine dinucleotide phosphate (NADPH) oxidase–dependent mechanism.[22,23] RAGE activation drives proinflammatory cytokine production and osteogenic gene expression in valve interstitial cells (VICs) in vitro.[24] Although mechanisms contributing to increased oxidative stress differ dramatically between the aorta and aortic valve (discussed later),[25,26] numerous studies have shown that RAGE activation is strongly associated with increases in TNF-α,[27,28] which may be a point of convergence in inflammatory signals driving calcification in the aortic valve and aorta.

Third, addition of exogenous TNF-α to cultured aortic VICs amplifies bone morphogenetic protein (BMP) signaling and accelerates calcium accumulation in vitro. TNF-α accelerated calcification only in cells from patients with calcific aortic valve disease (i.e., not in cells from nonstenotic control valves), suggesting that phenotypic and/or epigenetic changes that occur in vivo may persist in cultured VICs in vitro.[29] The molecular mechanisms by which TNF-α promotes VIC calcification are still being investigated, but work in aortic myofibroblasts suggests that reactive oxygen species (ROS) generated by TNF receptor 1 activation may be integral.[30,31]

Angiogenesis

Active inflammatory processes are sustained by angiogenesis, the process by which new blood vessels form from existing capillaries. This becomes particularly important when the valve becomes grossly thickened and the central components become relatively ischemic. Angiogenesis is seen in 85% of valve leaflets in patients with aortic valve disease and co-localizes to areas of inflammation, fibrosis, and ossification.[32–34]

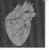

Angiogenesis is regulated by angiogenic factors such as vascular endothelial growth factor (VEGF), and fibroblast growth factor 2 (FGF2) and by several inhibitors.[35] The balance of proangiogenic and antiangiogenic factors is altered in calcific valve disease. For example, the antiangiogenic glycoprotein chondromodulin 1 is downregulated in the extracellular matrix (ECM) of diseased valves, which is then associated with angiogenesis.[36] New vessels that develop in calcific aortic valve disease are leaky and prone to rupture. This can cause valve leaflet hemorrhage, a potentially important trigger for further valve calcification.[37,38]

Matrix Remodeling and Fibrosis

Substantial changes in the composition, organization, and mechanical properties of the ECM are observed in stenotic aortic valves.[39] Progressive fibrosis leads to leaflet thickening and is characterized by increased deposition of collagen in all valve layers, along with associated remodeling and disorganization.[32] This pattern appears to be mediated in part by increased activity of matrix metalloproteinases (MMP1, MMP2, MMP3, and MMP9), their tissue inhibitors (TIMP1 and TIMP2),[40,41] and cathepsins, which are potent elastolytic enzymes.[42,43]

Progressive fibrosis of the valve contributes alongside calcification to increases in aortic valve stiffness, thereby directly resulting in progressive stenosis of the valve. In a small minority of often younger patients with aortic stenosis, fibrosis appears to be the predominant process responsible for valve narrowing with minimal or absent calcification[44,45] (Fig. 3.3). However, much more commonly extensive valvular calcification is associated with increases in ECM accumulation and turnover.[46,47] The profibrotic processes that occur in the valve are thought to play a role similar to that observed in skeletal bone formation, providing a scaffold on which subsequent calcification occurs. Fibrosis and calcification therefore appear to be closely linked and the major drivers of aortic stenosis progression.

Angiotensin II

Activation of the renin-angiotensin system is implicated at multiple levels in the pathogenesis of aortic stenosis in the valve and in the myocardium. The renin-angiotensin system is involved in the development of hypertension and may therefore accelerate valve disease progression by associated increases in valvular mechanical stress.[48] Angiotensin II also has proinflammatory and fibrotic effects at the local valve level, where profibrotic effects appear to be mediated by the angiotensin II type 1 (AT1) receptor. Although angiotensin II can have antiinflammatory and fibrotic effects by type 2 (AT2) receptors, they are downregulated in calcific aortic valve disease. Similarly, angiotensin-converting enzyme type 2 (ACE2), which mediates antifibrotic and antiinflammatory effects by the Ang(1-7)/MAS pathway is also downregulated.[49] Overall, the renin-angiotensin system plays a predominantly profibrotic and proinflammatory role in stenotic aortic valves.

Angiotensin II is upregulated in two ways. First, there is increased ACE activity in calcific aortic valve disease, which is likely delivered to the valve by its natural vehicle, LDL, after endothelial injury. Second, infiltrating macrophages are abundant and can act as primary sources of increased tissue angiotensin II concentrations due to their expression of chymase, which converts angiotensin I to angiotensin II.[50]

Although retrospective clinical studies suggest that ACE inhibition may slow progression of aortic valve disease,[51] there is a lack of randomized, controlled trial data, and their lack of effect on chymase activity makes ACE inhibition a less appealing target. Preclinical experiments in hypercholesterolemic rabbits showed that angiotensin I receptor blockade attenuates aortic VIC activation, endothelial disruption, and valvular inflammation in early stages of valve disease,[52] suggesting that direct angiotensin inhibition may also be useful.

Valve Interstitial Cell and Matrix Interaction

VICs are similar to activated myofibroblasts and appear to be the key coordinators of valvular fibrosis and later calcification. The interactions between VICs and their environment appears important in the regulation of fibrosis and calcification, and they can be functionally categorized as matricellular signaling, matricrine signaling, mechanical signaling through changes in matrix elasticity, and mechanical signaling due to changes in external forces (Fig. 3.4).

Matricellular signaling refers to induction of signals within the VIC by direct interactions with ECM components.[39] An example of matricellular signaling is the interaction between VICs and tenascin C. Although tenascin C levels are low in normal valves, expression is markedly upregulated, and location shifts from the subendothelium to the valve interstitium as the severity of calcific aortic valve disease progresses. It has been suggested that matricellular signals initiated by tenascin C upregulate MMP expression and alkaline phosphatase (ALP) activity in VICs.[53,54]

Matricrine signaling refers to the ability of the matrix to modulate the bioavailability and binding of growth factors through their sequestration and localization.[39] Examples of matricrine signaling are the regulation of latent transforming growth factor-β (TGF-β) assembly, the storage by fibronectin and binding of TNF-α by biglycan,[55] and the release of proinflammatory and procalcific elastin degradation products by cathepsins.[56] Upregulation of ECM molecules may play a key role in the localization of profibrotic and proinflammatory molecules to sites of calcification and injury in the valve.[57]

Mechanical signaling refers to changes in external mechanical forces that are ultimately transmitted to aortic VICs by the ECM.[39] Hypertension, which is a major risk factor for development of calcific aortic valve disease, increases myofibroblast activation and appears to accelerate the differentiation of cells to an osteoblast-like phenotype.[30,58-60] Detailed studies of changes in VIC biology in experimental models of hypertension (e.g., with or without genetic alterations in ECM proteins) are needed to understand the role of the ECM in the integration of physiologic and biochemical cues in vivo.

The stiffness of the ECM can have a profound effect on the differentiation of cells in response to various lineage-directing cues.[61] Reports clearly demonstrate that matrix stiffness is an independent determinant of cellular differentiation and determines whether cells undergo apoptosis or osteogenesis after specific stimuli (e.g., TGF-β).[39,57,62] Collectively, increases in matrix stiffness with progression of calcific aortic valve disease are likely to perpetuate osteogenesis, apoptosis, and calcification in an independent manner. This may be a major mechanism underlying the propagation phase of the disease process whereby calcification appears to beget further calcification.

PROPAGATION PHASE

Although inflammation and lipid deposition are implicated in the initiation of aortic stenosis, calcification appears to be the key process driving progressive valve narrowing and disease progression in the propagation phase. Atherosclerotic risk factors do not predict disease progression; rather, it is most closely associated with markers of valve calcification, whether measured using echocardiography, computed tomography, or positron emission tomography.[63-65] When devising strategies to slow disease progression in aortic stenosis, calcification is a key target.[5]

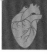

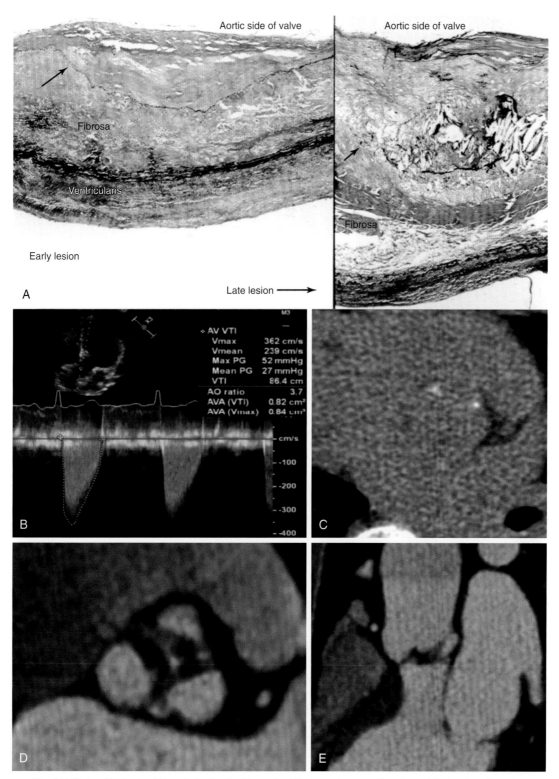

Fig. 3.3 Role of Valvular Fibrosis in Aortic Stenosis. (A) In most cases, fibrosis contributes to valve cusp thickening *(left)* alongside calcification with the latter predominating *(right,* massive calcium deposit), particularly in later stages of disease. (B–E) Investigations of a 58-year-old woman with tricuspid valve morphology. Echocardiography (B) showed a peak aortic velocity of 3.6 m/s and valve area by continuity equation of 0.8 cm², indicating moderate to severe aortic stenosis. However, noncontrast CT calcium scoring (C) showed minimal valvular calcification (calcium score 37 AU). Further contrast-enhanced sequences (D and E) revealed thickened leaflets with reduced signal, suggesting leaflet fibrosis. *AO,* Aorta; *AV,* aortic valve; *AVA,* aortic valve area; *PG,* pressure gradient; *VTI,* velocity time integral. (A from Freeman RV, Otto CM. Spectrum of calcific aortic valve disease: pathogenesis, disease progression, and treatment strategies. Circulation 2005;111:3316. B–E from Cartlidge TR, Pawade TA, Dweck MR. Aortic stenosis and CT calcium scoring: is it for everyone? Heart 20171;103:8-9.)

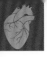

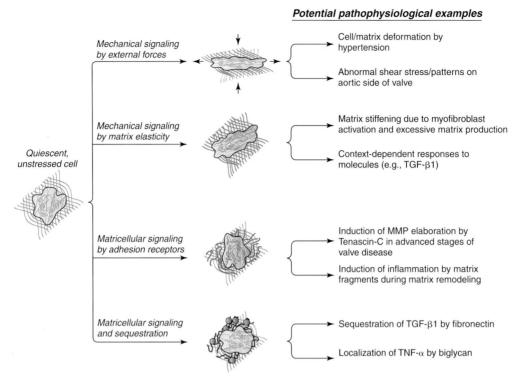

Potential pathophysiological examples

Mechanical signaling by external forces
- Cell/matrix deformation by hypertension
- Abnormal shear stress/patterns on aortic side of valve

Mechanical signaling by matrix elasticity
- Matrix stiffening due to myofibroblast activation and excessive matrix production
- Context-dependent responses to molecules (e.g., TGF-β1)

Quiescent, unstressed cell

Matricellular signaling by adhesion receptors
- Induction of MMP elaboration by Tenascin-C in advanced stages of valve disease
- Induction of inflammation by matrix fragments during matrix remodeling

Matricellular signaling and sequestration
- Sequestration of TGF-β1 by fibronectin
- Localization of TNF-α by biglycan

Fig. 3.4 Interactions between valve interstitial cells and their surrounding matrix and potential pathophysiologic stimuli that may promote development of calcific aortic valve disease. *MMP,* Matrix metalloproteinase; *TGF,* tumor growth factor; *TNF,* tumor necrosis factor. (Modified from Chen JH, Simmons CA. Cell-matrix interactions in the pathobiology of calcific aortic valve disease: critical roles for matricellular, matricrine, and matrix mechanics cues. Circ Res 2011;108:1510-1524.)

The propagation phase of aortic valve calcification appears to be a closely regulated process that depends on the influence of osteoblast-like cells that develop an osteogenic phenotype. Approximately 20% of stenotic aortic valves have evidence of bone matrix at the time of valve surgery. Histologically, the bone matrix has been associated with cells that resembled osteoblasts and osteoclasts (Fig. 3.5).[33] This finding suggests that this pathologic process is organized and regulated and that it may also be modifiable with targeted therapy.

The similarity between skeletal bone formation and aortic stenosis is further supported by gene-profiling studies showing increased expression of the runt-related transcription factor 2 gene *(RUNX2)* (i.e., core-binding factor subunit α1 *[CBFA1])* in aortic valve tissue, an essential component of osteoblastic differentiation and regulation.[66–68] Subsequent work demonstrated upregulation of several other ECM proteins closely involved in osteoblastic processes, including osteopontin and bone sialoprotein, which have complex roles that include facilitating osteoblast attachment to bone matrix.[34]

The source of osteoblast-like cells remains unclear. Although several cell types in native valve tissue can undergo differentiation into an osteoblastic phenotype in vitro, the most plausible candidate is the VIC. Fibroblasts can become activated by a variety of cell signaling pathways, including angiotensin II,[69] to adopt the myofibroblast phenotype demonstrated by VICs and characterized by α-smooth muscle actin (α-SMA) expression and increased type I collagen synthesis. The percentage of VICs increases in calcific valve disease (up to 30%), and VICs are thought to develop an osteoblast-like phenotype.[69,70]

The transition of the VIC to an osteogenic phenotype may be the key step in establishing the propagation phase of the disease, and it is regulated by a growing list of signaling molecules and complex pathways. In the early stages, macrophage-derived proinflammatory cytokines appear to be important.[42,71,72] Later, self-perpetuating, procalcific pathways dominate, including bone morphogenetic protein, WNT/β-catenin, and receptor activator of nuclear κ-B (RANK)/ RANK ligand (RANKL)/osteoprotegerin (OPG) pathways. A vicious cycle of calcification producing osteogenic differentiation and further calcification appears to become established, in part driven by increased mechanical stresses and valvular injury related to the calcium deposition (Fig. 3.6).

Bone Morphogenetic Protein Signaling

BMP2 through BMP7 proteins are multifunctional cytokines belonging to the TGF-β superfamily. Numerous studies have reported increased expression of multiple BMP isoforms, including BMP2, BMP4, and BMP6, in diseased human valves.[73–76]

BMP appears to have a central role in driving differentiation of cells, including VICs, toward an osteoblast-like phenotype.[76,77] BMP elaboration is thought to originate from the endothelium on the aortic face of the valve[78] (Fig. 3.7), where shear forces are nonlaminar and inhibitors of BMP signaling are disproportionately low.[73] Binding of BMPs to their receptor complex on aortic VICs results in SMAD1/5/8 phosphorylation and subsequent translocation of the SMAD complex to the nucleus, where it drives pro-osteogenic gene expression through binding to SMAD-binding elements.[79,80] Although SMAD6 appears to play a major role in tonic suppression of BMP signaling,[81] the role of other inhibitory molecules in the regulation of aortic valve calcification (e.g., SMURF1/2) remains poorly understood.

Bone morphogenetic protein signaling is also elevated in experimental animal models of calcific aortic valve disease. Increases in SMAD1/5/8 phosphorylation precede aortic valve dysfunction in hypercholesterolemic mice,[82] suggesting that increases in BMP signaling

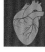

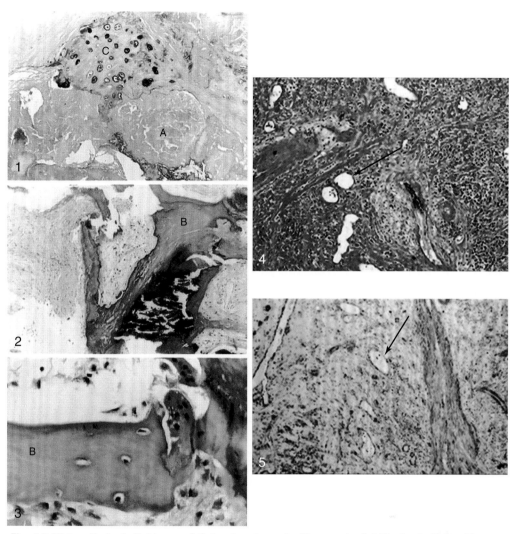

Fig. 3.5 Histopathologic Evidence of Osteochondrogenic Changes in Calcific Aortic Valve Disease. (1) Atheromatous *(A)* and chondrocyte-like *(C)* changes. (2 and 3) Mature bonelike structures *(B).* (4 and 5) Massive valvular collagen accumulation/fibrosis (Masson trichrome stain) and α-smooth muscle actin (immunohistochemistry) and areas of neovascularization *(arrows).* (Modified from Mohler ER 3rd, Gannon F, Reynolds C, et al. Bone formation and inflammation in cardiac valves. Circulation 2001;103:1522-1528; Rajamannan NM, Nealis TB, Subramaniam M, et al. Calcified rheumatic valve neoangiogenesis is associated with vascular endothelial growth factor expression and osteoblast-like bone formation. Circulation 2005;111:3296-1301.)

are not simply an epiphenomenon associated with end-stage valve calcification and stenosis.

WNT/β-Catenin Signaling

A second major osteogenic pathway activated in calcific aortic valve disease is WNT/β-catenin signaling (Fig. 3.8). The WNT family members are pleiotropic signaling proteins that affect embryonic development, cellular division, and differentiation. Activation of the canonical signaling pathway involves receptor binding of WNT ligands, which results in activation and nuclear translocation of β-catenin and increased pro-osteogenic gene expression.[83,84] Many components of this pathway have been implicated in calcified human and animal aortic valves, including WNT ligands (e.g., WNT3A, WNT7A),[57,85–87] lipoprotein receptor–related protein (LRP) receptor complex components (e.g., LRP5/6, frizzled receptors),[87,88] and nuclear translocation of the β-catenin transcription factor complex.[57,86,89]

WNT/β-catenin signaling can be negatively regulated at multiple levels, including through inhibition of WNT binding, inhibition of

β-catenin activation, and proteosomal degradation of β-catenin.[83,84] The role played by endogenous inhibitors of the WNT/β-catenin signaling pathway in aortic stenosis remains poorly understood.

Transforming Growth Factor-β Signaling

Like BMP signaling, canonical TGF-β signaling involves phosphorylation of SMAD proteins (SMAD2 and SMAD3 in particular) and translocation of the activated SMAD complex to the nucleus.[79,90] Although increases in TGF-β expression, SMAD2/3 phosphorylation, and multiple SMAD2/3 target genes have been demonstrated in humans and animals with calcific aortic valve disease[62,82,89,91] (Fig. 3.9), the true role of canonical TGF-β signaling in the initiation and progression of calcification in aortic valve disease remains controversial.

The key observation suggesting that TGF-β contributes to calcification is that cultured aortic VICs treated with exogenous TGF-β rapidly form calcified nodules by a caspase/apoptosis-dependent mechanism.[91] However, several other observations from animal models suggest instead that TGF-β does not accelerate aortic valve

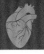

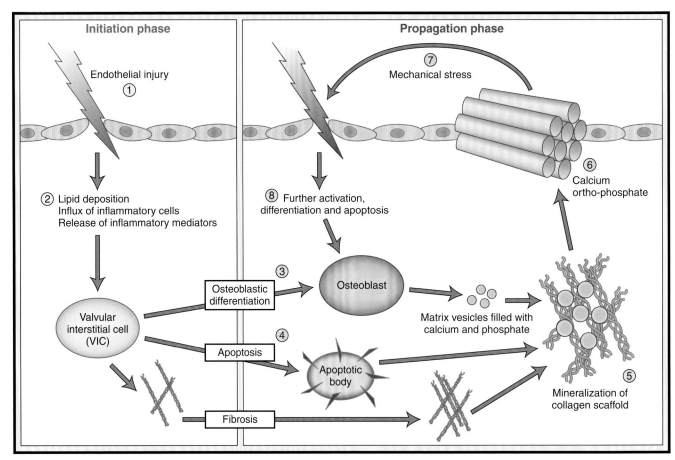

Fig. 3.6 The Propagation Phase. Initiation phase: endothelial injury *(1)* facilitates the infiltration of lipids and inflammatory cells into the valve, followed by release of proinflammatory mediators *(2)*. Endothelial injury and inflammation trigger the activation and differentiation of VICs to develop an osteoblast-like phenotype *(3)* and apoptosis of VICs and inflammatory cells *(4)*. Several mechanisms are implicated, such as RAS activation, BMP, and TGF-β signaling and the binding of RANKL to RANK. This accelerates collagen matrix deposition and upregulates other bone-related proteins, causing valvular thickening and stiffening. Calcium and phosphate are then deposited in the extracellular matrix by a combination of matrix vesicles and apoptotic bodies *(5)*. Calcification of the valve *(6)* results in altered valve hemodynamics and increased mechanical stress and injury *(7)*. This causes further calcification by osteogenic differentiation and apoptosis *(8)* and the development of a self-perpetuating cycle of calcification, valve injury, apoptosis, and osteogenic activation. *BMP,* Bone morphogenetic protein; *RANK,* receptor activator of nuclear κ-B; *RANKL,* receptor activator of nuclear κ-B ligand; *RAS,* renin-angiotensin system; *TGF-β,* transforming growth factor-β; *VIC,* valve interstitial cell. (Modified from Pawade TA, Newby DE, Dweck MR. Calcification in aortic stenosis: the skeleton key. J Am Coll Cardiol 2015;66:561-577.)

calcification. First, lipid lowering in mice with advanced aortic valve disease reduces osteogenic gene expression and does not reduce SMAD2/3 phosphorylation,[90] suggesting that TGF-β is not a primary driver of osteogenic gene expression in calcific aortic valve disease. Second, mice that are deficient in one copy of SMAD3 (i.e., Smad3[+/−] mice) have a higher bone mineral density than their wild-type littermates,[92] suggesting that TGF-β may suppress osteogenesis in bone.

Although canonical TGF-β signaling may not promote (or may even inhibit) valve calcification, emerging data suggest that TGF-β receptor activation may transactivate WNT/β-catenin signaling,[57] which is likely to promote VIC-mediated osteogenesis. Further studies with experimental manipulation of TGF-β signaling in robust, in vivo models of calcific aortic valve disease are essential to define its role in valve calcification and stenosis.

RANK, RANKL, and Osteoprotegerin

Calcium homeostasis exists under tight systemic regulation, with some factors appearing to have different effects on calcification in the skeleton and the vasculature, explaining the inverse correlation observed between these two processes. Patients with osteoporosis also have increased vascular and valvular calcification.[93] This phenomenon has been called the *calcification paradox* and may be explained in part by the activity of the RANK/RANKL/OPG pathway.

The cytokine RANKL, which is a member of the TNF family, binds to the transmembrane protein RANK. In skeletal bone, RANK is expressed on osteoclasts, which are activated by this receptor coupling, driving demineralization and bone resorption (Fig. 3.10). However, the opposite effect is seen in vascular tissue; RANKL appears to induce an osteoblast-like phenotype in human VICs in vitro, with increased expression of ALP and osteocalcin and the formation of calcific nodules.[94]

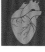

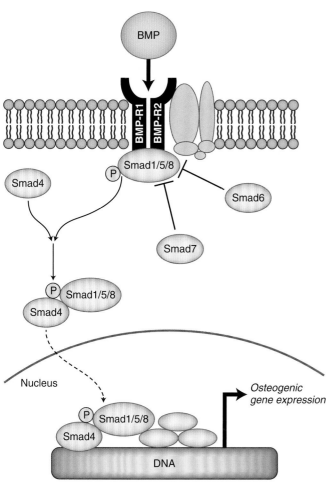

Fig. 3.7 Canonical Bone Morphogenetic Protein *(BMP)* Signaling. Binding of BMP ligand to its receptor complex results in phosphorylation *(P)* of SMAD1/5/8, translocation of the activated SMAD complex to the nucleus, and induction of osteogenic gene expression.

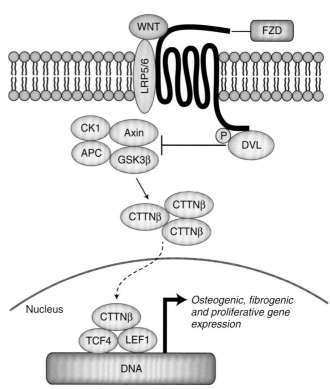

Fig. 3.8 Canonical WNT/β-catenin Signaling. WNT ligand binds to the lipoprotein-related protein receptor complex, leading to inhibition of β-catenin degradation. β-Catenin then undergoes translocation to the nucleus, where osteogenic gene expression is modulated. *APC,* Adenomatous polyposis coli tumor suppressor gene; *CK1,* c kinase 1; *CTTNβ,* β-catenin protein; *DVL,* disheveled proteins; *FZD,* frizzled proteins; *GSK3β,* glycogen synthetase kinase-3β; *LEF1,* lymphoid enhancer binding factor; *REV,* reversed; *TCF4,* transcription factor 4.

Immunohistochemical analysis of calcific aortic valves shows increased RANKL expression compared with controls, along with correspondingly lower levels of OPG, a soluble decoy receptor for RANKL that reduces RANKL/RANK signaling.[94] OPG-deficient mice develop osteoporosis and accelerated vascular calcification, along with an increase in RANKL levels.[95] The differential effects of RANKL in bone and vascular tissue are thought to be related to the cell types present: preosteoclasts are abundant in bone but absent in valvular tissue, in which the pro-osteoblastic VICs predominate.[96]

The RANK/RANKL/OPG axis is potentially modifiable using the monoclonal antibody denosumab, which is already approved for the treatment of osteoporosis. It may reduce valvular calcification while maintaining bone health.

Ectonucleotidases and Matrix Vesicles

Ectonucleotidases are a family of membrane-bound, nucleotide-metabolizing enzymes that modulate purinergic signaling and appear to be closely involved in vascular calcification. Activated myofibroblasts secrete matrix vesicles rich in ectonucleotidases, such as ectonucleotide pyrophosphatase/phosphodiesterase 1 (ENPP1) and ALP, which also contain large amounts of calcium and phosphate and other pro-osteogenic factors.[97] This process is better defined in atherosclerotic plaques,[4,42,98,99] in which matrix vesicles provide a nucleation site

for the formation of hydroxyapatite crystals.[97,100] However, similar mechanisms are thought to exist in aortic valve calcification, which also demonstrates high levels of ENPP1 and an ENPP1 polymorphism resulting in increased activity.[101]

The secretion of matrix vesicles is thought to be a key mechanism by which calcium, phosphate, and procalcific factors are delivered to areas of active osteogenesis in the valve. Secretion of matrix vesicles by macrophages has been described in atherosclerosis, establishing a potential link with inflammation and offering insights into the mechanisms of early calcium deposition in the valve.[102]

Cell Death as a Contributor to Non-osteogenic Calcification

Apoptotic bodies formed after cell death exhibit calcifying properties similar to those of matrix vesicles, suggesting a further link between calcification and cell death. Cell death can occur by apoptosis (in which the internal and external cell membranes are preserved so that the cell and its contents can be cleared by phagocytosis), necrosis (in which membrane lysis releases cellular contents and results in inflammation), or apoptosis followed by secondary necrosis.[103] The exact mechanisms by which cellular death promotes valve calcification have yet to be determined experimentally. However, cell death within the necrotic core is thought to be a potent stimulant of intimal calcification in atherosclerosis. Stippled microcalcification can be observed at an early stage in aortic stenosis, which appears to co-localize with areas of lipid deposition.[16]

Cell death and release of apoptotic bodies, which may contain calcium and inorganic phosphate ions, can facilitate the emergence of

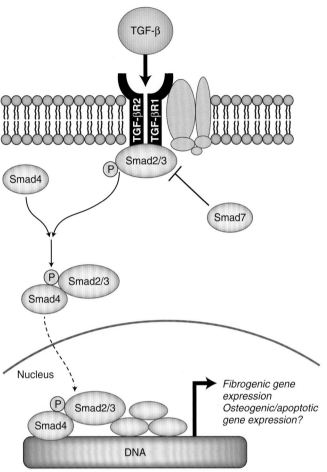

Fig. 3.9 Role of Tumor Growth Factor-β *(TGF-β)* Signaling in Calcific Aortic Valve Disease. In canonical TGF-β signaling, binding of TGF-β ligand to its receptor complex results in phosphorylation *(P)* of SMAD2/3, translocation of the activated SMAD complex to the nucleus, and induction of fibrogenic and osteogenic gene expression. *P,* Phosphorylation; *TGF-βR*, TGF-β receptor.

needlelike hydroxyapatite crystals inside the vesicles.[4,104] The hydroxyapatite crystals likely expand, piercing the outer vesicle membrane and acting as a nucleus for further calcium deposition in the extracellular environment in a process similar to that seen in bone.[105] Hydroxyapatite deposition is thought to lead to a further local macrophage-driven proinflammatory response, creating a positive feedback loop of inflammation and calcification.[106]

Several key observations indicate how this process occurs. First, calcified nodules that form after induction of cell death typically have a crystalline ultrastructure and lack live cells within the core of the calcified mass itself.[33] Second, TGF-β1–induced calcification is strongly associated with caspase activation and programmed cell death (apoptosis) in vitro, and cotreatment of cells with caspase inhibitors can markedly attenuate calcified nodule formation in vitro.[107] Treatments such as caspase inhibitors and molecules that attenuate cell necrosis may offer an efficacious alternative strategy to slow the progression of aortic stenosis.

ADDITIONAL MODULATORS OF OSTEOGENIC ACTIVITY

The previously described mechanisms are relatively well established as being involved in the pathogenesis of aortic valve calcification.

However, the situation is likely to be more complex, involving many other mechanisms and pathways. The most promising of these are summarized in the following sections.

Direct Inhibitors of Osteogenic Signaling
SMAD6
Reduced expression of osteogenic signaling inhibitors appears to play a significant role in the initiation and progression of calcific aortic valve disease. Genetic deletion of *SMAD6* results in cardiovascular calcification in the absence of additional exogenous stressors,[81] suggesting that tonic suppression of BMP signaling is critical for the prevention of valvular calcification.

Matrix GLA Protein
Tonic BMP ligand sequestration or neutralization appears to be important in preventing cardiovascular calcification because mice deficient in the matrix galactosidase-α (GLA) protein (which binds and inactivates BMP2) demonstrate spontaneous cardiovascular calcification early in life,[108] and mice overexpressing the matrix GLA protein (MGP) are protected against hypercholesterolemia-induced vascular calcification.[109] Although MGP levels are under transcriptional and translational regulation, the posttranslational γ-carboxylation of MGP is required for binding to BMP2.[110]

Several retrospective studies reported that drugs that inhibit γ-carboxylase (e.g., warfarin) have been associated with increased risk of cardiovascular calcification and aortic valve stenosis.[111,112] Along these lines, administration of warfarin to juvenile rats results in significant vascular calcification.[113] Collectively, tonic suppression of BMP signaling at the intracellular and extracellular levels appears to be an important potential strategy in slowing cardiovascular calcification, although the clinical effects of warfarin on vascular calcification requires further study.

Oxidative Stress
Although NADPH oxidase–derived free radicals have been implicated in the pathogenesis of atherosclerosis for many years,[114,115] the role of oxidative stress in calcific aortic valve disease is only beginning to be understood. However, oxidative stress does appear to have a key role in driving cell death and valve calcification.

Superoxide and hydrogen peroxide levels are dramatically increased in stenotic aortic valves[25,26,82,89] (Fig. 3.11). The increases occur almost exclusively in the calcified and pericalcific regions of the valve, and unlike atherosclerosis, they are predominantly the result of uncoupled nitric oxide synthase (NOS) activity and reductions in antioxidant enzyme expression.[25,26] Although NADPH oxidase–derived radicals appear to contribute to increased ROS levels in a subset of pericalcific regions,[116] global expression of most catalytic subunits of the oxidase are significantly reduced in human calcific aortic valve disease.[26]

Several observations suggest that ROS may play an important role in the pathogenesis of calcific aortic valve disease. First, increases in ROS occur before the onset of aortic valve dysfunction in hypercholesterolemic mice,[82] suggesting that elevations in ROS are not simply a consequence of aortic valve dysfunction. Second, a growing body of data demonstrates that ROS play a critical role in the transduction of multiple signaling cascades related to osteogenesis, including TGF-β and BMP signaling.[28,117,118] Third, increasing superoxide or hydrogen peroxide levels accelerates calcification of VICs in vitro.[117] Administration of α-lipoic acid (an antioxidant that reduces superoxide and hydrogen peroxide levels), but not tempol (which reduces only superoxide levels), reduces valvular calcification in a rabbit model of calcific aortic valve disease.[116]

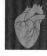

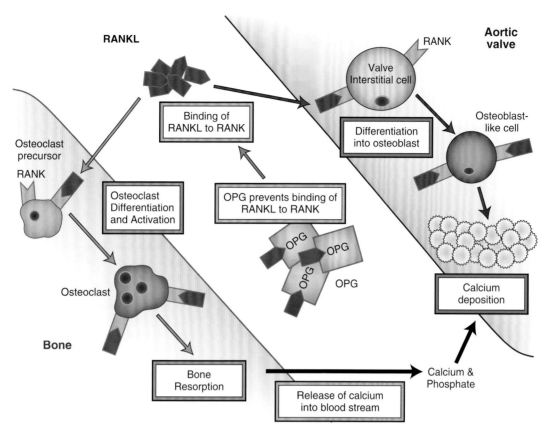

Fig. 3.10 Differential Mechanisms of RANK/RANKL Signaling in Bone and Valvular Tissue. RANKL binds to RANK on osteoclastic precursors in bone, leading to bone resorption and increased calcium and phosphate availability. It is thought that RANK/RANKL binding on valvular interstitial cells *(VICs)* leads to induction of an osteoblast-like phenotype, resulting in valvular osteogenesis. OPG binds and sequesters RANKL, reducing its activity in the bone and vasculature. *OPG,* Osteoprotegerin; *RANKL,* receptor activator of nuclear factor κ-B ligand; *RANK,* receptor activator of nuclear factor κ-B. (From Pawade TA, Newby DE, Dweck MR. Calcification in aortic stenosis: the skeleton key. J Am Coll Cardiol 2015;66:561-577.)

Other data suggest that ROS are not a primary driver of osteogenic signaling in calcific aortic valve disease. First, reduction of blood lipids in mice with severe valvular dysfunction and calcific aortic valve disease reduces BMP signaling, WNT signaling, and valvular calcification, but it does not lower ROS levels.[89] Second, although exogenous ROS do accelerate vascular smooth muscle cell (VSMC) calcification in vitro, increased ROS levels do not induce calcification in the absence of osteogenic stimuli.[119]

We are only beginning to understand the complex role of ROS in the pathogenesis of calcific aortic valve disease. Additional studies examining the role of different ROS-generating systems and the role of ROS in different subcellular compartments are needed for the development of complementary treatments to slow progression of valve disease.

Nitric Oxide Signaling

Nitric oxide (NO) is produced by the actions of NOS. Two of the three isoforms (endothelial and neuronal) are constitutively expressed and calcium dependent. The third isoform, inducible NOS, is calcium independent and involved in the immune response. As with oxidative stress, reductions in NO bioavailability and signaling play a major role in vasomotor dysfunction and atherosclerosis.[120,121] The precise role of NO in calcific aortic valve disease remains unclear, although NO signaling and ROS generation are intimately linked.

Endothelial NOS expression and protein levels are reduced in calcific aortic valve disease in animal models and humans.[122,123] The presence of ROS compounds any decrease in local NO production by the formation of peroxynitrite (ONOO⁻),[124] which further depletes local NO. ROS-mediated oxidation of soluble guanylate cyclase makes it insensitive to increases in NO levels, which further reduces downstream NO signaling.[125] There is a large increase in uncoupled NOS in calcific aortic valve disease, possibly by depletion of tetrahydobiopterin,[126] which results in further ROS production (mainly superoxide) and a self-perpetuating cycle of oxidative stress[26] (see Fig. 3.11).

Despite the strong association between calcific aortic valve disease and conditions that favor reduced NO signaling, few studies have experimentally examined the effects of NO bioavailability on osteogenic signaling and valve calcification. Early work suggested that treatment of hypercholesterolemic rabbits with statins was associated with increases in endothelial nitric oxide synthase (eNOS) levels and slower progression of calcific aortic valve disease.[122] Subsequent studies demonstrated that addition of exogenous NO slowed progression of VIC calcification in vitro.[127] Studies examining the role of NO in calcific aortic valve disease in vivo found that progression of aortic valve dysfunction was not accelerated in eNOS-deficient mice with tricuspid aortic valves but was in those with bicuspid aortic valves.[128]

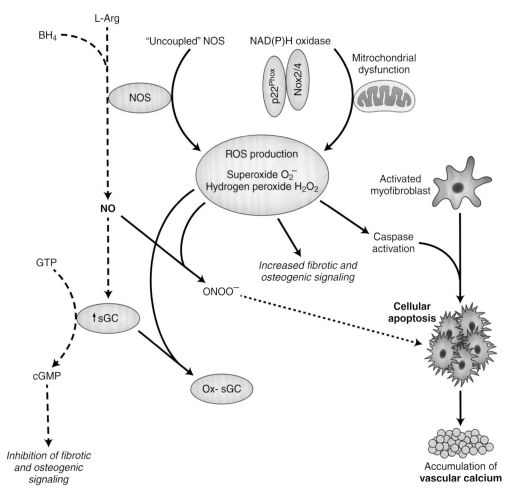

Fig. 3.11 Proposed Interplay Between Oxidative Stress and Nitric Oxide in Valvular Tissue. Superoxide and hydrogen peroxide levels are dramatically increased in stenotic aortic valves, predominantly as the result of uncoupled NOS activity (by depletion of tetrahydrobiopterin [BH$_4$]) and reductions in antioxidant enzyme expression. NADPH oxidase–derived radicals and ROS produced as a consequence of mitochondrial dysfunction contribute to a lesser degree. Endothelial nitric oxide synthase *(eNOS)* catalyzes the production of nitric oxide *(NO)* in the vasculature and valve tissue. NO causes vasodilatation and regulates endothelial function in the vasculature by increased cyclic GMP production. NO function in the aortic valve is not well understood, but decreased NO levels are associated with aortic valve disease. ROS can influence NO downstream signaling in several ways; for example, reacting with NO to form peroxynitrite *(ONOO⁻)* reduces NO bioavailability and oxidizes soluble guanylate cyclase *(sGC)*, making it insensitive to an increase in NO levels. ROS can drive myofibroblast apoptosis by the caspase pathway, leading to release of apoptotic bodies containing calcium, which provide a substrate for extracellular mineralization. *GMP*, Guanosine monophosphate; *GTP*, guanosine triphosphate; *L-Arg*, L-arginine; *NOS*, nitric oxide synthase; *Nox2*, NADPH oxidase catalytic subunit 2; *p22^{Phox}*, cytochrome b_{245} α polypeptide; *ROS*, reactive oxygen species. (Modified from Miller JD, Weiss RM, Serrano KM, et al. Lowering plasma cholesterol levels halts progression of aortic valve disease in mice. Circulation 2009;119:2693-2701.)

There are two potential interpretations of these data: (1) reductions in NO levels do not play a major role in progression of tricuspid calcific aortic valve disease because reducing NO production does not accelerate valve disease or (2) NO production already is dramatically reduced in calcific aortic valve disease, and further reducing NOS does not result in significant acceleration of valve dysfunction in an already compromised system.

Regardless of the effects of reducing NO on valve function, the preponderance of the evidence suggests that strategies aimed at increasing NO are worth exploring as a means of slowing the progression of calcific aortic valve disease. Dietary inorganic nitrites such as found in beetroot juice have been used to supplement NO in patients with heart failure and peripheral arterial disease,[129,130] but their utility in aortic stenosis has not been explored.

Peroxisome Proliferator–Activated Receptor-γ Signaling

During the differentiation of multipotent cells (e.g., mesenchymal stem cells, aortic VICs), there is a critical decision point at which cells enter an osteoblast-like lineage or an adipocyte-like lineage.[131] The decision is typically governed by the balance between RUNX2, a master regulator of osteogenesis, and peroxisome proliferator–activated receptor-γ (PPARγ), a master regulator of adipogenesis.[131,132]

PPARγ is potentially modifiable using thiazolidinediones (TZDs), which activate PPARγ and attenuate aortic valve calcification and dysfunction in hypercholesterolemic rabbits and mice.[24,133] However TZDs also inhibit osteogenic differentiation in bone so that administration of these agents is likely to require careful dose modulation to reduce cardiovascular calcification without negatively affecting skeletal ossification.

NOTCH1/Cadherin 11 Signaling

NOTCH1 belongs to a family of cell surface receptors that appear to be essential for cardiac development and remodeling. Several years ago, loss-of-function mutations in NOTCH1 were shown to be strongly associated with bicuspid valve formation and severe valve cusp calcification in humans.[134] This observation provided the impetus for a series of studies in experimental animals and in vitro model systems examining the role of NOTCH1 in the initiation and progression of calcific aortic valve disease.

Findings from these studies can be distilled to two key points. First, the developmental consequences of loss-of-function mutations in *NOTCH1* are highly context dependent because deletion of one copy in mice (i.e., *Notch1*$^{+/-}$) does not result in bicuspid valve formation.[135] Second, NOTCH1 appears to offer tonic suppression of valvular calcification; reducing NOTCH1 levels accelerates aortic VIC calcification in vitro and in vivo.[135] Mechanistically, this finding appears to be attributed to permissive increases in RUNX2-, BMP2-, and β-catenin–dependent signaling.[134,136]

Notch1$^{+/-}$ mice overexpress cadherin 11,[136] a cell junction protein that is upregulated by TGF-β1. Cadherin 11 is a potent driver of myofibroblast differentiation[137] and has been associated with calcific nodule formation in aortic valve tissue in vitro.[138] One study demonstrated that the procalcific NOTCH1$^{+/-}$ phenotype in VICs in vitro can be eliminated by administration of a cadherin 11–blocking antibody, making this a promising therapeutic target for future research.[139]

Galectin 3

Galectin 3 is a protein belonging to the β-galactoside lectin-binding family, and it is involved in a wide variety of cell processes, including cell division, inflammation, and fibrosis. In carotid arteries, galectin 3 drives osteogenic differentiation of VSMCs by means of the WNT/β-catenin pathway. Galectin 3 appears to be necessary for a complete transdifferentiation of VSMCs to an osteoblastic phenotype. Galectin 3–deficient VSMCs showed blunted expression of RUNX2 and ALP.[140]

Galectin 3 co-localizes to markers of inflammation, activated myofibroblasts, and calcification in human aortic valves and induces expression of IL-1β, IL-6, collagen type I, TGF-β, BMP2, and BMP4 by the ERK1/2 pathway.[141] Co-administration of MCP, a galectin inhibitor, appears to attenuate galectin 3–induced profibrotic and procalcific signaling. These findings require further investigation in larger clinical trials but suggest that galectin 3 is a potential therapeutic target.

Dipeptidyl Peptidase 4 Inhibition

Dipeptidyl peptidase 4 (DPP4) is an enzyme that inactivates glucagon-like peptide 1 (GLP1). The use of DPP4 inhibitors in patients with type 2 diabetes mellitus increases GLP1 levels and improves glycemic control. The proposed mechanism of action is modulation of the ERK1/2 pathway, which attenuates the alterations in proliferation, apoptosis, and calcification observed in high-glucose states.[142] In one study, DPP4 inhibition blocked osteogenic differentiation in human VICs and produced lower levels of aortic valve calcification in a murine model.[143] Slower progression of aortic valve stenosis in a rabbit model was observed, and further clinical studies investigating DPP4 inhibitors are warranted.[143]

Fetuin-A

Fetuin-A is a hepatic glycoprotein that is constitutively secreted into the circulation and prevents accumulation of calcification at ectopic sites.[144,145] Evidence that fetuin-A is a major inhibitor of soft tissue calcification comes from fetuin-A–deficient mice, in which massive calcified deposits develop throughout the body,[146] and which shows dramatic increases in intimal plaque calcification when crossed with apolipoprotein E (ApoE)–deficient mice.[147]

Degradation of fetuin-A by MMPs significantly reduces its ability to attenuate calcium accumulation.[148] Clinically, reductions in serum fetuin-A levels are strongly associated with vascular and valvular calcification,[149] although further clinical investigation is required.

Epigenetic Regulation of Osteogenic Signaling

Epigenetic modifications are emerging as major regulators of transcription factor binding and gene expression in numerous pathophysiologic conditions. Although little is known about epigenetic regulation of gene expression in calcific aortic valve disease, data from the literature on aging and other cardiovascular diseases suggest that alterations in histone acetylation and DNA methylation may play a significant role in the pathogenesis of valvular calcification and fibrosis.

Histone acetylation, which alters transcription factor binding and affinity, is regulated by class I to class IV histone deacetylases.[150] Class I deacetylases (e.g., histone deacetylase 3 [HDAC3]) and class III deacetylases (e.g., sirtuin proteins [SIRTs]) have been implicated in the regulation of proteins known to drive cardiovascular calcification. HDAC3 suppresses activity of RUNX2 and prevents osteoblastic differentiation[151] (i.e., exerts a protective effect), and SIRT1 tonically suppresses vascular inflammation and endothelial cell activation.[152] Experimental reductions in SIRT1 and SIRT6 increased histone acetylation, promoted genomic instability, and increased NF-κB binding in the nucleus.[153,154] Although age-related reductions in HDAC3 and/or SIRT1 or SIRT6 would be anticipated to increase cardiovascular calcification, it is not clear whether expression of these deacetylase isoforms is altered in the stenotic valve.

Histone acetylation is thought to alter gene expression on a relatively large scale, but changes in DNA methylation appear to alter gene expression in a more discrete manner.[155] Evidence that DNA methylation may play a role in regulation of aortic valve calcification can be drawn from the field of vascular calcification, in which induction of an osteogenic phenotype is associated with hypermethylation of the α-SMA promoter and the addition of DNA demethylating agents (e.g., procaine) markedly reduces VSMC calcification in vitro.[156] Whether DNA methylation silences expression of anticalcific genes in calcific aortic valve disease is unknown, but it remains an exciting area of future investigation.

SUMMARY OF MOLECULAR MECHANISMS IN THE VALVE

The initiation phase of aortic stenosis is characterized by endothelial damage, lipid deposition, and inflammation, with considerable overlap with atherosclerosis, including common risk factors. Once established, the disease enters the propagation phase, in which progression becomes dominated by advancing calcification of the aortic valve. The propagation phase involves many pathways that are more commonly associated with skeletal bone formation and that provide potential targets for therapeutic intervention. Fibrosis is also an important

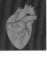

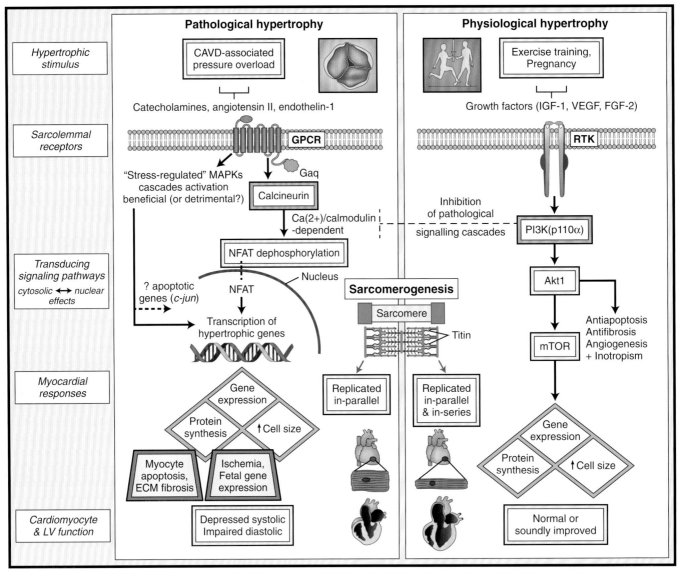

Fig. 3.12 Pathways Involved in Physiologic and Pathologic LV Hypertrophy. In physiologic hypertrophy, growth factors activate receptor tyrosine kinases *(RTK)*, which modify gene expression through the PI3K-AKT-mTOR pathway. This leads to eccentric or concentric hypertrophy, with sarcomeric expansion in series and in parallel and increased systolic performance. In contrast, pressure overload leads to induction of maladaptive changes by the Gαq/phospholipase pathway, an increase in cytosolic calcium ions, and activation of the MAPK and calcineurin/NFAT signaling cascades. This leads to sarcomeric replication in parallel only, with increased extracellular matrix *(ECM)* remodeling and fibrosis, subendocardial ischemia, and apoptosis. This ultimately results in systolic and diastolic dysfunction with chamber dilatation and clinical heart failure. *FGF-2*, fibroblast growth factor 2; *IGF*, insulinlike growth factor 1; *VEGF*, vascular endothelial growth factor. (From Pasipoularides A. Calcific aortic valve disease. Part 2. Morphomechanical abnormalities, gene reexpression, and gender effects on ventricular hypertrophy and its reversibility. J Cardiovasc Transl Res 2016;9:374-399.)

contributor to progressive valve stiffness and is involved in the transition from hypertrophy to heart failure in the myocardium.

MYOCARDIAL RESPONSE TO PRESSURE OVERLOAD

Progressive valvular stenosis is accompanied by compensatory hypertrophy of the LV. This occurs in response to pressure overload, normalizes LV wall stress, and maintains stroke volume. Pathologic hypertrophy is driven by a distinct cellular and molecular profile compared with physiologic hypertrophy, which occurs during

normal development or in response to physical exercise (Fig. 3.12 and Table 3.4).[157]

The hypertrophic response maintains wall stress and LV performance for many years or decades, but decompensation eventually occurs, and patients transition to heart failure, symptoms, and adverse events. This transition appears to be driven by two processes in particular: myocyte cell death and myocardial fibrosis.

Left Ventricular Hypertrophy

Restoration of wall stress in the presence of pressure overload is achieved by myocyte hypertrophy, the pattern of which is highly

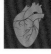

TABLE 3.4 Differences Between Physiologic and Pathologic Left Ventricular Myocardial Hypertrophy.

	Physiologic Hypertrophy	Pathologic Hypertrophy due to Pressure Overload
Stimulus	Exercise Pregnancy	Aortic stenosis Hypertension
Signaling pathways	PI3K-AKT-mTOR pathway	Calcineurin-NFAT and MAPK signaling cascades
Cardiomyocyte morphology	Increase myocyte length and width	Myocytes increase in width only
Sarcomeric replication	In series and in parallel	In parallel only
Remodeling	Eccentric or concentric	Usually concentric Increased relative wall thickness
Morphological changes	Normal extracellular matrix remodeling	Diffuse interstitial fibrosis Focal replacement fibrosis
Fetal gene expression	Normal	Upregulated
ATP production	Appropriate	Reduced
Ischemia	No	Subendocardial progressing to global
Cell turnover	Normal	Balance favors myocyte apoptosis
Long-term consequences	Normal or improved myocardial function Readily reversible upon removal of stimulus	Diastolic dysfunction Systolic dysfunction Less reversible Heart failure symptoms Predisposition to cardiac arrhythmia

From Pasipoularides A. Calcific aortic valve disease. Part 2. Morphomechanical abnormalities, gene reexpression, and gender effects on ventricular hypertrophy and its reversibility. J Cardiovasc Transl Res 2016;9:374-399.

heterogeneous. Concentric hypertrophy, concentric remodeling, and eccentric hypertrophy are classically described, with asymmetric patterns of wall thickening also increasingly appreciated.[158] Factors influencing the pattern and magnitude of the hypertrophic response are incompletely described but appear to include age, sex, obesity, and the metabolic syndrome.[159–161] Genetic factors are also implicated such as the ACE1/D polymorphism.[162] Systemic hypertension is often a major contributor to the total afterload experienced by the LV, and it therefore influences the hypertrophic response.

Individual variation in all of these factors explain why there is poor correlation between the magnitude of the hypertrophic response and the degree of aortic valve narrowing.[158] The duration of disease is likely to be important, although it remains almost impossible to establish this with accuracy because the disease can remain unrecognized for many years or decades before a diagnosis is established.

Physiologic cardiac hypertrophy in response to exercise is mediated by growth factors such as insulinlike growth factor 1 (IGF1), VEGF, and FGF2. This leads to activation of receptor tyrosine kinases and the PI3K-AKT-mTOR pathway and ultimately causes hypertrophy with a proportional increase in capillary density. The myocardium is therefore not rendered ischemic and is characterized by a lack of fetal gene reexpression or myocardial fibrosis.[163]

In contrast, the pathologic LV hypertrophy phenotype is driven by a mixture of direct mechanical forces, ischemia, and increased levels of catecholamines (i.e., angiotensin II and endothelin 1). These are potent hypertrophic stimuli, activating the Gαq/phospholipase pathway, MAPK and calcineurin/NFAT signaling cascades and an increase in cytosolic calcium ions.[164] The result is an increase in sarcomeric elements arranged in parallel[157] and development of concentric hypertrophy, which restores normal wall tension but preferentially subjects the subendocardial layers to higher mechanical stress. This leads to raised energy demands, higher intramural pressures, increased coronary resistance, and supply-demand ischemia predominantly in subendocardium.

Several genes are activated that are normally expressed only during fetal development. This includes the β isoform of the myosin heavy chain, which exhibits poorer contractile function and less efficient energy use compared with the α type.[165]

Diffuse Interstitial Fibrosis

The myocardial ECM serves a vital function in supporting the 3D arrangement of myocytes and capillaries and providing anchoring for the generation of contractile forces during ventricular systole. The predominant components are collagen I and III. Myofibroblasts are largely absent from the normal heart, which contrasts with valvular tissue.[166] However cardiac fibroblasts appear to transition to active myofibroblasts during pathologic hypertrophy influenced by factors such as MMP, TGF-β, and angiotensin II.[166]

Similar to their actions in valvular tissue, myofibroblasts are active secretors of ECM components and lead to pathologic remodeling with increased, disorganized deposition of collagen and proteoglycans. The physiologic consequences of this are increased myocardial stiffness, diastolic dysfunction, a reduction in cardiomyocyte electrical coupling, and eventually impaired systolic function.

Cell Death and Replacement Fibrosis

Historically, the heart has been viewed as a postmitotic, terminally differentiated organ in which growth occurs by hypertrophy rather than hyperplasia and cell renewal. However, current evidence supports a dynamic view of the myocardium, in which cell death by apoptosis and regeneration by endogenous and exogenous cardiac progenitor cells are vital ongoing processes.[167] This paradigm shift was spurred in 2009 by Bergman et al, who used ¹⁴C dating to show that the human heart renews approximately 50% of its myocytes during its lifetime.[168] Myocyte apoptosis can occur by two mechanisms; the type 1 (extrinsic) pathway involves exogenous ligands binding to death receptors, and the type 2 (intrinsic) pathway is characterized by cytochrome c release from mitochondria as a consequence of cellular energy depletion. A complicated sequence of events ensues, culminating in caspase 3 activation and cellular apoptosis.

Although hemodynamic loading in pathologic hypertrophy initiates proapoptotic and antiapoptotic signaling, the balance appears to favor apoptosis, with an increased rate of 5% to 10% per year and a net loss of myocytes.[169] Apoptosis is driven by a combination of direct, extreme mechanical forces, the actions of angiotensin II,[170] and subendocardial ischemia. This occurs from a combination of increased intramural pressure increasing coronary resistance, higher myocyte energy demand due to increased LV wall tension, and a failure of the coronary microvascular network to expand sufficiently, leading to increased capillary-to-myocyte distance.[171] The end result of cell death is focal collagen deposition (i.e., replacement fibrosis) under the influence of angiotensin II and TGF-β.[172]

Transition to Heart Failure

The loss of contractile units through apoptosis, increased myocardial fibrosis, and ongoing subendocardial ischemia eventually lead to cardiac decompensation, impaired systolic and diastolic function, and the transition to heart failure. Collagen accumulation also interferes with the normal electrophysiologic properties of the myocardium, potentially increasing the propensity to arrhythmia.[173]

It is becoming increasingly possible to detect cell death and myocardial fibrosis in patients by surrogate markers. High-sensitivity troponin assay results are linked with cell death, and cardiovascular magnetic resonance imaging provides assessment of diffuse and replacement myocardial fibrosis.[174–176] Dysregulation of calcium handling is also thought to play a role in LV decompensation, with downregulation and dysfunction of SERCA2A leading to increased cytosolic calcium concentrations that contribute to contractile dysfunction and arrhythmia.[177]

TRANSLATION TO THERAPEUTIC INTERVENTIONS AND FUTURE DIRECTIONS

As our understanding of the pathophysiology of aortic stenosis has changed in recent years, so have our targets for developing interventions that slow and ultimately reverse valvular fibrosis and calcification. Because of the similarities of the initiation phase of aortic stenosis with atherosclerosis, there was hope that lipid-lowering therapies would prove effective. This idea was supported by data from hypercholesterolemic animal models. However, several large, randomized clinical trials showed that statins did not effectively slow disease progression in patients with calcific aortic valve disease.[178–180] This suggests that once the propagation phase has been established, treatments that target the initiation phase are unlikely to be successful and that calcification should instead be more directly targeted.

The link between skeletal bone formation and calcific aortic valve disease suggests several targets for intervention. However, any treatment aimed at slowing the progression of valve calcification must not negatively affect skeletal ossification. Most patients with calcific aortic valve disease are elderly, and emerging data suggest that many patients with this disease have lower bone mineral density than age-matched patients without valve disease.[181] Treatments that may indiscriminately reduce osteoblast activity in cardiovascular and skeletal systems (e.g., many PPARγ agonists) may slow progression of calcific aortic valve disease but accelerate osteoporosis.

Development of drugs that drive specific subcomponents of specific signaling cascades (e.g., the antiinflammatory effects of PPARγ

agonists) or preferentially activate signaling cascades in specific tissues may overcome previous limitations. One promising candidate is a humanized murine antibody targeting cadherin 11, which is being investigated in a phase 1 clinical trial for the treatment of rheumatoid arthritis, but which could have anticalcific effects on the aortic valve in vivo (see Peroxisome Proliferator-Activated Receptor-γ Signaling).[139]

Other drugs that appear to have different effects on calcium metabolism in the skeleton and the vasculature have shown promise in preclinical and small observational studies. For example, bisphosphonates inhibit osteoclastic bone resorption, resulting in reduced systemic calcium and phosphate levels for valvular osteogenesis.[182] Bisphosphonates also appear to downregulate key inflammatory cytokines (e.g., IL-1β, IL-6, TNF-α), reduce MMP expression, and attenuate VICs from developing an osteoblastic phenotype. Bisphosphonate use has been associated with reduced valvular calcification[183] and reduced aortic stenosis progression[181,184] in observational studies.

Denosumab is a human monoclonal antibody to RANKL that reduces RANK signaling, which has reduced aortic valve calcification in a murine model[185] while simultaneously increasing skeletal bone mineralization. Bisphosphonate and denosumab are being tested on patients with aortic stenosis in a double-blind, randomized, controlled trial, SALTIRE 2.[178]

Modulation of LV hypertrophy from a pathologic to physiologic response is desirable. Targeting pathologic transcriptional pathways is attractive because they are controlled by a relatively small number of molecules (e.g., NFAT). However, such attempts would have limited efficacy if progressive valve stenosis and consequent worsening pressure overload is not treated simultaneously. For this reason, drugs targeting the renin-angiotensin-aldosterone axis hold particular promise in tackling valvular and myocardial fibrosis.

Application of new technologies may also help identify novel therapeutic targets. Genome-wide association studies (GWAS) have previously highlighted biologic processes involved in aortic stenosis.[186,187] However, integrating GWAS data with transcriptomics data from human aortic valve tissue has allowed identification of novel potential drivers of aortic stenosis. The palmdelphin gene (*PALMD*) on chromosome 1p21.2 was identified as a candidate causal gene in a large study, which showed that reduced *PALMD* expression had a strong association with the presence and severity of aortic valve disease and that a common *PALMD* single nucleotide polymorphism (SNP) accounted for more than 12.5% of the population-attributable risk.[188] These findings were then validated in the UK Biobank cohort. Further work is required to explore the exact mechanism of action and potential therapeutic targets.

CONCLUSIONS

Aortic stenosis is a complex and highly regulated disease process that is characterized by progressive valve narrowing and the deleterious effects on the LV myocardium. We currently lack medical therapies for modifying the natural history of this disease process, highlighting the need for a greater understanding of the molecular mechanisms underpinning aortic stenosis so that suitable therapeutic targets can be identified.

ACKNOWLEDGMENTS

We thank Professor J. Miller for the use of figures and tables from the previous iteration of this chapter.

REFERENCES

1. Nkomo VT, Gardin JM, Skelton TN, et al. Burden of valvular heart diseases: a population-based study. Lancet 2006;368(9540):1005-1011.

2. Osnabrugge RLJ, Mylotte D, Head SJ, et al. Aortic stenosis in the elderly: disease prevalence and number of candidates for transcatheter aortic valve replacement: a meta-analysis and modeling study. J Am Coll Cardiol 2013;62(11):1002-1012.

3. Rajamannan NM, Evans FJ, Aikawa E, et al. Calcific aortic valve disease: not simply a degenerative process: a review and agenda for research from the National Heart and Lung and Blood Institute Aortic Stenosis Working Group. Executive summary: calcific aortic valve disease-2011 update. Circulation 2011;124(16):1783-1791.

4. New SEP, Aikawa E. Molecular imaging insights into early inflammatory stages of arterial and aortic valve calcification. Circu Res 2011;108(11):1381-1391.

5. Pawade TA, Newby DE, Dweck MR. Calcification in aortic stenosis: the skeleton key. J Am Coll Cardiol 2015;66(5):561-577.

6. Freeman RV, Otto CM. Spectrum of calcific aortic valve disease: pathogenesis, disease progression, and treatment strategies. Circulation 2005;111(24):3316-3326.

7. Pachulski RT, Chan KL. Progression of aortic valve dysfunction in 51 adult patients with congenital bicuspid aortic valve: assessment and follow up by Doppler echocardiography. Br Heart J 1993;69(3):237-240.

8. Roberts WC, Ko JM. Frequency by decades of unicuspid, bicuspid, and tricuspid aortic valves in adults having isolated aortic valve replacement for aortic stenosis, with or without associated aortic regurgitation. Circulation 2005;111(7):920-925.

9. Stewart BF, Siscovick D, Lind BK, et al. Clinical factors associated with calcific aortic valve disease. Cardiovascular Health Study. J Am Coll Cardiol 1997;29(3):630-634.

10. Stritzke J, Linsel-Nitschke P, Markus MRP, et al. Association between degenerative aortic valve disease and long-term exposure to cardiovascular risk factors: results of the longitudinal population-based KORA/MONICA survey. Eur Heart J 2009;30(16):2044-2053.

11. Thanassoulis G, Massaro JM, Cury R, et al. Associations of long-term and early adult atherosclerosis risk factors with aortic and mitral valve calcium. J Am Coll Cardiol 2010;55(22):2491-2498.

12. Thanassoulis G, Campbell CY, Owens DS, et al. Genetic associations with valvular calcification and aortic stenosis. N Engl J Med 2013;368(6):503-512.

13. Raal FJ, Giugliano RP, Sabatine MS, et al. PCSK9 inhibition-mediated reduction in Lp(a) with evolocumab: an analysis of 10 clinical trials and the LDL receptor's role. J Lipid Res 2016;57(6):1086-1096.

14. Langsted A, Nordestgaard BG, Benn M, et al. PCSK9 R46L loss-of-function mutation reduces lipoprotein(a), LDL cholesterol, and risk of aortic valve stenosis. J Clin Endocrinol Metab 2016;101(9):3281-3287.

15. Wang W-G, He Y-F, Chen Y-L, et al. Proprotein convertase subtilisin/kexin type 9 levels and aortic valve calcification: a prospective, cross sectional study. J Int Med Res 2016;44(4):865-874.

16. Otto CM, Kuusisto J, Reichenbach DD, et al. Characterization of the early lesion of "degenerative" valvular aortic stenosis. Histological and immunohistochemical studies. Circulation 1994;90(2):844-853.

17. Isoda K, Matsuki T, Kondo H, et al. Deficiency of interleukin-1 receptor antagonist induces aortic valve disease in BALB/c mice. Arterioscler Thromb Vasc Biol 2010;30(4):708-715.

18. Coté N, Mahmut A, Bossé Y, et al. Inflammation is associated with the remodeling of calcific aortic valve disease. Inflammation 2013;36(3):573-581.

19. Lommi JI, Kovanen PT, Jauhiainen M, et al. High-density lipoproteins (HDL) are present in stenotic aortic valves and may interfere with the mechanisms of valvular calcification. Atherosclerosis 2011;219(2):538-544.

20. Mohty D, Pibarot P, Després J-P, et al. Association between plasma LDL particle size, valvular accumulation of oxidized LDL, and inflammation in patients with aortic stenosis. Arterioscler Thromb Vasc Biol 2008;28(1):187-193.

21. Kapadia SR, Yakoob K, Nader S, et al. Elevated circulating levels of serum tumor necrosis factor-alpha in patients with hemodynamically significant pressure and volume overload. J Am Coll Cardiol 2000;36(1):208-212.

22. Cecil DL, Terkeltaub RA. Arterial calcification is driven by RAGE in Enpp1-/- mice. J Vasc Res 2011;48(3):227-235.

23. Hofmann Bowman MA, Gawdzik J, Bukhari U, et al. S100A12 in vascular smooth muscle accelerates vascular calcification in apolipoprotein E-null mice by activating an osteogenic gene regulatory program. Arterioscler Thromb Vasc Biol 2011;31(2):337-344.

24. Li F, Cai Z, Chen F, et al. Pioglitazone attenuates progression of aortic valve calcification via down-regulating receptor for advanced glycation end products. Basic Res Cardiol 2012;107(6):306.

25. Miller JD, Weiss RM, Heistad DD. Calcific aortic valve stenosis: methods, models, and mechanisms. Circ Res 2011;108(11):1392-1412.

26. Miller JD, Chu Y, Brooks RM, et al. Dysregulation of antioxidant mechanisms contributes to increased oxidative stress in calcific aortic valvular stenosis in humans. J Am Coll Cardiol 2008;52(10):843-850.

27. Zhang H, Park Y, Wu J, et al. Role of TNF-alpha in vascular dysfunction. Clin Sci 2009;116(3):219-230.

28. Csiszar A, Ungvari Z. Endothelial dysfunction and vascular inflammation in type 2 diabetes: interaction of AGE/RAGE and TNF-alpha signaling. Am J Physiol Heart Circ Physiol 2008;295(2):H475-H476.

29. Yu Z, Seya K, Daitoku K, et al. Tumor necrosis factor-α accelerates the calcification of human aortic valve interstitial cells obtained from patients with calcific aortic valve stenosis via the BMP2-Dlx5 pathway. J Pharmacol Exp Ther 2011;337(1):16-23.

30. Warnock JN, Nanduri B, Pregonero Gamez CA, et al. Gene profiling of aortic valve interstitial cells under elevated pressure conditions: modulation of inflammatory gene networks. Int J Inflam 2011;2011(1):176412-176410.

31. Lai C-F, Shao J-S, Behrmann A, et al. TNFR1-activated reactive oxidative species signals up-regulate osteogenic Msx2 programs in aortic myofibroblasts. Endocrinology 2012;153(8):3897-3910.

32. Mazzone A, Epistolato MC, De Caterina R, et al. Neoangiogenesis, T-lymphocyte infiltration, and heat shock protein-60 are biological hallmarks of an immunomediated inflammatory process in end-stage calcified aortic valve stenosis. J Am Coll Cardiol 2004;43(9):1670-1676.

33. Mohler ER, Gannon F, Reynolds C, et al. Bone formation and inflammation in cardiac valves. Circulation 2001;103(11):1522-1528.

34. Pohjolainen V, Taskinen P, Soini Y, et al. Noncollagenous bone matrix proteins as a part of calcific aortic valve disease regulation. Hum Pathol 2008;39(11):1695-1701.

35. Hanahan D, Folkman J. Patterns and emerging mechanisms of the angiogenic switch during tumorigenesis. Cell 1996;86(3):353-364.

36. Yoshioka M, Yuasa S, Matsumura K, et al. Chondromodulin-I maintains cardiac valvular function by preventing angiogenesis. Nat Med 2006;12(10):1151-1159.

37. Akahori H, Tsujino T, Naito Y, et al. Intraleaflet haemorrhage as a mechanism of rapid progression of stenosis in bicuspid aortic valve. Int J Cardiol 2013;167(2):514-518.

38. Akahori H, Tsujino T, Naito Y, et al. Intraleaflet haemorrhage is associated with rapid progression of degenerative aortic valve stenosis. Eur Heart J 2011;32(7):888-896.

39. Chen J-H, Simmons CA. Cell-matrix interactions in the pathobiology of calcific aortic valve disease: critical roles for matricellular, matricrine, and matrix mechanics cues. Circ Res 2011;108(12):1510-1524.

40. Soini Y, Satta J, Määttä M, Autio-Harmainen H. Expression of MMP2, MMP9, MT1-MMP, TIMP1, and TIMP2 mRNA in valvular lesions of the heart. J Pathol 2001;194(2):225-231. doi:10.1002/path.850.

41. Fondard O, Detaint D, Iung B, et al. Extracellular matrix remodelling in human aortic valve disease: the role of matrix metalloproteinases and their tissue inhibitors. Eur Heart J 2005;26(13):1333-1341. doi:10.1093/eurheartj/ehi248.

42. Aikawa E, Aikawa M, Libby P, et al. Arterial and aortic valve calcification abolished by elastolytic cathepsin S deficiency in chronic renal disease. Circulation 2009;119(13):1785-1794.

43. Helske S, Syväranta S, Kupari M, et al. Possible role for mast cell-derived cathepsin G in the adverse remodelling of stenotic aortic valves. Eur Heart J 2006;27(12):1495-1504.

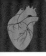

44. Shen M, Tastet L, Capoulade R, et al. Effect of age and aortic valve anatomy on calcification and haemodynamic severity of aortic stenosis. Heart 2017;103(1):32-39.

45. Cartlidge TRG, Pawade TA, Dweck MR. Aortic stenosis and CT calcium scoring: is it for everyone? Heart 2017;103(1):8-9.

46. Côté C, Pibarot P, Després J-P, et al. Association between circulating oxidised low-density lipoprotein and fibrocalcific remodelling of the aortic valve in aortic stenosis. Heart 2008;94(9):1175-1180.

47. Edep ME, Shirani J, Wolf P, Brown DL. Matrix metalloproteinase expression in nonrheumatic aortic stenosis. Cardiovasc Pathol 2000;9(5):281-286.

48. Capoulade R, Clavel M-A, Mathieu P, et al. Impact of hypertension and renin-angiotensin system inhibitors in aortic stenosis. Eur J Clin Invest 2013;43(12):1262-1272.

49. Peltonen T, Näpänkangas J, Ohtonen P, et al. (Pro)renin receptors and angiotensin converting enzyme 2/angiotensin-(1-7)/Mas receptor axis in human aortic valve stenosis. Atherosclerosis 2011;216(1):35-43.

50. Helske S, Lindstedt KA, Laine M, et al. Induction of local angiotensin II-producing systems in stenotic aortic valves. J Am Coll Cardiol 2004;44(9):1859-1866.

51. O'Brien KD, Probstfield JL, Caulfield MT, et al. Angiotensin-converting enzyme inhibitors and change in aortic valve calcium. Arch Intern Med 2005;165(8):858-862.

52. Arishiro K, Hoshiga M, Negoro N, et al. Angiotensin receptor-1 blocker inhibits atherosclerotic changes and endothelial disruption of the aortic valve in hypercholesterolemic rabbits. J Am Coll Cardiol 2007;49(13):1482-1489.

53. Jian B, Jones PL, Li Q, et al. Matrix metalloproteinase-2 is associated with tenascin-C in calcific aortic stenosis. Am J Pathol 2001;159(1):321-327.

54. Satta J, Melkko J, Pöllänen R, et al. Progression of human aortic valve stenosis is associated with tenascin-C expression. J Am Coll Cardiol 2002;39(1):96-101.

55. Macri L, Silverstein D, Clark RAF. Growth factor binding to the pericellular matrix and its importance in tissue engineering. Adv Drug Deliv Rev 2007;59(13):1366-1381.

56. Simionescu A, Simionescu DT, Vyavahare NR. Osteogenic responses in fibroblasts activated by elastin degradation products and transforming growth factor-beta1: role of myofibroblasts in vascular calcification. Am J Pathol 2007;171(1):116-123.

57. Chen J-H, Chen WLK, Sider KL, et al. β-catenin mediates mechanically regulated, transforming growth factor-β1-induced myofibroblast differentiation of aortic valve interstitial cells. Arterioscler Thromb Vasc Biol 2011;31(3):590-597.

58. Merryman WD, Youn I, Lukoff HD, et al. Correlation between heart valve interstitial cell stiffness and transvalvular pressure: implications for collagen biosynthesis. Am J Physiol Heart Circ Physiol 2006;290(1):H224-H231.

59. Carruthers CA, Alfieri CM, Joyce EM, et al. Gene expression and collagen fiber micromechanical interactions of the semilunar heart valve interstitial cell. Cell Mol Bioeng 2012;5(3):254-265.

60. Thayer P, Balachandran K, Rathan S, et al. The effects of combined cyclic stretch and pressure on the aortic valve interstitial cell phenotype. Ann Biomed Eng 2011;39(6):1654-1667.

61. Engler AJ, Sen S, Sweeney HL, Discher DE. Matrix elasticity directs stem cell lineage specification. Cell 2006;126(4):677-689.

62. Yip CYY, Chen J-H, Zhao R, Simmons CA. Calcification by valve interstitial cells is regulated by the stiffness of the extracellular matrix. Arterioscler Thromb Vasc Biol 2009;29(6):936-942.

63. Rosenhek R, Binder T, Porenta G, et al. Predictors of outcome in severe, asymptomatic aortic stenosis. N Engl J Med 2000;343(9):611-617.

64. Clavel M-A, Pibarot P, Messika-Zeitoun D, et al. Impact of aortic valve calcification, as measured by MDCT, on survival in patients with aortic stenosis: results of an international registry study. J Am Coll Cardiol 2014;64(12):1202-1213.

65. Jenkins WSA, Vesey AT, Shah ASV, et al. Valvular (18)F-fluoride and (18)F-fluorodeoxyglucose uptake predict disease progression and clinical outcome in patients with aortic stenosis. J Am Coll Cardiol 2015;66(10):1200-1201.

66. Ducy P. Cbfa1: a molecular switch in osteoblast biology. Dev Dyn 2000;219(4):461-471. doi:10.1002/1097-0177(2000)9999:9999<::AID-DVDY1074>3.0.CO;2-C.

67. Rajamannan NM, Subramaniam M, Rickard D, et al. Human aortic valve calcification is associated with an osteoblast phenotype. Circulation 2003;107(17):2181-2184.

68. Nagy E, Eriksson P, Yousry M, et al. Valvular osteoclasts in calcification and aortic valve stenosis severity. Int J Cardiol 2013;168(3):2264-2271.

69. Xie C, Shen Y, Hu W, et al. Angiotensin II promotes an osteoblast-like phenotype in porcine aortic valve myofibroblasts. Aging Clin Exp Res 2016;28(2):181-187.

70. Osman L, Yacoub MH, Latif N, et al. Role of human valve interstitial cells in valve calcification and their response to atorvastatin. Circulation 2006;114(1 Suppl):I547-I552.

71. Watson KE, Boström K, Ravindranath R, et al. TGF-beta 1 and 25-hydroxycholesterol stimulate osteoblast-like vascular cells to calcify. J Clin Invest 1994;93(5):2106-2113.

72. Aikawa E, Otto CM. Look more closely at the valve: imaging calcific aortic valve disease. Circulation 2012;125(1):9-11.

73. Ankeny RF, Thourani VH, Weiss D, et al. Preferential activation of SMAD1/5/8 on the fibrosa endothelium in calcified human aortic valves—association with low BMP antagonists and SMAD6. PLoS One 2011;6(6):e20969.

74. Seya K, Yu Z, Kanemaru K, et al. Contribution of bone morphogenetic protein-2 to aortic valve calcification in aged rat. J Pharmacol Sci 2011;115(1):8-14.

75. Yanagawa B, Lovren F, Pan Y, et al. miRNA-141 is a novel regulator of BMP-2-mediated calcification in aortic stenosis. J Thorac Cardiovasc Surg 2012;144(1):256-262.

76. Yang X, Meng X, Su X, et al. Bone morphogenic protein 2 induces Runx2 and osteopontin expression in human aortic valve interstitial cells: role of Smad1 and extracellular signal-regulated kinase 1/2. J Thorac Cardiovasc Surg 2009;138(4):1008-1015.

77. Yang X, Fullerton DA, Su X, et al. Pro-osteogenic phenotype of human aortic valve interstitial cells is associated with higher levels of Toll-like receptors 2 and 4 and enhanced expression of bone morphogenetic protein 2. J Am Coll Cardiol 2009;53(6):491-500.

78. Simmons CA, Grant GR, Manduchi E, Davies PF. Spatial heterogeneity of endothelial phenotypes correlates with side-specific vulnerability to calcification in normal porcine aortic valves. Circ Res 2005;96(7):792-799.

79. Massagué J, Wotton D. Transcriptional control by the TGF-beta/Smad signaling system. EMBO J 2000;19(8):1745-1754.

80. Heldin CH, Miyazono K, Dijke ten P. TGF-beta signalling from cell membrane to nucleus through SMAD proteins. Nature 1997;390(6659):465-471.

81. Galvin KM, Donovan MJ, Lynch CA, et al. A role for Smad6 in development and homeostasis of the cardiovascular system. Nat Genet 2000;24(2):171-174.

82. Miller JD, Weiss RM, Serrano KM, et al. Lowering plasma cholesterol levels halts progression of aortic valve disease in mice. Circulation 2009;119(20):2693-2701.

83. Clevers H. Wnt/beta-catenin signaling in development and disease. Cell 2006;127(3):469-480.

84. Logan CY, Nusse R. The Wnt signaling pathway in development and disease. Annu Rev Cell Dev Biol 2004;20(1):781-810.

85. Al-Aly Z, Shao J-S, Lai C-F, et al. Aortic Msx2-Wnt calcification cascade is regulated by TNF-alpha-dependent signals in diabetic Ldlr-/- mice. Arterioscler Thromb Vasc Biol 2007;27(12):2589-2596.

86. Alfieri CM, Cheek J, Chakraborty S, Yutzey KE. Wnt signaling in heart valve development and osteogenic gene induction. Dev Biol 2010;338(2):127-135.

87. Caira FC, Stock SR, Gleason TG, et al. Human degenerative valve disease is associated with up-regulation of low-density lipoprotein receptor-related protein 5 receptor-mediated bone formation. J Am Coll Cardiol 2006;47(8):1707-1712.

88. Rajamannan NM, Subramaniam M, Caira F, et al. Atorvastatin inhibits hypercholesterolemia-induced calcification in the aortic valves via the Lrp5 receptor pathway. Circulation 2005;112(9 Suppl):I229-I234.

89. Miller JD, Weiss RM, Serrano KM, et al. Evidence for active regulation of pro-osteogenic signaling in advanced aortic valve disease. Arterioscler Thromb Vasc Biol 2010;30(12):2482-2486.

90. Derynck R, Zhang YE. Smad-dependent and Smad-independent pathways in TGF-beta family signalling. Nature 2003;425(6958):577-584.

91. Clark-Greuel JN, Connolly JM, Sorichillo E, et al. Transforming growth factor-beta1 mechanisms in aortic valve calcification: increased alkaline phosphatase and related events. Ann Thorac Surg 2007;83(3):946-953.

92. Balooch G, Balooch M, Nalla RK, et al. TGF-beta regulates the mechanical properties and composition of bone matrix. Proc Natl Acad Sci USA 2005;102(52):18813-18818.

93. Kado DM, Browner WS, Blackwell T, et al. Rate of bone loss is associated with mortality in older women: a prospective study. J Bone Miner Res 2000;15(10):1974-1980.

94. Kaden JJ, Bickelhaupt S, Grobholz R, et al. Receptor activator of nuclear factor kappaB ligand and osteoprotegerin regulate aortic valve calcification. J Mol Cell Cardiol 2004;36(1):57-66.

95. Bucay N, Sarosi I, Dunstan CR, et al. Osteoprotegerin-deficient mice develop early onset osteoporosis and arterial calcification. Genes Dev 1998;12(9):1260-1268.

96. Tintut Y, Demer L. Role of osteoprotegerin and its ligands and competing receptors in atherosclerotic calcification. J Investig Med 2006;54(7):395-401.

97. Bertazzo S, Gentleman E, Cloyd KL, et al. Nano-analytical electron microscopy reveals fundamental insights into human cardiovascular tissue calcification. Nat Mater 2013;12(6):576-583.

98. Bobryshev YV, Killingsworth MC, Huynh TG, et al. Are calcifying matrix vesicles in atherosclerotic lesions of cellular origin? Basic Res Cardiol 2007;102(2):133-143.

99. Kapustin AN, Chatrou MLL, Drozdov I, et al. Vascular smooth muscle cell calcification is mediated by regulated exosome secretion. Circ Res 2015;116(8):1312-1323.

100. Dweck MR, Aikawa E, Newby DE, et al. Noninvasive molecular imaging of disease activity in atherosclerosis. Circ Res 2016;119(2):330-340.

101. Coté N, Husseini El D, Pépin A, et al. ATP acts as a survival signal and prevents the mineralization of aortic valve. J Mol Cell Cardiol 2012;52(5):1191-1202.

102. New SEP, Goettsch C, Aikawa M, et al. Macrophage-derived matrix vesicles: an alternative novel mechanism for microcalcification in atherosclerotic plaques. Circ Res 2013;113(1):72-77.

103. Kanduc D, Mittelman A, Serpico R, et al. Cell death: apoptosis versus necrosis (review). Int J Oncol 2002;21(1):165-170.

104. Proudfoot D, Skepper JN, Hegyi L, et al. Apoptosis regulates human vascular calcification in vitro: evidence for initiation of vascular calcification by apoptotic bodies. Circ Res 2000;87(11):1055-1062.

105. Kim KM. Calcification of matrix vesicles in human aortic valve and aortic media. Fed Proc 1976;35(2):156-162.

106. Nadra I, Mason JC, Philippidis P, et al. Proinflammatory activation of macrophages by basic calcium phosphate crystals via protein kinase C and MAP kinase pathways: a vicious cycle of inflammation and arterial calcification? Circ Res 2005;96(12):1248-1256.

107. Jian B, Narula N, Li Q-Y, et al. Progression of aortic valve stenosis: TGF-beta1 is present in calcified aortic valve cusps and promotes aortic valve interstitial cell calcification via apoptosis. Ann Thorac Surg 2003;75(2):457-465, discussion 465-466.

108. Luo G, Ducy P, McKee MD, et al. Spontaneous calcification of arteries and cartilage in mice lacking matrix GLA protein. Nature 1997;386(6620):78-81.

109. Yao Y, Bennett BJ, Wang X, et al. Inhibition of bone morphogenetic proteins protects against atherosclerosis and vascular calcification. Circ Res 2010;107(4):485-494.

110. Wallin R, Cain D, Hutson SM, et al. Modulation of the binding of matrix Gla protein (MGP) to bone morphogenetic protein-2 (BMP-2). Thromb Haemost 2000;84(6):1039-1044.

111. Lerner RG, Aronow WS, Sekhri A, et al. Warfarin use and the risk of valvular calcification. J Thromb Haemost 2009;7(12):2023-2027.

112. Danziger J. Vitamin K-dependent proteins, warfarin, and vascular calcification. Clin J Am Soc Nephrol 2008;3(5):1504-1510.

113. Howe AM, Webster WS. Warfarin exposure and calcification of the arterial system in the rat. Int J Exp Pathol 2000;81(1):51-56.

114. Lassègue B, Griendling KK. NADPH oxidases: functions and pathologies in the vasculature. Arterioscler Thromb Vasc Biol 2010;30(4):653-661.

115. Rivera J, Sobey CG, Walduck AK, Drummond GR. Nox isoforms in vascular pathophysiology: insights from transgenic and knockout mouse models. Redox Rep 2010;15(2):50-63.

116. Liberman M, Bassi E, Martinatti MK, et al. Oxidant generation predominates around calcifying foci and enhances progression of aortic valve calcification. Arterioscler Thromb Vasc Biol 2008;28(3):463-470.

117. Branchetti E, Sainger R, Poggio P, et al. Antioxidant enzymes reduce DNA damage and early activation of valvular interstitial cells in aortic valve sclerosis. Arterioscler Thromb Vasc Biol 2013;33(2):e66-e74.

118. Jain M, Rivera S, Monclus EA, et al. Mitochondrial reactive oxygen species regulate transforming growth factor-beta signaling. J Biol Chem 2013;288(2):770-777.

119. Byon CH, Sun Y, Chen J, et al. Runx2-upregulated receptor activator of nuclear factor κB ligand in calcifying smooth muscle cells promotes migration and osteoclastic differentiation of macrophages. Arterioscler Thromb Vasc Biol 2011;31(6):1387-1396.

120. Anderson TJ. Nitric oxide, atherosclerosis and the clinical relevance of endothelial dysfunction. Heart Fail Rev 2003;8(1):71-86.

121. Channon KM, Qian H, George SE. Nitric oxide synthase in atherosclerosis and vascular injury: insights from experimental gene therapy. Arterioscler Thromb Vasc Biol 2000;20(8):1873-1881.

122. Rajamannan NM, Subramaniam M, Stock SR, et al. Atorvastatin inhibits calcification and enhances nitric oxide synthase production in the hypercholesterolaemic aortic valve. Heart 2005;91(6):806-810.

123. Aicher D, Urbich C, Zeiher A, et al. Endothelial nitric oxide synthase in bicuspid aortic valve disease. Ann Thorac Surg 2007;83(4):1290-1294.

124. Fukai T, Ushio-Fukai M. Superoxide dismutases: role in redox signaling, vascular function, and diseases. Antioxid Redox Signal 2011;15(6):1583-1606.

125. Stasch J-P, Pacher P, Evgenov OV. Soluble guanylate cyclase as an emerging therapeutic target in cardiopulmonary disease. Circulation 2011;123(20):2263-2273.

126. McNeill E, Channon KM. The role of tetrahydrobiopterin in inflammation and cardiovascular disease. Thromb Haemost 2012;108(5):832-839.

127. Kennedy JA, Hua X, Mishra K, et al. Inhibition of calcifying nodule formation in cultured porcine aortic valve cells by nitric oxide donors. Eur J Pharmacol 2009;602(1):28-35.

128. Rajamannan NM. Oxidative-mechanical stress signals stem cell niche mediated Lrp5 osteogenesis in eNOS(-/-) null mice. J Cell Biochem 2012;113(5):1623-1634.

129. Eggebeen J, Kim-Shapiro DB, Haykowsky M, et al. One week of daily dosing with beetroot juice improves submaximal endurance and blood pressure in older patients with heart failure and preserved ejection fraction. JACC Heart Fail 2016;4(6):428-437.

130. Kenjale AA, Ham KL, Stabler T, et al. Dietary nitrate supplementation enhances exercise performance in peripheral arterial disease. J Appl Physiol 2011;110(6):1582-1591.

131. Kawai M, Sousa KM, MacDougald OA, Rosen CJ. The many facets of PPARgamma: novel insights for the skeleton. Am J Physiol Endocrinol Metab 2010;299(1):E3-E9.

132. Takada I, Kouzmenko AP, Kato S. Wnt and PPARgamma signaling in osteoblastogenesis and adipogenesis. Nat Rev Rheumatol 2009;5(8):442-447.

133. Chu Y, Lund DD, Weiss RM, et al. Pioglitazone attenuates valvular calcification induced by hypercholesterolemia. Arterioscler Thromb Vasc Biol 2013;33(3):523-532.

134. Garg V, Muth AN, Ransom JF, et al. Mutations in Notch-1 cause aortic valve disease. Nature 2005;437(7056):270-274.

135. Nigam V, Srivastava D. Notch1 represses osteogenic pathways in aortic valve cells. J Mol Cell Cardiol 2009;47(6):828-834.

136. Chen J, Ryzhova LM, Sewell-Loftin MK, et al. Notch1 mutation leads to valvular calcification through enhanced myofibroblast mechanotransduction. Arterioscler Thromb Vasc Biol 2015;35(7):1597-1605.

137. Hinz B, Pittet P, Smith-Clerc J, et al. Myofibroblast development is characterized by specific cell-cell adherens junctions. Mol Biol Cell 2004;15(9):4310-4320.

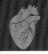
138. Hutcheson JD, Chen J, Sewell-Loftin MK, et al. Cadherin-11 regulates cell-cell tension necessary for calcific nodule formation by valvular myofibroblasts. Arterioscler Thromb Vasc Biol 2013;33(1):114-120.

139. Clark CR, Bowler MA, Snider JC, Merryman WD. Targeting cadherin-11 prevents Notch1-mediated calcific aortic valve disease. Circulation 2017;135(24):2448-2450.

140. Menini S, Iacobini C, Ricci C, et al. The galectin-3/RAGE dyad modulates vascular osteogenesis in atherosclerosis. Cardiovasc Res 2013;100(3):472-480.

141. Sádaba JR, Martínez-Martínez E, Arrieta V, et al. Role for galectin-3 in calcific aortic valve stenosis. J Am Heart Assoc 2016;5(11):e004360.

142. Shi L, Ji Y, Liu D, et al. Sitagliptin attenuates high glucose-induced alterations in migration, proliferation, calcification and apoptosis of vascular smooth muscle cells through ERK1/2 signal pathway. Oncotarget 2017;8(44):77168-77180.

143. Choi B, Lee S, Kim S-M, et al. Dipeptidyl peptidase-4 induces aortic valve calcification by inhibiting insulin-like growth factor-1 signaling in valvular interstitial cells. Circulation 2017;135(20):1935-1950.

144. Mori K, Emoto M, Inaba M. Fetuin-A and the cardiovascular system. Adv Clin Chem 2012;56:175-195.

145. Jahnen-Dechent W, Heiss A, Schäfer C, Ketteler M. Fetuin-A regulation of calcified matrix metabolism. Circ Res 2011;108(12):1494-1509.

146. Schäfer C, Heiss A, Schwarz A, et al. The serum protein alpha 2-Heremans-Schmid glycoprotein/fetuin-A is a systemically acting inhibitor of ectopic calcification. J Clin Invest 2003;112(3):357-366.

147. Westenfeld R, Schäfer C, Krüger T, et al. Fetuin-A protects against atherosclerotic calcification in CKD. J Am Soc Nephrol 2009;20(6):1264-1274.

148. Schure R, Costa KD, Rezaei R, et al. Impact of matrix metalloproteinases on inhibition of mineralization by fetuin. J Periodont Res 2013;48(3):357-366.

149. Burke AP, Kolodgie FD, Virmani R. Fetuin-A, valve calcification, and diabetes: what do we understand? Circulation 2007;115(19):2464-2467.

150. de Ruijter AJM, van Gennip AH, Caron HN, et al. Histone deacetylases (HDACs): characterization of the classical HDAC family. Biochem J 2003;370(Pt 3):737-749.

151. Schroeder TM, Kahler RA, Li X, Westendorf JJ. Histone deacetylase 3 interacts with runx2 to repress the osteocalcin promoter and regulate osteoblast differentiation. J Biol Chem 2004;279(40):41998-42007.

152. Stein S, Schäfer N, Breitenstein A, et al. SIRT1 reduces endothelial activation without affecting vascular function in ApoE–/– mice. Aging (Albany NY) 2010;2(6):353-360.

153. Yang B, Zwaans BMM, Eckersdorff M, Lombard DB. The sirtuin SIRT6 deacetylates H3 K56Ac in vivo to promote genomic stability. Cell Cycle 2009;8(16):2662-2663.

154. Yuan J, Pu M, Zhang Z, Lou Z. Histone H3-K56 acetylation is important for genomic stability in mammals. Cell Cycle 2009;8(11):1747-1753.

155. Jaenisch R, Bird A. Epigenetic regulation of gene expression: how the genome integrates intrinsic and environmental signals. Nat Genet 2003;33(Suppl 3):245-254.

156. Montes de Oca A, Madueño JA, Martinez-Moreno JM. High-phosphate-induced calcification is related to SM22α promoter methylation in vascular smooth muscle cells. J Bone Miner Res 2010;25(9):1996-2005.

157. Pasipoularides A. Calcific aortic valve disease: part 2-morphomechanical abnormalities, gene reexpression, and gender effects on ventricular hypertrophy and its reversibility. J Cardiovasc Transl Res 2016;9(4):374-399.

158. Dweck MR, Joshi S, Murigu T, et al. Left ventricular remodeling and hypertrophy in patients with aortic stenosis: insights from cardiovascular magnetic resonance. J Cardiovasc Magn Reson 2012;14(1):50.

159. Pagé A, Dumesnil JG, Clavel M-A, et al. Metabolic syndrome is associated with more pronounced impairment of left ventricle geometry and function in patients with calcific aortic stenosis: a substudy of the ASTRONOMER (Aortic Stenosis Progression Observation Measuring Effects of Rosuvastatin). J Am Coll Cardiol 2010;55(17):1867-1874.

160. Lund BP, Gohlke-Bärwolf C, Cramariuc D, et al. Effect of obesity on left ventricular mass and systolic function in patients with asymptomatic aortic stenosis (a Simvastatin Ezetimibe in Aortic Stenosis [SEAS] substudy). Am J Cardiol 2010;105(10):1456-1460.

161. Lindman BR, Arnold SV, Madrazo JA, et al. The adverse impact of diabetes mellitus on left ventricular remodeling and function in patients with severe aortic stenosis. Circ Heart Fail 2011;4(3):286-292.

162. Orlowska-Baranowska E, Placha G, Gaciong Z, et al. Influence of ACE I/D genotypes on left ventricular hypertrophy in aortic stenosis: gender-related differences. J Heart Valve Dis 2004;13(4):574-581.

163. DeBosch B, Treskov I, Lupu TS, et al. Akt1 is required for physiological cardiac growth. Circulation 2006;113(17):2097-2104.

164. Dorn GW, Force T. Protein kinase cascades in the regulation of cardiac hypertrophy. J Clin Invest 2005;115(3):527-537.

165. Miyata S, Minobe W, Bristow MR, Leinwand LA. Myosin heavy chain isoform expression in the failing and nonfailing human heart. Circ Res 2000;86(4):386-390.

166. Chen W, Frangogiannis NG. Fibroblasts in post-infarction inflammation and cardiac repair. Biochim Biophys Acta 2013;1833(4):945-953.

167. Leri A, Kajstura J, Anversa P. Role of cardiac stem cells in cardiac pathophysiology: a paradigm shift in human myocardial biology. Circ Res 2011;109(8):941-961.

168. Bergmann O, Bhardwaj RD, Bernard S, et al. Evidence for cardiomyocyte renewal in humans. Science 2009;324(5923):98-102.

169. Bishopric NH, Andreka P, Slepak T, Webster KA. Molecular mechanisms of apoptosis in the cardiac myocyte. Curr Opin Pharmacol 2001;1(2):141-150.

170. Leri A, Claudio PP, Li Q, et al. Stretch-mediated release of angiotensin II induces myocyte apoptosis by activating p53 that enhances the local renin-angiotensin system and decreases the Bcl-2-to-Bax protein ratio in the cell. J Clin Invest 1998;101(7):1326-1342.

171. Marcus ML, Harrison DG, Chilian WM, et al. Alterations in the coronary circulation in hypertrophied ventricles. Circulation 1987;75(1 Pt 2):I19-I25.

172. Dweck MR, Boon NA, Newby DE. Calcific aortic stenosis: a disease of the valve and the myocardium. J Am Coll Cardiol 2012;60(19):1854-1863.

173. Fielitz J, Hein S, Mitrovic V, et al. Activation of the cardiac renin-angiotensin system and increased myocardial collagen expression in human aortic valve disease. J Am Coll Cardiol 2001;37(5):1443-1449.

174. Chin CWL, Shah ASV, McAllister DA, et al. High-sensitivity troponin I concentrations are a marker of an advanced hypertrophic response and adverse outcomes in patients with aortic stenosis. Eur Heart J 2014;35(34):2312-2321.

175. Dweck MR, Joshi S, Murigu T, et al. Midwall fibrosis is an independent predictor of mortality in patients with aortic stenosis. J Am Coll Cardiol 2011;58(12):1271-1279.

176. Flett AS, Hayward MP, Ashworth MT, et al. Equilibrium contrast cardiovascular magnetic resonance for the measurement of diffuse myocardial fibrosis: preliminary validation in humans. Circulation 2010;122(2):138-144.

177. Lancel S, Qin F, Lennon SL, et al. Oxidative posttranslational modifications mediate decreased SERCA activity and myocyte dysfunction in Galphaq-overexpressing mice. Circ Res 2010;107(2):228-232.

178. Cowell SJ, Newby DE, Prescott RJ, et al. A randomized trial of intensive lipid-lowering therapy in calcific aortic stenosis. N Engl J Med 2005;352(23):2389-2397.

179. Chan KL, Teo K, Dumesnil JG, et al. Effect of lipid lowering with rosuvastatin on progression of aortic stenosis results of the Aortic Stenosis Progression Observation: Measuring Effects of Rosuvastatin (ASTRONOMER) Trial. Circulation 2010;121(2):306-314.

180. Rossebø AB, Pedersen TR, Boman K, et al. Intensive lipid lowering with simvastatin and ezetimibe in aortic stenosis. N Engl J Med 2008;359(13):1343-1356.

181. Skolnick AH, Osranek M, Formica P, Kronzon I. Osteoporosis treatment and progression of aortic stenosis. Am J Cardiol 2009;104(1):122-124.

182. Price PA, Faus SA, Williamson MK. Bisphosphonates alendronate and ibandronate inhibit artery calcification at doses comparable to those that inhibit bone resorption. Arterioscler Thromb Vasc Biol 2001;21(5):817-824.

183. Elmariah S, Delaney JAC, O'Brien KD, Budoff MJ, et al. Bisphosphonate use and prevalence of valvular and vascular calcification in women MESA (The Multi-Ethnic Study of Atherosclerosis). J Am Coll Cardiol 2010;56(21):1752-1759. doi:10.1016/j.jacc.2010.05.050.

184. Innasimuthu AL, Katz WE. Effect of bisphosphonates on the progression of degenerative aortic stenosis. Echocardiography 2011;28(1):1-7. doi:10.1111/j.1540-8175.2010.01256.x.

185. Helas S, Goettsch C, Schoppet M, et al. Inhibition of receptor activator of NF-kappaB ligand by denosumab attenuates vascular calcium deposition in mice. Am J Pathol 2009;175(2):473-478. doi:10.2353/ajpath.2009.080957.

186. Bossé Y, Miqdad A, Fournier D, et al. Refining molecular pathways leading to calcific aortic valve stenosis by studying gene expression profile of normal and calcified stenotic human aortic valves. Circ Cardiovasc Genet 2009;2(5):489-498.

187. Guauque-Olarte S, Droit A, Tremblay-Marchand J, et al. RNA expression profile of calcified bicuspid, tricuspid, and normal human aortic valves by RNA sequencing. Physiol Genomics 2016;48(10):749-761.

188. Thériault S, Gaudreault N, Lamontagne M, et al. A transcriptome-wide association study identifies PALMD as a susceptibility gene for calcific aortic valve stenosis. Nat Commun 2018;9(1):988.

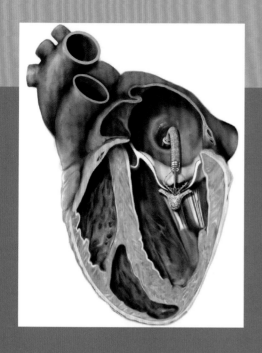

第4章
钙化性瓣膜病——临床与
遗传危险因素

当今，全球钙化性瓣膜病疾病负担较重，其是发达国家最常见的瓣膜病病因，主要病变部位为主动脉瓣瓣叶，同时二尖瓣瓣环也会受累。瓣膜组织钙化和纤维化持续进展，最终会导致瓣叶弹性丧失和瓣膜狭窄。目前，该疾病的临床和遗传危险因素尚未完全了解，亦无有效的治疗手段来预防疾病进展，除传统动脉粥样硬化的危险因素外，新发现的危险因素包括脂蛋白a水平、矿物质代谢水平（磷酸盐水平）和骨质疏松。

随着人口老龄化加剧，对疾病危险因素的研究，包括基因遗传学的研究，使我们对该疾病具有更深的认识。全基因组关联分析研究发现，NOTCH1和LPA是钙化性主动脉瓣疾病的强相关致病位点。孟德尔随机化研究发现脂蛋白a和低密度脂蛋白是主动脉瓣钙化的危险因素，甘油三酯是二尖瓣瓣环钙化的危险因素，并指明早期疾病的潜在治疗靶点。未来的工作将继续探究钙化性瓣膜病的致病因素，并通过阐述疾病的发生和发展过程，更好地预防和治疗钙化性瓣膜病。

李子昂

Clinical and Genetic Risk Factors for Calcific Valve Disease

George Thanassoulis

KEY POINTS

- Despite a large burden of disease, understanding of the clinical and genetic risk factors for the development and calcific valve disease remains incomplete, and no medical treatment exists to prevent disease progression.
- In addition to the traditional atherosclerotic risk factors that have been associated with the development of calcific valve disease, emerging risk factors include lipoprotein(a), mineral metabolism (e.g. phosphate levels), and osteoporosis.
- Genetic studies have identified *NOTCH1* and *LPA* as robust disease-associated loci for calcific aortic valve disease. Additional loci have also been identified.

- Mendelian randomization studies have provided evidence in support of circulating lipoprotein(a) and low-density lipoprotein as causal factors in calcific aortic valve disease and for triglycerides in mitral annular calcification, pointing to potential therapeutic targets in early disease.
- Work to identify clinical and genetic risk factors and to provide evidence for causality for the development and progression of calcific valve disease is ongoing.

Calcific valve disease is the most common cause of valvular heart disease in the developed world.[1] It affects predominantly the aortic valve leaflets, but also affects the mitral annulus and leads to progressive calcification and fibrosis, culminating in loss of leaflet elasticity, restriction of blood flow, and valvular stenosis. Despite the large burden of disease, understanding of the risks factors and the underlying causes of the initiation and progression of calcific valve disease remain incomplete. Nonetheless, with the aging of the population and the increasing numbers of individuals affected, research into the risk factors, including the role of genetics, has led to insights into this disease. It is hoped that these findings will pave the way for new approaches to prevent and treat aortic stenosis (AS) and other calcific valve disease.

CALCIFIC AORTIC VALVE DISEASE

Calcific aortic valve disease (CAVD) represents a continuum of disease that begins with aortic sclerosis, which is asymptomatic but can be detected noninvasively by echocardiography or by cardiac computed tomography (CT) (Fig. 4.1), and progresses to AS, which is characterized by obstruction to flow and the development of symptoms when stenosis becomes severe.

The natural history of CAVD consists of a long, clinically silent phase of valve calcification and hardening (i.e., sclerosis), which usually lasts at least a decade and heralds the clinical disease. Aortic valve sclerosis is exceedingly common, with a prevalence of 26% after 65 years of age, 40% after 75 years of age, and 75% after 85 years of age.[2] Aortic valve sclerosis, which was long deemed a benign consequence of aging, is now known to confer a 40% increase in the risk of death and a 66% increase in the risk of cardiovascular death, independent of age and cardiovascular risk factors.[3]

AS is the most common form of valve disease in the developed world, affecting more than 2.5 million individuals in the United States alone.[1] Approximately 2% of the population older than 65 years of age have AS, a figure that increases to almost 7% of those older than 80 years of age.[4,5] It is estimated that the direct health care costs of advanced AS in the United States exceed 1 billion dollars per year.[6]

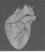

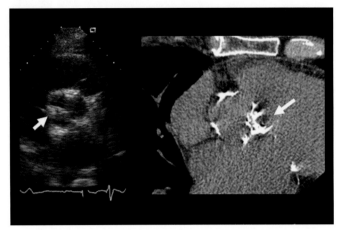

Fig. 4.1 Aortic Valve Calcification. Depiction of a patient with severe aortic stenosis shows the appearance of calcium on echocardiography (*left*) and computed tomography (*right*). The regions of valvular calcium are shown (*arrows*). Annular calcium also can be seen.

TABLE 4.1 Strength of Associations Seen in Observational and Epidemiologic Studies Between Clinical Risk Factors and Calcific Aortic Valve Disease.

Risk Factors	CAVD ANALYSES		
	Cross-Sectional	Incident	Progression
Age	+++	+++	+++
Male gender	++/−	++	0
Height	++	++	0
BMI	++	++	0
Hypertension	++	++	0
Diabetes	+++	+++	0
Metabolic syndrome	++	++	+
Lipoprotein(a)	+++	NA	++
Dyslipidemia	++	++	0
Smoking	++	++	+
Renal dysfunction	+	0	0
Inflammatory markers	+	0	0
Phosphorus	++	0	NA
Calcium levels	0	0	NA
Baseline calcium score	NA	NA	+++

BMI, Body mass index; *NA*, insufficient data available; +, weak positive association; ++, modest positive association; +++, strong positive association; −, weak negative association; 0, no association seen.

With the aging of the population, the prevalence of AS is projected to increase by more than twofold by 2040 and by threefold by 2060.[1,7] Although CAVD is poised to become a major contributor to health care expenditures, death, and disability, there are no medical treatments known to retard or arrest the progression of this disease.

Although CAVD has long been considered a degenerative condition of older age, research over the past 3 decades has demonstrated that the calcification and fibrosis, which characterizes this condition, are tightly regulated and likely occur in response to several risk factors that are shared with atherosclerosis. Although there is significant overlap between the early initiating lesion and certain shared risk factors,[8–11] there are major differences in the underlying pathophysiology of these diseases, including a much more prominent mineralization phase in early disease and other histopathologic differences.

Among individuals undergoing aortic valve replacement for (non-congenital) AS, only 40% have significant coronary disease requiring bypass,[12] suggesting unique pathologic processes in CAVD compared with coronary atherosclerosis. Lipid-lowering agents which have been remarkably effective for preventing atherosclerosis have also not demonstrated any benefit in randomized trials for CAVD[13–15] further demonstrating that atherosclerosis and CAVD are related but separate diseases.

Clinical Risk Factors
Older Age

Older age is the most important risk factor for the development of CAVD and its major clinical manifestation, AS (Table 4.1). The prevalence of CAVD (which includes sclerosis) based on echocardiography in the Cardiovascular Health Study (CHS) was determined to be 21% among individuals 65 to 74 years of age, 38% among those 75 to 84 years of age, and 52% among those older than 85 years.[10]

In multivariable models, each 10-year increment in age was associated with an adjusted odds ratio of 2.18 (95% confidence interval [CI]: 2.15–2.20, $P < 0.001$) for CAVD. For AS, estimates from a meta-analysis suggest that approximately 12% of individuals older than 75 years of age have AS and that almost 4% have severe AS.[16] Based on longitudinal data from the Multi-Ethnic Study of Atherosclerosis (MESA) using CT to measure valve calcium, age appears to influence progression of calcification and the development of new calcification in otherwise unaffected valves.[17] Although age has been shown to be a key risk factor, it remains unclear whether age is a marker for the

exposure time of other risk factors acting on the leaflets or whether aging itself predisposes to calcification and fibrosis.

Male Sex

Similar to the preponderance of coronary artery disease in men, a similar sex difference exists in CAVD. Male sex has been demonstrated to be a risk factor for CAVD in several studies. This may be related to the higher prevalence of bicuspid aortic valves in men, greater burden of cardiovascular risk factors, and lack of possible protective factors (e.g., estrogens). In multivariable analysis, male sex was shown to increase the odds of valve calcium by 1.56 (95% CI: 1.19–2.12, $P = 0.005$) in the Framingham Offspring Study cohorts, even after considering other possible risk factors.[11] In the CHS, male sex was an important predictor of progression to AS (odds ratio [OR] = 3.05, 95% CI: 1.76–5.27, $P < 0.001$).[10]

Race and Ethnicity

Limited data exist about whether race, ethnicity, or both, affect the prevalence of CAVD. In MESA, the baseline prevalence was 14% among white, 7% among Chinese, 11% among black, and 12% among Hispanic participants.[18] However, none of these differences persisted after multivariable adjustment for other risk factors, suggesting no independent contribution from race or ethnic background.

A large study using electronic health records identified a much lower prevalence of AS among African-American patients due to CAVD or bicuspid aortic valve compared with white patients (adjusted OR = 0.41, 95% CI: 0.33–0.50, $P < 0.001$).[19] Severe AS was also lower in African Americans (adjusted OR = 0.47, 95% CI: 0.36–0.61,

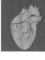

$P < 0.05$). These results were independent of traditional risk factors. To demonstrate that the results were not due to bias (e.g., referral), the study authors showed no racial difference in the prevalence rates of mitral regurgitation. African Americans also demonstrated reduced progression to AS in the CHS (OR = 0.49, 95% CI: 0.25–0.95, $P = 0.035$).[10] Whether these observations demonstrate true race-related differences due to genetic or other causes will require validation in future studies.

Cigarette Smoking

Cigarette smoking has been associated with CAVD in several studies. In the CHS, Stewart et al reported an adjusted odds ratio of 1.35 (95% CI: 1.1–1.7, $P = 0.006$) for current cigarette smoking.[10] Similarly, in Framingham Offspring, cigarette smoking was associated with an adjusted odds ratio 1.22 for aortic valve calcium (AVC). (95% CI: 1.06–1.39, $P = 0.005$).[11] In MESA, cigarette smoking was also a strong risk factor for incident aortic valve calcification (OR = 2.49, 95% CI: 1.49–4.15, $P = 0.001$).[17]

Blood Pressure, Hypertension, and Vascular Stiffness

Hypertension has been associated with CAVD in several studies. Lindroos et al, using cross-sectional data, reported a 74% (95% CI: 19%–155%) increased odds of valve calcification in hypertensive individuals (defined as a blood pressure > 165/95 mmHg) compared with normotensives.[20] Similarly, in a much larger study of 5201 participants of the CHS, Stewart et al observed that hypertension was found in 48% of individuals with valve calcification, compared with 43% among individuals with normal aortic valves (adjusted OR = 1.23; 95% CI: 1.1–1.4, $P = 0.002$).[10]

In a small, retrospective echographic study, Capoulade et al observed faster disease progression in hypertensives compared with normotensives (annualized progression peak aortic velocity [Vpeak]: (0.26 ± 0.23 m/s/yr vs. 0.17 ± 0.20 m/s/yr; $P < 0.01$).[21] Using CT, Linefsky et al observed an increasing prevalence of AVC across hypertension stages as defined by the Seventh Report of the Joint National Committee on Prevention, Detection, Evaluation, and Treatment of High Blood Pressure (JNC 7).[22] Valve calcium was observed in 6% of normotensives, 11% of individuals with borderline hypertension, 17% of those with stage I hypertension, and 16% of those with stage II hypertension. After multivariable adjustment, stage I or II hypertension was strongly associated with valve calcium (OR = 2.31, 95% CI: 1.35–3.94), but this was observed only in individuals younger than 65 years of age. A modest nonsignificant association (OR = 1.33, 95% CI: 0.96–1.85) was observed for participants older than 65 years of age. In keeping with these findings, Tastet et al demonstrated that hypertensive patients had faster 2-year AVC progression compared with normotensives (change in median AVC [25th percentile − 75th percentile]: +370 [126–824] vs. +157 [58–303]; $P = 0.007$).[23]

Hypertension was confirmed to be a strong risk factor for AS in 1.12 million Canadians followed for a median of 13 years (hazard ratio [HR] = 1.71, 95% CI: 1.66–1.76, $P < 0.001$).[24] In a large U.K. cohort of more than 5 million individuals (with 20,680 AS cases), Razimi et al provided strong evidence in favor of a continuous association between hypertension and AS. For each 20 mmHg increment in systolic blood pressure, 10 mmHg increment in diastolic blood pressure, and 15 mmHg in pulse pressure, there was an associated 41% (HR = 1.41, 95% CI: 1.38 to 1.45), 24% (HR = 1.24, CI: 1.19–1.29), and 46% greater risk of AS (HR = 1.46, CI: 1.42–1.50), respectively.[25]

Linefsky also reported that the strongest association with AVC across blood pressure measures was observed for pulse pressure.[22] For each 10 mmHg increase in pulse pressure, the odds ratio for AVC was

1.41 (CI: 1.21–1.64) among those younger than 65 years of age and 1.14 (CI: 1.05–1.23) among those older than 65 years. Pulse pressure is a known marker for vascular stiffness and may suggest that abnormal central aortic hemodynamics (i.e., increased stiffness and wave reflection) may be a risk factor for CAVD. This may be relevant because the pressure transmitted to the aortic cusps (i.e., tensile stress) may be implicated in matrix remodeling in the aortic valve leaflets and may promote thickening and calcification of the aortic valve. One study showed that the augmentation index (i.e., measure of arterial wave reflection) was an independent predictor of AVC after adjustment for traditional risk factors (OR = 1.08 per percent increment in augmentation index, 95% CI: 1.02–1.14, $P = 0.005$).[26]

In keeping with the previous findings, Sverdlov et al showed that the augmentation index and platelet nitric oxide responsiveness (i.e., measure of endothelial dysfunction) were also associated with disease progression, highlighting the importance of the central and peripheral vasculature in the development and progression of valve calcification.[27]

Despite these intriguing observational studies, no randomized trials have specifically evaluated the role of blood pressure lowering for the prevention of CAVD. However, several observational studies have suggested a possible link between antihypertensive drugs and reduced valve calcification. O'Brien demonstrated reduced progression of valve calcification in individuals receiving angiotensin-converting enzyme (ACE) inhibitors with or without angiotensin receptor blockers (ARBs), with 42% of individuals who received ACE inhibitors or ARBs showing evidence of progression, compared with 75% in individuals not receiving these drugs.[28] After multivariable adjustment, the odds ratio for progression was 0.29 (95% CI: 0.11–0.75, $P = 0.01$). In contrast, Rosenhek et al[29] observed no difference in disease progression among individuals with evidence of at least mild AS, a more advanced stage of disease than the subclinical valve disease evaluated by O'Brien et al.

In a later study of 338 patients with AS, ARB (but not ACE inhibitor) use was associated with a reduction in disease progression.[21] All of these results have been generated by observational, retrospective studies and therefore are prone to several biases, including confounding. Without a randomized trial, these results can only be considered hypothesis generating but suggest a possible role of the renin-angiotensin axis in this disease.

Dyslipidemia and Lipoprotein(a)

Dyslipidemia has been linked with AVC and AS in several observational studies and has spurred testing of lipid-lowering therapies to prevent disease progression. In seminal pathologic studies, Otto et al demonstrated that apolipoprotein B and lipoprotein(a) (Lp[a]) co-localized to areas of calcification in explanted aortic valves.[8,9] Individuals with familial hypercholesterolemia (see Genetic Factors in Calcific Aortic Valve Disease) have demonstrated severe valve calcification and AS, suggesting a possible association between LDL-C levels and AS. In a seminal study of the CHS, Stewart et al demonstrated that increased LDL-C levels were cross-sectionally associated with CAVD (OR [per mg/dL] = 1.12, 95% CI: 1.03–1.23, $P = 0.008$).[10]

Novaro et al demonstrated that LDL-C levels were a predictor of progression to aortic sclerosis in the CHS.[30] Thanassoulis et al showed that total cholesterol in young adulthood was a strong predictor of AVC measured more than 20 years later.[11] Similarly, Owens et al observed an association between the total cholesterol/HDL-C ratio and AVC at all ages, but they also found that the association with LDL-C levels was most strongly associated with valve calcium in individuals younger than 65 years of age.[18]

The association between LDL-C levels and CAVD has not been consistent across all studies, and several studies found no association

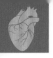

between the two, suggesting that the association between LDL-C and CAVD is likely heterogeneous and based on age, disease severity, and other factors. Several observational studies have also shown that statin use was associated with lower rates of AS and valve calcification.

Despite the many limitations of these observational studies and the degree of heterogeneity observed in the associations between LDL-C levels and AS, a strong hypothesis emerged (supported by animal studies) that lowering LDL-C levels with statins could prevent progression of AS. This hypothesis served as the impetus for three randomized, controlled trials that tested the effect of lipid lowering on CAVD[13–15] (Table 4.2). The Scottish Aortic Stenosis and Lipid Lowering Trial, Impact on Regression (SALTIRE)[14] tested whether 80 mg of atorvastatin could slow progression among 155 patients with moderate or more severe AS over 25 months but found no significant effect. The Simvastatin and Ezetimibe in Aortic Stenosis (SEAS) trial included 1873 patients (with characteristics similar to those of SALTIRE) randomized to 40 mg of simvastatin and 10 mg of ezetimibe daily for 56 months. SEAS demonstrated a reduction in ischemic events but not valve progression.[15] The Aortic Stenosis Progression Observation: Measuring Effects of Rosuvastatin (ASTRONOMER) trial randomized 269 patients with mild to moderate AS to 40 mg of rosuvastatin daily for 42 months but also failed to demonstrate any change in progression.[13]

The failure to reduce disease activity in AS, as observed in these trials, has significantly dampened enthusiasm for the LDL hypothesis of CAVD, but two caveats deserve mention. First, all trials included participants with relatively advanced valve disease (mean aortic valve area ≤1.5 cm², with increased transvalvular gradients). It remains possible that the role of lipids becomes less important after significant valve gradients develop and that further progression at this advanced stage is governed by hemodynamics of turbulent flow across the valve. Evidence supporting an early role for LDL-C in valve calcification was demonstrated in a large mendelian randomization study from the Cohorts for Heart and Aging Research in Genomic Epidemiology (CHARGE) Consortium, which showed that individuals genetically predisposed to higher LDL-C levels had a higher incidence of AVC and greater risk of AS (see Genome-Wide Association Studies and Mendelian Randomization).[31]

Second, due to ethical requirements, all three trials only enrolled individuals with low to moderate LDL-C levels who were not otherwise candidates for lipid-lowering therapy. Individuals with high LDL-C levels, who would be the most likely to demonstrate benefit from lipid-lowering therapy, were specifically excluded from such trials. Although these trials have proved that lipid-lowering agents do not slow the progression of advanced CAVD in individuals with low to moderate LDL-C levels, it remains unknown whether lipid lowering could prevent calcification at the earliest stages of disease (i.e., aortic sclerosis) in individuals with high levels of LDL-C.

Although LDL-C has garnered the most attention as a target of therapy for calcific valve disease for several decades, emerging data suggest that another lipoprotein, Lp(a), may be equally or more relevant in CAVD. Lp(a) is an LDL-like molecule that consists of an apolipoprotein B molecule covalently bound to an apo(a) moiety. Lp(a) levels are largely explained by genetics, and an elevated level is the most common genetic dyslipidemia worldwide, affecting one of five individuals.

Elevated Lp(a) levels have been associated with coronary heart disease and myocardial infarction for several decades, but few studies have evaluated its role in valve calcification and AS. Prior studies examining the association between Lp(a) and AS were usually limited by small sample sizes and cross-sectional associations. However, in 2013, the CHARGE Consortium reported that variants in the *LPA* locus, which control circulating plasma Lp(a) levels, were strongly associated with CAVD in several cohorts, including prospective analyses in large cohorts from Sweden and Denmark.[32] These results have been replicated by several independent groups and provide strong support for a possible causal association between Lp(a) and CAVD (see Genome-Wide Association Studies and Mendelian Randomization).

Diabetes, Obesity, and the Metabolic Syndrome

Independent associations of plasma glucose levels, measurements of insulin resistance, and the metabolic syndrome with CAVD have been inconsistent and heterogenous. In MESA, metabolic syndrome and diabetes were associated with AVC (OR = 1.4, 95% CI: 1.1–1.9 for metabolic syndrome and OR = 2.1, 95% CI: 1.5–2.9) and with

TABLE 4.2   Randomized, Controlled Trials Testing Statin Therapy for Slowing Progression of Calcific Aortic Valve Disease.

	SALTIRE[48]	SEAS[49]	ASTRONOMER[50]
AS severity			
AV jet velocity	3.7 m/s	3.1 m/s	3.2 m/s
AV area	1.0 cm²	1.3 cm²	1.5 cm²
Number of subjects	155	1873	269
Mean age	68 yr	67 yr	58 yr
BAV prevalence	3%	5%	49%
Baseline LDL	135±32 mg/dL	139±35 mg/dL	122±26 mg/dL
Statin tested	Atorvastatin 80 mg	Simvastatin 40 mg + ezetimibe 10 mg	Rosuvastatin 40 mg
Median follow up	25 mo	52 mo	42 mo
Valve outcomes assessed	1. AV jet velocity 2. AV calcium score	1. AV events 2. AV jet velocity	1. AV peak gradient 2. AV area
Results	No benefit	Reduction in ischemic but not AV events	No benefit

AS, Aortic stenosis; *ASTRONOMER*, Aortic Stenosis Progression Observation: Measuring Effects of Rosuvastatin trial; *AV*, aortic valve; *BAV*, bicuspid aortic valve; *LDL*, low-density lipoprotein cholesterol; *SALTIRE*, Scottish Aortic Stenosis and Lipid Lowering Trial, Impact on Regression; *SEAS*, Simvastatin and Ezetimibe in Aortic Stenosis trial.

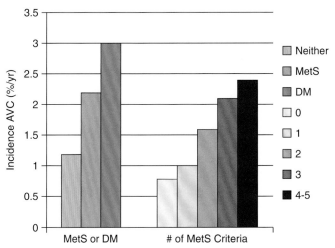

Fig. 4.2 Rates of Incident Aortic Valve Calcification *(AVC)* Related to Diabetes Mellitus *(DM)* and Metabolic Syndrome *(MetS)*. Data are shown for the 5723 participants in the Multi-Ethnic Study of Atherosclerosis who had metabolic syndrome (by criteria of the Third Report of the Expert Panel on Detection, Evaluation, and Treatment of High Blood Cholesterol in Adults [ATP-III]) or diabetes *(left)* and the number of metabolic syndrome criteria *(right)*. (Modified from Katz R, Budoff MJ, Takasu J, et al. Relationship of metabolic syndrome with incident aortic valve calcium and aortic valve calcium progression: the Multi-Ethnic Study of Atherosclerosis (MESA). Diabetes 2009;58:813-819.)

progression of valve calcium[33,34] (Fig. 4.2). However, similar associations were not identified in the CHS or the Framingham Offspring Study. However, an increasing body mass index (BMI) was associated with a trend toward increased AVC prevalence in the Framingham study (OR = 1.15, 95% CI: 0.99–1.33, $P = 0.06$).[11]

In a substudy of the ASTRONOMER trial, metabolic syndrome was associated with faster CAVD progression (0.25 m/s/yr vs. 0.19 m/s/yr, $P = 0.03$).[35] In a large Canadian cohort study that included more than 21,000 AS cases, diabetes was associated with an increased risk of AS (HR = 1.49, 95% CI: 1.44–1.54, $P < 0.001$).[24] Larsson et al demonstrated in two separate cohorts, which included 1297 incident AS cases, that compared with normal weight, overweight (BMI $\geq$ 25 to <30 kg/m^2) and obesity (BMI $\geq$ 30 kg/m^2) were associated with AS (HR = 1.24, 95% CI: 1.05–1.48 for overweight and HR = 1.81, 95% CI: 1.47–2.23).[36]

The disparate associations with obesity, diabetes, and metabolic syndrome across cohorts may be due to the analytic strategy in which body mass index or lipids are adjusted, which may attenuate the association with diabetes and metabolic syndrome. Together, the available data indicate that obesity is an important risk factor for AS, and this may be mediated partially by dysglycemia, lipid abnormalities, and perhaps other direct effects.

Chronic Kidney Disease and Mineral Metabolism

Advanced chronic kidney disease has been linked with rapid and progressive calcification of the cardiovascular system, including valve structures.[37–45] Several mechanisms have been implicated, including increases in blood pressure and lipoproteins and dysregulated mineral metabolism. Maher et al demonstrated a high prevalence of AVC and stenosis (28%) among hemodialysis patients younger than 70 years of age.[39,40] The strongest predictor for valve calcification was a high calcium-phosphate product level. End-stage renal disease also indicates more rapid progression of AS, compared with normal controls (−0.19 vs. −0.07 cm^2/yr, $P < 0.001$).[42]

In milder forms of chronic kidney disease, the associations with valve calcification have been less consistent. However, the lack of association may be due to the low prevalence of kidney dysfunction among many population cohorts and insufficient power. Evidence from the Chronic Renal Insufficiency Cohort demonstrated a clear association between lower glomerular filtration rate and both greater prevalence and severity of valve calcification.[46] This association was further demonstrated in a large cohort from Sweden with more than 1.2 million individuals (with 5850 incident AS cases). Compared with normal estimated glomerular filtration rates (eGFRs), lower eGFRs were associated with higher hazards of AS, ranging from a relative risk of 1.14 (95% CI: 1.05–1.25) for mild kidney disease (eGFR of 60 to 90 ml/min/1.73 m^2) to a relative risk of 1.56 (95% CI: 1.29–1.87) for advanced kidney disease (eGFR of 30 mL/min/1.73 m^2). These associations were shown to be independent from traditional cardiovascular risk factors.[47]

Several studies have implicated phosphate concentrations with AVC. Linefsky et al. demonstrated in MESA[48] and the CHS[49] that higher serum phosphate levels were associated with a greater prevalence of AVC (OR = 1.3 per 1-mg/dL increment in phosphate concentration, 95% CI: 1.1–1.5, $P < 0.001$ in CHS and 1.4 per 1-mg/dL increment, 95% CI: 1.1–1.7, $P = 0.01$ in MESA).[49] These associations were independent of traditional risk factors and renal function. Whether dysregulated phosphate metabolism represents a major causal pathway that is independent of renal dysfunction and could represent a target of therapy will require further study.

Osteoporosis and Bone Metabolism

Valve calcification shares many features with bone formation and follows a similar process of collagen deposition, followed by calcium deposition. The processes in the leaflets are thought to share the same regulating factors and signaling pathways seen in bone (e.g., osteoblastic differentiation, extracellular matrix remodeling).[50–59] Conditions of rapid bone turnover, including advanced kidney disease and primary bone disorders such as Paget disease, have been linked with increased cardiovascular calcification, suggesting a calcification paradox.[60] This has prompted an evaluation of possible links between bone health and CAVD.

Studies evaluating the links between osteoporosis and osteopenia have shown interesting, albeit inconsistent, results. In a small cohort of 114 participants, Aksoy et al demonstrated an association between reduced bone mineral density and valve calcification (OR = 0.59 per unit, 95% CI: 0.41–0.87, $P = 0.007$).[61] Similarly, in the European Prospective Investigation of Cancer–Norfolk (EPIC-Norfolk) study of more than 25,000 individuals (with 122 incident cases of AS), higher bone mineral density was associated with reduced incidence of AS (HR = 0.80 per SD in bone mineral density, 95% CI: 65–1.0, $P = 0.046$).[62] However, no association was observed between bone mineral density and valve calcium in 1317 Framingham Offspring study participants.[63]

Hekimian et al provided some mechanistic data showing that markers of bone resorption (i.e., terminal peptide of type 1 collagen and osteocalcin), parathyroid hormone levels, and vitamin D levels were each predictors of AS progression.[64] However, Dweck et al, using an elegant molecular imaging approach, provided evidence that valve calcification and bone resorption may represent parallel but separate processes.[65] They showed poor correlation between bone mineral density and valve calcium. More importantly, they showed that ^{18}F-labeled sodium fluoride (NaF) activity, an in vivo measure of active calcium deposition, was more strongly correlated with new valve calcification than activity measured at the bone (with almost no correlation between NaF activity at the valve and bone). These results indicate that the calcification occurring in bone and in the valve, although possibly

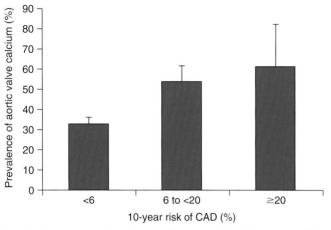

Fig. 4.3 Framingham Risk Score in Early Adulthood Compared With Prevalence of Aortic Valve Calcium (AVC) After a Median 27-Year Follow-Up. Categories are divided into low (<6%), intermediate (6% to <20%), and high (≥20%) 10-year risk for coronary artery disease (CAD). Higher aggregate risk scores were associated with a greater prevalence of AVC (*P* < 0.001 for trend across groups). *Error bars* represent 95% confidence intervals. (From Thanassoulis G, Massaro JM, Cury R, et al. Associations of long-term and early adult atherosclerosis risk factors with aortic and mitral valve calcium. J Am Coll Cardiol 2010; 55:2491-2498.)

linked by common mechanisms, may be entirely independent processes at their respective locations (i.e., bone vs. valve).

Building on these possible links, several studies have suggested a protective association between antiresorptive agents (e.g., bisphosphonates) and protection of CAVD.[66–69] Although these studies have suggested that antiresorptive agents could be used to prevent AS, only carefully performed, randomized trials can ultimately address this question.

Aortic Valve Calcium

The presence and extent of AVC and baseline hemodynamics (e.g., valve gradients) are among the best markers of disease progression and clinical outcome.[17,70] In MESA, a strong correlation was identified between baseline AVC and the annualized progression rate over 2 years, with a higher baseline AVC level strongly associated with a significantly more rapid progression (two to five times faster).[17]

Multiple Risk Factors and Risk Scores

Few studies have examined the joint effects of having one or more risk factors (i.e., risk factor score) on the development of AS. Framingham investigators demonstrated a graded relationship between both the presence and severity of AVC with the traditional Framingham cardiovascular disease risk score[11] (Fig. 4.3). Similarly, Yan et al demonstrated that the number of risk factors (including hypertension, dyslipidemia, and diabetes) was strongly associated with the presence of AS. Individuals with one, two, or three risk factors had hazard ratios of 1.73 (95% CI: 1.67–1.79), 2.31 (95% CI: 2.22–2.40), and 2.77 (95% CI: 2.57–2.98), respectively.[24]

Genetic Factors
Heritability

Although bicuspid aortic valve is highly heritable (with estimates of heritability of about 90%),[71] there have been no reported estimates of heritability for calcific AS. However, several lines of evidence suggest a

potential heritable component. First, using data from the Utah Population Database, which includes more than 2 million individual records with detailed genealogic data, individuals who died of (nonrheumatic) aortic valve diseases were found to have a much higher average relatedness than population controls.[72] Average relatedness among cases remained higher than population controls, even beyond second- and third-degree relatives, which are much less likely to share common environments.

Second, calcific AS cases cluster within close geographic regions. LeGal et al., using data from the region of Finistere, France, demonstrated a nonrandom distribution of cases throughout this region with several specific high-risk clusters.[73] Given that the population of this region is relatively static (with little population movement) and is relatively homogeneous with regard to lifestyle and other environmental influences, these data provide some support, albeit weak, for a possible genetic component for AS.

Third, using geographic data from France, Probst et al identified five families with a higher than expected prevalence of AS.[74] The largest family, consisting of 135 members, had 13 individuals with severe AS and another 20 individuals with milder forms of aortic valve disease. None of the AS cases had familial hypercholesterolemia or renal failure. Candidate gene analysis for apolipoprotein E (ApoE) and vitamin D receptor gene polymorphisms were also negative. Further analysis of hospital records identified 15 additional patients operated for severe AS from the same region as this family. An additional 199 individuals from this region were subsequently screened for AS, leading to the identification of 20 additional AS cases and 11 milder aortic valve abnormalities. The study authors performed a detailed 400-year genealogic analysis and identified a common ancestor born in 1650, providing a clear familial link between the 48 individuals with severe AS. Using this cluster of cases, the study authors estimated a 33% first-degree recurrence rate for severe AS, providing compelling evidence for a possible genetic cause.

Mendelian Disorders of Calcific Aortic Stenosis

Familial hypercholesterolemia has long been associated with the development of aortic valve disease with marked involvement of the aorta and aortic valve.[75,76] Valvular and supravalvular AS have been documented in patients with familial hypercholesterolemia, with supravalvular AS being much more frequent. Although these observations have been confirmed in animal models of hypercholesterolemia,[77,78] suggesting a probable role for increased cholesterol in AS, these disorders lead to extremely high LDL values and are rare in the general population, occurring in roughly 1 in 250 individuals.

Alkaptonuria is another rare disorder due to deficiency of homogentisic acid (HGA) dioxygenase, which metabolizes tyrosine, resulting in the accumulation of HGA in the tissues. AS is the most frequent complication, with a prevalence of 17% during the first 7 decades of life.[79] Calcification appears to closely correlate with areas of HGA-derived pigment deposition; however, the exact mechanisms of calcification remain unknown. These rare genetic disorders constitute an extremely small fraction of calcific AS cases and may have little in common with the calcific AS frequently encountered clinically.

In addition to the rare forms of AS, a linkage study of a large family with aortic valve disease identified the first bona fide genetic mechanism for it.[80] Garg et al identified a large family spanning five generations with 11 cases of congenital heart defects (i.e., nine had aortic valve abnormalities, of which six had bicuspid aortic valve). Seven family members also had evidence of accelerated AVC, including two individuals with a normal trileaflet valve.

A genome-wide scan of the family identified a linkage signal at a single locus on chromosome 9q34-35. Detailed analysis of this region

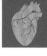

identified *NOTCH1* as a strong candidate for the causal gene. Sequencing of the *NOTCH1* gene identified a nonsense mutation at position 1108 (R1108X), which was subsequently found in all affected subjects (but not in unaffected family members), demonstrating an autosomal dominant inheritance pattern with complete penetrance. A second variant of *NOTCH1* was identified in a second family with bicuspid aortic valve and aortic calcification.

Although *NOTCH1* has been shown to be integral for cardiac and specifically for aortic valve development, this gene appears to also play a separate and equally important role in regulating AVC postnatally. The NOTCH1 protein is a potent repressor of RUNX2, which is upregulated in animal models of valvular calcification and is directly responsible for the expression of osteoblast-specific genes.[80] NOTCH1 also represses BMP2, a potent inducer of osteoblastic differentiation.[81] Although severe *NOTCH1* mutations predispose to accelerated calcification, the mutations are rare and likely play a very limited role in sporadic cases of calcific AS.

Candidate Genes for Calcific Aortic Stenosis

Several smaller genetic association studies have been performed to evaluate candidate genes thought to be involved in calcific AS. However, most were performed in the early 2000s, before current standards for genetic association studies. Genetic studies from this era must be interpreted cautiously due to the inconsistent results and the very high false-positive rate that has emerged, which is in large part attributable to the small sample sizes, lack of independent replication, and strong publication bias for positive results.[82]

Ortlepp et al performed one of the first candidate gene studies for AS. They examined a single common vitamin D receptor polymorphism.[83] In 100 cases of severe calcific AS and 100 carefully matched controls, the B allele was found to be significantly more frequent among cases than controls (56% vs. 40%, *P* < 0.001), but this finding failed to replicate in two subsequent case-control studies with much larger sample sizes.

Similarly, Nordstrom et al studied polymorphisms in the estrogen receptor-α (ER-α) gene *(ESR1)* and in the transforming-growth factor-β1 (TGF-β1) gene *(TGFB1)* for associations with aortic sclerosis in 41 people who underwent aortic valve replacement for AS and 41 controls.[84] The PvuII polymorphism in ER-α was more prevalent among cases than controls (OR = 03.38, 95% CI: 1.13–10.09; *P* = 0.03). No differences were seen for the TGF-β polymorphism. However, these findings were never subsequently confirmed or refuted.

Candidate genes in lipoprotein metabolism pathways have received significant attention as potential genetic causes of calcific AS. Several studies have studied polymorphisms in the *APOE*, *APOB*, and *APOA1* genes and reported conflicting results. Avakian et al evaluated polymorphisms in these three genes in 62 AS cases and 62 controls.[85] The *APOE* e2 allele and a polymorphism in *APOB* (X-X-) were associated with AS case status. No signal was observed at the *APOA1* gene. However, in 43 cases and 759 controls, Novaro et al failed to replicate the association with the *APOE* e2 allele, but they identified a different *APOE* allele (e4) that was associated with AS.[86] In a later study, Ortlepp et al found no evidence for an association between the *APOE* locus (including *APOE4*) and AS in more than 500 cases and 500 controls.[87] Gaudreault et al confirmed this null result and reported no significant association between *APOE* genotypes in a large AS case-control study.[88]

Based on the totality of the evidence, there does not appear to be any discernible signal at the *APOE* locus with AS, but this requires confirmation in larger studies. Gaudreault et al, using contemporary methods and strict criteria for statistical significance, did find evidence

for an association with polymorphisms in the *APOB* gene,[88] which would implicate LDL in the development of AS. However, the associated polymorphism in *APOB* was different from (and not in linkage disequilibrium with) the X-X- polymorphism in *APOB*, which was previously identified.[85]

Ortlepp et al also investigated the role of proinflammatory and antiinflammatory gene polymorphisms in AVC in several genes: interleukin-10 *(IL10)*, connective tissue growth factor *(CTGF,* now designated *CCN2)*, and *CCR5*.[89] Although *CCR5* and *CTGF/CCN2* polymorphisms were not associated, the high *IL10*-producing haplotype was significantly associated with valve calcification, suggesting somewhat paradoxically that antiinflammatory cytokines may be involved in valve calcification.

Gaudreault et al reported completely contradictory results, demonstrating that the low *IL10*-producing haplotype was most strongly associated with AS.[88] Although more biologically plausible and identified with more rigorous methods, the importance of this finding remains unclear, highlighting the conflicting nature of many association studies of candidate genes in AS.

A case-control study of 265 cases of AS and 961 controls, which used a two-step discovery and validation design with stringent criteria for statistical significance, evaluated a large panel of CAVD candidate genes and 29 additional SNPs from 8 AS candidate genes.[90] Of the 29 candidate SNPs for AS, none was found to be statistically significant, but three polymorphisms from the CAVD candidate genes were associated with AS case status at the following loci: *MYO7A*, which codes for an unconventional myosin; *AGTR2*, which codes for the angiotensin 2 receptor, type II; and *ELN*, which codes for elastin. Although the finding of an association with *AGTR2* variants is interesting due to other lines of evidence that angiotensin pathways may be involved in AS, the lack of replication in independent cohorts, the small sample used, and the low pretest odds for association preclude any important conclusions regarding this and other candidate genes for AS.

Genome-Wide Association Studies and Mendelian Randomization

Genome-wide association studies (GWAS) have been conducted since 2005 and have demonstrated robust and replicable associations with many human diseases. The GWAS approach consists of genotyping several hundred thousand SNPs throughout the genome (which are frequently used to impute genotypes for more than 15 million polymorphisms) of each individual. Each of these polymorphisms is then tested for association with disease using a case-control approach. Given the multiplicity of statistical tests, only very stringent evidence of association (i.e., genome-wide significance $P < 5 \times 10^{-8}$) is thought to indicate new disease-associated loci.

To ensure only true positive findings are identified, replication of each genome-wide polymorphism is normally obtained from independent cohorts demonstrating consistent association with a disease. This rigorous approach has only started to be applied to CAVD but has already been successful in identifying key genetic variants associated with disease.

As part of the CHARGE Consortium, Thanassoulis et al evaluated 6942 individuals in three cohorts with CT assessment of AVC and replicated the results in several additional large cohorts.[32] A SNP in intron 25 of the apolipoprotein(a) gene *(LPA)* reached genome-wide significance and was replicated across several ethnicities (Fig. 4.4). Forty-four additional SNPs were identified with some evidence for association but did not reach genome-wide significance; most of these were not within 60 kB of the candidate genes previously discussed.

The rs10455872 variant was observed to double the odds of AVC in all cohorts tested (Table 4.3). This SNP, which is a major determinant

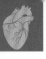

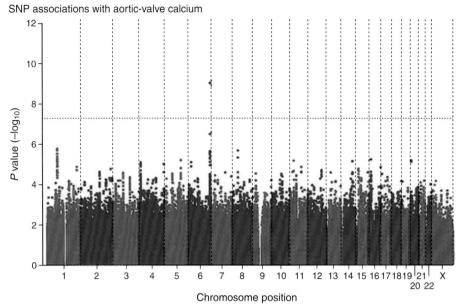

SNP associations with aortic-valve calcium

Fig. 4.4 Associations Between Each Single-Nucleotide Polymorphism *(SNP)* and Aortic Valve Calcium According to Chromosomal Position. The Manhattan plot provides evidence of association with aortic valve calcium (based on negative logarithm of the *P* value on the y-axis) across all available SNPs in the genome (chromosome location on x-axis). Higher peaks indicate lower *P* values. The peak seen on chromosome 6 is for the *LPA* locus, which is strongly associated with the finding of valve calcium. (From Thanassoulis G, Campbell CY, Owens DS, et al. Genetic associations with valvular calcification and aortic stenosis. N Engl J Med 2013;368:503-512.)

TABLE 4.3 SNP rs10455872 in *LPA* and Its Association With Aortic-Valve Calcium in White Europeans in the Discovery and Replication Cohorts.

Cohort	Minor Allele Frequency	No. of Participants	Odds Ratio (95% CI)	P Value
Discovery				
FHS	0.07	1298	2.33 (1.42–3.81)	7.9×10^{-4}
AGES-RS	0.06	3120	2.04 (1.52–2.74)	1.9×10^{-6}
MESA	0.06	2527	1.80 (1.09–2.97)	0.022
Pooled FHS, AGES-RS, and MESA cohorts	0.07	6942	2.05 (1.63–2.57)	9.0×10^{-10}
Replication				
HNR	0.06	745	2.04 (1.13–3.67)	0.018
Pooled FHS, AGES-RS, MESA, and HNR cohorts	0.07	7687	2.05 (1.66–2.53)	2.8×10^{-11}

AGES-RS, Age, Gene/Environment Susceptibility–Reykjavík Study; *FHS*, Framingham Heart Study; *HNR*, Heinz Nixdorf Recall study; *MESA*, Multi-Ethnic Study of Atherosclerosis.
From Thanassoulis G, Campbell CY, Owens DS, et al. Genetic associations with valvular calcification and aortic stenosis. N Engl J Med 2013; 368:503-512.

of circulating plasma Lp(a), was also validated prospectively in two cohorts, demonstrating a marked increased risk of incident AS. Based on the known biology of this SNP and using a mendelian randomization analysis, which leverages the inherent randomization of genetic material, the study authors demonstrated that the "genetically increased" Lp(a) level, as determined by the *LPA* genotype, was strongly associated with AS, with a hazard ratio of 1.68 per risk allele.

The *LPA* association with AS has been robustly replicated and validated by several independent groups.[91–93] The findings support a

true causal relationship between circulating Lp(a) levels and the development of AS, and for the first time, point to a potential novel therapeutic strategy to reduce aortic valve disease. Although limited options currently exist to lower Lp(a) levels, novel therapies are in development, including apo(a) antisense agents that lead to a more than 90% reduction in Lp(a) levels and that eventually may be used in randomized trials to test efficacy of Lp(a) lowering in AS.[94,95]

Recent evidence also supports the role of Lp(a) in AS progression. Capoulade et al, in an ancillary study of the ASTRONOMER trial, demonstrated that individuals in the highest Lp(a) tertile had a higher

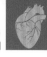

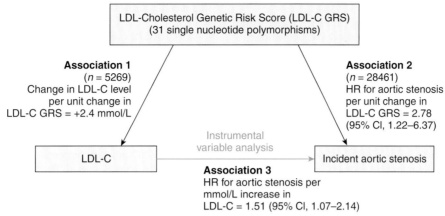

Fig. 4.5 Mendelian Randomization of Low-Density Lipoprotein Cholesterol *(LDL-C)* and Risk of Aortic Stenosis in the Malmö Diet and Cancer Study. Mendelian randomization is provides a robust test of the association between LDL-C and aortic stenosis (i.e., association 3). Association 3 can be tested by using standard epidemiologic methods, but these methods may be biased (e.g., confounding, reverse causality). To overcome this bias, mendelian randomization indirectly tests association 3 by first establishing by linear regression that LDL-C–related single nucleotide polymorphisms (SNPs) increase LDL-C (i.e., association 1). The LDL-C SNPs are then tested for an association with aortic stenosis (i.e., association 2). Under the assumption that the entire effect of the LDL-C SNPs on aortic stenosis (i.e., association 2) is mediated by their effect on increasing LDL-C (i.e., association 1), an unconfounded assessment of association 3 can be obtained (i.e., instrumental variable estimate). *HR,* Hazard ratio. (From Smith JG, Luk K, Schulz C-A, et al. Association of low-density lipoprotein cholesterol-related genetic variants with aortic valve calcium and incident aortic stenosis. JAMA 2014;312:1764-1771.

progression rate, especially younger participants.[96] Individuals with high Lp(a) levels (>58.5 mg/dL) had a 2.6-fold increase in the odds of having rapid progression (95% CI: 1.4–5.0, $P = 0.003$) and a 2-fold increase (95% CI: 1.0–3.4, $P = 0.04$) in the composite end point of aortic valve replacement or cardiac death. Among individuals older than 57 years of age, the odds ratio was 4.9 (95% CI: 1.8–13.7, $P = 0.002$) for rapid progression and 5.5 (95% CI: 1.7–17.5, $P = 0.004$) for valve replacement/cardiac death.

To further evaluate the role of other lipids, the CHARGE Consortium reported a large-scale, mendelian randomization study that examined the role of LDL-C, high-density lipoprotein cholesterol (HDL-C), and triglycerides using strongly associated genetic variants from throughout the genome. They demonstrated that a genetic predisposition to elevated LDL-C, but not other lipids, was associated with AVC (OR per genetic score increment = 1.38, 95% CI: 1.09–1.74, $P = 0.007$) and AS (HR per genetic score increment = 2.78, 95% CI: 1.22–6.37, $P = 0.02$) (Figs. 4.5 and 4.6).[31]

These results strongly support a causal role for elevated LDL-C levels in the development of CAVD and suggest that lowering LDL-C levels may be a therapeutic strategy for prevention. Given the failure of statin therapy for AS, these results also suggest the importance of starting lipid interventions earlier in the disease process, before significant calcification occurs.

Two additional genetic loci with robust associations with AS have been identified. A variant on chromosome 1 near the *PALMD* gene and a second variant on chromosome 2 near the *TEX41* gene have been associated with AS in two large-scale studies.[97,98] Both variants were also associated with other congenital malformations, which may suggest a role in cardiac valve development.

MITRAL ANNULAR CALCIFICATION

Mitral annular calcium (MAC) is defined as evidence of calcium deposition in the fibrous base of the mitral valve. MAC more frequently

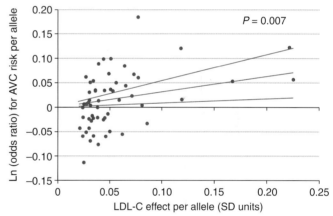

Fig. 4.6 Magnitude of Genetic Increase in Single Low-Density Lipoprotein Cholesterol *(LDL-C)* and Odds of Aortic Valve Calcium *(AVC)* Across All LDL-C Single Nucleotide Polymorphisms (SNPs) in the Cohorts for Heart and Aging Research (CHARGE) Consortium Participants. Each *dot* represents a single LDL-C SNP. Across all 57 LDL-C–associated SNPs, a given genetic increase in LDL-C correlated with a concomitant increase in the odds of AVC. The *solid line* represents the best line of fit, and the *dashed lines* represent the 95% confidence interval for this relationship; the *P* value reported is for the linear association. (From Smith JG, Luk K, Schulz C-A, et al. Association of low-density lipoprotein cholesterol-related genetic variants with aortic valve calcium and incident aortic stenosis. JAMA 2014;312:1764-1771.)

affects the posterior annulus than the anterior and is easily observed by echocardiography and cardiac CT. From population cohorts, the prevalence of MAC was determined to be 9% to 20%, depending on the age and prevalence of cardiovascular risk factors.[11,99] MAC has been associated with increased cardiovascular events (including increased cardiovascular mortality), increased risk of coronary artery disease and stroke, mitral regurgitation, and occasionally mitral stenosis.[100–105]

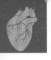

Risk Factors

The cause of MAC is not well established but appears to have many risk factors similar to those for atherosclerosis and AVC but with some potential differences. Similar to CAVD, the most important risk factor for MAC is advanced age.[11,81,99,106] Other risk factors shared with CAVD include cigarette smoking, diabetes, and increased BMI. Hypertension and left ventricular hypertrophy have been associated with MAC, suggesting that increased hemodynamic stress may play a role in calcification of the annulus.[107]

As seen in CAVD, renal dysfunction and abnormal calcium-phosphate metabolism has been associated with MAC.[108] In contrast to CAVD, LDL-C and HDL-C have not been strongly associated with MAC in most cohorts, and female sex (as opposed to male sex) is more strongly associated with MAC.[99,109] In the Framingham Heart Study, high-sensitivity C-reactive protein (CRP), a marker of inflammation, was associated with MAC, which was not observed for AVC.[11]

Genetic Factors

Our understanding of the genetics of MAC is limited. MAC in early adulthood has been associated with Marfan syndrome, which is caused by mutations in the *FBN1* gene, but whether this is directly attributable to loss of fibrillin-1 or secondary to hemodynamic stresses due to abnormalities in valve function remains unknown. Individuals with Hurler syndrome may develop MAC as children, but the pathophysiology is not well understood.[110]

The only genome-wide association study of MAC was performed by the CHARGE Consortium, who identified a common variant that achieved genome-wide significance near the *IL36G* gene (previously called *IL1F9*), which codes for interleukin-36γ (Fig. 4.7). The variant conferred a 1.66 increase in the odds of MAC (95% CI: 1.39–1.98, $P = 1.5 \times 10^{-8}$).[32] However, this variant was replicated only in MESA Hispanic Americans. Although this finding is interesting because it invokes a possible proinflammatory pathway that could be targeted by

drug therapy, further work is required to validate the finding in other cohorts.

The CHARGE Consortium reported the first mendelian randomization study of MAC that examined plasma lipids. They demonstrated that genetic predisposition to elevated triglyceride levels, but not LDL-C or HDL-C, was strongly associated with MAC (OR per unit of the genetic risk score = 1.73, 95% CI: 1.24–2.41).[111] These results were replicated among MESA Hispanic Americans and were robust in several sensitivity analyses addressing genetic pleiotropy. The results provide evidence that circulating triglycerides are causal in the development of MAC and may represent a therapeutic target to prevent MAC and its complications. The association may also explain the strong link between MAC and obesity, metabolic syndrome, and diabetes, which are all characterized by elevated triglyceride levels.

SUMMARY

Calcific mitral and aortic valve diseases are common conditions frequently seen in the aging population and are associated with significant morbidity and mortality as they advance to overt, symptomatic valve disease. Although the causes of and risk factors for calcific valve diseases are not well established, available evidence suggests a strong overlap with traditional atherosclerotic risk factors and with emerging risk factors such as vascular stiffness, inflammation, and mineral metabolism. Genetic evidence points to Lp(a) and LDL-C for CAVD and triglycerides and inflammation for MAC as causal factors and therefore as therapeutic targets for these diseases. Whether earlier intense modification of lipid levels and inflammation with novel lipid-lowering therapy (e.g., PCSK9i, *LPA* antisense molecules) or antiinflammatory agents can reduce the incidence of valve disease remains to be seen. However, ongoing investigation, especially in the genetics of CAVD, will undoubtedly point to novel therapeutic strategies.

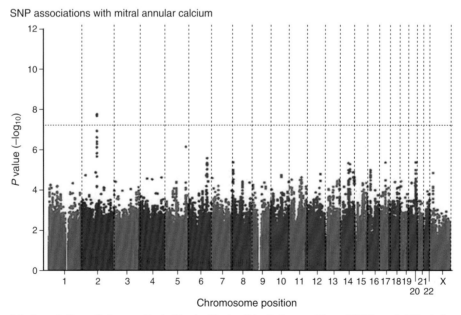

Fig. 4.7 Associations Between Each Single Nucleotide Polymorphism (SNP) and Mitral Annular Calcium According to Chromosomal Position. The Manhattan plot provides evidence of association with mitral annular calcium (based on negative logarithm of the *P* value on the y-axis) across all available SNPs in the genome (chromosome location on x-axis). Higher peaks indicate lower *P* values. The peak seen on chromosome 2 is for the *IL1F9* locus, which is strongly associated with mitral annular calcium. (From Thanassoulis G, Campbell CY, Owens DS, et al. Genetic associations with valvular calcification and aortic stenosis. N Engl J Med 2013;368:503-512.)

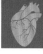

REFERENCES

1. Yutzey KE, Demer LL, Body SC, et al. Calcific aortic valve disease: a consensus summary from the Alliance of Investigators on Calcific Aortic Valve Disease. Arterioscler Thromb Vasc Biol 2014;34:2387-2393.

2. Lindroos M, Kupari M, Heikkilä J, Tilvis R. Prevalence of aortic valve abnormalities in the elderly: an echocardiographic study of a random population sample. J Am Coll Cardiol 1993;21:1220-1225.

3. Otto CM, Lind BK, Kitzman DW, et al. Association of aortic-valve sclerosis with cardiovascular mortality and morbidity in the elderly. N Engl J Med 1999;341:142-147.

4. Eveborn GW, Schirmer H, Heggelund, et al. The evolving epidemiology of valvular aortic stenosis. The Tromsø study. Heart 2013;99:396-400.

5. Roger VL, Go AS, Lloyd-Jones DM, et al. Heart disease and stroke statistics—2012 update: a report from the American Heart Association. Circulation 2012;125:e2-e220.

6. Clark MA, Arnold SV, Duhay FG, et al. Five-year clinical and economic outcomes among patients with medically managed severe aortic stenosis: results from a Medicare claims analysis. Circ Cardiovasc Qual Outcomes 2012;5:697-704.

7. Danielsen R, Aspelund T, Harris TB, Gudnason V. The prevalence of aortic stenosis in the elderly in Iceland and predictions for the coming decades: the AGES-Reykjavík study. Int J Cardiol 2014;176:916-922.

8. O'Brien KD, Reichenbach DD, Marcovina SM, et al. Apolipoproteins B, (a), and E accumulate in the morphologically early lesion of "degenerative" valvular aortic stenosis. Arterioscler Thromb Vasc Biol 1996;16:523-532.

9. Otto CM, Kuusisto J, Reichenbach DD, et al. Characterization of the early lesion of "degenerative" valvular aortic stenosis. Histological and immunohistochemical studies. Circulation 1994;90:844-853.

10. Stewart BF, Siscovick D, Lind BK, et al. Clinical factors associated with calcific aortic valve disease. Cardiovascular Health Study. J Am Coll Cardiol 1997;29:630-634.

11. Thanassoulis G, Massaro JM, Cury R, et al. Associations of long-term and early adult atherosclerosis risk factors with aortic and mitral valve calcium. J Am Coll Cardiol 2010;55:2491-2498.

12. García-Rubira JC, López V, Cubero J. Coronary arterial disease in patients with severe isolated aortic stenosis. Int J Cardiol 1992;35:121-122.

13. Chan KL, Teo K, Dumesnil JG, et al. Effect of lipid lowering with rosuvastatin on progression of aortic stenosis: results of the aortic stenosis progression observation: measuring effects of rosuvastatin (ASTRONOMER) trial. Circulation 2010;121:306-314.

14. Cowell SJ, Newby DE, Prescott RJ, et al. A randomized trial of intensive lipid-lowering therapy in calcific aortic stenosis. N Engl J Med 2005;352:2389-2397.

15. Rossebø AB, Pedersen TR, Boman K, et al. Intensive lipid lowering with simvastatin and ezetimibe in aortic stenosis. N Engl J Med 2008;359:1343-1356.

16. Osnabrugge RLJ, Mylotte D, Head SJ, et al. Aortic stenosis in the elderly: disease prevalence and number of candidates for transcatheter aortic valve replacement: a meta-analysis and modeling study. J Am Coll Cardiol 2013;62:1002-1012.

17. Owens DS, Katz R, Takasu J, et al. Incidence and progression of aortic valve calcium in the Multi-Ethnic Study of Atherosclerosis (MESA). Am J Cardiol 2010;105:701-708.

18. Owens DS, Katz R, Johnson E, et al. Interaction of age with lipoproteins as predictors of aortic valve calcification in the multi-ethnic study of atherosclerosis. Arch Intern Med 2008;168:1200-1207.

19. Patel DK, Green KD, Fudim M, et al. Racial differences in the prevalence of severe aortic stenosis. J Am Heart Assoc 2014;3:e000879.

20. Lindroos M, Kupari M, Valvanne J, et al. Factors associated with calcific aortic valve degeneration in the elderly. Eur Heart J 1994;15:865-870.

21. Capoulade R, Clavel M-A, Mathieu P, et al. Impact of hypertension and renin-angiotensin system inhibitors in aortic stenosis. Eur J Clin Invest 2013;43:1262-1272.

22. Linefsky J, Katz R, Budoff M, et al. Stages of systemic hypertension and blood pressure as correlates of computed tomography-assessed aortic valve calcium (from the Multi-Ethnic Study of Atherosclerosis). Am J Cardiol 2011;107:47-51.

23. Tastet L, Capoulade R, Clavel M-A, et al. Systolic hypertension and progression of aortic valve calcification in patients with aortic stenosis: results from the PROGRESSA study. Eur Heart J Cardiovasc Imaging 2017;18:70-78.

24. Yan AT, Koh M, Chan KK, et al. Association between cardiovascular risk factors and aortic stenosis: the CANHEART aortic stenosis study. J Am Coll Cardiol 2017;69:1523-1532.

25. Rahimi K, Mohseni H, Kiran A, et al. Elevated blood pressure and risk of aortic valve disease: a cohort analysis of 5.4 million UK adults. Eur Heart J 2018;39:3596-3603.

26. Sera F, Russo C, Iwata S, et al. Arterial wave reflection and aortic valve calcification in an elderly community-based cohort. J Am Soc Echocardiogr 2015;28:430-436.

27. Sverdlov AL, Ngo DTM, Chan WPA, et al. Determinants of aortic sclerosis progression: implications regarding impairment of nitric oxide signalling and potential therapeutics. European Heart Journal 2012;33:2419-2425.

28. O'Brien KD, Probstfield JL, Caulfield MT, et al. Angiotensin-converting enzyme inhibitors and change in aortic valve calcium. Arch Intern Med 2005;165:858-862.

29. Rosenhek R, Rader F, Loho N, et al. Statins but not angiotensin-converting enzyme inhibitors delay progression of aortic stenosis. Circulation 2004;110:1291-1295.

30. Novaro GM, Katz R, Aviles RJ, et al. Clinical factors, but not C-reactive protein, predict progression of calcific aortic-valve disease: the Cardiovascular Health Study. J Am Coll Cardiol 2007;50:1992-1998.

31. Smith JG, Luk K, Schulz C-A, et al. Association of low-density lipoprotein cholesterol-related genetic variants with aortic valve calcium and incident aortic stenosis. JAMA 2014;312:1764-1771.

32. Thanassoulis G, Campbell CY, Owens DS, et al. Genetic associations with valvular calcification and aortic stenosis. N Engl J Med 2013;368:503-512.

33. Katz R, Budoff MJ, Takasu J, et al. Relationship of metabolic syndrome with incident aortic valve calcium and aortic valve calcium progression: the Multi-Ethnic Study of Atherosclerosis (MESA). Diabetes 2009;58:813-819.

34. Katz R, Wong ND, Kronmal R, et al. Features of the metabolic syndrome and diabetes mellitus as predictors of aortic valve calcification in the Multi-Ethnic Study of Atherosclerosis. Circulation 2006;113:2113-2119.

35. Capoulade R, Clavel M-A, Dumesnil JG, et al. Impact of metabolic syndrome on progression of aortic stenosis: influence of age and statin therapy. J Am Coll Cardiol 2012;60:216-223.

36. Larsson SC, Wolk A, Håkansson N, Bäck M. Overall and abdominal obesity and incident aortic valve stenosis: two prospective cohort studies. Eur Heart J 2017;38:2192-2197.

37. Michel PL. Aortic stenosis in chronic renal failure patients treated by dialysis. Nephrol Dial Transplant 1998;13(Suppl 4):44-48.

38. Straumann E, Meyer B, Misteli M, et al. Aortic and mitral valve disease in patients with end stage renal failure on long-term haemodialysis. Br Heart J 1992;67:236-239.

39. Maher ER, Young G, Smyth-Walsh B, et al. Aortic and mitral valve calcification in patients with end-stage renal disease. The Lancet 1987;2:875-877.

40. Maher ER, Pazianas M, Curtis JR. Calcific aortic stenosis: a complication of chronic uraemia. Nephron 1987;47:119-122.

41. Hoshina M, Wada H, Sakakura K, et al. Determinants of progression of aortic valve stenosis and outcome of adverse events in hemodialysis patients. J Cardiol 2012;59:78-83.

42. Perkovic V, Hunt D, Griffin SV, et al. Accelerated progression of calcific aortic stenosis in dialysis patients. Nephron Clin Pract 2003;94:c40-c45.

43. Ureña P, Malergue MC, Goldfarb B, et al. Evolutive aortic stenosis in hemodialysis patients: analysis of risk factors. Nephrologie 1999;20:217-225.

44. Mills WR, Einstadter D, Finkelhor RS. Relation of calcium-phosphorus product to the severity of aortic stenosis in patients with normal renal function. Am J Cardiol 2004;94:1196-1198.

45. Ix JH, Shlipak MG, Katz R, et al. Kidney function and aortic valve and mitral annular calcification in the Multi-Ethnic Study of Atherosclerosis (MESA). Am J Kidney Dis 2007;50:412-420.

46. Guerraty MA, Chai B, Hsu JY, et al. Relation of aortic valve calcium to chronic kidney disease (from the Chronic Renal Insufficiency Cohort Study). Am J Cardiol 2015;115:1281-1286.

47. Vavilis G, Bäck M, Occhino G, et al. Kidney dysfunction and the risk of developing aortic stenosis. J Am Coll Cardiol 2019;73:305-314.

48. Linefsky JP, O'Brien KD, Sachs M, et al. Serum phosphate is associated with aortic valve calcification in the Multi-Ethnic Study of Atherosclerosis (MESA). Atherosclerosis 2014;233:331-337.

49. Linefsky JP, O'Brien KD, Katz R, et al. Association of serum phosphate levels with aortic valve sclerosis and annular calcification: the Cardiovascular Health Study. J Am Coll Cardiol 2011;58:291-297.

50. Boström KI, Rajamannam NM, Towler DA. The regulation of valvular and vascular sclerosis by osteogenic morphogens. Circ Res 2011;109:564-577.

51. Mohler ER, Kaplan FS, Pignolo RJ. Boning-up on aortic valve calcification. J Am Coll Cardiol 2012;60:1954-1955.

52. Rajamannam NM, Subramaniam M, Rickard D, et al. Human aortic valve calcification is associated with an osteoblast phenotype. Circulation 2003;107:2181-2184.

53. Mohler ER, Gannon F, Reynolds C, et al. Bone formation and inflammation in cardiac valves. Circulation 2001;103:1522-1528.

54. Miller JD, Weiss RM, Serrano KM, et al. Evidence for active regulation of pro-osteogenic signaling in advanced aortic valve disease. Arterioscler Thromb Vasc Biol 2010;30:2482-2486.

55. Kaden JJ, Bickelhaupt S, Grobholz R, et al. Receptor activator of nuclear factor kappaB ligand and osteoprotegerin regulate aortic valve calcification. J Mol Cell Cardiol 2004;36:57-66.

56. Hofbauer LC, Schoppet M. Clinical implications of the osteoprotegerin/RANKL/RANK system for bone and vascular diseases. JAMA 2004;292:490-495.

57. Venuraju SM, Yerramasu A, Corder R, Lahiri A. Osteoprotegerin as a predictor of coronary artery disease and cardiovascular mortality and morbidity. J Am Coll Cardiol 2010;55:2049-2061.

58. Kiechl S, Schett G, Wenning G, et al. Osteoprotegerin is a risk factor for progressive atherosclerosis and cardiovascular disease. Circulation 2004;109:2175-2180.

59. Kiechl S, Werner P, Knoflach M, et al. The osteoprotegerin/RANK/RANKL system: a bone key to vascular disease. Expert Rev Cardiovasc Ther 2006;4:801-811.

60. Persy V, D'Haese P. Vascular calcification and bone disease: the calcification paradox. Trends Mol Med 2009;15:405-416.

61. Aksoy Y, Yagmur C, Tekin GO, et al. Aortic valve calcification: association with bone mineral density and cardiovascular risk factors. Coron Artery Dis 2005;16:379-383.

62. Pfister R, Michels G, Sharp SJ, et al. Inverse association between bone mineral density and risk of aortic stenosis in men and women in EPIC-Norfolk prospective study. Int J Cardiol 2015;178:29-30.

63. Chan JJ, Cupples LA, Kiel DP, et al. QCT volumetric bone mineral density and vascular and valvular calcification: the Framingham Study. J Bone Miner Res 2015;30:1767-1774.

64. Hekimian G, Boutten A, Flamant M, et al. Progression of aortic valve stenosis is associated with bone remodelling and secondary hyperparathyroidism in elderly patients—the COFRASA study. Eur Heart J 2013;34:1915-1922.

65. Dweck MR, Khaw HJ, Sng GKZ, et al. Aortic stenosis, atherosclerosis, and skeletal bone: is there a common link with calcification and inflammation? Eur Heart J 2013;34:1567-1574.

66. Aksoy O, Cam A, Goel SS, et al. Do bisphosphonates slow the progression of aortic stenosis? J Am Coll Cardiol 2012;59:1452-1459.

67. Elmariah S, Delaney JAC, O'Brien KD, et al. Bisphosphonate use and prevalence of valvular and vascular calcification in women MESA (the Multi-Ethnic Study of Atherosclerosis). J Am Coll Cardiol 2010;56:1752-1759.

68. Skolnick AH, Osranek M, Formica P, Kronzon I. Osteoporosis treatment and progression of aortic stenosis. Am J Cardiol 2009;104:122-124.

69. Sterbakova G, Vyskocil V, Linhartova K. Bisphosphonates in calcific aortic stenosis: association with slower progression in mild disease—a pilot retrospective study. Cardiology 2010;117:184-189.

70. Messika-Zeitoun D, Bielak LF, Peyser PA, et al. Aortic valve calcification: determinants and progression in the population. Arterioscler Thromb Vasc Biol 2007;27:642-648.

71. Cripe L, Andelfinger G, Martin LJ, et al. Bicuspid aortic valve is heritable. J Am Coll Cardiol 2004;44:138-143.

72. Horne BD, Camp NJ, Muhlestein JB, Cannon-Albright LA. Evidence for a heritable component in death resulting from aortic and mitral valve diseases. Circulation 2004;110:3143-148.

73. Le Gal G, Bertault V, Bezon E, et al. Heterogeneous geographic distribution of patients with aortic valve stenosis: arguments for new aetiological hypothesis. Heart 2005;91:247-249.

74. Probst V, Le Scouarnec S, Legendre A, et al. Familial aggregation of calcific aortic valve stenosis in the western part of France. Circulation 2006;113:856-860.

75. Barr DP, Rothbard S, Eder HA. Atherosclerosis and aortic stenosis in hypercholesteremic xanthomatosis. J Am Med Assoc 1954;156:943-947.

76. Rajamannam NM, Edwards WD, Spelsberg TC. Hypercholesterolemic aortic-valve disease. N Engl J Med 2003;349:717-718.

77. Miller JD, Weiss RM, Serrano KM, et al. Lowering plasma cholesterol levels halts progression of aortic valve disease in mice. Circulation 2009;119:2693-2701.

78. Weiss RM, Ohashi M, Miller JD, et al. Calcific aortic valve stenosis in old hypercholesterolemic mice. Circulation 2006;114:2065-2069.

79. Hannoush H, Introne WJ, Chen MY, et al. Aortic stenosis and vascular calcifications in alkaptonuria. Mol Genet Metab 2012;105:198-202.

80. Garg V, Muth AN, Ransom JF, et al. Mutations in NOTCH1 cause aortic valve disease. Nature 2005;437:270-274.

81. Nigam V, Srivastava D. Notch1 represses osteogenic pathways in aortic valve cells. J Mol Cell Cardiol 2009;47:828-834.

82. Morgan TM, Krumholz HM, Lifton RP, Spertus JA. Nonvalidation of reported genetic risk factors for acute coronary syndrome in a large-scale replication study. JAMA 2007;297:1551-1561.

83. Ortlepp JR, Hoffmann R, Ohme F, et al. The vitamin D receptor genotype predisposes to the development of calcific aortic valve stenosis. Heart 2001;85:635-638.

84. Nordström P, Glader CA, Dahlén G, et al. Oestrogen receptor alpha gene polymorphism is related to aortic valve sclerosis in postmenopausal women. J Intern Med 2003;254:140-146.

85. Avakian SD, Annicchino-Bizzacchi JM, Grinberg M, et al. Apolipoproteins AI, B, and E polymorphisms in severe aortic valve stenosis. Clin Genet 2001;60:381-384.

86. Novaro GM, Sachar R, Pearce GL, et al. Association between apolipoprotein E alleles and calcific valvular heart disease. Circulation 2003;108:1804-1808.

87. Ortlepp JR, Pillich M, Mevissen V, et al. APOE alleles are not associated with calcific aortic stenosis. Heart 2006;92:1463-1466.

88. Gaudreault N, Ducharme V, Lamontagne M, et al. Replication of genetic association studies in aortic stenosis in adults. Am J Cardiol 2011;108:1305-1310.

89. Ortlepp JR, Schmitz F, Mevissen V, et al. The amount of calcium-deficient hexagonal hydroxyapatite in aortic valves is influenced by gender and associated with genetic polymorphisms in patients with severe calcific aortic stenosis. Eur Heart J 2004;25:514-522.

90. Ellis SG, Dushman-Ellis S, Luke MM, et al. Pilot candidate gene analysis of patients ≥60 years old with aortic stenosis involving a tricuspid aortic valve. Am J Cardiol 2012;110:88-92.

91. Arsenault BJ, Boekholdt SM, Dubé M-P, et al. Lipoprotein(a) levels, genotype, and incident aortic valve stenosis: a prospective Mendelian randomization study and replication in a case-control cohort. Circ Cardiovasc Genet 2014;7:304-310.

92. Cairns BJ, Coffey S, Travis RC, et al. A replicated, genome-wide significant association of aortic stenosis with a genetic variant for lipoprotein(a): meta-analysis of published and novel data. Circulation 2017;135:1181-1183.

93. Kamstrup PR, Tybjaerg-Hansen A, Nordestgaard BG. Elevated lipoprotein(a) and risk of aortic valve stenosis in the general population. J Am Coll Cardiol 2014;63:470-477.

94. Tsimikas S, Viney NJ, Hughes SG, et al. Antisense therapy targeting apolipoprotein(a): a randomised, double-blind, placebo-controlled phase 1 study. Lancet 2015;386:1472-1483.

95. Viney NJ, van Capelleveen JC, Geary RS, et al. Antisense oligonucleotides targeting apolipoprotein(a) in people with raised lipoprotein(a): two randomised, double-blind, placebo-controlled, dose-ranging trials. Lancet 2016;388:2239-2253.

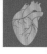

96. Capoulade R, Chan KL, Yeang C, et al. Oxidized phospholipids, lipoprotein(a), and progression of calcific aortic valve stenosis. J Am Coll Cardiol 2015;66:1236-1246.

97. Helgadottir A, Thorleifsson G, Gretarsdottir S, et al. Genome-wide analysis yields new loci associating with aortic valve stenosis. Nat Commun 2018;9:987.

98. Thériault S, Gaudreault N, Lamontagne M, et al. A transcriptome-wide association study identifies PALMD as a susceptibility gene for calcific aortic valve stenosis. Nat Commun 2018;9:988.

99. Kanjanauthai S, Nasir K, Katz R, et al. Relationships of mitral annular calcification to cardiovascular risk factors: the Multi-Ethnic Study of Atherosclerosis (MESA). Atherosclerosis 2010;213:558-562.

100. Fox CS, Vasan RS, Parise H, et al. Mitral annular calcification predicts cardiovascular morbidity and mortality: the Framingham Heart Study. Circulation 2003;107:1492-1496.

101. Völzke H, Haring R, Lorbeer R, et al. Heart valve sclerosis predicts all-cause and cardiovascular mortality. Atherosclerosis 2010;209:606-610.

102. Ramaraj R, Manrique C, Hashemzadeh M, Movahed M-R. Mitral annulus calcification is independently associated with all-cause mortality. Exp Clin Cardiol 2013;18:e5–e7.

103. Atar S, Jeon DS, Luo H, Siegel RJ. Mitral annular calcification: a marker of severe coronary artery disease in patients under 65 years old. Heart 2003;89:161-164.

104. Benjamin EJ, Plehn JF, D'Agostino RB, et al. Mitral annular calcification and the risk of stroke in an elderly cohort. N Engl J Med 1992;327:374-379.

105. Kizer JR, Wiebers DO, Whisnant JP, et al. Mitral annular calcification, aortic valve sclerosis, and incident stroke in adults free of clinical cardiovascular disease: the Strong Heart Study. Stroke 2005;36:2533-2537.

106. Sell S, Scully RE. Aging changes in the aortic and mitral valves. Histologic and histochemical studies, with observations on the pathogenesis of calcific aortic stenosis and calcification of the mitral annulus. Am J Pathol 1965;46:345-365.

107. Elmariah S, Delaney JAC, Bluemke DA, et al. Associations of LV hypertrophy with prevalent and incident valve calcification: Multi-Ethnic Study of Atherosclerosis. JACC Cardiovasc Imaging 2012;5:781-788.

108. Umana E, Ahmed W, Alpert MA. Valvular and perivalvular abnormalities in end-stage renal disease. Am J Med Sci 2003;325:237-242.

109. Elmariah S, Budoff MJ, Delaney JAC, et al. Risk factors associated with the incidence and progression of mitral annulus calcification: the Multi-Ethnic Study of Atherosclerosis. Am Heart J 2013;166:904-912.

110. Schieken RM, Kerber RE, Ionasescu VV, Zellweger H. Cardiac manifestations of the mucopolysaccharidoses. Circulation 1975;52:700-705.

111. Afshar M, Luk K, Do R, et al. Association of triglyceride-related genetic variants with mitral annular calcification. J Am Coll Cardiol 2017;69:2941-2948.

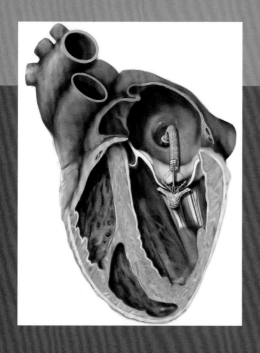

第5章
瓣膜性心脏病的左心室和血管变化

左心室和血管的适应性改变和后果是左心瓣膜疾病发病率和死亡率的基础。适应性改变是指瓣膜病变如何影响左心室的大小、重塑和功能。随着病情进展，左心室的结构和功能以不同的方式适应压力超负荷和容量超负荷。为优化以患者为中心的长期结局，阐明这些心室和血管变化的病理生理学，并了解其短期和长期后果，在更恰当的时间进行瓣膜干预以终止瓣膜进一步病变，对确定血管和左心室辅助药物治疗的新靶点具有重要作用。

熟悉压力-容量环是了解瓣膜性心脏病左心室反应的基础，核心概念包括前负荷、后负荷和收缩能力。瓣膜性心脏病引起前负荷、后负荷及心肌收缩能力不同程度改变，影响每搏输出量和心排量，表现为压力-容量环不同程度的变化。本章重点介绍了以下内容。

1.动脉粥样硬化压力超负荷、二尖瓣关闭不全容量超负荷和主动脉瓣反流压力超负荷和容量超负荷的综合作用。

2.左心室肥厚性重塑主要有4种类型：①正常几何形状；②同心性重塑；③向心性肥大；④离心性肥厚。肥厚性心室重塑的模式、程度和时间，除受特定瓣膜病变类型影响之外，还受年龄、性别、遗传、代谢因素、冠状动脉疾病和血压等多种因素的影响。

3.心室结构和功能的变化既可以是适应代偿性改变，也可以是失代偿性改变，并且在重度瓣膜病变修复后，可有不同程度的逆转。

4.左心室整体纵向应变检测可识别亚临床左心室收缩功能障碍，并与死亡率增加有关。

5.肺动脉高压在瓣膜疾病患者中很常见，并且与症状发作、症状严重程度和较低的生存率密切相关。

6.左心瓣膜疾病患者的肺静脉压通常会升高，肺血管重塑和（或）血管收缩，引起肺血管阻力增加，进一步升高肺动脉压。肺动脉高压的存在和严重程度及其在瓣膜手术后的可逆性具有预后意义。

7.全身性血管系统参与了瓣膜病（包括主动脉瓣狭窄）患者左心室的后负荷形成，影响瓣膜病变引起的左心室重塑和功能改变。

从病理生理和临床的角度，将肺血管、左心房、左心室、二尖瓣、主动脉瓣及全身血管系统视为一个整体，各组成部分之间相互影响，这种相互作用对症状的发作和严重程度、瓣膜的干预时机及进行瓣膜手术后预期的临床改善均有影响。

谢慕蓉

Left Ventricular and Vascular Changes in Valvular Heart Disease

Brian R. Lindman

CHAPTER OUTLINE

KEY POINTS

- In patients with significant valve disease, symptom onset, morbidity, and mortality after fixing the valve lesion are influenced by ventricular and vascular factors.
- The structure and function of the left ventricle adapt differently over time to pressure overload (e.g., aortic stenosis) and volume overload (e.g., mitral regurgitation).
- Changes to ventricular structure and function can be both adaptive and maladaptive and reverse to various degrees after significant valvular abnormalities are fixed.
- The pattern, extent, and timing of hypertrophic ventricular remodeling are influenced by numerous factors beyond the specific valve abnormality.

- Pulmonary hypertension is common in patients with valve disease and associated with symptom onset, symptom severity, and lower survival.
- In patients with left-sided valve disease, pulmonary venous pressures are commonly elevated, but reactive changes in the pulmonary vasculature can also cause concomitant increases in pulmonary vascular resistance.
- The systemic vasculature contributes to the afterload on the left ventricle in patients with valve disease, including aortic stenosis.
- From a pathophysiologic and clinical perspective, it is helpful to think of the pulmonary vasculature, left atrium and ventricle, mitral and aortic valves, and systemic vasculature as an integrated unit in which the components have bidirectional influences on one another.

The adaptations to and consequences of left-sided valve lesions underlie the morbidity and mortality that accompany them. Commonly, the adaptive response is conceptualized in terms of how it affects the size, remodeling, and function of the left ventricle (LV). Overgeneralizing, mitral regurgitation (MR) is a volume overload lesion that over time produces LV dilation and eccentric hypertrophy, whereas aortic stenosis (AS) is a pressure overload lesion that initially induces a smaller LV cavity and concentric hypertrophy. These changes in LV size and remodeling are accompanied by changes in diastolic and systolic function that become more abnormal if the valve lesion is not fixed.

While not diminishing the importance of these changes in LV structure and function in response to valve lesions, it is increasingly clear that the pulmonary and systemic vasculature changes in response to valve lesions plays an important role in the manifestations of valve disease and their clinical consequences.[1-4] It is likely best to take a more integrative perspective of the relationships of the pulmonary vasculature, left atrium (LA), mitral and aortic valves, LV, and systemic vasculature. The relationships within the valvular-ventricular-vascular unit are not linear or unidirectional, but bidirectional (Fig. 5.1). These complex interactions are modified by genetics, environment, sex, metabolic health, age, coronary artery disease, and other factors.

Dynamic changes brought on by activity or exercise also influence these interactions and the consequences of left-sided valve lesions.

Although some of the structural and functional changes in the LV and vasculature may not manifest overtly (e.g., reduced LV ejection fraction [EF]) before valve treatment, they may be maladaptive and only partially reversible, making the patient more vulnerable to heart failure or other adverse consequences after valve interventions.[5] To optimize long-term patient-centered outcomes, it is important to elucidate the pathophysiology of these ventricular and vascular changes and understand their short-term and long-term consequences to more appropriately time interventions to fix valve pathology and to identify novel targets for adjunctive medical therapy in the vasculature and the LV.[6]

LEFT VENTRICULAR HEMODYNAMICS: PRESSURE-VOLUME LOOPS

Familiarity with pressure-volume (PV) loops is foundational for understanding the LV response to stenosis or regurgitation of the mitral or aortic valves.[7] Core concepts include preload, afterload, and contractility. Fig. 5.2 shows a generic PV loop, with labels describing each part of the loop and important lines.

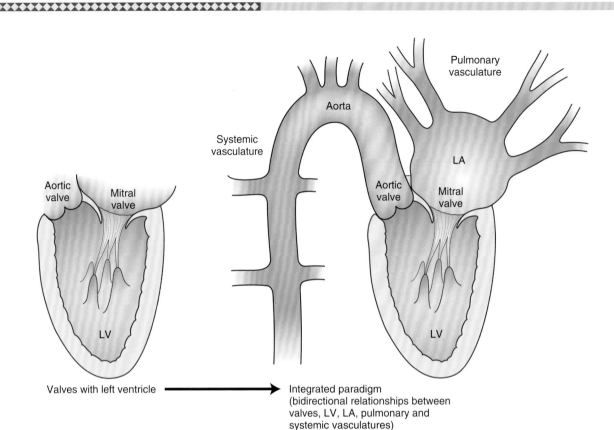

Fig. 5.1 Integrated Paradigm of Valvular, Ventricular, and Vascular Interactions. Rather than the aortic and mitral valves interacting with the LV in isolation, there are bidirectional interactions among the aortic and mitral valves, LV, LA, and pulmonary and systemic vasculatures.

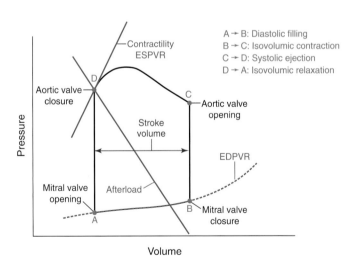

Fig. 5.2 Pressure-Volume Loop. Mitral valve opening *(A)*, mitral valve closure *(B)*, aortic valve opening *(C)*, aortic valve closure *(D)*, diastolic filling *(A to B)*, isovolumic contraction *(B to C)*, systolic ejection *(C to D)*, and isovolumic relaxation *(D to A)* are shown. The end-systolic pressure-volume relationship *(ESPVR)* line represents contractility. The end-diastolic pressure-volume relationship *(EDPVR)* line represents the compliance of the ventricle. Afterload is represented by the line connecting the maximum end-diastolic point on the x-axis intersection and the point representing aortic valve closure on the pressure-volume loop. Stroke volume is shown. The y-axis is the LV pressure. The x-axis is the LV volume.

Preload is the stretch of the sarcomeres in the myocardium at end-diastole before contraction. Preload is proportional to the volume of blood in the ventricle at end-diastole, but it is also influenced by the pressure required to achieve that volume. Preload is increased by increased blood volume or increased vasomotor tone in the venous system that increases blood return to the heart. An increase in preload, specifically an increase in end-diastolic volume, is associated with a rise in stroke volume if afterload and contractility remain constant (Fig. 5.3).

In contrast, a decrease in preload is associated with a decrease in stroke volume (see Fig. 5.3). Pertinent to this chapter, valve disease that alters the normal flow of blood through and out of the heart may also increase LV end-diastolic volume (e.g., MR, aortic regurgitation [AR]). Moreover, changes in the diastolic properties of the heart may increase preload, even at the same end-diastolic volume. Hypertrophic remodeling that decreases the compliance of the heart shifts the end-diastolic PV curve, or compliance curve, upward and to the left, and for any given LV end-diastolic volume, the end-diastolic pressure is higher (Fig. 5.4).

Afterload is the resistance to muscle fiber shortening during the systolic, or ejection, phase of the cardiac cycle. Muscle fiber tension, or wall stress, is quantified by the law of Laplace, which states that wall stress equals the intraventricular pressure multiplied by the radius of the LV cavity, divided by twice the thickness of the LV wall. Usually, the intraventricular pressure is essentially equal to aortic pressure. Increased pressure in the aorta (e.g., hypertension) and increased LV chamber dilation increase afterload, whereas an increase in wall thickness reduces wall stress and afterload.

On a PV loop, afterload, or arterial elastance, is represented by the line between the maximum LV end-diastolic point on the x-axis and the point of aortic valve closure at end-systole (Fig. 5.5). An increase in the slope of this line reflects an increase in afterload, which is accompanied by a decrease in stroke volume for a given preload and contractility

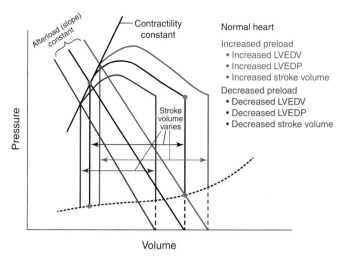

Fig. 5.3 Changes in Preload. An increase in preload (increased LV end-diastolic volume *[LVEDV]*) is associated with an increase in LV end-diastolic pressure *(LVEDP)* and increased stroke volume *(blue)*. A decrease in preload (decreased LVEDV) is associated with a decrease in LVEDP and decreased stroke volume *(red)*.

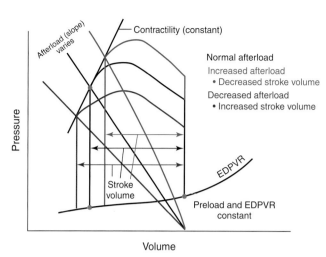

Fig. 5.5 Changes in Afterload. An increase in afterload, which is represented as a steeper angle of the afterload line, is associated with a decreased stroke volume when preload and contractility remain constant *(blue)*. A decrease in afterload, which is represented as a less steep angle of the afterload line, is associated with an increased stroke volume when preload and contractility remain constant *(red)*. *EDPVR*, End-diastolic pressure-volume relationship.

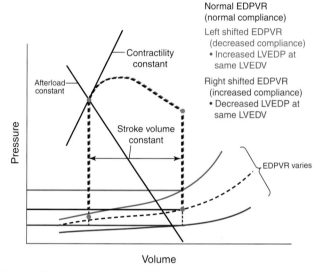

Fig. 5.4 Changes in Ventricular Compliance. A decrease in ventricular compliance is shown by the movement of the end-diastolic pressure-volume relationship *(EDPVR)* curve upward and to the left *(blue)*. This is associated with an increase in the LV end-diastolic pressure *(LVEDP)*. An increase in ventricular compliance is shown by the movement of the EDPVR curve downward and to the right *(red)*. This is associated with a decrease in the LVEDP. *LVEDV*, Left ventricular end-diastolic volume.

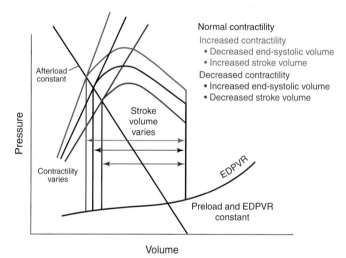

Fig. 5.6 Changes in Contractility. An increase in contractility, which is represented as a steeper angle of the end-systolic pressure-volume relationship *(EDPVR)* line, is associated with an increased stroke volume when preload and afterload remain constant *(blue)*. A decrease in contractility, which is represented as a less steep angle of the EDPVR, is associated with a decreased stroke volume when preload and afterload remain constant *(red)*.

(see Fig. 5.5). In contrast, a decrease in the slope of the line, perhaps related to administration of a vasodilator, reflects a decrease in afterload, which is accompanied by an increase in stroke volume for a given preload and contractility (see Fig. 5.5). An LV outflow tract obstruction, such as AS, adds resistance to LV emptying. The pressure gradient across the obstructed valve yields a much higher intraventricular pressure than aortic pressure, contributing to higher wall stress that is magnified as the severity of valve stenosis progresses.

Contractility is the calcium-dependent ability of muscle to contract, or generate force, at a given fiber length. In terms of PV loops, the contractility of the ventricle as a whole is considered, and it may be altered by multiple factors, including inotropes, acidosis, and exercise. However,

myocardial contractility may differ across the heart due to infarction, nonmyocyte infiltration, variation in electrical activation, and other regional differences. On a PV loop, contractility is represented by the line connecting the intersection of the x-axis and y-axis and the point representing end-systole (i.e., end-systolic PV line) (Fig. 5.6). This is also referred to as *end-systolic elastance*.

For a given preload and afterload, an increase in contractility leads to a decrease in the LV end-systolic volume and a resulting increase in stroke volume (see Fig. 5.6). In contrast, a decrease in contractility is associated with an increase in end-systolic volume and decrease in stroke volume (see Fig. 5.6). For patients with valve disease, compensatory mechanisms in place that alter contractility to preserve hemodynamics

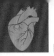

in the face of increased afterload or preload may begin to fail over time, which may precede or accompany the clinical decline of the patient.

LEFT VENTRICULAR HYPERTROPHIC REMODELING

The heart can undergo hypertrophic remodeling in response to a variety of stimuli.[8] Depending on the stimulus, this hypertrophic growth may be partially or completely reversible. Hypertrophic growth can be adaptive, as in the case of exercise, or pathologic, as in the case of hypertrophic cardiomyopathy.

The four principal categories of hypertrophic remodeling are (1) normal geometry; (2) concentric remodeling; (3) concentric hypertrophy; and (4) eccentric hypertrophy (Fig. 5.7).[9] The patterns of hypertrophic remodeling associated with each left-sided valve lesion are shown in Fig. 5.7. Numerous factors influence the type and degree of remodeling that may occur in a given individual, including age, sex, genetics, metabolic factors, coronary disease, and blood pressure.[10] Pressure or volume overload, or both, from heart valve disease can have an important effect on hypertrophic remodeling of the LV.

CHANGES TO THE LEFT VENTRICLE WITH LEFT-SIDED VALVE DISEASE

Aortic Stenosis
Pressure Overload
A simplified PV loop for AS may show the increase in afterload (due to an increase in ventricular pressure associated with the valvular

obstruction) and a resulting decrease in stroke volume (Fig. 5.8). However, several adaptive and maladaptive mechanisms influence preload, afterload, and contractility in patients with AS, yielding a more complex hemodynamic reality.

In most patients with AS, stroke volume is maintained at normal levels, even when AS is severe. The increased afterload often leads to an

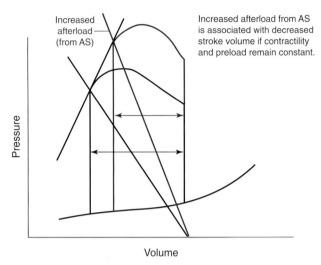

Fig. 5.8 Aortic Stenosis *(AS)* on a Pressure-Volume Loop. AS imposes increased afterload on the LV, which is shown by a steeper angle of the afterload line. Stroke volume is decreased when preload and contractility remain constant.

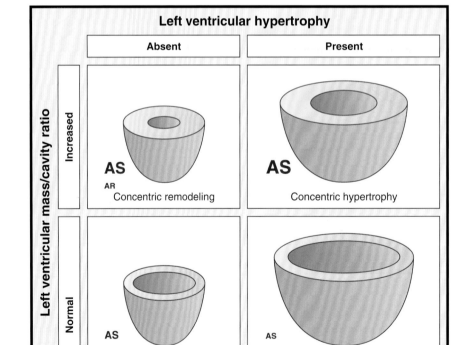

Fig. 5.7 LV Hypertrophic Remodeling. Patterns of LV hypertrophy are shown based on LV mass and the relative increase in mass versus cavity dimension. The patterns of remodeling for each left-sided valve lesion are shown with approximate proportions according to font size of the valve lesion. *AS,* Aortic stenosis; *AR,* atrial aortic regurgitation; *MR,* mitral regurgitation. (Modified from Lindman BR, Clavel MA, Mathieu P, et al. Calcific aortic stenosis. Nat Rev Dis Primers 2016;3.2:16006.)

increased end-diastolic volume and pressure (i.e., right side of the PV loop moves rightward). Hypertrophic remodeling impairs LV compliance, causing the LV end-diastolic PV curve to move upward and to the left. Increased preload activates Frank-Starling mechanisms, which along with increased circulating catecholamines increases contractility. Increased LV wall thickness may mitigate the increase in wall stress caused by the increased intraventricular pressure. Higher resistance and stiffness in the systemic vasculature of older adults with AS may cause higher systemic pressures and increased impedance to LV ejection, which together increase the vascular contribution to afterload beyond the valvular obstruction (Fig. 5.9).

Depending on the severity of AS and the extent of adaptive and maladaptive ventricular and vascular changes, the PV loops for individual patients with AS can look somewhat different and can evolve over time for a given patient as AS progresses and compensatory mechanisms develop and then fail.

Effects on Left Ventricular Remodeling and Function

Based on the principles of Ohm's law, as resistance to flow out of the LV increases due to progressive narrowing of the aortic valve, pressure inside the ventricle must increase to maintain flow. In 1975, Grossman et al used echocardiography and careful hemodynamic measurements to show that despite higher LV pressures, patients with AS had a wall stress comparable to normal controls.[11] They also observed that the patients with AS had increased absolute and relative wall thickness and had increased LV mass index. Based on Laplace's law, they hypothesized that initially increased wall stress resulting from increased LV pressures was a stimulus for a hypertrophic response that increased wall thickness, normalizing wall stress. Because LV ejection performance is directly affected by afterload (i.e., wall stress), this hypertrophic remodeling was seen as an important compensatory mechanism of the heart in the face of pressure overload from AS, but the physiology is not that simple.[12]

Hypertrophic remodeling in response to pressure overload occurs at a macroscopic and microscopic level. At a macro level, LV wall thickness and mass increase, manifesting most commonly as concentric

remodeling (i.e., increase in wall thickness but not LV mass) or concentric hypertrophy (i.e., increase in wall thickness and LV mass) and less commonly as eccentric hypertrophy (see Fig. 5.7).[13] Underlying these gross changes is myocyte hypertrophy, apoptosis, and replacement and interstitial fibrosis.[10] Details on the molecular mechanisms implicated in these changes can be found in Chapter 3, particularly Table 3.4.

Individuals with AS have impaired coronary flow reserve, and the amount of LV hypertrophy is associated with the degree of impairment.[14-16] Combined with more myocardial mass and increased intraventricular pressures, this can result in subendocardial ischemia. Although pressure overload is a stimulus for hypertrophic remodeling, the severity of AS does not closely correlate with the degree of hypertrophy.[17,18] Sex, genetics, vascular load, metabolic abnormalities, and numerous other factors influence the hypertrophic response to pressure overload.[18-21]

Structural changes in the myocardium (particularly fibrosis), increased myocyte passive tension, advanced glycation end products, abnormalities in calcium handling and metabolism, and titin isoenzyme shifts and hypophosphorylation are associated with impaired relaxation and increased stiffness that characterize diastolic dysfunction in the pressure-overloaded ventricle.[22-26]

Abnormal LV diastolic function accounts for most of the heart failure symptoms experienced by patients with AS and portends a worse prognosis for symptomatic and asymptomatic patients with AS.[27-29] Although there may be some improvements in diastolic function, it may also worsen after valve replacement.[30,31]

Assessment of LV systolic function by EF may be misleading in patients with LV remodeling. Global longitudinal strain detects subclinical systolic dysfunction, which is associated with increased mortality.[32-34] Eventually, if severe valve obstruction is not treated, overt systolic dysfunction manifested by a reduced EF will develop. Accumulating clinical evidence shows that although LV hypertrophy can decrease wall stress, more advanced hypertrophic remodeling is associated with worse systolic function, worse heart failure symptoms, and worse perioperative and long-term clinical outcomes after valve replacement.[35-41]

Preclinical studies have demonstrated that blocking the hypertrophic response to pressure overload does not have deleterious effects on LV performance despite increased wall stress.[42,43] Not only is the more marked increase in myocardial mass deleterious, but a more specific aspect of hypertrophic remodeling (i.e., cardiac fibrosis) has been identified as an adverse prognostic marker.[44] Increased midwall fibrosis (not fibrosis due to previous myocardial infarction) is an independent predictor of death for patients with moderate or severe AS and is associated with less improvement in LV function after valve replacement.[45-47] Weidemann et al reported that patients with severe fibrosis, despite an EF that was preserved, were more likely to have worse pre-operative heart failure symptoms and did not experience an improvement in their symptoms 9 months after valve replacement, whereas those with none or minimal fibrosis generally improved.[48] The amount of fibrosis does not appear to be related (at least not strongly) to the degree of hypertrophic remodeling.[45,48]

Hypertrophic remodeling of the heart can be maladaptive or adaptive, and in patients with AS, it may represent a combination of both.[8,20,49] The degree to which LV hypertrophic remodeling is maladaptive or adaptive and its consequent functional and clinical effects are not simply issues of how much muscle there is. The mass and geometry are only part of the story; the composition and energetics of the muscle matter.[49]

This could have implications for decisions on optimal timing of valve replacement. Perhaps some patients with severe asymptomatic AS or even moderate AS but clear evidence of maladaptive hypertrophic remodeling might benefit from valve replacement before symptoms

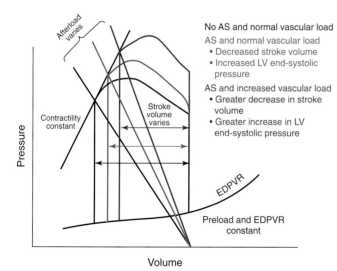

Fig. 5.9 Aortic Stenosis *(AS)* **With Different Vascular Loads.** AS with normal vascular load is associated with a decreased stroke volume and increased end-systolic pressure. Increased pulsatile and resistive load in the systemic vasculature further increases afterload beyond the increased afterload caused by valve obstruction, further decreasing stroke volume and increasing end-systolic pressure. These changes assume that preload and contractility remain constant. *EDPVR,* End-systolic pressure-volume relationship.

develop and the hypertrophic remodeling becomes less reversible. Simplistic cutpoints to trigger surgical referral based on the mass or geometry of the LV are likely too insensitive and nonspecific because the composition of the muscle undoubtedly matters. Further research is needed to determine whether circulating biomarkers or cardiac imaging with cardiac magnetic resonance could help in this regard.[50–52]

After relief of pressure overload with valve replacement, hypertrophic remodeling of the LV tends to reverse and is usually accompanied by improvements in LV function.[5,53] However, among patients, this reverse remodeling progresses at different rates and to various extents.[5,41,54,55] Multiple factors likely contribute to the pace and degree of reversibility in hypertrophic remodeling, but the reversal has clinical consequences.[5,56,57] In a series of patients with severe LV hypertrophy undergoing transcatheter aortic valve replacement (TAVR), those with a greater decrease in LV mass index at 30 days after TAVR had one half of the rate of hospitalizations over the subsequent year.[5] Further studies are needed to determine whether particular medical therapies may augment regression of LV hypertrophy after valve replacement and whether this may be clinically beneficial.[58]

Mitral Regurgitation
Volume Overload
In patients with MR, because of incomplete closure of the mitral valve and because LV pressure exceeds LA pressure during the period that the aortic valve is closed, there is no isovolumic contraction or relaxation phase. During what would normally be isovolumic contraction, before aortic valve opening, blood begins to leak from the LV into the LA, decreasing the LV volume. After the aortic valve closes, during what would normally be isovolumic contraction, blood continues to leak backward from the ventricle into the atrium, continuing to decrease LV volume. These phases therefore contribute to the regurgitant volume along with that occurring during the systolic ejection phase.

Due to the regurgitant volume, the LV then fills with an increased blood volume during diastole. The individual with MR shows an increased LV end-diastolic volume, which occurs at an increased end-diastolic pressure. Compensatory remodeling (i.e., LV dilation) tends to lower the end-diastolic PV curve due to improved LV compliance. There is an increase in LV end-diastolic volume, but there is a decrease in end-systolic volume. Together, there is an increase in total stroke volume. The amount that represents forward versus regurgitant stroke volume depends on the effective regurgitant orifice area and systemic blood pressure and arterial load. The shape of the PV loop for patients with MR differs based on a variety of factors, some of which may evolve over time, including the severity of MR, LV remodeling and compensation, total-body volume status, and systemic vascular pressure and load (Fig. 5.10).

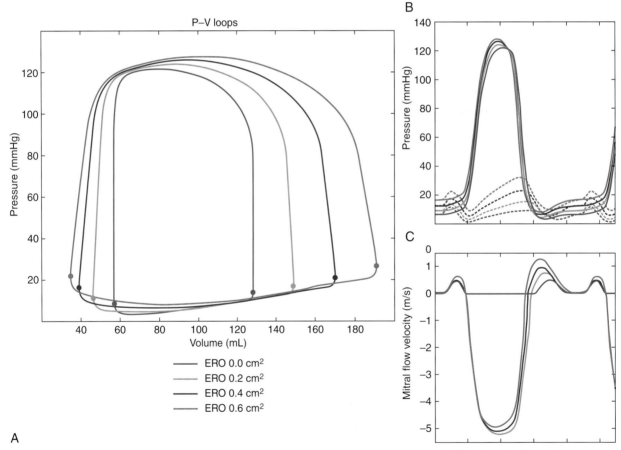

Fig. 5.10 Mitral Regurgitation on a Pressure-Volume Loop. The disappearance of isovolumic phases is visualized as the progressive angulation of the vertical segments of the pressure-volume *(P-V)* loops as the effective regurgitant orifice *(ERO)* exceeds 0.0 cm²; *bullets* depict the onset and end of the regurgitant period (A). LV *(solid lines)* and atrial *(dashed lines)* pressure evolution with time (B). Transmitral flow velocity, showing progressive shortening of the regurgitant time with increasing degrees of mitral regurgitation (C). (From Martinez-Legazpi P, Yotti R, Bermejo J. How heavy is the load? The ventricular mechanics of mitral regurgitation revisited in the era of percutaneous therapies. Heart 2017;103:567-569.)

Effects on Left Ventricular Remodeling and Function

MR increases the amount of blood that flows into the LV during diastole in proportion to the regurgitant volume. Based on the LV end-diastolic PV relationship, this increase in volume tends to increase LV end-diastolic pressure. However, in the presence of chronic volume overload, there is an increase in LV cavity compliance. The increase in compliance allows the ventricle to accommodate higher diastolic volumes while maintaining normal or near-normal end-diastolic pressure. Related to this, total stroke volume is increased, and forward stroke volume is maintained. This is explained by a larger volume of blood at end-diastole and increased preload by means of the Frank-Starling mechanism. Increases in sympathetic tone may also increase contractility initially.[59] Together, these adaptive changes enable many patients with significant MR to maintain a normal forward stroke volume and achieve expected levels of peak exercise capacity.[60]

The effects of MR on afterload are more complex. MR is often conceptualized as a state of reduced afterload due to a low impedance leak into the LA.[61,62] In this regard, terminology is important. Impedance is a hydraulic opposition, obstruction, or resistance to blood flow, whereas afterload is related to myocardial mechanics and the forces resisting myocardial shortening (i.e., wall stress).

Gaasch et al elegantly address the myth that blood flow into the LA represents a low impedance pathway.[63] In a double-outlet model, they showed that impedance to retrograde flow into the LA was greater than forward flow into the aorta over a range of regurgitant fractions up to 57% (Fig. 5.11). Although the pressure in the LA is relatively low compared with the aorta, yielding a larger downward pressure gradient between the ventricle and atrium compared with that between the ventricle and aorta, the effective regurgitant orifice area through the mitral valve is relatively small compared with a normal aortic valve orifice. Smaller holes cause greater obstruction to flow. Until the effective regurgitant orifice becomes quite large, impedance to retrograde flow is relatively greater than to forward flow. The total impedance to flow out of the double-outlet LV, however, was lower than normal impedance to LV flow.

Afterload is quantified by Laplace's law, in which wall stress equals LV pressure multiplied by the radius of the LV chamber, divided by twice the wall thickness. The study by Gaasch and many other studies have demonstrated that afterload in patients with chronic compensated MR is normal but is abnormally elevated in the decompensated phase due to progressive enlargement of the LV chamber.[63–67]

As a measure of LV performance or function, given its load dependence, EF is a misleading and poor tool.[68] Prior studies have demonstrated that a preoperative EF below 60% to 64% is associated with increased mortality rates and a greater incidence of postoperative LV dysfunction.[69,70] Despite a preserved EF, many patients with MR demonstrate reduced contractility.[71,72] Later studies have shown that rest and exercise measures of global longitudinal strain, a more sensitive measure of systolic function, can predict cardiovascular events and postoperative LV dysfunction in patients with primary MR (Fig. 5.12).[73–76] In contrast, preoperative EF was not a good predictor of postoperative LV function in any of these studies.[77] Insofar as monitoring LV function is a primary focus of following patients with MR to determine the optimal timing of surgery in asymptomatic patients, only following LV EF appears to be insufficient.

Changes in LV EF after mitral valve surgery are due to alterations in preload, afterload, contractility, and LV chamber size. It is commonly assumed that EF decreases after surgery because elimination of the regurgitant orifice has removed the low resistance path for flow out of the ventricle and afterload has increased. However, unless the regurgitant orifice is very large, the retrograde flow into the LA is actually the higher impedance path. Instead, before repair, the double outlet (i.e., forward and retrograde) from the LV yields an overall impedance

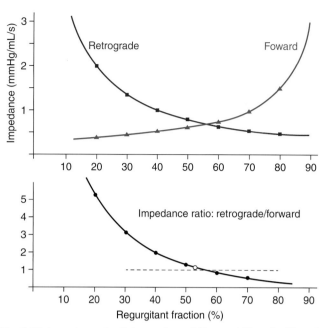

Fig. 5.11 Impedance to Retrograde and Forward Flow in Chronic Mitral Regurgitation. The model is based on an end-diastolic volume of 180 mL, an ejection fraction of 60%, and a LV mean systolic pressure of 100 mmHg. The durations of retrograde and forward flow were taken as 400 and 300 ms, respectively. In the upper panel, the impedance to retrograde flow (*solid squares*) is plotted against regurgitant fraction; the coordinates were calculated over a wide range of regurgitant fractions (at intervals of 10%). The impedance to forward flow (*solid triangles*) is plotted against regurgitant flow over the same range of regurgitant fractions. The impedance to retrograde flow is greater than forward flow over a wide range of regurgitant fractions up to 57%. Only when the regurgitant fraction exceeds 57% is the impedance to retrograde flow less than to forward flow. In the lower panel, the ratio of retrograde to forward impedance (*solid circles*) is plotted against regurgitant fraction. The model indicates that a ratio exceeding 1 (*broken line*) reflects a higher impedance to retrograde flow than to forward flow. The average ratio (1.22 ± 0.19) of the patient group with a regurgitant fraction of 53% ± 4% (*open circle*) is superimposed on the model. (From Gaasch WH, Shah SP, Labib SB, Meyer TE. Impedance to retrograde and forward flow in chronic mitral regurgitation and the physiology of a double outlet ventricle. Heart 2017;103:581-585.)

to flow out of the ventricle that is lower than normal. When one of the outlets is removed, the impedance to flow increases. Initially, there may be a reduction in EF, but as LV end-diastolic and end-systolic volumes decrease, EF quickly returns to normal as long as the chordal apparatus is maintained and contractile function is preserved.[68,72]

After correction of MR, the reverse remodeling of the LV and its optimal long-term function depend on microstructural and macrostructural changes and impairment of contractility that might have occurred in response to chronic volume overload. For example, evidence of increased oxidative stress has been observed in the myocardium of patients undergoing surgery for primary MR, which can have implications for postoperative ventricular performance.[71] To optimize postprocedural LV performance and freedom from heart failure, future research needs to identify more sophisticated tools to provide a window into the biology of the myocardium. A greater sensitivity is needed for the detection of early signs of maladaptive, prognostic changes in the ventricle to refine decision making about the optimal timing of surgical correction.

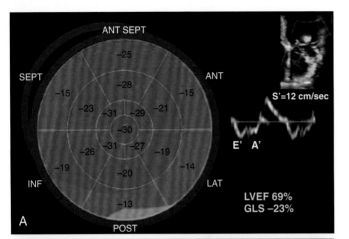

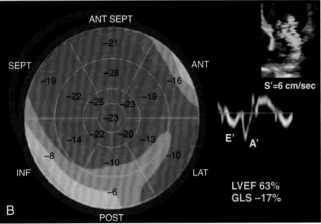

Fig. 5.12 Global Longitudinal Strain in Patients With Severe Primary Mitral Regurgitation and Preserved LV Ejection Fraction. The bull's eyes show the difference in global longitudinal strain *(GLS)* for two patients with severe primary mitral regurgitation *(MR)* and normal LV ejection fraction *(LVEF)*. The reduced GLS observed in patient B can be attributed to more advanced disease with subclinical LV dysfunction. (From Galli E, Lancellotti P, Sengupta PP, Donal E. LV mechanics in mitral and aortic valve diseases: value of functional assessment beyond ejection fraction. JACC Cardiovasc Imaging 2014;7:1151-1166.)

Aortic Regurgitation: Mixed Pressure and Volume Overload

AR is associated with combined volume and pressure overload on the LV. During diastole, normal diastolic filling through the mitral valve is augmented by regurgitant flow through the aortic valve from the higher-pressure aorta, resulting in a higher LV end-diastolic volume (Fig. 5.13). The LV responds by dilating to increase compliance and accommodate the increased volume at a lower LV end-diastolic pressure. By Frank-Starling mechanisms, this increased preload is accompanied by increased contractility, yielding a normal end-systolic volume when the ventricle is compensated. According to Laplace's law, however, the LV dilation is accompanied by an increase in wall stress.[66] This triggers hypertrophic remodeling, characterized by myocyte hypertrophy and increased interstitial fibrosis.[78] Although patients with AS tend to develop concentric hypertrophy and patients with MR develop eccentric hypertrophy, those with AR usually develop eccentric hypertrophy, but with greater wall thickness than observed with MR.

As with MR, there is no isovolumic relaxation or contraction phase in patients with AR (see Fig. 5.13). Immediately after systole, because aortic pressure exceeds LV pressure, blood begins to flow from the

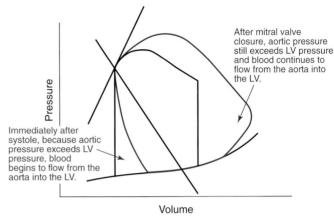

Fig. 5.13 Aortic Regurgitation on a Pressure-Volume Loop. Aortic regurgitation initially imposes an increased volume load on the LV. Due to regurgitant flow after the aortic valve should have closed, the LV volume is already increased when the mitral valve opens. After mitral valve closure, the LV volume continues to increase due to regurgitant flow through the aortic valve. Stroke volume is increased as a result of the increased LV volume. Compensatory mechanisms include dilation of the LV, which can also increase afterload over time (not shown).

aorta into the ventricle. At end-diastole, when the mitral valve closes, the aortic pressure still exceeds LV pressure, and blood continues to flow from the aorta into the LV.

Over time and with increasing severity of AR, the LV end-diastolic volumes can become markedly enlarged (Fig. 5.14). The systolic wall stress increases, and contractile function begins to decline, yielding increases in LV end-systolic volume and LV end-diastolic pressure. Unloading the heart with aortic valve replacement lowers wall stress and improves LV ejection performance, although contractile dysfunction may remain impaired.[79]

VASCULAR PROPERTIES AND LOAD

The properties of the pulmonary and systemic vasculature have an important influence on the pathophysiology and clinical manifestations of valvular heart disease. Often only considered in terms of pressure, the physiology is more complex. Total vascular hydraulic load, or opposition to flow, must be considered in terms of steady or resistive load (e.g., systemic vascular resistance) and pulsatile load (i.e., impedance) related to wave reflections and vascular stiffness (Table 5.1).[80-82] Although there are associations between pressure and pulsatile and resistive load, they are not equivalent and are often discordant. For example, the patient in shock is hypotensive but may have very high (e.g., cardiogenic shock) or very low (e.g., distributive shock) systemic vascular resistance.

Vascular resistance can be calculated with Ohm's law ($V = IR$; voltage = electrical current × resistance) in mind. Resistance equals the pressure drop across a vascular bed divided by the flow. For example, systemic vascular resistance is related to the pressure difference from the proximal aorta (i.e., mean arterial pressure) to the right atrium divided by cardiac output. Vascular resistance is related in part to smooth muscle tone and is usually responsive to pharmacologic interventions (e.g., vasopressors, vasodilators).

Impedance is the ratio of the pulsatile change in pressure divided by the pulsatile change in flow in a given vessel.[81] It is directly related to vessel stiffness, which is often measured by pulse wave velocity and indirectly to the cross-sectional area of the blood vessel. Pulsatile load, or impedance, is less dynamic because it is related to the stiffness of the vessel (often due to calcification and fibrosis) that is less responsive to pharmacologic interventions.[83]

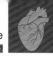

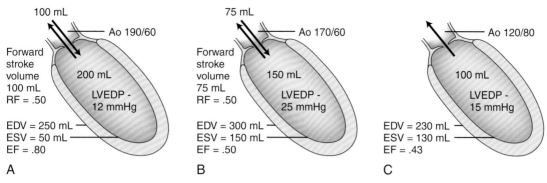

Fig. 5.14 Hemodynamics of Aortic Regurgitation. Hemodynamic changes occur in chronic compensated aortic regurgitation (AR). Eccentric hypertrophy produces increased end-diastolic volume *(EDV)*, which permits an increase in total and forward stroke volume. The volume overload is accommodated, and LV filling pressure is normalized. Ventricular emptying and end-systolic volume *(ESV)* remain normal (A). In chronic decompensated AR, impaired LV emptying produces an increase in ESV and a fall in ejection fraction *(EF)*, total stroke volume, and forward stroke volume. Further cardiac dilation and recurrent elevation of LV filling pressure occur (B). Immediately after valve replacement, preload estimated by EDV decreases, as does filling pressure. ESV also is decreased, but to a lesser extent; the result is an initial fall in EF. Despite these changes, elimination of AR leads to an increase in forward stroke volume, and with time, EF increases (C). *Ao,* Aortic pressure; *LVEDP,* left ventricular end-diastolic pressure; *RF,* regurgitant fraction.

TABLE 5.1 Vascular Load Parameters.

Type of Vascular Load	Definition	Terms Used	Measurement
Resistive load	Nonoscillatory (steady) opposition to flow; related to vasomotor properties and vascular smooth muscle cell proliferation	Systemic vascular resistance, pulmonary vascular resistance	Can be measured invasively or by combining echocardiographic measurements and sphygmomanometer readings
Pulsatile load	Opposition to pulsatile flow; change in pressure divided by change in flow; related to vessel stiffness and size and wave travel and reflections	Characteristic impedance, input impedance, arterial stiffness, pulse wave velocity, compliance, distensibility, elasticity	Can be measured invasively or noninvasively using echocardiographic measurements and sphygmomanometer readings, magnetic resonance imaging, or tonometry-based techniques

Pulmonary Vascular Changes

Pulmonary hypertension (PH) is defined as a mean pulmonary artery pressure $\geq$ 25 mmHg.[84] Precapillary PH is characterized by a pulmonary capillary wedge pressure or LV end-diastolic pressure $\leq$ 15 mmHg, whereas postcapillary PH is characterized by a pulmonary capillary wedge pressure or LV end-diastolic pressure $\geq$ 15 mmHg.[84] Postcapillary PH may be isolated (i.e., diastolic pulmonary artery pressure minus pulmonary artery wedge pressure < 7 mmHg) or combined with precapillary PH (i.e., diastolic pulmonary artery pressure minus pulmonary artery wedge pressure $\geq$ 7 mmHg).[85]

Other terminology used to distinguish patients with postcapillary PH includes passive PH (i.e., transpulmonary gradient $\leq$ 12 mmHg; pulmonary vascular resistance [PVR] < 3 Wood units) versus reactive or mixed PH (i.e., transpulmonary gradient >12 mmHg; PVR $\geq$ 3 Wood units).[84,86] Postcapillary PH, or PH due to left-sided heart disease, is classified as WHO group II and is the most common cause of PH.[86,87]

Mitral and aortic valve diseases are among the many causes of increased LA pressure, which is transmitted to the pulmonary vasculature, causing increased pulmonary pressures. Even without any changes in the pulmonary vasculature, an elevated pulmonary venous pressure is associated with an elevation in the pulmonary artery pressure. Remodeling or vasoconstriction, or both, of the pulmonary vasculature can lead to an increase in the PVR, further elevating the pulmonary arterial pressure. Although the pulmonary venous pressure is mostly related to adaptations in the LA and LV in response to the valvular lesion, the response of the pulmonary vasculature in patients with left-sided valve disease is less predictable. Changes in vasomotor tone and vascular remodeling are likely related to multiple factors, including the chronicity of pulmonary venous hypertension, sex, genetics, lung disease, the metabolic milieu, endothelial dysfunction, desensitization to natriuretic peptide–induced vasodilation, and decreased nitric oxide availability.[85,88]

Although the connection between PH and valve disease is most commonly attributed to mitral stenosis, PH is also found in patients with MR and AS. In younger, healthier patients undergoing surgical aortic valve replacement, PH has been observed in approximately one half of patients, whereas in older and sicker patients undergoing TAVR, PH is present in 64% to 75% and is moderate to severe in 25%.[4,89,90] In MR, the prevalence is fairly similar.[91,92]

In patients with left-sided valve disease, the presence and severity of PH has clinical consequences, most importantly an association with increased mortality rates.[4,89,91,92] Those with elevated PVR may be at greater risk.[89,90] Some patients may not have PH at rest, but an exercise study may uncover exercise-induced PH that has prognostic implications. Among asymptomatic patients with severe primary MR, exercise-induced PH was observed in almost one half of the patients and was a predictor of symptom-free survival.[93] Similarly, among asymptomatic patients with severe AS, exercise-induced PH was observed in 55% of patients and was associated with reduced cardiac event-free survival.

PH often improves, even normalizes, after treatment of the left-sided valve lesion.[94–97] However, due to a variety of factors, including prosthesis-patient mismatch and increased preoperative PVR, pulmonary artery pressure may remain elevated after valve surgery.[90,98,99] Residual PH is associated with increased mortality after aortic valve replacement.[89,100]

Because the presence and severity of PH and its reversibility after valve surgery have prognostic implications, it may influence decisions on the timing of valve surgery. Even in the absence of symptoms, the U.S. and European valve guidelines recommend treatment of primary MR when PH is present.[101] If the PH is severe or there is evidence of a very elevated PVR, there could be a question of whether PH is reversible and whether a valve procedure is futile. Although nitroprusside is sometimes used in a vasodilator challenge to assess the reversibility of PH and elevated PVR, it is not clear that the presence or lack of acute responsiveness to nitroprusside predicts reversibility after a valve procedure or long-term clinical outcomes. Patients who appear to have fixed PH when tested with one drug (e.g., prostaglandin E_1) may have

reversible PVR when tested with another (e.g., phosphodiesterase type 5 [PDE5] inhibitor).[102] The pulmonary hemodynamic response to a vasodilator should be assessed in the context of other clinical information and should not be the only factor considered in determining whether to proceed with surgery, keeping in mind that most patients experience an improvement in pulmonary pressures and PVR.[94]

Given the availability of drugs targeting PH, adjunctive medical therapy could potentially improve clinical outcomes of patients with valve disease and PH. Medical therapy administered before a valve procedure may decrease procedural risk, whereas medications given after a valve procedure may augment reversal of PH.

The immediate hemodynamic response to PDE5 inhibitors has been evaluated in patients with severe symptomatic AS. A single dose of sildenafil was shown to unload the left heart with a modest decrease in systemic pressures and unload the right heart (i.e., decreased PVR and increased pulmonary arterial compliance), resulting in consistently lower pulmonary artery pressures (i.e., median decrease of 25%) (Fig. 5.15).[6] In those with combined postcapillary

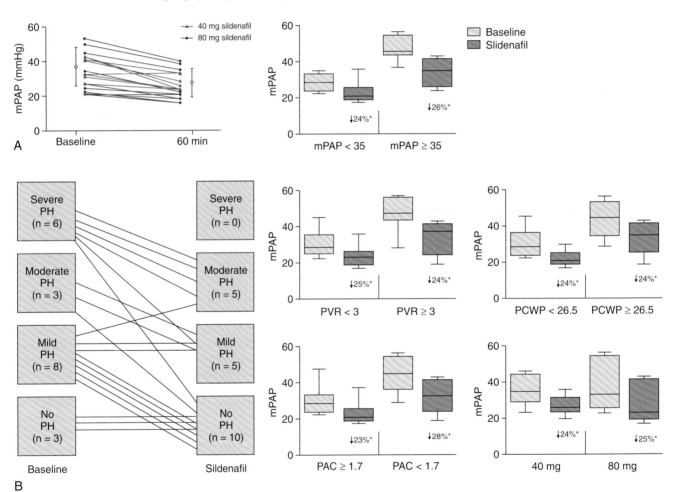

Fig. 5.15 Effect of Sildenafil on Pulmonary Vascular Hemodynamics in Patients With Severe Aortic Stenosis.* The change in mean pulmonary artery pressure *(mPAP)* from baseline to 60 minutes is shown for each patient by dose; error bars (SD) (A). The change from baseline to 60 minutes in the category of severity of pulmonary hypertension *(PH)* is shown for each subject; no PH (mPAP < 25), mild PH (25–34), moderate PH (35–44), severe PH (≥45) (B). Change in mPAP with sildenafil from baseline to 60 minutes according to dose or baseline hemodynamics with median percent change reported; the cutpoints for the pulmonary artery pressure *(PAC)* and pulmonary capillary wedge pressure *(PCWP)* groups were determined by the median value for the whole cohort (C). *Based on Wilcoxon signed-ranks test of the percent change from baseline to 60 minutes; indicates significance at *P* < 0.05. *PVR*, Pulmonary vascular resistance. (From Lindman BR, Zajarias A, Madrazo JA, et al. Effects of phosphodiesterase type 5 inhibition on systemic and pulmonary hemodynamics and ventricular function in patients with severe symptomatic aortic stenosis. Circulation 2012;125:2353-2362.)

and precapillary PH (PVR ≥3 Wood units), a single dose of sildenafil acutely reduced the PVR by a median of 52%. For the small subset of patients with severe AS and decompensated heart failure with significant PH, a few days or weeks on a PDE5 inhibitor could unload their heart and improve their pulmonary vascular hemodynamics, potentially reducing procedural risk. In a similar vain, in patients with persistent PH after a valve procedure, PDE5 inhibitors may improve the residual PH and improve clinical outcomes, although one report suggests potential harm from this strategy.[103] The clinical efficacy of these potential approaches with PDE5 inhibitors and other drugs targeting PH needs to be tested in prospective studies.

Systemic Vascular Changes

The systemic vasculature contributes to the afterload on the LV in patients with mitral or aortic valve disease, influencing the LV remodeling and functional changes that occur in response to these valve lesions. Even in patients with AS, the LV afterload is not fixed due to valve obstruction. Instead, the valve and systemic vasculature each contribute impedance to blood flow out of the LV (Fig. 5.16). The systemic vascular load manifests in terms of pressure, stiffness (i.e., pulsatile load), and resistance (i.e., resistive load).[1,81,82]

Pharmacologic agents targeting the vasculature can cause acute changes in cardiac pressures and performance, even in patients with severe calcific AS. Despite the long-standing teaching of a fixed LV afterload in patients with significant AS and concern about the potential for severe hypotension with vasodilators, Khot et al administered intravenous nitroprusside to patients with severe AS, LV dysfunction, and decompensated heart failure.[104] As expected, administration of nitroprusside was associated with a significant decline in systemic vascular resistance, but the decline in mean arterial pressure was modest because there was an accompanying marked increase in the stroke volume despite no change in the aortic valve area. Similarly, when patients with severe symptomatic AS were administered oral sildenafil, stroke volume increased despite a decrease in the pulmonary capillary wedge pressure.[6] These subjects moved to a different Frank-Starling curve because their LV afterload was decreased. The increase in stroke volume strongly correlated with a decrease in systemic vascular resistance and increase in systemic arterial compliance, whereas there was no clinically meaningful change in the aortic valve area. The anticipated favorable effects of sildenafil on the right side were accompanied by unloading of the left heart.[6]

For a similar severity of aortic valve obstruction, patients with stiffer vessels as measured by systemic arterial compliance more

commonly have LV systolic dysfunction.[105] Stiffening of the vasculature seems to play a role in the development of the paradoxical low-flow, low-gradient phenotype. Dahl et al compared patients with paradoxical low-flow, low-gradient, severe AS with patients with normal-flow, high-gradient, severe AS. They compared echocardiographic and hemodynamic data for them at the time of the index echocardiogram and looked at changes in these parameters over the 5 years before the index examination.

At the time of the index echocardiogram, aortic valve area index was similar for these patient groups. However, in patients with paradoxical low-flow, low-gradient, severe AS, the vasculature started modestly stiffer and became progressively more stiff over that 5-year period (i.e., systemic arterial compliance of 0.83 to 0.63 mL/m^2/mmHg), whereas vascular stiffness did not change over those 5 years in patients with high-gradient AS (i.e., systemic arterial compliance of 0.91 to 0.96 mL/m^2/mmHg). At the time of the index echocardiogram, the systemic arterial compliance was one-third lower in patients with paradoxical low-flow, low-gradient AS than in those with high-gradient AS. The progressive reduction in systemic arterial compliance over the 5 years in patients who would go on to develop paradoxical low-flow, low-gradient, severe AS was accompanied by a decline in LV EF and stroke volume, a decline in deceleration time, and an increase in pulmonary artery pressures, whereas there were no changes in these parameters in patients who would develop high-gradient, severe AS.

Although somewhat counterintuitive, emerging data suggest that valve function may influence systemic vascular function. Using high-fidelity sensors in the proximal aorta to make measurements of pressure and flow before and immediately after TAVR, Yotti et al demonstrated acute changes in pressure and indices of vascular function after TAVR (Fig. 5.17).[2] Valve obstruction dampened forward and backward compression waves, and immediately after valve obstruction was relieved, the systemic vasculature exhibited stiffer behavior. Valve lesions may mask and valve interventions may unmask and influence functional characteristics of the vasculature.

The potential clinical importance of blood pressure levels and vascular properties is highlighted by a recent analysis from the PARTNER trial. Evaluating patients at 30 days after transcatheter aortic valve replacement, after the valve problem had been fixed, Lindman et al observed that patients with lower systolic blood pressure had increased mortality rates (specifically cardiovascular mortality rates) between 30 days and 1 year.[1] Increased pulsatile load, but not resistive load, was associated with increased mortality. When combining systolic blood pressure and pulsatile load, patients with lower systolic blood pressure and stiffer vessels had a threefold higher mortality rate between 30 days and 1 year compared with patients with a higher blood pressure and less stiff vessels.[1]

This interplay between the valve, vasculature, and ventricle has implications for symptom onset and severity, timing of intervention on the valve, and anticipated clinical improvement after a valve procedure is performed. For example, a stiff vasculature or high systemic vascular resistance may be associated with dyspnea on exertion in a patient with moderate AS. Alternatively, a patient with low-flow, low-gradient AS and a stiff systemic vasculature may not experience the same degree of symptom improvement after the valve is replaced. This interplay also has potential implications for how we think about therapy for patients with valve disease. Perhaps, therapeutic interventions targeting the vasculature before valve intervention could mitigate maladaptive changes in the ventricle or interventions after a valve intervention might aid in reverse remodeling in the ventricle and improve clinical outcomes.

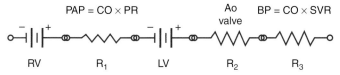

$$PAP = CO \times PR \qquad \begin{array}{c} Ao \\ valve \end{array} \qquad BP = CO \times SVR$$

RV   R$_1$ LV   R$_2$ R$_3$

Fig. 5.16 Diagram of the Circulation as an Electric Circuit. *Ao,* Aortic; *BP,* systemic blood pressure; *CO,* cardiac output; *LV,* left ventricle; *PAP,* pulmonary artery pressure; *PR,* pulmonary resistance; *R$_1$,* total pulmonary resistance; *R$_2$,* aortic valve resistance; *R$_3$,* systemic vascular resistance; *RV,* right ventricle; *SVR,* systemic vascular resistance. (From Carabello BA. Georg Ohm and the changing character of aortic stenosis: it's not your grandfather's Oldsmobile. Circulation 2012;125:2295-2297.)

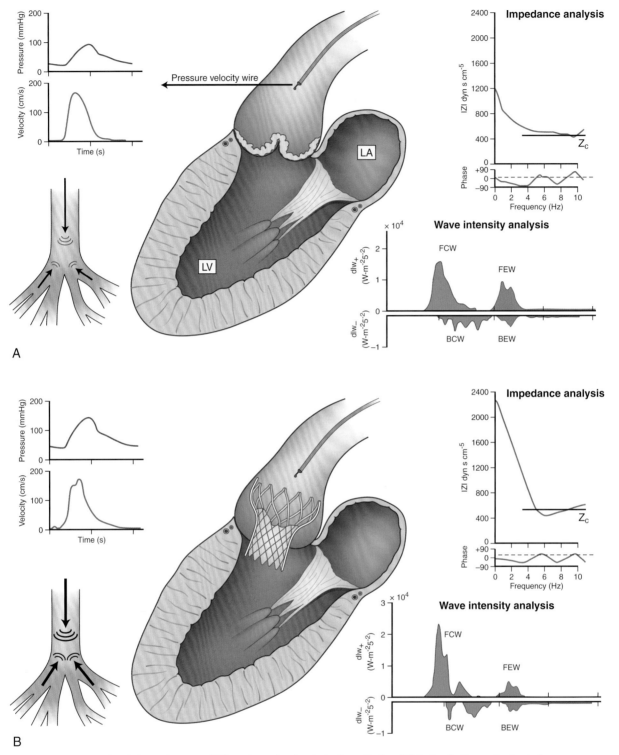

Fig. 5.17 Aortic Impedance and Wave Intensity Analysis for a Patient With Aortic Stenosis. Aortic impedance and wave intensity analysis are shown for a patient before (A) and after (B) transcatheter aortic valve replacement (TAVR). Aortic systolic and pulse pressures increased after TAVR. Fourier decomposition of the simultaneous aortic pressure and velocity signals shows that SVR and the first 3 harmonic frequencies of the impedance spectrum *(Z)* increase after TAVR. Wave intensity analysis was used to separate total wave intensity into contributions from the forward *(dlw₊)* and backward *(dlw₋)* traveling waves. Compression waves *(salmon)* increase pressure, and expansion waves *(green)* decrease aortic pressure. The forward compression wave *(FCW)* increases immediately after TAVR. *BCW,* Backward compression wave; *BEW,* backward compression wave; *dlw,* wave intensity; *FEW,* forward expansion wave; *LA,* left atrium; *LV,* left ventricle; *SVR,* systemic vascular resistance. (From Yotti R, Bermejo J, Gutierrez-Ibanes E, et al. Systemic vascular load in calcific degenerative aortic valve stenosis: insight from percutaneous valve replacement. J Am Coll Cardiol 2015;65:423-433.)

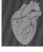

REFERENCES

1. Lindman BR, Otto CM, Douglas PS, et al. Blood pressure and arterial load after transcatheter aortic valve replacement for aortic stenosis. Circ Cardiovasc Imaging 2017;10(7). pii: e006308.

2. Yotti R, Bermejo J, Gutierrez-Ibanes E, et al. Systemic vascular load in calcific degenerative aortic valve stenosis: insight from percutaneous valve replacement. J Am Coll Cardiol 2015;65(5):423-433.

3. Carabello BA. Georg Ohm and the changing character of aortic stenosis: it's not your grandfather's Oldsmobile. Circulation 2012;125(19):2295-2297.

4. Lindman BR, Zajarias A, Maniar HS, et al. Risk stratification in patients with pulmonary hypertension undergoing transcatheter aortic valve replacement. Heart 2015;101(20):1656-1664.

5. Lindman BR, Stewart WJ, Pibarot P, et al. Early regression of severe left ventricular hypertrophy after transcatheter aortic valve replacement is associated with decreased hospitalizations. JACC Cardiovasc Interv 2014;7(6):662-673.

6. Lindman BR, Zajarias A, Madrazo JA, et al. Effects of phosphodiesterase type 5 inhibition on systemic and pulmonary hemodynamics and ventricular function in patients with severe symptomatic aortic stenosis. Circulation 2012;125(19):2353-2362.

7. Fukuta H, Little WC. The cardiac cycle and the physiologic basis of left ventricular contraction, ejection, relaxation, and filling. Heart Fail Clin 2008;4(1):1-11.

8. Hill JA, Olson EN. Cardiac plasticity. N Engl J Med 2008;358(13):1370-1380.

9. Lang RM, Badano LP, Mor-Avi V, et al. Recommendations for cardiac chamber quantification by echocardiography in adults: an update from the American Society of Echocardiography and the European Association of Cardiovascular Imaging. J Am Soc Echocardiogr 2015;28(1):1-39;e14.

10. Burchfield JS, Xie M, Hill JA. Pathological ventricular remodeling: mechanisms: part 1 of 2. Circulation 2013;128(4):388-400.

11. Grossman W, Jones D, McLaurin LP. Wall stress and patterns of hypertrophy in the human left ventricle. J Clin Invest 1975;56(1):56-64.

12. Schiattarella GG, Hill TM, Hill JA. Is load-induced ventricular hypertrophy ever compensatory? Circulation 2017;136(14):1273-1275.

13. Lindman BR, Clavel M-A, Mathieu P, et al. Calcific aortic stenosis. Nat Rev Dis Primers 2016;2:16006.

14. Mahmod M, Francis JM, Pal N, et al. Myocardial perfusion and oxygenation are impaired during stress in severe aortic stenosis and correlate with impaired energetics and subclinical left ventricular dysfunction. J Cardiovasc Magn Reson 2014;16:29.

15. Steadman CD, Jerosch-Herold M, Grundy B, et al. Determinants and functional significance of myocardial perfusion reserve in severe aortic stenosis. JACC Cardiovasc Imaging 2012;5(2):182-189.

16. Garcia D, Camici PG, Durand LG, et al. Impairment of coronary flow reserve in aortic stenosis. J Appl Physiol 2009;106(1):113-121.

17. Dweck MR, Joshi S, Murigu T, et al. Left ventricular remodeling and hypertrophy in patients with aortic stenosis: insights from cardiovascular magnetic resonance. J Cardiovasc Magn Reson 2012;14:50.

18. Lindman BR, Arnold SV, Madrazo JA, et al. The adverse impact of diabetes mellitus on left ventricular remodeling and function in patients with severe aortic stenosis. Circ Heart Fail 2011;4(3):286-292.

19. Lorell BH, Carabello BA. Left ventricular hypertrophy: pathogenesis, detection, and prognosis. Circulation 2000;102(4):470-479.

20. Petrov G, Dworatzek E, Schulze TM, et al. Maladaptive remodeling is associated with impaired survival in women but not in men after aortic valve replacement. JACC Cardiovasc Imaging 2014;7(11):1073-1080.

21. Page A, Dumesnil JG, Clavel MA, et al. Metabolic syndrome is associated with more pronounced impairment of left ventricle geometry and function in patients with calcific aortic stenosis: a substudy of the ASTRONOMER (Aortic Stenosis Progression Observation Measuring Effects of Rosuvastatin). J Am Coll Cardiol 2010;55(17):1867-1874.

22. Zaid RR, Barker CM, Little SH, Nagueh SF. Pre- and post-operative diastolic dysfunction in patients with valvular heart disease: diagnosis and therapeutic implications. J Am Coll Cardiol 2013;62(21):1922-1930.

23. Borbely A, Falcao-Pires I, van Heerebeek L, et al. Hypophosphorylation of the Stiff N2B titin isoform raises cardiomyocyte resting tension in failing human myocardium. Circ Res 2009;104(6):780-786.

24. Falcao-Pires I, Hamdani N, Borbely A, et al. Diabetes mellitus worsens diastolic left ventricular dysfunction in aortic stenosis through altered myocardial structure and cardiomyocyte stiffness. Circulation 2011;124(10):1151-1159.

25. Falcao-Pires I, Palladini G, Goncalves N, et al. Distinct mechanisms for diastolic dysfunction in diabetes mellitus and chronic pressure-overload. Basic Res Cardiol 2011;106(5):801-814.

26. Williams L, Howell N, Pagano D, et al. Titin isoform expression in aortic stenosis. Clin Sci 2009;117(6):237-242.

27. Biner S, Rafique AM, Goykhman P, Morrissey RP, Naghi J, Siegel RJ. Prognostic value of E/E' ratio in patients with unoperated severe aortic stenosis. JACC Cardiovasc Imaging 2010;3(9):899-907.

28. Lund O, Flo C, Jensen FT, et al. Left ventricular systolic and diastolic function in aortic stenosis. Prognostic value after valve replacement and underlying mechanisms. Eur Heart J 1997;18(12):1977-1987.

29. Asami M, Lanz J, Stortecky S, et al. The impact of left ventricular diastolic dysfunction on clinical outcomes after transcatheter aortic valve replacement. JACC Cardiovasc Interv 2018;11(6):593-601.

30. Hess OM, Ritter M, Schneider J, Grimm J, Turina M, Krayenbuehl HP. Diastolic stiffness and myocardial structure in aortic valve disease before and after valve replacement. Circulation 1984;69(5):855-865.

31. Lamb HJ, Beyerbacht HP, de Roos A, et al. Left ventricular remodeling early after aortic valve replacement: differential effects on diastolic function in aortic valve stenosis and aortic regurgitation. J Am Coll Cardiol 2002;40(12):2182-2188.

32. Kearney LG, Lu K, Ord M, et al. Global longitudinal strain is a strong independent predictor of all-cause mortality in patients with aortic stenosis. Eur Heart J Cardiovasc Imaging 2012;13(10):827-833.

33. Dahl JS, Videbaek L, Poulsen MK, Rudbaek TR, Pellikka PA, Moller JE. Global strain in severe aortic valve stenosis: relation to clinical outcome after aortic valve replacement. Circ Cardiovasc Imaging 2012;5(5):613-620.

34. Delgado V, Tops LF, van Bommel RJ, et al. Strain analysis in patients with severe aortic stenosis and preserved left ventricular ejection fraction undergoing surgical valve replacement. Eur Heart J 2009;30(24):3037-3047.

35. Beach JM, Mihaljevic T, Rajeswaran J, et al. Ventricular hypertrophy and left atrial dilatation persist and are associated with reduced survival after valve replacement for aortic stenosis. J Thorac Cardiovasc Surg 2014;147(1):362-369.

36. Kupari M, Turto H, Lommi J. Left ventricular hypertrophy in aortic valve stenosis: preventive or promotive of systolic dysfunction and heart failure? Eur Heart J 2005;26(17):1790-1796.

37. Mihaljevic T, Nowicki ER, Rajeswaran J, et al. Survival after valve replacement for aortic stenosis: implications for decision making. J Thorac Cardiovasc Surg 2008;135(6):1270-1278; discussion 1278-1279.

38. Duncan AI, Lowe BS, Garcia MJ, et al. Influence of concentric left ventricular remodeling on early mortality after aortic valve replacement. Ann Thorac Surg 2008;85(6):2030-2039.

39. Mehta RH, Bruckman D, Das S, et al. Implications of increased left ventricular mass index on in-hospital outcomes in patients undergoing aortic valve surgery. J Thorac Cardiovasc Surg 2001;122(5):919-928.

40. Dinh W, Nickl W, Smettan J, et al. Reduced global longitudinal strain in association to increased left ventricular mass in patients with aortic valve stenosis and normal ejection fraction: a hybrid study combining echocardiography and magnetic resonance imaging. Cardiovasc Ultrasound 2010;8:29.

41. Taniguchi K, Takahashi T, Toda K, et al. Left ventricular mass: impact on left ventricular contractile function and its reversibility in patients undergoing aortic valve replacement. Eur J Cardiothorac Surg 2007;32(4):588-595.

42. Esposito G, Rapacciuolo A, Naga Prasad SV, et al. Genetic alterations that inhibit in vivo pressure-overload hypertrophy prevent cardiac dysfunction despite increased wall stress. Circulation 2002;105(1):85-92.

43. Hill JA, Karimi M, Kutschke W, et al. Cardiac hypertrophy is not a required compensatory response to short-term pressure overload. Circulation 2000;101(24):2863-2869.

44. Musa TA, Treibel TA, Vassiliou VS, et al. Myocardial scar and mortality in severe aortic stenosis: data from the BSCMR Valve Consortium. Circulation 2018. Jul 12. pii: CIRCULATIONAHA.117.032839

45. Dweck MR, Joshi S, Murigu T, et al. Midwall fibrosis is an independent predictor of mortality in patients with aortic stenosis. J Am Coll Cardiol 2011;58(12):1271-1279.

46. Herrmann S, Stork S, Niemann M, et al. Low-gradient aortic valve stenosis myocardial fibrosis and its influence on function and outcome. J Am Coll Cardiol 2011;58(4):402-412.

47. Azevedo CF, Nigri M, Higuchi ML, et al. Prognostic significance of myocardial fibrosis quantification by histopathology and magnetic resonance imaging in patients with severe aortic valve disease. J Am Coll Cardiol 2010;56(4):278-287.

48. Weidemann F, Herrmann S, Stork S, et al. Impact of myocardial fibrosis in patients with symptomatic severe aortic stenosis. Circulation 2009;120(7):577-584.

49. Carabello BA. Is cardiac hypertrophy good or bad? The answer, of course, is yes. JACC Cardiovasc Imaging 2014;7(11):1081-1083.

50. Lindman BR, Breyley JG, Schilling JD, et al. Prognostic utility of novel biomarkers of cardiovascular stress in patients with aortic stenosis undergoing valve replacement. Heart 2015;101(17):1382-1388.

51. Chin CW, Shah AS, McAllister DA, et al. High-sensitivity troponin I concentrations are a marker of an advanced hypertrophic response and adverse outcomes in patients with aortic stenosis. Eur Heart J 2014;35(34):2312-2321.

52. Dweck MR, Boon NA, Newby DE. Calcific aortic stenosis: a disease of the valve and the myocardium. J Am Coll Cardiol 2012;60(19):1854-1863.

53. Kamperidis V, Joyce E, Debonnaire P, et al. Left ventricular functional recovery and remodeling in low-flow low-gradient severe aortic stenosis after transcatheter aortic valve implantation. J Am Soc Echocardiogr 2014;27(8):817-825.

54. Lund O, Emmertsen K, Dorup I, Jensen FT, Flo C. Regression of left ventricular hypertrophy during 10 years after valve replacement for aortic stenosis is related to the preoperative risk profile. Eur Heart J 2003;24(15):1437-1446.

55. Monrad ES, Hess OM, Murakami T, Nonogi H, Corin WJ, Krayenbuehl HP. Time course of regression of left ventricular hypertrophy after aortic valve replacement. Circulation 1988;77(6):1345-1355.

56. Ali A, Patel A, Ali Z, et al. Enhanced left ventricular mass regression after aortic valve replacement in patients with aortic stenosis is associated with improved long-term survival. J Thorac Cardiovasc Surg 2011;142(2):285-291.

57. Lessick J, Mutlak D, Markiewicz W, Reisner SA. Failure of left ventricular hypertrophy to regress after surgery for aortic valve stenosis. Echocardiography 2002;19(5):359-366.

58. Kjeldsen SE, Dahlof B, Devereux RB, et al. Effects of losartan on cardiovascular morbidity and mortality in patients with isolated systolic hypertension and left ventricular hypertrophy: a Losartan Intervention for Endpoint Reduction (LIFE) substudy. JAMA 2002;288(12):1491-1498.

59. Hankes GH, Ardell JL, Tallaj J, et al. Beta1-adrenoceptor blockade mitigates excessive norepinephrine release into cardiac interstitium in mitral regurgitation in dog. Am J Physiol Heart Circ Physiol 2006;291(1):H147-151.

60. Messika-Zeitoun D, Johnson BD, Nkomo V, et al. Cardiopulmonary exercise testing determination of functional capacity in mitral regurgitation: physiologic and outcome implications. J Am Coll Cardiol 2006;47(12):2521-2527.

61. Ross J, Jr. Afterload mismatch in aortic and mitral valve disease: implications for surgical therapy. J Am Coll Cardiol 1985;5(4):811-826.

62. Schuler G, Peterson KL, Johnson A, et al. Temporal response of left ventricular performance to mitral valve surgery. Circulation 1979;59(6):1218-1231.

63. Gaasch WH, Shah SP, Labib SB, Meyer TE. Impedance to retrograde and forward flow in chronic mitral regurgitation and the physiology of a double outlet ventricle. Heart 2017;103(8):581-585.

64. Zile MR, Gaasch WH, Levine HJ. Left ventricular stress-dimension-shortening relations before and after correction of chronic aortic and mitral regurgitation. Am J Cardiol 1985;56(1):99-105.

65. Corin WJ, Monrad ES, Murakami T, Nonogi H, Hess OM, Krayenbuehl HP. The relationship of afterload to ejection performance in chronic mitral regurgitation. Circulation 1987;76(1):59-67.

66. Wisenbaugh T, Spann JF, Carabello BA. Differences in myocardial performance and load between patients with similar amounts of chronic aortic versus chronic mitral regurgitation. J Am Coll Cardiol 1984;3(4):916-923.

67. Gaasch WH, Meyer TE. Left ventricular response to mitral regurgitation: implications for management. Circulation 2008;118(22):2298-2303.

68. Carabello BA. A tragedy of modern cardiology: using ejection fraction to gauge left ventricular function in mitral regurgitation. Heart 2017;103(8):570-571.

69. Enriquez-Sarano M, Tajik AJ, Schaff HV, Orszulak TA, Bailey KR, Frye RL. Echocardiographic prediction of survival after surgical correction of organic mitral regurgitation. Circulation 1994;90(2):830-837.

70. Tribouilloy C, Rusinaru D, Szymanski C, et al. Predicting left ventricular dysfunction after valve repair for mitral regurgitation due to leaflet prolapse: additive value of left ventricular end-systolic dimension to ejection fraction. Eur J Echocardiogr 2011;12(9):702-710.

71. Ahmed MI, Gladden JD, Litovsky SH, et al. Increased oxidative stress and cardiomyocyte myofibrillar degeneration in patients with chronic isolated mitral regurgitation and ejection fraction >60%. J Am Coll Cardiol 2010;55(7):671-679.

72. Starling MR, Kirsh MM, Montgomery DG, Gross MD. Impaired left ventricular contractile function in patients with long-term mitral regurgitation and normal ejection fraction. J Am Coll Cardiol 1993;22(1):239-250.

73. Lancellotti P, Cosyns B, Zacharakis D, et al. Importance of left ventricular longitudinal function and functional reserve in patients with degenerative mitral regurgitation: assessment by two-dimensional speckle tracking. J Am Soc Echocardiogr 2008;21(12):1331-1336.

74. Magne J, Mahjoub H, Dulgheru R, Pibarot P, Pierard LA, Lancellotti P. Left ventricular contractile reserve in asymptomatic primary mitral regurgitation. Eur Heart J 2014;35(24):1608-1616.

75. Mascle S, Schnell F, Thebault C, et al. Predictive value of global longitudinal strain in a surgical population of organic mitral regurgitation. J Am Soc Echocardiogr 2012;25(7):766-772.

76. Witkowski TG, Thomas JD, Debonnaire PJ, et al. Global longitudinal strain predicts left ventricular dysfunction after mitral valve repair. Eur Heart J Cardiovasc Imaging 2013;14(1):69-76.

77. Galli E, Lancellotti P, Sengupta PP, Donal E. LV mechanics in mitral and aortic valve diseases: value of functional assessment beyond ejection fraction. JACC Cardiovasc Imaging 2014;7(11):1151-1166.

78. Taniguchi K, Kawamoto T, Kuki S, et al. Left ventricular myocardial remodeling and contractile state in chronic aortic regurgitation. Clin Cardiol 2000;23(8):608-614.

79. Taniguchi K, Nakano S, Kawashima Y, et al. Left ventricular ejection performance, wall stress, and contractile state in aortic regurgitation before and after aortic valve replacement. Circulation 1990;82(3):798-807.

80. Laskey WK, Kussmaul WG, Martin JL, Kleaveland JP, Hirshfeld JW Jr, Shroff S. Characteristics of vascular hydraulic load in patients with heart failure. Circulation 1985;72(1):61-71.

81. Chirinos JA, Segers P. Noninvasive evaluation of left ventricular afterload: part 1: pressure and flow measurements and basic principles of wave conduction and reflection. Hypertension 2010;56(4):555-562.

82. Chirinos JA, Segers P. Noninvasive evaluation of left ventricular afterload: part 2: arterial pressure-flow and pressure-volume relations in humans. Hypertension 2010;56(4):563-570.

83. Kass DA. Ventricular arterial stiffening: integrating the pathophysiology. Hypertension 2005;46(1):185-193.

84. Galie N, Hoeper MM, Humbert M, et al. Guidelines for the diagnosis and treatment of pulmonary hypertension: the Task Force for the Diagnosis and Treatment of Pulmonary Hypertension of the European Society of Cardiology (ESC) and the European Respiratory Society (ERS), endorsed by the International Society of Heart and Lung Transplantation (ISHLT). Eur Heart J 2009;30(20):2493-2537.

85. Vachiery JL, Adir Y, Barbera JA, et al. Pulmonary hypertension due to left heart diseases. J Am Coll Cardiol 2013;62(25 Suppl):D100-D108.

86. Rosenkranz S, Gibbs JS, Wachter R, De Marco T, Vonk-Noordegraaf A, Vachiery JL. Left ventricular heart failure and pulmonary hypertension. Eur Heart J 2016;37(12):942-954.

87. Simonneau G, Robbins IM, Beghetti M, et al. Updated clinical classification of pulmonary hypertension. J Am Coll Cardiol 2009;54(1 Suppl):S43-S54.

88. Guazzi M, Borlaug BA. Pulmonary hypertension due to left heart disease. Circulation 2012;126(8):975-990.

89. Melby SJ, Moon MR, Lindman BR, Bailey MS, Hill LL, Damiano RJ, Jr. Impact of pulmonary hypertension on outcomes after aortic valve replacement for aortic valve stenosis. J Thorac Cardiovasc Surg 2011;141(6):1424-1430.

90. O'Sullivan CJ, Wenaweser P, Ceylan O, et al. Effect of pulmonary hypertension hemodynamic presentation on clinical outcomes in patients with severe symptomatic aortic valve stenosis undergoing transcatheter aortic valve implantation: insights from the new proposed pulmonary hypertension classification. Circ Cardiovasc Interv 2015;8(7):e002358.

91. Barbieri A, Bursi F, Grigioni F, et al. Prognostic and therapeutic implications of pulmonary hypertension complicating degenerative mitral regurgitation due to flail leaflet: a multicenter long-term international study. Eur Heart J 2011;32(6):751-759.

92. Matsumoto T, Nakamura M, Yeow WL, et al. Impact of pulmonary hypertension on outcomes in patients with functional mitral regurgitation undergoing percutaneous edge-to-edge repair. Am J Cardiol 2014;114(11):1735-1739.

93. Magne J, Lancellotti P, Pierard LA. Exercise pulmonary hypertension in asymptomatic degenerative mitral regurgitation. Circulation 2010;122(1):33-41.

94. Braunwald E, Braunwald NS, Ross J Jr, Morrow AG. Effects of mitral-valve replacement on the pulmonary vascular dynamics of patients with pulmonary hypertension. N Engl J Med 1965;273:509-514.

95. Ben-Dor I, Goldstein SA, Pichard AD, et al. Clinical profile, prognostic implication, and response to treatment of pulmonary hypertension in patients with severe aortic stenosis. Am J Cardiol 2011;107(7):1046-1051.

96. Tracy GP, Proctor MS, Hizny CS. Reversibility of pulmonary artery hypertension in aortic stenosis after aortic valve replacement. Ann Thorac Surg 1990;50(1):89-93.

97. Dalen JE, Matloff JM, Evans GL, et al. Early reduction of pulmonary vascular resistance after mitral-valve replacement. N Engl J Med 1967;277(8):387-394.

98. Walls MC, Cimino N, Bolling SF, Bach DS. Persistent pulmonary hypertension after mitral valve surgery: does surgical procedure affect outcome? J Heart Valve Dis 2008;17(1):1-9; discussion 9.

99. Li M, Dumesnil JG, Mathieu P, Pibarot P. Impact of valve prosthesis-patient mismatch on pulmonary arterial pressure after mitral valve replacement. J Am Coll Cardiol 2005;45(7):1034-1040.

100. Sinning JM, Hammerstingl C, Chin D, et al. Decrease of pulmonary hypertension impacts on prognosis after transcatheter aortic valve replacement. EuroIntervention 2014;9(9):1042-1049.

101. Nishimura RA, Otto CM, Bonow RO, et al. 2014 AHA/ACC guideline for the management of patients with valvular heart disease: a report of the American College of Cardiology/American Heart Association Task Force on Practice Guidelines. Circulation 2014;129(23):e521-e643.

102. Melenovsky V, Al-Hiti H, Kazdova L, et al. Transpulmonary B-type natriuretic peptide uptake and cyclic guanosine monophosphate release in heart failure and pulmonary hypertension: the effects of sildenafil. J Am Coll Cardiol 2009;54(7):595-600.

103. Bermejo J, Yotti R, Garcia-Orta R, et al. Sildenafil for improving outcomes in patients with corrected valvular heart disease and persistent pulmonary hypertension: a multicenter, double-blind, randomized clinical trial. Eur Heart J 2018;39(15):1255-1264.

104. Khot UN, Novaro GM, Popovic ZB, et al. Nitroprusside in critically ill patients with left ventricular dysfunction and aortic stenosis. N Engl J Med 2003;348(18):1756-1763.

105. Briand M, Dumesnil JG, Kadem L, et al. Reduced systemic arterial compliance impacts significantly on left ventricular afterload and function in aortic stenosis: implications for diagnosis and treatment. J Am Coll Cardiol 2005;46(2):291-298.

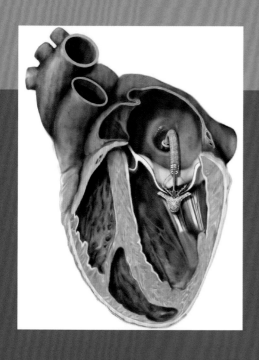

中文导读

第6章
瓣膜性心脏病的治疗原则

　　本章对瓣膜性心脏病的整体治疗原则进行了详细阐述。首先，强调瓣膜性心脏病患者应在由多学科团队（心内科专家、心外科专家、影像学专家、老年病学专家、介入心脏病专家、麻醉医师）组成的心脏瓣膜中心接受最佳治疗。心脏瓣膜中心负责患者病情的精准评估、治疗方案的制定、定期随访、患者教育等。超声心动图（经胸超声心动图或经食管超声心动图）仍然是瓣膜性心脏病的重要检查方式，对于可疑、确诊的瓣膜性心脏病，术中引导及监测、人工瓣术后随访均具有重要意义。CT、心脏MRI和心导管检查也可提供更多补充诊断价值。风湿热的一级及二级预防可明显减少风湿性心脏病的发生，同时应遵循"合理应用抗生素、足疗程"原则。感染性心内膜炎预防指南不推荐对原发性瓣膜性心脏病患者在牙科手术前预防使用抗生素，仅推荐将抗生素用于人工瓣术后、发绀型先天性心脏病、心脏移植术后等患者。目前尚无特定药物能预防钙化性心脏瓣膜疾病进展。指南建议自身瓣膜病（主动脉瓣疾病、三尖瓣疾病或二尖瓣反流）、生物瓣术后或二尖瓣修复术后合并房颤患者，应采用抗凝治疗，直接口服抗凝剂或维生素K拮抗剂均适用于这些患者。房颤合并风湿性二尖瓣狭窄或机械瓣术后的患者，应使用维生素K拮抗剂进行抗凝治疗。瓣膜性心脏病患者保持整体健康状态非常重要，包括冠心病风险因素控制、定期运动、标准免疫接种和最佳牙科护理。对瓣膜性心脏病患者应进行定期评估，动态观察瓣膜病严重程度和左心室对慢性容量和压力超负荷的反应，以优化外科手术和经皮介入干预的时机。对于接受非心脏手术的瓣膜病患者，管理重点是准确评估瓣膜病变程度和有无症状，并在围手术期进行适当的血流动力学监测和容量负荷优化。最后，对瓣膜性心脏病患者进行教育是坚持定期随访、预防并发症和早期识别症状的关键。

叶蕴青

Principles of Medical Therapy for Patients With Valvular Heart Disease

John P. Erwin III, Catherine M. Otto

CHAPTER OUTLINE

KEY POINTS

- Patients with valvular heart disease (VHD) are best cared for in the context of a multidisciplinary heart valve clinic.
- Many adverse outcomes for adults with VHD are caused by sequelae of the disease process, including atrial fibrillation (AF), embolic events, left ventricular (LV) dysfunction, pulmonary hypertension, and endocarditis.
- Medical treatment of adults with VHD focuses on prevention and treatment of complications because there are no specific therapies to prevent progression of valve disease.
- Infective endocarditis (IE) prophylaxis guidelines recommend antibiotics before dental or other procedures associated with bacteremia for adults with prosthetic valves but not for patients with native valve disease.
- Periodic evaluation of disease severity and the LV response to chronic volume and pressure overload allows optimal timing of surgical and percutaneous interventions.
- General health maintenance is important, including evaluation and treatment of coronary disease risk factors, regular exercise, standard immunizations, and optimal dental care.

- Management of concurrent cardiovascular disease follows standard approaches with modification as needed, based on the potential confounding effects of valve hemodynamics.
- Standard guidelines for anticoagulation are appropriate in patients with AF and native aortic valve disease, tricuspid valve disease, or mitral regurgitation. In patients with AF and a bioprosthetic valve or mitral valve repair, anticoagulation is recommended regardless of risk score. Either a direct oral anticoagulant or a vitamin K antagonist is appropriate in these patients.
- In AF patients with rheumatic mitral stenosis or a mechanical heart valve, vitamin K antagonists should be used for anticoagulation.
- For patients with valvular disease undergoing noncardiac surgery, management focuses on an accurate assessment of disease severity and symptom status, with appropriate hemodynamic monitoring and optimization of loading conditions in the perioperative period.
- Evaluation of coronary anatomy usually is needed before valve surgery because of the high prevalence of coronary disease and improved surgical outcomes with concurrent coronary revascularization.

THE HEART VALVE CLINIC

For patients with valvular heart disease (VHD), the basic principles of management include the following:

- Obtain an accurate diagnosis of the specific valvular lesion and quantitative disease severity using the history, physical examination, Doppler echocardiography, and other advanced imaging modalities.

- Monitor asymptomatic patients who have moderate or severe valve disease.
- Prevent and manage complications of the disease process, such as endocarditis, atrial fibrillation (AF), and embolic events.
- Periodically re-evaluate ventricular size and function to identify early ventricular dysfunction and optimize the timing of surgical or percutaneous intervention.
- Provide optimal management of associated conditions.

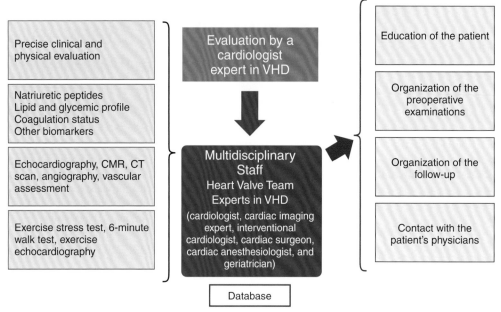

Organizational Aspects of a Heart Valve Clinic

Precise clinical and physical evaluation

Natriuretic peptides
Lipid and glycemic profile
Coagulation status
Other biomarkers

Echocardiography, CMR, CT scan, angiography, vascular assessment

Exercise stress test, 6-minute walk test, exercise echocardiography

Evaluation by a cardiologist expert in VHD

Multidisciplinary Staff
Heart Valve Team
Experts in VHD
(cardiologist, cardiac imaging expert, interventional cardiologist, cardiac surgeon, cardiac anesthesiologist, and geriatrician)

Database

Education of the patient

Organization of the preoperative examinations

Organization of the follow-up

Contact with the patient's physicians

Fig. 6.1 Functioning of the Advanced Heart Valve Clinic. Optimal decision making requires input from cardiologists, imaging specialists, cardiovascular surgeons, and other experts, such as neurologists, anesthesiologists, and palliative care specialists. *CMR*, Cardiac magnetic resonance; *CT*, computed tomography; *VHD*, valvular heart disease. (From Lancellotti P, Rosenhek R, Pibarot P, et al. ESC Working Group on Valvular Heart Disease position paper—heart valve clinics: organization, structure, and experiences. Eur Heart J 2013; 34:1597-1606.)

- Set and maintain standards for valve interventions, including surgical valve repair and replacement and percutaneous techniques.
- Provide patient education regarding the disease process, expected outcomes, symptom surveillance, and potential medical or surgical therapies.
- Assess before noncardiac surgery or pregnancy.

These goals are best met with an interdisciplinary health care team structured as a heart valve clinic. Many general cardiologists have little experience in managing these complex patients despite the fact that moderate or severe heart valve disease occurs in 13% of persons 75 years of age or older as a result of degenerative diseases reflecting increasing life spans.[1] Data from the Euro Heart Surveys shows that many patients are not treated according to current guidelines. Some are inappropriately denied interventions that would improve survival and quality of life, whereas others undergo intervention earlier in the disease course than necessary.[2]

Optimal decision making requires input from cardiologists with expertise in valve disease, interventional cardiologists, imaging specialists, and cardiovascular surgeons. Other experts, such as neurologists, anesthesiologists, and palliative care specialists, may also need to be involved with the heart team in certain circumstances (Fig. 6.1). There is also an emerging role in the management of patients with cardiac implanted device infections for individuals with expertise in removal of pacemaker or defibrillator leads and generators. With the use of telemedicine, it may be reasonable to manage patients with lower-acuity VHD in a center without on-site multispecialty care through telecommunication with a heart valve team. The European Society of Cardiology published a position paper on the need for heart valve clinics, with specific recommendations for goals, patient population, clinic structure, and the tasks for each member of the heart valve clinic team.[3]

DIAGNOSIS OF VALVE DISEASE

VHD may first be diagnosed in the setting of an acute medical event, such as heart failure, pulmonary edema, AF, or infective endocarditis (IE). More often, the diagnosis of VHD is suspected before the onset of overt symptoms, based on the physical examination finding of a cardiac murmur, screening of relatives in a family with a history of a genetic disorder, or abnormal findings on an electrocardiograph, chest radiograph, or echocardiogram requested for unrelated reasons (Box 6.1). Worldwide, many patients are first diagnosed with VHD when a cardiac murmur is heard during an episode of acute rheumatic fever.

In patients with a cardiac murmur, the first step is clinical assessment based on the history and physical examination.[4] If clinical evaluation indicates a high likelihood of significant valvular disease, the next step is echocardiography to confirm the diagnosis and evaluate valve anatomy and function.[5–6]

For a patient with cardiac or respiratory symptoms and a cardiac murmur on auscultation, it is prudent to obtain an echocardiogram to evaluate for possible valvular disease. When symptoms exist, it is difficult to reliably exclude significant valvular disease by physical examination because the findings may be subtle.[7] For example, some patients with severe aortic stenosis have only a grade 2 or 3 murmur on examination, and the carotid upstroke may appear normal due to coexisting atherosclerosis.[8] With the growing prevalence of obesity and decline in physical examination skills in many societies, the examination has also lost some sensitivity.[9,10] Diagnosis can be even more difficult in other situations. For example, many patients with acute mitral regurgitation have no audible murmur.[11]

Among *asymptomatic* patients with a murmur detected on physical examination, those with a benign flow murmur should be distinguished

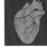

BOX 6.1   Echocardiographic Indications for Adults With Suspected or Known Valvular Heart Disease

Suspected Valvular Disease
- Cardiac murmur in a patient with cardiorespiratory symptoms
- Murmur suggesting structural heart disease, even if asymptomatic
  - Diastolic murmur
  - Continuous murmur
  - Holosystolic or late systolic murmur
  - Murmur associated with an ejection click or irradiation of neck or back
  - Grade 3 or louder mid-peaking systolic murmur

Known Native Valve Disease
- Stenosis
  - Initial diagnosis and assessment of hemodynamic severity
  - Assessment of left and right ventricular size, function, and hemodynamics
  - Re-evaluation for changing signs or symptoms
  - Assessment of changes in valve or ventricular function during pregnancy
  - Periodic re-evaluation
  - Assessment of pulmonary pressures with exercise in mitral stenosis patients when there is a discrepancy between symptoms and resting hemodynamics
  - TEE before percutaneous valvotomy in patients with mitral stenosis
- Regurgitation
  - Initial diagnosis and assessment of hemodynamic severity
  - Initial evaluation of left and right ventricular size, function, and hemodynamics
  - Assessment of aortic regurgitation in cases of aortic root enlargement
  - Re-evaluation with a change in symptoms
  - Periodic re-evaluation even in asymptomatic patients
  - Re-assessment of valve and ventricular function during pregnancy
- Mitral valve prolapse
  - Assessment of leaflet morphology, hemodynamic severity, and ventricular compensation

- Infective endocarditis[a]
- Detection of valvular vegetations with or without positive blood cultures
- Characterization of hemodynamic severity with known endocarditis
- Detection of complications such as abscesses, fistulas, and shunts
- Re-evaluation of high-risk patients (e.g., virulent organism, clinical deterioration, persistent or recurrent fever, new murmur, persistent bacteremia)

Interventions for Valvular Disease
- Selection of alternate therapies for mitral valve disease (e.g., balloon valvuloplasty, surgical valve repair vs. replacement, percutaneous approaches)[a]
- Monitoring interventional techniques in the catheterization laboratory (i.e., 3D TEE, ICE, or TTE)
- Intraoperative TEE for valve repair surgery
- Intraoperative TEE for stentless bioprosthetic, homograft, autograft, or trans-aortic, transapical, or veno-aortic valve replacement interventions
- Intraoperative TEE for valve surgery of infective endocarditis

Prosthetic Valves
- Baseline postoperative study (i.e., hospital discharge or 6–8 weeks)
- Annual evaluation of bioprosthetic valves beginning 5 years after implantation
- Changing clinical signs and symptoms or suspected prosthetic valve dysfunction[a]
- Prosthetic valve endocarditis
  - Detection of endocarditis and characterization of valve and ventricular function
  - Detection of endocarditis complications and re-evaluation in complex endocarditis[a]
  - Persistent fever without bacteremia or a new murmur[a]
  - Bacteremia without a known source[a]

[a]TEE is usually required.
ICE, Intracardiac echocardiography; *TEE*, transesophageal echocardiography; *TTE*, transthoracic echocardiography; *3D*, three-dimensional.
Modified from Nishimura RA, Otto CM, Bonow RO, et al. 2014 AHA/ACC guideline for the management of patients with valvular heart disease: a report of the American College of Cardiology/American Heart Association Task Force on Practice Guidelines. J Am Coll Cardiol 2014;63:e57-e185.

---

from those with a pathologic murmur.[12] Although there are no absolutely reliable criteria for making this distinction, a reasonable estimate of the pretest likelihood of disease can be derived from the history and physical examination findings. Flow murmurs, defined as audible systolic murmurs in the absence of structural heart disease, are most common in younger patients and in those with high output states. A flow murmur is a normal finding in pregnancy and is appreciated in 90% of pregnant women.[13] Flow murmurs also are likely in patients who are anemic or febrile.

Typically, a flow murmur is systolic, is of low intensity (grade 1 to 2), is loudest at the base with little radiation, ends before the second heart sound, and has a crescendo-decrescendo or ejection shape with an early systolic peak. These murmurs are related to rapid ejection into the aorta or pulmonary artery in patients with normal valve function, high flow rates, and good transmission of sound to the chest wall.[11] The yield of echocardiography is very low for asymptomatic patients with a typical flow murmur on examination, no cardiac history, and no cardiac symptoms on careful questioning.

Echocardiographic examination usually is appropriate in asymptomatic patients who have a diastolic or continuous murmur, a systolic murmur of grade 3 or higher, an ejection click or mid-systolic click, a holosystolic (rather than ejection) murmur, or an atypical pattern of radiation, even if the patient is asymptomatic. To some extent, the loudness of the murmur correlates with disease severity, but this is not

reliable for decision making about an individual patient.[14,15] Echocardiography allows differentiation of valve disease from a flow murmur, identification of the specific valve involved, definition of the cause of valve disease, and quantitation of the hemodynamic severity of the lesion along with left ventricular (LV) size and function. Based on these data, the expected prognosis, need for preventive measures, and timing of subsequent examinations (if any) can be determined.

Distinguishing a benign from a pathologic murmur is more difficult in older rather than younger patients; many older patients have some degree of aortic valve sclerosis or mild mitral regurgitation that can be appreciated on auscultation, and many have mild symptoms that may or may not be related to heart disease.[16,17] In this setting, a baseline echocardiogram may be prudent. The finding of aortic sclerosis is associated with an increased risk of adverse cardiovascular events, and some patients have progressive valve obstruction. A soft mitral regurgitant murmur is most likely associated with mild to moderate regurgitation due to mitral annular calcification, but establishing the diagnosis with a baseline echocardiogram and excluding other causes of mitral regurgitation, such as ischemic disease or mitral valve prolapse, is appropriate.

Although echocardiography is the primary diagnostic modality used for evaluation of valve disease, cardiac magnetic resonance (CMR) imaging and computed tomography (CT) are useful in some cases (see Chapters 8 and 15). Diagnostic cardiac catheterization continues to be

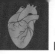

useful in selected patients, particularly when echocardiographic data are nondiagnostic or discrepant with other clinical data.

PREVENTIVE MEASURES

Diagnosis and Prevention of Rheumatic Fever

Rheumatic fever is a multiorgan inflammatory disease that occurs 10 days to 3 weeks after group A streptococcal pharyngitis. The clinical diagnosis is based on the conjunction of an antecedent streptococcal throat infection and classic manifestations of the disease, including carditis, polyarthritis, chorea, erythema marginatum, and subcutaneous nodules.[18] Clinical guidelines for the diagnosis of rheumatic fever provide increased specificity because many of the manifestations of rheumatic fever are also seen in other conditions (Box 6.2).[19] Although these guidelines are helpful in the initial diagnosis of rheumatic fever, exceptions do occur, and consideration of the diagnosis is important in the recognition of this disease. Poststreptococcal reactive arthritis has some overlap in symptoms and signs with acute rheumatic fever but is not associated with cardiac involvement.[20]

The carditis associated with rheumatic fever is a pancarditis; the pericardium, myocardium, and valvular tissue may be involved. Rheumatic disease preferentially affects the mitral valve; mitral regurgitation is characteristic of the acute episode, whereas mitral stenosis is characteristic of the long-term effect of the disease process.[21] Although echocardiography can increase the sensitivity of an early diagnosis of rheumatic fever, a slight degree of mitral regurgitation is common in normal individuals, and this is therefore not a specific finding.[22]

Primary prevention of rheumatic fever is based on treatment of streptococcal pharyngitis with appropriate antibiotics for a sufficient length of time (Table 6.1).[23] Patients with a history of rheumatic fever are at high risk for recurrent disease leading to repeated episodes of valvulitis and increased damage to the valvular apparatus. Because recurrent streptococcal infections may be asymptomatic, secondary prevention is based on the use of continuous antibiotic therapy (Table 6.2). The risk of recurrent disease is related to the number of previous episodes, time interval since the last episode, risk of exposure to streptococcal infections (i.e., contact with children or crowded situations), and patient age. A longer duration of secondary prevention is recommended for patients with evidence of carditis or persistent valvular disease than for those with no evidence of valvular damage.

There are gaps in the implementation of medical and surgical interventions of proven effectiveness for rheumatic heart disease in low- and middle-income countries. They include the suboptimal use of penicillin for secondary prophylaxis, inadequate monitoring and control of oral anticoagulant therapy, the dearth of reproductive services for women with rheumatic heart disease, and disparities in the use of percutaneous and surgical interventions between different countries.[24]

Prevention of Infective Endocarditis

IE occurs when bacteremia results in bacterial adherence and proliferation at sites of platelet and fibrin deposition on disrupted endothelial surfaces. Patients with native or prosthetic VHD are at increased risk for IE due to endothelial disruption on the valve leaflets by high-velocity and turbulent blood flow patterns (see Chapter 22). About 50% of patients with endocarditis have underlying native valve disease, and endocarditis may precipitate the diagnosis of valve disease in a previously asymptomatic patient.

Prevention of bacterial endocarditis is based on short-term antibiotic therapy at times of anticipated bacteremia in patients who are at the highest risk for endocarditis. The American Heart Association and American College of Cardiology published revised guidelines for groups of patients at highest risk, the procedures for which IE prophylaxis is indicated (Box 6.3), and the appropriate antibiotic regimens for dental procedures (Table 6.3).[7] Prophylaxis for other procedures should include antibiotics active against the most likely organisms, as detailed in the guidelines. Antibiotics also are recommended at the time of surgical implantation of prosthetic cardiac valves or other intracardiac material such as cardiac implantable electronic devices.

Current guidelines no longer recommend endocarditis prophylaxis for patients with native VHD based on a careful review of the published literature and expert opinion. The key elements underlying the current recommendations are (1) the recognition that bacteremia due to normal daily activities, such as tooth brushing, flossing, and chewing, is much more frequent than bacteremia related to dental procedures; (2) there are no controlled studies showing that short-term antibiotics at the time of anticipated bacteremia prevents endocarditis and estimates of total benefit are exceedingly small; (3) the risk of an adverse reaction to the antibiotic is higher than any potential benefit; and (4) the most important factor in reducing daily bacteremia is maintaining optimal oral health and hygiene, including regular dental care.[25,26]

The current recommendations resulted in a decrease of approximately 80% in the use of antibiotic prophylaxis with no evidence for an increase in endocarditis cases in large datasets from the United Kingdom and the United States.[27,28] A systematic review published in 2016 identified seven observational studies that provided estimates of IE diagnostic rates before and after changes to national guideline recommendations.[29] The quality of the studies varied but was generally insufficient to resolve uncertainty about how these changes had affected rates of incident IE. One of the studies reported a small rate increase, whereas the others reported no significant change compared with the period antedating guideline changes. Add to this the increasing prevalence of staphylococcal endocarditis in recent years, and it is clear that studies of almost unprecedented scale would be required to confidently identify changes in rates of incident IE in response to the antibiotic guideline changes.

BOX 6.2   Updated Jones Criteria for the Diagnosis of Initial Rheumatic Fever Attacks

Major criteria
- Carditis (may involve endocardium, myocardium, and pericardium)
- Polyarthritis (most frequent manifestation, usually migratory)
- Chorea (documentation of recent group A streptococcal infection may be difficult)
- Erythema marginatum (distinctive, evanescent rash on trunk and proximal extremities)
- Subcutaneous nodules (firm, painless nodule on extensor surfaces of elbows, knees, and wrists)

Minor criteria
- Clinical findings (arthralgia, fever)
- Laboratory findings (elevated erythrocyte sedimentation rate or C-reactive protein level)
- Electrocardiography (prolonged PR interval)

Evidence of antecedent group A streptococcal infection
- Positive throat culture or rapid streptococci antigen test
- Elevated or rising streptococcal antibody titer

High probability of rheumatic fever
- 2 major criteria or 1 major criterion plus 2 minor criteria

PLUS
- evidence of preceding group A streptococcal infection

Modified from Ferrieri P, Jones Criteria Working Group. Proceedings of the Jones Criteria workshop. Circulation 2002;106:2521-2523.

TABLE 6.1   Recommendations for Prevention of Rheumatic Fever.

Medication	Adults	Children (≤27 kg)
For Primary Prevention (i.e., Treatment of Group A Streptococcal Tonsillopharyngitis)		
Oral penicillin V[a] (phenoxymethyl penicillin)	500 mg two to three times daily for 10 days	250 mg two to three times daily for 10 days
IM penicillin, single dose	Penicillin G benzathine and penicillin G procaine (Bicillin C-R) 2.4 million units **or** penicillin G benzathine (Bicillin L-A) 1.2 million units	Penicillin G benzathine and penicillin G procaine (Bicillin C-R 900/300) 1.2 million units (consists of benzathine penicillin G 900,000 units mixed with procaine penicillin G 300,000 units)[b]
Amoxicillin[c,d]	875 mg orally twice daily or 500 mg three times daily for 10 days	50 mg/kg/day orally (maximum 1000 mg/day); may be administered once daily or in two or three equally divided doses; duration is 10 days
Cephalexin[d,e]	500 mg orally twice daily for 10 days	25–50 mg/kg/day orally in two equally divided doses (maximum 1000 mg/day) for 10 days
For Potentially Severe Hypersensitivity to β-Lactam Antibiotics (e.g., Penicillin, Cephalosporins)		
Azithromycin[f]	500 mg orally on day 1 followed by 250 mg daily on days 2 through 5	12 mg/kg orally once daily for 5 days
Clarithromycin	250 mg orally twice daily for 10 days	7.5 mg/kg/dose twice daily for 10 days
Clindamycin	28–70 kg: 20 mg/kg/day orally in three equally divided doses for 10 days >70 kg: 450–600 mg/day orally three times daily for 10 days	20 mg/kg/day orally in three equally divided doses for 10 days
Cefadroxil	—	30 mg/kg once daily (maximum 1000 mg/day) for 10 days

[a]Oral penicillin V is the drug of choice for group A streptococcal pharyngitis.
[b]Penicillin G benzathine and penicillin G procaine (Bicillin C-R 900/300) requires further study before routine use in adults or large adolescents is acceptable. Bicillin L-A (benzathine penicillin G 600,000 units IM) is an acceptable alternative regimen for patients < 27 kg.
[c]Although single-dose amoxicillin is recommended by the 2009 American Health Association guidelines, its superiority over the doses listed has not been proved definitively, and it is not approved for children younger than 12 years of age.
[d]Dose alteration needed for severe renal insufficiency.
[e]Other cephalosporins (i.e., cefadroxil, cefprozil, cefaclor, cefuroxime, loracarbef, cefdinir, cefpodoxime, cefixime, and ceftibuten) are acceptable. Cefpodoxime and cefdinir are U.S. FDA approved for 5 days of therapy; all other cephalosporins require 10 days of therapy.
[f]Erythromycin or clarithromycin is acceptable (10 days of therapy).
Modified from Shulman ST, Bisno AL, Clegg HW, et al. Clinical practice guideline for the diagnosis and management of group A streptococcal pharyngitis: 2012 update by the Infectious Diseases Society of America. Clin Infect Dis 2012;55:1279-1282.

TABLE 6.2   Secondary Prevention of Recurrent Rheumatic Fever.

Drug	Adults	Children (≤27 kg)
Penicillin G benzathine	1.2 million units IM every 4 weeks (or every 3 weeks in high-risk situations)	600,000 units every 4 weeks[a] (or every 3 weeks in high-risk situations)
Penicillin V	500 mg twice daily	250 mg orally twice daily
Sulfadiazine	1000 mg orally once daily	500 mg orally once daily
For Patients Allergic to Penicillin and Sulfadiazine		
Azithromycin	250 mg orally once daily[b]	5 mg/kg orally once daily (maximum 250 mg/day)
Duration of Secondary Prophylaxis (Whichever Is Longer) in Rheumatic Fever Patients		
With carditis and residual valve disease (including after valve surgery): 10 years or until 40 years of age; sometimes lifelong		
With carditis but no residual valve disease: 10 years or until 21 years of age		
Without carditis: 5 years or until 21 years of age		

[a]For small children and infants: 25,000 units/kg intramuscularly every 4 weeks (or every 3 weeks in high-risk situations).
[b]Macrolide susceptibility testing should be pursued before use of this drug class. Erythromycin is an acceptable alternative to azithromycin, although the latter has fewer adverse effects and permits once-daily dosing. Erythromycin dosing for adults: 250 mg orally twice daily. Erythromycin dosing for children: 20 mg/kg/day divided twice daily (maximum 500 mg/day).
Modified from Gerber MA, Baltimore RS, Eaton CB, et al. Prevention of rheumatic fever and diagnosis and treatment of acute streptococcal pharyngitis: a scientific statement from the American Heart Association Rheumatic Fever, Endocarditis, and Kawasaki Disease Committee of the Council on Cardiovascular Disease in the Young, the Interdisciplinary Council on Functional Genomics and Translational Biology, and the Interdisciplinary Council on Quality of Care and Outcomes Research. Circulation 2009;119:1541-1551. Copyright © 2009 Lippincott Williams & Wilkins.

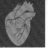

BOX 6.3 Cardiac Conditions for Which Endocarditis Prophylaxis for Dental Procedures Is Reasonable

Benefit

1. Prosthetic cardiac valves, including transcatheter-implanted prostheses and homografts
2. Prosthetic material used for cardiac valve repair, such as annuloplasty rings and chords
3. Previous infective endocarditis (IE)
4. Unrepaired cyanotic congenital heart disease or repaired congenital heart disease with residual shunts or valvular regurgitation
5. Cardiac transplant with valve regurgitation due to a structurally abnormal valve

No Benefit

Prophylaxis against endocarditis is not recommended for patients with valvular heart disease who are at risk for IE for nondental procedures (e.g., TEE, esophagogastroduodenoscopy, colonoscopy, or cystoscopy) in the absence of active infection (class III, level of evidence B)

From Nishimura RA, Otto CM, Bonow RO, et al. 2017 AHA/ACC focused update of the 2014 AHA/ACC guideline for the management of patients with valvular heart disease: a report of the American College of Cardiology/American Heart Association Task Force on Clinical Practice Guidelines. J Am Coll Cardiol 2017;70:252-289.

Prevention of Embolic Events

Prevention of embolic events in patients with VHD, particularly those with prosthetic valves, mitral stenosis, or AF, is a key component of optimal medical therapy[23,30] (Table 6.4). Anticoagulation in patients with prosthetic valves is discussed in Chapter 26; this section discusses anticoagulation in adults with native valve disease. The consequences of a systemic embolic event can be devastating and may occur even in previously asymptomatic patients.

In the era before surgery and anticoagulant therapy, mitral stenosis was estimated to be responsible for 25% of all deaths from systemic embolism.[32] Studies on the prevalence of thromboembolism in mitral regurgitation have yielded contrasting results, most likely due to the multiple mechanisms of mitral regurgitation. Mitral valve prolapse is a common, sometimes congenital form of mitral valve disease. Although early evidence from case series and control studies suggested an association with stroke, more robust studies failed to replicate this finding.[31,32] Systemic embolism usually is caused by left atrial (LA) thrombus formation in patients with low blood flow in a dilated LA chamber, with or without concurrent AF (Fig. 6.2).[35-40]

Aortic stenosis has not been demonstrated to confer a higher additional risk of thromboembolism beyond the risk from AF, which frequently coexists with this valvulopathy. The same applies to aortic insufficiency. Embolic events caused by calcific debris from the aortic or mitral valve are much less common but may occur when a catheter is passed across the valve.[41]

Therapy for prevention of embolic events in patients with VHD typically includes antiplatelet agents, vitamin K antagonists (VKA) such as warfarin, and direct oral anticoagulants (DOACs). DOACs should not be used in patients with mechanical prosthetic valves because of a higher incidence of thromboembolic events in several case reports and early termination of the RE-ALIGN trial due to an increased rate of valve thrombosis, stroke, and myocardial infarction in those randomized to dabigatran compared with VKA therapy.[42-44] These findings prompted the U.S. Food and Drug Administration to issue a black box warning against the use of dabigatran with mechanical heart valves.[35]

Native Valve Disease With Atrial Fibrillation

Paroxysmal, persistent, or permanent AF should be treated with anticoagulation as stated in the current AF guidelines when the patient has native aortic valve or nonrheumatic mitral valve disease.[35,36,45] There was initial concern that DOACs might not be appropriate for patients with valve disease and AF because the clinical trials purported to have

TABLE 6.3 American Heart Association Recommendations for Endocarditis Prophylaxis for Dental Procedures.

Situation	Agent	REGIMEN: SINGLE DOSE 30–60 MINUTES BEFORE PROCEDURE	
		Adults	**Children**
Oral	Amoxicillin	2.0 g	50 mg/kg
Unable to take oral medications	Ampicillin	2.0 g IM or IV	50 mg/kg IM or IV
	or		
	Cefazolin or ceftriaxone	1.0 g IM or IV	50 mg/kg IM or IV
Allergic to penicillins or ampicillin, oral	Cephalexin[a,b]	2.0 g	50 mg/kg
	or		
	Clindamycin	600 mg	20 mg/kg
	or		
	Azithromycin or clarithromycin	Adults 500 mg; Children 15 mg/kg orally 1 hr before procedure	15 mg/kg
Allergic to penicillins or ampicillin and unable to take oral medications	Cefazolin or ceftriaxone[b]	1.0 g IM or IV	50 mg/kg IM or IV
	or		
	Clindamycin	600 mg IM or IV	20 mg/kg IM or IV

[a]Or other first- or second-generation oral cephalosporin in equivalent adult or pediatric dosage.
[b]Cephalosporins should not be used in an individual with anaphylaxis, angioedema, or urticaria; instead, use penicillin or ampicillin.
IM, Intramuscularly; *IV*, intravenously.
From Wilson W, Taubert KA, Gewitz M, et al. Prevention of infective endocarditis: guidelines from the American Heart Association. Circulation 2007;116:1736-1754.

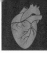

TABLE 6.4   Recommendations for Anticoagulation in Patients With Native Valvular Heart Disease or Bioprosthetic Valves.

Valve Lesion	Recommendation
Rheumatic Mitral Valve Stenosis	
Paroxysmal, persistent or permanent AF	Warfarin, INR 2.0–3.0
Previous embolic event or left atrial thrombus (even with normal sinus rhythm)	Warfarin, INR 2.0–3.0
Recurrent systemic emboli despite adequate anticoagulation	Add aspirin 80–100 mg once daily **OR** dipyridamole 400 mg once daily **OR** ticlopidine 250 mg twice daily
Native Valve Aortic Stenosis, Aortic Regurgitation, Mitral Regurgitation, or Tricuspid Regurgitation	
Paroxysmal, persistent or permanent AF and a CHA2DS2-VASc score ≥ 2 in the setting of native aortic valve disease, tricuspid valve disease, or mitral regurgitation	Antithrombotic therapy with a DOAC or VKA (INR 2.0–3.0). The indication for anticoagulation in these patients should follow guideline-directed therapy using the CHA2DS2-VASc score.
Bioprosthetic Valve, Mitral Valve Repair, or Ring Annuloplasty[a]	
Paroxysmal, persistent or permanent AF	Antithrombotic therapy with a DOAC or VKA (INR 2.0–3.0). Patients with a bioprosthetic valve or mitral repair are at higher risk for embolic events with AF and should undergo anticoagulation irrespective of the CHA2DS2-VASc score.
Infective Endocarditis	
Native valve or tissue prosthesis	Anticoagulation therapy contraindicated
Mechanical valve	Continue or restart anticoagulation (heparin or warfarin) as soon as neurologic condition allows
Nonbacterial Thrombotic Endocarditis	
With systemic emboli	Heparin anticoagulation
Debilitating disease with aseptic vegetations on echocardiography	Heparin anticoagulation

[a]Irrespective of whether open surgical arrhythmia procedures or surgical left atrial appendage surgery has been performed. Open surgical arrhythmia procedures do not reduce the risk of stroke in patients with atrial arrhythmias and valvular heart disease. This includes surgical maze procedures, pulmonary vein isolation, and ligation of the left atrial appendage. These procedures should not be employed to obviate long-term oral anticoagulation. The decision about-long term anticoagulation should be made according to the AHA/ACC/HRS guidelines for the management of patients with AF based on the risk of embolic events versus the risk of bleeding and not predicated on whether a surgical arrhythmia procedure was performed.

AF, Atrial fibrillation; *AHA*, American Heart Association; *CHA2DS2-VASc score*, an updated algorithm for stroke risk assessment in AF (Congestive heart failure, Hypertension, Age [>65 = 1 point, >75 = 2 points], Diabetes, previous Stroke or transient ischemic attack [2 points], VAScular disease [peripheral arterial disease, previous myocardial infarction, aortic atheroma] and sex category [female gender]); *DOAC*, direct-acting oral anticoagulant; *INR*, international normalized ratio; *VKA*, vitamin K antagonist.

Data from Bonow RO, Carabello BA, Kanu C, et al. ACC/AHA 2006 guidelines for the management of patients with valvular heart disease: a report of the American College of Cardiology/American Heart Association Task Force on Practice Guidelines (writing committee to revise the 1998 Guidelines for the Management of Patients With Valvular Heart Disease): developed in collaboration with the Society of Cardiovascular Anesthesiologists: endorsed by the Society for Cardiovascular Angiography and Interventions and the Society of Thoracic Surgeons. Circulation 2006;114:e84-e231; Whitlock RP, Sun JC, Fremes SE, et al. Antithrombotic and thrombolytic therapy for valvular disease: Antithrombotic Therapy and Prevention of Thrombosis, 9th ed: American College of Chest Physicians Evidence-Based Clinical Practice Guidelines. Chest 2012;141(Suppl):e576S-e600S; January CT, Wann LS, Calkins H, et al. 2019 AHA/ACC/HRS focused update of the 2014 AHA/ACC/HRS guideline for the management of patients with atrial fibrillation: a report of the American College of Cardiology/American Heart Association Task Force on Clinical Practice Guidelines and the Heart Rhythm Society. J Am Coll Cardiol 2019;74:104-132.

excluded patients with VHD. However, in the ARISTOTLE study comparing apixaban with VKA therapy for prevention of embolic events in patients with AF, detailed echocardiographic information on VHD severity was not collected, and the classification of valvular lesion and severity relied on clinical data from the case report forms.[36] Patients with clinically significant (moderate to severe) mitral stenosis and those with mechanical prosthetic heart valves were excluded, but patients with any other form of VHD were enrolled, including those with mild mitral stenosis, mitral regurgitation, aortic stenosis or regurgitation, tricuspid valve disease, and previous valve surgery.[37] A subgroup analysis of these data suggested that apixaban compared with warfarin resulted in reductions in stroke or systemic embolism, caused less

bleeding, and reduced mortality rates similarly for patients with and without VHD (Table 6.5).

Most experts think that patients with AF and aortic valve disease or nonrheumatic mitral valve disease should be treated using the same guidelines as for management of AF in patients without valve disease, particularly if the valve disease is only mild or moderate in severity.[38,39] However, VKA therapy continues to be recommended for patients with AF associated with rheumatic mitral valve disease. The risk of atrial thrombus and embolism is particularly high for AF in adults with mitral stenosis; an international normalized ratio (INR) of 2.0 to 3.0 is recommended for these patients. Treatment with a DOAC is contraindicated for those with rheumatic mitral stenosis. Anticoagulation also is

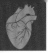

recommended for patients with mitral stenosis and a previous embolic event or a LA thrombus, even if they are currently in sinus rhythm.[7,40]

The optimal choice and need for anticoagulation after mitral valve repair is less clear.[46] Registry data suggest that VKA treatment during the first 3 months after mitral valve repair is associated with a lower risk of stroke or death without excess major bleeding risk.[47] There is a

pressing need for a randomized trial to guide therapy and to ascertain the potential for resource conservation.[48]

Other Indications for Anticoagulation

Some data support the use of VKA anticoagulation in patients with mitral stenosis who are in sinus rhythm with an LA dimension greater than 55 mm and those with prominent spontaneous contrast on echocardiography because of the high risk of atrial thrombus formation even in the absence of AF,[49] but this clinical decision is influenced by the severity of stenosis and the existence of comorbid conditions.

In the absence of AF, anticoagulation is not indicated for patients with aortic valve disease or asymptomatic mitral valve prolapse because of the low risk of embolic events with these lesions. Although elderly patients with mitral annular calcification appear to be at higher risk for embolic events, there is no evidence that anticoagulation is beneficial in the absence of concurrent AF.[7,49–51] If patients with mitral prolapse have unexplained transient ischemic attacks, treatment with aspirin is recommended. Long-term VKA anticoagulation is indicated for patients with mitral valve prolapse with or without a documented systemic embolic event who are in AF if there is at least one other risk factor (i.e., age > 65 years, mitral regurgitation, or LA thrombus).[52]

For younger patients (<65 years) with mitral prolapse and AF, aspirin therapy is recommended unless there is a history of stroke, hypertension, mitral regurgitation, or LA thrombus—situations for which VKA is appropriate. However, some clinicians also consider VKA therapy for patients who have mitral prolapse with a stroke and excessive leaflet thickening (>5 mm) or redundancy (even without AF or other risk factors) and for those with persistent transient ischemic

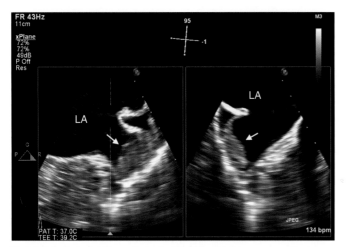

Fig. 6.2 Left Atrial Thrombus. In this 45-year-old woman with severe mitral stenosis referred for balloon valvotomy, transesophageal biplane orthogonal images of the left atrial *(LA)* appendage show an irregular mass *(arrows)* consistent with atrial thrombus. (From Otto CM. Textbook of clinical echocardiography. 5th ed. Philadelphia: Elsevier; 2013.)

TABLE 6.5   Definitions of Nonvalvular Atrial Fibrillation as Exclusion Criteria in Phase II and III Trials With Direct Oral Anticoagulants for Atrial Fibrillation.

Study	Study Drug	Atrial Fibrillation Exclusion Criteria
SPORTIF-III[152]	Ximelagatran	Mitral stenosis, previous valvular heart surgery, active infective endocarditis
SPORTIF-IV[153]	Ximelagatran	Mitral stenosis, previous valvular heart surgery, active infective endocarditis
PETRO[154]	Dabigatran etexilate	Mitral stenosis, prosthetic valves
RE-LY[155,156]	Dabigatran etexilate	History of heart valve disorder (including hemodynamically relevant valve disease and prosthetic valve)
ROCKET-AF[157]	Rivaroxaban	Hemodynamically significant mitral valve stenosis, prosthetic heart valve (annuloplasty with or without prosthetic ring, commissurotomy, and valvuloplasty are permitted)
J-ROCKET AF[158]	Rivaroxaban	Hemodynamically significant mitral valve stenosis, prosthetic heart valve
AVERROES[159,160]	Apixaban	Valvular disease requiring surgery
ARISTOTLE[36]	Apixaban	Clinically significant (moderate or severe) mitral stenosis
ARISTOTLE-J[161]	Apixaban	Valvular heart disease
Edoxaban phase II study[162,163]	Edoxaban	Comorbid rheumatic valvular disease, history of valvular surgery, infective endocarditis
ENGAGE AF-TIMI 48[164]	Edoxaban	Moderate or severe mitral stenosis, unresected atrial myxoma, mechanical heart valve (bioprosthetic heart valve and valve repair are permitted)
EXPLORE-Xa[165]	Betrixaban	Conditions other than atrial fibrillation that required chronic anticoagulation

ARISTOTLE: Apixaban for Reduction in Stroke and Other Thromboembolic Events in Atrial Fibrillation; *ARISTOTLE-J:* Safety and efficacy of the oral direct factor Xa inhibitor apixaban in Japanese patients with nonvalvular atrial fibrillation; *AVERROES:* apixaban versus acetylsalicylic acid to prevent stroke in atrial fibrillation patients who have failed or are unsuitable for vitamin K antagonist treatment; *Edoxaban phase II study:* randomized, parallel-group, multicenter, multinational, phase 2 study comparing edoxaban, an oral factor Xa inhibitor, with warfarin for stroke prevention in patients with atrial fibrillation; *ENGAGE AF-TIMI 48:* Effective Anticoagulation with Factor Xa Next Generation in Atrial Fibrillation–Thrombolysis in Myocardial Infarction 48; *EXPLORE-Xa:* phase II study of the safety, tolerability and pilot efficacy of oral factor Xa inhibitor betrixaban compared with warfarin; *J-ROCKET AF:* Japanese Rivaroxaban Once daily oral direct factor Xa inhibition Compared with vitamin K antagonism for prevention of stroke and Embolism Trial in Atrial Fibrillation; *PETRO:* dabigatran with or without concomitant aspirin compared with warfarin alone in patients with nonvalvular atrial fibrillation; *RE-LY:* Randomized Evaluation of Long-Term Anticoagulation Therapy; *ROCKET-AF:* rivaroxaban versus warfarin in nonvalvular atrial fibrillation; *SPORTIF-III:* stroke prevention with the oral direct thrombin inhibitor ximelagatran compared with warfarin in patients with nonvalvular atrial fibrillation; *SPORTIF-IV:* ximelagatran compared with warfarin for prevention of thromboembolism in patients with nonvalvular atrial fibrillation: rationale, objectives, and design of a pair of clinical studies and baseline patient characteristics.
Modified from De Caterina R, Camm AJ. What is 'valvular' atrial fibrillation? A reappraisal. Eur Heart J 2014;35:3328-3335.

attacks despite aspirin.[53] In addition to the standard practice of short-duration electrocardiographic (ECG) monitoring, noninvasive ambulatory ECG monitoring for a target of 30 days should be considered to improve the detection of AF in these situations.[54]

For patients with IE, anticoagulation should be avoided in general due to the increased risk of hemorrhagic transformation of embolic stroke and the lack of evidence of benefit.[55,56] The major exception to the avoidance of anticoagulation in endocarditis cases is the presence of a mechanical valve. In this situation, most studies suggest that chronic anticoagulation should be continued unless the patient develops a stroke.[57] The choice of intravenous heparin (which allows anticoagulation to be promptly stopped in the event of a stroke) versus VKA therapy is controversial and depends on the specific clinical circumstances of each case. If VKA is used, close monitoring is needed because many antibiotics affect its metabolism.

Anticoagulation Clinics

When VKA therapy is needed, management by hospital-based anticoagulation clinics results in lower complication rates compared with standard care, with a higher percentage of patients being in the therapeutic window and at a lower cost than with traditional physician-based management[58,59] (Fig. 6.3). The typical anticoagulation clinic is staffed by pharmacists with special expertise in anticoagulation management who use written policies and procedures developed in collaboration with the responsible physicians to monitor and adjust the medication dose based on the blood INR.

At the initiation of therapy, a target INR and acceptable range are defined by the referring physician for each patient based on published guidelines and clinical factors unique to the patient. The pharmacist interviews each patient with specific attention to current medications, diet, lifestyle, and any other factors that may affect long-term anticoagulation therapy. Patient education about anticoagulation, possible dietary and drug interactions, recognition of complications of therapy, and the need for careful monitoring of the INR is provided verbally and with the use of a variety of media.

Typically, the INR is measured weekly or more frequently after the initiation of therapy, with a typical interval of 4 weeks for patients on a stable therapeutic regimen. At each visit, the timing of the next INR measurement is determined based on the current INR and any trends over the past several visits. Further patient education and counseling are provided as needed. The pharmacist monitors concurrent medical therapy for any potential drug interactions, and the patient or physician can contact the pharmacist before starting new prescription or nonprescription medications to avoid possible interactions by choosing an alternate agent or to alert the pharmacist of the need for more frequent INR determinations if an effect is likely.

Minor bleeding complications can be managed by the anticoagulation clinic in consultation with the physician, depending on the specific protocol at each institution. Patients with major bleeding episodes or thromboembolic events are triaged promptly for acute medical care. The anticoagulation clinic manages changes in therapy necessitated by

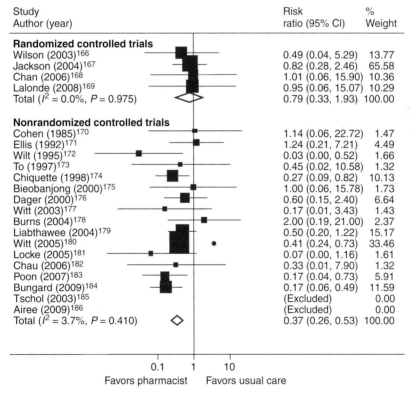

Fig. 6.3 Effect of Pharmacist-Led Clinical Care Versus Usual Care on Thromboembolic Events. Data from a meta-analysis of 24 studies with 728,377 patients show the relative benefit of a pharmacist-led anticoagulation clinic versus standard care in terms of the incidence of thromboembolic events. Patients in these studies were receiving warfarin anticoagulation for a variety of indications, including atrial fibrillation and mechanical heart valves. *Diamonds* indicate the summary risk ratios and 95% confidence intervals *(CIs)*. The size of each *square* is proportional to the reciprocal of the variance of the study. (From Saokaew S, Permsuwan U, Chaiyakunapruk N, et al. Effectiveness of pharmacist-participated warfarin therapy management: a systematic review and meta-analysis. J Thromb Haemost 2010;8:2418-2427.)

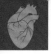

surgical or invasive procedures using procedures developed in conjunction with the referring physician (Figs. 6.4 and 6.5).

Another option is self-management of anticoagulation by the patient using a small home monitoring device that analyzes a fingerstick blood sample. In randomized trials, conventional therapy and home management showed similar rates of anticoagulation control, with an INR in the therapeutic range about two thirds of the time for both groups, but the rate of major complications was lower for the home management group.[60] A meta-analysis of 14 randomized studies of home monitoring of VKA therapy demonstrated lower rates of thromboembolic events, all-cause mortality, and major hemorrhage.[61] All of the study authors emphasized that home monitoring was appropriate only for selected patients and that it required careful education and supervision.[62]

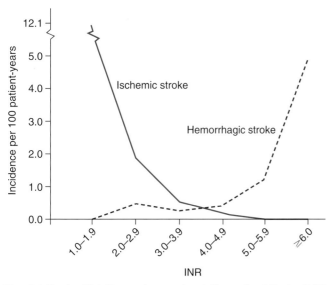

Fig. 6.4 Stroke Risk Versus International Normalized Ratio *(INR)*. Incidence of ischemic and hemorrhagic stroke among patients with mechanical heart valves according to INR category. (From Cannegieter SC, Rosendaal FR, Wintzen AR, et al. Optimal oral anticoagulant therapy in patients with mechanical heart valves. N Engl J Med 1995;333:11-17.)

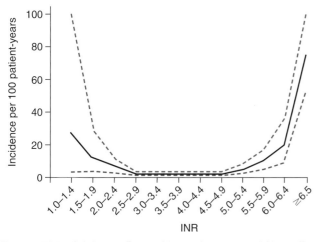

Fig. 6.5 Risk of Adverse Events Versus International Normalized Ratio *(INR)* Among Patients on Oral Anticoagulation. INR-specific incidence of all adverse events (i.e., all episodes of thromboembolism, all major bleeding episodes, and unclassified stroke). The *dotted lines* indicate the 95% confidence interval. (From Cannegieter SC, Rosendaal FR, Wintzen AR, et al. Optimal oral anticoagulant therapy in patients with mechanical heart valves. N Engl J Med 1995;333:11-17.)

BOX 6.4 Recommendations for Participation in Competitive Sports by Adults With Asymptomatic Valvular Heart Disease[a]

- Should not participate in any competitive sports
  - Severe MS
  - MS of any degree with an exercise PA pressure > 50 mmHg
  - Severe MR with pulmonary hypertension, LV dilation (EDD ≥ 60 mm) or LV systolic dysfunction
  - Severe AS
  - Severe AR and LV dilation (EDD ≥ 65 mm)
- Avoid sports with risk of bodily contact
  - All patients with valvular heart disease on long-term anticoagulation
- Can participate in all competitive sports
  - Mild MS in NSR and an exercise PA pressure < 50 mmHg
  - Mild to moderate MR in NSR with normal LV size and function
  - Mild AS (with annual evaluation of AS severity; with periodic aortic root assessment in bicuspid aortic valve cases)
  - Mild to moderate AR with normal LV size

[a]Recommendations for patients with moderate asymptomatic valve disease are individualized depending on the type and level of activity and objective measures of the patient's exercise response.
AR, Atrial regurgitation; *AS,* atrial stenosis; *EDD,* end-diastolic left ventricular dimension; *LV,* left ventricular; *MR,* mitral regurgitation; *MS,* mitral stenosis; *NSR,* normal sinus rhythm; *PA,* pulmonary artery. Modified from Bonow RO, Cheitlin MD, Crawford JH, et al. Task Force 3: valvular heart disease. J Am Coll Cardiol 2005;45:1334-1340.

General Health Maintenance

Adults with mild to moderate asymptomatic VHD should be encouraged to maintain a normal body weight and to remain physically fit with regular dynamic physical activity. There are no restrictions on participation in competitive sports in asymptomatic patients with VHD who are in sinus rhythm, have normal LV size and systolic function, and have normal pulmonary pressures at rest and with exercise. Even those with severe asymptomatic valve disease should be encouraged to participate in regular low-level aerobic activity, although participation in competitive sports and strenuous activity should be avoided, as summarized in Box 6.4.[63] Recommendations regarding competitive sports are more problematic for patients with moderate disease and should be individualized based on the existence of LV dilation or dysfunction and the patient's hemodynamic response to exercise (Fig. 6.6). Patients on chronic anticoagulation for AF or a prosthetic valve should avoid sports with the potential for bodily contact or falls.

Pneumococcal and annual influenza vaccinations are recommended for all adults older than 65 years of age and are especially important for patients with valvular disease because the increased hemodynamic demands of an acute infection may lead to cardiac decompensation. For younger patients with valve disease, routine immunization is indicated only if they have coexisting conditions associated with immunocompromise.

Patients with valvular disease should have an assessment of risk factors for coronary artery disease and aggressive risk factor modification as appropriate. Because aortic valve sclerosis is associated with an increased risk of myocardial infarction and cardiac death, the finding of aortic sclerosis on echocardiography should prompt a careful evaluation and initiation of treatment for known cardiac risk factors.[64,65] Many patients with valvular disease need eventual surgical intervention, and surgical mortality and morbidity rates are markedly increased when coronary disease complicates VHD. The negative impact of coexisting coronary disease is particularly striking for mitral regurgitation, with coronary disease conferring a fourfold increase in the surgical mortality rate, although this varies by surgical center.[66–68] In aortic

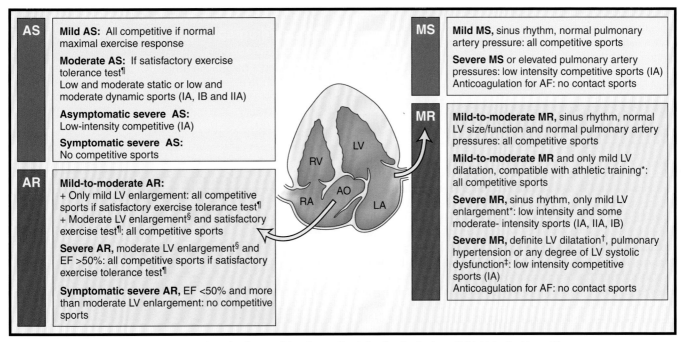

Fig. 6.6 Recommendations for Competitive Sports Participation by Patients With Valvular Heart Disease. Parameters include satisfactory exercise capacity without symptoms, ST depression, ventricular tachyarrhythmias and normal blood pressure response (¶); left ventricular end-systolic dimension (LVESD) < 50 mm in men, < 40 mm in women, or < 25 mm/m² in either sex (§); left ventricular end-diastolic dimension (LVEDD) < 60 mm or < 35 mm/m² in men or < 40 mm/m² in women (*); LVEDD ≥ 65 mm or ≥ 35.3 mm/m² in men or ≥ 40 mm/m² in women (†); and ejection fraction (EF) < 60% or LVESD > 40 mm (‡). *AF,* Atrial fibrillation; *AR,* aortic regurgitation; *AS,* aortic stenosis; *AV,* aortic valve; *LA,* left atrium; *LV,* left ventricle; *MR,* mitral regurgitation; *MS,* mitral stenosis; *MV,* mitral valve. (From D'Silva A, Sharma S. Management of young competitive athletes with cardiovascular conditions. Heart 2017;103:463-473.)

stenosis, concurrent coronary disease is associated with an approximate doubling of the surgical mortality rate.[69–71]

Registry data show that, with improvement in surgical techniques and team-based care in the setting of concomitant coronary artery disease and valvular disease, many centers have greatly narrowed the mortality risk gap for these patients' short-term outcomes when adjusted for age and other comorbidities, although perioperative complications still remain quite high.[72] Knowledge of the outcomes of these conditions in the physician's medical community is important to adequately counsel the patient and allow well-informed, shared decision making. As treatment options expand beyond traditional surgical interventions, it is necessary to understand the importance of concomitantly and appropriately treating the coronary artery disease

burden in VHD patients; the prognostic importance of revascularization in this population should influence decisions regarding the revascularization strategy for patients undergoing valve therapy.[73]

MONITORING DISEASE PROGRESSION

Periodic history taking, physical examination, and noninvasive monitoring are essential for optimal timing of interventions in patients with VHD. Disease progression may be evident as changes in valve anatomy or motion; an increase in the severity of valve stenosis or regurgitation; LV dilation, hypertrophy, or dysfunction in response to pressure or volume overload; or secondary effects of the valvular lesion, such as pulmonary hypertension or AF (Table 6.6).

TABLE 6.6 Stages of Progression of Valvular Heart Disease.

Stage	Definition	Description
A	At risk	Patients with risk factors for the development of VHD
B	Progressive	Patients with progressive VHD (mild to moderate severity and asymptomatic) Asymptomatic patients who have reached the criteria for severe VHD
C	Asymptomatic severe	C1: Asymptomatic patients with severe VHD in whom the left or right ventricle remains compensated C2: Asymptomatic patients who have severe VHD with decompensation of the left or right ventricle
D	Symptomatic severe	Patients who have developed symptoms as a result of VHD

VHD, Valvular heart disease.
Adapted from Nishimura RA, Otto CM, Bonow RO, et al. 2014 AHA/ACC guideline for the management of patients with valvular heart disease: a report of the American College of Cardiology/American Heart Association Task Force on Practice Guidelines. J Am Coll Cardiol. 2014;63:e57-e185.

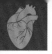
The frequency of periodic evaluations is tailored to each case and depends on the severity of the lesion at the initial evaluation, the known natural history of the disease, indications for surgical intervention, and other clinical factors for each patient.

No simple set of rules defines the optimal or most cost-effective frequency of evaluation. However, based on our understanding of the natural history of valve disease, a framework for periodic evaluation can be devised (Table 6.7). An initial complete diagnostic echocardiographic study is performed to define disease severity, LV size and systolic function, pulmonary pressures, and associated abnormalities. Next, a basic frequency of repeat examination is suggested for each valve lesion depending on the severity of valve disease and, for valve regurgitation, the LV response to chronic volume overload.

The specific timing of repeat studies may need to be modified depending on interim changes in symptoms or physical examination findings, new-onset AF, evidence of progressive LV dilation or early contractile dysfunction, or evidence of increasing pulmonary pressures. For example, an apparent increase in ventricular dimensions in a patient with chronic regurgitation prompts a repeat evaluation at a shorter time interval to distinguish a pathologic change from normal physiologic or measurement variation. Similarly, a change in symptom status for a patient with myxomatous mitral valve disease warrants re-evaluation because a sudden change in regurgitant severity due to chordal rupture may have occurred. More frequent examinations are warranted when quantitative parameters are approaching the values defined as optimal for timing of surgical intervention.

In other clinical situations, re-evaluation may be indicated to assess hemodynamics under changing physiologic conditions (e.g., during pregnancy), to assess other affected structures (e.g., aortopathy associated with a bicuspid valve),[74] to guide a surgical or interventional procedure, or to assess results and complications after an intervention.[75] For patients with comorbid diseases, such as those undergoing noncardiac surgery, a repeat echocardiographic examination may be needed to assist in medical or surgical management.

MEDICAL THERAPY

Prevention of Progressive Valve Disease

Ideally, the treatment of VHD should be directed toward the underlying disease process affecting valve anatomy and function. Worldwide, primary prevention of rheumatic heart disease would have a dramatic impact on the incidence of VHD.[22] For patients with rheumatic heart disease, prevention of recurrent episodes of rheumatic fever is critical for preventing further valve damage and progressive disease. However, no specific therapies are available to prevent or reverse the primary disease processes in other types of valve disease.

Recognition that calcific valve disease is an active disease process with similarities to atherosclerosis led to the hypothesis that disease progression might be prevented by lipid-lowering therapy (see Chapters 3 and 4). However, well-designed, randomized prospective trials of lipid-lowering therapy in adults with mild to moderate calcific aortic valve disease have shown no effect on disease progression or the need for valve replacement.[18,76–78] Hopefully, further research will lead to targeted therapy to prevent disease progression in adults with calcific valve disease.[79,80]

Prevention of Left Ventricular Contractile Dysfunction

As discussed in Chapter 5, the basic response of the LV to the chronic volume overload imposed by aortic or mitral regurgitation is an increase in chamber size. Initially, LV systolic function is normal, but

TABLE 6.7　Framework for Periodic Echocardiography in Patients With Valvular Heart Disease.

Step 1: Initial Diagnostic Study
Comprehensive baseline echocardiographic and Doppler examination. Transesophageal imaging should be considered if transthoracic images are nondiagnostic.

Step 2: Frequency of Examination
The basic frequency of echocardiographic examination provides a starting point for each patient; it is modified as appropriate in steps 3 and 4.

Valve Lesion	Severity	Basic Frequency
Aortic stenosis	Mild (V_{max} < 3.0 m/s)	3–5 years
	Moderate (V_{max} 3–4 m/s)	1–2 years
	Severe (V_{max} > 4.0 m/s)	Annually
Aortic regurgitation	Mild	2–3 years
	Moderate, normal LV size	1–2 years
	Severe, normal LV size	Annually
	Severe, LV dilation	6–12 months
Mitral stenosis	Mild (MVA > 2.0 cm²)	2–3 years
	Moderate (MVA 1–2 cm²)	Annually
	Severe (MVA < 1.0 cm²)	6–12 months
Mitral regurgitation	Mild	2–3 years
	Moderate	1–2 years
	Severe, normal LV size	Annually
	Severe, change in LV size or function	6 months

Step 3: Modifiers of Examination Frequency
Increase frequency:
- Interim change in symptoms or physical examination findings
- New-onset atrial fibrillation
- Evidence for progressive LV dilation and/or early contractile dysfunction
- Evidence for increasing pulmonary pressures
- Rising BNP levels

Decrease frequency:
- Stable findings over 2–3 examination intervals

Step 4: Special Situations
Preoperative for noncardiac surgery
Pregnancy
Monitoring of interventional procedures
Assessment of complications and hemodynamic results after an intervention
Intraoperative transesophageal monitoring

BNP, Brain natriuretic peptide; *MVA*, mitral valve area; V_{max}, maximal velocity across the valve.
Adapted from Nishimura RA, Otto CM, Bonow RO, et al. 2014 AHA/ACC guideline for the management of patients with valvular heart disease: a report of the American College of Cardiology/American Heart Association Task Force on Practice Guidelines. J Am Coll Cardiol 2014;63:e57-e185.

with long-standing disease, contractile dysfunction may supervene and may not improve after intervention to correct the regurgitant lesion. Whereas most patients develop symptoms that prompt consideration of valve surgery, in a subset of patients, LV dysfunction occurs before symptom onset.[81] A major focus of the medical management of patients with chronic valvular regurgitation is periodic noninvasive evaluation to monitor LV size and systolic function. The rationale for sequential monitoring is that surgical intervention can be performed just before or soon after the onset of contractile dysfunction.

Although no value of brain natriuretic peptide (BNP) is agreed on as mandating a valvular intervention, an increasing BNP level on sequential follow-up examinations is worrisome and may help to steer management.[82] However, caution should be used in the use of BNP to follow VHD. Although it is recognized that BNP concentrations are elevated in patients with valvular heart lesions, significant adverse cardiac remodeling can occur in VHD despite plasma BNP concentrations within the normal range.[83,84]

A more elusive goal in the medical therapy for patients with chronic regurgitation is to prevent or delay progressive LV dilation and contractile dysfunction, thereby delaying the need for surgical intervention. Afterload reduction therapy improves acute hemodynamics, but clinical studies have yielded varied results on the potential benefit of afterload reduction to prevent progressive LV dilation in response to chronic aortic or mitral regurgitations (see Chapters 12 and 19). There are no class I indications for afterload reduction therapy in non-hypertensive adults with chronic asymptomatic aortic or mitral regurgitation.[7,82,85] However, adults with chronic regurgitation and an elevated blood pressure, which is common in this patient group, should receive appropriate antihypertensive therapy.

Instead of altering systemic vascular resistance, another approach to therapy is to prevent adverse effects on the LV myocardium. A pilot study of β-blocker therapy for patients with mitral regurgitation showed a favorable trend in prevention of LV systolic dysfunction compared with placebo.[86] These data may stimulate larger prospective trials of therapy directed toward preserving LV function in adults with VHD.[87]

In patients with asymptomatic valvular aortic stenosis, the development of LV contractile dysfunction is uncommon, occurring in less than 1%,[88] and the timing of surgical intervention is based on symptom onset and severity of stenosis rather than on changes in LV geometry or function.[89–91] There are no known medical therapies to prevent or modify the development of LV hypertrophy in adults with aortic stenosis, and it is not clear that preventing this adaptive response would improve outcome. However, speckle-tracking strain imaging has shown that subclinical changes in LV longitudinal shortening occur early in the disease process.[92]

There has been considerable interest in the changes in diastolic ventricular dysfunction that occur in patients with aortic stenosis.[93,94] It has been hypothesized that surgical intervention before the development of irreversible changes in the myocardium might improve long-term clinical outcome.[95–97] However, there is no medical therapy known to prevent early systolic or diastolic dysfunction in patients with pressure overload hypertrophy.

Prevention of Left Atrial Enlargement and Atrial Fibrillation

Progressive LA enlargement and AF typically complicate the clinical course of mitral valve disease. Mitral regurgitation and mitral stenosis are associated with LA dilation due to the pressure and volume overload of the LA.[98–100] AF occurs frequently, particularly in older patients and in those with severe and long-standing disease. Atrial enlargement and fibrillation occasionally complicate aortic valve disease, typically late in the disease course, and may worsen hemodynamics substantially due to loss of the atrial contribution to ventricular filling.[101,102]

Medically, there is no specific therapy to prevent these complications of the disease process, although it has been proposed that earlier surgical or percutaneous intervention might prevent atrial enlargement and eventual AF. Surgical intervention for mitral regurgitation soon after the onset of AF (within 3 months) is more likely to restore

sinus rhythm than in patients with AF of longer duration, but it still is not uniformly successful.[63] In patients with mitral stenosis, AF usually recurs or persists after intervention.

Prevention of Pulmonary Hypertension

The chronic elevation in LA pressure associated with mitral valve disease results in a passive increase in pulmonary pressures that resolves when LA pressure decreases after surgical or percutaneous intervention. However, reactive changes in the pulmonary vasculature may become superimposed on this passive rise in pressure, with secondary histologic changes leading to irreversible pulmonary hypertension. Intervention before the onset of irreversible changes is desirable to avoid long-term complications of right-sided heart failure. In some patients, an excessive rise in pulmonary pressures with exercise may be the first clue that intervention is needed to prevent further irreversible changes in the pulmonary vasculature.[103–105]

For adults with aortic valve disease, pulmonary hypertension is a risk factor for increased operative mortality and decreased long-term survival.[106] Preliminary studies suggest that phosphodiesterase type 5 inhibitors may be beneficial in reducing systemic and pulmonary vascular resistance in aortic stenosis patients.[107]

Symptoms Caused by Valve Disease

Although the goal in management of patients with valvular disease is to avoid symptoms and the need for medical therapy by optimizing the timing of surgical intervention, some patients have persistent symptoms after surgery, have symptoms only in response to a superimposed hemodynamic stress (e.g., pregnancy), or are not candidates for surgical intervention. In these situations, medical therapy is based primarily on adjustment of loading conditions and control of heart rate and rhythm.

Patients with pulmonary congestion are treated with diuretics to decrease LA and pulmonary venous pressures, whether elevated LA pressures are due to LV dysfunction, mitral regurgitation, or mitral stenosis. However, when mitral stenosis exists, care is needed to ensure that LA pressures allow adequate LV diastolic filling across the narrowed valve. In patients with aortic stenosis, diuretics should be used cautiously because pulmonary congestion often is caused by diastolic dysfunction rather than volume overload. The further decrease in ventricular diastolic volume induced by diuretics may worsen symptoms as mid-cavity ventricular obstruction develops in the small, hypertrophied, hyperdynamic LV.

Afterload reduction is most beneficial for the treatment of heart failure symptoms in patients with acute aortic or mitral regurgitation. With acute regurgitation, a continuous intravenous infusion of nitroprusside may be used. Intraaortic balloon counterpulsation provides effective afterload reduction while maintaining coronary diastolic perfusion pressures in patients with acute mitral regurgitation. However, an intraaortic balloon is contraindicated with aortic regurgitation because the increase in aortic diastolic pressure results in more severe valve regurgitation. In symptomatic patients with chronic regurgitation, standard therapy for heart failure is reasonable, including afterload reduction, only if surgery is not an option or if heart failure occurs in the setting of a reversible hemodynamic stress. In patients with mitral stenosis, afterload reduction is not helpful because the ventricle typically is small with normal systolic function.

In the past, there was concern that afterload reduction in adults with severe aortic stenosis might result in a precipitous fall in blood pressure due to peripheral vasodilation because only a fixed stroke volume can be pumped though the rigid orifice.[108,109] However, other studies suggested that cautious use of afterload reduction is well tolerated and could be beneficial until definitive therapy can be performed.[110,111] Most likely, the benefit of afterload reduction is a greater

degree of leaflet motion and increase in functional valve area when cardiac output is increased.[112,113] Particularly when there is coexisting LV dysfunction, the decrease in systemic vascular resistance may lead to improved LV contractility and an increase in LV output due to increased opening of the valve leaflets[114]; however, with the increasing options of interventional/surgical approaches, most patients in this situation need to be treated in a specialized valve center if aggressive therapy is the wish of the patient. Chapter 12 discusses acute mechanical interventional approaches in the decompensated aortic valve patient. The mortality rate is high for these patients, and it is prudent to include a discussion of palliative and hospice care for those not wanting aggressive mechanical management at this phase of the disease process.[115,116]

MANAGEMENT OF CONCURRENT CARDIOVASCULAR CONDITIONS

Hypertension

Concurrent hypertension is common in adults with VHD, with prevalence close to 50% after 65 years of age. Elevated blood pressure is a risk factor for development of aortic and mitral valve disease.[117,118] Many patients with VHD also have hypertension, which should be treated according to established guidelines. Treatment of hypertension is well tolerated by patients with mitral valve disease, and modification in therapy because of the valve lesions is rarely needed.

Treatment of hypertension in patients with aortic valve disease is especially important to reduce total ventricular afterload, which includes the load imposed by the valve lesions and the systemic vascular resistance. With aortic regurgitation, two factors are important in the treatment of hypertension. First, severe aortic regurgitation is characterized by a wide pulse pressure; overtreatment of the high systolic pressure caused by a large total stroke volume may result in excessively low diastolic pressures. In theory, this could compromise diastolic coronary blood flow. Second, therapy that lowers heart rate may result in a higher systolic blood pressure due to an even larger stroke volume with a longer diastolic filling period. If a β-blocker is used, additional therapy with an afterload reducing agent may be need.

With aortic stenosis, treatment of hypertension should follow standard approaches except that therapy should be initiated at low doses and slowly titrated to the therapeutic dose to avoid hypotension. Diuretics should be avoided, particularly in elderly women with aortic stenosis, who typically have a small, hypertrophied ventricle, because any decrease in preload reduces forward cardiac output. Despite concerns in the past that systemic vasodilation might result in hypotension due to lack of a compensatory increase in stroke volume across the narrowed valve as systemic resistance decreases, angiotensin-converting enzyme inhibitor therapy is well tolerated in adults with moderate aortic stenosis.[119,120] Afterload reduction therapy has been proposed as having potential but unproven benefit for preservation of ventricular systolic and diastolic function in aortic stenosis.[121] The presence of hypertension may affect the accuracy of measures of aortic stenosis severity, and blood pressure should be controlled before valve disease severity is assessed.[122–125]

Coronary Artery Disease

Coronary artery disease is common in adults with VHD, as expected based on age, sex, and clinical risk factors in this patient group.[126] Coronary angiography is needed for most patients undergoing valve surgery because concurrent coronary artery bypass grafting is recommended if significant disease is detected. Similarly, the timing of valve

intervention may be affected by the presence and severity of coronary disease, particularly when a patient with asymptomatic aortic stenosis is referred for valve surgery.

For adults with asymptomatic valve disease, prevention of coronary disease based on risk factor evaluation and modification is essential. When symptoms occur, particularly angina, it may be difficult to distinguish whether they are the result of coronary or valve disease.[127] The resting ECG often shows LV hypertrophy and ST changes due to valve disease. Exercise and pharmacologic stress tests are less accurate for detection of coronary stenoses when valve disease exists because exercise duration may be limited by valve, not coronary, disease, and coronary flow patterns are affected by valve hemodynamics.[128]

Direct imaging of coronary anatomy, usually by coronary angiography but alternatively with high-resolution coronary computed tomographic angiography (CCTA) imaging, may be needed.[129] If the cause of symptoms remains unclear after consideration of the severity of valve and coronary disease, it may be appropriate to consider a percutaneous coronary intervention. If symptoms resolve, continued treatment of coronary disease is reasonable; persistent symptoms suggest that the cause is the valve disease. Standard approaches to percutaneous and medical therapy for coronary disease are appropriate for adults with VHD.[130]

Aortic Disease

Aortic valve dysfunction may be caused by or associated with abnormalities of the aortic root. In adults with a bicuspid valve, dilation of the aortic sinuses or ascending aorta is common, and patients with a bicuspid aortic valve have an increased risk of aortic dissection (see Chapter 13). In adults with a primary abnormality of the aorta such as Marfan syndrome, aortic regurgitation may be the result of aortic dilation with relatively normal valve anatomy. Tomographic imaging with a wide field of view (i.e., cardiac CT or CMR) typically is needed in addition to echocardiography for evaluation and monitoring of the location and degree of aortic dilation because echocardiography cannot reliably evaluate the entire length of the aorta. In cases of aortic dilation, the severity of aortic involvement may be the primary driver for repeat imaging and for the timing of surgical intervention.[131,132]

Arrhythmias

For patients with VHD and AF, restoration and maintenance of sinus rhythm is essential to prevent atrial thrombus formation and preserve the atrial contribution to LV diastolic filling. Approaches to restoring and maintaining sinus rhythm are no different for these patients than for those without valve disease other than the increased awareness of embolic risk and need for appropriate anticoagulation (see Table 6.4).[38]

There is increasing interest in concurrent procedures, such as the maze procedure, to restore sinus rhythm at the time of surgical intervention for mitral valve disease.[133,134] AF ablation is unlikely to be successful in cases of significant valve disease unless the hemodynamic abnormality also is corrected.[135] Often, the onset of AF is the first sign of hemodynamic decompensation in patients with chronic, slowly progressive valve disease. Concomitant use of procedures such as the maze procedure has never been shown to decrease the risk of thromboembolic events, and restoration of sinus rhythm with these types of procedures does not obviate the need for chronic anticoagulation based on the best current data.[38,136,137]

When sinus rhythm cannot be maintained, the ventricular rate is controlled with the use of standard approaches. Rate control is especially important for patients with mitral stenosis because a shortened diastolic filling time may result in a symptomatic decrease in forward cardiac output.[138,139]

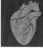

Even with sinus rhythm, heart rate control may be needed in patients with VHD. For example, the increased heart rate (and shortened diastolic filling time) associated with pregnancy in a patient with mitral stenosis leads to inadequate ventricular filling and a reduced cardiac output. Slowing the heart rate with a β-blocker improves diastolic filling and restores a normal cardiac output.[140] Another example is the elderly patient with aortic stenosis. The patient may develop bradycardia due to calcification of the conduction system with heart block or due to sick sinus syndrome; this further reduces the total cardiac output across the stenotic valve, leading to cardiac symptoms.

It is important to understand the risk of heart block with procedures to replace the aortic valve. Whether traditional surgical approaches or newer, less invasive means are used, the necessity of permanent pacing therapy after aortic valve replacement ranges from 3% to 7%.[141,142] Planning for these procedures should consider that severe mitral annular calcification detected preoperatively is associated with a higher risk (odds ratio = 2.83) of requiring permanent pacing periprocedurally and with a higher overall mortality rate.[143] Symptoms due to bradycardia resolve after placement of a pacer, possibly allowing deferral of aortic valve surgery.

There is an increased risk of sudden death of patients with VHD and significant LV dilation or dysfunction due to chronic aortic regurgitation,[144] which can be ameliorated by aortic valve replacement. Mitral valve prolapse also is associated with an increased risk of sudden death, but anti-arrhythmic therapy or placement of an automated implanted defibrillator is based on standard indications for these procedures, not on the existence of valve disease alone.[145]

Heart Failure

Heart failure due to valve stenosis or regurgitation is an indication for surgical or percutaneous intervention in cases of aortic or mitral valve disease. When valve disease is severe, it is likely that heart failure is a result of the valve lesion. For example, severe aortic regurgitation results in LV dilation and systolic dysfunction. With prompt valve replacement, ventricular size and function return to normal.

If valve disease is mild to moderate and there is evidence of heart failure, evaluation for other causes is appropriate. The combination of moderate to severe aortic stenosis and moderate to severe LV dysfunction is a particular clinical challenge because it can be difficult to distinguish whether aortic stenosis resulted in ventricular dysfunction or the poor ventricular function contributed to reduced aortic valve opening (see Chapter 11).

If heart failure is not caused by valve dysfunction, standard approaches to medical therapy and continued sequential monitoring of the valve disease are reasonable. Therapy may need to be started at low doses and titrated slowly upward in cases of aortic stenosis to avoid hypotension due to an abrupt change in systemic vascular resistance. Evaluation of volume status should include consideration of the effects of valve dysfunction on ventricular filling and standard parameters. For example, in mitral stenosis, the LV may still be underfilled if central venous and pulmonary venous pressures are elevated.

Heart failure may be the cause of valve dysfunction. For example, primary ventricular dilation and dysfunction result in secondary (functional) mitral regurgitation due to distortion of the normal mitral annular-ventricular geometry, even when the mitral valve is structurally normal. Primary and secondary forms of mitral regurgitation are distinguished by the relative time courses of ventricular and valvular dysfunction, valve anatomy, and evaluation for other causes of myocardial dysfunction. In patients with secondary mitral regurgitation, treatment of ventricular dysfunction may decrease regurgitant severity (see Chapter 19).

NONCARDIAC SURGERY IN PATIENTS WITH VALVE DISEASE

Most adults with VHD can safely undergo noncardiac surgery, particularly when they have only mild or moderate disease.[146,147] Key principles in management of patients with VHD undergoing noncardiac surgery are
- Accurate assessment of the severity of valve disease
- Symptom status
- Hemodynamic monitoring in the perioperative period
- Optimization of loading conditions

Most adverse outcomes after noncardiac surgery in adults with VHD are caused by failure to recognize valve disease preoperatively.[148] If VHD is suspected based on the history or physical examination findings, echocardiography is appropriate to identify and define the severity of valve lesions.

In asymptomatic patients, valve regurgitation, even if severe, is generally well tolerated during noncardiac surgery. However, patients with moderate to severe left-sided valve obstruction are at higher risk because an elevated preload results in pulmonary edema, whereas a low preload results in hypotension due to a low cardiac output. Peripheral vasodilation is poorly tolerated because of the inability to increase stroke volume when systemic vascular resistance falls.

In asymptomatic patients with stenotic lesions, invasive hemodynamic monitoring often is helpful beginning in the preoperative setting to allow optimization of loading conditions, and continuing for 48 to 72 hours postoperatively during the period of major changes in volume status. Intraoperative echocardiography and participation of an experienced cardiac anesthesiologist also are recommended. When left-sided valve obstruction is very severe, relief of stenosis before noncardiac surgery may be considered, depending on the urgency of the noncardiac surgery and whether a percutaneous approach to relief of valve obstruction is possible.[149]

Symptoms due to valve disease are an indication for a corrective valve procedure. Elective noncardiac surgery should be deferred until after treatment of the valve lesions, whenever possible. With urgent surgery, symptomatic valve regurgitation is managed with the use of standard heart failure regimens based on hemodynamic parameters. Symptomatic severe left-sided valve obstruction can sometimes be managed with the combination of invasive hemodynamic monitoring, intraoperative echocardiography, and consultation with an experienced cardiac anesthesiologist. However, in the case of mitral stenosis, percutaneous valvotomy should be considered if valve anatomy is suitable and there is no LA thrombus. In cases of severe symptomatic aortic stenosis, balloon valvotomy or percutaneous valve implantation may be considered for severe stenosis and an urgent noncardiac surgical procedure. Management of VHD during pregnancy is discussed in Chapter 27.

PATIENT EDUCATION

Patient education is the key to adherence with periodic noninvasive monitoring, prevention of complications, and early recognition of symptoms in patients with VHD. Each patient should understand the expected long-term prognosis, potential complications, typical symptoms, rationale for sequential monitoring, and indications for surgical intervention. Appropriate education avoids needless concern and prompts early reporting of symptoms, allowing optimal timing of surgical intervention. Increasingly, patients are actively involved in decisions about whether to intervene, timing of surgery, and choice of intervention.[150,151]

Patients also should be knowledgeable about the risk of IE and the importance of maintaining optimal oral hygiene, including regular dental care. Education about the clinical presentation of endocarditis and the importance of obtaining blood cultures before antibiotics are started allows the patient to make sure primary care physicians consider the possibility of endocarditis with a febrile illness. Patients with a prosthetic valve should be aware of situations in which endocarditis prophylaxis is needed and the specific antibiotic regimen to be taken.

Patients on long-term anticoagulation need education and a reliable, available source for consultation regarding VKA dose, interactions with other medications, and prompt evaluation of any complications.

All patients with VHD should be evaluated for risk factors for coronary artery disease and should receive education and appropriate therapy for coronary risk factor reduction. Although certain situations may call for modification of exercise habits, most patients with VHD can exercise safely.

Because the risk of pregnancy in patients with VHD ranges from normal to very high, the risk should be estimated and discussed with the patient (see Chapter 27). In patients with very-high-risk valve lesions, surgical correction before a planned pregnancy should be considered. For women on long-term anticoagulation, the issue of VKA versus heparin anticoagulation during pregnancy should be addressed. Contraception options should be reviewed with all women with valvular disease.

For patients with inherited forms of valve disease such as Marfan syndrome, the physician should make every effort to ensure that other family members are screened for the disease. Because of increased understanding of the genetic basis of myxomatous mitral valve disease and bicuspid aortic valve, screening of family members may be appropriate for patients with these conditions, particularly if there is a family history of sudden death or aortic dissection.

REFERENCES

1. Nkomo VT, Gardin JM, Skelton TN, et al. Burden of valvular heart diseases: a population-based study. Lancet 2006;368:1005-11.
2. Iung B, Cachier A, Baron G, et al. Decision-making in elderly patients with severe aortic stenosis: why are so many denied surgery? Eur Heart J 2005;26(24):2714-20.
3. Lancellotti P, Rosenhek R, Pibarot P, et al. ESC Working Group on Valvular Heart Disease position paper—heart valve clinics: organization, structure, and experiences. Eur Heart J 2013;34:1597-606.
4. Perloff JK. Physical examination of the heart and circulation. 4th ed. MD People's Medical Publishing House; 2009.
5. Spencer KT, Kimura BJ, Korcarz CE, et al. Focused cardiac ultrasound: recommendations from the American Society of Echocardiography. J Am Soc Echocardiogr 2013;26(6):567-581.
6. Otto CM. Textbook of clinical echocardiography. 5th ed. Philadelphia: Elsevier; 2013.
7. Nishimura RA, Otto CM, Bonow RO, et al. 2014 AHA/ACC guideline for the management of patients with valvular heart disease: a report of the American College of Cardiology/American Heart Association Task Force on Practice Guidelines. J Am Coll Cardiol 2014;63(22):e57-e185.
8. Premkumar P. Utility of echocardiogram in the evaluation of heart murmurs. Med Clin North Am 2016;100(5):991-1001
9. Zacharias SK, Goldstein JA. Clinical assessment of the severity of aortic stenosis. Aortic stenosis. London: Springer; 2015. p. 21-28.
10. Morrell ED, Katz WE, Tulsky AA. Morbid obesity: obscuring the diagnosis of aortic stenosis in a patient with cardiogenic wheezing. J Gen Int Med 2013;28(1):155-159.
11. Verghese A, Charlton B, Kassirer JP, Ramsey M, Ioannidis JP. Inadequacies of physical examination as a cause of medical errors and adverse events: a collection of vignettes. Am J Med 2015;128(12):1322-1324.
12. Bursi F, Enriquez-Sarano M, Nkomo VT, et al. Heart failure and death after myocardial infarction in the community: the emerging role of mitral regurgitation. Circulation 2005;111:295-301.
13. Barrett MJ, Ayub B, Martinez MW. Cardiac auscultation in sports medicine: strategies to improve clinical care. Curr Sports Med Rep 2012;11(2):78-84.
14. Sanghavi M, Rutherford JD. Cardiovascular physiology of pregnancy. Circulation 2014;130(12):1003-1008.
15. Desjardins VA, Enriquez-Sarano M, Tajik AJ, Bailey KR, Seward JB. Intensity of murmurs correlates with severity of valvular regurgitation. Am J Med 1996;100(2):149-56.
16. Munt B, Legget ME, Kraft CD, Miyake-Hull CY, Fujioka M, Otto CM. Physical examination in valvular aortic stenosis: correlation with stenosis severity and prediction of clinical outcome. Am Heart J 1999;137(2):298-306.
17. Kueh S-H, Pasley T, Wheeler M, Pemberton J. The not so innocent heart murmur: a five year experience. Intern Med J 2016. Accepted Author Manuscript. doi:10.1111/imj.13331.
18. Lindman BR, Bonow RO, Otto CM. Current management of calcific aortic stenosis. Circ Res 2013;113(2):223-237.
19. Gewitz, MH, Baltimore RS, Tani LY, et al. Revision of the Jones Criteria for the diagnosis of acute rheumatic fever in the era of Doppler echocardiography a scientific statement from the American Heart Association. Circulation 2015;131:1806-1818. doi: 10.1161/CIR.0000000000000205.
20. Barash J, Mashiach E, Navon-Elkan P, et al. Differentiation of post-streptococcal reactive arthritis from acute rheumatic fever. J Pediatr 2008;153(5):696-9.
21. van Bemmel JM, Delgado V, Holman ER, et al. No increased risk of valvular heart disease in adult poststreptococcal reactive arthritis. Arthritis Rheum 2009;60(4):987-93.
22. Marijon E, Mirabel M, Celermajer DS, Jouven X. Rheumatic heart disease. Lancet 2012;379(9819):953-964.
23. Reményi B, Wilson N, Steer A, et al. World Heart Federation criteria for echocardiographic diagnosis of rheumatic heart disease—an evidence-based guideline. Nat Rev Cardiol 2012;9(5):297-309.
24. Shulman ST, Bisno AL, Clegg HW, et al. Clinical practice guideline for the diagnosis and management of group A streptococcal pharyngitis: 2012 update by the Infectious Diseases Society of America. Clinical Infectious Dis 2012;cis629.
25. Zühlke L, Engel ME, Karthikeyan G, et al. Characteristics, complications, and gaps in evidence-based interventions in rheumatic heart disease: the Global Rheumatic Heart Disease Registry (the REMEDY study). Eur Heart J 2015;36(18):1115-22.
26. Seto TB. The case for infectious endocarditis prophylaxis: time to move forward. Arch Intern Med 2007;167(4):327-30.
27. Morris AM. Coming clean with antibiotic prophylaxis for infective endocarditis. Arch Intern Med 2007;167(4):330-332.
28. Thornhill MH, Dayer MJ, Forde JM, et al. Impact of the NICE guideline recommending cessation of antibiotic prophylaxis for prevention of infective endocarditis: before and after study. BMJ 2011;342:d2392.
29. Desimone DC, Tleyjeh IM, Correa de Sa DD, et al. Incidence of infective endocarditis caused by viridans group streptococci before and after publication of the 2007 American Heart Association's endocarditis prevention guidelines. Circulation 2012;126(1):60-4.
30. Khan O, Shafi AMA, Timmis A. International guideline changes and the incidence of infective endocarditis: a systematic review. Open Heart 2016;3:e000498. doi:10.1136/openhrt-2016-000498.
31. Vahanian A, Alfieri O, Andreotti F, et al. Guidelines on the management of valvular heart disease (version 2012). Eur Heart J 2012;33(19):2451-96.
32. De Caterina R, Camm AJ. What is 'valvular'atrial fibrillation? A reappraisal. Eur Heart J 2014;35(47):3328-3335.
33. Gilon D, Buonanno FS, Joffe MM, et al. Lack of evidence of an association between mitral-valve prolapse and stroke in young patients. N Engl J Med 1999;341:8-13.
34. Freed LA, Levy D, Levine RA, et al. Prevalence and clinical outcome of mitral-valve prolapse. N Engl J Med 1999;341:1-7.

35. FDA drug safety communication: Pradaxa (dabigatran etexilate mesylate) should not be used in patients with mechanical prosthetic heart valves. http://www fda gov/Drugs/DrugSafety/ucm332912 htm 2012.

36. Granger CB, Alexander JH, McMurray JJ, et al. Apixaban versus warfarin in patients with atrial fibrillation. N Engl J Med 2011;365:981-992.

37. Avezum A, Lopes RD, Schulte PJ, et al. Apixaban in comparison with warfarin in patients with atrial fibrillation and valvular heart disease findings from the apixaban for reduction in stroke and other thromboembolic events in atrial fibrillation (ARISTOTLE) trial. Circulation 2015;132(8): 624-32.

38. January CT, Wann LS, Alpert JS, et al. American College of Cardiology/ American Heart Association Task Force on Practice Guidelines. 2014 AHA/ACC/HRS guideline for the management of patients with atrial fibrillation: a report of the American College of Cardiology/American Heart Association Task Force on Practice Guidelines and the Heart Rhythm Society. J Am Coll Cardiol 2014;64(21):e1-e76.

39. Wann LS, Curtis AB, Ellenbogen KA, et al. 2011 ACCF/AHA/HRS focused update on the management of patients with atrial fibrillation (update on Dabigatran): a report of the American College of Cardiology Foundation/ American Heart Association Task Force on practice guidelines. Circulation 2011;123(10):1144-50.

40. De Caterina R, Husted S, Wallentin L, et al. Vitamin K antagonists in heart disease: current status and perspectives (Section III). Thromb Haemostasis 2013;110(6):1087-107.

41. Hamon M, Lipiecki J, Carrié D, et al. Silent cerebral infarcts after cardiac catheterization: a randomized comparison of radial and femoral approaches. Am Heart J 2012;164(4):449-54.

42. Chu JW, Chen VH, Bunton R. Thrombosis of a mechanical heart valve despite dabigatran. Ann Intern Med 2012;157(4):304.

43. Price J, Hynes M, Labinaz M, Ruel M, Boodhwani M. Mechanical valve thrombosis with dabigatran. J Am Coll Cardiol 2012;60(17):1710-1711.

44. Stewart RA, Astell H, Young L, White HD. Thrombosis on a mechanical aortic valve whilst anti-coagulated with dabigatran. Heart Lung Circ 2012;21(1):53-5.

45. Erwin JP 3rd, Iung B. Current recommendations for anticoagulant therapy in patients with valvular heart disease and atrial fibrillation: the ACC/ AHA and ESC/EACTS guidelines in harmony…but not lockstep! Heart 2018;104(12):968-970.

46. Suri RM, Thourani VH, He X, et al. Variation in warfarin thromboprophylaxis after mitral valve repair: does equipoise exist and is a randomized trial warranted?. Ann Thorac Surg 2013;95(6):1991-9.

47. Valeur N, Mérie C, Hansen ML, et al. Risk of death and stroke associated with anticoagulation therapy after mitral valve repair. Heart 2016;102(9): 687-93.

48. Paparella D, Di Mauro M, Worms KB, et al. Antiplatelet versus oral anticoagulant therapy as antithrombotic prophylaxis after mitral valve repair. J Thorac Cardiovasc Surg 2016;151(5):1302-8.

49. Colli A, Verhoye JP, Heijmen R, et al. Low-dose acetyl salicylic acid versus oral anticoagulation after bioprosthetic aortic valve replacement. Final report of the ACTION registry. Int J Cardiol 2013;168(2):1229-36.

50. Otto CM, Prendergast B. Aortic-valve stenosis—from patients at risk to severe valve obstruction. N Engl J Med 2014;371(8):744-756.

51. Riaz H, Alansari SA, Khan MS, et al. Safety and use of anticoagulation after aortic valve replacement with bioprostheses a meta-analysis. Circ Cardiovasc Qual Outcomes 2016;9(3):294-302.

52. Hart RG, Diener HC, Coutts SB, et al. Embolic strokes of undetermined source: the case for a new clinical construct. Lancet Neurol 2014;13(4):429-38.

53. Stroke Prevention in Atrial Fibrillation Study Group Investigators. Preliminary report of the stroke prevention in atrial fibrillation study. N Engl J Med 1990;1990(322):863-8.

54. Gladstone DJ, Spring M, Dorian P, et al. Atrial fibrillation in patients with cryptogenic stroke. N Engl J Med 2014;370(26):2467-77.

55. Chan KL, Tam J, Dumesnil JG, et al. Effect of long-term aspirin use on embolic events in infective endocarditis. Clin Infect Dis 2008;46(1):37-41.

56. Baddour LM, Wilson WR, Bayer AS, et al. Infective endocarditis in adults: diagnosis, antimicrobial therapy, and management of complications: a

scientific statement for healthcare professionals from the American Heart Association. Circulation 2015;132(15):1435-1486.

57. García-Cabrera E1, Fernández-Hidalgo N, Almirante B, et al. Neurological complications of infective endocarditis risk factors, outcome, and impact of cardiac surgery: a multicenter observational study. Circulation 2013;127:2272-2284.

58. Saokaew S, Permsuwan U, Chaiyakunapruk N, et al. Effectiveness of pharmacist-participated warfarin therapy management: a systematic review and meta-analysis. J Thromb Haemost 2010;8:2418-2427.

59. Aziz F, Corder M, Wolffe J, Comerota AJ. Anticoagulation monitoring by an anticoagulation service is more cost-effective than routine physician care. J Vasc Surg 2011;54(5):1404-7.

60. Menendez-Jandula B, Souto JC, Oliver A, et al. Comparing self-management of oral anticoagulant therapy with clinic management: a randomized trial. Ann Intern Med 2005;142(1):1-10.

61. Heneghan C, Alonso-Coello P, Garcia-Alamino JM, Perera R, Meats E, Glasziou P. Self-monitoring of oral anticoagulation: a systematic review and meta-analysis. Lancet 2006;367(9508):404-11.

62. Ansell J, Jacobson A, Levy J, Voller H, Hasenkam JM. Guidelines for implementation of patient self-testing and patient self-management of oral anticoagulation. International consensus guidelines prepared by International Self-Monitoring Association for Oral Anticoagulation. Int J Cardiol 2005;99(1):37-45.

63. Gillinov AM, Gelijns AC, Parides MK, et al. Surgical ablation of atrial fibrillation during mitral-valve surgery. N Engl J Med 2015;372(15): 1399-1409.

64. Otto CM, Lind BK, Kitzman DW, Gersh BJ, Siscovick DS. Association of aortic-valve sclerosis with cardiovascular mortality and morbidity in the elderly. N Engl J Med 1999;341(3):142-7.

65. Owens DS, Budoff MJ, Katz R, et al. Aortic valve calcium independently predicts coronary and cardiovascular events in a primary prevention population. JACC Cardiovasc Imaging 2012;(6):619-625.

66. Smith PK, Puskas JD, Ascheim DD, et al. Surgical treatment of moderate ischemic mitral regurgitation. N Engl J Med 2014;371:2178-2188. DOI: 10.1056/NEJMoa1410490.

67. Pieri M, Belletti A, Monaco F, et al. Outcome of cardiac surgery in patients with low preoperative ejection fraction. BMC Anesthesiol 2016;16(1):97.

68. Rankin JS, Badhwar V, He X, et al. The Society of Thoracic Surgeons mitral valve repair/replacement plus coronary artery bypass grafting composite score: a report of the Society of Thoracic Surgeons quality measurement task force. Ann Thorac Surg 2017;103(5):1475-1481.

69. Hamm CW, Möllmann H, Holzhey D, et al. The German aortic valve registry (GARY): in-hospital outcome. Eur Heart J 2014;35(24):1588-98.

70. Dewey TM, Brown DL, Herbert MA, et al. Effect of concomitant coronary artery disease on procedural and late outcomes of transcatheter aortic valve implantation. Ann Thorac Surg 2010;89(3):758-67.

71. Rosenhek R, Iung B, Tornos P, et al. ESC working group on valvular heart disease position paper: assessing the risk of interventions in patients with valvular heart disease. Eur Heart J 2012;33:822-828.

72. Li Z, Anderson I, Amsterdam EA, Young JN, Parker J, Armstrong EJ. Effect of coronary artery disease extent on contemporary outcomes of combined aortic valve replacement and coronary artery bypass graft surgery. Ann Thorac Surg 2013;96(6):2075-82.

73. Thalji NM, Suri RM, Daly RC, et al. The prognostic impact of concomitant coronary artery bypass grafting during aortic valve surgery: implications for revascularization in the transcatheter era. J Thorac Cardiovasc Surg 2015;149(2):451-60.

74. Hiratzka LF, Creager MA, Isselbacher EM, et al. Surgery for aortic dilatation in patients with bicuspid aortic valves: a statement of clarification from the American College of Cardiology/American Heart Association task force on clinical practice guidelines. Circulation 2016;133(7):680-6.

75. Sinning JM, Vasa-Nicotera M, Chin D, et al. Evaluation and management of paravalvular aortic regurgitation after transcatheter aortic valve replacement. J Am Coll Cardiol 2013;62(1):11-20.

76. Cowell SJ, Newby DE, Prescott RJ, et al. A randomized trial of intensive lipid-lowering therapy in calcific aortic stenosis. N Engl J Med 2005; 352(23):2389-97.

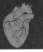
77. Rossebo AB, Pedersen TR, Boman K, et al. Intensive lipid lowering with simvastatin and ezetimibe in aortic stenosis. N Engl J Med 2008; 359(13):1343-56.

78. Chan KL, Teo K, Dumesnil JG, Ni A, Tam J. Effect of lipid lowering with rosuvastatin on progression of aortic stenosis: results of the aortic stenosis progression observation: measuring effects of rosuvastatin (ASTRONOMER) trial. Circulation 2010;121(2):306-14.

79. Thanassoulis G. Lipoprotein (a) in calcific aortic valve disease: from genomics to novel drug target for aortic stenosis. J Lipid Res 2016;57(6): 917-24.

80. Marquis-Gravel G, Redfors B, Leon MB, Généreux P. Medical treatment of aortic stenosis. Circulation 2016;134(22):1766-1784.

81. Carabello B. How to follow patients with mitral and aortic valve disease. Med Clin N Am 2015;99(4):739-57.

82. Steadman CD, Ray S, Ng LL, McCann GP. Natriuretic peptides in common valvular heart disease. J Am Coll Cardiol 2010;55(19):2034-48.

83. Gotzmann M, Czauderna A, Aweimer A, et al. B-type natriuretic peptide is a strong independent predictor of long-term outcome after transcatheter aortic valve implantation. J Heart Valve Dis 2014;23(5):537-44.

84. Sharma V, Stewart RA, Lee M, et al. Plasma brain natriuretic peptide concentration in patients with valvular heart disease. Open Heart 2016;3(1):e000184. doi:10.1136/epenhrt-2014-000184

85. Evangelista A, Tornos P, Sambola A, et al. Long-term vasodilator therapy in patients with severe aortic regurgitation. N Engl J Med 2005;353(13): 1342-1349.

86. Ahmed MI, Aban I, Lloyd SG, et al. A randomized controlled phase IIb trial of beta(1)-receptor blockade for chronic degenerative mitral regurgitation. J Am Coll Cardiol 2012;60(9):833-838.

87. Carabello BA. Beta-blockade for mitral regurgitation: could the management of valvular heart disease actually be moving into the 21st century? J Am Coll Cardiol 2012;60(9):839-840.

88. Henkel DM, Malouf JF, Connolly HM, et al. Asymptomatic left ventricular systolic dysfunction in patients with severe aortic stenosis: characteristics and outcomes. J Am Coll Cardiol 2012;60(22):2325-9.

89. Otto CM, Burwash IG, Legget ME, et al. A prospective study of asymptomatic valvular aortic stenosis: clinical, echocardiographic, and exercise predictors of outcome. Circulation 1997;95:2262-70.

90. Egbe AC, Poterucha JT, Warnes CA. Mixed aortic valve disease: midterm outcome and predictors of adverse events. Eur Heart J 2016;37(34): 2671-2678.

91. Zilberszac R, Gabriel H, Schemper M, Laufer G, Maurer G, Rosenhek R. Asymptomatic severe aortic stenosis in the elderly. JACC Cardiovasc Imaging 2017;10(1):43-50.

92. Kearney LG, Lu K, Ord M, et al. Global longitudinal strain is a strong independent predictor of all-cause mortality in patients with aortic stenosis. Eur Heart J Cardiovasc Imaging 2012;13(10):827-833.

93. Losi MA, Izzo R, Stabile E, et al. Diastolic dysfunction reduces stroke volume during daily's life activities in patients with severe aortic stenosis. Int J Cardiol 2015;195:64-5.

94. Dahl JS, Christensen NL, Videbæk L, et al. Left ventricular diastolic function is associated with symptom status in severe aortic valve stenosis. Circ Cardiovasc Imaging 2014;7(1):142-8.

95. Zaid RR, Barker CM, Little SH, Nagueh SF. Pre- and post-operative diastolic dysfunction in patients with valvular heart disease: diagnosis and therapeutic implications. J Am Coll Cardiol 2013;62(21):1922-30.

96. Kang DH, Park SJ, Rim JH, et al. Early surgery versus conventional treatment in asymptomatic very severe aortic stenosis. Circulation 2010;121(13):1502-9.

97. Gada H, Scuffham PA, Griffin B, Marwick TH. Quality-of-life implications of immediate surgery and watchful waiting in asymptomatic aortic stenosis: a decision-analytic model. Circ Cardiovasc Qual Outcomes 2011;4(5):541-8.

98. Pape LA, Price JM, Alpert JS, Ockene IS, Weiner BH. Relation of left atrial size to pulmonary capillary wedge pressure in severe mitral regurgitation. Cardiology 1991;78(4):297-303.

99. Burwash IG, Blackmore GL, Koilpillai CJ. Usefulness of left atrial and left ventricular chamber sizes as predictors of the severity of mitral regurgitation. Am J Cardiol 1992;70(7):774-9.

100. Sanfilippo AJ, Abascal VM, Sheehan M, et al. Atrial enlargement as a consequence of atrial fibrillation. A prospective echocardiographic study. Circulation 1990;82(3):792-7.

101. Kottkamp H. Human atrial fibrillation substrate: towards a specific fibrotic atrial cardiomyopathy. Eur Heart J 2013;34(35):2731-8.

102. Braunwald E, Frahm CJ. Studies on Starling's law of the heart. IV. Observations on the hemodynamic functions of the left atrium in man. Circulation 1961;24:633.

103. Leavitt JI, Coats MH, Falk RH. Effects of exercise on transmitral gradient and pulmonary artery pressure in patients with mitral stenosis or a prosthetic mitral valve: a Doppler echocardiographic study. J Am Coll Cardiol 1991;17(7):1520-6.

104. Lewis GD, Bossone E, Naeije R, et al. Pulmonary vascular hemodynamic response to exercise in cardiopulmonary diseases. Circulation 2013; 128(13):1470-9.

105. Magne J, Donal E, Mahjoub H, et al. Impact of exercise pulmonary hypertension on postoperative outcome in primary mitral regurgitation. Heart 2015;101(5):391-6.

106. Melby SJ, Moon MR, Lindman BR, Bailey MS, Hill LL, Damiano RJ, Jr. Impact of pulmonary hypertension on outcomes after aortic valve replacement for aortic valve stenosis. J Thorac Cardiovasc Surg 2011;141(6):1424-30.

107. Lindman BR, Bonow RO, Otto CM. Current management of calcific aortic stenosis. Circ Res 2013;113(2):223-37.

108. Richards AM, Nicholls MG, Ikram H, Hamilton EJ, Richards RD. Syncope in aortic valvular stenosis. Lancet 1984;2(8412):1113-6.

109. Johnson AM. Aortic stenosis, sudden death, and the left ventricular baroceptors. Br Heart J 1971;33(1):1-5.

110. Khot UN, Novaro GM, Popovic ZB, et al. Nitroprusside in critically ill patients with left ventricular dysfunction and aortic stenosis. N Engl J Med 2003;348(18):1756-63.

111. Marquis-Gravel G, Redfors B, Leon MB, Généreux P. Medical treatment of aortic stenosis. Circulation 2016;134(22):1766-84.

112. Bermejo J, Antoranz JC, Burwash IG, et al. In-vivo analysis of the instantaneous transvalvular pressure difference-flow relationship in aortic valve stenosis: implications of unsteady fluid-dynamics for the clinical assessment of disease severity. J Heart Valve Dis 2002;11(4):557-66.

113. Burwash IG, Thomas DD, Sadahiro M, et al. Dependence of Gorlin formula and continuity equation valve areas on transvalvular volume flow rate in valvular aortic stenosis. Circulation 1994;89:827-35.

114. Zile MR, Gaasch WH. Heart failure in aortic stenosis - improving diagnosis and treatment. N Engl J Med 2003;348(18):1735-6.

115. Hu K, Wan Y, Hong T, et al. Therapeutic decision-making for elderly patients with symptomatic severe valvular heart diseases. Int Heart J 2016;57(4):434-40.

116. Kirkpatrick JN, Hauptman PJ, Swetz KM, et al. Palliative care for patients with end-stage cardiovascular disease and devices: a report from the palliative care working group of the geriatrics section of the American College of Cardiology. JAMA Int Med 2016;176(7):1017-9.

117. Rahimi K, Mohseni H, Kiran A, et al. Elevated blood pressure and risk of aortic valve disease: a cohort analysis of 5.4 million UK adults. Eur Heart J 2018;39(39):3596-3603. doi: 10.1093/eurheartj/ehy486.

118. Rahimi K, Mohseni H, Otto CM, et al. Elevated blood pressure and risk of mitral regurgitation: A longitudinal cohort study of 5.5 million United Kingdom adults. PLoS Med 2017;14(10):e1002404. doi: 10.1371/journal.pmed.1002404.

119. O'Brien KD, Zhao XQ, Shavelle DM, et al. Hemodynamic effects of the angiotensin-converting enzyme inhibitor, ramipril, in patients with mild to moderate aortic stenosis and preserved left ventricular function. J Investig Med 2004;52(3):185-91.

120. Marquis-Gravel G, Redfors B, Leon MB, Généreux P. Medical treatment of aortic stenosis. Circulation 2016;134(22):1766-84.

121. Nadir MA, Wei L, Elder DH, et al. Impact of renin-angiotensin system blockade therapy on outcome in aortic stenosis. J Am Coll Cardiol 2011;58(6):570-6.

122. Kadem L, Dumesnil JG, Rieu R, Durand LG, Garcia D, Pibarot P. Impact of systemic hypertension on the assessment of aortic stenosis. Heart 2005;91(3):354-61.

123. Otto CM. Valvular aortic stenosis: disease severity and timing of intervention. J Am Coll Cardiol 2006;47(11):2141-51.

124. Bermejo J. The effects of hypertension on aortic valve stenosis. Heart 2005;91(3):280-2.

125. Little SH, Chan KL, Burwash IG. Impact of blood pressure on the Doppler echocardiographic assessment of severity of aortic stenosis. Heart 2007; 93(7):848-55.

126. Emren ZY, Emren SV, Kılıçaslan B, et al. Evaluation of the prevalence of coronary artery disease in patients with valvular heart disease. J Cardiothorac Surg 2014;9:153.

127. Carabello BA. Introduction to aortic stenosis. Circ Res 2013;113(2):179-85.

128. Fletcher GF, Ades PA, Kligfield P, et al. Exercise standards for testing and training a scientific statement from the American Heart Association. Circulation 2013;128(8):873-934.

129. Larsen LH, Kofoed KF, Dalsgaard M, et al. Assessment of coronary artery disease using coronary computed tomography angiography in patients with aortic valve stenosis referred for surgical aortic valve replacement. Int J Cardiol 2013;168(1):126-31.

130. Di Gioia G, Pellicano M, Toth GG, et al. Clinical outcome of patients with aortic stenosis and coronary artery disease not treated according to current recommendations. J Cardiovasc Transl Res 2016;9(2):145-52.

131. Verma S, Siu SC. Aortic dilatation in patients with bicuspid aortic valve. N Engl J Med 2014;370(20):1920-9.

132. Hiratzka LF, Creager MA, Isselbacher EM, et al. Surgery for aortic dilatation in patients with bicuspid aortic valves: a statement of clarification from the American College of Cardiology/American Heart Association task force on clinical practice guidelines. Circulation 2016;133(7):680-686. doi: 10.1161/CIR.0000000000000331.

133. Gillinov AM, Bhavani S, Blackstone EH, et al. Surgery for permanent atrial fibrillation: impact of patient factors and lesion set. Ann Thorac Surg 2006;82(2):502-13.

134. Doty JR, Doty DB, Jones KW, et al. Comparison of standard Maze III and radiofrequency Maze operations for treatment of atrial fibrillation. J Thorac Cardiovasc Surg 2007;133(4):1037-44.

135. Iung B, Leenhardt A, Extramiana F. Management of atrial fibrillation in patients with rheumatic mitral stenosis. Heart 2018;104(13):1062-1068. doi: 10.1136/heartjnl-2017-311425. Epub 2018 Feb 16. Review. PMID:29453328

136. Oral H, Chugh A, Ozaydin M, et al. Risk of thromboembolic events after percutaneous left atrial radiofrequency ablation of atrial fibrillation. Circulation 2006;114:759-65.

137. Gillinov AM, Gelijns AC, Parides MK, et al. Surgical ablation of atrial fibrillation during mitral-valve surgery. N Engl J Med 2015;372:1399-409.

138. Chandrashekhar Y, Westaby S, Narula J. Mitral stenosis. Lancet 2009;374(9697):1271-83.

139. Agrawal V, Kumar N, Lohiya B, et al. Metoprolol vs ivabradine in patients with mitral stenosis in sinus rhythm. Int J Cardiol 2016;221:562-566.

140. al Kasab SM, Sabag T, al Zaibag M, et al. Beta-adrenergic receptor blockade in the management of pregnant women with mitral stenosis. Am J Obstet Gynecol 1990;163(1 Pt 1):37-40.

141. Huynh H, Dalloul G, Ghanbari H, et al. Permanent pacemaker implantation following aortic valve replacement: current prevalence and clinical predictors. Pacing Clin Electrophysiol 2009;32(12):1520-5.

142. Fadahunsi OO, Olowoyeye A, Ukaigwe A, et al. Incidence, predictors, and outcomes of permanent pacemaker implantation following transcatheter aortic valve replacement: analysis from the US Society of Thoracic Surgeons/American College of Cardiology TVT Registry. JACC Cardiovasc Interv 2016;9(21):2189-99.

143. Abramowitz Y, Kazuno Y, Chakravarty T, et al. Concomitant mitral annular calcification and severe aortic stenosis: prevalence, characteristics and outcome following transcatheter aortic valve replacement. Eur Heart J 2016;38(16):1194-1203.

144. Brinkley DM, Gelfand EV. Valvular heart disease: classic teaching and emerging paradigms. Am J Med 2013;126(12):1035-1042.

145. Nalliah CJ, Mahajan R, Haqqani H, et al. Mitral valve prolapse and sudden death: a systematic review. Circulation 2015;132(Suppl 3):A13720-guideline update on perioperative cardiovascular evaluation for noncardiac surgery.

146. Fleisher LA, Beckman JA, Brown KA, et al. ACC/AHA 2006 guideline update on perioperative cardiovascular evaluation for noncardiac surgery: focused update on perioperative beta-blocker therapy: a report of the American College of Cardiology/American Heart Association Task Force on Practice Guidelines (Writing Committee to Update the 2002 Guidelines on Perioperative Cardiovascular Evaluation for Noncardiac Surgery): developed in collaboration with the American Society of Echocardiography, American Society of Nuclear Cardiology, Heart Rhythm Society, Society of Cardiovascular Anesthesiologists, Society for Cardiovascular Angiography and Interventions, and Society for Vascular Medicine and Biology. Circulation 2006;113(22):2662-74.

147. Fleisher LA, Beckman JA, Brown KA, et al. ACC/AHA 2006 guideline update on perioperative cardiovascular evaluation for noncardiac surgery: focused update on perioperative beta-blocker therapy: a report of the American College of Cardiology/American Heart Association Task Force on Practice Guidelines (Writing Committee to Update the 2002 Guidelines on Perioperative Cardiovascular Evaluation for Noncardiac Surgery): developed in collaboration with the American Society of Echocardiography, American Society of Nuclear Cardiology, Heart Rhythm Society, Society of Cardiovascular Anesthesiologists, Society for Cardiovascular Angiography and Interventions, and Society for Vascular Medicine and Biology. Circulation 2006;113(22): 2662-74.

148. Heiberg J, El-Ansary D, Canty DJ, Royse AG, Royse CF. Focused echocardiography: a systematic review of diagnostic and clinical decision-making in anaesthesia and critical care. Anaesthesia 2016;71(9):1091-100.

149. Pislaru SV, Abel MD, Schaff HV, Pellikka PA. Aortic stenosis and noncardiac surgery: managing the risk. Curr Prob Cardiol 2015;40(11):483-503.

150. Hussain AI, Garratt AM, Brunborg C, Aakhus S, Gullestad L, Pettersen KI. Eliciting patient risk willingness in clinical consultations as a means of improving decision-making of aortic valve replacement. J Am Heart Assoc 2016 Mar 1;5(3):e002828.

151. Lauck SB, Gibson JA, Baumbusch J, et al. Transition to palliative care when transcatheter aortic valve implantation is not an option: opportunities and recommendations. Curr Opin Support Palliat Care 2016;10(1):18-23.

152. Olsson SB. Stroke prevention with the oral direct thrombin inhibitor ximelagatran compared with warfarin in patients with non-valvular atrial fibrillation (SPORTIF III): randomised controlled trial. Lancet 2003; 362:1691-1698.

153. Halperin JL. Ximelagatran compared with warfarin for prevention of thromboembolism in patients with nonvalvular atrial fibrillation: rationale, objectives, and design of a pair of clinical studies and baseline patient characteristics (SPORTIF III and V). Am Heart J 2003;146:431-438.

154. Ezekowitz MD, Reilly PA, Nehmiz G, et al. Dabigatran with or without concomitant aspirin compared with warfarin alone in patients with nonvalvular atrial fibrillation (PETRO Study). Am J Cardiol 2007;100: 1419-1426.

155. Ezekowitz MD, Connolly S, Parekh A, et al. Rationale and design of RE-LY: randomized 3334 evaluation of long-term anticoagulant therapy, warfarin, compared with dabigatran. Am Heart J 2009;157:805-810, 810.e1-2

156. Connolly SJ, Ezekowitz MD, Yusuf S, et al. Dabigatran versus warfarin in patients with atrial fibrillation. N Engl J Med 2009;361:1139-1151.

157. Patel MR, Mahaffey KW, Garg J, et al. Rivaroxaban versus warfarin in nonvalvular atrial fibrillation. N Engl J Med 2011;365:883-891.

158. Hori M, Matsumoto M, Tanahashi N, et al. Rivaroxaban vs warfarin in Japanese patients with atrial fibrillation - the J-ROCKET AF study. Circ J 2012;76:2104-2111.

159. Eikelboom JW, O'Donnell M, Yusuf S, et al. Rationale and design of AVERROES: apixaban versus acetylsalicylic acid to prevent stroke in atrial fibrillation patients who have failed or are unsuitable for vitamin K antagonist treatment. Am Heart J 2010;159:348-353.e1.

160. Connolly SJ, Eikelboom J, Joyner C, et al. Apixaban in patients with atrial fibrillation. N Engl J Med 2011;364:806-817.

161. Ogawa S, Shinohara Y, Kanmuri K. Safety and efficacy of the oral direct factor Xa inhibitor apixaban in Japanese patients with non-valvular atrial fibrillation: The ARISTOTLE-J study. Circ J 2011;75:1852-1859.

162. Yamashita T, Koretsune Y, Yasaka M, et al. Randomized, multicenter, warfarin-controlled phase II study of edoxaban in Japanese patients with non-valvular atrial fibrillation. Circ J 2012;76:1840-1847.

163. Giugliano RP, Ruff CT, Braunwald E, et al. Edoxaban versus warfarin in patients with atrial fibrillation. N Engl J Med 2013;369:2093-2104.

164. Ruff CT, Giugliano RP, Antman EM, et al. Evaluation of the novel factor Xa inhibitor edoxaban compared with warfarin in patients with atrial fibrillation: design and rationale for the Effective aNticoaGulation with factor xA next GEneration in Atrial Fibrillation-Thrombolysis In Myocardial Infarction study 48 (ENGAGE AF-TIMI 48). Am Heart J 2010;160:635-641.

165. Connolly SJ, Eikelboom J, Dorian P, et al. Betrixaban compared with warfarin in patients with atrial fibrillation: results of a phase 2, randomized, dose-ranging study (Explore-Xa). Eur Heart J 2013;34:1498-1505.

166. Wilson SJ, Wells PS, Kovacs MJ, et al. Comparing the quality of oral anticoagulant management by anticoagulation clinics and by family physicians: a randomized controlled trial. Can Med Assoc J 2003;169:293-298.

167. Jackson SL, Peterson GM, Vial JH, Jupe DML. Improving the outcomes of anticoagulation: an evaluation of home follow up of warfarin initiation. J Intern Med 2004;256:137-44.

168. Chan FWH, Wong RSM, Lau WH, et al. Management of Chinese patients on warfarin therapy in two models of anticoagulation service – a prospective randomized trial. Br J Clin Pharmacol 2006;62:601-609.

169. Lalonde L, Martineau J, Blais N, et al. Is long term pharmacist managed anticoagulation service efficient? A pragmatic randomized controlled trial. Am Heart J 2008;156:148-154.

170. Cohen IA, Hutchison TA, Kirking DM, Shue ME. Evaluation of a pharmacist managed anticoagulation clinic. J Clin Hosp Pharm 1985; 10:167-175.

171. Ellis RF, Stephens MA, Sharp GB. Evaluation of a pharmacy managed warfarin monitoring service to coordinate inpatient and outpatient therapy. Am J Hosp Pharm 1992;49:3873-394.

172. Wilt VM, Gums JG, Ahmed OI, Moore LM. Outcome analysis of a pharmacist managed anticoagulation service. Pharmacotherapy 1995;15:732-735.

173. To EK, Pearson GJ. Implementation and evaluation of a pharmacist assisted warfarin dosing program. Can J Hosp Pharm 1997;50:169-175.

174. Chiquette E, Amato MG, Bussey HI. Comparison of an anticoagulation clinic with usual medical care: anticoagulation control, patient outcomes, and health care costs. Arch Intern Med 1998;158:1641-1647.

175. Bieobanjong S. The Clinical Outcomes of Pharmaceutical Care on Warfarin in Out Patients at Chiangrai Regional Hospital. Chiang Mai: Chiang Mai University, 2000.

176. Dager WE, Branch JM, King JH, et al. Optimization of inpatient warfarin therapy: impact of daily consultation by a pharmacist managed anticoagulation service. Ann Pharmacother 2000;34:567-572

177. Witt DM, Humphries TL. A retrospective evaluation of the management of excessive anticoagulation in an established clinical pharmacy anticoagulation service compared to traditional care. J Thromb Thrombolysis 2003;15:113-118.

178. Burns N. Evaluation of warfarin dosing by pharmacists for elderly medical in-patients. Pharm World Sci 2004;26:232-237.

179. Liabthawee W. Impact of Education and Conseling by Clinical Pharmacists on Anticoagulation Therapy in Patients With Mechanical Heart Valves. Bangkok: Mahidol University, 2004.

180. Witt DM, Sadler MA, Shanahan RL, et al. Effect of a centralized clinical pharmacy anticoagulation service on the outcomes of anticoagulation therapy. Chest 2005;127:1515-1522.

181. Locke C, Ravnan SL, Patel R, Uchizono JA. Reduction in warfarin adverse events requiring patient hospitalization after implementation of a pharmacist managed anticoagulation service. Pharmacotherapy 2005;25:685-689.

182. Chau T, Rotbard M, King S, Li MM, Leong WA. Implementation and evaluation of a warfarin dosing service for rehabilitation medicine: report from a pilot project. Can J Hosp Pharm 2006;59:136-147.

183. Poon IO, Lal L, Brown EN, Braun UK. The impact of pharmacist managed oral anticoagulation therapy in older veterans. J Clin Pharm Ther 2007;32:21-29.

184. Bungard TJ, Gardner L, Archer SL, et al. Evaluation of a pharmacist managed anticoagulation clinic: improving patient care. Open Med 2009;3:16-21.

185. Tschol N, Lai DSK, Tilley JA, Wong H, Brown GR. Comparison of physician and pharmacist managed warfarin sodium treatment in open heart surgery patients. Can J Cardiol 2003;19:1413-1417.

186. Airee A, Guirguis AB, Mohammad RA. Clinical outcomes and pharmacists' acceptance of a community hospital's anticoagulation management service utilizing decentralized clinical staff pharmacists. Ann Pharmacother 2009;43:621-628.

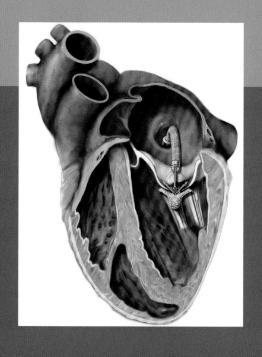

第7章
瓣膜病患者干预治疗的风险评估

　　成年人主动脉瓣狭窄的治疗多采用外科手术或经胸导管介入的方式开展，治疗前对患者进行有效的风险预测具有重要意义。要做到通过风险评估对患者临床结局进行个体化预测，高质量的临床数据库及风险模型缺一不可。风险评估系统常通过使用逻辑回归模型对临床结局事件发生的可能性进行计算分析。用于设计风险评估系统的患者样本由建模样本与验证样本构成，前者的数据用来确定模型的变量与系数，后者的数据用来评价模型的拟合度、区分度与标定度。使用风险评估体系预测结局事件同样存在局限性：其评估结果的精准性受到患者群体特点、治疗方式及时间的影响；此外，临床常用的评估体系往往缺乏罕见、未知变量之于临床结局影响的考量；评估体系中所选取的危险因素往往难以同时兼顾与结局事件的相关性和在实际临床场景下相关数据的易获得性。目前，已设计出多个风险评估体系来预测不同患者群体在接受外科主动脉瓣置换术后多个时期的临床结局，其中，1995年基于超过15 000名欧洲国家患者的临床数据分析研发出的Logistic EuroSCORE风险评估系统涵盖了12个心脏术后早期死亡事件的危险因素，因其操作的简便性而被广泛使用，2010年在其基础上覆盖了更多样化的患者群体及危险因素，设计出了EuroSCORE II风险评估系统。2002年—2006年，通过研究美国接受单一主动脉瓣置换术患者群体的临床数据设计出了STS-PROM风险预测模型，该模型囊括24个术后死亡的危险因素，其对于高危患者主动脉瓣置换术后早期死亡风险的预测价值优于Logistic EuroSCORE。以往在预测经导管主动脉瓣置换术后的临床结局时多借用外科手术的风险预测模型，但是由于接受两种治疗的患者存在差异性，且原有的风险评估体系尚存在局限性，因此产生了German Aortic Valve Score、FRANCE 2 Risk Model等预测模型来提高风险评估的准确性。目前推荐运用多种风险评价体系，结合患者的功能状态及所接受的特殊操作等临床信息对患者临床结局进行个体化的综合评估。

牛冠男　　陈乔凡

Surgical and Procedural Risk Assessment of Patients With Valvular Heart Disease

Mohanad Hamandi, Michael J. Mack

KEY POINTS

- Accurate risk assessment is a critical component of informed consent.
- Risk scores are predicted probabilities calculated from a multivariable logistic regression model that is calibrated using data on a specific treatment from a fixed period. They are accurate only for a specific population and treatment over the time frame in which they are developed and validated.
- The Society of Thoracic Surgeons' Predicted Risk of Mortality (STS-PROM) and the European System for Cardiac Operative Risk Evaluation (EuroSCORE) are the most common risk prediction models used to assess candidates for surgical and transcatheter valve procedures.

- The analysis of patients' limitation of functional capacity, or frailty, is an important consideration in clinical decision making.
- Frailty measures are gait speed, grip strength, serum albumin level, and activities of daily living.
- An integrative approach to risk assessment is recommended before surgical or transcatheter valve procedures.
- Risk assessment includes a comprehensive clinical evaluation, measures of frailty and functional status, use of risk scores, and consideration of procedure-specific impediments.

Analysis of adult patients with aortic stenosis undergoing surgical and transcatheter procedures is a rich area of outcomes and comparative effectiveness research. Although a single universal risk prediction model based on the minimal number of important risk factors that is applicable to all patients undergoing treatment of valvular heart disease is desirable, the reality is that multiple algorithms have been proposed that measure different outcomes. These risk tools must be continuously updated as calibration drift occurs and as treatment strategies, patient selection, procedures, and procedure performance evolve (Fig. 7.1).

RISK ALGORITHMS

Goals

Outcomes data from medical procedures are commonly used to compare treatments or providers. Early databases were originally used to assess outcomes from cardiac surgical procedures, most commonly coronary artery bypass grafting (CABG). In the United States, these registries were first constructed from administrative claims data from the Health Care Financing Administration (HCFA), which was the precursor of the Center for Medicare and Medicaid Services (CMS). The purpose of these databases was to assess outcomes in various clinical programs, but they did not account for patient-specific factors

that could influence outcomes.[1,2] The need for patient-specific predictions of procedural outcomes led to the development of several high-quality clinical databases and risk models for patients undergoing cardiac surgery.[3,4]

Patient outcomes are influenced by severity of illness, treatment effectiveness, and chance, and comparisons between groups must account for differences in prevalence of risk factors, a concept called *case mix*.[5–9] Outcome variations due to case mix can be reduced or eliminated by several methods, most rigorously by randomization, which balance known and unknown risk factors. However, outcomes from randomized, controlled clinical trials may not be generalizable to the larger, unselected population of patients.

Registry data are important for comparing outcomes among various treatments or providers with covariate matching or propensity score matching techniques to account for case mix.[10,11] With the use of statistical modeling techniques, most commonly multivariable regression analysis, the association between individual risk factors, known as *predictor variables* or *covariates,* and outcomes can be determined.[12] After the impact of each risk factor is determined (called *weighting*) from a given population sample, it becomes possible to estimate the probability of the outcome for patients having particular combinations of these risk factors.[13]

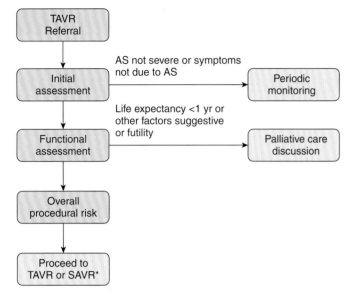

*Per current AHA/ACC guideline for the management of patients with valvular heart disease

Fig. 7.1 Timing and Sequence of Risk Assessment in Patients Referred for TAVR. *AS*, Aortic stenosis, *AVR*, aortic valve replacement; *SAVR*, surgical aortic valve replacement; *TAVR*, transcatheter aortic valve replacement.

Construction of Risk Models

Risk scores are predicted probabilities calculated from a multivariable logistic regression model calibrated on data from a fixed time. The first element in constructing a robust risk model is a clinical database with as complete and accurate data as possible.[14] The second element is risk modeling by experienced statisticians to ensure development of a relevant multivariable model.[15]

Logistic regression modeling has been used for development of the Society of Thoracic Surgeons (STS) risk score and for models constructed by New York State,[16] the Veterans Administration,[17] and the Northern New England Cardiovascular Disease Study Group.[18] Other models, such as the Parsonnet score[19] and the European System for Cardiac Operative Risk Evaluation (EuroSCORE),[20] used simple additive scores with weights derived from logistic regression models. Some evidence indicates that logistic regression models perform better.[21]

For development of a risk model, the study population is usually divided into a development or training sample and a validation or test sample. For the STS Isolated Valve Risk model, the study population was randomly divided into a 60% development sample and a 40% validation sample. The development sample was then used to identify predictor variables and estimate model coefficients. Data from the validation sample were used to assess model fit, discrimination, and calibration.[22]

Discrimination refers to the model's ability to separate two groups studied, such as survivors and nonsurvivors. An area under the receiver operating characteristic curve (AUROC) is calculated using the concordance statistic (i.e., C-index), with ranges between 0.5 and 1.0. The higher the value of the C-index, the better the discrimination, whereas values closer to 0.5 indicate that the model's ability to discriminate is no better than random chance or the flip of a coin.[23] In most risk prediction models used for cardiac surgery, the AUROC is between 0.75 and 0.80.

Limitations

In the employment of risk adjustment, important limitations have to be taken into account to ensure that valid information rather than misinformation is obtained from the correction.[24] First, risk algorithms are accurate only for the population and in the time frame in which they are developed and validated.

Second, risk adjustment loses accuracy at the extremes of the population studied, where there are too few patients on which to build a statistically valid model. This tail of the bell-shaped curve is where high-risk patients with aortic stenosis reside, accounting for some of the overestimation of risk seen with many models.[25,26]

Third, risk algorithms cannot reliably be applied directly to populations and treatments other than those in which they were developed. The implication is that although both surgical aortic valve replacement (SAVR) and transcatheter aortic valve implantation (TAVI) are used in treating patients with aortic stenosis, AVR risk algorithms are based only on SAVR outcomes and therefore may not to be directly applicable to TAVI.

Fourth, risk algorithms cannot account for variables not collected or analyzed. This lack of accounting has one of two causes: (1) the occurrence of the factor or condition (e.g., porcelain aorta, liver disease) is so infrequent that its impact cannot be measured, or (2) the factor might have not been previously known to be a factor that was causal or cannot be accurately measured or quantified. The role of frailty and its impact on outcomes of treatment is a case in point.

Fifth, all risk predictors fall prey to the phenomenon of "garbage in equals garbage out." Unless the factors on which the algorithm is formulated are based on complete and accurate data, an inaccurate predictor will result. A corollary is that the risk predictor must be user friendly. The greater number of variables collected in formulation of the risk algorithm, the more accurate the prediction of risk; however, the more burdensome the collection of data required, the less complete and accurate will be the information. There must be a balance between including all information that is likely to be a factor in causing risk and user-friendliness by being least burdensome to facilitate complete and accurate collection and ensure that the tool is routinely employed in decision making. One risk algorithm for aortic stenosis, the Age, Creatinine, Ejection Fraction (ACEF) score, provides reasonable prediction using only the three factors in its name: age, serum creatinine level, and ejection fraction.[27]

Clinical Utility

Profiling risk for patients undergoing medical procedures serves many purposes.[28] First, it allows outcomes prediction for individual patients, enabling the patient and caregiver to be better informed in making decisions regarding the advisability and risks of a specific medical procedure. Second, patients undergoing medical procedures frequently have comorbidities that cause various levels of risk, and they therefore can adversely affect the outcomes of a procedure. When different modalities of treatment or different caregivers are compared, risk adjustment allows a balanced analysis of outcomes (i.e., comparative effectiveness) by accounting for the risk factor variation among different patient cohorts. This correction allows for a more level playing field of outcomes assessment, and the ability to achieve an apples-to-apples comparison is one of the advantages of clinical outcomes databases over administrative databases, which have limited ability to adjust risk.

Risk adjustment allows a more meaningful analysis of hospitals or therapies for comparative safety and effectiveness of treatment (Table 7.1). For example, it is possible to compare two standard procedures (e.g., CABG surgery compared with percutaneous coronary intervention) or a new procedure with an existing standard (e.g., TAVI compared with SAVR) for outcomes comparisons in different centers. Public reporting of surgical outcomes in the

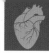

TABLE 7.1 Risk Assessment Combining Clinical Data, STS Risk Estimate, Frailty, Major Organ System Dysfunction, and Procedure-Specific Impediments.

Step 1: Initial Assessment

Valve-related symptoms and severity	Symptoms	Intensity, acuity
	AS severity	Echocardiography and other imaging
Baseline clinical data	Cardiac history	Prior cardiac interventions
	Physical examination and laboratory results	Routine blood tests, pulmonary function tests
	Chest irradiation	Access issues other cardiac effects
	Dental evaluation	Treat dental issues before TAVR
	Allergies	Contrast, latex, medications
	Social support	Recovery, transportation, postdischarge planning
Major CV comorbidity	Coronary artery disease	Coronary angiography
	LV systolic dysfunction	LV ejection fraction
	Concurrent valve disease	Severe MR or MS
	Pulmonary hypertension	Assess pulmonary pressures
	Aortic disease	Porcelain aorta (CT scan)
	Chest or vascular access	Prohibitive reentry after previous open heart surgery (CT scan)
		Hostile chest
		Peripheral vascular disease
Major noncardiovascular comorbidity	Malignancy	Remote or active, life expectancy
	Gastrointestinal and liver disease, bleeding	IBD, cirrhosis, varices, GIB—ability to take antiplatelets/anticoagulation
	Kidney disease	eGFR < 30 mL/min/1.73 m^2 or dialysis
	Pulmonary disease	Oxygen requirement, FEV1 $< 50\%$ predicted or D$_{LCO}$ $< 50\%$ predicted
	Neurologic disorders	Movement disorders, dementia

Step 2: Functional Assessment

Frailty and disability	Frailty assessment	Gait speed (<0.5 m/s or <0.83 m/s with disability/cognitive impairment)
		Frailty (not frail or frail by assessments)
	Nutritional risk/status	Nutritional risk status (BMI < 21 kg/m^2, albumin < 3.5 mg/dL, $>$10-lb weight loss in past year, or $\leq$11 on MNA)
Physical function	Physical function and endurance	6-min walk <50 m or unable to walk
	Independent living	Dependent in $\geq$1 activities
Cognitive function	Cognitive impairment	MMSE < 24 or dementia
	Depression	Depression history or positive screen
	Prior disabling stroke	
Futility	Life expectancy	<1 year of life expectancy
	Lag-time to benefit	Survival with benefit of $< 25\%$ at 2 years

Step 3: Overall Procedural Risk

Risk categories	Low risk	STS-PROM $< 4\%$ and
		No frailty and
		No comorbidity and
		No procedure-specific impediments
	Intermediate risk	STS-PROM 4%–8% or
		Mild frailty or
		1 major organ system compromise not to be improved postoperatively or
		A possible procedure-specific impediment
	High risk	STS-PROM $> 8\%$ or
		Moderate-severe frailty or
		>2 major organ system compromises not to be improved postoperatively or
		A possible procedure-specific impediment
	Prohibitive risk	PROM $> 50\%$ at 1 year or
		$\geq$3 major organ system compromises not to be improved postoperatively or
		Severe frailty or
		Severe procedure-specific impediments

AS, Aortic stenosis; *D*LCO, carbon dioxide diffusing capacity; *eGFR*, estimated glomerular filtration rate; *FEV*, forced expiratory volume; *GIB*, gastrointestinal bleeding; *IBD*, irritable bowel syndrome; *MMSE*, Mini-Mental Status Exam; *MNA*, Mini Nutritional Assessment; *MR*, mitral regurgitation; *MS*, mitral stenosis; *STS-PROM*, Society of Thoracic Surgeons' Predicted Risk of Mortality; *TAVR*, transcatheter aortic valve replacement.
Data from Otto CM, Kumbhani DJ, Alexander KP, et al. 2017 ACC expert consensus decision pathway for transcatheter aortic valve replacement in the management of adults with aortic stenosis: a report of the American College of Cardiology Task Force on Clinical Expert Consensus Documents. J Am Coll Cardiol 2017;69:1313-1346.

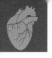
United States is done by risk-adjusted results, in which the observed outcome divided by the expected outcome is based on known patient risk factors. This approach creates an observed-to-expected ratio (O/E) that is a multiplier of the observed mortality. An O/E ratio of less than 1 indicates a better-than-expected outcome, whereas a ratio greater than 1 means the outcome is worse than expected on the basis of the patient's existing comorbidities or risk factors. Without the risk adjustment that takes into account the patient-specific factors that may adversely affect outcomes, meaningful comparison is not possible.

Predicted Outcomes

The earliest and most common use of risk prediction was for evaluating early mortality after isolated CABG. Because the procedure was performed commonly and outcomes were publicly reported, risk prediction for an apples-to-apples comparison among surgical centers performing CABG became common. *Early mortality*, as defined by the STS, includes all deaths occurring before 30 days in or out of the hospital and any death occurring in the hospital at any time. Other risk prediction models for early mortality include only in-hospital mortality, which misses between 10% and 40% of the early deaths. The advantage of reporting in-hospital mortality is that the data are more easily collected and probably more accurate. The disadvantage, however, is that very ill postoperative patients who are quite likely to die are frequently discharged to long-term acute care or skilled nursing facilities less than 30 days after surgery and therefore may not be counted. In a 2012 analysis of EuroSCORE II outcome data, in which hospital mortality is about 4%, adding 30-day mortality increases the reported mortality by about 0.6% (relative increase of 15%), and adding 90-day mortality increases it further by about 0.9%.[29] When comparing various risk predictors, it is important to ensure that the same data definitions are being used by each model.

Risk prediction models for early mortality after cardiac surgery have been expanded to use for other procedures. Isolated CABG (C-index = 0.78) risk prediction is available for isolated SAVR, isolated mitral valve repair or replacement, CABG combined with AVR, and CABG with mitral valve repair or replacement. Weighting of the various risk factors is recalibrated with each new version of the STS Adult Cardiac Database according to the most recent data uploaded by the 1005 cardiac surgery programs in the United States that participate in the database.

Rankin et al[30] published a risk prediction for multiple valve operations, including aortic and mitral valve operation; mitral, tricuspid, and aortic valve operation; and mitral and tricuspid operation, which has acceptable discrimination (C-index = 0.711 to 0.727).[30] In addition to early mortality, the STS risk prediction algorithm predicted long-term survival for isolated CABG, with survival at 1, 3, 5, and 10 years having AUROC values similar to the value of 30-day survival (0.794).[31]

A composite score of mortality and major morbidity after SAVR also was published.[32] The STS AVR composite score is based solely on outcomes, including risk-standardized mortality and any-or-none risk-standardized morbidity (i.e., occurrence of sternal infection, reoperation, stroke, renal failure, or prolonged ventilation). The STS online risk calculator can calculate major morbidity and mortality after SAVR.[33]

RISK ALGORITHMS FOR SURGICAL AORTIC VALVE REPLACEMENT

At least 12 risk algorithms have been constructed for various populations and different periods to predict outcomes after SAVR. The two most widely used are the Logistic EuroSCORE and the STS Predicted Risk of Mortality (STS-PROM).[28,34,35]

Logistic EuroSCORE

The Logistic EuroSCORE was developed in 1995 as an additive score (i.e., Additive EuroSCORE) and later converted to a logistic regression model. It was derived from a data set from eight European countries and was based on a population sample of almost 15,000 patients undergoing all types of cardiac operations. The 12 covariates identified were predictive of early mortality. The benefit of the Logistic EuroSCORE is its user-friendliness because it requires only 18 data fields for the calculation. The shortcoming for use in the United States is that the algorithm is calculated on a relatively small sample size from almost 20 years ago for a population outside the country. These factors make the applicability of the risk model to the current patients undergoing SAVR, especially in the United States, quite questionable. The Logistic EuroSCORE has been repeatedly demonstrated to overpredict actual risk in the assessment of patients for whom surgery poses a high risk.[25,26] This problem results from factors mentioned previously, including too few patients at high risk to be accurately analyzed and the fact that they underwent surgery in an earlier time. To address some of these shortcomings, the Logistic EuroSCORE has been updated as the EuroSCORE II[36] (Table 7.2).

This updated risk predictor was derived from more than 22,000 patients operated on in 2010 in 43 countries. It includes all cardiac procedures and has 18 covariates predictive of surgical aortic valve mortality. Whether the accuracy of the EuroSCORE II model has been improved is a subject of debate. Pooling contemporaneous multi-institutional data, Grant et al[37] found that EuroSCORE II performed well overall in the United Kingdom and was an acceptable contemporary generic cardiac surgery risk model. However, they also found that the model was poorly calibrated for isolated CABG surgery and for the highest-risk and lowest-risk patients. The investigators recommended that regular revalidation of EuroSCORE II will be needed to identify calibration drift or clinical inconsistencies, which commonly emerge in clinical prediction models.

Chalmers et al[38] applied the model to a 5500-patient cohort and concluded that EuroSCORE II was globally better calibrated than the EuroSCORE and found better overall discrimination, with a C-index of 0.79 (old model = 0.77), and found that its best performance was in mitral (0.87) and coronary (0.79) surgery; Euro SCORE II was weakest in isolated AVR (C-index 0.69), which was only marginally better than the old model (0.67).[38] A third study also found better performance of the EuroSCORE II model[39] (see Table 7.1).

TABLE 7.2 Comparison of Logistic EuroSCORE, STS-PROM, and EuroSCORE II.

Characteristic	Logistic EuroSCORE	STS-PROM	EuroSCORE II
Year of population analysis	1995	2002–2006	May–July 2010
Place	Europe (8 countries)	United States	43 countries worldwide
Number of operations	14,799	67,292	22,381
Type of operations	All cardiac	Aortic valve only	All cardiac
Covariates for aortic valve mortality	12	24	18

STS-PROM Risk Model

The STS-PROM model has generally correlated better with clinical outcomes. The model was developed in a later era (2002–2006) in the United States with use of data from 67,000 patients undergoing only isolated AVR.[22] Twenty-four covariates for mortality were identified. At least two series found the STS-PROM was a better predictor of early mortality than the Logistic EuroSCORE, especially for higher-risk patients undergoing AVR.[40,41] However, there still is the tendency for the STS instrument to underpredict risk.

The STS-PROM was updated from version 2.61 to version 2.73. The updated version includes multiple potential risk factors not previously collected, such as previous radiation exposure, liver disease, and frailty as measured by gait speed. As with all risk algorithms, calibration drift occurs as the original data set becomes dated, and the algorithm will need to be updated after sufficient numbers of patients are available for the new version that has captured the new possible predictors. Many other risk prediction models have been constructed but are not widely used.[42–46]

RISK ALGORITHMS FOR TRANSCATHETER AORTIC VALVE IMPLANTATION

Predictive modeling for the management of patients with aortic stenosis initially was developed for surgical intervention. With the introduction of TAVI, these risk algorithms were used for applications for which they were not developed nor originally intended[47] (Table 7.3). However, given the lack of other options, this approach was reasonable at the time. However, use of a surgical risk model may unintentionally inflate the apparent value of TAVI because of the observed early post-TAVI mortality, which is better than the expected postoperative mortality based on surgical predictive models, particularly with of the Logistic EuroSCORE. One factor leading to inaccuracy of applying surgical risk score to the TAVI procedure is the inclusion of patients being assessed for TAVI who are at the extremes of risk, where the current surgical risk models fail because there are too few patients at very high risk to develop risk discrimination. Surgical risk models also do not take into account several variables that may play significant roles in surgical and TAVI risk, such as a heavily calcific or porcelain aorta, previous chest radiation therapy, liver disease, and frailty. These factors were not considered in the original models because the data were not collected or there were too few occurrences of the factor to accurately incorporate it

into the risk modeling. There are many studies attesting to the inaccuracies of the Logistic EuroSCORE in CABG and AVR populations,[36,48–55] and its use in TAVI further compounds the inaccuracy.

German Aortic Valve Score

To help address some of the inadequacies of the current risk prediction models for adults undergoing TAVI and SAVR, the German Aortic Valve Registry (GARY) group developed the German Aortic Valve Score.[56] Based on 11,794 patients undergoing SAVR or TAVI in Germany in 2008, Kötting et al[55] identified 15 risk factors influencing in-hospital mortality using multiple logistic regression. The most important risk predictors were age, body mass index, renal disease, urgency status, and left ventricular function. This risk model had a high degree of discrimination, with an AUROC of 0.808.

The German Aortic Valve Score is the first attempt to develop a risk algorithm that can be applied with some degree of accuracy to patients who are considering TAVI or SAVR. One limitation of this model is the rapid evolution of TAVI, which means that predictions based on patients treated in 2008 already may be not applicable to current treatment options. Second, patients undergoing TAVI constituted only 5.1% (573 of 11,147) of the study population, reducing the validity of risk prediction for TAVI. TAVI also was performed in only 25 of the 81 participating institutions, limiting generalizability of the score. Third, the model was developed for interhospital comparisons only and therefore can predict only overall outcomes in German hospitals and cannot discriminate among different procedures, approaches, or devices.

The German Aortic Risk Score unfortunately cannot determine whether SAVR or TAVI is preferable in an individual patient. It is also likely that different factors constitute different risk profiles for different procedures. For example, frailty may be weighted more when considering SAVR compared with TAVI. The risks may not be the same for the different approaches for TAVI because severe lung disease may be a significant factor impacting outcomes with the transapical approach but not the transfemoral approach.

Another limitation of the German Aortic Valve Score is the methodology with which the risk model was constructed. Most risk models are developed with a portion of the overall population, usually 50% to 60% of the study group, to construct a weighted risk model. The remaining portion of the study population then is used for validation. This approach was not used because of the small number of TAVI procedures

TABLE 7.3	Comparison of TAVI-Specific Risk Models.					
	German Aortic Valve Score	FRANCE 2	TAVI2-SCORe	OBSERVANT	CoreValve U.S. Program	STS/ACC TVT
Valve	5% TAVI SAPIEN, 95% SAVR	CoreValve (67%) SAPIEN (33%)	CoreValve (2%) SAPIEN (98%)	CoreValve (52%) SAPIEN (48%)	CoreValve	CoreValve, SAPIEN
Patient cohort	11,794	3,833	511	1,878	3,687	20,586
C-statistic	0.81	0.67	0.72	0.73	0.75 30 day 0.79 1 year	0.67
Covariates for TAVI mortality	15	9	8	7	4 for 30 day, 4 for 1 year	9
Mortality measure	In-hospital	In-hospital, 30 day,	1 year	30-day	30 day 1 year	In-hospital
Place	Germany	France	France and Netherlands	Italy	United States	United States
Year of population analysis	2008	2010–2011	2007–2012	2010–2012	2010–2014	2011–2014

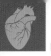

in the study, and external validation in other populations is needed. This model was based on in-hospital mortality, which is lower than the 30-day definition of mortality used by the STS algorithm.

FRANCE 2 Risk Model

The French Aortic National CoreValve and Edwards 2 (FRANCE 2) investigators[57] developed a TAVI-specific risk score based on a population of 3833 patients who underwent TAVI between January 1, 2010, and December 31, 2011. The study population was randomly divided into two groups, with 2552 patients used to develop the score and 1281 patients used for validation. The FRANCE 2 model considers eight patient-related and one procedure-related predictors of all-cause in-hospital or 30-day mortality. However, the C-statistics of the development and validation groups were 0.67 and 0.59, respectively, which limits their value compared with established risk scores.

TAVI2-SCORe

Development of the Transcatheter Aortic Valve Replacement–System for Cardiac Operative Risk Evaluation II (TAVI2-SCORe) score was based on 511 patients who underwent TAVI at two centers in the Netherlands and Italy between 2007 and 2012.[58] This score uses eight patient-related predictors of 1-year mortality. This derivative model had a C-statistic of 0.715, compared with C-statistics of 0.609 for EuroSCORE-I, 0.633 for Euro-SCORE-II, and 0.50 for the STS-PROM score in the same population. The study population for the TI1-SCORe model outperformed established risk models in this population, but 98% of the patient cohort received balloon-expandable Edwards SAPIEN prosthesis, whereas only 2% received self-expandable CoreValve prosthesis, limiting prediction of outcomes for patients being considered for a self-expandable prosthesis, which was confirmed subsequently in a single center study.[59]

OBSERVANT Risk Model

The OBSERVANT risk score was developed from the TAVI cohort in the Observational Study of Appropriateness, Efficacy, and Effectiveness of AVR-TAVI Procedures for the Treatment of Severe Symptomatic Aortic Stenosis (OBSERVANT).[60] The score was derived from 1256 patients and validated on 622 patients who underwent TAVI in Italy between 2010 and 2012. Seven variables were identified to be predictive of 30-day mortality. The investigators found that renal dysfunction (defined as a glomerular filtration rate [GFR] < 45 mL/min) was the single most powerful predictor of 30-day mortality. The model showed good discrimination in the development and validation data sets (C-statistics = 0.73 and 0.71, respectively). However, the internal validation and the small size of the patient cohort may limit its accuracy. Multiple independent studies showed that the OBSERVANT risk model did not perform well compared with the established risk models.[59,61]

CoreValve U.S. Risk Score

Another TAVI-specific risk model was developed to predict 30-day and 1-year mortality for the extreme-risk and high-risk patients enrolled in the CoreValve U.S. Pivotal Trial and continued access registry.[62] This score was developed and validated from a population of 2482 and 1205 patients, respectively. What is unique about this risk model is the addition of frailty and disability assessments. Significant predictors of 30-day mortality included age older than 85 years, home oxygen use, residence in an assisted living facility, and albumin level <3.3 g/dL, whereas 1-year mortality predictors included home oxygen use, albumin level <3.3 g/dL, STS-PROM score >7%, and a high Charlson comorbidity index score.

The CoreValve U.S. Risk Score highlighted the need to incorporate current risk models with frailty to predict early and late mortality.

Limitations of the CoreValve risk model are the inclusion only of patients receiving this specific valve type and the wide 95% confidence intervals (CIs). It is likely that expanding TAVI to include lower-risk patients would further limit the applicability of this risk model.

STS/ACC TVT Risk Model

The STS/ACC TVT risk model was based entirely on the Society of Thoracic Surgeons/American College of Cardiology Transcatheter Valve Therapy registry (STS/ACC TVT) data from 2011 to 2014.[63] This score was derived from a patient population of 13,718 and validated on 6868 different patients in a subsequent time period. Strengths of this model are inclusion of all commercially available valves in the United States and the use of nine variables to predict in-hospital mortality. Although the C-statistic of 0.66 in the validation cohort for this model presented an improvement over the previously reported C-statistic for STS-PROM, EuroSCORE, and FRANCE 2 risk models, the investigators emphasized that this model should not dictate which patients are candidate for TAVI even though it does provides useful information on procedural mortality to use in shared decision making. However, this model does not predict longer-term mortality beyond the hospital course, and frailty indices and quality of life measures were not included in the model.

In a study of 946 consecutive patients who underwent TAVI in Germany between 2013 and 2015, the TVT risk model for prediction of in-hospital mortality was found to have a similar c-statistic compared with the TVT cohort.[64] The STS-PROM and TVT scores performed similarly and were superior to the German Aortic Valve Score, EuroSCORE I, and EuroSCORE II for prediction of 30-day mortality (Fig. 7.2).

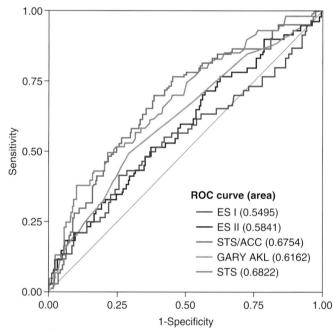

Fig. 7.2 Ability of Five Risk Scores to Predict 30-Day Mortality. *ACC,* American College of Cardiology; *AKL,* aortic valve (*Aortenklappe* in German) score; *ES I,* EuroSCORE I; *ES II,* EuroSCORE I; *GARY,* German Aortic Valve Registry; *ROC,* receiver operating characteristic; *STS,* Society of Thoracic Surgeons. (From Arsalan M, Maren W, Hecker F, et al. TAVI risk scoring using established versus new scoring systems: role of the new STS/ACC model. EuroIntervention 2018;13:1520-1526; Otto CM, Kumbhani DJ, Alexander KP, et al. 2017 ACC expert consensus decision pathway for transcatheter aortic valve replacement in the management of adults with aortic stenosis: a report of the American College of Cardiology Task Force on Clinical Expert Consensus Documents. J Am Coll Cardiol 2017;69:1313-1346.)

ROC curve (area)
— ES I (0.5495)
— ES II (0.5841)
— STS/ACC (0.6754)
— GARY AKL (0.6162)
— STS (0.6822)

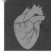

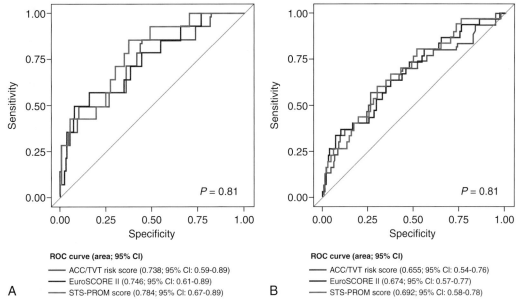

Fig. 7.3 **Comparison of the Discrimination Ability of Three Risk Scores.** (A) In-hospital mortality. (B) Thirty-day mortality. *ACC*, American College of Cardiology; *ROC*, receiver operating characteristic; *STS-PROM*, Society of Thoracic Surgeons' Predicted Risk of Mortality, *TVT*, Transcatheter Valve Therapy registry. (From Codner P, Malick W, Kouz R, et al. Mortality risk after transcatheter aortic valve implantation: analysis of the predictive accuracy of the Transcatheter Valve Therapy registry risk assessment model. EuroIntervention 2018;14:405-412.)

In another study of 3491 consecutive patients who underwent TAVI from 2011 to 2016 in Switzerland, Pilgrim et al[65] found that the TVT risk model had a moderate discrimination C-statistic of 0.66 for in-hospital mortality and C-statistic of 0.67 for 30-day mortality. The TVT risk model also showed improved calibration for in-hospital and 30-day mortality compared with the STS-PROM score.

In a population of 1068 consecutive patients who underwent TAVI from 2014 to 2016 in the United States, Codner et al[66] reported a high level of discrimination for in-hospital mortality (C-statistic = 0.74, 95% CI: 0.59–0.88). However, when compared with STS-PROM and EuroSCORE II, the TVT risk score was not significantly different for prediction of in-hospital and 30-day mortality (Fig. 7.3).

The STS/ACC TVT Registry is about to launch the 30-day predictive risk model for mortality that will include frailty assessment. Other models in development from the 60,000+ database of TAVI patients include predictors of stroke and of mortality and major morbidity at 30 days. Additional models are being developed for 1-year mortality and a patient-reported outcome of being alive and with an improved quality of life at 1 year. Because the current TAVI trials include outcome measures other than mortality, it is possible to envision the eventual construction of risk models that can predict composite outcomes, including mortality, stroke, and functional quality of life.

FRAILTY AND PROCEDURAL ASSESSMENT

Current risk prediction models for patients with valvular heart disease fail to include frailty despite increasing recognition of the importance of limited functional capacity (i.e., frailty) in short-term and long-term clinical outcomes (Table 7. 4). The most commonly used metric in assessing frailty of patients with cardiovascular disease is the 5-m walk test, but other measures also have been proposed.[67,68]

TABLE 7.4 Risk Factors Not Included in the Current Risk Scores.	
Procedural variables	Chest irradiation
	Previous coronary bypass surgery with patent graft
	Porcelain aorta
Baseline	Liver disease
	Frailty
	Nutritional status
	Debility

Green et al[69] developed a composite frailty score that included gait speed, grip strength, serum albumin level, and activities of daily living. A high score was associated with a threefold higher 1-year mortality rate compared with nonfrail patients (Table 7.5). Hermiller et al[62] found that home oxygen use, assisted living, a serum albumin level less than 3.3 g/dL, a history of falls in the past 6 months, and age older than 85 years were predictors of mortality at 30-days.[62,70] Novel metrics of frailty such as sarcopenia, thoracic aortic calcification, and mental health have been suggested for comprehensive risk stratification.[70]

In addition to frailty, procedure-specific impediments affect the decision about SAVR, TAVI, and palliative care. For example, multiple factors area associated with an increased risk of the surgical approach, including porcelain aorta, prior chest irradiation, and patent bypass graft that might be jeopardized at the time of surgery.[71–76]

Postprocedural or in-hospital stroke remains a significant complication after TAVI. Thourani et al[77] developed a risk prediction model to estimate in-hospital strokes using 97,600 cases from the TVT registry. It has created a benchmark for the rate and relevant patient risk factors for in-hospital strokes after TAVR.

TABLE 7.5 Frailty Assessment Tools.

	Frailty Index (0–7 Points)[73]	Essential Frailty Toolset (0–5 Points)[74]	"Fried Scale" (0–5 Points)[75]	Rockwood CFS (Multipoint Scale, ≥7 Points)[76]
Assessment tools	Timed get up and go test Mini Mental State Exam Mini Nutritional Assessment Activities of daily living Decreased frequency in walking 200 m or climbing stairs during the preceding 6 mo	Time to stand 5 times without using arms Mini Mental State Exam Hemoglobin Serum Albumin Mini Nutritional Assessment	5-m walk test Dominant hand grip strength (average of three trials) Unintentional weight loss ≥5 lb in preceding 6 mo Response to question six in SF-12 questionnaire (5-category scale)	Semiquantitative evaluation of accumulated health deficits based on mobility, inactivity, exhaustion, and disability of activities of daily life

INTEGRATIVE APPROACH

- An integrative approach to risk assessment is recommended for patients being considered for a surgical or transcatheter valve procedure.

- Risk assessment includes a comprehensive clinical evaluation, measures of frailty and functional status, use of risk scores, and consideration of procedure-specific impediments.

REFERENCES

1. Chassin MR, Hannan EL, DeBuono BA. Benefits and hazards of reporting medical outcomes publicly. N Engl J Med 1996;334:394-8.
2. Grover FL, Hammermeister KE, Shroyer ALW. Quality initiatives and the power of the database: what they are and how they run. Ann Thorac Surg 1995;60:1514-21.
3. Clark RE. The development of The Society of Thoracic Surgeons voluntary national database system: genesis, issues, growth, and status. Best Pract Benchmarking Healthc 1996;1:62-9.
4. Hammermeister KE, Johnson R, Marshall G, et al. Continuous assessment and improvement in quality of care: a model from the Department of Veterans Affairs cardiac surgery. Ann Surg 1994;219:281-90.
5. Daley J. Criteria by which to evaluate risk-adjusted outcomes programs in cardiac surgery. Ann Thorac Surg 1994;58:1827-35.
6. Iezzoni LI. The risks of risk adjustment. JAMA 1997;278:1600-7.
7. Iezzoni LI. Risk adjustment for measuring healthcare outcomes. Chicago: Health Administration Press; 1997.
8. Tu JV, Sykora K, Naylor CD. Assessing the outcomes of coronary artery bypass graft surgery: how many risk factors are enough? Steering Committee of the Cardiac Care Network of Ontario. J Am Coll Cardiol 1997;30:1317-23.
9. Luft HS, Romano PS. Chance, continuity, and change in hospital mortality rates. Coronary artery bypass graft patients in California hospitals, 1983 to 1989. JAMA 1993;270:331-7.
10. Grunkemeier GL, Payne N, Jin R, et al. Propensity score analysis of stroke after off-pump coronary artery bypass grafting. Ann Thorac Surg 2002;74:301-5.
11. Blackstone EH. Comparing apples and oranges. J Thorac Cardiovasc Surg 2002;123:8-15.
12. Harrell FE Jr. Regression modeling strategies with applications to linear models, logistic regression, and survival analysis. New York: Springer-Verlag; 2001.
13. Kouchoukos NT, Ebert PA, Grover FL, et al. Report of the Ad Hoc Committee on Risk Factors for Coronary Artery Bypass Surgery. Ann Thorac Surg 1988;45:348-9.
14. Edwards FH. Evolution of The Society of Thoracic Surgeons National Cardiac Surgery Database. J Invasive Cardiol 1998;10:485-8.
15. Shahian DM, Blackstone EH, Edwards FH, et al. Cardiac surgery risk models: a position article. Ann Thorac Surg 2004;78:1868-77.
16. Hannan EL, Kilburn H Jr, O'Donnell JF, et al. Adult open heart surgery in New York State: an analysis of risk factors and hospital mortality rates. JAMA 1990;264:2768-74.
17. Grover FL, Shroyer AL, Hammermeister KE. Calculating risk and outcome: the Veterans Affairs database. Ann Thorac Surg 1996;62:S6–11.
18. O'Connor GT, Plume SK, Olmstead EM, et al. Multivariate prediction of in-hospital mortality associated with coronary artery bypass graft surgery. Northern New England Cardiovascular Disease Study Group. Circulation 1992;85:2110-18.
19. Parsonnet V, Dean D, Bernstein AD. A method of uniform stratification of risk for evaluating the results of surgery in acquired adult heart disease. Circulation 1989;79:I3–I12.
20. Nashef SA, Roques F, Michel P, et al. European system for cardiac operative risk evaluation (EuroSCORE). Eur J Cardiothorac Surg 1999;16:9-13.
21. Marshall G, Grover FL, Henderson WG, et al. Assessment of predictive models for binary outcomes: an empirical approach using operative death from cardiac surgery. Stat Med 1994;13:1501-11.
22. O'Brien SM, Shahian DM, Filardo G. The Society of Thoracic Surgeons 2008 Cardiac Surgery Risk Models: Part 2—Isolated Valve Surgery. Ann Thorac Surg 2009;88:S23–42.
23. Zou KH, O'Malley AJ, Mauri L. Receiver-operating characteristic analysis for evaluating diagnostic tests and predictive models. Circulation 2007;115:654-7.
24. Nashef SA, Sharples LD, Roques F, et al. EuroSCORE II and the art and science of risk modeling. Eur J Cardiothorac Surg 2013;43:695-6.
25. Osswald BR, Gegouskov V, Badowski-Zyla D, et al. Overestimation of aortic valve replacement risk by EuroSCORE: implications for percutaneous valve replacement. Eur Heart J 2009;30:74-80.
26. Leontyev S, Walther T, Borger MA, et al. Aortic valve replacement in octogenarians: utility of risk stratification with EuroSCORE. Ann Thorac Surg 2009;87:1440-5.
27. Ranucci M, Castelvecchio S, Conte M, et al. The easier, the better: age, creatinine, ejection fraction score for operative mortality risk stratification in a series of 29,659 patients undergoing elective cardiac surgery. J Thorac Cardiovasc Surg 2011;142:581-6.
28. Kappetein AP, Head SJ. Predicting prognosis in cardiac surgery: a prophecy? Eur J Cardiothorac Surg 2012;41:732-3.
29. Nashef SA, Roques F, Sharples LD, et al. EuroSCORE II. Eur J Cardiothorac Surg 2012;41:734-44.
30. Rankin SJ, He X, O'Brien SM. The Society of Thoracic Surgeons risk model for operative mortality after multiple valve surgery. Ann Thorac Surg 2013;95:1484-90.
31. Puskas JD, Kilgo PD, Thourani VH, et al. The Society of Thoracic Surgeons 30-Day Predicted Risk of Mortality score also predicts long-term survival. Ann Thorac Surg 2012;93:26-35.

32. Shahian DM, He X, Jacobs JP. The Society of Thoracic Surgeons Isolated Aortic Valve Replacement (AVR) Composite Score: a report of the STS Quality Measurement Task Force. Ann Thorac Surg 2012;94:2166-71.

33. Online STS Risk Calculator. Available at <http://riskcalc.sts.org>.

34. Roques F, Nashef SAM, Michel P, et al. Risk factors and outcome in European cardiac surgery: analysis of the EuroSCORE multinational database of 19,030 patients. Eur J Cardiothorac Surg 1999;15:816-23.

35. Roques F, Michel P, Goldstone AR, et al. The logistic EuroSCORE. Eur Heart J 2003;24:881-2.

36. EuroSCORE Interactive Calculator. Available at <http://www.euroscore.org/calc>.

37. Grant SW, Hickey GL, Dimarakis I, et al. How does EuroSCORE II perform in UK cardiac surgery; an analysis of 23,740 patients from the Society for Cardiothoracic Surgery in Great Britain and Ireland National Database. Heart 2012;98:1566-72.

38. Chalmers J, Pullan M, Fabri B, et al. Validation of EuroSCORE II in a modern cohort of patients undergoing cardiac surgery. Eur J Cardiothorac Surg 2013;43:688-94.

39. Di Dedda U, Pelissero G, Agnelli B, et al. Accuracy, calibration and clinical performance of the new EuroSCORE II risk stratification system. Eur J Cardiothorac Surg 2013;43:27-32.

40. Dewey T, Brown D, Ryan WH, et al. Reliability of risk algorithms in predicting early and late operative outcomes in high risk patients undergoing aortic valve replacement. J Thorac Cardiovasc Surg 2008;135:180-7.

41. Conradi L, Seiffert M, Treede H, et al. Transcatheter aortic valve implantation versus surgical aortic valve replacement: a propensity score analysis in patients at high surgical risk. J Thorac Cardiovasc Surg 2012;143:64-71.

42. Ambler G, Omar RZ, Royston P, et al. Generic, simple risk stratification model for heart valve surgery. Circulation 2005;112:224-31.

43. Nowicki ER, Birkmeyer NJ, Weintraub RW, et al. Multivariable prediction of in-hospital mortality associated with aortic and mitral valve surgery in Northern New England. Ann Thorac Surg 2004;77:1966-77.

44. Ranucci M, Castelvecchio S, Menicanti L, et al. Risk of Assessing mortality risk in elective cardiac operations: age, creatinine, ejection fraction, and the Law of Parsimony. Circulation 2009;119:3041-3.

45. Ranucci M, Castelvecchio S, Conte M. The easier, the better: age, creatinine, ejection fraction score for operative mortality risk stratification in a series of 29,659 patients undergoing elective cardiac surgery. J Thorac Cardiovasc Surg 2011;142:581-6.

46. Ariyaratne TV, Billah B, Yap CH, et al. An Australian risk prediction model for determining early mortality following aortic valve replacement. Eur J Cardiothorac Surg 2011;39:815-21.

47. Sergeant P, Meuris B, Pettinari M. EuroSCORE II, illum qui est gravitates magni observe. Eur J Cardiothorac Surg 2012;41:729-31.

48. Gummert JF, Funkat A, Osswald B, et al. EuroSCORE overestimates the risk of cardiac surgery: results from the national registry of the German Society of Thoracic and Cardiovascular Surgery. Clin Res Cardiol 2009;98:363-9.

49. Biancari F, Kangasniemi OP, Aliasim Mahar M, et al. Changing risk of patients undergoing coronary artery bypass surgery. Interact Cardiovasc Thorac Surg 2009;8:40-4.

50. Nilsson J, Algotsson L, Höglund P, et al. Comparison of 19 pre-operative risk stratification models in open-heart surgery. Eur Heart J 2006;27:867-74.

51. Bridgewater B, Neve H, Moat N, et al. Predicting operative risk for coronary artery surgery in the United Kingdom: a comparison of various risk prediction algorithms. Heart 1998;79:350-5.

52. Bhatti F, Grayson AD, Grotte G, et al. The logistic EuroSCORE in cardiac surgery: how well does it predict operative risk? Heart 2006;92:1817-20.

53. Bode C, Kelm M. EuroSCORE: still gold standard or less? Clin Res Cardiol 2009;98:353-4.

54. Zheng Z, Li Y, Zhang S, et al, Chinese CABG Registry Study. The Chinese coronary artery bypass grafting registry study: how well does the EuroSCORE predict operative risk for Chinese population? Eur J Cardiothorac Surg 2009;35:54-8.

55. Grossi EA, Schwartz CF, Yu PJ, et al. High-risk aortic valve replacement: are the outcomes as bad as predicted? Ann Thorac Surg 2008;85:102-6.

56. Kötting J, Schiller W, Beckmann A, et al. German Aortic Valve Score: a new scoring system for prediction of mortality related to aortic valve procedures in adults. Eur J Cardiothorac Surg 2013;43:971-7.

57. Iung B, Laouénan C, Himbert D, et al. Predictive factors of early mortality after transcatheter aortic valve implantation: individual risk assessment using a simple score. Heart 2014;100:1016-23.

58. Debonnaire P, Fusini L, Wolterbeek R, et al. Value of the "TAVI2-SCORe" versus surgical risk scores for prediction of one year mortality in 511 patients who underwent transcatheter aortic valve implantation. Am J Cardiol 2015;115:234-42.

59. Collas VM, Van De Heyning CM, Paelinck BP, et al. Validation of transcatheter aortic valve implantation risk scores in relation to early and mid-term survival: a single-centre study. Interact Cardiovasc Thorac Surg 2016;22:273-9.

60. Capodanno D, Barbanti M, Tamburino C, et al. A simple risk tool (the OBSERVANT score) for prediction of 30-day mortality after transcatheter aortic valve replacement. Am J Cardiol 2014;113:1851-8.

61. Halkin A, Steinvil A, Witberg G, et al. Mortality prediction following transcatheter aortic valve replacement: a quantitative comparison of risk scores derived from populations treated with either surgical or percutaneous aortic valve replacement. The Israeli TAVR Registry Risk Model Accuracy Assessment (IRRMA) study. Int J Cardiol 2016;215:227-31.

62. Hermiller JB, Jr., Yakubov SJ, Reardon MJ, et al. Predicting early and late mortality after transcatheter aortic valve replacement. J Am Coll Cardiol 2016;68:343-352.

63. Edwards FH, Cohen DJ, O'Brien SM, et al. Development and validation of a risk prediction model for in-hospital mortality after transcatheter aortic valve replacement. JAMA Cardiol 2016;1:46-52.

64. Arsalan M, Maren W, Hecker F, et al. TAVI risk scoring using established versus new scoring systems: role of the new STS/ACC model. EuroIntervention 2018;13:1520-6.

65. Pilgrim T, Franzone A, Stortecky S, et al. Predicting mortality after transcatheter aortic valve replacement: external validation of the transcatheter valve therapy registry model. Circ Cardiovasc Interv 2017;10:1-9.

66. Codner P, Malick W, Kouz R, et al. Mortality risk after transcatheter aortic valve implantation: analysis of the predictive accuracy of the Transcatheter Valve Therapy registry risk assessment model. EuroIntervention 2018;14:405-12.

67. Mack MJ, Holper EM. TAVR risk assessment: does the eyeball test have 20/20 vision, or can we do better? J Am Coll Cardiol 2016;68:353

68. Afilalo J, Eisenberg MJ, Morin JF, et al. Gait speed as an incremental predictor of mortality and major morbidity in elderly patients undergoing cardiac surgery. J Am Coll Cardiol 2010;56: 1668–76.

69. Green P, Woglom AE, Genereux P., et al. Gait speed and dependence in activities of daily living in older adults with severe aortic stenosis. Clin Cardiol 2012;35:307-14.

70. Hebeler KR, Baumgarten H, Squiers JJ, et al. Albumin is predictive of 1-year mortality after transcatheter aortic valve replacement. Ann Thorac Surg 2018;106:1302-07.

71. Nishimura RA, Otto CM, Bonow RO, et al. 2014 AHA/ACC guideline for the management of patients with valvular heart disease: executive summary: a report of the American College of Cardiology/American Heart Association Task Force on Practice Guidelines. Circulation 2014;129:2440-2492.

72. Vahanian A, Otto CM. Risk stratification of patients with aortic stenosis. Eur Heart J 2010; 4:416-23.

73. Stortecky S, Schoenenberger AW, Moser A, et al. Evaluation of multidimensional geriatric assessment as a predictor of mortality and cardiovascular events after transcatheter aortic valve implantation. JACC Cardiovasc Interv 2012;5:489-496.

74. Afilalo J, Lauck S, Kim DH, et al. Frailty in older adults undergoing aortic valve replacement: the FRAILTY-AVR Study. J Am Coll Cardiol 2017;70:689-700.

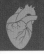

75. Arnold SV, Afilalo J, Spertus JA, et al. Prediction of poor outcome after transcatheter aortic valve replacement J Am Coll Cardiol 2016;68:1868-1877.

76. Shimura T, Yamamoto M, Kano S, et al. Impact of the clinical frailty scale on outcomes after transcatheter aortic valve replacement. Circulation 2017;135:2013-2024.

77. Thourani VH, O'Brien SM, Kelly JJ, et al. Development and application of a risk prediction model for in-hospital stroke after transcatheter aortic valve replacement: a report from the Society of Thoracic Surgeons/American College of Cardiology Transcatheter Valve Therapy Registry. Ann Thorac Surg 2019;107:1097-1103.

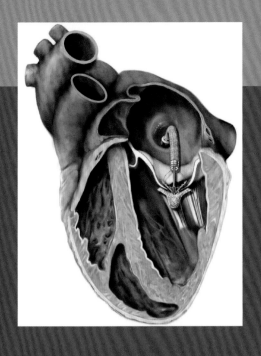

中文导读

第8章
主动脉瓣的影像评估

　　影像评估是结构性心脏病医师的另一双"眼睛"。众多影像学评估方式目前均被用于主动脉瓣及主动脉根部评估，如超声心动图、CT、心导管及心脏MRI检查。本章详细阐述了以上工具在主动脉瓣诊疗应用中的优缺点及选择建议。超声心动图因便携、易于掌握、可提供实时高分辨的心脏运动情况和心内结构功能血流状态，目前仍然是主动脉瓣疾病最重要的评估工具，对病因和疾病严重程度都可提供良好的判断。主动脉瓣狭窄的严重程度诊断依靠主动脉瓣峰值流速、平均压差和连续方程计算的瓣口面积。流出道和瓣口的速度时间积分比值也可用来体现主动脉瓣狭窄的严重程度，尤其在声窗不佳时。主动脉瓣反流的严重程度诊断应用缩流颈宽度、连续波多普勒的速度信号和反流束的表现进行评估。在特定情况下，推荐应用反流量和瓣口反流面积。与主动脉瓣疾病相关的主动脉扩张可通过超声诊断，但是完善的评估需要应用门控增强CT或心脏MRI检查。当超声检查不能明确诊断或超声检查发现与症状不符时，CT和MRI可用于评估主动脉瓣功能障碍的原因及严重程度。经食管超声心动图检查的主要应用指征包括：明确主动脉瓣形态，功能定量和评估主动脉根部解剖结构。准备进行经导管主动脉瓣置换术治疗的患者，经食管主动脉瓣环三维评估可作为门控CT评估的次选替代。CT目前已成为准备进行经导管主动脉瓣置换术的患者术前评估的重要工具。心脏MRI在检查跨瓣流速方面可能出现低估，但是对于心脏重构和纤维化的定量评估非常重要。

张　倩

Imaging the Aortic Valve

Rebecca T. Hahn, João L. Cavalcante

CHAPTER OUTLINE

KEY POINTS

- Echocardiography is the primary modality for determining the morphology of the aortic valve and the cause and severity of dysfunction.
- In addition to symptoms, quantitative echocardiographic evaluation of left ventricular size and systolic function is key in clinical decision making for adults with aortic valvular heart disease.
- Aortic stenosis severity is defined by maximum aortic jet velocity, mean gradient, and continuity equation valve area. The dimensionless velocity index should be also considered, particularly in the absence of good echocardiographic windows.
- Aortic regurgitant severity is defined by vena contracta width, the continuous-wave Doppler velocity signal, and presence of aortic flow reversal. In selected cases, calculation of regurgitant volume and regurgitant orifice area is recommended.

- Aortic dilation associated with aortic valve disease can be diagnosed by echocardiography, but cross-sectional imaging with gated computed tomography angiography or cardiac magnetic resonance necessary for complete evaluation.
- Computed tomography and cardiac magnetic resonance imaging can be used to determine the cause and severity of aortic valve dysfunction when echocardiography is nondiagnostic or there is discrepancy between symptoms and echocardiographic findings.
- Primary indications for transesophageal imaging include clarification of aortic valve morphology, quantification of function, and assessment of aortic root morphology. Three-dimensional evaluation of the aortic annulus by transesophageal imaging can be when gated computed tomography angiography is suboptimal for planning of transcatheter aortic valve implantation.

IMAGING AORTIC VALVE ANATOMY

Multiple imaging modalities are used to characterize the morphology and function of the aortic valve and aortic root. Echocardiography remains the primary imaging modality because of ease of use, portability, and high temporal resolution enabling accurate real-time assessment of moving structures and flow in two-dimensional (2D) and three-dimensional (3D) formats. Extensive outcomes data are associated with echocardiographic measurements of ventricular and valvular

function.[1,2] Nonetheless, cardiac computed tomography (CT) and cardiac magnetic resonance (CMR) imaging offer significant complementary information for the evaluation of patients with aortic valve disease. The advantages and limitations of each modality are discussed.

Normal Anatomy of the Aortic Valve and Aortic Root

An understanding of aortic valve and aortic root anatomy is essential to interpret imaging of these structures. The aortic valve complex is composed of the left ventricular outflow tract (LVOT), aortic valve

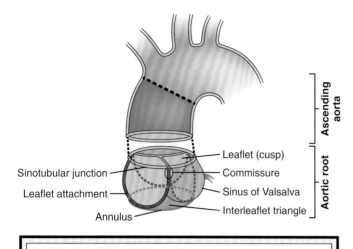

Aortic valve: Three leaflets only

Aortic root: All components (*Sinuses of Valsalva, interleaflet triangles, sinutubular junction, leaflet attachments, leaflets, annulus*)

Fig. 8.1 Proposed Terminology of the Aortic Root Components. The aortic valve complex is composed of the aortic valve (leaflets only) and aortic root. The aortic root is composed of the sinuses of Valsalva, interleaflet triangles, sinutubular junction, leaflet attachments, leaflets, and annulus. (From Sievers HH, Hemmer W, Beyersdorf F, et al. The everyday used nomenclature of the aortic root components: the tower of Babel. Eur J Cardio-Thorac Surg 2012;41:478-482.)

leaflets, and aortic root to the sinotubular junction (Fig. 8.1).[3] An understanding of the complexity of the normal and congenitally abnormal anatomy should start with early development.[4] Early in development, the outflow tract myocardium encases the developing aortic root and regresses as the valvar sinuses develop. The pericardial space no longer has direct continuity with the left ventricular (LV) cavity due to regression of the encasing myocardium, explaining the reflection of the visceral and parietal pericardial surfaces around the aortic root. The mitral-aortic curtain forms in part from the regression of the myocardium in this region, forming a fibrous connection between the mitral valve and the aortic root.

The aortic valve leaflets are semilunar structures supported by the aortic sinuses.[5] Each semilunar cusp is attached to the aortic wall in a curved manner, with the basal attachment located in the LV below the anatomic ventriculoaortic junction and the distal attachment at the sinotubular junction (STJ).[6] When the curved path of the aortic leaflet insertion points are tracked, the 3D spatial configuration of the aortic valve resembles a crown.[7] The STJ is the distal attachment of the leaflet zones of coaptation and is an essential component of valve function; dilation of this structure may lead to malcoaptation and aortic regurgitation (AR). The body of each leaflet extends from the semilunar hinge to the lunula or leaflet edge. Overlap of the lunula ensures a competent valve, but fenestrations may occur with aging and, depending on the extent and location, may result in regurgitation. The proximal and distal attachments of the leaflets are subject to the hemodynamic and anatomic cyclic changes of the ventricle and aorta, respectively.

Coaptation of the three leaflets occurs at no more than one half of the overall height of the aortic root.[4] The fibrous interleaflet triangles between the scalloped hinge lines of the leaflets have as their base the true ventriculoarterial junction, or the plane of mitral-aortic continuity. The top of the triangle is at the level of the STJ. The interleaflet

triangles can be easily imaged from the ventricular aspect of the aortic root but not from the aortic side. The membranous septum underlies the right interleaflet triangle between the right and noncoronary cusps. The interleaflet triangles form the boundary between the LV and the extracardiac space; the transverse sinus or the tissue plane separates the aortic root from the free-standing muscular subpulmonary infundibulum.

The aortic valve leaflets are supported by the sinuses of Valsalva. The left coronary sinus is typically the smallest sinus, the right coronary sinus is larger, and the noncoronary sinuses are the largest.[8] The larger sinuses experience increased stress and strain and more commonly exhibit calcification, dilation, or aneurysm formation. The noncoronary sinus also may be referred to as the nonadjacent sinus because it does not border the pulmonary root, unlike the right and left sinuses.

The largest interleaflet triangle is between the noncoronary and left coronary leaflets (triangle between the left and right leaflets is the smallest). There is myocardial support underneath the right and left coronary sinuses, with only fibrous support beneath the noncoronary leaflet. The fibrous support is composed of the central fibrous body (through which runs the atrioventricular bundle of His), the subaortic curtain (in continuity with the anterior mitral leaflet), and the left fibrous trigone. The aortic root changes shape throughout the cardiac cycle, starting as a cone, becoming a cylinder, and then becoming an inverted cone. This ability to change shapes is made possible by the fibrous interleaflet triangles.

Echocardiography of Normal Aortic Valve Anatomy

According to guidelines,[1] transthoracic echocardiography (TTE) is the diagnostic imaging modality recommended in the initial evaluation of patients with known or suspected aortic valve disease to confirm the diagnosis, establish cause, determine severity, assess hemodynamic consequences, determine prognosis, and evaluate for the timing of intervention.

The aortic valve and root are imaged from multiple standard 2D TTE imaging planes, including: parasternal long- and short-axis views, apical five- and three-chamber views, and subcostal views (Fig. 8.2). When TTE image quality is suboptimal, transesophageal echocardiography (TEE) or CMR may be appropriate. Standard TEE aortic valve imaging planes include: mid-esophageal short- and long-axis views, transgastric long-axis view, and deep transgastric five-chamber view (Fig. 8.3).[9]

The echocardiographic aortic annulus is a virtual anatomic structure. The plane of the annulus is defined by the three nadirs (most basal) of the semilunar hinge lines of the leaflets, but it has no other anatomic or histologic definition.[7] More than one half of the circumference of the annulus is formed by the base of the interleaflet triangles. The annulus expands by up to one sixth during ventricular ejection; it is the largest and most circular in mid-systole, becoming smallest and most elliptical at end-diastole.[10–13]

Accurate and reproducible measurement of the diameter of this virtual ring by 2D TTE is not feasible for two reasons. First, with a trileaflet aortic valve, any long-axis plane bisecting a cusp hinge point on one side does not image a hinge point on the other side, but rather images a region of fibrous tissue between the scalloped cusps. Second, the annulus is often asymmetric and oval, with annular diameters largest in the coronal plane and shortest in the sagittal plane.[12,14,15] Aligning long-axis views to bisect the largest diameter of the annulus or LVOT is essential to accurate measurement of these structures. The use of simultaneous biplane imaging, a 3D matrix probe function, can help identify the optimal location for these measurements.[16–18]

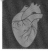

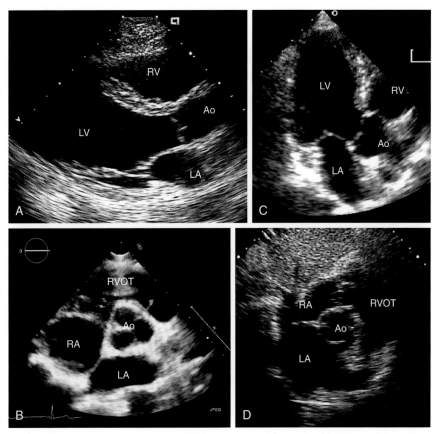

Fig. 8.2 Standard Transthoracic Echocardiographic Aortic Valve Imaging Planes. The aortic valve and root are imaged from multiple standard 2D TTE imaging planes, including parasternal long-axis (A) and short-axis views (B), apical five- and three-chamber views (C), and subcostal views (D). When TTE image quality is suboptimal, TEE may be appropriate. *Ao*, Aorta; *RVOT*, right ventricular outflow tract.

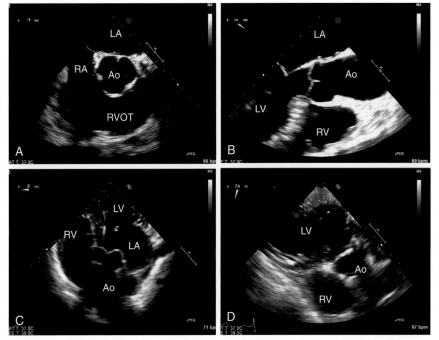

Fig. 8.3 Standard TEE Aortic Valve Imaging Planes. Standard transesophageal echocardiographic aortic valve imaging planes include the following. (A) Mid-esophageal short-axis view (rotation angle of 25 to 45 degrees). (B) Mid-esophageal long-axis view (rotation angle of 120 to 140 degrees). (C) Deep transgastric five-chamber view (rotation angle of 0 to 20 degrees). (D) Transgastric long-axis view (rotation angle of 120 to 140 degrees). *Ao*, Aorta; *RVOT*, right ventricular outflow tract.

ACQUISITION

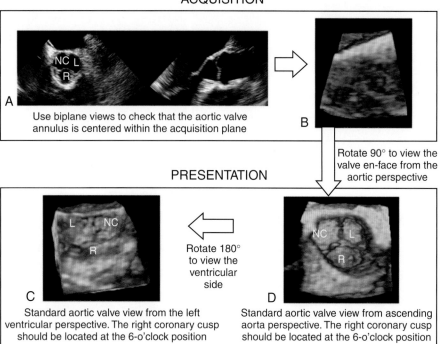

Use biplane views to check that the aortic valve
annulus is centered within the acquisition plane

Rotate 90° to view the
valve en-face from the
aortic perspective

PRESENTATION

Rotate 180°
to view the
ventricular
side

Standard aortic valve view from the left
ventricular perspective. The right coronary cusp
should be located at the 6-o'clock position

Standard aortic valve view from ascending
aorta perspective. The right coronary cusp
should be located at the 6-o'clock position

Fig. 8.4 Recommendations for Standard 3D Acquisition and Display of the Aortic Valve. American
Society of Echocardiography guidelines provide recommendations for standard 3D acquisition and display of the aortic valve. (A) Acquisition views from simultaneous biplane imaging. (B) Zoom volume that
is acquired from the mid-esophageal view. This volume is then rotated to show the aortic view of the
valve (C) or the ventricular view (D). *L*, Left cusp; *NC*, noncoronary cusp; *R*, right cusp. (From Hahn RT,
Abraham T, Adams MS, et al. Guidelines for performing a comprehensive transesophageal echocardiographic examination: recommendations from the American Society of Echocardiography and the
Society of Cardiovascular Anesthesiologists. J Am Soc Echocardiogr 2013;26:921-964.)

Several 3D echo studies have advanced our understanding of the
aortic valve complex anatomy, including the shape of the LVOT and
annulus,[10,12,14,19–22] aortic root,[23,24] and aortic valve leaflets.[25,26] The
American Society of Echocardiography produced guidelines for standard 3D acquisition and display of the aortic valve (Fig. 8.4).[17] After
the 2D image is optimized, narrow-angle or wide-angle (user-defined)
acquisition modes can be used to optimize the 3D image and to examine aortic valve and root anatomy. 3D TTE acquisitions are obtained
from the parasternal long-axis view with and without color (i.e., narrow angle and zoomed acquisitions). 3D TEE volumes are obtained
from a 60-degree, mid-esophageal, short-axis view with and without
color (i.e., zoomed or full-volume acquisition) and from a 120-degree,
mid-esophageal, long-axis view with and without color (i.e., zoomed
or full-volume acquisition).

After acquisition, when displayed *en face*, the aortic valve should be
oriented with the right coronary cusp located inferiorly, regardless
of whether the aortic or the LVOT perspective is presented. Color
Doppler 3D TEE imaging should also be performed to detect the initial
appearance of flow at the onset of systole.

Cross-Sectional Imaging of Normal Aortic Valves

The use of cross-sectional imaging for patients with normal aortic
valve is typically not recommended unless echocardiographic windows are suboptimal or there is a discrepancy between symptoms
or echocardiographic findings, or both. Both gated computed tomography angiography (CTA) and CMR can provide unparalleled
visualization of the aortic valve morphology and function, but CTA
requires intravenous access for contrast administration, a small

radiation dose, and heart rate control. CMR can visualize the aortic
valve without radiation, intravenous contrast, or heart rate control,
but it cannot visualize calcification well. Both imaging modalities
are excellent for visualization and quantification of aortopathy,
which can be seen in some cases even in the absence of significant
aortic valve pathology (Fig. 8.5).

Congenitally Abnormal Anatomy of the Aortic Valve

Bicuspid aortic valves (BAVs) are the most common congenital cardiovascular abnormality, affecting up to 2% of the population.[27]
Beyond the abnormal aortic valve morphology, which can facilitate
early degeneration (i.e., stenosis and regurgitation), patients with
BAV can also have other associated conditions, such as aortopathy
involving the aortic root or thoracic aorta and aortic coarctation.[28]
Despite the aortopathy, BAV patients tend to have a small risk of
aortic dissection compared with other cohorts with connective tissue
disorders.[27,29]

BAVs typically have a single line of coaptation, which extends to the
sinotubular junction at both ends with two well-defined interleaflet
triangles. Unicuspid valves have a single line of coaptation, which extends from the STJ to the centroid of the valvar orifice with a single,
well-defined, interleaflet triangle between the noncoronary and left
coronary leaflets.

Valvar morphology assessment by echocardiography requires on-
axis imaging from the short-axis views of the aortic valve. Distinguishing a raphe from a functional zone of apposition is difficult in diastole.
Imaging the valve from the short-axis view in systole allows appreciation of the zones of apposition versus fusion of the cusps.

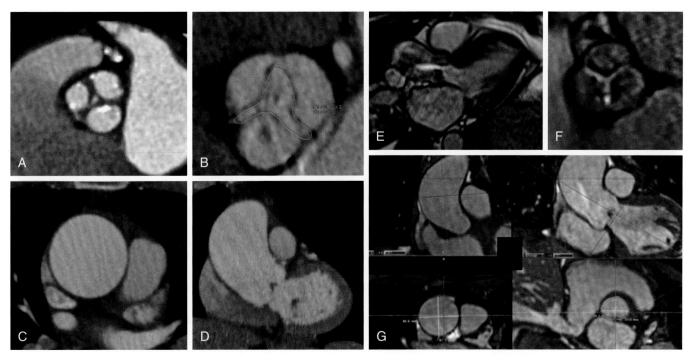

Fig. 8.5 Aortic Valve and Aortic Pathology on Computed Tomography (CT) and Cardiac Magnetic Resonance Imaging (CMR). Aortic valve (AoV) and associated aortopathy can be visualized by CT and CMR imaging. (A) CT short-axis reformat view of the AoV in diastole in patient with aortic regurgitation. (B) CT short-axis view of the AoV at the leaflet tips used for planimetry of the anatomic orifice area. Short-axis (C) and long-axis (D) views show a dilated ascending aorta in a patient with bicuspid aortic valve. Long-axis (E) and short-axis (F) views show CMR visualization of severe aortic stenosis. (G) Noncontrast 3D CMR data set allows multiplanar reformat and measurement of aortopathy and aortic annulus.

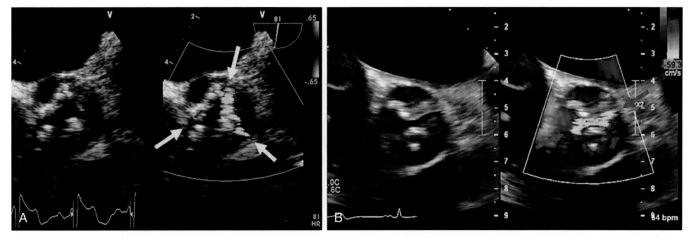

Fig. 8.6 Echocardiographic Diagnosis of Bicuspid Aortic Valve Stenosis. Color Doppler image of the aortic valve from a short-axis (SAX) view in systole may be helpful in distinguishing bicuspid from tricuspid aortic valve in the setting of severe aortic stenosis with reduced leaflet mobility. (A) SAX view of a tricuspid aortic valve without commissural fusion with color flow seen in three commissures *(yellow arrows)*. (B) Bicuspid aortic valve with a single commissure that extends to the sinutubular junction at both ends *(red arrows)*.

For patients with good-quality transthoracic images, who do not have dense bicuspid aortic valve calcification, diagnostic sensitivity and specificity are more than 70% and 90%, respectively.[30,31] However, diagnostic uncertainty may remain for 10% to 15% of patients after an echocardiogram.[29] Particularly in the setting of calcification, color Doppler in systole may be helpful in distinguishing immobile trileaflet aortic valves without commissural fusion from bicuspid valves with

fusion (Fig. 8.6). TEE and 3D modalities significantly improve the diagnostic and phenotyping accuracy for BAVs.[32–35]

Several classification systems have been used in the past. Most were based on the fusion of cusps and orientation or number of the raphae.[36–38] Some of these classification systems then identified patients with no raphe as pure BAV or type 0.[38] One classification system identifies only two BAV phenotypes: fusion of the right and left coronary

TABLE 8.1   Advantages and Limitations of Imaging Modalities for the Assessment of Valvular Disease.

Modality	Advantages	Disadvantages
Echocardiography	Readily available and portable Transthoracic and transesophageal approaches No iodinated intravenous contrast No radiation Excellent temporal resolution Good spatial resolution Functional and hemodynamic information Automated postprocessing tools are becoming available	Requires adequate training and technical skills for comprehensive examination Potentially more skill required for 3D and annular assessment Transesophageal echocardiography is semi-invasive, and sedation typically required Limitations of ultrasound physics (e.g., acoustic shadowing, far-field imaging) can compromise interpretation Lateral resolution × frame rate issues
Computed tomography	Excellent spatial resolution (gold standard for anatomic information and structural planning) Noninvasive and fast Comprehensive vascular assessment Easy to use/familiarity Automated postprocessing tools are available with comprehensive vascular assessment	Frequently requires iodinated intravenous contrast (elevated risk for patients with chronic kidney dysfunction) Radiation dose has improved, but high in 4D (functional) CT Poor temporal resolution (better with dual-source CT) Suboptimal in patients with increased heart rate/arrhythmia Not portable Blooming artifacts can occur with calcium, valve stent frames, intracardiac leads, and other conditions
Cardiac magnetic resonance	Good temporal and spatial resolution Minimal effect of body habitus Gold standard for ventricular volumes, mass, and ejection fraction (no contrast required) Excellent for valvular regurgitation (no contrast) Excellent myocardial tissue characterization No radiation and noninvasive Can assess anatomy without intravenous gadolinium Vascular assessment Hemodynamic information	Spatial resolution inferior to CT and 3D TEE (thick slices) Lower temporal resolution than echocardiography Requires adequate training for comprehensive examination acquisition and interpretation Longer examination (free-breathing cardiac magnetic resonance examination is possible) Claustrophobia Incompatible with certain intracardiac devices and cardiac resynchronization therapy; cases of older prosthesis–patient mismatch Suboptimal quantification can occur with fast and irregular cardiac arrhythmia (unless newer pulse sequences are available) Cannot visualize calcification well Peak velocities may be underestimated

cusps (BAV-AP) and fusion of the right or left coronary cusp and non-coronary cusp (BAV-RL).[39] These two phenotypes have some support from animal studies identifying defective development of different embryologic structures.[40]

Morphology may provide valuable data regarding risk stratification of BAV patients.[39,41,42] In a small population of 167 patients, Kang et al showed that moderate-to-severe aortic stenosis (AS) is more prevalent among patients with BAV-RL (66.2% vs. 46.2% in BAV-AP; $P = 0.01$), and moderate-to-severe AR is more prevalent among patients with in BAV-AP (32.3% vs. 6.8% in BAV-RL; $P < 0.0001$). The association with bicuspid aortic valve and dilation of the ascending aorta has been well-established.[43–45] Some investigators have suggested that the aortic abnormality is unrelated to the valvular pathology[43,45] and a primary anomaly is associated with this entity.

For a comprehensive evaluation of BAV morphology and function, in addition to other associated conditions, cross-sectional imaging with gated CTA or CMR is necessary.[1,46] Table 8.1 summarizes the advantages and disadvantages of each cross-sectional imaging method.

Although TTE is adequate for screening, cross-sectional imaging is required to guide timing of surveillance and aortic intervention. Cardiac gated CTA and CMR are the best imaging modalities due to their exquisite spatial resolution and 3D imaging reconstruction capabilities. To provide accurate measurements, adequate postprocessing using multiplanar reformatting with double oblique reconstructions is

necessary.[47] The thresholds for intervention and discussion of BAV outcomes can be found in Chapter 11.

Studies using advanced imaging techniques with 4D flow CMR have suggested that hemodynamic factors such as regional wall stress in the setting of eccentric outflow patterns contribute to the pattern of aortic dilation.[48–51]

AORTIC STENOSIS SEVERITY

The stages of valvular AS are defined by symptoms, valve hemodynamics, and the effect of valve obstruction on ventricular structure and function. Echocardiography remains the initial imaging modality for the diagnosis, phenotyping, and hemodynamic assessment of aortic valve dysfunction and the initial assessment of the thoracic aorta (Table 8.2). CTA and CMR have become important adjunctive imaging modalities for the evaluation of patients with AS, giving the growing complexity in assessing this valve pathology.

Echocardiography

According to guidelines, TTE is indicated when there is an unexplained systolic murmur, a single second heart sound, a history of a bicuspid aortic valve, or symptoms that may be due to AS.[1,2] The evaluation of aortic valve area (AVA) should include direct visualization, planimetry, and Doppler assessment. Doppler echocardiography assessment of AS can be categorized as flow-dependent measurements

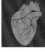

TABLE 8.2   Criteria for Assessing Severity of Aortic Stenosis.

	Mild	Moderate	Severe
Valve Anatomy			
	Mild-to-moderate leaflet calcification of a bicuspid or trileaflet valve with some reduction in systolic motion or Rheumatic valve changes with commissural fusion		Severe leaflet calcification or congenital stenosis with severely reduced leaflet opening
Quantitative Parameters (Flow Dependent)			
Peak velocity	<3 m/s	3–4 m/s	>4 m/s
Mean gradient	<20 mmHg	20–40 mmHg	>40 mmHg
Quantitative Parameters (Flow-Independent)			
Doppler velocity index	>0.5	0.25–0.5	<0.25
Aortic valve area (AVA)	>1.5 cm²	1.0–1.5 cm²	<1.0 cm²
AVA index	>0.85 cm²/m²	0.6–0.85 cm²/m²	≤0.6 cm²/m²

Data from Baumgartner H, Hung J, Bermejo J, et al. Recommendations on the echocardiographic assessment of aortic valve stenosis: a focused update from the European Association of Cardiovascular Imaging and the American Society of Echocardiography. Eur Heart J Cardiovasc Imaging 2017;18:254-275.

or flow-independent measurements. Flow-dependent measurements obtained from continuous-wave Doppler across the stenotic aortic valve, include jet velocity and peak and mean gradients. Relatively flow-independent measurements of aortic valve area include the AVA calculated from the continuity equation[52–55] and the dimensionless velocity or velocity-time integral (VTI) ratio, also known as the dimensionless index (DI).[56]

Direct Visualization and Planimetry

Direct visualization and estimation of location and severity of valve calcification (i.e., leaflet tips, commissures or sinuses of Valsalva) and mobility of the leaflets should not be underestimated as a tool for assessing AS severity.

Direct planimetry of a stenotic aortic orifice has been validated.[57–60] Okura et al[61] evaluated the reliability of 2D TTE AVA planimetry by comparing the planimetered inner leaflet edges from short-axis views at the time of maximal opening (i.e., early systole) with similar measurements made on TEE and with valve area by the continuity equation and the Gorlin formula. Correlation was high (r = 0.98, 0.9, and 0.89, respectively) with a very low standard error of the estimates (0.04 cm², 0.09 cm², and 0.10 cm², respectively). Multiple studies have suggested that 3D planimetered AVA is larger than 2D measurements,[58,62] but 3D measurements showed a lower mean difference with continuity equation calculations.[58]

In clinical practice, direct 2D planimetry using 2D TTE is not always feasible due to difficult windows and visualization of the aortic valve opening. The significant upward motion of the aortic annulus in systole makes it harder to define whether the plane is at the leaflet tips.

In these instances, use of simultaneous biplane imaging to define the short-axis level of the leaflet tips, or direct planimetry using 3D multiplanar reconstruction, may be helpful.

Velocity and Pressure Gradients

The maximum velocity of blood flow across the aortic valve (V_{max}) is measured by continuous-wave Doppler and is an important measure of AS disease severity. Natural history studies have shown that outcomes are determined by peak transaortic velocity, with progressively worse survival correlating with increasing velocities above 4 m/s.[63–65] The change in velocity over time is another parameter that predicts outcome. Rosenhek et al[64] found that in patients with moderately or severely calcified aortic valves whose aortic jet velocity increased by 0.3 m/s or more within 1 year, 79% underwent surgery or died within 2 years.

The pressure gradient across the valve (ΔP) is related to V_{max}, the proximal velocity (V_{prox}), and the mass density of blood (ρ), as stated in the Bernoulli equation, which includes terms for conversion of potential to kinetic energy (i.e., convective acceleration), the effects of local acceleration, and viscous (v) losses:

$$\Delta P = \tfrac{1}{2}\, \rho\left(V_{max^2} - V_{prox^2}\right) + \rho(dv/dt)dx + R(v)$$

where dv/dt is rate of change in velocity over time; dx is the time-varying velocity at each distance along the flow stream; and R is a constant describing the viscous losses for that fluid and orifice.

In clinical practice, the terms for acceleration and viscous losses are ignored, and $\tfrac{1}{2}\,\rho$ is converted to allow pressure to be measured in mmHg and velocity in m/s, so that

$$\Delta P = 4\left(V_{max^2} - V_{prox^2}\right)$$

When the proximal velocity is low (<1.5 m/s) and the jet velocity is high ($V_{prox^2} \ll V_{max^2}$), the equation can be further simplified as the modified Bernoulli equation:

$$\Delta P = 4\left(V_{max^2}\right)$$

The assumptions of the modified Bernoulli equation may not be valid in some circumstances (i.e., severe anemia, dynamic LVOT obstruction, or concomitant subvalvular stenosis when the proximal velocity cannot be assumed to be negligible).

Maximum instantaneous transaortic gradient is calculated from the maximum transvalvular velocity, whereas the mean gradient is calculated by averaging the instantaneous gradient over the systolic ejection period. A mean gradient of more than 40 mmHg is considered severely increased and is associated with a peak velocity of 4 m/s. However, large population-based studies have shown that the AVA cutpoint of 1.0 cm² corresponds to a mean gradient of 30 to 35 mmHg.[66]

Underestimating V_{max} (and pressure gradient) most frequently occurs in the setting of a nonparallel intercept angle between the continuous-wave Doppler beam and the direction of blood flow. Because of the asymmetric nature of the aortic root, with the greatest stress on the right and noncoronary cusps, greater calcification, particularly of the noncoronary cusp, may occur.[67] In addition to asymmetric calcification, acute angulation of the aortic root, which may be more prevalent in the elderly, is associated with anteriorly directed transaortic jets that can be best imaged from nonapical windows (Fig. 8.7).[68,69] Studies have shown that the V_{max} was most frequently obtained in the right parasternal window (50%), followed by the apical windows (39%).[68]

Patients with an acute LV–aortic root angle measured in the parasternal long-axis view, which is frequently seen with basal septal hypertrophy, had V_{max} obtained from the right parasternal window

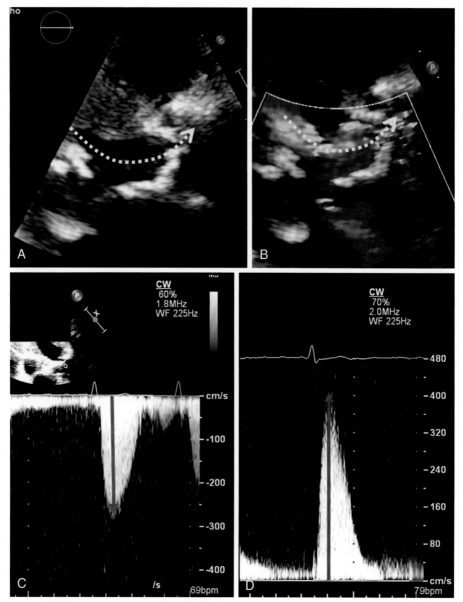

Fig. 8.7 Multiwindow Acquisition of Continuous-Wave Doppler Signal. In addition to asymmetric calcification, acute angulation of the aortic root (A) is more prevalent among the elderly and associated with anteriorly directed transaortic jets (B). The continuous-wave Doppler window, which captures the highest transaortic velocity, may not be from the apical window (C) but from a nonapical window. (D) Spectral Doppler from a nonimaging (Pedoff) probe captures the highest transaortic velocity.

more frequently than from apical windows (65% vs. 19%). Failure to capture the nonapical window V_{max} resulted in misclassification of the AS grade in 8% to 15% of patients. A multiwindow Doppler assessment is mandatory. To optimize the angle of insonation, a dedicated small dual-crystal continuous-wave Doppler transducer is frequently used.

Other sources of error in measuring V_{max} include incorrect identification of the flow signal (e.g., mistaking the mitral regurgitation signal for AS), respiratory motion, and measurement variation. Because velocity and gradient depend on flow, several physiologic situations can result in low-velocity/gradient, severe AS, including: tachycardia,[70] bradycardia,[71] hypertension,[72–74] small ventricular cavity,[75] severe diastolic dysfunction, severe mitral or tricuspid valve disease, pulmonary hypertension, and left or right ventricular dysfunction.[76]

Valve Area by the Continuity Equation

The flow-independent hemodynamic measurements of AVA include the AVA calculated from the continuity equation[52–55] and the Doppler index. The continuity equation is based on the conservation of mass principle, in which flow across any region of a continuous tube should be the constant. The stroke volume across the LVOT should be the same as the stroke volume across the aortic valve (Fig. 8.8). Because stroke volume is the product of cross-sectional area (CSA) and the velocity-time integral of flow (VTI), the stroke volume (in ml) across the LVOT (SV_{LVOT}) is calculated as

$$SV_{LVOT} = CSA_{LVOT} \times VTI_{LVOT}$$

where CSA_{LVOT} is the LVOT CSA in cm^2 and VTI_{LVOT} is the stroke distance (measured as the VTI) in cm at the LVOT by pulsed-wave

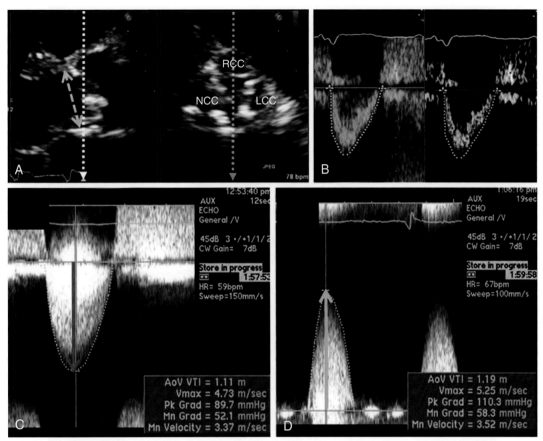

Fig. 8.8 Measurements Required for Calculation of the Aortic Valve Area by the Continuity Equation. Simultaneous biplane imaging of the left ventricular outflow tract (LVOT) (A) shows how the right coronary cusp *(RCC)* and the interleaflet triangle between the left *(LCC)* and noncoronary cusps *(NCC)* are imaged to measure the largest systolic LVOT diameter. To quantify stroke volume, the modal velocity of the pulsed-wave flow at the LVOT is measured while being careful not to measure the highest velocity spectral (B) but rather the most frequently sampled velocities (B, second beat, *red dots*). The peak transaortic velocity must be imaged, which for this patient was not from the apical view (C) but rather the right parasternal view (D).

Doppler. The CSA_{LVOT} is calculated as $\pi(D/2)^2$, where D is the diameter of the LVOT. Likewise, $SV_{aortic\ valve}$ is calculated as

$$SV_{aortic\ valve} = AVA \times VTI_{aortic\ valve}$$

where *AVA* is given in cm^2 and *$VTI_{aortic\ valve}$* is the stroke distance (measured as the VTI) in cm across the aortic valve by continuous-wave Doppler. Because $SV_{LVOT} = SV_{aortic\ valve}$, solving for AVA results in the continuity equation:

$$AVA = (CSA_{LVOT} \times VTI_{LVOT})/VTI_{aortic\ valve}$$

Because the cardiac output required in an individual depends on body size, indexing the AVA to body surface area (BSA) is another important measure of severity. Obese patients may not require the same amount of cardiac output as nonobese patients, and the American Society of Echocardiography[77] reported that indexing the valve area is particularly important in smaller patients with a height < 135 cm (<65 inches), a BSA < 1.5 m^2, or a body mass index (BMI) < 22 kg/m^2 using an indexed AVA of ≥ 0.6 cm^2/m^2 to define severe AS.

The greatest potential for error in the calculation of the AVA is the measurement of the LVOT diameter in systole because the assumption of the continuity equation is that the LVOT cross-sectional area is circular and this single dimension is squared to calculate the LVOT area. The LVOT diameter is measured by 2D TTE at peak systole, when the elliptical LVOT is more circular.[78]

There are two additional important caveats for measurement of the LVOT. First, although current echocardiographic guidelines recommend measuring the LVOT diameter 5 to 10 mm below the annulus to correlate with the location of the pulsed-wave sample volume, studies comparing 2D TTE and cardiac catheterization showed that calculation of the AVA using LVOT diameter measured below the aortic annulus underestimates catheter-derived AVA.[78,79] AVA calculated with LVOT diameter measured at the level of the aortic annulus is more accurate,[79–81] in part because the LVOT is more elliptical apical to the annulus.[78]

Second, the correct long-axis imaging window should bisect the maximum diameter of the aorta, and simultaneous multiplane imaging using simultaneous multiplane imaging allows imaging of the short-axis and long-axis planes to ensure imaging of the correct plane (Fig. 8.9). The right coronary cusp hinge point is imaged anteriorly, and the fibrous interleaflet trigone is imaged posteriorly. With appropriate

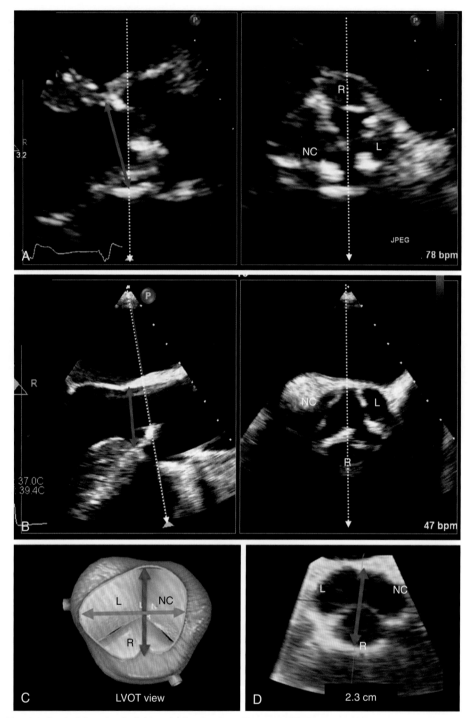

Fig. 8.9 Optimizing the Left Ventricular Outflow Tract *(LVOT)* **Diameter Measurement.** To accurately measure the LVOT diameter, the correct long-axis imaging window should bisect the maximum diameter of the aorta. In the simultaneous multiplane transthoracic example (A), simultaneous multiplane transesophageal example (B), cartoon image (C), and 3D cropped image (D), the middle of the right coronary cusp *(R)* is imaged anteriorly, and the fibrous interleaflet trigone (between the left cusp *[L]* and noncoronary cusp *[NC]*) posteriorly. This sagittal plane dimension *(red arrow)* usually represents the shorter of the two orthogonal dimensions of an elliptical annulus. The coronal plane (C, *blue line*) is typically the longest dimension. (C and D from Hahn RT, Abraham T, Adams MS, et al. Guidelines for performing a comprehensive transesophageal echocardiographic examination: recommendations from the American Society of Echocardiography and the Society of Cardiovascular Anesthesiologists. J Am Soc Echocardiogr 2013;26:921-964.)

gain and processing adjustments, the LVOT diameter is measured in the parasternal long-axis view using a zoomed freeze-frame at early to mid-systole, inner edge to inner edge, from where the anterior cusp meets the ventricular anteroseptum to the posterior virtual annulus, where the posterior interleaflet triangle meets the anterior mitral leaflet. Because there is no anatomic marker for the virtual annular plane within the interleaflet trigone, the correct annular diameter is measured by assuming the virtual annulus is approximately perpendicular to the long-axis of the aorta. Calcification of the scalloped lines of leaflet attachment within the sinuses (and defining the borders of the interleaflet trigone) should not be mistaken for the hinge point of the aortic cusp.

Although echocardiographic guidelines recommend a single-diameter measurement of the LVOT to calculate AVA,[77] planimetry of the valve orifice and LVOT area by real-time 3D (RT3D) methods has been shown to be accurate and reproducible,[59,82,83] and they compare favorably with CTA.[84,85] Studies have shown that the LVOT is elliptical[82,86,87] and that the long-axis (sagittal) plane diameter derived from 2D images may underestimate the true LVOT dimensions. Compared with CTA, 2D echo may underestimate LVOT area and therefore the AVA.[88,89]

Studies comparing standard 2D linear measurements with 3D planimetry of LVOT area show a 10% to 23% underestimation of cardiac output [90] or AVA using 2D TTE or TEE modalities.[21,22] However, other studies suggest that CTA overestimates the LVOT area compared with CMR imaging or 3D echo.[91] In a head-to-head comparison of CTA and Doppler echocardiography, Clavel et al showed that CTA for AVA calculation did not improve the correlation with transvalvular gradient, the concordance gradient-AVA, or mortality prediction compared with echocardiographic AVA.[92]

Thresholds for excess mortality differ between imaging modalities: AVA ≤ 1.0 cm² for echocardiographic methods versus ≤1.2 cm² for CTA methods. There are strong outcomes data using traditional 2D methods of measuring LVOT and calculating AVA.[92,93] The LVOT should be measured in systole from the clearest image that yields the largest diameter, excluding ectopic calcifications, at or very close to the level of the aortic annulus and distal to any septal bulge.[94]

In the setting of unreliable LVOT measurement data, using just the Doppler measurements in the continuity equation provides a more accurate measure of AVA severity and is associated with aortic valve events defined as aortic valve replacement, congestive heart failure due to AS, or death from cardiovascular causes.[95] Wiggers[96] reported decades ago that significant obstruction to flow occurred when a tube became limited to one third of its normal area, and this principle is reflected in the Doppler index, defined as the ratio of $VTI_{LVOT}/VTI_{aortic\ valve}$ or V_{LVOT}/V_{max}. Normal valve areas have a Doppler index of slightly less than 1, and a value of less than 0.25 indicates severe stenosis.[80] This index number is highly reproducible, simplifies the assessment of AS severity, and normalizes for body size because it represents the ratio of actual to expected valve area in each patient.

The next most common error is failure to correctly position the pulsed-wave Doppler sample volume and measure the modal velocity of LVOT flow (Fig. 8.10). Because of flow acceleration just proximal to the stenotic orifice, current guidelines suggest that the pulsed-wave sample volume be placed just apical to this region of turbulent flow. The VTI should be measured from the modal velocity, which is the most frequently sampled velocity in a spectral profile. To trace the VTI_{LVOT}, gains may need to be reduced so that only the densest spectral profile is seen.

Severe AS according the American College of Cardiology (ACC) guidelines is ≤1.0 cm², but this Gorlin-derived area cutoff represents the anatomic valve area. Doppler echocardiography measures the vena contracta of the transaortic jet stream, which typically is smaller than

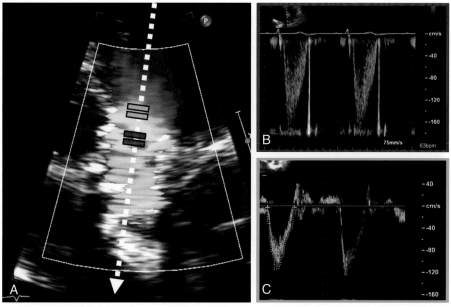

Fig. 8.10 Optimizing the Left Ventricular Outflow Tract (LVOT) Velocity-Time Integral Measurement. One source of error is the measurement of the velocity-time integral (VTI) of the LVOT. (A). The five-chamber view with color Doppler shows prominent flow acceleration *(yellow aliasing flow)* proximal to the valve plane. A sample volume placed at the level of the annulus (A, *red double line*) results in spectral broadening (B) and overestimation of stroke volume. A sample volume placed just proximal to the turbulent flow (A, *green double line*) results in a modal velocity profile (C) with very little spectral broadening.

the anatomic valve area. Nonetheless, numerous studies have shown that a continuity equation valve area of ≤ 1.0 cm^2 predicts outcomes and remains a reliable tool for diagnosis and management of these patients.[92,93]

Other Echocardiographic Measures of Stenosis Severity

Another measure of AVA accounts for the mechanical energy loss related to the valve and ascending aorta. The energy loss index (ELI) is calculated as: ELI = [AVA × A_A/A_A − AVA]/BSA, where A_A represents the ascending aorta diameter.[97] Similar to valve area, it is less flow dependent than gradient or peak velocity, takes into account pressure recovery, and is roughly equivalent to AVA measured by catheter.[77] Using ELI, a substudy of the Simvastatin Ezetimibe in AS (SEAS) trial reclassified 47.5% of patients from having severe to having nonsevere AS.[98] The energy loss is most significant in small aortas (<30 mm). An ELI of $\leq$ 0.5 to 0.6 cm^2/m^2 is consistent with severe AS.[98,99] In clinical practice, however, this measurement has not been widely adopted. The additional measurement of the ascending aorta and necessary calculation introduces further complexity, imprecision, and therefore variation to this parameter.

Cardiac Catheterization

Cardiac catheterization for hemodynamic assessment is not routinely used to diagnose aortic valve disease but is still helpful when there are discrepancies in symptoms, AVA, and gradients. According to ACC guidelines,[1] cardiac catheterization should be used only to assess AS severity in the setting of inadequate echocardiographic assessment or discrepant clinical or echo data. Although the risk of retrograde passage of a catheter across a narrowed and diseased aortic valve is small, a prospective, randomized study found that 3% of patients with suspected AS undergoing cardiac catheterization experienced a clinically significant neurologic event and that 22% had magnetic resonance imaging (MRI) evidence of an acute cerebral embolic event.[100] Nonetheless, catheterization can be useful in symptomatic patients when noninvasive tests are inconclusive or when there is a discrepancy between the findings on noninvasive testing and physical examination regarding the severity of the valve lesion. Cardiac catheterization assesses AS severity using three measurements: the transvalvular pressure gradient, the cardiac output, and the formula that relates the two variables (i.e., Gorlin formula).

Numerous methods for performing pressure gradient measurements across the aortic valve can be used and have been reviewed.[101] The single-catheter pullback technique is not recommended because spontaneous changes in cardiac cycle length, especially in the setting of atrial or ventricular arrhythmias, result in significant beat-to-beat variations in ventricular and aortic pressure tracings. Simultaneous LV and femoral pressures should never be used because there can be overestimation or underestimation of the true aortic valve gradient from large-vessel stenosis or peripheral amplification of the distal pressures. The optimal technique to assess aortic valve gradient is to record simultaneously obtained LV and ascending aortic pressures using a dual-lumen single catheter (i.e., Langston pigtail catheter) (Fig. 8.11).

The pressure gradient between the LV and the aorta can be described by three invasive measurements: (1) the maximum gradient, (2) the peak-to-peak gradient, and (3) the mean gradient. The maximum gradient represents the maximum difference that can be measured between the LV and aorta during systole and corresponds to the maximum instantaneous gradient measured by echocardiography. The maximum gradient occurs early during ventricular ejection, before the peak LV pressure.

The peak-to-peak gradient measures the difference between the peak LV pressure and the peak aortic pressure. Because these

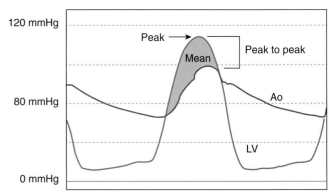

Fig. 8.11 Hemodynamic Measurement of Aortic Gradient. The optimal technique to assess aortic valve gradient is to record simultaneously obtained left ventricular *(LV)* and ascending aortic *(Ao)* pressures. The pressure gradient between the LV and the aorta can be described by three invasive measurements: (1) the peak instantaneous (i.e., maximum) gradient, (2) the peak-to-peak gradient, and (3) the mean gradient.

maximum pressures do not occur at the same time, this measure has no true physiologic meaning.

The mean gradient represents the area under the LV-aortic pressure curve and correlates well with the mean gradient measured by echocardiography.[102,103] It is recommended that the mean aortic valve gradient be used, which is the integrated gradient throughout the entire systolic ejection period and the optimal indicator of severity of obstruction.

Because gradients are flow dependent, a measure of cardiac output is essential for accurately assessing AS severity. The gold standard for cardiac output determination is the Fick principle, in which cardiac output is O_2 consumption divided by the difference between arterial and venous O_2. The direct measurement of O_2 consumption is often replaced by the use of standard tables for an assumed value, but these estimations may cause an error of as much as 40% in the determination of cardiac output.[101] Most laboratories now use thermodilution based on an indicator dilution method to measure cardiac output. Although usually accurate for patients with a normal or high output who are in normal sinus rhythm, it becomes inaccurate for patients with intracardiac shunts, low-cardiac-output states, significant tricuspid regurgitation, or irregular rhythms.

AVA is calculated using the flow equation as in echocardiography:

$$\text{Aortic valve area (in cm}^2) = \text{Flow (in cm}^3/\text{s)} \div \text{Velocity (in cm/s)}$$

Doppler interrogation of a valve measures flow velocity directly, whereas in the catheterization laboratory, velocity is imputed with the Torricelli law from the transvalvular pressure gradient:

$$\text{Velocity} = \sqrt{2g\Delta P}$$

where g is the velocity of acceleration resulting from gravity, and ΔP is the pressure gradient. The gravity acceleration term converts millimeters of mercury (the units of pressure) into the force that drives blood across the valve orifice.

The Gorlin equation for calculating AVA[104] uses two empirical constants. The coefficient of orifice contraction (C_c) accounts for the fact that fluids moving through an orifice tend to stream through its middle so that the physiologic orifice is smaller than the physical orifice. The velocity coefficient (C_v) accounts for the fact that not all of the pressure gradient is converted to flow because some of the velocity is lost to friction within the valve:

$$\text{Aortic valve area} = CO\Big/\Big(SEP \times HR \times 44.3 \times \sqrt{MG}\Big)$$

where *CO* is cardiac output, *SEP* is systolic ejection period, *HR* is heart rate, and *MG* is mean gradient.

The Gorlin equation has significant limitations because these coefficients have never been determined and have been assumed to be 1, a theoretical impossibility. Nonetheless, it remains one of the ways of assessing stenosis severity by catheterization. The simplified Hakki equation[105] (i.e., aortic valve area equals cardiac output divided by the square root of the transaortic pressure gradient) has a high correlation with the formal Gorlin equation. The correlation is unchanged when the peak gradient was used instead of the mean gradient in the simplified formula.

Discrepancies in gradient measurements may occur between catheterization and echocardiography. The peak LV-to-peak aortic pressure gradient measured by catheterization is not directly measured because these peak pressures do not occur simultaneously. Echocardiographically measured peak velocities correspond to the peak instantaneous pressure gradient.[103,106] Peak instantaneous gradients can be measured by catheterization and correspond to the echocardiographic peak Doppler gradient.

Differences in catheterization and echocardiographic measured gradients can also arise in the setting of downstream pressure recovery.[107–109] As blood crosses a narrow orifice, the jet stream continues to narrow just beyond the orifice and is referred to as the *vena contracta*. The highest jet velocities occur at the vena contracta, and this is measured by Doppler echocardiography. Because of conservation of energy, the kinetic energy of the jet stream beyond the vena contracta must be converted to potential energy or pressure. This downstream pressure recovery within the aorta can be measured by catheterization, resulting in a lower pressure gradient compared with that measured by Doppler.

Similar to echocardiographic measures of stenosis, the grading of severity by catheterization should integrate multiple measures such as valve gradient, AVA calculations, pressure contours (i.e., in fixed valvular obstruction, there is a reduction and delay [parvus et tardus]) in the upstroke of the central aortic pressure), and the contractile state of the ventricle.

Gated Computed Tomography Angiography

CTA has become in invaluable tool for assessing the aortic valve complex in the setting of AS[10,110] and has become an essential imaging modality before transcatheter aortic valve therapy.[111]

The prognostic importance of aortic valve calcium has long been recognized,[64,112] but CTA measures of aortic valve calcium burden (in Agatston units [AU]) has allowed determination of outcomes based directly on metrics.[113–115] CTA can aid in the determination of severity of disease by planimetry[110] (see Fig. 8.5B) and aortic valve calcium quantification[116] (Fig. 8.12). In patients with low-flow AS, the severity of calcification may help distinguish those patients with true AS from patients with pseudosevere AS.[116–118] Sex-specific criteria have been established with cutoffs of ≥ 1275 AU for women and ≥ 2065 AU for men, or aortic valve calcium indexed to body size of ≥ 637 AU/m² for women and 1067 AU/m² for men, and aortic valve calcium density (aortic valve calcium indexed to annular area) ≥ 292 AU/cm² for women and 476 AU/cm² for men.[116]

These thresholds for severe AS were validated in a large, multicenter registry, including more than 900 patients across eight international centers. Using different scanners but the same methodology with noncontrast, prospective gated CT acquisition, the values to define severe AS were almost identical to those established by Clavel et al (i.e., women: 1377 AU; men: 2062 AU). Aortic valve calcification predicted outcomes (i.e., death or need for AV replacement) better than echocardiographic variables.[119]

Careful exclusion of the aortic valve calcification that extends into the aortic annulus or mitral-aortic curtain, or both, is necessary and better confirmed with multiplanar reformatting rather than axial imaging. Taken together, this flow-independent method has shown its reproducibility and great clinical applicability to adjudicate AS severity and to guide procedure decision making in transcatheter aortic valve procedures (see Chapter 12).

Cardiac Magnetic Resonance Imaging

Although echocardiography remains the first-line modality for assessment of aortic valvular morphology and function,[2,120] CMR imaging

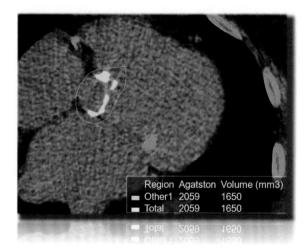

- **How to obtain AoV Ca2⁺ score and measure it**
  - Same approach as coronary artery calcium scoring.
  - Noncontrast, prospective gated CT (typically in diastole).
  - Axial scans, 2.5–3 mm slice thickness.
  - Circle the AoV calcium in all the contiguous slices.
  - Careful to not include calcification involving the sinotubular junction, LVOT, mitral annulus or coronaries.
  - Expressed as Agatston units (radiodensity + volume).

Region	Agatston	Volume (mm3)
Other1	2059	1650
Total	2059	1650

Fig. 8.12 CT Acquisition and Measurement of Aortic Valve *(AoV)* Calcium Score. AoV calcium score provides a flow-independent metric of aortic stenosis severity. In this example, a 74-year-old female with heavily calcified AoV has a calcium score that puts her in the severe aortic stenosis category. *LVOT,* Left ventricular outflow tract.

can be quite helpful in a number of circumstances (see Table 8.1), particularly when image quality is suboptimal, when there is discrepancy between symptoms and aortic valve area or gradients, or when there is a need to identify and quantify myocardial remodeling and fibrosis in AS.

In addition to providing a comprehensive assessment of global and regional biventricular remodeling, CMR can be used to perform quantification of LV and right ventricular (RV) volumes at end-diastole and end-systole, determining ventricular stroke volume and ejection fraction (EF) by summation of the method of discs, and to accurately quantify LV mass.[121]

CMR can be used to assess the aortic root, define aortic valve morphology, and confirm the location (e.g., valvular vs. subvalvular) and severity of AS. Severity of aortic valve stenosis can be determined by planimetry of the valve orifice using typical cine imaging with steady-state free precession sequences. For this acquisition, it is important to obtain two orthogonal cine views (e.g., three chamber and coronal) and then prescribe with a stack of contiguous 6-mm slices (0-mm gaps) from the LVOT through the sinotubular junction cutting the through the aortic valve plane. Using the crosshair navigator, the operator can identify the exact plane that intersects the aortic valve leaflet tips (Fig. 8.13)[122–124] and perform phase-contrast velocity mapping for stroke volume, peak velocity, peak gradient, and AR volume.[124,125]

For the quantification of aortic valve peak jet velocity and gradient, through-plane phase-contrast velocity mapping is used, typically with breath-held acquisition.[126] This method uses the rotational spin phase shift of moving protons (vs. stationary protons) with the magnitude of the shift proportional to the velocity. Velocities can be measured through plane (i.e., in a short-axis view of the valve) or in plane (i.e., the long-axis

view of the valve or jet). The latter permits visualization of the site of stenosis and measurement of the velocity along the course of the jet.

CMR has important limitations in measuring peak aortic valve gradients and velocities. First, unlike echocardiography, in which the Doppler angle of insonation should be ideally parallel to the main aortic valve jet velocity, the CMR imaging plane must be oriented as perpendicular as possible to the direction of the blood flow acceleration (i.e., use of through-plane method) and at the site of maximum velocity. Second, adjustment of encoding velocity must be performed before data acquisition to avoid aliasing, and TTE Doppler information is helpful to guide selection. Third, 2D phase-contrast imaging peak gradient and velocities, although correlating with TTE, can often underestimate the values due to several factors. Fourth, arrhythmias introduce significant variability, which typically requires changing the phase-contrast acquisition from breath-held to free-breathing forms, with an increased number of signal averages (minimum of three). Fifth, imaging artifacts and, more importantly, field inhomogeneities from intracardiac devices can produce changes in the magnetic field and further introduce imprecision for phase-contrast quantification.

Underestimation of velocities, particularly with severely stenotic valves, is caused by several factors: thicker image slice thickness that results in averaging of velocities in the slice volume, poor temporal resolution (typically 20 to 25 ms), and signal loss from jet turbulence. For these reasons, aortic valve 2D planimetry may be a more accurate method of assessing AS severity by CMR. For patients with cardiac arrhythmia, breath-held, prospective, triggered, or real-time cine acquisitions are recommended to avoid the typical blurring seen with cardiac arrhythmia using conventional segmented acquisition.

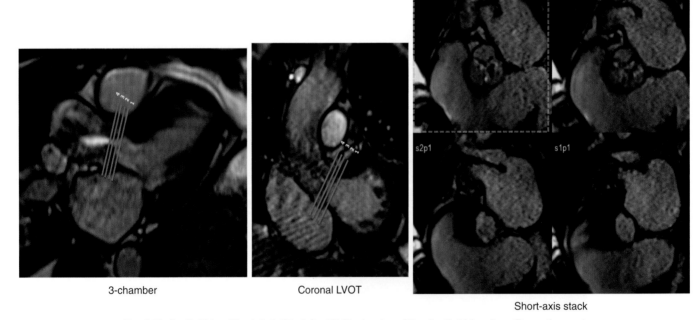

3-chamber   Coronal LVOT   Short-axis stack

Fig. 8.13 Aortic Valve Short-Axis Stack for 2D Planimetry of the Aortic Valve Area. Two orthogonal cine views (e.g., three-chamber and coronal) are used as reference, and then a short-axis prescription plan with a stack of contiguous 6-mm cine slices (0-mm gaps) from the left ventricular outflow tract *(LVOT)* through the sinotubular junction cutting the through the aortic valve (AoV) plane is obtained. Using the crosshair navigator, the clinician can identify the exact plane that intersects the AoV leaflet tips. In this case, it is line #4, which corresponds to the right panel highlighted box. If significant spin dephasing artifact created by the turbulent jet is observed, switch from standard steady-state free precession to gradient recall echo to improve visualization of the AoV area.

TABLE 8.3 Relative Utility of Imaging Modalities for the Assessment of Aortic Stenosis.

Aortic Stenosis	TTE	TEE	CMR	CT	Cath
Valve morphology	+++	++++	+++	++/+++	+
Cause of disease	+++	++++	++++	++++	++
Calcification	++	++	++	++++	+++
Valve hemodynamics/severity of stenosis	++++	++++	++	++	++++
Left ventricular response	+++	++	++++	+++	
Other modalities					
Pulmonary artery pressure	+++	+++	++	++	++++
RV size and function	++	++	++++	++++	—

CMR of patients with AS provides noninvasive quantification of replacement fibrosis with late gadolinium enhancement (LGE), diffuse interstitial myocardial fibrosis (MF) with T1-weighted mapping that correlates with myocardial collagen,[127] and subclinical myocardial dysfunction,[128] which plays a role in outcomes.[129] This topic is discussed in more detail later (see Cardiac Magnetic Resonance for Evaluating Left Ventricular Response to Aortic Valve Disease). The relative utility of each modality is summarized in Table 8.3.

AORTIC REGURGITATION SEVERITY

Identifying the cause and severity of AR is important, particularly when surgical intervention is being considered. The various causes of AR can be grossly divided into leaflet abnormalities and aortic root abnormalities. aortic valve repair may be considered for AR in the setting of pure annular dilation, single leaflet prolapse with otherwise normal or mildly reduced leaflet mobility, and small leaflet perforation or fenestration.[130,131]

The Carpentier classification, which was originally designed for the mitral valve,[132] has been adapted for AR[133] and can be used to guide repair techniques and predict recurrence of AR.[134] As for the mitral valve, this scheme classifies dysfunction based on the leaflet morphology (Fig. 8.14). Type 1 is associated with normal leaflet motion and can be subcategorized based on the exact pathology of the aortic root or valve: Type 1A AR occurs in the setting of STJ enlargement and dilation of the ascending aorta; type 1B is a result of dilation of the sinuses of Valsalva and the STJ; type IC is a result of dilation of the ventriculoarterial junction (i.e., aortic annulus); and type 1D results from cusp perforation or fenestration without a primary aortic annular lesion. Type II is associated with excessive leaflet motion from leaflet prolapse

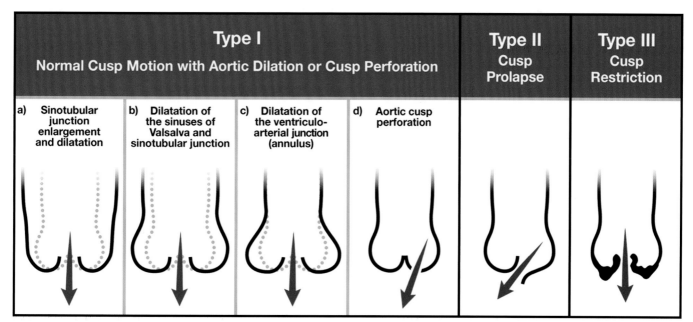

Fig. 8.14 Suggested Classification of Aortic Regurgitation (AR) Morphology. AR can be classified by morphology. Type Ia depicts sinotubular junction enlargement and dilation of the ascending aorta. Type Ib depicts dilation of the sinuses of Valsalva and sinotubular junction. Type Ic depicts dilation of the ventriculoarterial junction (annulus). Type Id denotes aortic cusp perforation. (From Zoghbi WA, Adams D, Bonow RO, et al. Recommendations for noninvasive evaluation of native valvular regurgitation: a report from the American Society of Echocardiography developed in collaboration with the Society for Cardiovascular Magnetic Resonance. J Am Soc Echocardiogr 2017;30:303-371.)

Grading the Severity of Chronic Aortic Regurgitation by Echocardiography[1]

Parameters	Mild	Moderate		Severe
Structural Parameters				
Aortic leaflets	Normal or abnormal	Normal or abnormal		**Abnormal/flail, or wide coaptation defect**
LV size	**Normal**[2]	Normal or dilated		Usually dilated[3]
Qualitative Doppler				
Jet width in LVOT, color flow	**Small in central jets**	Intermediate		**Large in central jets;** variable in eccentric jets
Flow convergence, color flow	**None or very small**	Intermediate		**Large**
Jet density, CW	**Incomplete or faint**	Dense		Dense
Jet deceleration rate, CW (PHT, msec)[4]	Incomplete or faint, Slow >500	Medium 500–200		**Steep <200**
Diastolic flow reversal in descending aorta, PW	**Brief, early diastolic reversal**	Intermediate		**Prominent holodiastolic reversal**
Semiquantitative[5]				
VCW (cm)	<0.3	0.3–0.6		>0.6
Jet width/LVOT width, central jets (%)	<25	25–45	46–64	≥65
Jet CSA/LVOT CSA, central jets (%)	<5	5–20	21–59	≥60
Quantitative parameters[6]				
RVol (mL/beat)	<30	30–44	45–59	≥60
RF	<30%	30–39%	40–49%	≥50%
EROA (cm²)	<0.10	0.10–0.19	0.20–0.29	≥0.30

PHT, Pressure half-time; *PW,* pulsed wave Doppler.
Color Doppler usually performed at Nyquist limit of 50–70 cm/sec.
1. Bolded signs are considered specific for their AR grade. All parameters have limitations, and an integrated approach must be used that weighs the strength of each echocardiographic measurement. All signs and measures should be interpreted in an individualized manner that accounts for body size, sex, and all other patient characteristics.

2. Unless there are other reasons for LV dilation.
3. Specific in normal LV function, in absence of causes of volume overload. Exception: acute AR, in which chambers have not had time to dilate.
4. PHT is shortened with increasing LV diastolic pressure and may be lengthened in chronic adaption to severe AR.
5. Quantitative parameters can subclassify the moderate regurgitation group.

Fig. 8.15 Summary of the Assessment of Aortic Regurgitant Severity. The assessment of aortic regurgitant severity with echocardiography used a multiparametric multiview and therefore an integrative approach.

as a result of excessive leaflet tissue or commissural disruption. Type III is associated with restricted leaflet motion, which is seen with congenitally abnormal valves, degenerative calcification, or any other cause of thickening or fibrosis or calcification of the valve leaflets.

The most common causes of acute AR are bacterial endocarditis, aortic dissection, and blunt chest trauma.[135–138] Less common causes of acute AR include spontaneous aortic dissection,[139–141] spontaneous rupture of leaflet fenestrations,[142,143] nonbacterial endocarditis,[144,145] and complications of invasive procedures such as aortic valvuloplasty[146,147] and percutaneous balloon dilation of aortic coarctation.[148]

Echocardiography

Echocardiography remains the primary initial diagnostic modality according to the American Heart Association (AHA) and ACC guidelines.[1] Because of the influence of hemodynamic factors, the blood pressure and heart rate must be recorded during the echocardiographic assessment of AR. Reports should include the mechanism of regurgitation. Assessment of aortic regurgitant severity with echocardiography

includes a multiparametric multiview and therefore is an integrative approach (Fig. 8.15).

The importance of this approach cannot be overemphasized. AR parameters depend on physiologic factors such as blood pressure, heart rate, and ventricular and aortic compliance. The regurgitant jet path is frequently nonlinear, and no single parameter has sufficient sensitivity, specificity, or accuracy to be diagnostic. Each parameter has advantages and limitations. Examples of the echocardiographic parameters used to assess AR severity are shown in Fig. 8.16.

Color Doppler Parameters

Several echocardiographic parameters can be used to assess the severity of AR and are well described in American and European guidelines.[149,150] One of the oldest echocardiographic signs of AR is high frequency oscillations on M-mode, with early closure of the mitral valve indicative of more significant disease. However, these single-dimension signs of AR have been replaced by the 2D, 3D, and Doppler assessment of disease severity.[149–152]

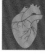

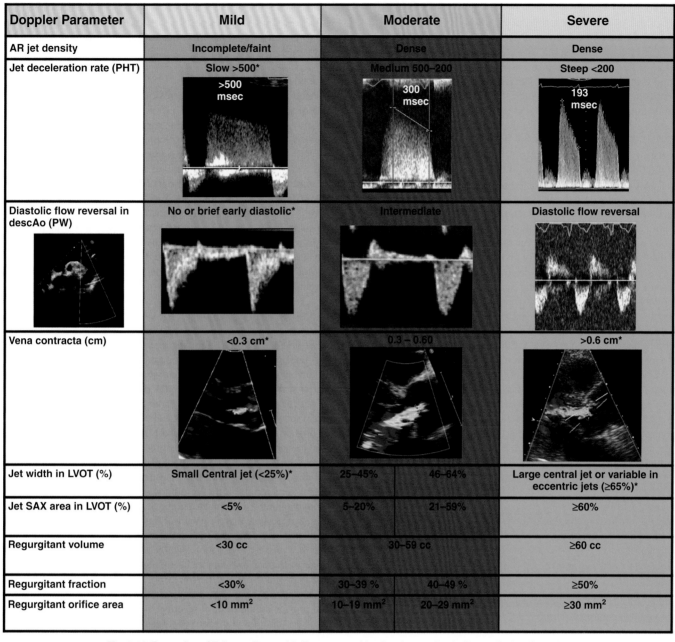

Doppler Parameter	Mild	Moderate		Severe
AR jet density	Incomplete/faint	Dense		Dense
Jet deceleration rate (PHT)	Slow >500* >500 msec	Medium 500–200 300 msec		Steep <200 193 msec
Diastolic flow reversal in descAo (PW)	No or brief early diastolic*	Intermediate		Diastolic flow reversal
Vena contracta (cm)	<0.3 cm*	0.3 – 0.60		>0.6 cm*
Jet width in LVOT (%)	Small Central jet (<25%)*	25–45%	46–64%	Large central jet or variable in eccentric jets (≥65%)*
Jet SAX area in LVOT (%)	<5%	5–20%	21–59%	≥60%
Regurgitant volume	<30 cc	30–59 cc		≥60 cc
Regurgitant fraction	<30%	30–39 %	40–49 %	≥50%
Regurgitant orifice area	<10 mm²	10–19 mm²	20–29 mm²	≥30 mm²

Fig. 8.16 Examples of Echocardiographic Parameters Used to Assess Aortic Regurgitation Severity. Several parameters are used to measure the severity of aortic regurgitation severity. *AR*, Atrial regurgitation; *LVOT*, left ventricular outflow tract; *PHT*, pressure half-time; *PW*, pulsed-wave Doppler, *SAX*, short-axis view.

Diastolic color-flow Doppler from the aorta into the LV defines AR. It is important to visualize the three components of the color jet (i.e., flow convergence, vena contracta, and jet area) for a better assessment of the origin and direction of the jet and its overall severity. Jet area and jet length should not be used to assess the severity of AR because of hemodynamic and physical characteristics of these jets. Color Doppler jets depend on the diastolic aortic pressure and on diastolic ventricular compliance. Aortic regurgitant jets are frequently eccentric, moving in or out of the plane of view, constrained by the LVOT, or entrained within the LVOT, leading to rapid jet broadening. Because of these variable characteristics, color Doppler jet length or jet area from any window should not be used for assessing severity of AR.

Visualizing the regurgitant jet from apical views is the most sensitive method of detection, but parasternal long- and short-axis views are essential for evaluating the origin of the jet and its semiquantitative characteristics. Despite jet broadening within the LVOT and LV, the proximal width of central AR jets (within the first 0.5 to 1.0 cm of the origin, just distal to the vena contracta) can be compared with the LVOT diameter and used to assess the severity of regurgitation semiquantitatively. A ratio of less than 25% usually indicates mild, a ratio of 25% to 64% indicates moderate, and one greater than 65% indicates severe AR. Similarly, the ratio of the area of the jet in cross section (i.e., short-axis view) to the LVOT area provides a measure of AR severity. However, this measurement is difficult without the use of simultaneous multilane imaging to confirm the location of the short-axis plane. In the setting of eccentric or multiple jets, these measurements are not valid.

The vena contracta is the narrowest portion of the color Doppler jet at or just distal to the anatomic regurgitant orifice and may be a valid measure of AR severity with eccentric and central jets. A vena contracta of less than 0.3 cm indicates mild, 0.3 to 0.6 cm indicates moderate, and greater than 0.6 cm indicates severe AR, and it can be assessed by TTE or TEE.[153,154] For the semiquantitative methods of assessing AR, a measurement greater than 0.6 cm has high sensitivity, specificity, and positive and negative predictive values.[155] In the setting of multiple jets, this measurement is not valid.

Proximal flow convergence can be used qualitatively and quantitatively for evaluation of AR severity.[156,157] The theory behind this method is that blood flow accelerates on the upstream side of a regurgitant valve, resulting in successively higher hemispheres of flow as blood approaches the regurgitant orifice. Color-flow imaging codes velocities and direction of flow by color maps, typically with blue representing flow away from the transducer and red representing flow toward the transducer. Because it is a pulsed-wave Doppler technology, color Doppler is subject to aliasing when velocities exceed the Nyquist limit as determined by instrument settings and depth. After flow has exceeded the Nyquist limit, the color display changes in color from blue to red (or vice versa). Changing the baseline of the color Doppler flow toward or away from transducer changes the velocity of the color shift. The visualization of the hemisphere of flow acceleration proximal to a regurgitant orifice represents an isovelocity surface area, where flow is equal to the aliasing velocity (v) on the color-flow image. By definition, the instantaneous flow rate (Q) at this site (e.g., regurgitant flow rate) is the cross-sectional area of flow times velocity. The area of flow can be calculated as the area of a hemisphere (with radius r), so that

$$Q = 2\pi r^2 v$$

Because of the conservation of mass theory, the continuity equation principle can be used:

$$\text{Regurgitant orifice area} \left(\text{in cm}^2\right) = \text{Flow} \left(\text{in cm}^3/\text{s}\right) \div \text{Velocity} \left(\text{in cm/s}\right)$$

where Velocity (V) is the maximal continuous-wave Doppler velocity through the regurgitant orifice:

$$\text{Regurgitant orifice area} = Q/V$$

From the regurgitant orifice area, the regurgitant stroke volume is calculated by multiplying by the velocity-time integral of the aortic regurgitant jet (VTI_{AR}):

$$\text{RSV} = \text{ROA} \times \text{VTI}_{AR}$$

Although this method is more difficult for AR, some technical tips may be helpful. Zooming in on the LVOT in the parasternal or preferably on the apical long-axis views provides the best windows for recording the proximal flow convergence, with a baseline shift of the Nyquist limit in the direction of the jet used to measure the flow convergence radius. Imaging from a slightly high parasternal window may improve the alignment of the insonation beam and regurgitant jet and optimize measurement of the radius using the proximal isovelocity surface area (PISA) method. Because the PISA-based quantitation relies on a single measurement of radius in early diastole

(at the same time as the measurement of peak AR velocity), noncircular, dynamic, or multiple jets may not be accurately assessed. Despite these limitations, PISA quantification in AR cases should be attempted.

Pulsed-Wave Doppler

Diastolic reversal of flow in the proximal descending aorta in the setting of a normal aorta valve is typically early and brief. Holodiastolic flow reversal within the descending aorta (just beyond the aortic isthmus) as detected by pulsed-wave Doppler is an abnormal finding that is typically consistent with at least moderate (i.e., proximal descending aorta) or severe (i.e., abdominal aorta) AR.[158] However, in the absence of AR, holodiastolic retrograde aortic flow can also be seen most commonly in hypertensive patients with reduced aortic compliance[159,160] and in other conditions such as a left-to-right shunt across a patent ductus arteriosus, upper extremity arteriovenous fistula, a ruptured sinus of Valsalva, or aortic dissection with diastolic flow into the false lumen. Use of a minimum end-diastolic velocity of the holodiastolic retrograde aortic flow of less than 25 cm/s may increase specificity.[150,158,161]

Continuous-Wave Doppler

Accurate assessment of AR severity using continuous-wave Doppler relies on aligning the regurgitant jet parallel to the insonation beam and imaging the spectral flow throughout the diastolic filling period. Unfortunately, most AR jets are curvilinear due to the eccentricity of the jet at the leaflet level or due to the shape of the LVOT, limiting the use of the apical views for continuous-wave Doppler imaging of the jet. In some instance, a high left or right parasternal view may align the insonation beam with the regurgitant jet.

The density of the continuous-wave Doppler signal is thought to reflect the volume of regurgitation, particularly when compared with the density of the forward flow. This is true, but only for the narrow lateral dimension of the continuous-wave Doppler sampling. Although a faint or incomplete jet may indicate mild or trace regurgitation, is it possible that a curvilinear but significant AR jet may appear less dense along the edges of the regurgitant jet. Similarly, a dense jet may be consistent with more significant regurgitation. However, because of the narrow Doppler beam, the density of the jet cannot differentiate moderate (i.e., narrow) from severe (i.e., wide) AR.

Measuring the pressure half-time of the AR spectral Doppler slope can provide an indicator of severity.[162] A steep slope indicates a more rapid equalization of pressures between the aorta and LV during diastole. A pressure half-time greater than 500 ms suggests mild AR, and one less than 200 ms indicates severe AR. However, because this parameter is affected by the compliance of the LV, patients with severe chronic regurgitation with well-compensated ventricular function may have a pressure half-time in the moderate range. In contrast, mild AR in patients with severe diastolic dysfunction may have short pressure half-time. A computational modeling study supports this theory.[163] Increasing LV and/or aortic stiffness led to faster decay of the transvalvular pressure gradient and therefore to faster decay of diastolic flow velocity across the aortic valve compared with normal stiffness, with the same effective regurgitant orifice area (EROA) resulting in a shorter pressure half-time but lower regurgitant fraction.

Quantitative Assessment

Quantitation of flow with pulsed-wave Doppler for the assessment of AR is based on measurement of total stroke volume across the regurgitant valve minus the forward stroke volume (i.e., amount of blood delivered to the body) across a normal valve. For AR, total stroke volume is measured in the LVOT, and forward stroke volume is measured across the mitral or pulmonic (PA) valve[164]:

$$RegurgVol_{AR} = (CSA_{LVOT} \times VTI_{LVOT}) - (CSA_{PA} \times VTI_{PA})$$

where *CSA* is the cross-sectional area of the respective structure. The regurgitant orifice is then calculated as follows:

$$EROA_{AR} = RegurgVol_{AR}/VTI_{AR}$$

Aortic regurgitant fraction then is the ratio of regurgitant stroke volume to total stroke volume:

$$RF = RegurgVol_{AR}/total\ stroke\ volume$$

This method is valid in the setting of noncircular, dynamic, or multiple regurgitant jets because it does not directly measure the orifice but rather the regurgitant volume. However, the errors inherent in the measurement of diameters (particularly of the mitral annulus) and the assumptions of a circular area used for each stroke volume calculation may also reduce the accuracy of this method. Echocardiographic quantitation of aortic regurgitant severity using relative stroke volumes across the aortic and mitral valves has a higher intraobserver and interobserver variation compared with CMR imaging.[165] Use of 3D measurements of the mitral annulus[166] may improve the calculation of forward stroke volume in this setting, but measurements have also validated the use of a single, four- or two-chamber diameter in a circular formula.

Regurgitation Quantitation by 3D Echocardiography

Direct planimetry of the AR vena contracta area with 3D color Doppler has been described.[167,168] For regurgitant jets, planimetry of short-axis view of the jet at the level of the vena contracta is feasible for native regurgitant valve disease[151,169–171] and after surgical[172] or transcatheter interventions.[173] This method requires using two orthogonal long-axis views of the jet, one with the narrowest and one with the broadest width of the jet, to identify the plane of the vena contracta. The vena contracta is then directly planimetered from this short-axis view (Fig. 8.17).

Calculation of regurgitant volume in native valvular disease using the PISA method[174] has known technical limitations, primarily the geometric assumptions of PISA shape required to calculate effective regurgitant orifice area. Many studies have validated the use of single-beat, real-time 3D echocardiographic color Doppler imaging, which allows the direct measurement of PISA without geometric assumptions for aortic, mitral, and tricuspid regurgitation assessment.[167,175–177]

Newer methods of determining relative flows within the heart make use of the velocity and direction of flow information inherent in color Doppler. Off-line software has been developed that uses 2D color Doppler images to determine the velocity, flow rate, and flow volume in any given region of the heart.[178] Extension of this technology to 3D

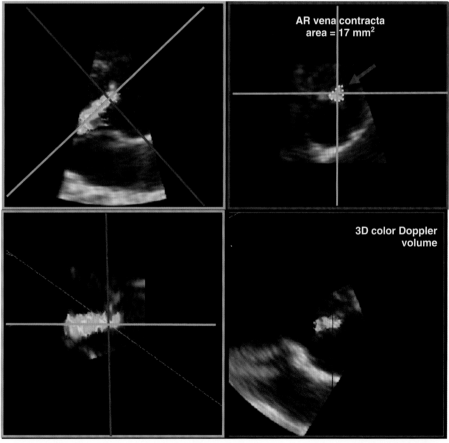

Fig. 8.17 Direct Planimetry of the Aortic Regurgitation *(AR)* Vena Contracta Area With 3D Color Doppler. Direct planimetry of the AR vena contracta area with 3D color Doppler requires multiplanar reconstruction of the short-axis view of the regurgitant jet. Two orthogonal long-axis views *(green and blue planes)* are used to identify plane of the vena contracta *(red plane)*. The vena contracta area is then directly planimetered from this short-axis view *(yellow dotted line)*.

color Doppler volume sets allows rapid, accurate, and reproducible quantitation of relative stroke volumes[179,180]

Thavendiranathan et al[180] used the velocity information encoded in the volume color Doppler data to target the appropriate region of interest by using the simultaneous 3D imaging of the mitral annulus and LVOT. Color Doppler velocity is multiplied by a known area of this cross section (i.e., voxel area), and the resulting spatially averaged flow rates are used to generate flow-time curves that resemble those obtained by MRI. The temporal integration of the flow-time curve generates the stroke volume. There was excellent correlation between the automated measured mitral inflow and aortic stroke volumes and the MRI stroke volume ($r = 0.91$, 95% CI, 0.83 to 0.95, and $r = 0.93$, 95% CI, 0.87 to 0.96, respectively, $P < 0.001$) and very low interobserver variation. Automation of the measurement process allowed calculations of mitral inflow and aortic stroke volumes to be performed very rapidly. Further validation of this method by other groups is necessary before it becomes the standard for measurement of aortic regurgitant volumes.

Cardiac Catheterization

Most patients with valve regurgitation can be fully evaluated by clinical and noninvasive testing, coming to the catheterization laboratory only for definition of the coronary anatomy before surgery or confirmation of hemodynamics (i.e., pulmonary artery pressures). However, for some patients for whom clinical and echocardiographic parameters are inconsistent, cardiac catheterization, specifically cineangiography, may be performed.

Cineangiographic or fluoroscopic assessment of regurgitation uses the time and density of contrast going back into a proximal chamber to grade valve regurgitation.[181] The method of Sellers et al[181] was initially described for a mixed population of valvular heart disease; only 251 had isolated aortic disease (i.e., stenosis and regurgitation). The technique used a catheter with multiple side holes and an end hole placed 2 to 3 cm above the aortic valve. The type of catheter used may influence the grading of severity, and others have suggested that a pigtail catheter without an end hole should be used.[182]

Sellers and colleagues interpreted the cineangiogram with a single projection using 35 to 40 mL of 75% Hypaque. Although biplane techniques may increase the accuracy of angiographic grading,[183,184] this technique remains highly subjective and depends the on observer's experience and numerous technical and physiologic factors. Technical factors include the intensity of fluoroscopy, the use of single or biplane imaging, the volume of the contrast medium injected, and the type and position of the catheter tip. Physiologic factors include heart rate, cardiac rhythm, preload, afterload, and LV function. These issues result in significant variation in grading, inconsistent correlation with quantitative assessment of AR, and significant overlap between angiographic grades.[185,186]

Hemodynamic measurements may provide additional information on the severity of AR. Unfortunately, there is poor correlation between AR severity and aortic pressure at end-diastole or pulse pressure.[187,188] The dicrotic notch on the down stroke of the arterial pressure waveform is thought to represent slight backward flow in the aorta on closure of the aortic valve; absence of the dicrotic notch is associated with severe AR but cannot be used to define lesser grades. Grading AR using hemodynamic tracings has been validated using measurement of the corrected diastolic pulse pressure (i.e., between the dicrotic notch and end-diastole) or the diastolic slope (i.e., slope of the pressure drop after the dicrotic notch),[189] with a direct relationship found between these measurements and larger regurgitant volumes.

Computed Tomography

CTA is typically not the primary cross-sectional imaging modality for the evaluation of native AR severity because of the need for intravenous contrast, radiation exposure, and an inability to directly quantify the aortic regurgitant volume.[190] Nonetheless, it can be considered in the context of suboptimal echocardiographic evaluation and for patients with AR but no access to a CMR scanner or with a strong contraindication for its performance.

A gated CTA data set should be acquired using the general principles of adequate heart rate control and left-sided chamber contrast opacification. Use of retrospective gated acquisition, which would cover the entire cardiac cycle, allows indirect quantification of AR as the difference between the LV stroke volume and the RV stroke volume.[191] Alternatively, prospective gating with increased padding (typically between 50 and 100 ms) allows lower radiation exposure and provides multiple diastolic phases for the visualization and measurement of the anatomic regurgitation orifice area (ROA) (Fig. 8.18).

Gated CTA can be helpful in evaluating the AR mechanism and providing comprehensive anatomic information for potential valve repair with an accuracy similar to that for direct surgical inspection.[192] Using a 64-slice CTA scanner, Alkadhi et al found a better discrimination between degrees of AR when cutoff ROAs (i.e., 25 mm^2 and 75 mm^2) were used compared with the semiquantitative TTE classification of mild, moderate, and severe AR.[193] Comparing newer dual-source CTA scanners, which provide superior temporal resolution, with superior quantitative CMR method of 2D phase-contrast, different cutoffs were proposed for CTA-derived ROAs to distinguish between mild and moderate and between moderate and severe AR (15 mm^2 and 23 mm^2, respectively).[194] This difference in cutoffs makes it imperative to perform a multimodality and preferably multicentric study to establish a robust and reproducible CTA-derived ROA grading scheme.

Cardiac Magnetic Resonance Imaging

The severity of AR can be assessed by CMR using three methods: (1) qualitative evaluation using visual assessment of the extent of signal loss due to spin dephasing on cine acquisitions,[195,196] (2) planimetry of the anatomic ROA from the cine acquisitions of the short-axis of the aortic valve,[197,198] or (3) quantitation of the aortic regurgitant volume and regurgitant fraction. Quantifying regurgitant volume can be accomplished by two methods: direct measurement using through-plane, 2D electrocardiogram-gated, phase-contrast velocity mapping for flow mapping and indirect quantitation using relative ventricular volumes (LV stroke volume − RV stroke volume).

Phase-contrast direct measurement of flow is accomplished by placing the imaging slice perpendicular to the aortic valve plane and just immediately above the aortic valve cups at the ST junction. Antegrade and retrograde flow across the orifice can be measured by assessing the proton phase shifts described in the previous discussion of AS (Fig. 8.19). The primary limitation of the method is the dynamism of the aortic root (i.e., motion toward the apex and expansion of the aortic in systole), which changes the level of the imaging plane during systole and diastole. Nonetheless, this is the method of choice in most instances and has been used to quantify regurgitant after transcatheter aortic valve replacement (TAVR).[199] Slice tracking is feasible but has not gained widespread use.[200]

Other methods for quantifying AR by CMR can be used to confirm the phase-contrast method. Measurements of relative RV and LV stroke volumes are accurate and reproducible by CMR, and subtracting the RV from the LV stroke volume should result in quantitation of aortic regurgitant volume.[201] This method, however, should be used only when there is a single regurgitant valve. The accuracy of the ventricular volume depends greatly on the correct contouring of the basal ventricular image slice, and differentiating atrial from ventricular chambers requires careful review frame by frame. Relative stroke

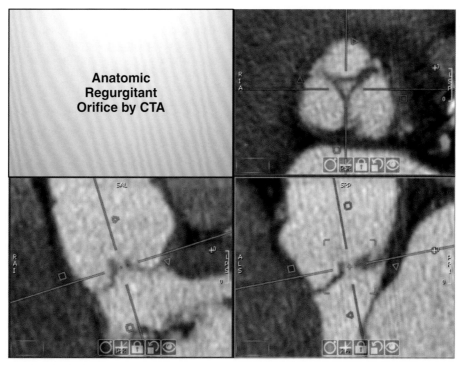

Fig. 8.18 Measurement of the Anatomical Regurgitant Orifice Area by Computed Tomography Angiography _(CTA)_ Using Multiplanar Reformat. The anatomic regurgitant orifice area is measured by CTA using multiplanar reformat. Crosshairs are aligned at the aortic valve leaflet tips in mid-diastole, and planimetry of the regurgitant orifice is performed.

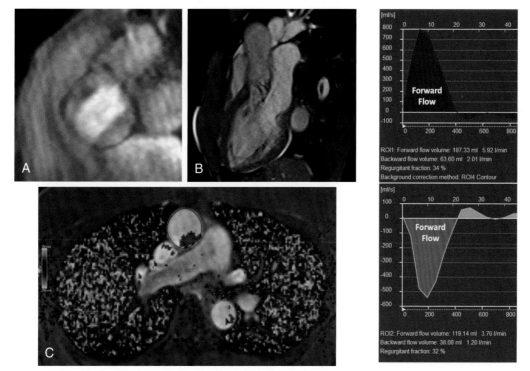

Fig. 8.19 Quantification of Aortic Regurgitation by Cardiac Magnetic Resonance (CMR). Using 2D phase contrast imaging, a perpendicular plane is applied to quantify the forward and backward aortic flow. This plane should be placed near the aortic valve (preferably at the sinus of Valsalva and sinotubular junction). (A) Young patient with bicuspid aortic valve. (B) Diastolic frame demonstrates an eccentric aortic regurgitation (AR) jet directed toward the anterior mitral valve leaflet. (C) Phase-contrast imaging with regions of interest at the proximal ascending aorta _(red)_ and descending thoracic aorta _(green)_. (D and E) Quantification of forward and backward flow, regurgitant volume, and regurgitant fraction, which are used for quantification of AR severity. In this case, moderately-severe AR is noted (regurgitant fraction = 34%) with almost an entire holodiastolic flow reversal in the ascending and descending thoracic aorta.

volume quantitation may overestimate regurgitation due to coronary artery flow.

Quantitation of RV volumes has been controversial because the RV outflow tract volume may be more difficult to define. In this setting, combining methods of direct measurements of total LV stroke volume and phase-contrast forward flow should allow quantitation of regurgitation volume.

Quantification of AR by CMR has good reproducibility and can predict outcomes. Myerson and colleagues studied a multicentric cohort of 113 patients with moderate to severe AR identified by echocardiography and followed them over a mean of 3 years. They found that a CMR aortic regurgitant fraction greater than 33% and/or LV end-diastolic volume grater than 246 ml were associated with a higher likelihood of aortic valve surgery.[202] In direct comparison with TTE, AR quantification by CMR was shown to be more reproducible (i.e., lower intraobserver and interobserver variation)[165] and more strongly associated with outcomes, including the need for aortic valve surgery.[203] CMR should be considered in AR when there are suboptimal echocardiographic images, discordance between clinical assessment and echocardiographic or Doppler findings, in patients with bicuspid aortic valves, or when aortopathy cannot be assessed accurately or fully with echocardiography.[204]

The through-plane slice location is recommended for flow quantification by 2D phase-contrast matters. It should be placed at the level of the ST junction and not higher (i.e., at the level of the main pulmonary artery).[205] Other supportive findings, such as holodiastolic flow reversal at the descending thoracic aorta by phase-contrast imaging, have been associated with significant AR.[206]

Technologic advances, such as the use of 4D flow imaging coupled with acceleration of image acquisition with compressed-sensing and parallel imaging,[207] have the potential to bring 4D phase-contrast acquisitions to standard CMR imaging of regurgitant jets, but further validation is necessary. The relative utility of each modality is summarized in Table 8.4.

Assessing the LV response in patients with aortic valve disease is an important component of the evaluation because timing of intervention may be influenced by these parameters. Although echocardiography remains the primary imaging modality for assessing ventricular size, mass, and function, emergence of evaluation of MF with the use of CMR imaging provides an opportunity to expand our understanding of the pathophysiology and perform better patient-selection.

ASSESSMENT OF PATHOPHYSIOLOGY

Aortic Stenosis

In chronic AS, the LV remodels by increasing wall thickness. Usually, the process is associated with increased LV mass (i.e., concentric hypertrophy), but in some cases, wall thickness increases while LV volume decreases, and LV mass remains static (i.e., concentric remodeling). These changes in LV geometry are both adaptive and pathologic. Laplace's law describes the physiologic relationships among increasing afterload, ventricular size, and wall thickness. Applying Laplace's law to a geometric ellipsoid,[208] the mean wall stress (σ) can be defined as follows:

$$\sigma = (P \times r)/2h$$

where P = LV pressure, r = LV radius, and h = LV thickness. LV ejection varies inversely with afterload, which is the force opposing ejection. As the pressure overload increases, an increase in LV wall thickness maintains normal wall stress and EF. Increased wall thickness in AS has been associated with impaired calcium handling, cytoskeletal changes, apoptosis, and increased collagen fiber deposition. These changes result in detectable reduced deformation characteristics and chamber compliance before any change in EF. This cascade of events eventually leads to decreased stroke volume and increased filling pressure, resulting in heart failure with a preserved EF. Long-standing and severe pressure overload often leads to excess afterload when LV hypertrophy is inadequate to normalize wall stress, reducing the EF and cardiac output. The prevalence of hypertension was 75% or higher in a series of older patients with AS,[209,210] with hypertension further increasing LV afterload, increasing the maladaptive effects of ventricular remodeling, and reducing function and survival.[211–213]

Aortic Regurgitation

AR places volume and pressure overloads on the LV. The blood flow regurgitated into the LV during diastole is compensated by increasing the total LV stroke volume. Regurgitation with resulting volume overload results in LV dilation, and an increase in stroke volume with diastolic runoff results in a widened pulse pressure. Increases in pressure and ventricular diameters should, according to the Laplace formula, result in very high wall stress.

LV remodeling in AR includes increased chamber volume and increased wall thickness. Over time, increased wall thickness and interstitial fibrosis of the myocardium reduces LV compliance, and the high diastolic volume of AR must also increase diastolic pressure, leading to pulmonary congestion and the symptoms of heart failure, including primarily dyspnea on exertion. Eventually, prolonged volume overload with increased afterload leads to systolic dysfunction. When LV end-systolic diameter (LVESD) is greater than 50 mm, the probability of death, symptoms, or LV dysfunction is 19% per year.[2] Current recommendations for intervention according to the AHA/ACC[1] and the European Society of Cardiology (ESC) and the European Association

TABLE 8.4 Relative Utility of Imaging Modalities for the Assessment of Aortic Regurgitation.					
Aortic Regurgitation	TTE	TEE	CMR	CT	Cath
Aortic morphology	++	+++	++++	++++	+
Valve morphology	+++	++++	++++	+++	+
Calcification	++	++	++	++++	+++
Valve hemodynamics/severity of regurgitation	+++	++++ (w/3D)	++++	+++	++/+++
Left ventricular response	+++	++	++++	+++	++
Other modalities					
Pulmonary artery pressure	+++	+++	++	++	++++
RV size and function	++	++	++++	++++	

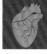

TABLE 8.5 Current Recommendations for Intervention According to the AHA/ACC[1] and the ESC/EACTS[2] Guidelines Using Left Ventricular Size or Function Criteria.

	AHA/ACC		ESC/EACTS	
	Indication for AVR	Class of Recommendation	Indication for AVR	Class of Recommendation
Asymptomatic severe AS	LVEF < 50%	I	LVEF < 50%	I
			Normal EF and low surgical risk, with excessive LV hypertrophy in the absence of hypertension	IIb
Symptomatic severe AS	LVEF < 50% with DSE-proven severe AS	IIa	LVEF < 50% with flow reserve	IIa
			LVEF < 50% without flow reserve	IIb
Asymptomatic severe AR	LVEF < 50%	I	LVEF ≤ 50%	I
	LVEF ≥ 50% with LVESD > 50 mm	IIa	EF > 50% with severe LVEDD > 70 mm, or LVESD > 50 mm or LVESD > 25 mm/m²	IIa
	LVEF ≥ 50% with LVEDD > 65 mm	IIb		
Symptomatic severe AR	With LV dilation	I		

AHA/ACC, American College of Cardiology/American Heart Association; *AR,* aortic regurgitation; *AS,* aortic stenosis; *AVR,* aortic valve replacement; *DSE,* dobutamine stress echocardiogram; *ESC/EACTS,* European Society of Cardiology/European Association for Cardio-Thoracic Surgery; *LVEDD,* left ventricular end-diastolic diameter; *LVEF,* left ventricular ejection fraction; *LVESD,* left ventricular end-systolic diameter.

for Cardio-Thoracic Surgery (EACTS)[2] guidelines using LV size or function criteria are listed in Table 8.5.

Left Ventricular Volumes and Size

Echocardiography is an indispensable imaging tool for the assessment of ventricular size and function. Multiple measures of size and function should be used. Although linear measurements and EF are the primary measurements used by current guidelines as indications for intervention, newer parameters such as 3D volumes and myocardial strain imaging may become important as outcomes data are accumulated. American Society of Echocardiography guidelines provide comprehensive recommendations for assessing chamber size and function.[214]

Linear Measurements

The most commonly used parameters to describe LV cavity size include linear internal dimensions and volumes. End-diastole and end-systole measurements should be recorded. They are then used to derive parameters of global LV function. To allow comparison among individuals with different body sizes, chamber measurements should be indexed to body size. Some studies suggest that indexing to height raised to allometric powers may have advantages over indexing to BSA, especially when attempting to predict events in obese patients.[215] However, other studies suggest no advantage in predicting outcomes in the general population.[216]

Linear measurements of the LV and its walls should be performed with the parasternal long-axis view with the following caveats: (1) electronic calipers should be positioned on the interface between the myocardial wall and LV cavity and the interface between the wall and the pericardium; (2) measurements should be performed perpendicular to the LV long axis; and (3) end-diastolic dimension measurements are performed at or just below the tips of the mitral leaflets, with end-systolic dimension measurements performed at the same level of myocardium as the diastolic measurements.

Although M-mode echocardiography has superior axial and temporal resolution, an oblique orientation of the M-mode beam or incorrect identification of endocardial borders leads to measurement errors. Internal dimensions can be obtained with a 2D-guided M-mode approach, although linear measurements obtained from 2D echocardiographic images are preferred by the guidelines, as long as they remain perpendicular to the long axis of the LV and are not oblique.

Although linear measurements fail to describe the 3D remodeling of the LV, numerous outcomes studies show the utility of using single 2D LV dimensions, and current guidelines are based on these measurements.[1] In the asymptomatic patient with severe AR and a normal EF (≥50%), severe LV dilation in systole (>50 mm) is a IIA indication for intervention, whereas severe diastolic dilation (>65 mm) is a IIB indication for intervention.[1]

The 2D thresholds have been questioned because of emerging data showing that risk of death is significantly and continuously increased beyond left LV end systolic dimension indexed to body surface area (iLVESD) greater than 2.0 cm/m², which is lower than currently recommended iLVESD of 2.5 cm/m² or greater that is used as the threshold for surgical intervention.[217] Global longitudinal strain, which is load dependent and therefore altered in patients with significant AR, can be used as an ancillary tool to stratify the risk of asymptomatic patients with preserved LVEF who may benefit from earlier aortic valve intervention.[218]

Volumetric Measurements

LV volumes are measured using 2D or 3D modalities. Because of the various shapes of the LV, particularly in the setting of cardiac disease, volume calculations derived from linear measurements assume a fixed geometric shape and can be inaccurate. The Teichholz and Quiñones methods for calculating LV volumes from LV linear dimensions are no longer recommended for clinical use, but they can be used with symmetric ventricular geometries as a quick check of more complex measurements of volume.

The guideline-recommended method for measuring 2D echocardiographic volume is the biplane method of disks summation (i.e., modified Simpson rule). Manual tracing of the endocardial borders requires experience, but automated border detection or newer approaches such as speckle tracking may become standard in the future. As long as the two apical orthogonal views have similar lengths, the algorithm creates a series of discs of equal height, with areas defined by the shape of the two orthogonal views. To optimize accuracy of volume measurements, (1) apical views should maximize the ventricular areas while avoiding foreshortening of the LV, (2) the interface between the compacted myocardium and ventricular cavity is traced (not the interface with the trabeculated myocardium), and (3) at the mitral valve level, the contour is closed by connecting the two opposite mitral annuli (medial and lateral) with a straight line.

The area-length method using short-axis mid-ventricular area and apical ventricular length provides an alternative for calculating LV volumes when endocardial tracing cannot be accurately performed. The shortcoming of this method is that it also relies on geometric assumptions of a symmetric, bullet-shaped ventricle.

Because the issue of foreshortening is less relevant in 3D data sets, 3D image acquisition should focus primarily on including the entire LV within the pyramidal data set. To ensure reasonably accurate identification of end-systole, the temporal resolution of 3D imaging should be maximized without compromising spatial resolution.

Despite these caveats, 2D volumes underestimate ventricular volumes compared with CMR, which is the gold standard. Ultrasound contrast agents enhance endocardial border detection, and volume measurements are larger with enhancement and are closer to those obtained with CMR.[219] Acoustic shadowing of the base of the LV occurs with high-density contrast in the near-field apex and can be avoided by allowing a short period of washout and distribution throughout the LV.[220]

3D echocardiographic volume measurements do not rely on geometric assumptions and are accurate and reproducible. Unfortunately, there are few data on the utility of 2D or 3D volume measurements for optimizing timing of intervention in patients with valvular heart disease.

Measures of Ventricular Function
Global Left Ventricular Systolic Function

Global LV function is usually assessed by measuring the EF:

$$EF = (ED_{vol} - ES_{vol})/ED_{vol}$$

where ED_{vol} is the end-diastolic volume and ES_{vol} is the end-systolic volume. The limitations of linear compared with volumetric methods for deriving ventricular volumes apply. The biplane method of disks (i.e., modified Simpson rule) is the recommended 2D method to assess LV EF.

Cardiac mechanics can be assessed with the use of tissue Doppler and speckle tracking for the measurement of myocardial displacement.[221] Lagrangian strain is the change in length of an object within a certain direction relative to its baseline length:

$$Strain = (L_t - L_0)/L_0$$

where L_t is the length at time t and L_0 is the initial length at time zero. The measurement of myocardial deformation, or strain, is the fractional change in the length of a myocardial segment (expressed as a percent of the baseline length). Strain rate is the rate of change in strain. The deformation of the myocardium is directional. Lengthening is represented by positive strain, and shortening by negative strain. The most commonly used strain-based measure of LV global systolic function is global longitudinal strain (GLS). It is usually assessed by speckle-tracking echocardiography, with a more negative number representing greater shortening in systole and better function. The preponderance of available data is for midwall GLS.

Numerous studies have shown the utility of strain imaging for assessing LV function in aortic valve disease. In the presence of a normal EF, increasing severity of AS was associated with a reduced GLS.[222,223] Subclinical improvement in global and regional systolic function assessed by tissue Doppler and speckle strain also occurs after TAVR,[224–226] even in the absence of a significant change in EF.[227] Regional strain abnormalities in patients with severe AS may be able to further substratify patients with concomitant infiltrative diseases such as amyloid[228] or coronary disease. In patients with cardiac amyloid, relative apical sparing (with preserved apical longitudinal strain) was sensitive (93%) and specific (82%) in differentiating amyloid from controls, some of whom had severe AS. In patients with moderate or severe AS and concomitant coronary disease, worse apical and mid-longitudinal strain parameters predicted significant coronary stenosis.[229]

Because mortality is significantly associated with symptom development,[230] GLS has been postulated as a possible early marker of ventricular dysfunction in asymptomatic patients with severe AS and may be a useful tool in determining the timing of intervention in this population. Carasso et al[231] showed that longitudinal strain was low in asymptomatic patients with severe AS with supernormal apical circumferential strain and rotation. In symptomatic patients, however, longitudinal strain was significantly lower, with no compensatory circumferential myocardial mechanics. Other investigators suggest that after adjusting for AS severity and ejection fraction, only basal longitudinal strain (not GLS) was an independent predictor of symptomatic status.[232] After TAVR, the improvement in GLS may be a result of basal and mid-segment improvement only.[233]

Strain imaging may be particularly useful for predicting outcomes of patients with discordant measures or nonsevere stenosis. In patients with low-flow, low-gradient AS with a normal EF, one study showed that stroke volume index ($\leq$35 mL/m^2) and GLS ($>$−15%) were independently associated with worse survival.[234] In patients with low-flow, low-gradient AS with reduced EF, GLS is independently associated with mortality, and dobutamine stress GLS may provide incremental prognostic value beyond GLS measured at rest.[235] 3D GLS may be a better predictor of outcome compared with 2D strain.[236] Kusunose et al studied 395 patients with moderate to severe AS (AVA < 1.3 cm^2) and found that GLS was an independent predictor of mortality in this population. A GLS greater than −12% was associated with the lowest survival rate.[237]

Deformation characteristics have been studied in patients with AR.[238–242] In a prospective study of young patients (<18 years old) with AR, the only significant predictor of progression of disease on multivariable analysis was GLS ($P = 0.04$), with a cutoff value greater than −19.5%, sensitivity of 77.8%, specificity of 94.1%, and area under the curve of 0.89.[238] Prospective studies of adult patients have shown that strain parameters by speckle tracking can detect early myocardial systolic and diastolic dysfunction.[240] Lower strain values were associated with disease progression in medically managed patients and with impaired outcomes for surgically treated patients. A systolic radial strain rate of <1.82/s was a predictor of postoperative LV dysfunction.[241] In a prospective study of 60 patients with chronic AR who were followed for 64 months, global longitudinal strain (four-chamber view only) was an independent predictor of mortality (hazards ratio = 1.313, 95% CI 1.010 to 1.706, $P = 0.042$).[242]

Left Ventricular Mass

LV mass is an important risk factor for and a strong predictor of cardiovascular events in aortic valve disease.[243–246] Several methods can be used to calculate LV mass by echocardiography. The methods that use linear measurements of LV diastolic diameter and wall thickness rely on measuring non-oblique images and on geometric formulas to calculate the volume of the LV myocardium. 2D-guided M-mode imaging or measurements from 2D echocardiographic images are preferred over blind M-mode imaging, and measurements using this method have robust normative data with well-established cutoffs for normal and hypertrophied ventricles. Direct 2D measures of wall thickness may yield smaller values than the M-mode technique, and LV mass calculated using this formula may not be directly interchangeable with other measures. Despite advances in image quality (i.e., harmonics) and 3D modalities, normative data for LV mass in the modern era is lacking.

All methods then convert the volume to mass by multiplying the volume of myocardium by the myocardial density (approximately 1.05 g/mL). It is important to use the same method and to measure the walls at the same level of the ventricle to follow patients over time. Calculation of relative wall thickness (RWT):

$$RWT = (2 \times \text{posterior wall thickness})/(\text{LV internal diameter at end-diastole})$$

This permits categorization of an increase in LV mass as concentric (RWT > 0.42) or eccentric (RWT < 0.42) hypertrophy and allows the identification of concentric remodeling (i.e., normal LV mass with increased RWT).

Cardiac Magnetic Resonance for Evaluating Left Ventricular Response to Aortic Valve Disease

CMR has been increasingly used for evaluating patients with aortic valve disease, particularly those being consider for aortic valve intervention, for characterization of the myocardial response in pressure and volume overload. The Expert Consensus Decision Pathway for TAVR for Adults with AS suggests the use of CMR for the identification of cardiomyopathy, myocardial ischemia and scar, and quantification of MF.[204] However, given the traditional reliance on bedside assessments and echocardiography and the required expertise and relatively diminished availability, the incorporation of CMR into routine clinical practice and decision making for AS remains limited.

Over the past few years, CMR for patients with AS has provided remarkable insights into the myocardial response, which was found to be heterogeneous and gender specific.[247] CMR with LGE imaging allows visualization and quantification of MF unlike any other clinical tool, with reliable precision and prognostic capabilities over and above traditional predictors such as age, LV EF, and echocardiographic measures of AS severity. LV hypertrophy comes at a cost of increased MF, which can be type 1, diffuse reactive fibrosis that tends to be associated with heightened interstitial collagen deposition and is potentially reversible with aortic valve replacement, or type 2, replacement fibrosis, which is not reversible[248] and is independently associated with poor outcomes.

A large CMR registry from six centers un the United Kingdom includes 674 patients who underwent a CMR study before surgical aortic valve replacement (SAVR) or TAVR revealed important findings. First, preoperative MF is common, with 51% of the cohort affected, and it was predominantly nonischemic in origin (33% nonischemic vs. 18% ischemic). Patients with MF had a more advanced AS phenotype with worse symptoms, greater myocardial infarction, more LV hypertrophy, and a lower LV EF. Second, regardless of the aortic valve intervention (SAVR or TAVR), MF was independently associated with a twofold higher rate of all-cause mortality and a threefold higher rate of cardiac death over a median follow-up of only 3.6 years. This hazard was

evident for ischemic and nonischemic types. The risk of MF was not just binary (i.e., present vs. absent); it was dose dependent. For every 1% increase in MF, all-cause and cardiovascular mortality rates increased by 11% and 8%, respectively.[249]

These observations are provocative and reflect the prognostic importance of the ventricular response to AS. There is always the potential for selection bias with confounding variables in retrospective analyses. Patients with MF were sicker. Nonetheless, early, subclinical alterations in the myocardial architecture are known to occur in AS, even before the valvular lesion is severe, and we need the ability to detect these changes and a greater understanding of their implications. Moreover, these findings support the mechanistic concept that once MF is established by CMR, there is the potential for progression and even irreversibility despite aortic valve replacement.

CMR and bone scintigraphy have other utility for the aging cardiovascular system. There is increased recognition of common disease overlaps with AS, such as wild-type transthyretin cardiac amyloidosis in patients receiving SAVR[250] or TAVR.[251–253] The prevalence appears to be high (13% to 16%) and may be prognostically relevant, which has raised questions about potential futility of intervention.[250,252] Evidence of concomitant cardiac amyloidosis can better inform and frame shared decision-making discussions regarding expectations after aortic valve interventions.

The myocardial response to volume overload due to significant AR is associated with significant MF detected by CMR. A small study by Azevedo and colleagues reported a 69% prevalence of LGE, mostly in a multifocal pattern[254] and associated it with outcomes. Larger multicentric studies are necessary to define the role of identification and quantification of MF in patients with AR and its relation to outcomes.

REFERENCES

1. Nishimura RA, Otto CM, Bonow RO, et al. 2014 AHA/ACC Guideline for the management of patients with valvular heart disease: a report of the American College of Cardiology/American Heart Association Task Force on practice guidelines. J Am Coll Cardiol 2014;63(22):e57-e185.
2. Vahanian A, Alfieri O, Andreotti F, et al. Guidelines on the management of valvular heart disease (version 2012): The Joint Task Force on the Management of Valvular Heart Disease of the European Society of Cardiology (ESC) and the European Association for Cardio-Thoracic Surgery (EACTS). Eur J Cardiothorac Surg 2012;42(4):S1-S44.
3. Sievers HH, Hemmer W, Beyersdorf F, et al. The everyday used nomenclature of the aortic root components: the tower of Babel? Eur J Cardiothorac Surg 2012;41(3):478-482.
4. Tretter JT, Spicer DE, Mori S, et al. The significance of the interleaflet triangles in determining the morphology of congenitally abnormal aortic valves: implications for noninvasive imaging and surgical management. J Am Soc Echocardiogr 2016;29(12):1131-1143.
5. Loukas M, Bilinsky E, Bilinsky S, et al. The anatomy of the aortic root. Clin Anat 2014;27(5):748-756.
6. Anderson RH. Clinical anatomy of the aortic root. Heart 2000;84(6):670-673.
7. Piazza N, de Jaegere P, Schultz C, et al. Anatomy of the aortic valvar complex and its implications for transcatheter implantation of the aortic valve. Circ Cardiovasc Interv 2008;1(1):74-81.
8. Schafers HJ, Schmied W, Marom G, Aicher D. Cusp height in aortic valves. J Thorac Cardiovasc Surg 2013;146(2):269-274.
9. Hahn RT, Abraham T, Adams MS, et al. Guidelines for performing a comprehensive transesophageal echocardiographic examination: recommendations from the American Society of Echocardiography and the Society of Cardiovascular Anesthesiologists. J Am Soc Echocardiogr 2013;26(9):921-964.

10. Hamdan A, Guetta V, Konen E, et al. Deformation dynamics and mechanical properties of the aortic annulus by 4-dimensional computed tomography insights into the functional anatomy of the aortic valve complex and implications for transcatheter aortic valve therapy. J Am Coll Cardiol 2012;59(2):119-127.

11. Koos R, Altiok E, Mahnken AH, et al. Evaluation of aortic root for definition of prosthesis size by magnetic resonance imaging and cardiac computed tomography: implications for transcatheter aortic valve implantation. Int J Cardiol 2012;158(3):353-358.

12. Altiok E, Koos R, Schroder J, et al. Comparison of two-dimensional and three-dimensional imaging techniques for measurement of aortic annulus diameters before transcatheter aortic valve implantation. Heart 2011;97(19):1578-1584.

13. Murphy DT, Blanke P, Alaamri S, et al. Dynamism of the aortic annulus: effect of diastolic versus systolic CT annular measurements on device selection in transcatheter aortic valve replacement (TAVR). J Cardiovasc Comput Tomogr 2016;10(1):37-43.

14. Tzikas A, Schultz CJ, Piazza N, et al. Assessment of the aortic annulus by multislice computed tomography, contrast aortography, and trans-thoracic echocardiography in patients referred for transcatheter aortic valve implantation. Catheter Cardiovasc Interv 2011;77(6):868-875.

15. Koos R, Altiok E, Mahnken AH, et al. Evaluation of aortic root for definition of prosthesis size by magnetic resonance imaging and cardiac computed tomography: implications for transcatheter aortic valve implantation. Int J Cardiol 2011.

16. Bloomfield GS, Gillam LD, Hahn RT, et al. A practical guide to multimodality imaging of transcatheter aortic valve replacement. JACC Cardiovasc Imaging 2012;5(4):441-455.

17. Lang RM, Badano LP, Tsang W, et al. EAE/ASE recommendations for image acquisition and display using three-dimensional echocardiography. Eur Heart J Cardiovasc Imaging 2012;13(1):1-46.

18. Goldstein SA, Evangelista A, Abbara S, et al. Multimodality imaging of diseases of the thoracic aorta in adults: from the American Society of Echocardiography and the European Association of Cardiovascular Imaging: endorsed by the Society of Cardiovascular Computed Tomography and Society for Cardiovascular Magnetic Resonance. J Am Soc Echocardiogr 2015;28(2):119-182.

19. Messika-Zeitoun D, Serfaty JM, Brochet E, et al. Multimodal assessment of the aortic annulus diameter: implications for transcatheter aortic valve implantation. J Am Coll Cardiol 2010;55(3):186-194.

20. Gurvitch R, Webb JG, Yuan R, et al. Aortic annulus diameter determination by multidetector computed tomography: reproducibility, applicability, and implications for transcatheter aortic valve implantation. JACC Cardiovasc Interv 2011;4(11):1235-1245.

21. Gaspar T, Adawi S, Sachner R, et al. Three-dimensional imaging of the left ventricular outflow tract: impact on aortic valve area estimation by the continuity equation. J Am Soc Echocardiogr 2012;25(7):749-757.

22. Saitoh T, Shiota M, Izumo M, et al. Comparison of left ventricular outflow geometry and aortic valve area in patients with aortic stenosis by 2-dimensional versus 3-dimensional echocardiography. Am J Cardiol 2012;109(11):1626-1631.

23. Akhtar M, Tuzcu EM, Kapadia SR, et al. Aortic root morphology in patients undergoing percutaneous aortic valve replacement: evidence of aortic root remodeling. J Thorac Cardiovasc Surg 2009;137(4):950-956.

24. Buellesfeld L, Stortecky S, Kalesan B, et al. Aortic root dimensions among patients with severe aortic stenosis undergoing transcatheter aortic valve replacement. JACC Cardiovasc Interv 2013;6(1):72-83.

25. Ewe SH, Ng AC, Schuijf JD, et al. Location and severity of aortic valve calcium and implications for aortic regurgitation after transcatheter aortic valve implantation. Am J Cardiol 2011;108(10):1470-1477.

26. Colli A, D'Amico R, Kempfert J, et al. Transesophageal echocardiographic scoring for transcatheter aortic valve implantation: impact of aortic cusp calcification on postoperative aortic regurgitation. J Thorac Cardiovasc Surg 2011;142(5):1229-1235.

27. Michelena HI, Prakash SK, Della Corte A, et al. Bicuspid aortic valve: identifying knowledge gaps and rising to the challenge from the International Bicuspid Aortic Valve Consortium (BAVCon). Circulation 2014;129(25):2691-2704.

28. Biner S, Rafique AM, Ray I, et al. Aortopathy is prevalent in relatives of bicuspid aortic valve patients. J Am Coll Cardiol 2009;53(24):2288-2295.

29. Michelena HI, Khanna AD, Mahoney D, et al. Incidence of aortic complications in patients with bicuspid aortic valves. JAMA 2011;306(10):1104-1112.

30. Ocak I, Lacomis JM, Deible CR, et al. The aortic root: comparison of measurements from ECG-gated CT angiography with transthoracic echocardiography. J Thorac Imaging 2009;24(3):223-226.

31. Brandenburg RO, Jr., Tajik AJ, Edwards WD, et al. Accuracy of 2-dimensional echocardiographic diagnosis of congenitally bicuspid aortic valve: echocardiographic-anatomic correlation in 115 patients. Am J Cardiol 1983;51(9):1469-1473.

32. Malagoli A, Barbieri A, Modena MG. Bicuspid aortic valve regurgitation: quantification of anatomic regurgitant orifice area by 3D transesophageal echocardiography reconstruction. Echocardiography 2008;25(7):797-798.

33. Koh TW. Diagnosis of bicuspid aortic valve: role of three-dimensional transesophageal echocardiography and multiplane review analysis. Echocardiography 2013;30(3):360-363.

34. Unsworth B, Malik I, Mikhail GW. Recognising bicuspid aortic stenosis in patients referred for transcatheter aortic valve implantation: routine screening with three-dimensional transoesophageal echocardiography. Heart 2010;96(8):645.

35. Shibayama K, Harada K, Berdejo J, et al. Comparison of aortic root geometry with bicuspid versus tricuspid aortic valve: real-time three-dimensional transesophageal echocardiographic study. J Am Soc Echocardiogr 2014;27(11):1143-1152.

36. Schaefer BM, Lewin MB, Stout KK, et al. The bicuspid aortic valve: an integrated phenotypic classification of leaflet morphology and aortic root shape. Heart 2008;94(12):1634-1638.

37. Buchner S, Hulsmann M, Poschenrieder F, et al. Variable phenotypes of bicuspid aortic valve disease: classification by cardiovascular magnetic resonance. Heart 2010;96(15):1233-1240.

38. Sievers HH, Schmidtke C. A classification system for the bicuspid aortic valve from 304 surgical specimens. J Thorac Cardiovasc Surg 2007;133(5):1226-1233.

39. Kang JW, Song HG, Yang DH, et al. Association between bicuspid aortic valve phenotype and patterns of valvular dysfunction and bicuspid aortopathy: comprehensive evaluation using MDCT and echocardiography. JACC Cardiovasc Imaging 2013;6(2):150-161.

40. Fernandez B, Duran AC, Fernandez-Gallego T, et al. Bicuspid aortic valves with different spatial orientations of the leaflets are distinct etiological entities. J Am Coll Cardiol 2009;54(24):2312-2318.

41. Tzemos N, Therrien J, Yip J, et al. Outcomes in adults with bicuspid aortic valves. JAMA 2008;300(11):1317-1325.

42. Michelena HI, Prakash SK, Della Corte A, et al. Bicuspid aortic valve: identifying knowledge gaps and rising to the challenge from the International Bicuspid Aortic Valve Consortium (BAVCon). Circulation 2014;129(25):2691-2704.

43. Hahn RT, Roman MJ, Mogtader AH, Devereux RB. Association of aortic dilation with regurgitant, stenotic and functionally normal bicuspid aortic valves. J Am Coll Cardiol 1992;19(2):283-288.

44. Keane MG, Wiegers SE, Plappert T, et al. Bicuspid aortic valves are associated with aortic dilatation out of proportion to coexistent valvular lesions. Circulation 2000;102(19 Suppl 3):III35-III39.

45. Beroukhim RS, Kruzick TL, Taylor AL, et al. Progression of aortic dilation in children with a functionally normal bicuspid aortic valve. Am J Cardiol 2006;98(6):828-830.

46. Svensson LG, Adams DH, Bonow RO, et al. Aortic valve and ascending aorta guidelines for management and quality measures. Ann Thorac Surg 2013;95(Suppl 6):S1-S66.

47. Mendoza DD, Kochar M, Devereux RB, et al. Impact of image analysis methodology on diagnostic and surgical classification of patients with thoracic aortic aneurysms. Ann Thorac Surg 2011;92(3):904-912.

48. Bissell MM, Hess AT, Biasiolli L, et al. Aortic dilation in bicuspid aortic valve disease: flow pattern is a major contributor and differs with valve fusion type. Circ Cardiovasc Imaging 2013;6(4):499-507.

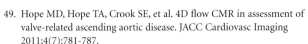
49. Hope MD, Hope TA, Crook SE, et al. 4D flow CMR in assessment of valve-related ascending aortic disease. JACC Cardiovasc Imaging 2011;4(7):781-787.

50. Meierhofer C, Schneider EP, Lyko C, et al. Wall shear stress and flow patterns in the ascending aorta in patients with bicuspid aortic valves differ significantly from tricuspid aortic valves: a prospective study. Eur Heart J Cardiovasc Imaging 2013;14(8):797-804.

51. Mahadevia R, Barker AJ, Schnell S, et al. Bicuspid aortic cusp fusion morphology alters aortic three-dimensional outflow patterns, wall shear stress, and expression of aortopathy. Circulation 2014;129(6):673-682.

52. Hatle L. Assessment of aortic blood flow velocities with continuous wave Doppler ultrasound in the neonate and young child. J Am Coll Cardiol 1985;5(Suppl 1):113S-119S.

53. Skjaerpe T, Hegrenaes L, Hatle L. Noninvasive estimation of valve area in patients with aortic stenosis by Doppler ultrasound and two-dimensional echocardiography. Circulation 1985;72(4):810-818.

54. Otto CM, Pearlman AS, Comess KA, et al. Determination of the stenotic aortic valve area in adults using Doppler echocardiography. J Am Coll Cardiol. 1986;7(3):509-517.

55. Zoghbi WA, Farmer KL, Soto JG, et al. Accurate noninvasive quantification of stenotic aortic valve area by Doppler echocardiography. Circulation 1986;73(3):452-459.

56. Baumgartner H, Hung J, Bermejo J, et al. Recommendations on the echocardiographic assessment of aortic valve stenosis: a focused update from the European Association of Cardiovascular Imaging and the American Society of Echocardiography. J Am Soc Echocardiogr 2017;30(4):372-392.

57. Blot-Souletie N, Hebrard A, Acar P, et al. Comparison of accuracy of aortic valve area assessment in aortic stenosis by real time three-dimensional echocardiography in biplane mode versus two-dimensional transthoracic and transesophageal echocardiography. Echocardiography 2007;24(10):1065-1072.

58. Nakai H, Takeuchi M, Yoshitani H, et al. Pitfalls of anatomical aortic valve area measurements using two-dimensional transoesophageal echocardiography and the potential of three-dimensional transoesophageal echocardiography. Eur J Echocardiogr 2010;11(4):369-376.

59. Goland S, Trento A, Iida K, et al. Assessment of aortic stenosis by three-dimensional echocardiography: an accurate and novel approach. Heart 2007;93(7):801-807.

60. Machida T, Izumo M, Suzuki K, et al. Value of anatomical aortic valve area using real-time three-dimensional transoesophageal echocardiography in patients with aortic stenosis: a comparison between tricuspid and bicuspid aortic valves. Eur Heart J Cardiovasc Imaging 2015;16(10):1120-1128.

61. Okura H, Yoshida K, Hozumi T, et al. Planimetry and transthoracic two-dimensional echocardiography in noninvasive assessment of aortic valve area in patients with valvular aortic stenosis. J Am Coll Cardiol 1997;30(3):753-759.

62. Saura D, de la Morena G, Flores-Blanco PJ, et al. Aortic valve stenosis planimetry by means of three-dimensional transesophageal echocardiography in the real clinical setting: feasibility, reliability and systematic deviations. Echocardiography 2015;32(3):508-515.

63. Otto CM, Pearlman AS, Gardner CL. Hemodynamic progression of aortic stenosis in adults assessed by Doppler echocardiography. J Am Coll Cardiol 1989;13(3):545-550.

64. Rosenhek R, Binder T, Porenta G, et al. Predictors of outcome in severe, asymptomatic aortic stenosis. N Engl J Med 2000;343(9):611-617.

65. Rosenhek R, Zilberszac R, Schemper M, et al. Natural history of very severe aortic stenosis. Circulation 2010;121(1):151-156.

66. Minners J, Allgeier M, Gohlke-Baerwolf C, et al. Inconsistencies of echocardiographic criteria for the grading of aortic valve stenosis. Eur Heart J 2008;29(8):1043-1048.

67. Masjedi S, Amarnath A, Baily KM, Ferdous Z. Comparison of calcification potential of valvular interstitial cells isolated from individual aortic valve cusps. Cardiovasc Pathol 2016;25(3):185-194.

68. Thaden JJ, Nkomo VT, Lee KJ, Oh JK. Doppler imaging in aortic stenosis: the importance of the nonapical imaging windows to determine severity in a contemporary cohort. J Am Soc Echocardiogr 2015;28(7):780-785.

69. Cho EJ, Kim SM, Park SJ, et al. Identification of factors that predict whether the right parasternal view is required for accurate evaluation of aortic stenosis severity. Echocardiography 2016;33(6):830-837.

70. Parker JO, Mark AL, Sanghvi VR, et al. Hemodynamic effects of pacing-induced tachycardia in valvular aortic stenosis. Can Med Assoc J 1983;129(1):38-41.

71. Kadem L, Pibarot P, Dumesnil JG, et al. Independent contribution of left ventricular ejection time to the mean gradient in aortic stenosis. J Heart Valve Dis 2002;11(5):615-623.

72. Kadem L, Dumesnil JG, Rieu R, et al. Impact of systemic hypertension on the assessment of aortic stenosis. Heart 2005;91(3):354-361.

73. Little SH, Chan KL, Burwash IG. Impact of blood pressure on the Doppler echocardiographic assessment of severity of aortic stenosis. Heart 2007;93(7):848-855.

74. Eleid MF, Nishimura RA, Sorajja P, Borlaug BA. Systemic hypertension in low-gradient severe aortic stenosis with preserved ejection fraction. Circulation 2013;128(12):1349-1353.

75. Barasch E, Fan D, Chukwu EO, et al. Severe isolated aortic stenosis with normal left ventricular systolic function and low transvalvular gradients: pathophysiologic and prognostic insights. J Heart Valve Dis 2008;17(1):81-88.

76. Pibarot P, Dumesnil JG. Low-flow, low-gradient aortic stenosis with normal and depressed left ventricular ejection fraction. J Am Coll Cardiol 2012;60(19):1845-1853.

77. Baumgartner H, Hung J, Bermejo J, et al. Echocardiographic assessment of valve stenosis: EAE/ASE recommendations for clinical practice. J Am Soc Echocardiogr 2009;22(1):1-23; quiz 101-102.

78. Mehrotra P, Flynn AW, Jansen K, et al. Differential left ventricular outflow tract remodeling and dynamics in aortic stenosis. J Am Soc Echocardiogr 2015;28(11):1259-1266.

79. LaBounty TM, Miyasaka R, Chetcuti S, et al. Annulus instead of LVOT diameter improves agreement between echocardiography effective orifice area and invasive aortic valve area. JACC Cardiovasc Imaging 2014;7(10):1065-1066.

80. Oh JK, Taliercio CP, Holmes DR, Jr., et al. Prediction of the severity of aortic stenosis by Doppler aortic valve area determination: prospective Doppler-catheterization correlation in 100 patients. J Am Coll Cardiol 1988;11(6):1227-1234.

81. Michelena HI, Margaryan E, Miller FA, et al. Inconsistent echocardiographic grading of aortic stenosis: is the left ventricular outflow tract important? Heart 2013;99(13):921-931.

82. Doddamani S, Bello R, Friedman MA, et al. Demonstration of left ventricular outflow tract eccentricity by real time 3D echocardiography: implications for the determination of aortic valve area. Echocardiography 2007;24(8):860-866.

83. Shahgaldi K, Manouras A, Brodin LA, Winter R. Direct measurement of left ventricular outflow tract area using three-dimensional echocardiography in biplane mode improves accuracy of stroke volume assessment. Echocardiography 2010;27(9):1078-1085.

84. Jilaihawi H, Doctor N, Kashif M, et al. Aortic annular sizing for transcatheter aortic valve replacement using cross-sectional 3-dimensional transesophageal echocardiography. J Am Coll Cardiol 2013;61(9):908-916.

85. Khalique OK, Kodali SK, Paradis JM, et al. Aortic annular sizing using a novel 3-dimensional echocardiographic method: use and comparison with cardiac computed tomography. Circ Cardiovasc Imaging 2014;7(1):155-163.

86. Burgstahler C, Kunze M, Loffler C, et al. Assessment of left ventricular outflow tract geometry in non-stenotic and stenotic aortic valves by cardiovascular magnetic resonance. J Cardiovasc Magn Reson 2006;8(6):825-829.

87. De Vecchi C, Caudron J, Dubourg B, et al. Effect of the ellipsoid shape of the left ventricular outflow tract on the echocardiographic assessment of aortic valve area in aortic stenosis. J Cardiovasc Comput Tomogr 2014;8(1):52-57.

88. Halpern EJ, Mallya R, Sewell M, et al. Differences in aortic valve area measured with CT planimetry and echocardiography (continuity equation) are related to divergent estimates of left ventricular outflow tract area. AJR Am J Roentgenol 2009;192(6):1668-1673.

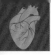

89. O'Brien B, Schoenhagen P, Kapadia SR, et al. Integration of 3D imaging data in the assessment of aortic stenosis: impact on classification of disease severity. Circ Cardiovasc Imaging 2011;4(5):566-573.

90. Montealegre-Gallegos M, Mahmood F, Owais K, et al. Cardiac output calculation and three-dimensional echocardiography. J Cardiothorac Vasc Anesth 2014;28(3):547-550.

91. Tsang W, Bateman MG, Weinert L, et al. Accuracy of aortic annular measurements obtained from three-dimensional echocardiography, CT and MRI: human in vitro and in vivo studies. Heart 2012;98(15):1146-1152.

92. Clavel MA, Malouf J, Messika-Zeitoun D, et al. Aortic valve area calculation in aortic stenosis by CT and Doppler echocardiography. JACC Cardiovasc Imaging 2015;8(3):248-257.

93. Malouf J, Le Tourneau T, Pellikka P, et al. Aortic valve stenosis in community medical practice: determinants of outcome and implications for aortic valve replacement. J Thorac Cardiovasc Surg 2012;144(6):1421-1427.

94. Pibarot P, Clavel MA. Left ventricular outflow tract geometry and dynamics in aortic stenosis: implications for the echocardiographic assessment of aortic valve area. J Am Soc Echocardiogr 2015;28(11):1267-1269.

95. Jander N, Hochholzer W, Kaufmann BA, et al. Velocity ratio predicts outcomes in patients with low gradient severe aortic stenosis and preserved EF. Heart 2014;100(24):1946-1953.

96. Wiggers CJ. Physiology in Health and Disease. Philadelphia, PA: Lea & Febiger; 1945:733.

97. Heinrich RS, Marcus RH, Ensley AE, et al. Valve orifice area alone is an insufficient index of aortic stenosis severity: effects of the proximal and distal geometry on transaortic energy loss. J Heart Valve Dis 1999;8(5):509-515.

98. Bahlmann E, Cramariuc D, Gerdts E, et al. Impact of pressure recovery on echocardiographic assessment of asymptomatic aortic stenosis: a SEAS substudy. JACC Cardiovasc Imaging 2010;3(6):555-562.

99. Garcia D, Dumesnil JG, Durand LG, et al. Discrepancies between catheter and Doppler estimates of valve effective orifice area can be predicted from the pressure recovery phenomenon: practical implications with regard to quantification of aortic stenosis severity. J Am Coll Cardiol 2003;41(3):435-442.

100. Meine TJ, Harrison JK. Should we cross the valve: the risk of retrograde catheterization of the left ventricle in patients with aortic stenosis. Am Heart J 2004;148(1):41-42.

101. Nishimura RA, Carabello BA. Hemodynamics in the cardiac catheterization laboratory of the 21st century. Circulation 2012;125(17):2138-2150.

102. Smith MD, Dawson PL, Elion JL, et al. Systematic correlation of continuous-wave Doppler and hemodynamic measurements in patients with aortic stenosis. Am Heart J 1986;111(2):245-252.

103. Currie PJ, Hagler DJ, Seward JB, et al. Instantaneous pressure gradient: a simultaneous Doppler and dual catheter correlative study. J Am Coll Cardiol 1986;7(4):800-806.

104. Gorlin R, Gorlin SG. Hydraulic formula for calculation of the area of the stenotic mitral valve, other cardiac valves, and central circulatory shunts. I. Am Heart J 1951;41(1):1-29.

105. Hakki AH, Iskandrian AS, Bemis CE, et al. A simplified valve formula for the calculation of stenotic cardiac valve areas. Circulation 1981;63(5):1050-1055.

106. Hatle L, Angelsen BA, Tromsdal A. Non-invasive assessment of aortic stenosis by Doppler ultrasound. Br Heart J 1980;43(3):284-292.

107. Bonow RO, Carabello BA, Chatterjee K, et al. 2008 Focused update incorporated into the ACC/AHA 2006 guidelines for the management of patients with valvular heart disease: a report of the American College of Cardiology/American Heart Association Task Force on Practice Guidelines (Writing Committee to Revise the 1998 Guidelines for the Management of Patients With Valvular Heart Disease): endorsed by the Society of Cardiovascular Anesthesiologists, Society for Cardiovascular Angiography and Interventions, and Society of Thoracic Surgeons. Circulation 2008;118(15):e523-e661.

108. Niederberger J, Schima H, Maurer G, Baumgartner H. Importance of pressure recovery for the assessment of aortic stenosis by Doppler ultrasound. Role of aortic size, aortic valve area, and direction of the stenotic jet in vitro. Circulation 1996;94(8):1934-1940.

109. Chambers JB, Sprigings DC, Cochrane T, et al. Continuity equation and Gorlin formula compared with directly observed orifice area in native and prosthetic aortic valves. Br Heart J 1992;67(2):193-199.

110. Feuchtner GM, Dichtl W, Friedrich GJ, et al. Multislice computed tomography for detection of patients with aortic valve stenosis and quantification of severity. J Am Coll Cardiol 2006;47(7):1410-1417.

111. Achenbach S, Delgado V, Hausleiter J, et al. SCCT expert consensus document on computed tomography imaging before transcatheter aortic valve implantation (TAVI)/transcatheter aortic valve replacement (TAVR). J Cardiovasc Comput Tomogr 2012;6(6):366-380.

112. Otto CM, Lind BK, Kitzman DW, et al. Association of aortic-valve sclerosis with cardiovascular mortality and morbidity in the elderly. N Engl J Med 1999;341(3):142-147.

113. Messika-Zeitoun D, Aubry MC, Detaint D, et al. Evaluation and clinical implications of aortic valve calcification measured by electron-beam computed tomography. Circulation 2004;110(3):356-362.

114. Feuchtner GM, Muller S, Grander W, et al. Aortic valve calcification as quantified with multislice computed tomography predicts short-term clinical outcome in patients with asymptomatic aortic stenosis. J Heart Valve Dis 2006;15(4):494-498.

115. Clavel MA, Pibarot P, Messika-Zeitoun D, et al. Impact of aortic valve calcification, as measured by MDCT, on survival in patients with aortic stenosis: results of an international registry study. J Am Coll Cardiol 2014;64(12):1202-1213.

116. Clavel MA, Messika-Zeitoun D, Pibarot P, et al. The complex nature of discordant severe calcified aortic valve disease grading: new insights from combined Doppler echocardiographic and computed tomographic study. J Am Coll Cardiol 2013;62(24):2329-2338.

117. Aksoy O, Cam A, Agarwal S, et al. Significance of aortic valve calcification in patients with low-gradient low-flow aortic stenosis. Clin Cardiol 2014;37(1):26-31.

118. Cueff C, Serfaty JM, Cimadevilla C, et al. Measurement of aortic valve calcification using multislice computed tomography: correlation with haemodynamic severity of aortic stenosis and clinical implication for patients with low ejection fraction. Heart 2011;97(9):721-726.

119. Pawade T, Clavel MA, Tribouilloy C, et al. Computed tomography aortic valve calcium scoring in patients with aortic stenosis. Circ Cardiovasc Imaging 2018;11(3):e007146.

120. Nishimura RA, Otto CM, Bonow RO, et al. 2014 AHA/ACC guideline for the management of patients with valvular heart disease: executive summary: a report of the American College of Cardiology/American Heart Association Task Force on Practice Guidelines. J Am Coll Cardiol 2014;63(22):2438-2488.

121. Schulz-Menger J, Bluemke DA, Bremerich J, et al. Standardized image interpretation and post processing in cardiovascular magnetic resonance: Society for Cardiovascular Magnetic Resonance (SCMR) board of trustees task force on standardized post processing. J Cardiovasc Magn Reson 2013;15:35.

122. Kramer CM, Barkhausen J, Flamm SD, et al. Standardized cardiovascular magnetic resonance imaging (CMR) Society for Cardiovascular Magnetic Resonance: board of trustees task force on standardized protocols. J Cardiovasc Magn Reson 2008;10:35.

123. Reant P, Lederlin M, Lafitte S, et al. Absolute assessment of aortic valve stenosis by planimetry using cardiovascular magnetic resonance imaging: comparison with transesophageal echocardiography, transthoracic echocardiography, and cardiac catheterisation. Eur J Radiol 2006;59(2):276-283.

124. Cavalcante JL, Lalude OO, Schoenhagen P, Lerakis S. Cardiovascular magnetic resonance imaging for structural and valvular heart disease interventions. JACC Cardiovasc Interv 2016;9(5):399-425.

125. Tanaka K, Makaryus AN, Wolff SD. Correlation of aortic valve area obtained by the velocity-encoded phase contrast continuity method to direct planimetry using cardiovascular magnetic resonance. J Cardiovasc Magn Reson 2007;9(5):799-805.

126. Gatehouse PD, Keegan J, Crowe LA, et al. Applications of phase-contrast flow and velocity imaging in cardiovascular MRI. Eur Radiol 2005;15(10):2172-2184.

127. Kockova R, Kacer P, Pirk J, et al. Native T1 relaxation time and extracellular volume fraction as accurate markers of diffuse myocardial fibrosis in heart valve disease- comparison with targeted left ventricular myocardial biopsy. Circ J 2016;80(5):1202-1209.

128. Lee SP, Lee W, Lee JM, et al. Assessment of diffuse myocardial fibrosis by using MR imaging in asymptomatic patients with aortic stenosis. Radiology 2015;274(2):359-369.

129. Herrmann S, Stork S, Niemann M, et al. Low-gradient aortic valve stenosis myocardial fibrosis and its influence on function and outcome. J Am Coll Cardiol 2011;58(4):402-412.

130. Carr JA, Savage EB. Aortic valve repair for aortic insufficiency in adults: a contemporary review and comparison with replacement techniques. Eur J Cardiothorac Surg 2004;25(1):6-15.

131. Saczkowski R, Malas T, de Kerchove L, et al. Systematic review of aortic valve preservation and repair. Ann Cardiothorac Surg 2013; 2(1):3-9.

132. Carpentier A. Cardiac valve surgery—the "French correction". J Thorac Cardiovasc Surg 1983;86(3):323-337.

133. El Khoury G, Glineur D, Rubay J, et al. Functional classification of aortic root/valve abnormalities and their correlation with etiologies and surgical procedures. Curr Opin Cardiol 2005;20(2):115-121.

134. Boodhwani M, de Kerchove L, Glineur D, et al. Repair-oriented classification of aortic insufficiency: impact on surgical techniques and clinical outcomes. J Thorac Cardiovasc Surg 2009;137(2):286-294.

135. Mann T, McLaurin L, Grossman W, Craige E. Assessing the hemodynamic severity of acute aortic regurgitation due to infective endocarditis. N Engl J Med 1975;293(3):108-113.

136. Gustavsson CG, Gustafson A, Albrechtsson U, et al. Diagnosis and management of acute aortic dissection, clinical and radiological follow-up. Acta Med Scand 1988;223(3):247-253.

137. Obadia JF, Tatou E, David M. Aortic valve regurgitation caused by blunt chest injury. Br Heart J 1995;74(5):545-547.

138. Pretre R, Faidutti B. Surgical management of aortic valve injury after nonpenetrating trauma. Ann Thorac Surg 1993;56(6):1426-1431.

139. Yeo TC, Ling LH, Ng WL, Chia BL. Spontaneous aortic laceration causing flail aortic valve and acute aortic regurgitation. J Am Soc Echocardiogr 1999;12(1):76-78.

140. Ha JW, Chang BC, Lee DI, et al. Flail aortic valve and acute aortic regurgitation due to spontaneous localized intimal tear of ascending aorta. Echocardiography 2001;18(5):381-383.

141. Newcomb AE, Rowland MA. Nontraumatic localized dehiscence of the proximal ascending aorta through an aortic valve commissure. Ann Thorac Surg 2004;78(1):321-323.

142. Akiyama K, Ohsawa S, Hirota J, Takiguchi M. Massive aortic regurgitation by spontaneous rupture of a fibrous strand in a fenestrated aortic valve. J Heart Valve Dis 1998;7(5):521-523.

143. Irisawa Y, Itatani K, Kitamura T, et al. Aortic regurgitation due to fibrous strand rupture in the fenestrated left coronary cusp of the tricuspid aortic valve. Int Heart J 2014;55(6):550-551.

144. Kardaras FG, Kardara DF, Rontogiani DP, et al. Acute aortic regurgitation caused by non-bacterial thrombotic endocarditis. Eur Heart J 1995;16(8):1152-1154.

145. Niclauss L, Letovanec I, Chassot PG, et al. Acute aortic valve insufficiency and cardiogenic shock due to an isolated giant cell inflammation of the aortic valve leaflets: case report and review of the literature. J Heart Valve Dis 2008;17(3):343-347.

146. Dall'Ara G, Saia F, Moretti C, et al. Incidence, treatment, and outcome of acute aortic valve regurgitation complicating percutaneous balloon aortic valvuloplasty. Catheter Cardiovasc Interv 2015.

147. Ben-Dor I, Pichard AD, Satler LF, et al. Complications and outcome of balloon aortic valvuloplasty in high-risk or inoperable patients. JACC Cardiovasc Interv 2010;3(11):1150-1156.

148. McCrindle BW, Jones TK, Morrow WR, et al. Acute results of balloon angioplasty of native coarctation versus recurrent aortic obstruction are equivalent. Valvuloplasty and Angioplasty of Congenital Anomalies

(VACA) Registry Investigators. J Am Coll Cardiol 1996;28(7): 1810-1817.

149. Zoghbi WA, Enriquez-Sarano M, Foster E, et al. Recommendations for evaluation of the severity of native valvular regurgitation with two-dimensional and Doppler echocardiography. J Am Soc Echocardiogr 2003;16(7):777-802.

150. Lancellotti P, Tribouilloy C, Hagendorff A, et al. European Association of Echocardiography recommendations for the assessment of valvular regurgitation. Part 1: aortic and pulmonary regurgitation (native valve disease). Eur J Echocardiogr 2010;11(3):223-244.

151. Fang L, Hsiung MC, Miller AP, et al. Assessment of aortic regurgitation by live three-dimensional transthoracic echocardiographic measurements of vena contracta area: usefulness and validation. Echocardiography 2005;22(9):775-781.

152. Sato H, Ohta T, Hiroe K, et al. Severity of aortic regurgitation assessed by area of vena contracta: a clinical two-dimensional and three-dimensional color Doppler imaging study. Cardiovasc Ultrasound 2015;13:24.

153. Tribouilloy CM, Enriquez-Sarano M, Bailey KR, et al. Assessment of severity of aortic regurgitation using the width of the vena contracta: a clinical color Doppler imaging study. Circulation 2000;102(5): 558-564.

154. Willett DL, Hall SA, Jessen ME, et al. Assessment of aortic regurgitation by transesophageal color Doppler imaging of the vena contracta: validation against an intraoperative aortic flow probe. J Am Coll Cardiol 2001;37(5):1450-1455.

155. Messika-Zeitoun D, Detaint D, Leye M, et al. Comparison of semiquantitative and quantitative assessment of severity of aortic regurgitation: clinical implications. J Am Soc Echocardiogr 2011;24(11):1246-1252.

156. Reimold SC, Ganz P, Bittl JA, et al. Effective aortic regurgitant orifice area: description of a method based on the conservation of mass. J Am Coll Cardiol 1991;18(3):761-768.

157. Vandervoort PM, Rivera JM, Mele D, et al. Application of color Doppler flow mapping to calculate effective regurgitant orifice area. An in vitro study and initial clinical observations. Circulation 1993;88(3):1150-1156.

158. Tribouilloy C, Avinee P, Shen WF, et al. End diastolic flow velocity just beneath the aortic isthmus assessed by pulsed Doppler echocardiography: a new predictor of the aortic regurgitant fraction. Br Heart J 1991;65(1):37-40.

159. Svedlund S, Wetterholm R, Volkmann R, Caidahl K. Retrograde blood flow in the aortic arch determined by transesophageal Doppler ultrasound. Cerebrovasc Dis 2009;27(1):22-28.

160. Hashimoto J, Ito S. Aortic stiffness determines diastolic blood flow reversal in the descending thoracic aorta: potential implication for retrograde embolic stroke in hypertension. Hypertension 2013;62(3):542-549.

161. Reimold SC, Maier SE, Aggarwal K, et al. Aortic flow velocity patterns in chronic aortic regurgitation: implications for Doppler echocardiography. J Am Soc Echocardiogr 1996;9(5):675-683.

162. Teague SM, Heinsimer JA, Anderson JL, et al. Quantification of aortic regurgitation utilizing continuous wave Doppler ultrasound. J Am Coll Cardiol 1986;8(3):592-599.

163. Palau-Caballero G, Walmsley J, Gorcsan J, 3rd, et al. Abnormal ventricular and aortic wall properties can cause inconsistencies in grading aortic regurgitation severity: a computer simulation study. J Am Soc Echocardiogr 2016;29(11):1122-1130.e1124.

164. Enriquez-Sarano M, Bailey KR, Seward JB, et al. Quantitative Doppler assessment of valvular regurgitation. Circulation 1993;87(3): 841-848.

165. Cawley PJ, Hamilton-Craig C, Owens DS, et al. Prospective comparison of valve regurgitation quantitation by cardiac magnetic resonance imaging and transthoracic echocardiography. Circ Cardiovasc Imaging 2013;6(1):48-57.

166. Hyodo E, Iwata S, Tugcu A, et al. Accurate measurement of mitral annular area by using single and biplane linear measurements: comparison of conventional methods with the three-dimensional planimetric method. Eur Heart J Cardiovasc Imaging 2012;13(7):605-611.

167. Pirat B, Little SH, Igo SR, et al. Direct measurement of proximal isovelocity surface area by real-time three-dimensional color Doppler for quantitation of aortic regurgitant volume: an in vitro validation. J Am Soc Echocardiogr 2009;22(3):306-313.

168. Thavendiranathan P, Liu S, Datta S, et al. Automated quantification of mitral inflow and aortic outflow stroke volumes by three-dimensional real-time volume color-flow Doppler transthoracic echocardiography: comparison with pulsed-wave Doppler and cardiac magnetic resonance imaging. J Am Soc Echocardiogr 2012;25(1):56-65.

169. Mori Y, Shiota T, Jones M, et al. Three-dimensional reconstruction of the color Doppler-imaged vena contracta for quantifying aortic regurgitation: studies in a chronic animal model. Circulation 1999;99(12):1611-1617.

170. Perez de Isla L, Zamorano J, Fernandez-Golfin C, et al. 3D color-Doppler echocardiography and chronic aortic regurgitation: a novel approach for severity assessment. Int J Cardiol 2013;166(3):640-645.

171. Chen TE, Kwon SH, Enriquez-Sarano M, et al. Three-dimensional color Doppler echocardiographic quantification of tricuspid regurgitation orifice area: comparison with conventional two-dimensional measures. J Am Soc Echocardiogr 2013;26(10):1143-1152.

172. Franco E, Almeria C, de Agustin JA, et al. Three-dimensional color Doppler transesophageal echocardiography for mitral paravalvular leak quantification and evaluation of percutaneous closure success. J Am Soc Echocardiogr 2014;27(11):1153-1163.

173. Altiok E, Hamada S, Brehmer K, et al. Analysis of procedural effects of percutaneous edge-to-edge mitral valve repair by 2D and 3D echocardiography. Circ Cardiovasc Imaging 2012;5(6):748-755.

174. Zoghbi WA, Enriquez-Sarano M, Foster E, et al. Recommendations for evaluation of the severity of native valvular regurgitation with two-dimensional and Doppler echocardiography. J Am Soc Echocardiogr 2003;16(7):777-802.

175. Little SH, Igo SR, Pirat B, et al. In vitro validation of real-time three-dimensional color Doppler echocardiography for direct measurement of proximal isovelocity surface area in mitral regurgitation. Am J Cardiol 2007;99(10):1440-1447.

176. de Agustin JA, Marcos-Alberca P, Fernandez-Golfin C, et al. Direct measurement of proximal isovelocity surface area by single-beat three-dimensional color Doppler echocardiography in mitral regurgitation: a validation study. J Am Soc Echocardiogr 2012;25(8):815-823.

177. de Agustin JA, Viliani D, Vieira C, et al. Proximal isovelocity surface area by single-beat three-dimensional color Doppler echocardiography applied for tricuspid regurgitation quantification. J Am Soc Echocardiogr 2013;26(9):1063-1072.

178. Li C, Zhang J, Li X, et al. Quantification of chronic aortic regurgitation by vector flow mapping: a novel echocardiographic method. Eur J Echocardiogr 2010;11(2):119-124.

179. Little SH, Igo SR, McCulloch M, et al. Three-dimensional ultrasound imaging model of mitral valve regurgitation: design and evaluation. Ultrasound Med Biol 2008;34(4):647-654.

180. Thavendiranathan P, Liu S, Datta S, et al. Automated quantification of mitral inflow and aortic outflow stroke volumes by three-dimensional real-time volume color-flow Doppler transthoracic echocardiography: comparison with pulsed-wave Doppler and cardiac magnetic resonance imaging. J Am Soc Echocardiogr 2012;25(1):56-65.

181. Sellers RD, Levy MJ, Amplatz K, Lillehei CW. Left retrograde cardioangiography in acquired cardiac disease: technic, indications and interpretations in 700 cases. Am J Cardiol 1964;14:437-447.

182. Kiemeneij F, Suwarganda JSM, De Jong IH, Schuilenburg RM. Cineaortography in the assessment of aortic regurgitation: a comparison of different catheter types. Eur Heart J 1986;7(6):509-511.

183. Arvidsson H, Karnell J. Quantitative assessment of mitral and aortic insufficiency by angiocardiography. Acta Radiol Diagn (Stockh) 1964;2:105-119.

184. Sandler H, Dodge HT, Hay RE, Rackley CE. Quantitation of valvular insufficiency in man by angiocardiography. Am Heart J 1963;65:501-513.

185. Michel PL, Vahanian A, Besnainou F, Acar J. Value of qualitative angiographic grading in aortic regurgitation. Eur Heart J 1987;8(Suppl C):11-14.

186. Croft CH, Lipscomb K, Mathis K, et al. Limitations of qualitative angiographic grading in aortic or mitral regurgitation. Am J Cardiol 1984;53(11):1593-1598.

187. Frank MJ, Casanegra P, Migliori AJ, Levinson GE. The clinical evaluation of aortic regurgitation, with special reference to a neglected sign: the popliteal-brachial pressure gradient. Arch Intern Med 1965;116:357-365.

188. Cohn LH, Mason DT, Ross J, Jr., et al. Preoperative assessment of aortic regurgitation in patients with mitral valve disease. Am J Cardiol 1967;19(2):177-182.

189. Judge TP, Kennedy JW. Estimation of aortic regurgitation by diastolic pulse wave analysis. Circulation 1970;41(4):659-665.

190. LaBounty TM, Glasofer S, Devereux RB, et al. Comparison of cardiac computed tomographic angiography to transesophageal echocardiography for evaluation of patients with native valvular heart disease. Am J Cardiol 2009;104(10):1421-1428.

191. Feuchtner GM, Spoeck A, Lessick J, et al. Quantification of aortic regurgitant fraction and volume with multi-detector computed tomography comparison with echocardiography. Acad Radiol 2011;18(3):334-342.

192. Koo HJ, Kang JW, Kim JA, et al. Functional classification of aortic regurgitation using cardiac computed tomography: comparison with surgical inspection. Int J Cardiovasc Imaging 2018;34(8):1295-1303.

193. Alkadhi H, Desbiolles L, Husmann L, et al. Aortic regurgitation: assessment with 64-section CT. Radiology 2007;245(1):111-121.

194. Ko SM, Park JH, Shin JK, Kim JS. Assessment of the regurgitant orifice area in aortic regurgitation with dual-source CT: comparison with cardiovascular magnetic resonance. J Cardiovasc Comput Tomogr 2015;9(4):345-353.

195. Debl K, Djavidani B, Buchner S, et al. Assessment of the anatomic regurgitant orifice in aortic regurgitation: a clinical magnetic resonance imaging study. Heart 2008;94(3):e8.

196. Buchner S, Debl K, Poschenrieder F, et al. Cardiovascular magnetic resonance for direct assessment of anatomic regurgitant orifice in mitral regurgitation. Circ Cardiovasc Imaging 2008;1(2):148-155.

197. Chatzimavroudis GP, Oshinski JN, Franch RH, et al. Evaluation of the precision of magnetic resonance phase velocity mapping for blood flow measurements. J Cardiovasc Magn Reson 2001;3(1):11-19.

198. Hundley WG, Li HF, Hillis LD, et al. Quantitation of cardiac output with velocity-encoded, phase-difference magnetic resonance imaging. Am J Cardiol 1995;75(17):1250-1255.

199. Ribeiro HB, Orwat S, Hayek SS, et al. Cardiovascular magnetic resonance to evaluate aortic regurgitation after transcatheter aortic valve replacement. J Am Coll Cardiol 2016;68(6):577-585.

200. Kozerke S, Scheidegger MB, Pedersen EM, Boesiger P. Heart motion adapted cine phase-contrast flow measurements through the aortic valve. Magn Reson Med 1999;42(5):970-978.

201. Sondergaard L, Lindvig K, Hildebrandt P, et al. Quantification of aortic regurgitation by magnetic resonance velocity mapping. Am Heart J 1993;125(4):1081-1090.

202. Myerson SG, d'Arcy J, Mohiaddin R, et al. Aortic regurgitation quantification using cardiovascular magnetic resonance: association with clinical outcome. Circulation 2012;126(12):1452-1460.

203. Harris AW, Krieger EV, Kim M, et al. Cardiac magnetic resonance imaging versus transthoracic echocardiography for prediction of outcomes in chronic aortic or mitral regurgitation. Am J Cardiol 2017;119(7):1074-1081.

204. Doherty JU, Kort S, Mehran R, et al. ACC/AATS/AHA/ASE/ASNC/HRS/SCAI/SCCT/SCMR/STS 2017 appropriate use criteria for multimodality imaging in valvular heart disease: a report of the American College of Cardiology appropriate use criteria task force, American Association for Thoracic Surgery, American Heart Association, American Society of Echocardiography, American Society of Nuclear Cardiology, Heart Rhythm Society, Society for Cardiovascular Angiography and Interventions, Society of Cardiovascular Computed Tomography, Society for Cardiovascular Magnetic Resonance, and Society of Thoracic Surgeons. J Am Coll Cardiol 2017;70(13):1647-1672.

205. Gabriel RS, Renapurkar R, Bolen MA, et al. Comparison of severity of aortic regurgitation by cardiovascular magnetic resonance versus

transcthoracic echocardiography. Am J Cardiol 2011;108(7):
1014-1020.

206. Bolen MA, Popovic ZB, Rajiah P, et al. Cardiac MR assessment
of aortic regurgitation: holodiastolic flow reversal in the descending
aorta helps stratify severity. Radiology 2011;260(1):98-104.

207. Hsiao A, Lustig M, Alley MT, et al. Evaluation of valvular insufficiency
and shunts with parallel-imaging compressed-sensing 4D phase-contrast
MR imaging with stereoscopic 3D velocity-fusion volume-rendered
visualization. Radiology 2012;265(1):87-95.

208. Mirsky I. Left ventricular stresses in the intact human heart. Biophys J
1969;9(2):189-208.

209. Popma JJ, Adams DH, Reardon MJ, et al. Transcatheter aortic valve
replacement using a self-expanding bioprosthesis in patients with severe
aortic stenosis at extreme risk for surgery. J Am Coll Cardiol 2014;63(19):
1972-1981.

210. Rodes-Cabau J, Webb JG, Cheung A, et al. Transcatheter aortic valve
implantation for the treatment of severe symptomatic aortic stenosis
in patients at very high or prohibitive surgical risk: acute and late
outcomes of the multicenter Canadian experience. J Am Coll Cardiol
2010;55(11):1080-1090.

211. Briand M, Dumesnil JG, Kadem L, et al. Reduced systemic arterial
compliance impacts significantly on left ventricular afterload and
function in aortic stenosis: implications for diagnosis and treatment.
J Am Coll Cardiol 2005;46(2):291-298.

212. Hachicha Z, Dumesnil JG, Pibarot P. Usefulness of the valvuloarterial
impedance to predict adverse outcome in asymptomatic aortic stenosis.
J Am Coll Cardiol 2009;54(11):1003-1011.

213. Rieck AE, Cramariuc D, Boman K, et al. Hypertension in aortic stenosis:
implications for left ventricular structure and cardiovascular events.
Hypertension 2012;60(1):90-97.

214. Lang RM, Badano LP, Mor-Avi V, et al. Recommendations for cardiac
chamber quantification by echocardiography in adults: an update from
the American Society of Echocardiography and the European Association
for Cardiovascular Imaging. J Am Soc Echocardiogr 2015;28(1):1-39.e14.

215. de Simone G, Kizer JR, Chinali M, et al. Normalization for body size and
population-attributable risk of left ventricular hypertrophy: the Strong
Heart Study. Am J Hypertens 2005;18(2 Pt 1):191-196.

216. Cuspidi C, Facchetti R, Bombelli M, et al. Prognostic value of left
ventricular mass normalized to different body size indexes: findings from
the PAMELA population. J Hypertens 2015;33(5):1082-1089.

217. Mentias A, Feng K, Alashi A, et al. Long-Term outcomes in patients with
aortic regurgitation and preserved left ventricular ejection fraction. J Am
Coll Cardiol 2016;68(20):2144-2153.

218. Alashi A, Mentias A, Abdallah A, et al. Incremental prognostic utility of
left ventricular global longitudinal strain in asymptomatic patients with
significant chronic aortic regurgitation and preserved left ventricular
ejection fraction. JACC Cardiovasc Imaging 2018;11(5):673-682.

219. Hundley WG, Kizilbash AM, Afridi I, et al. Administration of an
intravenous perfluorocarbon contrast agent improves echocardiographic
determination of left ventricular volumes and ejection fraction:
comparison with cine magnetic resonance imaging. J Am Coll Cardiol
1998;32(5):1426-1432.

220. Porter TR, Mulvagh SL, Abdelmoneim SS, et al. Clinical applications of
ultrasonic enhancing agents in echocardiography: 2018 American
Society of Echocardiography guidelines update. J Am Soc Echocardiogr
2018;31(3):241-274.

221. Mor-Avi V, Lang RM, Badano LP, et al. Current and evolving
echocardiographic techniques for the quantitative evaluation of cardiac
mechanics: ASE/EAE consensus statement on methodology and
indications endorsed by the Japanese Society of Echocardiography. J Am
Soc Echocardiogr 2011;24(3):277-313.

222. Miyazaki S, Daimon M, Miyazaki T, et al. Global longitudinal strain in
relation to the severity of aortic stenosis: a two-dimensional speckle-
tracking study. Echocardiography 2011;28(7):703-708.

223. Ng AC, Delgado V, Bertini M, et al. Alterations in multidirectional myocardial
functions in patients with aortic stenosis and preserved ejection fraction: a
two-dimensional speckle tracking analysis. Eur Heart J 2011;32(12):1542-1550.

224. Sengupta PP, Tajik AJ, Chandrasekaran K, Khandheria BK. Twist
mechanics of the left ventricle: principles and application. JACC
Cardiovasc Imaging 2008;1(3):366-376.

225. Bauer F, Eltchaninoff H, Tron C, et al. Acute improvement in global and
regional left ventricular systolic function after percutaneous heart valve
implantation in patients with symptomatic aortic stenosis. Circulation
2004;110(11):1473-1476.

226. Delgado M, Ruiz M, Mesa D, et al. Early improvement of the regional
and global ventricle function estimated by two-dimensional speckle
tracking echocardiography after percutaneous aortic valve implantation
speckle tracking after CoreValve implantation. Echocardiography
2013;30(1):37-44.

227. Kamperidis V, Joyce E, Debonnaire P, et al. Left ventricular functional
recovery and remodeling in low-flow low-gradient severe aortic stenosis
after transcatheter aortic valve implantation. J Am Soc Echocardiogr
2014;27(8):817-825.

228. Phelan D, Collier P, Thavendiranathan P, et al. Relative apical sparing of
longitudinal strain using two-dimensional speckle-tracking
echocardiography is both sensitive and specific for the diagnosis of
cardiac amyloidosis. Heart 2012;98(19):1442-1448.

229. Carstensen HG, Larsen LH, Hassager C, et al. Association of ischemic
heart disease to global and regional longitudinal strain in asymptomatic
aortic stenosis. Int J Cardiovasc Imaging 2015;31(3):485-495.

230. Ross J, Jr., Braunwald E. Aortic stenosis. Circulation 1968;38(Suppl 1):
61-67.

231. Carasso S, Mutlak D, Lessick J, et al. Symptoms in severe aortic stenosis
are associated with decreased compensatory circumferential myocardial
mechanics. J Am Soc Echocardiogr 2015;28(2):218-225.

232. Attias D, Macron L, Dreyfus J, et al. Relationship between longitudinal
strain and symptomatic status in aortic stenosis. J Am Soc Echocardiogr
2013;26(8):868-874.

233. Logstrup BB, Andersen HR, Thuesen L, et al. Left ventricular global
systolic longitudinal deformation and prognosis 1 year after femoral and
apical transcatheter aortic valve implantation. J Am Soc Echocardiogr
2013;26(3):246-254.

234. Kamperidis V, van Rosendael PJ, Ng AC, et al. Impact of flow and left
ventricular strain on outcome of patients with preserved left ventricular
ejection fraction and low gradient severe aortic stenosis undergoing
aortic valve replacement. Am J Cardiol 2014;114(12):1875-1881.

235. Dahou A, Bartko PE, Capoulade R, et al. Usefulness of global left
ventricular longitudinal strain for risk stratification in low ejection
fraction, low-gradient aortic stenosis: results from the multicenter
True or Pseudo-Severe Aortic Stenosis study. Circ Cardiovasc Imaging
2015;8(3):e002117.

236. Nagata Y, Takeuchi M, Wu VC, et al. Prognostic value of LV deformation
parameters using 2D and 3D speckle-tracking echocardiography in
asymptomatic patients with severe aortic stenosis and preserved LV
ejection fraction. JACC Cardiovasc Imaging 2015.

237. Kusunose K, Goodman A, Parikh R, et al. Incremental prognostic value
of left ventricular global longitudinal strain in patients with aortic
stenosis and preserved ejection fraction. Circ Cardiovasc Imaging
2014;7(6):938-945.

238. Di Salvo G, Rea A, Mormile A, et al. Usefulness of bidimensional strain
imaging for predicting outcome in asymptomatic patients aged ≤ 16
years with isolated moderate to severe aortic regurgitation. Am J Cardiol
2012;110(7):1051-1055.

239. Iida N, Seo Y, Ishizu T, et al. Transmural compensation of myocardial
deformation to preserve left ventricular ejection performance in chronic
aortic regurgitation. J Am Soc Echocardiogr 2012;25(6):620-628.

240. Olsen NT, Sogaard P, Larsson HB, et al. Speckle-tracking
echocardiography for predicting outcome in chronic aortic regurgitation
during conservative management and after surgery. JACC Cardiovasc
Imaging 2011;4(3):223-230.

241. Onishi T, Kawai H, Tatsumi K, et al. Preoperative systolic strain rate
predicts postoperative left ventricular dysfunction in patients with
chronic aortic regurgitation. Circ Cardiovasc Imaging 2010;3(2):
134-141.

242. Park SH, Yang YA, Kim KY, et al. Left ventricular strain as predictor of chronic aortic regurgitation. J Cardiovasc Ultrasound 2015;23(2): 78-85.

243. Capoulade R, Clavel MA, Le Ven F, et al. Impact of left ventricular remodelling patterns on outcomes in patients with aortic stenosis. Eur Heart J Cardiovasc Imaging 2017;18(12):1378-1387.

244. Duncan AI, Lowe BS, Garcia MJ, et al. Influence of concentric left ventricular remodeling on early mortality after aortic valve replacement. Ann Thorac Surg 2008;85(6):2030-2039.

245. Dweck MR, Joshi S, Murigu T, et al. Left ventricular remodeling and hypertrophy in patients with aortic stenosis: insights from cardiovascular magnetic resonance. J Cardiovasc Magn Reson 2012;14:50.

246. Debry N, Marechaux S, Rusinaru D, et al. Prognostic significance of left ventricular concentric remodeling in patients with aortic stenosis. Arch Cardiovasc Dis 2017;110(1):26-34.

247. Treibel TA, Kozor R, Fontana M, et al. Sex dimorphism in the myocardial response to aortic stenosis. JACC Cardiovasc Imaging 2018;11(7):962-973.

248. Everett RJ, Tastet L, Clavel MA, et al. Progression of hypertrophy and myocardial fibrosis in aortic stenosis: a multicenter cardiac magnetic resonance study. Circ Cardiovasc Imaging 2018;11(6):e007451.

249. Musa TA, Treibel TA, Vassiliou VS, et al. Myocardial scar and mortality in severe aortic stenosis: data from the BSCMR valve consortium. Circulation 2018;138(18):1935-1947.

250. Treibel TA, Fontana M, Gilbertson JA, et al. Occult transthyretin cardiac amyloid in severe calcific aortic stenosis: prevalence and prognosis in patients undergoing surgical aortic valve replacement. Circ Cardiovasc Imaging 2016;9(8).

251. Scully PR, Treibel TA, Fontana M, et al. Prevalence of cardiac amyloidosis in patients referred for transcatheter aortic valve replacement. J Am Coll Cardiol 2018;71(4):463-464.

252. Cavalcante JL, Rijal S, Abdelkarim I, et al. Cardiac amyloidosis is prevalent in older patients with aortic stenosis and carries worse prognosis. J Cardiovasc Magn Reson 2017;19(1):98.

253. Castano A, Narotsky DL, Hamid N, et al. Unveiling transthyretin cardiac amyloidosis and its predictors among elderly patients with severe aortic stenosis undergoing transcatheter aortic valve replacement. Eur Heart J 2017;38(38):2879-2887.

254. Azevedo CF, Nigri M, Higuchi ML, et al. Prognostic significance of myocardial fibrosis quantification by histopathology and magnetic resonance imaging in patients with severe aortic valve disease. J Am Coll Cardiol 2010;56(4):278-287.

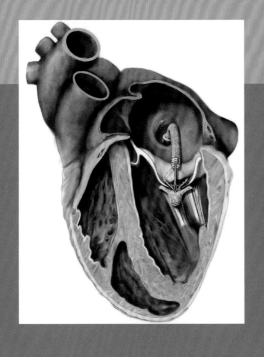

第9章
主动脉瓣狭窄：临床表现、疾病阶段和干预时机

　　主动脉瓣狭窄是老年人的常见疾病，75岁以上患病率约为12%，随着人口老龄化，该病的患病率将进一步增加。尽管在了解疾病的临床、遗传学和分子机制方面已经取得了一定进展，但尚无有效的药物治疗可以延缓血流动力学的进展，因此主动脉瓣置换术仍然是严重主动脉瓣狭窄的标准治疗方法，经导管主动脉瓣置换术的出现为不能或不愿接受外科主动脉瓣置换术的患者提供了新的治疗选择。目前经导管主动脉瓣置换术可安全地应用于中危和高危患者，但尚需更长期的随访结果来确定预后。在本章中，作者将主动脉瓣狭窄的临床表现、评估方法及疾病分期进行细致阐述。超声心动图是评估主动脉瓣狭窄的金标准，当严重主动脉瓣狭窄患者的症状史不明确，或由于低流量状态导致血流动力学严重程度不确定时，可考虑进行激发试验；主动脉瓣狭窄的分期是结合血流动力学评估、解剖学特点、症状特征和射血分数测量进行的分层，旨在强调更好的临床分期能够让早期患者和晚期伴有多种合并症的患者更准确及时地选择合适的主动脉瓣置换术时机和策略。

李　喆

Aortic Stenosis: Clinical Presentation, Disease Stages, and Timing of Intervention

Jason P. Linefsky, Catherine M. Otto

CHAPTER OUTLINE

KEY POINTS

- Aortic stenosis is an active, progressive disease that involves inflammatory and bone mineralization pathways.
- The stages of aortic stenosis combine hemodynamic assessment, anatomic findings, symptomatic status, and ejection fraction measurements to help categorize management strategies.
- Echocardiography is the gold standard for evaluating aortic stenosis.
- Stress testing is considered for patients with severe aortic stenosis when the symptom history is equivocal or hemodynamic severity is uncertain due to low-flow states.

- No medical therapy has reduced hemodynamic progression, but research is ongoing to identify novel therapeutic targets.
- Aortic valve replacement remains standard treatment for severe aortic stenosis when there are symptoms or a reduced ejection fraction.
- Transcatheter aortic valve replacement can be performed safely in patients who are at intermediate or high risk of surgical mortality, but definitive long-term durability outcomes beyond 5 years remains lacking.

Aortic stenosis (AS) is common among the elderly. with an estimated prevalence of 12% after 75 years of age.[1] Severe disease occurs in 1% to 3% of those older than 65 years of age, and the rate is expected to increase as the population ages.[2] Despite the rising estimates, temporal trends over 2 decades in the Swedish population have shown lower age-adjusted incidence rates for AS.[3] The decreasing incidence seen over 20 years despite the aging population suggests that better cardiovascular health and modification of risk factors are associated with a lower rate of development of calcific valve disease (see Chapter 4).

Although there has been significant advancement in understanding the clinical, genetic, and molecular mechanisms for disease, the treatment for AS remains aortic valve replacement (AVR). The advent of Transcatheter aortic valve replacement (TAVR) provides treatment options for patients who are not candidates or unwilling to undergo surgical aortic valve replacement (SAVR).[4] Continuous improvement in transcatheter techniques and prosthetic valve design, declining SAVR and TAVR morbidity and mortality rates, and better risk stratification are fostering a paradigm shift toward AVR in more patients earlier in the disease course and in those with end-stage disease or multiple comorbidities.

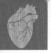

STAGES OF DISEASE

Morbidity from left ventricular (LV) outflow obstruction does not occur until very late in the disease process (Fig. 9.1), and traditional parameters of AS severity often are based on valve hemodynamics.[5] However, AS is an active disease process that is better characterized by the combination of valve leaflet changes, hemodynamics, LV function, and clinical symptoms as defined in the 2014 American College/American Heart Association (ACC/AHA) Guidelines for the Management of Patients with Valvular Heart Disease.[6] Similar to stages of heart failure, AS disease stages are classified using a progressive categorization of patients who are at risk (stage A) to end-stage disease (stage D) (Table 9.1).

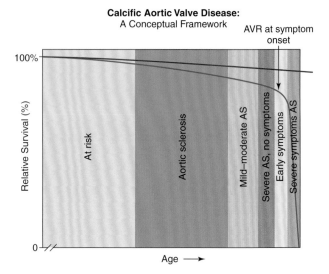

Calcific Aortic Valve Disease:
A Conceptual Framework

Fig. 9.1 Slow Progression of Aortic Stenosis (AS). Conceptual framework for the natural history of calcific aortic valve disease illustrates the spectrum of disease from the at-risk patient to the patient with end-stage, severe, symptomatic AS. After aortic sclerosis is detectable, there is an increased risk of cardiovascular events, as shown by deviation of the survival curve *(purple line)* from the expected event-free survival *(light blue line)*. At the onset of even mild symptoms, survival deviates even more from expected, with a dramatic decline in survival with severe, symptomatic AS. Aortic valve replacement *(AVR)* at the onset of early symptoms prevents these late adverse outcomes. (From Otto CM. Calcific aortic valve disease: outflow obstruction is the end stage of a systemic disease process. Eur Heart J 2009;30:1940-1942.)

TABLE 9.1 Definitions and Management by Aortic Stenosis Stage.

Stage	Symptom Description	Anatomic Features	Key Hemodynamics	LV Function	Management
A	At risk (asymptomatic)	Congenitally abnormal (bicuspid) Mild sclerosis or calcification Normal opening	$V_{max} < 2$ m/s	Normal	Atherosclerotic risk factor control Family screening, counseling (congenital valve disease) Antibiotic prophylaxis (rheumatic disease)
B	Progressive (asymptomatic)	Mild to moderate calcification Mildly restricted opening	2 m/s $\leq V_{max} < 4$ m/s 20 mmHg $\leq \Delta P < 40$ mmHg	EF $\geq 50\%$ DD	Echo surveillance 1–2 yr for moderate AS 3–5 yr for mild AS
C	Asymptomatic severe	Severe calcification and restricted opening	$V_{max} \geq 4$ m/s $\Delta P \geq 40$ mmHg		
C1	Asymptomatic severe with normal EF			EF $\geq 50\%$ LVH	Echo surveillance 6–12 mo Clinical evaluation for symptom identification Consider stress testing
C2	Asymptomatic severe with low EF			EF $< 50\%$	AVR
D	Symptomatic severe	Severe calcification and restricted opening			
D1	High gradient		$V_{max} \geq 4$ m/s $\Delta P \geq 40$ mmHg	LVH DD PHT	AVR
D2	LG reduced EF		AVA ≤ 1 cm^2 $V_{max} < 4$ m/s $\Delta P < 40$ mmHg	EF $< 50\%$	DSE to rule-out pseudosevere AS and determine contractile reserve Possible AVR Evaluate for other causes of ↓LVEF
D3	LG normal EF		AVA ≤ 1 cm^2 AVAi ≤ 0.6 cm^2/m^2 $V_{max} < 4$ m/s $\Delta P < 40$ mmHg SVI < 35 mL/m^2	EF $\geq 50\%$ Significant LVH Restrictive DD	Blood pressure control (<140 mmHg) Rule out measurement error Index AVA for small body size Consider valve calcium scoring Possible AVR

AS, Aortic stenosis; *AVA*, aortic valve area; *AVAi*, aortic valve area indexed for body surface area; *AVR*, aortic valve replacement; *DD*, diastolic dysfunction; *ΔP*, mean aortic gradient; *DSE*, dobutamine stress echocardiography; *EF*, ejection fraction; *LV*, left ventricular; *LG*, low-gradient; *LVH*, left ventricular hypertrophy; *PHT*, pulmonary hypertension; *SVI*, stroke volume index; *V$_{max}$*, maximum transvalvular aortic velocity.

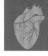

ETIOLOGY

The most common causes of AS are calcific disease, a congenital bicuspid valve, and rheumatic heart disease (Table 9.2). Echocardiography allows an accurate diagnosis with characterization of the number of valve cusps, degree of leaflet calcification, and evidence for commissural fusion in rheumatic valve disease (Fig. 9.2). Calcific disease of a trileaflet valve is rare before the age of 50 years; in older adults, bicuspid valve disease still accounts for most cases of severe AS before the seventh to eighth decade.[7]

Bicuspid aortic valve disease often is associated with ascending aortic aneurysms and, less commonly, with aortic coarctation (see Chapter 11). Rheumatic aortic valve disease is rare in Europe and North America, but it is still prevalent in other world regions and is invariably accompanied by mitral valve involvement.[8-10]

CLINICAL PRESENTATION

Clinical History

The most common AS presentation is an asymptomatic systolic murmur during physical examination or an incidental finding on echocardiography. Symptoms due to AS do not appear until significant hemodynamic obstruction occurs, although the exact degree of stenosis resulting in symptoms varies between patients.[11] When outflow obstruction is only mild to moderate, alternative causes of symptoms should be sought.

The classic symptoms of angina, syncope, and heart failure were first described in middle-aged adults with rheumatic heart disease and now are rarely seen in patients who are educated about the disease process and followed prospectively. However, a detailed history is important to identify functional changes over time and to distinguish symptoms of AS from other medical conditions such as coronary disease, pulmonary disease, and deconditioning.

Dyspnea on exertion or decreased exercise tolerance is the most common initial symptom due to AS and is often related to diastolic dysfunction and elevated LV filling pressures.[12] A recent study found that dyspnea was the primary concern in 70% of symptomatic patients and was independently associated with higher Doppler-derived E/e′ ratios.[13] In the elderly, decreased exercise tolerance is not always recognized by the patient as an important symptom because disease progression is insidious, and other comorbidities often contribute to impaired functional status. Approximately 18% to 37% of patients with severe AS initially categorized as asymptomatic have symptoms when performing exercise.[14-16]

Angina is the second most common symptom of patients with AS. Angina results from a myocardial oxygen supply-demand mismatch and it more often occurs with coexisting coronary artery disease (CAD) and hypertension. Approximately 20% to 50% of patients with AS have coexisting CAD, and the likelihood of coronary disease increases with presence of atherosclerotic risk factors.[17] Myocardial ischemia in AS results from a unique combination of left ventricular hypertrophy (LVH) and associated hemodynamic changes, including

	Clinical	Associated
Cause	**Presentation**	**Findings**
Common		
Calcific aortic valve disease	Advanced age Atherosclerotic risk factors	Atherosclerotic coronary disease Frailty
Congenital valve disease	Family history Earlier presentation than calcific aortic valve disease	Aortic aneurysms or coarctation
Rheumatic	Endemic areas Rheumatic fever	Mitral valve disease
Uncommon		
Metabolic	Alkaptonuria (arthritis, high levels of homogentisic acid) Lupus (rash, joint pains, kidney disease)	Brown or blue pigment deposition Leaflet thickening and verrucous vegetations Antiphospholipid antibodies
Radiation	Hodgkin's lymphoma Breast cancer Mediastinal irradiation	Premature coronary disease Pericardial and myocardial disease Fibrosis/calcification of other valves and annulus
Subvalvular	Asymptomatic with a murmur Subaortic membrane or fibromuscular ridge	Aortic regurgitation Associated congenital defects (VSD, coarctation, PS)
Supravalvular	Williams syndrome Homozygous FH	Short stature, elfin facies Renal abnormalities Impaired cognition Tuberous xanthomas LDL-cholesterol > 500 mg/dL

TABLE 9.2 Causes of Aortic Stenosis With Distinguishing Features.

FH, Familial hypercholesterolemia; *LDL*, low-density lipoprotein; *PS*, pulmonic stenosis; *VSD*, ventricular septal defect.

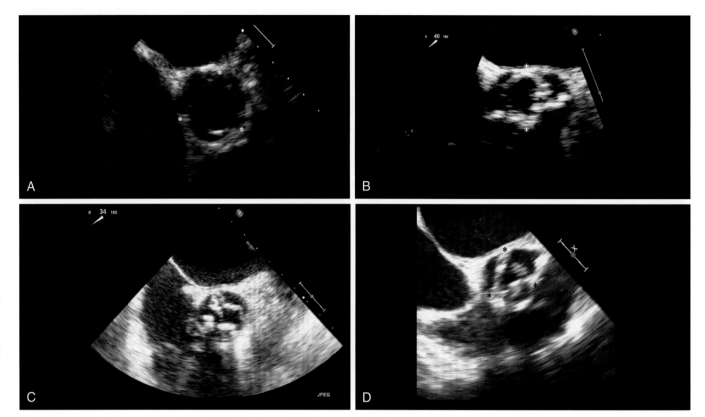

Fig. 9.2 Anatomic Features of Aortic Stenosis for Different Causes During Systole. (A) Short-axis transesophageal view of a normal trileaflet aortic valve with three commissures *(asterisk)*. The aortic valve opens widely with thin leaflets (Video 9.2A ▶). (B) A congenital bicuspid valve with only two commissures *(asterisk)* in an anteroposterior orientation. The opening of the valve is restricted, with thickened leaflets and an oval fish-mouth orifice (Video 9.2B ▶). (C) Calcific aortic valve in a trileaflet valve. There is an irregular calcification, thickening, and opening (Video 9.2C ▶). (D) Rheumatic aortic stenosis has significant commissural fusion *(asterisk)* and diffuse leaflet thickening leading to a reduced triangular orifice (Video 9.2D ▶)

a decreased diastolic coronary perfusion pressure, impaired myocardial relaxation, decreased coronary vessel density, shorter diastolic filling times, and microvascular dysfunction.[18] Lower coronary flow reserve also occurs in AS, resulting in exertional angina symptoms.[19]

Syncope or exertional dizziness is the least frequent component of the classic symptom triad. Causes of syncope in AS patients include cardiac arrhythmias, reduced cardiac output due to the narrowed obstructive valve, or a baroreceptor-mediated vasodilatory and bradycardic reflex during high LV wall stress. AS patients with severe stenosis and syncope are reported to have higher LV wall stress and lower stroke volumes.[20] Ectopic ventricular beats are more common when LVH occurs in AS.[21]

Physical Examination

The cardiovascular examination for AS focuses on cardiac auscultation and carotid pulse palpation. No single physical examination finding completely excludes AS or predicts severity, but it instead identifies individuals who need further noninvasive testing. The published diagnostic accuracy for physical findings in AS are usually based on highly trained cardiology experts; less experienced examiners may not identify these abnormalities with the same acumen.[22,23]

A systolic ejection murmur is found almost universally in AS. It results from turbulent flow across the narrowed aortic orifice.[24,25]

The murmur typically is loudest at the base of the heart along the right second intercostal space, but the site of maximum intensity in some people is closer to the apex. Radiation of the murmur to the right clavicular area and carotid artery often is detected; less commonly the murmur radiates toward the apex. The intensity of the murmur does not reliably exclude severe obstruction because most patients with severe AS have only a grade 2 or 3 murmur. However, a very loud murmur (≥grade 4 with a palpable thrill) is very specific for severe AS. Late systolic peaking of the murmur intensity correlates with more severe disease, but the auscultation properties of the murmur in any individual can vary greatly due to individual body habitus, LV function, and coexisting aortic regurgitation.

A soft or single second heart sound (S_2) occurs in AS due to the rigidity of the aortic valve cusps, and leaflet closure does not result in an audible sound. The presence of a normally split S^2 in an adult with AS reliability excludes severe valve obstruction.

The carotid arterial pulse is examined for timing and amplitude. A normal carotid pulse is easily palpable with light pressure and occurs simultaneously with precordial apex pulsation. Obstruction to blood flow from AS produces a weak and slowly rising carotid pulse (i.e., pulsus parvus et tardus). However, when there is coexisting hypertension or atherosclerosis, the carotid upstroke is relatively normal in timing and magnitude, reflecting reduced vascular compliance rather than the absence of severe AS.

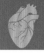

EVALUATION

Echocardiography

Echocardiography is the primary diagnostic modality for the evaluation of AS, allowing determination of the cause, disease severity, hemodynamic consequences, and prognosis for clinical decision making. Transthoracic echocardiography is recommended for initial assessment, periodic surveillance, and occurrence of new symptoms or physical examination changes.[6] Blood pressure and heart rate are reported on the echocardiogram at the time of the study because valvular gradients are influenced by hypertension and volume flow rate.

Two-dimensional (2D) transthoracic echocardiography provides imaging of morphology and calcification of the aortic valve (see Fig. 9.2). Restricted opening of the aortic valve leaflets is observed, but measuring the anatomic valve area by 2D or 3D echocardiography is limited by irregular 3D surfaces and calcification shadowing artifacts (Fig. 9.3). The severity of calcification is categorized because more severe calcification is associated with more advanced disease (Fig. 9.4). Severity of stenosis is determined from hemodynamic assessment with Doppler echocardiography (see Chapter 8). Continuous-wave (CW) Doppler through the aortic valve measures maximum transaortic jet velocity and mean gradient. Severity categories correlate with prognosis (Fig. 9.5), with severe AS defined as maximum velocity above 4 m/s (mean gradient of 40 mmHg), and mild AS is defined as a maximum velocity below 3 m/s (mean gradient of 20 mmHg).

When AS velocity is less than 4 m/s but there is concern about severe AS, the stroke volume index is calculated, and functional aortic valve area (AVA) is calculated using the continuity equation (Fig. 9.6). A low-flow state is defined as a stroke volume index of 35 mL/m^2 or less, and low-flow, low-gradient (LFLG) AS is defined low-flow with a low-gradient (velocity <4.0 m/s) but a valve area of less than 1.0 cm^2.

The two main causes of LFLG AS are a reduced LV ejection fraction (EF) (i.e., stage D2 or classic LFLG severe AS) or a small LV chamber size due to concentric LVH with a preserved EF (i.e., stage D3 or paradoxical LFLG severe AS). It also is important to ensure measurement accuracy and avoid an erroneous diagnosis of severe low-flow AS when only moderate AS is present. Potential pitfalls in echocardiographic diagnosis include a nonparallel alignment of the Doppler probe with the aortic jet, incorrect positioning of the sample volume for LV outflow velocities, and underestimation of the LV outflow tract diameter. Oblique image planes result in a smaller measured outflow tract diameter, which is then squared, leading to large errors in the calculated AVA. In adults, LV outflow tract size does not change over time. Changes between studies distinguish between disease progression and measurement variation.

In cases of LFLG severe AS with a low EF (<50%), the next step is low-dose dobutamine stress echocardiography (see Low-Dose Dobutamine Stress Echocardiography). Diagnosis of paradoxical LFLG AS with discordance between gradients and valve area but a preserved EF often is a diagnostic dilemma.[26] Although diastolic dysfunction, concentric LVH, and reduced LV longitudinal shortening may result in a reduced stroke volume despite a normal EF, meticulous evaluation for possibilities of measurement error should be considered, especially when there is minimal LVH and only mild diastolic changes.

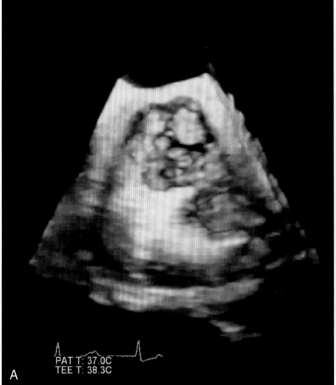
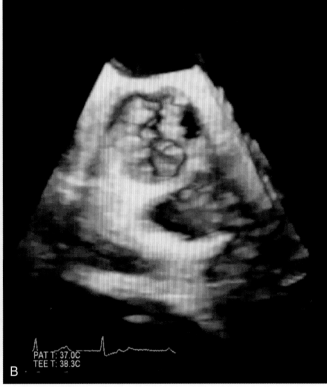

Fig. 9.3 Three-Dimensional (3D) Echocardiography in Aortic Stenosis (Video 9.3 ▶). Short-axis, 3D zoom mode shows the aortic valve in systole (A) and diastole (B). Thickening, calcification, and restricted opening are seen. Dropout artifact of the aortic cusp body is prominent during diastole, as is commonly seen using 3D echocardiography.

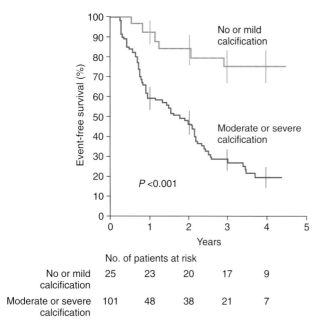

Fig. 9.4 Effect of Leaflet Calcification on Outcome in Asymptomatic Severe Aortic Stenosis. Kaplan-Meier estimates of event-free survival among 25 patients with no or mild aortic valve calcification compared with that among 101 patients with moderate or severe calcification. All patients had an aortic jet velocity of at least 4 m/s at study entry. The *vertical bars* indicate standard errors. (From Rosenhek R, Binder T, Porenta G, et al. Predictors of outcome in severe, asymptomatic aortic stenosis. N Engl J Med 2000;343:611-617.)

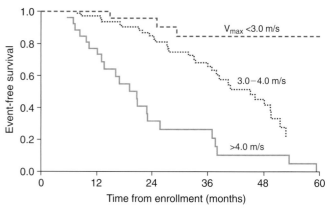

Fig. 9.5 Impact of Aortic Jet Velocity on Outcome in Asymptomatic Aortic Stenosis. Cox regression analysis shows event-free survival for 123 initially asymptomatic adults with valvular aortic stenosis, defined by maximum aortic jet velocity (V_{max}) at entry ($P < 0.001$ by log-rank test). (From Otto CM, Burwash IG, Legget ME, et al. Prospective study of asymptomatic valvular aortic stenosis. Clinical, echocardiographic, and exercise predictors of outcome. Circulation 1997;95:2262-2270.)

Other possible causes of low flow through the aortic valve, such as mitral regurgitation, atrial fibrillation, significant hypertension, and right heart failure, should be ruled out. In patients with small body sizes, the AVA may be proportionally smaller and can be indexed for body surface area; conversely, AVA does not increase with obesity, and indexing should be used cautiously for patients with a large body size.[27]

When aortic jet velocity is higher than normal (>2 m/s), but the valve does not appear significantly thickened or calcified, other conditions need to be considered. Coexisting aortic regurgitation and other high-flow states produce elevated aortic velocities without obstruction. The level of obstruction must be confirmed because a high outflow velocity may be due to a subaortic membrane or hypertrophic cardiomyopathy. Valvular AS is distinguished from dynamic subvalvular obstruction based on the shape of the CW Doppler velocity curve (Fig. 9.7) and color Doppler evidence for the anatomic site of obstruction. Supravalvular AS is very uncommon and associated with certain congenital conditions such as Williams syndrome and familial hypercholesterolemia. Supravalvular stenosis is identified by high aortic velocity and a very narrow aorta with a normal-appearing valve in susceptible patient populations.

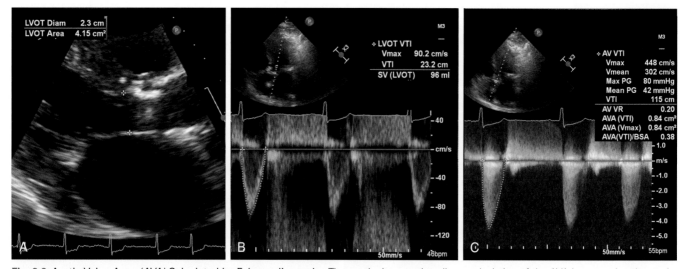

Fig. 9.6 Aortic Valve Area (AVA) Calculated by Echocardiography. The continuity equation allows calculation of the AVA by assuming the stroke volume through the left ventricular outflow tract (LVOT) is the same as through the aortic valve. The volume of blood is estimated by measuring a velocity-time integral (VTI) in the LVOT using pulse-wave Doppler (A) and then multiplying the LVOT area, assumed as a circular orifice with the diameter of the outflow tract (B) (Video 9.6 ⬤). Dividing this product by the VTI through the aortic valve using continuous-wave Doppler (C) gave an AVA in this patient of 0.84 cm².

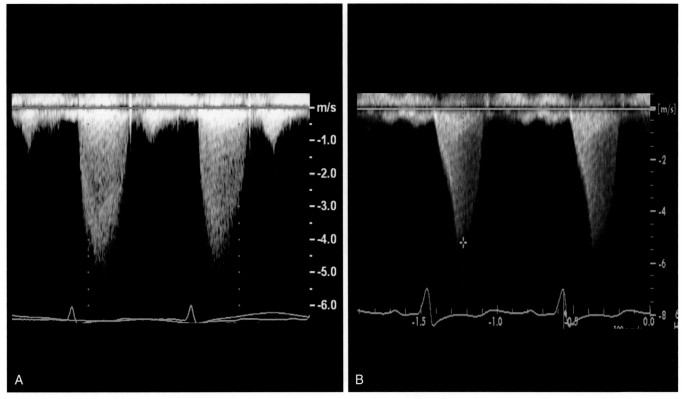

Fig. 9.7 Comparison of Aortic Stenosis and Hypertrophic Cardiomyopathy Spectral Waveform. Shown are continuous-wave Doppler spectral waveforms from a patient with fixed obstruction in severe aortic stenosis (A) and a dynamic obstruction in hypertrophic cardiomyopathy (B). The hypertrophic cardiomyopathy dynamic obstruction is distinguished from aortic stenosis by the middle to late peaking *(dagger shape)* of the waveform and change in gradient with loading conditions (see Fig. 9.6).

Cardiac Catheterization

Invasive evaluation for AS is rarely necessary but is helpful in selected cases with discrepant clinical and imaging findings. Care is needed because there is a risk of cerebral emboli with retrograde catheterization across a stenotic aortic valve, although this has not been a major issue in patients undergoing TAVR.[28] Key findings from hemodynamic catheterization include hemodynamic verification of the level of obstruction (i.e., subvalvular or valvular), measurement of the mean systolic pressure gradient, AVA calculation with the Gorlin formula, and the timing and shape of the pressure tracing waveforms.[29] Similar to echocardiography, technical factors with hemodynamic catheterization should be taken into account when interpreting severity.

Pressure tracings are recorded simultaneously in the midcavity of the LV and in the proximal ascending aorta, using 6-Fr or larger catheters with side holes, flushed with saline to optimize the pressure waveform contour in terms of overdumping and underdumping (Fig. 9.8). Less ideal, but a commonly practiced technique, is a single pullback measurement of pressure tracings from the LV to the aorta. The difference between the peak LV and peak aortic pressures (i.e., peak-to-peak gradient) is easy to measure but does not have an echocardiographic correlation because those two pressures do not occur at the same point in time. The maximum instantaneous gradient at catheterization correlates best with the maximum velocity by Doppler echocardiography; mean gradients by both techniques correlate well if loading conditions are matched between the echocardiogram and cardiac catheterization.

Because AVA calculation depends on measurement of transaortic volume flow rate and pressure measurements, variation in cardiac output techniques affects determination of AVA at cathterization.[30] In clinical practice, cardiac output is measured by thermodilution technique or Fick equation estimates, with potential measurement variations and limitations of each approach.[31] Recognizing the technical pitfalls, echocardiography and catheterization aid in reconciling discrepancies when present.

Stress Testing

Stress testing is useful when the decision for AVR remains indeterminate despite the clinical history and resting hemodynamic assessment. The indolent nature of AS often leads patients to consider themselves asymptomatic because they discount symptoms with declining activity. Conversely, symptomatic patients may have low gradients, and the contribution and benefit of correction of the valvular disease may be uncertain. Dynamic assessment with stress testing is performed using exercise or pharmacologic protocols depending on the clinical scenario. Stress testing provides prognostic information by identifying subsets of AS patients who are at high risk for adverse clinical events or AVR (Table 9.3).[11,15,16,32–37]

Exercise Treadmill Stress Testing

The most common indication for stress testing of AS patients is to verify that those with severe AS (stage C) are truly asymptomatic. Exercise testing in apparently asymptomatic AS is safe when supervised by highly trained personnel and if terminated at the onset of

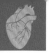

rrssrrrrsrrsrsssrsrsrrrrr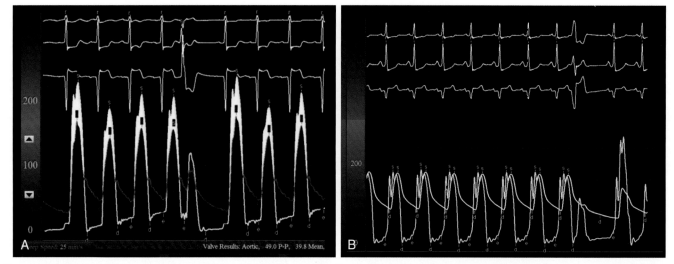

Fig. 9.8 Comparison of Aortic Stenosis (AS) and Hypertrophic Cardiomyopathy During Hemodynamic Catheterization. (A) Simultaneous pressure-wave contours in AS demonstrate a delayed and reduced aortic upstroke with a mean gradient at 40 mmHg *(shaded area)*. An increase in aortic pulse pressure *(red pressure curve)* after a pause from a premature ventricular contraction is seen. (B) A dynamic obstruction in hypertrophic cardiomyopathy occurs with an augmented ventricular beat after a premature ventricular contraction. Unlike AS, there is a decreased arterial pulse pressure *(white pressure curve)* with a spike and dome configuration.

TABLE 9.3 Selected Outcome Studies on Exercise Testing in Asymptomatic Aortic Stenosis.

Study	Mean Follow-Up (N)	Protocol	AS Criteria	Abnormal Criteria	Outcome	Key Findings
Otto et al, 1997[11]	30 mo (104)	Bruce	$V_{max} \geq$ 2.5 m/s	↓SBP > 10 mmHg ↓ST segment > 2 mm Ventricular arrhythmia	AVR or death	Exercise not predictive of outcome with adjustment for baseline rest hemodynamics
Amato et al, 2001[15]	14.8 mo (66)	Ellestad (treadmill)	AVA ≤ 1 cm²	↓ST segment ≥ 1 mm (men) or ≥ 2 mm (women) Chest pain/presyncope Ventricular arrhythmia ↑SBP < 20 mmHg	Symptoms or death	HR = 7.43 for + ET 6% sudden death in cohort (all had abnormal test)
Alborino et al, 2002[35]	36 mo (30)	Upright bicycle	ΔP ≥ 30 mmHg	Limiting breathlessness (at < 5 METs) Angina or syncope ECG criteria for ischemia ↑SBP < 20 mmHg Ventricular arrhythmia	CV death or AVR	60% rate of + ET Event-free survival at 3 years: 33% for + ET 83% for − ET No CV deaths occurred
Das et al, 2005[32]	12 mo (125)	Modified Bruce (treadmill)	AVA ≤ 1.4 cm²	Limiting breathlessness Chest discomfort Dizziness	Symptoms or death	HR 7.73 (95% CI: 2.8–21.4) No deaths occurred
Lancellotti et al, 2005[16]	15 mo (69)	Semisupine bicycle (↑25 W/2 min)	AVA ≤ 1 cm²	Angina or dyspnea ↓ST segment ≥ 2 mm ↑SBP < 20 mmHg Ventricular arrhythmia	Symptoms, HF, CV death, or AVR	78% of patients with outcome had + ET ↑P ≥ 18 mmHg predictor of outcome
Maréchaux et al, 2010[33]	20 mo (186)	Semisupine bicycle (↑25 W/3 min)	AVA ≤ 1.5 cm²	Limiting symptoms SBP fall from baseline Ventricular arrhythmia	CV death or AVR	27% had + ET Patients with − ET had HR = 1.67 (95% CI: 1.32–2.13) per 10 mmHg increase of ΔP
Lancellotti et al, 2012[34]	19 mo (105)	Semisupine bicycle (↑25 W/2 min)	AVAi ≤ 0.6 cm²/m²	Limiting breathlessness (at < 75 W exercise) Angina/dizziness/syncope ↓ST segment ≥ 2 mm ↑SBP < 20 mmHg Ventricular arrhythmia	CV death or AVR	HR = 2.0 (95% CI:1.1–3.6) for PHT 7 deaths occurred, all had PHT

Continued

>> **186**

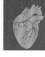

	Mean		AS			
Study	Follow-Up (N)	Protocol	Criteria	Abnormal Criteria	Outcome	Key Findings
Levy et al, 2014[36]	28 mo (43)	Upright cycle (↑20 W/min)	AVA ≤ 1 cm² or AVAi ≤ 0.6 cm²/m²	Limiting breathlessness Angina/dizziness/syncope SBP fall from baseline Ventricular arrhythmia	AVR referral due to symptoms	28% had + ET HR = 3.1 (95% CI: 1–8.7) for Vo₂ ≥ 14 mL/kg/min HR = 3.7 (95% CI: 1.3–10.3) for VE/Vco₂ slope > 34
Saeed et al, 2018[37]	35 mo (316)	Modified Bruce (treadmill)	AVA ≤ 1.5 cm	Significant symptom ↑SBP < 20 mmHg Sustained tachyarrhythmia	AVR or death	Annual ETT performed 1st ETT: 29% had symptoms Event-free survival at 2 years: 46% for + ET 70% for − ET

TABLE 9.3 **Selected Outcome Studies on Exercise Testing in Asymptomatic Aortic Stenosis.—cont'd**

AS, Aortic stenosis; *AVA*, aortic valve area; *AVAi*, aortic valve area indexed for body surface area; *AVR*, aortic valve replacement; *CI*, confidence interval; *CV*, cardiovascular; *ΔP*, mean aortic gradient; *ET*, symptom-limited exercise test; *ETT*, exercise tolerance test; *HF*, heart failure; *HR*, hazard ratio; *−*, negative; *METs*, metabolic equivalents for task; *N*, number of patients; *PHT*, pulmonary hypertension (exercise-induced pulmonary artery systolic pressure > 60 mmHg); *+*, positive; *SBP*, systolic blood pressure; *VE/Vco₂*, ventilation/carbon dioxide output; *Vo₂*, peak oxygen consumption; *W*, watt.

symptoms or with a fall in blood pressure. Exercise testing is risky in symptomatic severe AS (stage D1) and is not recommended. A careful history immediately before stress testing is mandatory.

Abnormal exercise findings are usually defined by breathlessness at low workloads, chest pain, dizziness, systolic blood pressure failing to rise more than 20 mmHg or falling from baseline, horizontal or downsloping ST-segment depression of 2 mm or greater, or more than 3 consecutive ventricular beats. Distinguishing limiting symptoms from normal exercise fatigue is challenging, but patients with symptoms at low workloads (<75 watts or 5 metabolic equivalents for task [METs]) are considered to be symptomatic. Patients with fatigue near 80% of their predicted maximum workload that resolves quickly with rest are considered to have a normal response.

Low-Dose Dobutamine Stress Echocardiography

Low-flow states are defined as an indexed stroke volume less than or equal to 35 mL/m², most often due to LV systolic dysfunction, which is called classic low-flow, low-gradient AS.[38] Others have defined low flow based on a peak flow rate of 200 mL/s or less and suggest that stress testing is not helpful when the flow rate is higher than this value.[39] Systolic dysfunction may result from severe valvular disease or from an underlying cardiomyopathy (frequently ischemic in nature). Impaired contractility in combination with a higher afterload on the myocardium leads to reduced opening of a moderately diseased aortic valve (i.e., pseudosevere AS). In symptomatic patients with an AVR of 1.0 cm² or less with a low gradient (mean gradient < 40 mmHg, velocity < 4.0 m/s) and EF less than 50%, low-dose dobutamine stress echocardiography (DSE) is safe and reliably identifies whether the reduced AVA is due to severe valve obstruction or only moderate AS in the setting of primary myocardial disease.

Dobutamine protocols usually begin at 5 μg/kg/min and titrate 5 μg/kg/min every 5 minutes to a target dose of 20 μg/kg/min. Dobutamine doses above 20 μg/kg/min do not usually raise transvalvular flow rates; they instead augment cardiac output by increasing heart rates.[40] Measures of stroke volume, valve gradients, EF, and wall motion are made at each stage. DSE is diagnostic for severe AS if the aortic velocity reaches 4 m/s with a simultaneous AVA of 1 cm² or less at any point during the test. An AVA above 1 cm² or a failure of velocity to increase to more than 4 m/s is consistent with pseudosevere AS.

In some patients, the transaortic volume flow rate fails to increase in response to dobutamine. These individuals usually have a severe cardiomyopathy and very poor prognosis with or without AVR. The inability to increase stroke volume or lack of contractile reserve is defined as an increase in stroke volume of less than 20%. It may be helpful for patients with a lower increase in stroke volume to calculate the estimated AVA if the flow rate is normal.[41] This projected AVA performed better in the diagnosis of severe AS than traditional DSE measures in a multicenter observational study.[41]

The use of stress echocardiography in patients with LFLG AS with preserved EF has been evaluated in few studies and is not recommended in current guidelines. Clavel et al[42] suggest that projected valve area at a normal flow rate on stress echocardiography identifies those with severe AS, based on clinical outcomes. Although there were no complications of stress testing in this small study, there is concern that use of dobutamine in patients with a small hypertrophied ventricle might result in even further reduction in LV volumes and forward stroke volume.

Computed Tomography

CT is useful for two situations in adults with AS: prosthetic aortic valve sizing before TAVR (see Chapter 13) and quantification of aortic valve calcium (AVC) to assess disease severity in the setting of low gradients (Fig. 9.9). AVC is scored with Agatston scoring methods that are similar to those used for coronary artery calcium scoring.[43] Some researchers suggest normalizing AVC by the valve area, producing AVC density measurements, but total scores and density show similar diagnostic and prognostic abilities.

There is a close linear correlation (R = 0.81, P < 0.0001) between valve weight and AVC scores, as demonstrated in a study of 126 severe AS patients who underwent AVC scoring within 6 months of AVR.[44] However, despite a mean AVA of 0.77 cm² and a mean gradient of 55 mmHg, AVC scores exhibited a very wide variation (59–11,000 AU). AVC scores do not follow a normal distribution in population studies, and progression of AVC has been associated only with male sex and baseline calcification.[45] Males have consistently had more calcification and higher valve weights despite similar amounts of hemodynamic obstruction from AS.[44,46] Studies defining optimal AVC cutoff values are sex specific, with more than 1200 AU for women (>300 AU/cm² for AVC density) and more than 2000 for men (>500 AU/cm² for AVC density) for severe AS.[47]

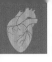

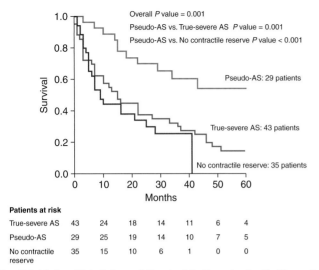

Fig. 9.9 Higher Risk-Adjusted Survival in Pseudo–Aortic Stenosis (AS). Kaplan–Meier survival estimates in low-flow, low-gradient AS undergoing conservative treatment according to the results of dobutamine testing. (From Fougères E, Tribouilloy C, Monchi M, et al. Outcomes of pseudo-severe aortic stenosis under conservative treatment. Eur Heart J 2012;33:2426-2433.)

The utility of AVC in clinical decision making remains unclear. Some experts suggest using AVC scores in classic low-flow AS (stage D2) when there is a lack of flow reserve or for stage D3 disease.[47,48] However, AVC cutoffs were validated for severe AS by echocardiography during normal flow conditions (stage D1), and different treatment strategies have not been studied with the use of AVC scores.

The prognostic value of severe AVC density is clear, with a 2.5-fold increased risk of mortality independent of clinical and hemodynamic parameters.[49] Increased cardiovascular risk associated with AVC also has been well established in patients without valvular obstruction.[50,51]

Biomarkers

The role of biomarkers in AS remains a subject of much interest, but studies have not yet confirmed a definitive role for them in evaluating AS patients. The best-studied biomarkers, brain natriuretic peptide (BNP) and troponin (Tn), associate with pathologic alterations in LV geometry and function. However, changes with LV pathology are not specific for AS and can exhibit interindividual variation. European, but not American, guidelines provide a weak recommendation for the use of BNP in the evaluation of AS, stating that markedly elevated BNP levels in an asymptomatic AS patient with low surgical risk may be considered for AVR.[52] BNP levels are associated more strongly with LV mass, systolic function, and symptomatic status, rather than hemodynamic severity.[53]

Although some studies have reported a moderate association between BNP and clinical outcomes, other studies have demonstrated limited usefulness due to significant interindividual variation. Cimadevilla et al[54] prospectively followed 142 asymptomatic severe AS patients for 2 years, and after adjustment for age, sex, and AVA, N-terminal-pro-BNP (NT-pro-BNP) was not associated with AS-related events.

In the largest study on BNP in AS, Clavel et al[55] followed 1953 patients with at least moderate AS for an average of 3.8 ± 2.4 years and analyzed BNP level ratios indexed to age and sex upper limits of normal. BNP ratios were strongly associated with mortality in the cohort (Fig. 9.10) after accounting for clinical parameters, hemodynamic severity, LV function, and AVR. However, the beneficial impact of BNP as a determinant for AVR in asymptomatic AS remains unknown.

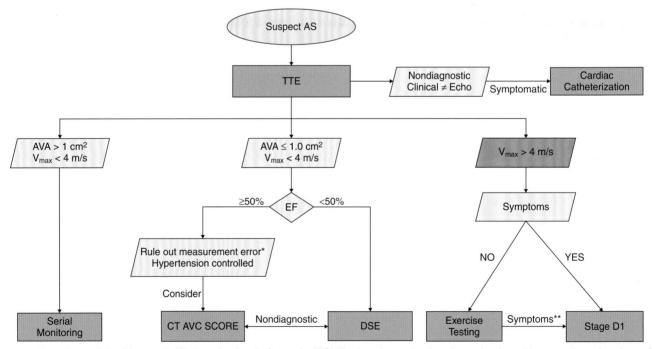

Fig. 9.10 Flowchart of the Diagnostic Workup for Aortic Stenosis (AS). Noninvasive evaluation always begins with a transthoracic echocardiogram. Invasive evaluation with catheterization is reserved for when the echocardiographic images are nondiagnostic or there are discrepant clinical symptoms and signs of severe AS exist despite nonsevere echocardiographic findings. Technical issues (asterisk) such as underestimation of outflow tract diameter or nonparallel alignment of Doppler should be considered. Evaluation includes calculations to adjust for body size with the stroke volume index <35 mL/m^2, indexed aortic valve area <0.6 cm^2/m^2. Symptoms (double asterisk) with exercise testing are defined as AS symptoms (e.g., angina, syncope, dyspnea) at very low workloads. AVA, Aortic valve area; AVC, aortic valve calcification; CT, computed tomography; DSE, dobutamine stress echocardiography; EF, ejection fraction; TTE, transthoracic echocardiography; V$_{max}$, maximum aortic jet velocity.

High-sensitivity Tn assays detected elevated Tn concentrations in patients with AS. The ability of Tn, a marker of myocyte necrosis, to identify a transition from compensated LVH to a decompensated ventricle with fibrosis can help identify high-risk patients warranting AVR. In a study by Chin et al with more than 250 patients with AS,[56] Tn I concentrations were associated with LV mass and midwall fibrosis as detected by cardiac magnetic resonance imaging (MRI). In the same study, Tn I levels were associated with AVR and death after adjustment for demographics, EF, and mean gradients. Tn levels were not associated with CAD. However, similar to BNP, there is significant overlap in Tn levels with LVH and fibrosis, and the demographically adjusted risk for AS events was only fairly modest, with a hazard ratio of 1.6 per logarithmic increase of Tn.

Given the conflicting evidence for a single biomarker to definitively aid in clinical decision making, novel biomarkers of cardiovascular stress have been studied collectively with BNP and Tn in AS. Lindman et al studied eight known heart failure biomarkers in 345 severe AS patients at a single center and reported incremental survival discrimination with elevations above median values for growth differentiation factor 15, soluble ST2, and NT-pro-BNP.[57] For each biomarker elevation, there was a 60% increase in the relative risk of mortality. High-sensitivity Tn T levels were associated with fibrosis and inflammation in surgical biopsy specimens but were not additive with the biomarker model on prognosis. The utility of using diverse biomarkers representing various pathologic pathways in AS risk stratification is promising but awaits further validation studies before clinical application.

CLINICAL COURSE

AS is a slowly progressive, active disease process with a long, asymptomatic early phase, followed by a later phase in which hemodynamic obstruction accelerates more rapidly, leading to significant complications and high mortality rates if not treated promptly. Symptoms herald ominous problems such as heart failure, arrhythmia, and sudden death. Serial clinical and imaging evaluations are necessary, with interval timing determined by baseline hemodynamic severity, comorbidities, and changes over time. Guideline recommendations for echocardiography intervals are based on the average progression from clinical studies, but they must be individualized because some patients can progress rapidly. Changes in clinical status always warrant a repeat evaluation.

At Risk for Aortic Stenosis (Stage A)

Risk factors for calcific aortic valve disease include clinical factors, a congenital bicuspid aortic valve, and older age (see Chapter 4).[58] Adults with detectable areas of focal leaflet thickening or calcification on echocardiography (i.e., aortic valve sclerosis) have a higher risk of adverse cardiovascular outcomes even in the absence of hemodynamic obstruction to LV outflow.[51] Many of these patients progress to more severe leaflet disease, with a velocity greater than 2.0 m/s and a measurable pressure gradient across the valve. Initial retrospective, single-center studies reported rates of progression to AS of up to 66% over 5 years,[59] but population based studies have shown a lower rate of approximately 2% per year.[60] In the Cardiovascular Health Study, aortic sclerosis was identified at baseline in 29% of patient older than 65 years, but only 9% developed AS over 5 years.[61]

Progressive Mild to Moderate Aortic Stenosis (Stage B)

Over the past 2 decades, several studies have documented the hemodynamic progression of AS using noninvasive echocardiography evaluations (Table 9.4).[11,62-71] Average reported yearly progression for maximum velocity, mean gradients, and AVA are between 0.15 and 0.3 m/s, 3 and 4 mmHg, and 0.1 and 0.2 cm^2, respectively, but with wide individual variation in progression rates. Accurate prediction of the rate of

TABLE 9.4   Contemporary Studies on Hemodynamic Progression of Aortic Stenosis.

Study	Study Design	Follow-Up (N)	AS Criteria	$\Delta V_{max}/\Delta P/\Delta AVA$	Associated Predictors
Otto et al, 1997[11]	Prospective cohort	2.5 years, (123)	$V_{max} \geq 2.5$	0.32/7.0/−0.12	None identified
Rosenhek et al, 2004[63]	Retrospective university cohort	4.0 years, (176)	$2.5 \leq V_{max} < 4$	0.24/X/X	AVC, age, CAD
Rossebø et al, 2008[62]	Multicenter RCT	4.3 years, (1873)	$2.5 \leq V_{max} < 4$	0.16/2.8/−0.03	X
Kamalesh et al, 2009[64]	Retrospective university cohort	2.5 years, (166)	$AVA \geq 1.5$ cm^2	X/3.0/−0.22	DM
Chan et al, 2010[65]	Multicenter RCT	3.5 years, (269)	$2.5 \leq V_{max} < 4$	0.24/3.9/−0.08	Age, AVC
Nistri et al, 2012[66]	Retrospective PCP-referred cohort	2.9 years, (153)	Any degree of AS	0.26/X/X	LVEDD
Kearney et al, 2012[67]	Prospective cohort	6.5 years, (147)	$P \geq 10$	X/5.0/−0.11	AVC, baseline P, eGFR < 30
Eveborn et al, 2013[68]	Population based	6.4 years, (118)	$P \geq 15$	X/3.2/X	Baseline P > 30
Nguyen et al, 2015[69]	Prospective cohort	2.9 years, (149)	$P \geq 10$	X/3.0/X	Baseline P, AVC
de Oliveira Moraes et al, 2015[70]	Retrospective university cohort	2.4 years, (125)	$V_{max} > 2.5$	0.14/4.1/−0.07	Baseline P, DM, heart rate
Ersboll et al, 2015[71]	Retrospective university cohort	3.1 years, (1240)	$10 \leq P \leq 40$	X/6.8%,[a] 7.1%[b]/X	Age, baseline P, CKD, HL

[a]Reported as percent change from baseline values for mild AS.
[b]Reported as percent change from baseline values for moderate AS; estimated to be 2.2 mmHg change.
AS, Aortic stenosis; *AVA*, aortic valve area; *AVC*, moderate or severe aortic valve calcification; *CKD*, chronic kidney disease; Δ, yearly average change; *ΔAVA*, yearly decrease in aortic valve area (cm^2); *CAD*, coronary artery disease; *DM*, diabetes mellitus; *eGFR*, estimated glomerular filtration rate (mL/min); *HL*, hyperlipidemia; *LVEDD*, left ventricular end-diastolic diameter; *N*, number of patients; *P*, mean aortic gradient (mmHg); *PCP*, primary care provider; *RCT*, randomized, controlled trial; *V_{max}*, maximum aortic jet velocity (m/s); *X*, not reported.

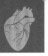

progression in an individual patient is not possible but consistently reported risk factors for faster hemodynamic progression include older age and more severe disease at baseline. A small reduction in a more narrowed orifice leads to a higher gradient change compared with the same reduction in orifice area with a larger initial valve area.

The severity of leaflet calcification predicts progression rates. However, quantification of AVC by echocardiography is not reliable and the utility of CT-measured AVC scores awaits further study.

Asymptomatic Severe Aortic Stenosis (Stage C)

Many adults with hemodynamically severe AS remain asymptomatic, sometimes for years, suggesting that the exact degree of obstruction is not the only factor determining symptom onset.[72] The interaction of the degree of valve obstruction, LV performance, systemic vascular compliance, and metabolic demands in each patient likely interact in determining whether patients perceive exercise limitation or other symptoms. In the absence of symptoms, adverse clinical outcomes are rare unless there is concurrent LV systolic dysfunction.

Exercise testing to confirm symptom status is helpful in risk stratification. Asymptomatic AS patients with severe AS who have a normal exercise stress test result have a good prognosis, with no reported sudden death after 1 year of follow-up, as opposed to a 5% sudden death rate for those with abnormal stress results.[32,73] ST depression is very common during exercise testing with AS, but when analyzed independently, it does not discriminate people into a higher risk for AS events or obstructive coronary disease. Ventricular arrhythmias, although abnormal, happen only rarely in contemporary series.

Some investigators suggest there is additive value in measuring stress hemodynamics. Although transvalvular velocity and gradient are expected to increase with increasing transvalvular flow across a restrictive orifice during stress, Lancellotti et al found that an increase in the mean transvalvular gradient at or above 18 mmHg best distinguished a higher-risk population.[16] Similarly, Maréchaux et al reported a 3.8-fold higher risk of AVR or cardiovascular death when mean gradients increased at least 20 mmHg with exercise.[33] Unfortunately, the predictive accuracy of the exercise increase in Doppler gradients for adverse outcomes is marginal, with a sensitivity of 70% and specificity of 62%.[34]

Otto et al highlighted significant overlap in exercise findings and found they did not alter risk models when accounting for baseline clinical and echocardiographic variables.[11] Although several risk markers used with stress testing have been identified, such as abnormal exercise tolerance, a blunted blood pressure response, increasing mean gradients, and exercise induced pulmonary hypertension, cardiac event rates over 1 to 3 years for all patients studied were 26% to 60%, highlighting the need for close follow-up regardless of negative stress testing results.

Symptomatic Severe Aortic Stenosis (Stage D)
Sudden Death
The risk of sudden death is high among patients with symptomatic severe AS; it approaches 2% per month. The prognosis is significantly better for patients without symptoms: less than 1% per year.[74] Higher rates of sudden death without preceding symptoms have been identified for patients with very severe AS (maximum velocity $\geq$5 m/s and mean gradient $\geq$60 mmHg).[75,76] The mechanism of sudden death in AS is not completely known, but possibilities include ventricular arrhythmia or baroreceptor reflex bradycardia and hypotension.[21] Arrhythmia causes are supported by association of sudden death with electrocardiographic evidence of QRS prolongation.[74]

Heart Failure
The pressure overload from AS leads to adaptive LV changes, most commonly concentric LVH, with eventual development of heart failure. Females, diabetics, and obese individuals with AS are more prone to develop concentric LVH. Global systolic function as measured by EF remains preserved until very late in the disease course, but preceding diastolic dysfunction, elevated filling pressures, and reduced LV longitudinal systolic function lead to symptomatic dyspnea and decreased functional capacity in advanced disease.[14]

Atrial Fibrillation
Atrial fibrillation (AF) is common among patients with AS with an increasing prevalence at later stages of disease. Patients with stage B disease have a reported prevalence of 9%, whereas 27% of stage D2 patients are affected. Almost one half of patients undergoing AVR develop some form of AF. LV changes leading to diastolic and systolic dysfunction result in elevated filling pressure, left atrial enlargement, and atrial stretch and fibrosis. AS directly leads to atrial substrate changes, and AS and AF share many common risk factors, mainly age and hypertension. Prognosis for AS is worse when AF occurs, with a fourfold risk of heart failure and a 2.5-fold excess mortality risk.[77,78]

Other
Bleeding in the gastrointestinal tract (i.e., Heyde syndrome) has been reported 1% to 3% of adults with AS due to angiodysplastic vessels in the colon and small intestine. The bleeding tendency results from an acquired von Willebrand factor (VWF) deficiency that results from loss of high-molecular-weight multimers of VWF. VWF is necessary for platelet adhesion and activation in subendothelial connective tissue. High shear stress from AS enhances VWF susceptibility to proteolysis, reducing the ratio of VWF activity to antigen.[79]

AVR improves bleeding outcomes and restores VWF activity. However, residual factors maintaining high shear stress, such as patient-prosthesis mismatch, biological valve deterioration, or paravalvular leak can lead to recurrence of bleeding and VWF loss.[80]

MEDICAL THERAPY

Despite an increasing understanding of the active pathology in AS, medical therapies have not prevented disease progression.[81] Experimental evidence has shown promising targets in inflammatory and mineralization pathways (see Chapters 3 and 4), but they have not translated to clinical benefits. Although there is a lack of clinical evidence, promising investigations are ongoing.[82] Although therapy specifically targeting AS is unavailable, medical care commonly used for comorbid conditions found in AS patients is tailored to the unique AS physiology.

Prevention of Disease Progression
AS and CAD share many clinical risk factors, and valvular lesions have similarities to atherosclerosis in terms of lipid deposition and oxidation. Animal models demonstrate that lipid deposition in AS can trigger inflammation and mineralization in the valves. Although it seems plausible that statin therapy could reduce AS progression, multiple clinical trials comparing a statin with placebo for stage B AS found no difference in the rates hemodynamic progression or AS-related clinical events.[62,83,84] The AHA/ACC guideline recommendations do not endorse statin therapy for the prevention of AS progression.[6]

There are several possible explanations for the lack of positive findings with statin therapy. First, it is possible that lipid inflammation is more important in the earlier disease process (stage A) before hemodynamic and aggressive calcification occurs. Second, although lipid reduction may reduce inflammatory pathways, it also enhances calcification, as seen in coronary atherosclerosis. It is likely that animal models, which rely on severe hypercholesterolemia to develop AS, may not accurately reflect the human disease process.

Although statin therapies have not shown benefit, further investigations into targeting lipoprotein(a) (LPA) in AS are ongoing. A large genome-wide association study found that genetic polymorphisms along with LPA levels were associated with incident AS and AVR.[85] The use of niacin and other inhibitors to LPA synthesis to hinder AS progression remains speculative. Also, therapies targeting dysregulated bone metabolism, such as bisphosphonates and denosumab, are being evaluated based on associations of osteoporosis with ectopic calcification.

Comorbid Conditions

Although statin therapy is not indicated for AS progression, patients with AS benefit from medical therapy for cardiovascular risk prevention. Almost one half of AS patients have coexisting CAD that warrants statin therapy. Symptomatic CAD in stage A and stage B AS is managed the same way as in a patient without AS. Because angina can result from obstructive CAD or AS, symptomatic angina patients with hemodynamic severe AS are considered stage D and have AVR and concurrent revascularization planned. Given the high rate of CAD in AS, coronary angiography is recommended for all AS patients needing AVR, except for the very young (<40 years of age) with congenital AS.

High blood pressure frequently accompanies AS and imposes a double load on the LV, leading to LVH. Analysis from the simvastatin ezetimibe in AS trial found that AS patients with hypertension were three times more likely to develop LVH and twice as likely to die. Low systolic and pulse pressures were also associated with higher mortality rates. Optimal risk was found to be a systolic blood pressure of 120 to 139 mmHg and diastolic pressure of 70 to 89 mmHg.[86]

Treatment of high blood pressure with guideline-directed medical therapy is a class I indication in the AHA/ACC guidelines, with a caveat that starting doses are low and gradual titration occurs with monitoring.[6] High vascular afterload affects evaluation of AS hemodynamic severity with overestimation or underestimation of the AVA and gradients, depending on the specific patient characteristics.[87] Systemic hypertension should be adequately controlled before assessing hemodynamic severity of AS.

The choice of antihypertensive therapy must be individualized. Diuretic use is cautioned against when there is severe LVH and small LV volumes due to concern about reducing preload and cardiac output in AS. In acute decompensated heart failure and severe AS, blood pressure lowering with nitroprusside may be considered for hemodynamic management of low cardiac output with high vascular resistance when active invasive monitoring is undertaken. Small studies have investigated inhibition of the renin-angiotensin-aldosterone system for chronic management of blood pressure in AS (see Chapter 3). One study randomized 100 asymptomatic AS patients to ramipril or placebo and found significant regression of LV mass along with trends for reduced AS progression.[88] Larger studies with longer follow-up are needed to determine benefits in clinical outcomes with antihypertensive therapy.

Anticoagulation management of AF with AS continues to evolve. Native-valve AS patients have been included in trials of target-specific oral anticoagulants with no difference in efficacy for apixaban or dabigatran compared with traditional warfarin management.[89,90] Valvular AF has had various definitions in clinical trials. The AHA/ACC definition includes bioprosthetic aortic valves. A single pilot study with limited follow-up found that use of dabigatran appeared similar to warfarin in preventing intracardiac thrombosis.[91] More definitive evaluation of direct thrombin oral anticoagulant effects with bioprosthetic valves and atrial fibrillation remain needed.[92]

Periodic Monitoring

For patients who do not have an indication for AVR, serial evaluation is required due to the progressive nature of the disease. Repeat echocardiography intervals depend on baseline hemodynamic severity. For patients with mild, moderate, and severe stenosis, repeat imaging is recommended every 3 to 5 years, 1 to 2 years, and 6 months to 1 year, respectively. For patients without prior echocardiographic evaluations, choosing a shorter duration within the recommended range is advised because some patients progress more rapidly than others. Conversely, if severity has been stable, a longer interval between imaging studies is reasonable. Regardless of the surveillance imaging, clinical follow-up is recommended on a minimum yearly basis to evaluate for clinical changes and provide patient education about potential symptoms. Repeat echocardiography is appropriate for changes in clinical status.

Exercise Limitations

Most patients with AS are elderly and no longer compete in competitive sports. For younger, active patients with congenital AS obstruction, significant dynamic exercise demanding high cardiac output increases valvular gradients, whereas heavy static exercise increases afterload to an already pressure overloaded LV. Avoidance of competitive athletics has been recommended by expert opinion for cases of severe AS, whereas no restrictions are required for mild AS.[93] Those with a moderate AS severity are allowed to compete in low-intensity sports and some moderate-intensity activities based on exercise testing results. Usually more relevant are activity restrictions related to comorbid conditions, such as ischemic heart disease or congestive heart failure.

Noncardiac Surgery

Patients with AS are at higher risk for perioperative complications when undergoing noncardiac surgery. Event rates for major adverse cardiovascular events are worse with more advanced AS.[94] Adverse events related to noncardiac surgery for patients with AS are associated with conditions similar to those for patients without AS undergoing operations, mainly coexisting coronary disease, renal failure, and the underlying risk of the surgical procedure.

Proceeding with needed elective surgery is reasonable for asymptomatic patients with AS if there are no indications for AVR. For patients with indications for AVR, postponing elective procedures is prudent until AVR has been performed because adverse event rates up to 30% have been reported in surgical series with undiagnosed severe AS. Balloon valvuloplasty is not routinely recommended before noncardiac surgery, except in selected patients who are hemodynamically unstable from their valve obstruction and require urgent noncardiac surgery before AVR.

Mild AS does not require any additional changes in management. Individuals with asymptomatic, moderate to severe AS can proceed with surgery; invasive hemodynamic monitoring 24 hours before and 48 hours after moderate-risk surgery is optional. Avoiding significant hypotension, bradycardia, and tachycardia is paramount in cases of significant AS. Invasive hemodynamic monitoring assists management of hemodynamic perturbations that occur with surgery, such as volume changes, vascular resistance changes from anesthetics, and reduced cardiac output with new-onset AF. In cases of stage C disease, preoperative invasive or CT coronary angiography is appropriate because noninvasive ischemia testing is less reliable for diagnosis and prognosis in AS.

AORTIC VALVE REPLACEMENT

Timing of Intervention

AVR is a class I (strong) recommendation for the treatment of symptomatic patients with severe AS due to the known grim prognosis

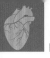

without AVR and the demonstrated success of AVR in prolonging life and relieving symptoms.[95] AVR with a surgical or transcatheter approach is recommended regardless of patient age and comorbidities, unless comorbidities or limited life expectancy suggest that a palliative care option is more appropriate (see Palliative Care). Even mild symptoms of exertional dyspnea or decreased exercise capacity are an indication for AVR for patients with severe AS. If symptom status is unclear, exercise testing is recommended.

The role of AVR in asymptomatic patients with AS has been debated for decades. Improvement in AVR techniques, with lower procedural risk and better prognostication in AS, allows consideration of AVR in asymptomatic patients with severe AS and LV systolic dysfunction, very severe valve obstruction, or evidence for rapid hemodynamic progression (Table 9.5 and Fig. 9.11).[52,96] Because almost all patients progress to severe valve obstruction and symptoms after even mild AS occurs, the primary factors limiting earlier AVR are the risk of the procedure, imperfect prosthetic valve hemodynamics, risks of anticoagulation with a mechanical AVR, and limited durability of bioprosthetic valves (see Chapter 26). Ongoing studies are assessing the role of TAVR earlier in the disease course of AS.

Symptomatic Severe Aortic Stenosis (Stage D1)

Severe AS is defined as a calcified valve with reduced systolic opening and a maximum aortic velocity of $\geq$ 4 m/s or a mean gradient of $\geq$ 40 mmHg, regardless of valve area, and it is an indication for AVR if the patient has symptoms. Valve area usually is less than 1 cm^2, but it often is greater in large individuals or when mixed stenosis and regurgitation exist.

Despite the known benefits of AVR for severe symptomatic AS, up to one third of patients are denied or have refused surgery.[97] The evolution of TAVR has made AVR accessible to those previously deemed inoperable.[98] Historically, AVR recommendations were based on observational surgical series, which found that patients with AVR lived

longer and with improved symptoms compared with those that did not undergo surgery. Several robust randomized studies of TAVR versus medical therapy have shown impressive mortality benefits (>25% absolute reduction) compared with other modern cardiovascular treatments (Fig. 9.12). Unfortunately, very-high-risk patients undergoing TAVR still have a very high mortality rate. Even TAVR is not recommended if the likelihood of beneficial survival is less than 25% over 2 years (see Chapter 7).

Asymptomatic Severe Aortic Stenosis (Stage C)

Pressure overload from AS leads to LVH and myocardial fibrosis, eventually causing heart failure with decreased LV diastolic or systolic function, or both. Intervening before significant irreversible LV systolic dysfunction is recommended because patients with significant reductions in EF who are unable to augment flow have dismal outcomes when they progress to stage D2. Operative outcomes are negatively influenced by continuously declining EF.[100] As soon as the EF falls below 50% (stage C2), AVR is indicated.[6,52] Although it makes sense that prevention of diastolic dysfunction would be beneficial, the risk-benefit ratio of earlier AVR for this indication has not been studies in clinical trials.

Some subgroups of patients with severe asymptomatic AS (stage C1) have high rates of adverse outcomes. Rosenhek et al found that asymptomatic AS patients with a maximum velocity greater than 5 m/s had only a 25% and 3% event-free survival after 3 years and 6 years, respectively (Fig. 9.13).[101]Another prospective registry study at a center with excellent surgical outcomes found that AS patients undergoing early surgery had better survival rates than propensity-matched controls under conventional management when maximum velocities were greater than 4.5 m/s.[75] A higher maximum aortic velocity has been repeatedly associated with escalating adverse event rates in a dose-response type of relationship. In heart centers with excellent surgical outcomes, it is reasonable to pursue early surgical AVR (class IIa) for

	STRENGTH OF RECOMMENDATION (LEVEL OF EVIDENCE)	
Recommendation	ACC/AHA[6]	ESC[52]
Symptomatic severe AS by patient history	I (B)	I (B)
Severe AS with symptoms on exercise testing	I (B)	I (C)
Asymptomatic severe AS (LVEF < 50%)	I (B)	I (C)
Severe AS undergoing cardiac surgery	I (B)	I (C)
Asymptomatic very severe AS[a] and low surgical risk	IIa (B)	IIa (C)
Asymptomatic severe AS with abnormal exercise test	IIa (B)	IIa (C)
Symptomatic LFLG severe AS (LVEF < 50%) and confirmatory DSE[b]	IIa (B)	Ia (C)
Symptomatic LFLG severe AS (LVEF < 50%) without flow reserve on DSE[b]		IIa (C)
Symptoms most likely due to LFLG severe AS (LVEF ≥ 50%) after careful confirmation of severe AS	IIa (C)	IIa (C)
Moderate AS undergoing cardiac surgery	IIa (C)	IIa (C)
Asymptomatic severe AS with rapid progression and low surgical risk	IIb (C)	IIa (C)
Asymptomatic severe AS with markedly elevated BNP		IIa (C)
Asymptomatic severe AS with mean gradient increase > 20 mmHg with exercise		IIb (C)
Asymptomatic severe AS with excessive LVH and no hypertension		IIb (C)

TABLE 9.5 Guideline Recommendations for Timing of Aortic Valve Replacement in Aortic Stenosis.

[a]Very severe defined as maximum velocity $\geq$ 5 m/s by ACC/AHA and $\geq$ 5.5 m/s by ESC.
[b]Maximum aortic velocity $\geq$ 4 m/s (mean gradient $\geq$ 40 mmHg) and valve area $\leq$ 1.0 cm^2 by ACC/AHA and > 20% increase in stroke volume by ESC.
ACC/AHA, American College of Cardiology/American Heart Association; *AS,* aortic stenosis; *BNP,* brain natriuretic peptide; *DSE,* dobutamine stress echocardiogram; *ESC,* European Society of Cardiology; *LFLG,* low-flow, low-gradient; *LVEF,* left ventricular ejection fraction; *LVH,* left ventricular hypertrophy.

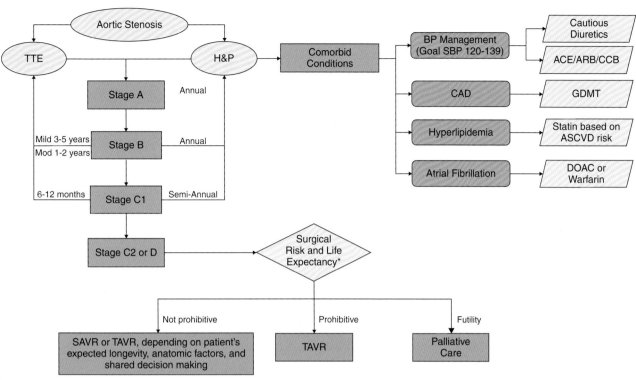

Fig. 9.11 Management of Aortic Stenosis. Serial monitoring with clinical examination and transthoracic echocardiography *(TTE)* occur more frequently for progressive stages of aortic stenosis. At each clinical evaluation, cardiovascular comorbidities are addressed. At end stages of aortic stenosis, determination of surgical risk for aortic valve replacement *(AVR)* is undertaken to determine the appropriate AVR strategy. Futility of AVR is a shared-decision process with a heart valve team and patient when life expectancy is less than 1 year or when there is a less than 25% likelihood of clinical benefit over 2 years due to other conditions not fixed with AVR. Surgical risk *(asterisk)* includes an integrated assessment of the Society of Thoracic Surgery predicted risk of mortality, frailty, major organ system dysfunction, and procedure-specific risks. The decision to perform SAVR versus TAVR in patients with an indication for AVR is continually evolving. Major considerations include expected patient longevity versus valve durability, valve and vascular anatomy, comorbidities, and patient preferences and values in the context of a shared decision making process (see Chapter 12). Strength of recommendation *(double asterisk)* in the American Heart Association/American College of Cardiology 2017 focused update of valvular guidelines.[96] *ACE,* Angiotensin-converting enzyme inhibitor; *ARB,* angiotensin receptor blocker; *ASCVD,* atherosclerotic cardiovascular disease; *BP,* blood pressure; *CAD,* coronary artery disease; *CCB,* calcium channel blocker; *DOAC,* direct oral anticoagulant; *GDMT,* guideline-directed medical therapy; *H&P,* history and physical examination; *Mod,* moderate; *SAVR,* surgical aortic valve replacement; *SBP,* systolic blood pressure; *TAVR,* transcatheter aortic valve replacement.

stage C1 patients with very severe stenosis ($V_{max} > 5$ m/s) and low surgical risk (Society of Thoracic Surgery score < 4 %).

An overall poorer prognosis has been documented for severe AS patients with abnormal stress testing (see Stress Testing), rapid progression of disease ($V_{max} \geq 0.3$ m/s/yr), severe LVH, or markedly elevated BNP levels (see Biomarkers) (see Fig. 9.9). However, absolute cutpoints for these parameters demonstrating benefit from early AVR have not been well studied.

Refinement of risk stratification combining clinical, imaging, and biomarker data to better identify risk in stage C1 patients has been undertaken. Monin et al proposed a combination risk score using maximum velocity, BNP, and sex and found that those in the highest quartile had an 80% risk of AVR or death in 2 years compared with only 7% in the lowest quartile.[102] External validation in another study found the score to perform less well.[103]

Chin et al created and externally validated a risk score for MRI-detected myocardial fibrosis and AS-related events using maximum velocity, sex, age, high-sensitivity Tn I, and LV strain pattern on electrocardiograms.[104] A nomogram was derived, and individuals deemed at high-risk (>57%) were found to have a 10-fold higher event rate compared with low-risk patients. The use of risk scores is promising, but they await further study to validate whether early AVR benefits those deemed at high risk.

A major concern about the current data related to early AVR for stage C1 disease is that surgical selection bias and residual confounding cannot be fully overcome with statistical techniques, especially in studies with small numbers of patients.[75,105] Although meta-analysis of the available studies has shown reduced associated risk with early AVR, there is significant heterogeneity between studies, high rates of noncardiac death, continued occurrence of sudden death after AVR, and a substantial lack of AVR in stage D patients in conventionally managed groups.[106–107] Most patients with stage C1 develop symptoms within 5 years of diagnosis, but the annual risk of sudden death is low, between 0.5% and 1.5%.[75,101,105,108,109]

To better evaluate these issues, a randomized, controlled trial, AVATAR, was begun to compare rates of major adverse cardiovascular events with early SAVR versus watchful waiting in cases of asymptomatic severe AS.[110] In the meantime, the best approach is to tailor decisions for individuals based on their risk factors, AS severity, procedural risk, and personal preference.[111]

Low-Flow, Low-Gradient Aortic Stenosis With Reduced Ejection Fraction (Stage D2)

For patients with apparent low-flow, low-gradient AS, when dobutamine stress testing indicates that AS is only moderate in severity, therapy focuses on improving LV systolic function. Moderate AS in systolic heart failure may adversely affect prognosis, but further data are needed to determine whether relief of AS can improve outcomes for this patient group.

In the largest study of conservative management for pseudosevere AS, 29 patients with pseudosevere AS without initial AVR had a 5-year

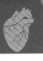

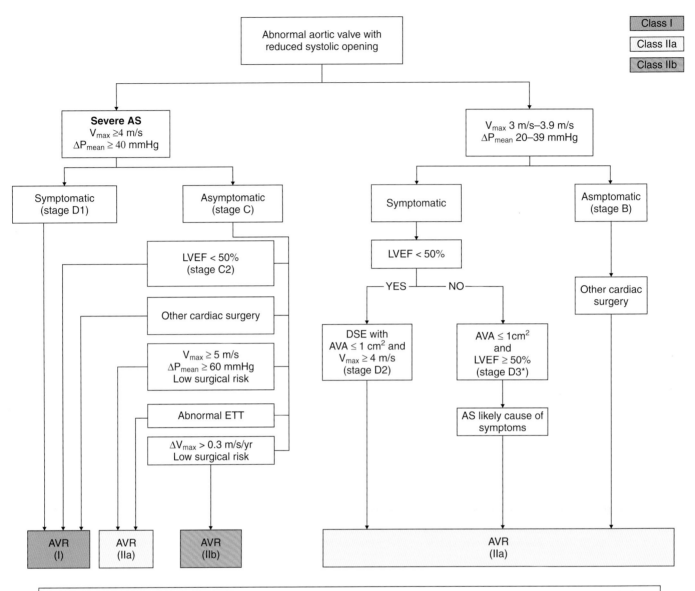

Fig. 9.12 Indications for Aortic Valve Replacement *(AVR)* in Patients With Aortic Stenosis *(AS)*. *Arrows* show the decision pathways that result in a recommendation for AVR. Periodic monitoring is indicated for all patients in whom AVR is not yet indicated, including those with asymptomatic AS (stage D or C) and those with low-gradient AS (stage D2 or D3) who do not meet the criteria for intervention. ΔP_{mean}, Mean pressure gradient; *AVA*, aortic valve area; *BP*, blood pressure; *DSE*, dobutamine stress echocardiogram; *ETT*, exercise tolerance test; *LVEF*, left ventricular ejection fraction; V_{max}, maximum aortic jet velocity. (From Nishimura RA, Otto CM, Bonow RO, et al. 2014 AHA/ACC guideline for the management of patients with valvular heart disease: a report of the American College of Cardiology/American Heart Association Task Force on Practice Guidelines. J Am Coll Cardiol 2014;63:e57-e185.)

survival comparable to that of propensity-matched patients with systolic heart failure but without valvular disease.[112] Patients with pseudosevere AS have a better risk-adjusted prognosis than those with severe AS who do not undergo initial AVR (Fig. 9.14). Some patients with pseudosevere AS inevitably undergo AVR over time because of progression to severe AS or a need for concomitant coronary bypass surgery.

Individuals with confirmed severe AS with low-flow pattern (stroke volume index $\leq$ 35 mL/m^2) due to LV systolic dysfunction have a worse prognosis compared with individuals with a normal-flow pattern. Several studies have shown dismal outcomes for stage D2 patients when treated medically. However, SAVR is high risk in this situation, with operative mortality rates between 9% and 16%.[99,113,114] Surgical mortality rates are even higher when there is absence of flow reserve, presence

of CAD, and mean gradients below 20 mmHg.[115] Surgical series over the past several decades have consistently shown that AS patients with the highest gradients have the best outcomes after AVR. However, for patients with low-gradient severe AS, AVR still should be pursued unless other comorbidities severely limit life expectancy over the next year.

Tribouilloy et al[115] showed a significant difference in 5-year survival with AVR compared with risk-adjusted matched controls for low-flow patients (65% vs. 11%, respectively). Alternatively, for high-risk and surgically inoperable patients, TAVR is an increasingly preferred option and may be reasonable in lower-risk patients. Subgroup analysis from the PARTNER study confirmed the comparable benefit of AVR in stage D2 patients to the overall benefit of the trial (HR = 0.43, 95% CI: 0.19–0.98; P = 0.04).[116]

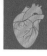

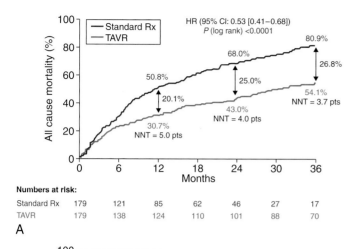

A

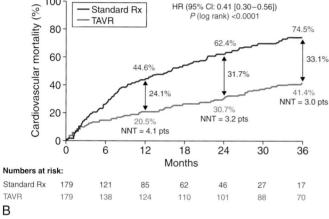

B

Fig. 9.13 Reduction in Mortality With Aortic Valve Replacement. Cumulative hazard curves compare all-cause (A) and cardiovascular-related (B) mortality between patients randomly assigned to transcatheter aortic valve replacement *(TAVR)* or standard therapy for surgically inoperable, severe aortic stenosis. *CI,* Confidence interval; *HR,* hazard ratio; *NNT,* number needed to treat; *pts,* patients; *Rx,* therapy. (Modified from Kapadia SR, Tuzcu EM, Makkar RR, et al. Long-term outcomes of inoperable patients with aortic stenosis randomly assigned to transcatheter aortic valve replacement or standard therapy. Circulation 2014;130:1483-1492.)

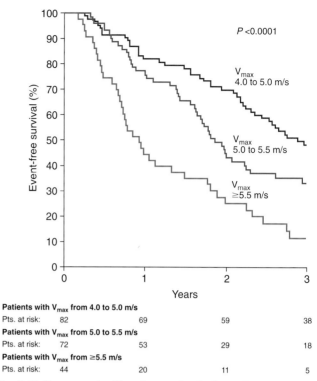

Fig. 9.14 Outcomes for Very Severe Aortic Stenosis. Kaplan-Meier event-free survival estimates for patients with a maximum aortic valve jet velocity *(V_max)* between 4.0 and 5.0 m/s (*yellow line*; n = 82), between 5.0 and 5.5 m/s (*blue line*; n = 72), and ≥5.5 m/s (*green line*; n = 44). (From Rosenhek R, Zilberszac R, Schemper M, et al. Natural history of very severe aortic stenosis. Circulation 2010;121:151-156.)

Low-Flow, Low-Gradient Aortic Stenosis With Preserved Ejection Fraction (Stage D3)

The prognosis for and management of patients with paradoxical low-flow, low-gradient AS (stage D3) continue to be debated. Studies examining outcomes of medically treated stage D3 patients have had mixed results compared with those for stage D1 and stage B patients (Table 9.6).[117–125] A meta-analysis reported no significant mortality difference between stage D3 and D1 patients (HR = 1.07, 95% CI: 0.83–1.38).[126] However, there is significant heterogeneity between small studies in regard to study types, population characteristics, symptom status, outcomes measured, rates of AVR, and follow-up duration. Stage D3 patients are on average older, more likely to be female, and have more comorbidities, including hypertension. When analyzed prospectively and with adjustment for confounding effects, the stage D3 patient's prognosis appears better than for AS with high gradients, but some authors of retrospective studies argue that natural history is worse when patients have symptoms and LVH.[117–119]

Patients selected to undergo AVR in stage D3 have better outcomes than those who are managed medically. A meta-analysis showed that low-flow, low-gradient AS patients with preserved EF have a lower rate of referral for AVR and have a 56% lower mortality rate than conservatively treated patients.[127] The best available data comes from subgroup analysis of the PARTNER trial, which showed a significant 21% absolute survival benefit for those who get TAVR compared with no AVR for stage D3 patients who were able achieve a high gradient (≥40 mmHg) during DSE.

It is challenging to determine whether AS is the cause of symptoms when the maximum gradient is below 40 mmHg and LV systolic function is normal. For these patients, the recommended approach is to verify echocardiographic measurements made while the patient is normotensive, visualize severe leaflet calcification with restricted valve opening, identify LVH with restrictive filling patterns, and exclude other potential causes of symptoms. When severe symptomatic AS with low gradient and preserved EF is confirmed, it is reasonable to consider AVR.

Undergoing Cardiac Surgery

When patients with asymptomatic, moderate to severe AS are scheduled to undergo other cardiac surgery (e.g., aortic root replacement, coronary bypass, other valve surgery), the risks and benefits of concurrent AVR must be evaluated. The natural history of AS is one of progression, and most patients with moderate or severe AS require AVR in 5 to 7 years and 2 to 4 years, respectively. Another factor supporting SAVR at the time of noncardiac surgery is that the SAVR mortality rate after previous coronary bypass surgery is up to 17%.[128] Current recommendations endorse SAVR at the time of noncardiac surgery for some stage B and all stage C patients.

The addition of AVR to bypass surgery increases cross-clamp time, stroke risks, and has a 1% to 3% higher operative mortality rate. The

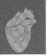

TABLE 9.6 Studies of Prognosis for Low-Flow, Low-Gradient Aortic Stenosis With Preserved Ejection Fraction.

Study	Study Design	Mean Follow-Up (N)	Mean V_{max}/ ΔP/AVA/SVi	End Point	Event-Free Survival	Survival Compared With HG/ LGNF/Mod
Jander et al, 2011[120]	Randomized clinical trial	3.8 years (223)	3.3/24/0.77/29.4	AVR, CHF, or CV death	53.8%	↑/↔/↔
Clavel et al, 2012[118]	Retrospective cohort	4.2 years (187)	3/22/0.82/30	AVR or death	24% at 5 yr	↓/X/↓
Lancellotti et al, 2012[34]	Prospective observational	2.3 years (11)	3.8/33/0.8/31	AVR or CV death	27% at 2 yr	↓/↓/X
Eleid et al, 2013[87]	Retrospective cohort	2.3 years (53)	3.6/30/0.87/31	All-cause mortality	60% at 2 yr	↓/↓/X
Mehrotra et al, 2013[122]	Retrospective cohort	3 years (38)	3.3/26/0.74/29.4	All-cause mortality	58% at 3 yr	X/↓/↓
Maes et al, 2014[123]	Prospective observational	2.3 years (115)	3.4/27/0.7/28	All-cause mortality	42% at 4 yr	↑/↔/X
Maor et al, 2014[124]	Retrospective cohort	2.9 years (136)	3.5/29/0.78/32	All-cause mortality	59% at 3 yr	X/↓/X
Tribouilloy et al, 2015[117]	Prospective observational	3.3 years (57)	3.3/30/0.8/30.1	All-cause mortality	65% at 4 yr	↑/↔/↔
Gonzalez Gomez et al, 2017[125]	Prospective observational	1.7 years (442)	3.3/25/<1/29	CV death or admission	82% at 2 yr	↓/X/X

AS, Aortic stenosis; *AVA*, aortic valve area (cm²); *AVR*, aortic valve replacement; *CHF*, congestive heart failure hospitalization; *CV*, cardiovascular; *HG*, high-gradient AS (P ≥ 40, AVA ≤ 1.0); *LGNF*, low-gradient, normal-flow, severe AS (AVA ≤ 1.0, P < 40, SVi > 35); *Mod*, moderate AS (AVA ≥ 1.0, P < 40); *N*, number of low-flow, low-gradient, preserved ejection fraction patients; *P*, mean aortic gradient (mmHg); *SVi*, stroke volume index (mL/m²); *Vmax*, maximum aortic jet velocity (m/s); *X*, not reported.

age of the patient and likelihood that AVR will be beneficial in an individual's lifetime need to be considered. Use of off-pump coronary bypass and the increasing availability of TAVR make it reasonable to defer AVR in some stage B patients. An individualized approach is warranted for moderate AS patients based on the additional operative risk, feasibility of future TAVR, likelihood of lifetime benefit of AVR, and prosthetic valve risks.

Choice of Valve

The choice of a prosthetic aortic valve must consider clinical, anatomic, and hemodynamic factors and patient preferences and values (Table 9.7).[6,52,96,129] The first decision is between a mechanical or bioprosthetic valve. Mechanical valves are very durable, and repeat valve replacement is unlikely to be needed, but they require surgical implantation and lifelong anticoagulation with a vitamin K antagonist. Bioprosthetic valves do not require anticoagulation and can be implanted using a transcatheter or surgical approach, but they have finite durability, and repeat intervention is likely to be needed if the valve fails during the patient's remaining lifetime (see Chapter 26).

Survival and long-term outcomes are similar for both valve types over a 15-year period for patients between 50 and 69 years of age.[130] The use of mechanical valves before the age of 50 continues to be recommended to avoid future need for a high-risk redo AVR, although this remains controversial.

When a bioprosthetic valve is appropriate, the decision between a transcatheter and surgical approach is based on a heart valve team approach,[131] depending on surgical risk, anatomic considerations, vascular accessibility, and patient preferences (see Chapter 12). TAVR is an option for individuals with AS regardless of surgical risk.[132] The major

considerations in the choice between TAVR and SAVR now are expected patient longevity (in relation to known valve durability) as well as anatomic valve and vascular factors. Informed shared decision making should take patient preferences and values into consideration in the context of a heart valve team (see Chapter 12).[132a–132d] Currently, the use of TAVR is not recommended for low-risk younger patients (<65 years), because TAVR durability beyond 5 years is less well established. In the future, the promising strategy of placing a TAVR valve in a failing bioprosthetic valve (valve-in-valve procedure) must be taken into account. The valve-in-valve technique appears to be comparable to redo SAVR, and mechanical valves may be avoided in some younger patients in the future.[133]

Rarely, other alternatives for AVR are considered such as aortic homografts, pulmonary autograft (Ross procedure), and aortic root replacement/enlargement (see Chapter 14). Patients with severe AS and a small aortic annulus sometimes require a surgical annular enlarging procedure. Conversely, patients with aortic valve disease and a dilated aortic typically require a composite valve and root replacement or concurrent graft replacement of the ascending aorta. These considerations may mandate surgical rather than transcatheter AVR in some patients. Basal septal hypertrophy is seen in up to 10% of those with AS, and it sometimes contributes to subaortic obstruction. When there are elements of dynamic obstruction or very severe hypertrophy requiring small prosthetic valve implants, myectomy has been performed with satisfactory outcomes when done by experienced hands.[134]

Outcomes After Aortic Valve Replacement
Clinical Outcomes
Survival after AVR is similar to that for age- and gender-matched adults over the subsequent 5 years, and the procedure significantly

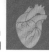

TABLE 9.7 Guideline Recommendations for Choice of Prosthetic Valve.

Recommendation	STRENGTH OF RECOMMENDATION (LEVEL OF EVIDENCE)		
	ACC/AHA[6]	ESC[52]	BMJ[129]
Choice of valve with shared decision-making process based on desire of informed patient	I (C-LD)	I (C)	
Mechanical Valve			
Mechanical valve in another position		I (C)	
Risk of accelerated valve deterioration (<40 years, ↑PTH)		I (C)	
Patients < 60 years of age (aortic) or 65 (mitral)	IIa (B)	IIa (C)	
Patients < 50 years of age	IIa (B-NR)		
Bioprosthetic Valve			
Patient of any age with inability to take anticoagulation	I (C)	I (C)	
Reoperation for mechanical valve thrombosis		I (C)	
Patients > 70 years of age	IIa (B)	IIa (C)	
Young women contemplating pregnancy		IIa (C)	
Transcatheter Aortic Valve			
Prohibitive risk of surgery	I (A)	I (B)	
High risk of surgery	I (A)	IIa (B)[a]	
Intermediate risk of surgery	IIa (B-R)	I (B)[a]	
Patients ≥ 85 years of age		+	Strong (moderate)
Patients 75–84 years of age		+	Weak (moderate)

[a]Elevated risk patients (STS or Euroscore II > 4%) with favorable patient characteristics assessed by a heart team, particularly for elderly patients with transfemoral access.
ACC/AHA, American College of Cardiology/American Heart Association; *BMJ*, British Medical Journal Rapid Recommendations; *ESC*, European Society of Cardiology; ↑*PTH*, hyperparathyroidism; +, favors transcatheter aortic valve.

alters the unfavorable natural history of severe AS.[135] However, excess mortality over expected 15-year survival has been reported.[136] AVR is a highly effective treatment for AS but not a cure because residual mortality and morbidity remains. Excess adjusted mortality has been associated with worsening functional heart failure classification, EF, AF, and associated regurgitation.[137] Improvement in heart failure symptoms and quality of life is fairly universal for AVR survivors when symptomatic disease is due to valvular obstruction. However, survival, quality of life, and functional status often improves little in very elderly patients with significant comorbidities and frailty.[138]

Perioperative outcomes for TAVR and SAVR have been fairly comparable for intermediate-risk and high-risk surgical patients in clinical trials (see Chapter 12),[132,139] but the TAVR technique continues to improve, resulting in better procedural outcomes over time. Among a cohort of high-risk and surgically inoperable patients, the 30-day mortality rate was only 2.5% using a third-generation balloon-expandable valve. The rates for 1-year cardiovascular survival and freedom from significant paravalvular leak in the cohort remained very high at 92% and 97%, respectively.[140] Transfemoral access is the first-line method when feasible for TAVR due to its association with better clinic outcomes compared with alternative access sites.[141]

Stroke remains a concern after AVR, with reported rates between 1% and 11%, depending on technique and the population studied. Initial PARTNER trial results demonstrated higher clinical stroke rates for TAVR compared with SAVR (4.6% and 2.4%, respectively). Subsequent registry and clinical trial data show equivalence of clinical neurologic events for both techniques.[142] The ability to mitigate stroke risk with cardioembolic protection devices, anticoagulation, and improved procedural techniques await additional investigation.

Hemodynamic Outcomes

The ability of AVR to unload the LV allows improvement in EF and regression of LVH. Patients with moderately reduced systolic function typically have a 10% to 13% improvement in EF after AVR.[143] No differences were found in the PARTNER trial between SAVR and TAVR in the ability to improve ventricular function. Unfortunately, not all patients have systolic improvement. Patients with very low gradients, EF less than 20%, pacemakers, and significant fibrosis with prior myocardial infarctions are less likely to augment EF. The ability to increase the EF when already above 50% (stage D3) is limited, but echocardiographic studies have shown mild improvements in global longitudinal strain after AVR.[144]

Regression of LV mass occurs over months to years after AVR, but it is attenuated by systemic hypertension and patient-prosthesis mismatch.[145,146] TAVR has been associated with less patient-prosthesis mismatch than SAVR and results in more LV mass reduction.[147] LVH regression is associated with improvement in diastolic function[148,149] and is associated with lower rates of hospitalization and heart failure.[150] The ability for the LV to remodel after AVR appears to be a marker of less myocardial fibrosis and a healthier ventricle.

PALLIATIVE CARE

The decision to proceed with AVR is shared by the heart valve team, patient, and patient's family. Elderly AS patients frequently have significant comorbidities that reduce quality of life or shorten life expectancy irrespective of AS. In the original PARTNER trial that enrolled prohibitive-risk AS patients, one half of the study population died or had no quality of life benefit 1 year after TAVR. TAVR is now an option

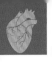
for prohibitive-risk surgical patients, but careful patient selection is needed to determine when AVR is futile.

Futility for TAVR is defined as a life expectancy of less than 1 year despite AVR or likelihood of less than 25% for symptomatic improvement of at least one class in New York Heart Association functional class or Canadian Cardiovascular Society angina.[131] The ability to predict futility remains an ongoing area of interest, but noncardiac comorbidities associated with poor outcomes include severe pulmonary disease requiring oxygen, advanced kidney disease, cirrhosis, advanced frailty, poor independent function, cognitive impairment, mood disorders, and malnutrition.[138]

The determination of futility is based on the patient's values and goals of care. Cognitive impairment and mood assessment screening with the Mini-Mental Status Exam and Geriatric Depression Scale tests assist in ensuing informed decision making by the patient with involvement of family or caregivers when appropriate. When the heart valve team determines futility of therapeutic benefit, palliative care services are offered to patients and their families. It is important to avoid abandonment and discuss palliative care as focused on improvements in quality of life instead of lengthening life.

Final stages of AS are similar to end-stage heart failure, and relief of pain, dyspnea, and nausea are paramount. Individuals with advanced heart failure have a high burden of symptoms and an interdisciplinary palliative care approach that includes medicine, nursing, psychology, spiritual services, and social work improves patient and family experience with end-of-life care.[151–153]

REFERENCES

1. Osnabrugge RL, Mylotte D, Head SJ, et al. Aortic stenosis in the elderly: disease prevalence and number of candidates for transcatheter aortic valve replacement: a meta-analysis and modeling study. J Am Coll Cardiol 2013;62:1002-1012.
2. d'Arcy JL, Coffey S, Loudon MA, et al. Large-scale community echocardiographic screening reveals a major burden of undiagnosed valvular heart disease in older people: the OxVALVE Population Cohort Study. Eur Heart J 2016;37(47):3515-3522.
3. Martinsson A, Li X, Andersson C, et al. Temporal trends in the incidence and prognosis of aortic stenosis: a nationwide study of the Swedish population. Circulation 2015;131:988-994.
4. Grover FL, Vemulapalli S, Carroll JD, et al. 2016 Annual Report of the Society of Thoracic Surgeons/American College of Cardiology Transcatheter Valve Therapy Registry. J Am Coll Cardiol 2017;69(10):1215-1230.
5. Otto CM. Calcific aortic valve disease: outflow obstruction is the end stage of a systemic disease process. Eur Heart J 2009;30:1940-1942.
6. Nishimura RA, Otto CM, Bonow RO, et al. 2014 AHA/ACC guideline for the management of patients with valvular heart disease: a report of the American College of Cardiology/American Heart Association Task Force on Practice Guidelines. J Am Coll Cardiol 2014;63:e57-e185.
7. Roberts WC, Janning KG, Ko JM, et al. Frequency of congenitally bicuspid aortic valves in patients ≥80 years of age undergoing aortic valve replacement for aortic stenosis (with or without aortic regurgitation) and implications for transcatheter aortic valve implantation. Am J Cardiol 2012; 109:1632-1636.
8. Lawrence JG, Carapetis JR, Griffiths K, et al. Acute rheumatic fever and rheumatic heart disease: incidence and progression in the Northern Territory of Australia, 1997 to 2010. Circulation 2013;128:492-501.
9. Mirabel M, Tafflet M, Noël B, et al. Newly diagnosed rheumatic heart disease among indigenous populations in the Pacific. Heart 2015;101: 1901-1906.
10. Sliwa K, Carrington MJ, Klug E, et al. Predisposing factors and incidence of newly diagnosed atrial fibrillation in an urban African community: insights from the Heart of Soweto Study. Heart 2010;96:1878-1882.
11. Otto CM, Burwash IG, Legget ME, et al. Prospective study of asymptomatic valvular aortic stenosis. Clinical, echocardiographic, and exercise predictors of outcome. Circulation 1997;95:2262-2270.
12. Nishizaki Y, Daimon M, Miyazaki S, et al. Clinical factors associated with classical symptoms of aortic valve stenosis. J Heart Valve Dis 2013;22: 287-294.
13. Park SJ, Enriquez-Sarano M, Chang SA, et al. Hemodynamic patterns for symptomatic presentations of severe aortic stenosis. JACC Cardiovasc Imaging 2013;6:137-146.
14. Lancellotti P, Donal E, Magne J, et al. Risk stratification in asymptomatic moderate to severe aortic stenosis: the importance of the valvular, arterial and ventricular interplay. Heart 2010;96:1364-1371.
15. Amato MC, Moffa PJ, Werner KE, Ramires JA. Treatment decision in asymptomatic aortic valve stenosis: role of exercise testing. Heart 2001;86:381-386.
16. Lancellotti P, Lebois F, Simon M, et al. Prognostic importance of quantitative exercise Doppler echocardiography in asymptomatic valvular aortic stenosis. Circulation 2005;112:I377-I382.
17. Larsen LH, Kofoed KF, Dalsgaard M, et al. Assessment of coronary artery disease using coronary computed tomography angiography in patients with aortic valve stenosis referred for surgical aortic valve replacement. Int J Cardiol 2013;168:126-131.
18. Broyd CJ, Sen S, Mikhail GW, et al. Myocardial ischemia in aortic stenosis: insights from arterial pulse-wave dynamics after percutaneous aortic valve replacement. Trends Cardiovasc Med 2013;23:185-191.
19. Wiegerinck EM, van de Hoef TP, Rolandi MC, et al. Impact of aortic valve stenosis on coronary hemodynamics and the instantaneous effect of transcatheter aortic valve implantation. Circ Cardiovasc Interv 2015; 8:e002443.
20. Harada K, Saitoh T, Tanaka J, et al. Valvuloarterial impedance, but not aortic stenosis severity, predicts syncope in patients with aortic stenosis. Circ Cardiovasc Imaging 2013;6:1024-1031.
21. Sorgato A, Faggiano P, Aurigemma GP, et al. Ventricular arrhythmias in adult aortic stenosis: prevalence, mechanisms, and clinical relevance. Chest 1998;113:482-491.
22. Das P, Pocock C, Chambers J. The patient with a systolic murmur: severe aortic stenosis may be missed during cardiovascular examination. QJM 2000;93:685-688.
23. Abe Y, Ito M, Tanaka C, et al. A novel and simple method using pocket-sized echocardiography to screen for aortic stenosis. J Am Soc Echocardiogr 2013;26:589-596.
24. Munt B, Legget ME, Kraft CD, et al. Physical examination in valvular aortic stenosis: correlation with stenosis severity and prediction of clinical outcome. Am Heart J 1999;137:298-306.
25. Aronow WS, Kronzon I. Prevalence and severity of valvular aortic stenosis determined by Doppler echocardiography and its association with echocardiographic and electrocardiographic left ventricular hypertrophy and physical signs of aortic stenosis in elderly patients. Am J Cardiol 1991; 67:776-777.
26. Hachicha Z, Dumesnil JG, Bogaty P, Pibarot P. Paradoxical low-flow, low-gradient severe aortic stenosis despite preserved ejection fraction is associated with higher afterload and reduced survival. Circulation 2007; 115:2856-2864.
27. Rogge BP, Gerdts E, Cramariuc D, et al. Impact of obesity and nonobesity on grading the severity of aortic valve stenosis. Am J Cardiol 2014;113: 1532-1535.
28. Omran H, Schmidt H, Hackenbroch M, et al. Silent and apparent cerebral embolism after retrograde catheterisation of the aortic valve in valvular stenosis: a prospective, randomised study. Lancet 2003;361:1241-1246.
29. Nishimura RA, Carabello BA. Hemodynamics in the cardiac catheterization laboratory of the 21st century. Circulation 2012;125:2138-2150.
30. Gertz ZM, Raina A, O'Donnell W, et al. Comparison of invasive and noninvasive assessment of aortic stenosis severity in the elderly. Circ Cardiovasc Interv 2012;5:406-414.
31. Yang CS, Marshall ES, Fanari Z, et al. Discrepancies between direct catheter and echocardiography-based values in aortic stenosis. Catheter Cardiovasc Interv 2016;87:488-497.
32. Das P, Rimington H, Chambers J. Exercise testing to stratify risk in aortic stenosis. Eur Heart J 2005;26:1309-1313.

33. Maréchaux S, Hachicha Z, Bellouin A, et al. Usefulness of exercise-stress echocardiography for risk stratification of true asymptomatic patients with aortic valve stenosis. Eur Heart J 2010;31:1390-1397.

34. Lancellotti P, Magne J, Donal E, et al. Determinants and prognostic significance of exercise pulmonary hypertension in asymptomatic severe aortic stenosis. Circulation 2012;126:851-859.

35. Alborino D, Hoffmann JL, Fournet PC, Bloch A. Value of exercise testing to evaluate the indication for surgery in asymptomatic patients with valvular aortic stenosis. J Heart Valve Dis 2002;11:204-209.

36. Levy F, Fayad N, Jeu A, et al. The value of cardiopulmonary exercise testing in individuals with apparently asymptomatic severe aortic stenosis: a pilot study. Arch Cardiovasc Dis 2014;107:519-528.

37. Saeed S, Rajani R, Seifert R, et al. Exercise testing in patients with asymptomatic moderate or severe aortic stenosis. Heart 2018.

38. Clavel MA, Magne J, Pibarot P. Low-gradient aortic stenosis. Eur Heart J 2015;37:2645-2657.

39. Chahal NS, Drakopoulou M, Gonzalez-Gonzalez AM, et al. Resting aortic valve area at normal transaortic flow rate reflects true valve area in suspected low-gradient severe aortic stenosis. JACC Cardiovasc Imaging 2015;8:1133-1139.

40. Pellikka PA, Roger VL, McCully RB, et al. Normal stroke volume and cardiac output response during dobutamine stress echocardiography in subjects without left ventricular wall motion abnormalities. Am J Cardiol 1995;76:881-886.

41. Clavel MA, Burwash IG, Mundigler G, et al. Validation of conventional and simplified methods to calculate projected valve area at normal flow rate in patients with low flow, low gradient aortic stenosis: the multicenter TOPAS (True or Pseudo Severe Aortic Stenosis) study. J Am Soc Echocardiogr 2010;23:380-386.

42. Clavel MA, Ennezat PV, Maréchaux S, et al. Stress echocardiography to assess stenosis severity and predict outcome in patients with paradoxical low-flow, low-gradient aortic stenosis and preserved LVEF. JACC Cardiovasc Imaging 2013;6:175-183.

43. Budoff M, Katz R, Wong N, et al. Effect of scanner type on the reproducibility of extracoronary measures of calcification: the multi-ethnic study of atherosclerosis. Acad Radiol 2007;14:1043-1049.

44. Thaden JJ, Nkomo VT, Suri RM, et al. Sex-related differences in calcific aortic stenosis: correlating clinical and echocardiographic characteristics and computed tomography aortic valve calcium score to excised aortic valve weight. Eur Heart J 2016;37:693-699.

45. Owens DS, Katz R, Takasu J, et al. Incidence and progression of aortic valve calcium in the Multi-Ethnic Study of Atherosclerosis (MESA). Am J Cardiol 2010;105:701-708.

46. Aggarwal SR, Clavel MA, Messika-Zeitoun D, et al. Sex differences in aortic valve calcification measured by multidetector computed tomography in aortic stenosis. Circ Cardiovasc Imaging 2013;6:40-47.

47. Clavel MA, Messika-Zeitoun D, Pibarot P, et al. The complex nature of discordant severe calcified aortic valve disease grading: new insights from combined Doppler-echocardiographic and computed tomographic study. J Am Coll Cardiol 2013;62(24):2329-2338.

48. Cueff C, Serfaty JM, Cimadevilla C, et al. Measurement of aortic valve calcification using multislice computed tomography: correlation with haemodynamic severity of aortic stenosis and clinical implication for patients with low ejection fraction Heart 2011;97:721-726.

49. Clavel MA, Pibarot P, Messika-Zeitoun D, et al. Impact of aortic valve calcification, as measured by MDCT, on survival in patients with aortic stenosis: results of an international registry study. J Am Coll Cardiol 2014;64:1202-1213.

50. Otto C, Lind B, Kitzman D, et al. Association of aortic-valve sclerosis with cardiovascular mortality and morbidity in the elderly. N Engl J Med 1999;341:142-147.

51. Owens DS, Budoff MJ, Katz R, et al. Aortic valve calcium independently predicts coronary and cardiovascular events in a primary prevention population. JACC Cardiovasc Imaging 2012;5:619-625.

52. Baumgartner H, Falk V, Bax JJ, et al. and Group ESD. 2017 ESC/EACTS Guidelines for the management of valvular heart disease. Eur Heart J 2017;38:2739-2791.

53. Steadman CD, Ray S, Ng LL, McCann GP. Natriuretic peptides in common valvular heart disease. J Am Coll Cardiol 2010;55:2034-2048.

54. Cimadevilla C, Cueff C, Hekimian G, et al. Prognostic value of B-type natriuretic peptide in elderly patients with aortic valve stenosis: the COFRASA-GENERAC study. Heart 2013;99:461-467.

55. Clavel MA, Malouf J, Michelena HI, et al. B-type natriuretic peptide clinical activation in aortic stenosis: impact on long-term survival. J Am Coll Cardiol 2014;63:2016-2025.

56. Chin CW, Shah AS, McAllister DA, et al. High-sensitivity troponin I concentrations are a marker of an advanced hypertrophic response and adverse outcomes in patients with aortic stenosis. Eur Heart J 2014;35:2312-2321.

57. Lindman BR, Breyley JG, Schilling JD, et al. Prognostic utility of novel biomarkers of cardiovascular stress in patients with aortic stenosis undergoing valve replacement. Heart 2015;101:1382-1388.

58. Rahimi K, Mohseni H, Kiran A, et al. Elevated blood pressure and risk of aortic valve disease: a cohort analysis of 5.4 million UK adults. Eur Heart J 2018;39:3596-3603.

59. Faggiano P, Antonini-Canterin F, Erlicher A, et al. Progression of aortic valve sclerosis to aortic stenosis. Am J Cardiol 2003;91:99-101.

60. Coffey S, Cox B, Williams MJ. The prevalence, incidence, progression, and risks of aortic valve sclerosis: a systematic review and meta-analysis. J Am Coll Cardiol 2014;63:2852-2861.

61. Novaro G, Katz R, Aviles R, et al. Clinical factors, but not C-reactive protein, predict progression of calcific aortic-valve disease: the Cardiovascular Health Study. J Am Coll Cardiol 2007;50:1992-1998.

62. Rossebø A, Pedersen T, Boman K, et al. Intensive lipid lowering with simvastatin and ezetimibe in aortic stenosis. N Engl J Med 2008;359:1343-1356.

63. Rosenhek R, Klaar U, Schemper M, et al. Mild and moderate aortic stenosis. Natural history and risk stratification by echocardiography. Eur Heart J 2004;25:199-205.

64. Kamalesh M, Ng C, El Masry H, et al. Does diabetes accelerate progression of calcific aortic stenosis? Eur J Echocardiogr 2009;10:723-725.

65. Chan KL, Teo K, Dumesnil JG, et al. Effect of Lipid lowering with rosuvastatin on progression of aortic stenosis: results of the aortic stenosis progression observation: measuring effects of rosuvastatin (ASTRONOMER) trial Circulation 2010;121:306-314.

66. Nistri S, Faggiano P, Olivotto I, et al. Hemodynamic progression and outcome of asymptomatic aortic stenosis in primary care. Am J Cardiol 2012;109:718-723.

67. Kearney LG, Ord M, Buxton BF, et al. Progression of aortic stenosis in elderly patients over long-term follow up. Int J Cardiol 2013;167:1226-1231.

68. Eveborn GW, Schirmer H, Heggelund G, et al. The evolving epidemiology of valvular aortic stenosis. The Tromsø study. Heart 2013;99:396-400.

69. Nguyen V, Cimadevilla C, Estellat C, et al. Haemodynamic and anatomic progression of aortic stenosis. Heart 2015;101:943-947.

70. de Oliveira Moraes AB, Stähli BE, Arsenault BJ, et al. Resting heart rate as a predictor of aortic valve stenosis progression. Int J Cardiol 2016;204:149-151.

71. Ersboll M, Schulte PJ, Al Enezi F, et al. Predictors and progression of aortic stenosis in patients with preserved left ventricular ejection fraction. Am J Cardiol 2015;115:86-92.

72. Lancellotti P, Magne J, Dulgheru R, et al. Outcomes of patients with asymptomatic aortic stenosis followed up in heart valve clinics. JAMA Cardiol 2018;3(11):1060-1068.

73. Rafique AM, Biner S, Ray I, et al. Meta-analysis of prognostic value of stress testing in patients with asymptomatic severe aortic stenosis. Am J Cardiol 2009;104:972-977.

74. Greve AM, Gerdts E, Boman K, et al. Impact of QRS duration and morphology on the risk of sudden cardiac death in asymptomatic patients with aortic stenosis: the SEAS (Simvastatin and Ezetimibe in Aortic Stenosis) Study. J Am Coll Cardiol 2012;59:1142-1149.

75. Kang DH, Park SJ, Rim JH, et al. Early surgery versus conventional treatment in asymptomatic very severe aortic stenosis. Circulation 2010;121:1502-1509.

76. Kitai T, Honda S, Okada Y, et al. Clinical outcomes in non-surgically managed patients with very severe versus severe aortic stenosis. Heart 2011;97:2029-2032.

77. Levy F, Rusinaru D, Maréchaux S, et al. Determinants and prognosis of atrial fibrillation in patients with aortic stenosis. Am J Cardiol 2015;116:1541-1546.

78. Greve AM, Gerdts E, Boman K, et al. Prognostic importance of atrial fibrillation in asymptomatic aortic stenosis: the Simvastatin and Ezetimibe in Aortic Stenosis study. Int J Cardiol 2013;166:72-76.

79. Natorska J, Mazur P, Undas A. Increased bleeding risk in patients with aortic valvular stenosis: from new mechanisms to new therapies. Thromb Res 2016;139:85-89.

80. Sedaghat A, Kulka H, Sinning JM, et al. Transcatheter aortic valve implantation leads to a restoration of von Willebrand factor (VWF) abnormalities in patients with severe aortic stenosis—incidence and relevance of clinical and subclinical VWF dysfunction in patients undergoing transfemoral TAVI. Thromb Res 2017;151:23-28.

81. Towler DA. Molecular and cellular aspects of calcific aortic valve disease. Circ Res 2013;113:198-208.

82. Marquis-Gravel G, Redfors B, Leon MB and Généreux P. Medical treatment of aortic stenosis. Circulation 2016;134:1766-1784.

83. Chan KL, Teo K, Dumesnil JG, Ni A, et al. Effect of lipid lowering with rosuvastatin on progression of aortic stenosis: results of the aortic stenosis progression observation: measuring effects of rosuvastatin (ASTRONOMER) trial. Circulation 2010;121:306-314.

84. Teo KK, Corsi DJ, Tam JW, et al. Lipid lowering on progression of mild to moderate aortic stenosis: meta-analysis of the randomized placebo-controlled clinical trials on 2344 patients. Can J Cardiol 2011; 27:800-808.

85. Thanassoulis G, Campbell CY, Owens DS, et al. Group CECW. Genetic associations with valvular calcification and aortic stenosis. N Engl J Med 2013;368:503-512.

86. Nielsen OW, Sajadieh A, Sabbah M, et al. Assessing optimal blood pressure in patients with asymptomatic aortic valve stenosis: the Simvastatin Ezetimibe in Aortic Stenosis study (SEAS). Circulation 2016;134: 455-468.

87. Eleid MF, Nishimura RA, Sorajja P, Borlaug BA. Systemic hypertension in low-gradient severe aortic stenosis with preserved ejection fraction. Circulation 2013;128:1349-1353.

88. Bull S, Loudon M, Francis JM, et al. A prospective, double-blind, randomized controlled trial of the angiotensin-converting enzyme inhibitor Ramipril In Aortic Stenosis (RIAS trial). Eur Heart J Cardiovasc Imaging 2015;16: 834-841.

89. Ezekowitz MD, Nagarakanti R, Noack H, et al. Comparison of dabigatran and warfarin in patients with atrial fibrillation and valvular heart disease: The RE-LY Trial (Randomized Evaluation of Long-Term Anticoagulant Therapy). Circulation 2016;134:589-598.

90. Avezum A, Lopes RD, Schulte PJ, et al. Apixaban in comparison with warfarin in patients with atrial fibrillation and valvular heart disease: findings from the Apixaban for Reduction in Stroke and Other Thrombo-embolic Events in Atrial Fibrillation (ARISTOTLE) Trial. Circulation 2015;132:624-632.

91. Durães AR, de Souza Roriz P, de Almeida Nunes B, et al. Dabigatran versus warfarin after bioprosthesis valve replacement for the management of atrial fibrillation postoperatively: DAWA pilot study. Drugs R D 2016;16: 149-154.

92. Tarantini G, Mojoli M, Urena M, Vahanian A. Atrial fibrillation in patients undergoing transcatheter aortic valve implantation: epidemiology, timing, predictors, and outcome. Eur Heart J 2017;38(17):1285-1293.

93. Bonow RO, Cheitlin MD, Crawford MH, Douglas PS. Task force 3: valvular heart disease. J Am Coll Cardiol 2005;45:1334-1340.

94. Tashiro T, Pislaru SV, Blustin JM, et al. Perioperative risk of major non-cardiac surgery in patients with severe aortic stenosis: a reappraisal in contemporary practice Eur Heart J 2014;35:2372-2381.

95. Braunwald E. On the natural history of severe aortic stenosis. J Am Coll Cardiol 1990;15:1018-1020.

96. Nishimura RA, Otto CM, Bonow RO, et al. 2017 AHA/ACC focused update of the 2014 AHA/ACC guideline for the management of patients with valvular heart disease: a report of the American College of Cardiology/American Heart Association Task Force on Clinical Practice Guidelines. Circulation 2017;135(25):e1159-e1195.

97. Bach DS, Siao D, Girard SE, et al. Evaluation of patients with severe symptomatic aortic stenosis who do not undergo aortic valve replacement: the potential role of subjectively overestimated operative risk. Circ Cardiovasc Qual Outcomes 2009;2:533-539.

98. Kapadia SR, Tuzcu EM, Makkar RR, et al. Long-term outcomes of inoperable patients with aortic stenosis randomly assigned to transcatheter aortic valve replacement or standard therapy. Circulation 2014;130: 1483-1492.

99. Monin JL, Quéré JP, Monchi M, et al. Low-gradient aortic stenosis: operative risk stratification and predictors for long-term outcome: a multicenter study using dobutamine stress hemodynamics. Circulation 2003;108:319-324.

100. Halkos ME, Chen EP, Sarin EL, et al. Aortic valve replacement for aortic stenosis in patients with left ventricular dysfunction. Ann Thorac Surg 2009;88:746-751.

101. Rosenhek R, Zilberszac R, Schemper M, et al. Natural history of very severe aortic stenosis. Circulation 2010;121:151-156.

102. Monin JL, Lancellotti P, Monchi M, et al. Risk score for predicting outcome in patients with asymptomatic aortic stenosis. Circulation 2009; 120:69-75.

103. Farré N, Gómez M, Molina L, et al. Prognostic value of NT-proBNP and an adapted monin score in patients with asymptomatic aortic stenosis. Rev Esp Cardiol (Engl Ed) 2014;67:52-57.

104. Chin CW, Messika-Zeitoun D, Shah AS, et al. A clinical risk score of myocardial fibrosis predicts adverse outcomes in aortic stenosis. Eur Heart J 2016;37:713-723.

105. Taniguchi T, Morimoto T, Shiomi H, et al. Initial surgical versus conservative strategies in patients with asymptomatic severe aortic stenosis. J Am Coll Cardiol 2015;66:2827-2838.

106. Généreux P, Stone GW, O'Gara PT, et al. Natural history, diagnostic approaches, and therapeutic strategies for patients with asymptomatic severe aortic stenosis. J Am Coll Cardiol 2016;67:2263-2288.

107. Lim WY, Ramasamy A, Lloyd G, Bhattacharyya S. Meta-analysis of the impact of intervention versus symptom-driven management in asymptomatic severe aortic stenosis. Heart 2017;103:268-272.

108. Pellikka PA, Sarano ME, Nishimura RA, et al. Outcome of 622 adults with asymptomatic, hemodynamically significant aortic stenosis during prolonged follow-up. Circulation 2005;111:3290-3295.

109. Lancellotti P, Donal E, Magne J, et al. Impact of global left ventricular afterload on left ventricular function in asymptomatic severe aortic stenosis: a two-dimensional speckle-tracking study. Eur J Echocardiogr 2010;11:537-543.

110. Banovic M, Iung B, Bartunek J, et al. Rationale and design of the Aortic Valve replAcemenT versus conservative treatment in Asymptomatic seveRe aortic stenosis (AVATAR trial): a randomized multicenter controlled event-driven trial. Am Heart J 2016;174:147-153.

111. Izumi C. Asymptomatic severe aortic stenosis: challenges in diagnosis and management. Heart 2016;102:1168-1176.

112. Fougères E, Tribouilloy C, Monchi M, et al. Outcomes of pseudo-severe aortic stenosis under conservative treatment. Eur Heart J 2012;33: 2426-2433.

113. Quere JP, Monin JL, Levy F, et al. Influence of preoperative left ventricular contractile reserve on postoperative ejection fraction in low-gradient aortic stenosis. Circulation 2006;113:1738-1744.

114. Levy F, Laurent M, Monin J, et al. Aortic valve replacement for low-flow/low-gradient aortic stenosis operative risk stratification and long-term outcome: a European multicenter study. J Am Coll Cardiol 2008;51: 1466-1472.

115. Tribouilloy C, Lévy F, Rusinaru D, et al. Outcome after aortic valve replacement for low-flow/low-gradient aortic stenosis without contractile reserve on dobutamine stress echocardiography. J Am Coll Cardiol 2009;53:1865-1873.

116. Herrmann HC, Pibarot P, Hueter I, et al. Predictors of mortality and outcomes of therapy in low-flow severe aortic stenosis: a Placement of Aortic Transcatheter Valves (PARTNER) trial analysis. Circulation 2013;127:2316-2326.

117. Tribouilloy C, Rusinaru D, Maréchaux S, et al. Low-gradient, low-flow severe aortic stenosis with preserved left ventricular ejection fraction: characteristics, outcome, and implications for surgery. J Am Coll Cardiol 2015;65:55-66.

118. Clavel MA, Dumesnil JG, Capoulade R, et al. Outcome of patients with aortic stenosis, small valve area, and low-flow, low-gradient despite preserved left ventricular ejection fraction. J Am Coll Cardiol 2012;60:1259-1267.

119. Lancellotti P, Magne J, Donal E, et al. Clinical outcome in asymptomatic severe aortic stenosis: insights from the new proposed aortic stenosis grading classification. J Am Coll Cardiol 2012;59:235-243.

120. Jander N, Minners J, Holme I, et al. Outcome of patients with low-gradient "severe" aortic stenosis and preserved ejection fraction. Circulation 2011; 123:887-895.

121. Eleid MF, Sorajja P, Michelena HI, et al. Flow-gradient patterns in severe aortic stenosis with preserved ejection fraction: clinical characteristics and predictors of survival. Circulation 2013;128:1781-1789.

122. Mehrotra P, Jansen K, Flynn AW, et al. Differential left ventricular remodelling and longitudinal function distinguishes low flow from normal-flow preserved ejection fraction low-gradient severe aortic stenosis. Eur Heart J 2013;34:1906-1914.

123. Maes F, Boulif J, Piérard S, et al. Natural history of paradoxical low-gradient severe aortic stenosis. Circ Cardiovasc Imaging 2014;7:714-722.

124. Maor E, Beigel R, Grupper A, et al. Relation between stroke volume index to risk of death in patients with low-gradient severe aortic stenosis and preserved left ventricular function. Am J Cardiol 2014;114:449-455.

125. González Gómez A, Fernández-Golfín C, Monteagudo JM, et al. Severe aortic stenosis patients with preserved ejection fraction according to flow and gradient classification: prevalence and outcomes. Int J Cardiol 2017; 248:211-215.

126. Bavishi C, Balasundaram K, Argulian E. Integration of flow-gradient patterns into clinical decision making for patients with suspected severe aortic stenosis and preserved LVEF: a systematic review of evidence and meta-analysis. JACC Cardiovasc Imaging 2016;9:1255-1263.

127. Dayan V, Vignolo G, Magne J, et al. Outcome and impact of aortic valve replacement in patients with preserved LVEF and low-gradient aortic stenosis. J Am Coll Cardiol 2015;66:2594-2603.

128. Yamashita K, Fujita T, Hata H, et al. Long-term outcome of isolated off-pump coronary artery bypass grafting in patients with coronary artery disease and mild to moderate aortic stenosis. J Cardiol 2017;70(1):48-54.

129. Vandvik PO, Otto CM, Siemieniuk RA, et al. Transcatheter or surgical aortic valve replacement for patients with severe, symptomatic, aortic stenosis at low to intermediate surgical risk: a clinical practice guideline. BMJ 2016;354:i5085.

130. Chiang YP, Chikwe J, Moskowitz AJ, et al. Survival and long-term outcomes following bioprosthetic vs mechanical aortic valve replacement in patients aged 50 to 69 years. JAMA 2014;312:1323-1329.

131. Otto CM, Kumbhani DJ, Alexander KP, et al. 2017 ACC expert consensus decision pathway for transcatheter aortic valve replacement in the management of adults with aortic stenosis: a report of the American College of Cardiology task force on clinical expert consensus documents. J Am Coll Cardiol 2017;69(10):1313-1346.

131a. Burke CR, Kirkpatrick JN, Otto CM. Goals of care in patients with severe aortic stenosis. Eur Heart J 2020;41(8):929-932.

132. Leon MB, Smith CR, Mack MJ, et al. Transcatheter or surgical aortic-valve replacement in intermediate-risk patients. N Engl J Med 2016; 374:1609-1620.

132a. Mack MJ, Leon MB, Thourani VH, et al. Transcatheter aortic-valve replacement with a balloon-expandable valve in low-risk patients. N Engl J Med 2019;380(18):1695-1705.

132b. Popma JJ, Deeb GM, Yakubov SJ, et al. Transcatheter aortic-valve replacement with a self-expanding valve in low-risk patients. N Engl J Med 2019;380(18):1706-1715.

132c. Testa L, Latib A, Brambilla N, et al. Long-term clinical outcome and performance of transcatheter aortic valve replacement with a self-expandable bioprosthesis. Eur Heart J 2020 Jan 6. pii: ehz925. doi: 10.1093/eurheartj/ehz925. [Epub ahead of print]

132d. Søndergaard L, Ihlemann N, Capodanno D, et al. Durability of transcatheter and surgical bioprosthetic aortic valves in patients at lower surgical risk. J Am Coll Cardiol 2019;73(5):546-553.

133. Ejiofor JI, Yammine M, Harloff MT, et al. Reoperative surgical aortic valve replacement versus transcatheter valve-in-valve replacement for degenerated bioprosthetic aortic valves. Ann Thorac Surg 2016;102:1452-1458.

134. Kayalar N, Schaff HV, Daly RC, et al. Concomitant septal myectomy at the time of aortic valve replacement for severe aortic stenosis. Ann Thorac Surg 2010;89:459-464.

135. Viktorsson SA, Helgason D, Orrason AW, et al. Favorable survival after aortic valve replacement compared to the general population. J Heart Valve Dis 2016;25:8-13.

136. Kvidal P, Bergström R, Hörte LG, Ståhle E. Observed and relative survival after aortic valve replacement. J Am Coll Cardiol 2000;35:747-756.

137. Goldberg JB, DeSimone JP, Kramer RS, et al. and Group NNECDS. Impact of preoperative left ventricular ejection fraction on long-term survival after aortic valve replacement for aortic stenosis. Circ Cardiovasc Qual Outcomes 2013;6:35-41.

138. Lindman BR, Alexander KP, O'Gara PT, Afilalo J. Futility, benefit, and transcatheter aortic valve replacement. JACC Cardiovasc Interv 2014; 7:707-716.

139. Adams DH, Popma JJ, Reardon MJ. Transcatheter aortic-valve replacement with a self-expanding prosthesis. N Engl J Med 2014;371:967-968.

140. Herrmann HC, Thourani VH, Kodali SK, et al. One-year clinical outcomes with SAPIEN 3 transcatheter aortic valve replacement in high-risk and inoperable patients with severe aortic stenosis. Circulation 2016;134:130-140.

141. Blackstone EH, Suri RM, Rajeswaran J, et al. Propensity-matched comparisons of clinical outcomes after transapical or transfemoral transcatheter aortic valve replacement: a placement of aortic transcatheter valves (PARTNER)-I trial substudy. Circulation 2015;131:1989-2000.

142. Gleason TG, Schindler JT, Adams DH, et al. The risk and extent of neurologic events are equivalent for high-risk patients treated with transcatheter or surgical aortic valve replacement. J Thorac Cardiovasc Surg 2016;152:85-96.

143. Elmariah S, Palacios IF, McAndrew T, et al. Outcomes of transcatheter and surgical aortic valve replacement in high-risk patients with aortic stenosis and left ventricular dysfunction: results from the Placement of Aortic Transcatheter Valves (PARTNER) trial (cohort A). Circ Cardiovasc Interv 2013;6:604-614.

144. Kamperidis V, Joyce E, Debonnaire P, et al. Left ventricular functional recovery and remodeling in low-flow low-gradient severe aortic stenosis after transcatheter aortic valve implantation. J Am Soc Echocardiogr 2014;27:817-825.

145. Lund O, Emmertsen K, Dørup I, et al. Regression of left ventricular hypertrophy during 10 years after valve replacement for aortic stenosis is related to the preoperative risk profile. Eur Heart J 2003;24:1437-1446.

146. Kandler K, Møller CH, Hassager C, et al. Patient-prosthesis mismatch and reduction in left ventricular mass after aortic valve replacement. Ann Thorac Surg 2013;96:66-71.

147. Pibarot P, Weissman NJ, Stewart WJ, et al. Incidence and sequelae of prosthesis-patient mismatch in transcatheter versus surgical valve replacement in high-risk patients with severe aortic stenosis: a PARTNER trial cohort—an analysis. J Am Coll Cardiol 2014;64:1323-1334.

148. Lamb HJ, Beyerbacht HP, de Roos A, et al. Left ventricular remodeling early after aortic valve replacement: differential effects on diastolic function in aortic valve stenosis and aortic regurgitation. J Am Coll Cardiol 2002;40:2182-2188.

149. Vizzardi E, D'Aloia A, Fiorina C, et al. Early regression of left ventricular mass associated with diastolic improvement after transcatheter aortic valve implantation. J Am Soc Echocardiogr 2012;25:1091-1098.

150. Lindman BR, Stewart WJ, Pibarot P, et al. Early regression of severe left ventricular hypertrophy after transcatheter aortic valve replacement is associated with decreased hospitalizations. JACC Cardiovasc Interv 2014;7:662-673.

151. Lauck SB, Gibson JA, Baumbusch J, et al. Transition to palliative care when transcatheter aortic valve implantation is not an option: opportunities and recommendations. Curr Opin Support Palliat Care 2016;10:18-23.

152. Kelley AS, Morrison RS. Palliative care for the seriously ill. N Engl J Med 2015;373:747-755.

153. Rosenhek R, Binder T, Porenta G, et al. Predictors of outcome in severe, asymptomatic aortic stenosis. N Engl J Med 2000;343:611-617.

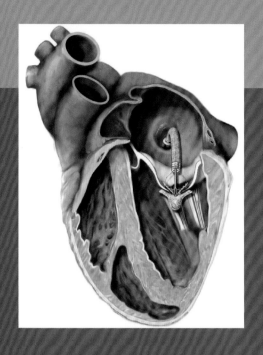

第10章
主动脉瓣反流：临床表现、疾病阶段和管理

　　本章主要围绕主动脉瓣反流的临床表现、分期和治疗等内容展开，主要内容概况：主动脉瓣反流病因；急性主动脉瓣反流的诊断、病理生理学和治疗；慢性主动脉瓣反流临床表现——病史、体格检查、心电图、胸部X线检查、超声心动图、其他影像检查和运动测试；慢性主动脉瓣反流疾病分期——病理生理学和进展；慢性主动脉瓣反流治疗——血管扩张治疗和心内膜炎预防；慢性主动脉瓣反流系统评估；慢性主动脉瓣反流手术适应证——主动脉瓣置换或修复，还应考虑升主动脉扩张及其伴随疾病。本章内容要点包括：主动脉瓣反流由主动脉瓣瓣叶、主动脉根部或升主动脉异常引起；主动脉瓣反流评估包括瓣叶形态、反流机制、严重程度和升主动脉扩张程度；超声心动图是评估主动脉瓣反流严重程度最有用的工具，测量指标包括彩色多普勒缩流颈宽度和降主动脉舒张期逆向血流持续时间，而近端血流等速面法对容量负荷不太敏感但技术要求更高；心脏MRI可定量分析主动脉瓣反流严重程度和左心室功能，主要用于超声心动图分析欠佳时；心脏MRI和CT可准确测量升主动脉内径，有利于分析功能性主动脉瓣反流机制、随访升主动脉内径和确定升主动脉手术最佳治疗时间和策略；临床症状是大多数慢性主动脉瓣反流患者的手术指征，但无症状心室收缩力受损，如左室射血分数<50%或左心室收缩末期内径>50 mm（>21 mm/m²）是治疗决策最有用的参数，当体表面积<1.65 m²，建议采用收缩末期内径指数；治疗重度主动脉瓣反流而保留主动脉瓣手术，包括保留瓣叶手术和主动脉瓣瓣叶修复手术；术中经食管超声心动图的应用非常必要，修复术后必须即刻评估瓣膜功能，并识别术后早期复发风险。

陈　阳

Aortic Regurgitation: Clinical Presentation, Disease Stages, and Management

Arturo Evangelista, Pilar Tornos, Robert O. Bonow

CHAPTER OUTLINE

KEY POINTS

- Aortic regurgitation (AR) may be caused by abnormalities of the aortic leaflets, aortic root, or ascending aorta. Evaluation of AR should include valve morphology, regurgitation mechanism, and severity and aortic dilation assessment.
- Color Doppler proximal jet width with measurement of the vena contracta and diastolic flow reversal in the descending aorta are the most useful echocardiographic methods to assess AR severity in clinical practice. The flow convergence method (i.e., proximal isovelocity surface area [PISA] method) is less sensitive to loading conditions but more technically demanding.
- Cardiac magnetic resonance (CMR) may be used in the quantitative assessment of regurgitant severity and left ventricular (LV) function when echocardiography is suboptimal. CMR and computed tomography provide accurate ascending aorta measurements, which are important for understanding functional AR

mechanisms, follow-up of aorta size, and targeting the optimal time and strategy for ascending aorta surgery.
- Symptoms are the indication for surgical intervention in most patients with chronic AR; but some patients have impaired ventricular contractility in the absence of symptoms. LV ejection fraction less than 50% and/or LV end-systolic diameter greater than 50 mm (>21 mm/m^2) are the most useful parameters for clinical decision making. Indexed end-systolic diameter is recommended when the body surface area is less than 1.65 m^2.
- Conservative aortic valve surgery, including valve-sparing operations, and aortic cusp repair should be considered in the management of severe AR. Intraoperative transesophageal echocardiography is mandatory after repair to assess the functional result and identify patients at risk for early AR recurrence.

Aortic regurgitation (AR) is characterized by diastolic reflux of blood from the aorta into the left ventricle (LV). The overall prevalence of AR detected by color Doppler echocardiography in an adult population was 4.9% in the Framingham Heart Study[1] and 10% in the Strong Heart Study.[2] Most cases were trace or mild AR; moderate or severe AR is less common (0.5%–2.7%).

ETIOLOGY

AR causes fall into two broad categories: primary abnormalities of the aortic valve leaflets and abnormalities of the aortic root and ascending

aorta (Table 10.1). The most frequent causes include congenital abnormalities of the aortic valve (most notably bicuspid valves, but also unicuspid, and quadricuspid valves), rheumatic disease, infective endocarditis, calcific degeneration, and myxomatous degeneration (Fig. 10.1). Other common causes of AR represent diseases of the aorta without direct involvement of the aortic valve, as in patients with aorta dilation secondary to genetic disorders such as Marfan syndrome, idiopathic annulo-aortic ectasia, degenerative aneurysms (more frequent in patients with systemic hypertension), and aortic dissection.[3,4]

With the development and clinical adoption of transcatheter aortic valve replacement (TAVR) techniques, TAVR has emerged as a common

TABLE 10.1	Causes of Aortic Regurgitation.
Leaflet abnormalities	Rheumatic disease
	Aortic valve sclerosis and calcification
	Congenital abnormalities (bicuspid, unicuspid, and quadricuspid valves; and aortic regurgitation associated with discrete subaortic stenosis and ventricular septal defect)
	Infective endocarditis
	Myxomatous valve disease
	Complicating balloon valvuloplasty and transcatheter aortic valve implantation
	Rare causes (drugs, leaflet fenestration, irradiation, nonbacterial endocarditis, trauma)
Aortic root abnormalities	Chronic hypertension
	Marfan syndrome
	Annulo-aortic ectasia
	Aortic dissection
	Ehlers-Danlos syndrome
	Osteogenesis imperfecta
	Atherosclerotic aneurysm
	Syphilitic aortitis
	Other systemic inflammatory disorders (giant cell aortitis, Takayasu disease, Reiter syndrome)
Combined valve and aortic root abnormalities	Bicuspid aortic valve
	Ankylosing spondylitis

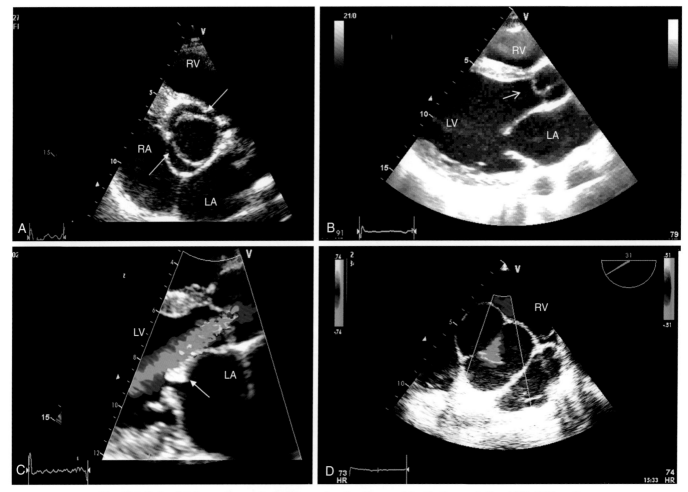

Fig. 10.1 Role of Echocardiography in Diagnosing the Cause of Aortic Regurgitation (AR). (A) Transthoracic parasternal short-axis view shows a bicuspid aortic valve (Video 10.1A ⏵). (B) Myxomatous aortic valve with prolapse of the right coronary cusp *(arrow)* (Video 10.1B ⏵). (C) Rheumatic valvular disease with mitral *(arrow)* and aortic involvement. (D) Transesophageal echocardiography shows a central regurgitant orifice due to an annulo-aortic ectasia. *Ao*, Aorta; *LA*, left atrium; *LV*, left ventricle; *RV*, right ventricle.

and potentially important cause of acute and chronic AR.[5] AR may also develop as a complication of balloon aortic valvuloplasty[6] or after LV assist device implantation.[7] However, in many cases of AR, the precise cause is unclear. In a pathologic study of a surgical series of excised aortic valves, up to 34% of pure AR cases, the cause was unclear.[3] In the Euro Heart Survey for Valvular Diseases, AR represented 13.3% of patients with single native left-sided disease: 15.2% had a congenital origin, and the same percentage was observed for rheumatic origin.[8]

Most of these lesions produce chronic AR, with slow, insidious LV dilation and a prolonged asymptomatic phase. Other lesions, particularly infective endocarditis, aortic dissection, and trauma, more often produce acute severe AR with sudden elevation of LV filling pressures, pulmonary edema, and reduced cardiac output.

ACUTE AORTIC REGURGITATION

Diagnosis

Acute severe AR may be misdiagnosed as another acute condition. Many of the characteristic physical findings of chronic volume overload are modified or absent when valvular regurgitation is acute, and the severity of AR can be underestimated. Due to acute hemodynamic deterioration, patients with acute AR are often tachycardic, tachypneic, and in pulmonary edema. However, LV size may be normal on physical examination, and cardiomegaly may be absent on the chest radiograph. Pulse pressure may not be increased because systolic pressure is reduced in relation to the decrease in forward stroke volume, and diastolic pressure equals the elevated LV diastolic pressure. In the absence of a widened pulse pressure, the characteristic peripheral signs of AR are absent. Although a diastolic murmur is usually present, it can be soft and short because the rapidly rising LV diastolic pressure reduces the aortic-ventricular pressure gradient. The murmur is often difficult to hear.

Echocardiography is indispensable in confirming the presence and severity of AR, assessing its cause, and determining whether there is a rapid equilibration of aortic and LV diastolic pressure. Evidence for rapid pressure equilibration includes a short AR diastolic half-time (<300 ms) and a short mitral deceleration time (<150 ms) (Fig. 10.2). Premature mitral valve closure is a specific and sensitive, noninvasive indicator of acute severe AR, and the extent of premature mitral valve closure correlates with the degree of increase in LV diastolic pressure.[9] In severe AR, the LV end-diastolic pressure can exceed the left atrial pressure and cause premature, presystolic closure of the mitral valve.

Transesophageal echocardiography (TEE) is indicated when aortic dissection, acute endocarditis, or trauma is suspected (Fig. 10.3). Computed tomography (CT) or cardiac magnetic resonance (CMR) can be

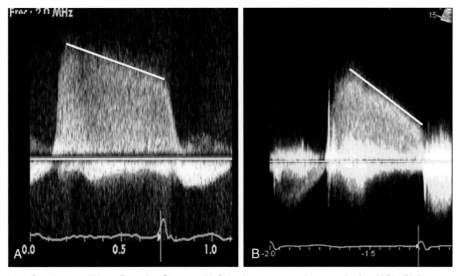

Fig. 10.2 Continuous-Wave Doppler Curves. (A) Chronic severe aortic regurgitation (AR). (B) Acute severe AR. Notice the steeper deceleration slope in the acute phase, which is due to the equalization of LV and aortic diastolic pressures.

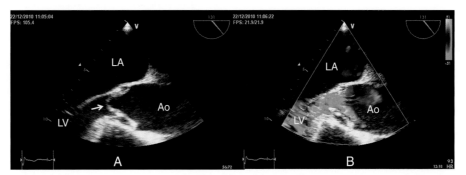

Fig. 10.3 Aortic Regurgitation (AR) in a Patient With Ascending Aorta Dissection. (A) Transesophageal echocardiography shows an intimal flap prolapsing through the aortic valve *(arrow)* (Video 10.3A ▶). (B) Severe AR is defined by color Doppler (Video 10.3B ▶). *Ao,* Aorta; *LA,* left atrium; *LV,* left ventricle.

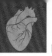
used in some settings when it can yield a more rapid diagnosis of aortic dissection than can be achieved by TEE.[10,11] Intraoperative TEE is indispensable for demonstrating the mechanism of AR in aortic dissection and can facilitate the choice of aortic valve surgical procedure (i.e., resuspension or replacement). Mechanisms include aortic root dilation, false lumen–produced annulus pressure on a cusp that causes asymmetric cusp coaptation, flail of an aortic cusp attributable to annular support disruption, and prolapse of a mobile intimal flap through the aortic valve.[12]

Pathophysiology

In acute severe AR, the abrupt development of a large regurgitant volume is imposed on a LV of normal size that has not had time to adapt to the volume overload. The acute increase in diastolic flow into the nondilated LV leads to a marked elevation in end-diastolic pressure due to a rightward shift along the normal LV diastolic pressure-volume curve. In severe cases, the increased ventricular pressures during the diastolic filling period in conjunction with the decrease in the aortic diastolic pressure leads to a rapid equalization of aortic and LV pressures at end-diastole.[9,13] With acute regurgitation, forward cardiac output is decreased because the total stroke volume of the nondilated ventricle includes the regurgitant and forward stroke volume. Compensatory tachycardia may partially correct this decline in forward stroke volume, but it is often insufficient to maintain cardiac output, and patients may present in cardiogenic shock. Pulmonary edema results from the markedly elevated LV end-diastolic pressure and concomitant elevation of pulmonary venous pressure. Acutely-diminished coronary flow reserve may lead to subendocardial ischemia. In patients with preexisting LV hypertrophy due to arterial hypertension or aortic stenosis, acute moderate AR (as may develop after TAVR) can cause severe hemodynamic changes due to a noncompliant LV with a reduced preload reserve.[14]

Management

Death due to pulmonary edema, ventricular arrhythmias, electromechanical dissociation, or circulatory collapse is common in acute, severe AR. Patients often require emergency or urgent aortic valve replacement (AVR) for correction of the underlying disease process and relief of the acute volume overload. Intraaortic balloon counterpulsation is contraindicated. In patients with acute AR due to an ascending aortic dissection, prompt surgical intervention with a composite replacement of the aorta along with aortic valve or a valve-sparing reimplantation technique is required.[15,16] In cases of severe acute AR due to infective endocarditis, patients need immediate antibiotics and aggressive medical treatment. If the hemodynamic situation does not improve immediately, emergent AVR may be lifesaving. If the clinical situation stabilizes, surgery may be postponed for a few days so that the patient, under strict medical supervision, can be treated with antibiotics before surgical correction.[17,18]

CHRONIC AORTIC REGURGITATION

Clinical Presentation

Clinical History

Many patients with AR are diagnosed before symptom onset based on the finding of a diastolic murmur on physical examination, discovery of an enlarged cardiac silhouette on the chest radiograph, or evidence of LV hypertrophy on electrocardiography. The most common initial symptom of patients with chronic severe AR is exertional dyspnea, most likely due to an elevated LV end-diastolic pressure with exercise.[19–21]

Because chronic AR has a slowly progressive course, the gradual decrease in exercise capacity may not be recognized as abnormal by the patient, and very careful questioning is often needed to elicit evidence of a subtle decline in functional status. In cases of doubtful or equivocal symptoms, exercise testing may be valuable for assessing functional capacity. In more advanced cases with severe LV dysfunction, patients can have symptoms of overt heart failure, including dyspnea at rest, orthopnea, and pulmonary edema. The acute onset of heart failure symptoms can occur in patients with chronic disease due to an acute increase in regurgitation severity, such as patients with infective endocarditis or aortic dissection.

Angina may occur, even in the absence of atherosclerotic coronary artery disease, due to lower myocardial perfusion pressure, increased myocardial oxygen demand, and a decreased ratio of coronary artery size to myocardial mass.[22] Syncope or sudden death, albeit rare, can occur in AR. Sudden death has been associated with extreme degrees of LV dilation.[23] Some patients may be uncomfortably aware of their heart beat or palpitations related to increased pulse pressure, which is the earliest symptom leading to the diagnosis of AR.

Physical Examination

In patients with mild or moderate AR, diastolic murmur may be the only finding on physical examination, but many patients also have a systolic outflow murmur related to increased stroke volume that is often more apparent than the diastolic murmur. The aortic regurgitant murmur is one of high frequency that begins immediately after S_2, continues to S_1, and decreases in intensity. When due to valve leaflet abnormalities, this murmur is best heard along the left sternal border in the third or fourth intercostal spaces, whereas when caused by aortic root disease, selective radiation along the right sternal border is common. However, the diastolic murmur often goes unnoticed on physical examination. Compared with Doppler echocardiography or aortic angiography, the sensitivity of auscultation for AR detection is 37% to 73%, with a specificity of 85% to 92%.[24–26]

The loudness of the murmur correlates with disease severity to some extent.[26] Another classic finding in patients with severe chronic AR is the Austin-Flint murmur, a low-pitched mid-diastolic rumble that mimics the murmur of mitral stenosis. Comparisons of Doppler echocardiographic findings with physical examination findings suggests that this diastolic murmur is related to AR severity, with a jet directed toward the anterior mitral leaflet or LV free wall, causing vibrations detected on auscultation as a low-pitched diastolic rumble.[27]

Physical examination can detect most cases of severe AR through the combination of the cardiac murmurs, widened pulse pressure on blood pressure measurement, and peripheral findings related to the widened pulse pressure. In severe AR, systolic arterial pressure is classically elevated, and diastolic pressure is abnormally low, although blood pressure may remain normal in many patients with severe AR.[28] Apical impulse is diffuse and hyperdynamic, and it is displaced laterally and inferiorly due to LV dilation. The carotid pulse may be bounding with a more rapid pressure increase rate in early systole and an increase in the amplitude of the systolic pressure curve followed by a rapid falloff. A bisferiens carotid pulse may be identified. In very severe cases, the head may bob forward with each heart beat (i.e., DuMusset sign).

The classic peripheral signs of AR occur only in cases of severe and chronic regurgitation and reflect the increased pulse pressure. They include the water-hammer or collapsing pulse (i.e., Corrigan pulse), systolic pulsation of the fingernail bed on gentle pressure (i.e., Quincke pulse), and a systolic and diastolic bruit over the femoral arteries on gentle compression by the stethoscope (i.e., Duroziez sign), a manifestation of the reversal of flow in the descending aorta. The physical findings in acute AR differ from those of chronic regurgitation in parallel with the different hemodynamics of acute versus chronic disease (Table 10.2).

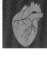

TABLE 10.2 Chronic Compensated, Chronic Decompensated, and Acute Aortic Regurgitation.

Characteristics	Chronic Compensated	Chronic Decompensated	Acute
Cause	Valvular or aortic root abnormalities	Valvular or aortic root abnormalities	Dissection, endocarditis, trauma
Physiology			
LV volume	Increased (ESD <55 mm)	Increased (ESD >55 mm)	Normal
Ejection fraction	Normal (>55%)	Normal or decreased	Normal or decreased
LV EDP	Normal	Normal or increased	Increased
Physical Examination			
Diastolic murmur	High-pitched, decrescendo, holodiastolic	High-pitched, decrescendo, holodiastolic	Low-pitched, harsh, early diastolic
Pulse pressure	Wide	Wide	Normal
LV impulse	Enlarged	Enlarged	Normal
Peripheral signs of AR	Present	Present	Absent
Clinical presentation	Asymptomatic	Gradual onset of symptoms, typically exertional	Sudden onset, pulmonary edema, and hypotension

AR, Aortic regurgitation; *EDP,* end-diastolic pressure; *ESD,* end-systolic dimension; *LV,* left ventricular.

Electrocardiography and Chest Radiography

The electrocardiogram (ECG) findings for patients with AR include voltage criteria for LV hypertrophy and associated repolarization abnormalities. A strain pattern on the resting ECG correlates strongly with abnormal LV dimensions, mass, and wall stress.[29] However, some patients with severe AR and pathologic LV hypertrophy do not meet ECG criteria for LV hypertrophy.[30] When the ECG is normal at rest, flat and/or downsloping ST-segment depression may develop with exercise, even in the absence of coronary artery disease, and it is associated with an increased LV systolic dimension. Ventricular ectopic beats and nonsustained ventricular arrhythmias are relatively common in AR and have a significant correlation with LV hypertrophy and function.[31]

The chest radiograph shows an enlarged silhouette due to LV dilation, and aortic root enlargement is also frequently seen. Evidence of LV hypertrophy on the ECG and cardiac size on the chest radiograph have been shown to be predictors of outcome after AVR. However, neither offers sufficiently precise data to be useful in clinical decision making or the sequential follow-up of patients with AR.

Echocardiography

Echocardiography is the primary imaging test for AR assessment because it provides accurate information on valve anatomy and proximal ascending aorta size, and it quantifies the severity of AR and LV size and function. Echocardiography is used to diagnose and estimate regurgitation severity using color Doppler (regurgitant jet width with vena contracta >6 mm)[32,33] (Fig. 10.4). Pulse-wave Doppler in the descending aorta also indicates severe AR when the diastolic velocity time integral of the diastolic flow reversal at the proximal descending thoracic aorta is 13 cm or greater, the end-diastolic flow velocity of the proximal descending aorta is more than 13 cm/s, or there is holodiastolic reversal of flow in the abdominal aorta[34,35] (Fig. 10.5).

Because these indices are influenced by loading conditions and the compliance of the ascending aorta and LV, the best way to evaluate AR severity is to integrate several Doppler methods.[33,36,37] Quantitative Doppler echocardiography using the continuity equation or analysis of proximal isovelocity surface area is less sensitive to loading conditions[38,39] and provides measurements of regurgitant volume, regurgitant fraction, and effective regurgitant orifice (Fig. 10.6). These measurements have become

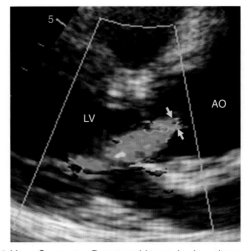

Fig. 10.4 Vena Contracta. Parasternal long-axis view shows the vena contracta *(arrows)* of the regurgitant flow by Doppler in a patient with severe aortic regurgitation. *AO,* Aorta; *LV,* left ventricle.

the preferred method for assessing AR severity.[33,40] The criteria for defining severe AR are shown in Table 10.3.

Echocardiography is performed to determine regurgitation mechanisms, describe valve anatomy, and determine the feasibility of valve repair. Analysis of the AR mechanism influences patient management, particularly when the ascending aorta is dilated or when conservative surgery is considered. Several functional classifications have been proposed. The adapted Carpentier classification for AR is the most widely used[41,42] (Fig. 10.7): type I, due to aortic root or sinotubular junction dilation; type II, when valvular dysfunction results from sigmoid prolapse or sigmoid flail; and type III, when AR is associated with thickened and rigid valves with reduced motion.

For some patients, TEE may be necessary if the cause and extent of the aortic valve and aortic root are not well defined by transthoracic imaging. AR quantification by TEE in patients with mechanical or bioprosthetic valves or TAVR can be challenging. Eccentric AR may be overestimated if there is broadening of the jet soon after the

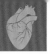

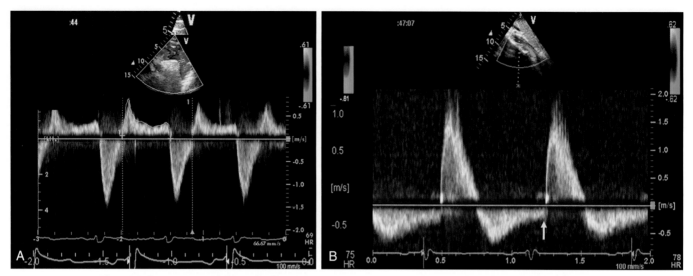

Fig. 10.5 **Assessment of Diastolic Flow Reversal in the Descending Aorta by Pulse-Wave Doppler.**
(A) Aorta flow in descending the thoracic aorta. The velocity-time integral is 22 cm, and end-diastolic velocity
is greater than 20 cm/s. (B) Abdominal aortic flow in the case of severe aortic regurgitation in which holodiastolic retrograde flow is observed *(arrow)*.

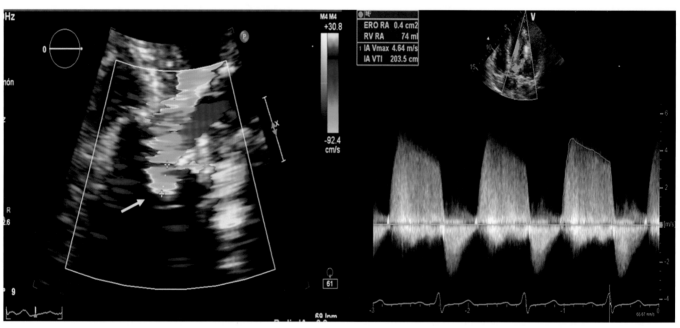

Fig. 10.6 **Assessment of Aortic Regurgitation Severity.** The quantitative assessment of aortic regurgitation
(AR) severity using the proximal isovelocity surface area (PISA) method shows severe aortic regurgitation
(EROA $\geq$ 0.30 cm^2 and regurgitant volume $\geq$ 60 mL/beat). EROA = 6.28 $\times$ r^2 $\times$ V$_{aliasing}$ /V$_{AR}$; EROA = 6.28 $\times$
(0.9 cm)^2 $\times$ 31 cm/s/464 cm/s = 0.4 cm^2; and regurgitant volume = EROA $\times$ VTI$_{AR}$; regurgitant volume =
EROA $\times$ VTI$_{AR}$ = 0.35 cm^2 $\times$ 203.5 cm= 71 cm^2. V$_{AR}$: maximum velocity of protodiastole of AR curve. *ERO,*
Effective regurgitant orifice; *EROA,* effective regurgitant orifice area; *VTI,* velocity-time integral.

vena contracta or underestimated if the jet courses along the anterior
septum or the anterior mitral leaflet. Less than 10% of the sewing ring
seen to be involved on the short-axis view suggests mild regurgitation,
10% to 20% indicates moderate regurgitation, and more than 20%
suggests severe regurgitation.[43]

Advances in three-dimensional (3D) echocardiography make it
possible to visualize the aortic anatomy better and to measure the vena
contracta area more accurately. Studies show that 3D color Doppler
measurement of the vena contracta area improves AR quantitation

compared with two-dimensional (2D) methods. Similarly, 3D color
Doppler proximal isovelocity surface area (PISA) methods also improve AR quantification compared with 2D methods.[44] Nevertheless,
technologic advances are required to resolve some limitations such as
frame rates or stitch artifacts.

An important role of echocardiography is to provide precise and
reproducible measures of LV dimensions, volumes, and systolic performance, and it is therefore the cornerstone of clinical decision making and
serial follow-up of patients with chronic AR. Indexing LV dimensions

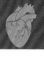

TABLE 10.3 Severity Grades of Aortic Regurgitation.

Parameters	Mild	Moderate	Severe
Qualitative			
Aortic valve morphology	Normal/abnormal	Normal/abnormal	Abnormal/flail/large coaptation defect
Color flow AR jet width[a]	Small in central jets	Intermediate	Large in central jet, varied eccentric jets
CW signal of AR jet	Incomplete/faint	Dense	Dense
Diastolic flow reversal in the descending aorta	Brief, protodiastolic flow reversal	Intermediate	Holodiastolic flow reversal (end-diastolic velocity >20 cm/s)
Diastolic flow reversal in the abdominal aorta	Absent	Absent	Present
Semiquantitative			
VC width (mm)	<3	Intermediate	≥6
Pressure half-time (ms)[b]	>500	Intermediate	<200
Quantitative			
EROA (mm^2)	<10	10–19, 20–29[d]	≥30
RVol (mL)	<30	30–44, 45–59[d]	≥60
+LV size[c]			

[a]At a Nyquist limit of 50–60 cm/s.

[b]Pressure half-time is shortened with increasing LV diastolic pressure, vasodilator therapy, and in patients with a dilated, compliant aorta or lengthened in chronic AR.

[c]Unless for other reasons, the LV size is usually normal in patients with mild AR. In acute severe AR, the LV size is often normal. Accepted cutoff values for nonsignificant LV enlargement: LV end-diastolic diameter < 56 mm, LV end-diastolic volume < 82 mL/m^2, LV end-systolic diameter < 40 mm, LV end-systolic volume < 30 mL/m^2.

[d]Grading of the severity of AR classifies regurgitation as mild, moderate, or severe and subclassifies the moderate regurgitation group as mild to moderate (EROA = 10–19 mm or an RVol of 20–44 mL) and moderate to severe (EROA = 20–29 mm^2 or an RVol of 45–59 mL).

AR, Aortic regurgitation; *CW*, continuous wave; *LA*, left atrium; *EROA*, effective regurgitant orifice area; *LV*, left ventricle; *RVol*, regurgitant volume; *VC*, vena contracta.

From Lancellotti P, Tribouilloy C, Hagendorff A, et al. Recommendations for the echocardiographic assessment of native valvular regurgitation: an executive summary from the European Association of Cardiovascular Imaging. Eur Heart J Cardiovasc Imaging 2013;14:611-644.

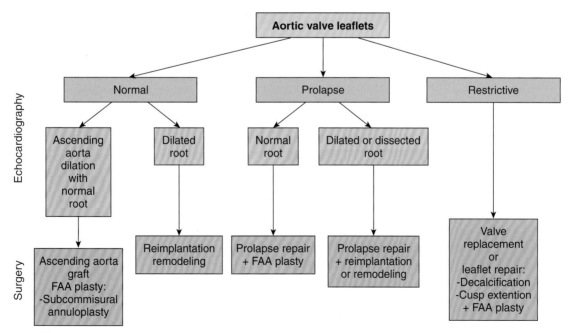

Fig. 10.7 Functional Classification of Aortic Regurgitation (AR). Repair-oriented functional classification of AR with description of disease mechanisms and repair techniques used. *FAA*, Functional aortic annulus.

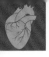
and volumes for body surface area is especially recommended for women and men of small body size.[45,46] Serial echocardiographic evaluation of LV size and function should take into account the potential of confounding factors of interval changes in instrumentation, variations in recording and measuring data and in loading conditions, and physiologic differences. When a change is detected, it is prudent to repeat the examination to confirm the magnitude and direction of the change.

Good-quality echocardiograms and data confirmation are essential before recommending surgery in asymptomatic patients. Advanced imaging methods such as speckle-tracking echocardiography may prove to be more sensitive than LV ejection fraction (LVEF) for the early detection of LV systolic and diastolic dysfunction in chronic AR and may play a role in determining surgical indications in the future. Because the subendocardial layer is the first to be affected in AR, the longitudinal alignment of myocardial fibers in this layer renders decreased longitudinal contraction an early sign of LV dysfunction. Subnormal LV longitudinal deformation detected by speckle-tracking echocardiography predicts disease progression in asymptomatic patients under conservative treatment and unfavorable postoperative outcomes of surgical candidates[47–50] (Fig. 10.8).

Aortic root and proximal ascending aorta diameters should be analyzed in all patients with AR. Measurements by 2D echocardiography should be reported at four levels: annulus, sinuses of Valsalva, sinotubular junction, and tubular ascending aorta. Measurements must be taken in the parasternal long-axis view from leading edge to leading edge at end-diastole, except for the aortic annulus, which is measured inner to inner at mid-systole.[51]

Other Imaging Modalities

Cardiac magnetic resonance. For patients with indeterminant echocardiographic findings, CMR is a reliable tool for assessment of AR severity.[52,53] Cine CMR sequences, such as steady-state free precession (SSFP) techniques, permit visualization of the aortic valve in a chosen plane with excellent image quality (Fig. 10.9). Magnetic resonance phase-contrast sequences perpendicular to the aortic valve allow accurate antegrade and retrograde blood flow measurements in the ascending aorta, enabling the severity of AR by calculation of regurgitant volume, peak velocity, and regurgitant fraction to be assessed (see Fig. 10.8).

Compared with TTE, CMR has lower intraobserver and interobserver variations in measuring regurgitant volume, suggesting that

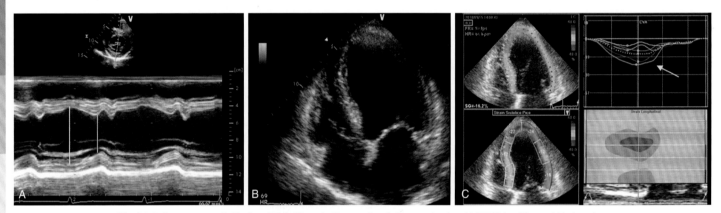

Fig. 10.8 Asymptomatic Patient With Chronic Severe Aortic Regurgitation (AR) With a Normal Estimation of LV Systolic Function by 2D Echocardiography. (A) Transthoracic parasternal short-axis view and M-mode show severe enlargement of LV diameters (end-diastolic diameter = 68 mm; end-systolic diameter = 48 mm) but normal systolic function. (B) Apical four-chamber view of the same patient shows moderate spherical enlargement of the LV with an ejection fraction of 53%. (C) 2D-strain reveals low values, unmasking subclinical myocardial dysfunction.

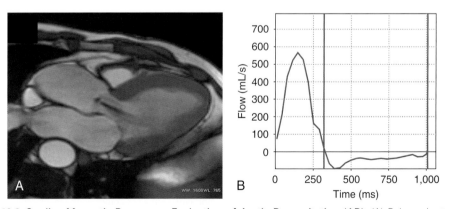

Fig. 10.9 Cardiac Magnetic Resonance Evaluation of Aortic Regurgitation (AR). (A) Balanced, steady-state free precession image. Oblique axial LV inflow/outflow view shows grade 3 AR. (B) Flow versus time plot for the ascending aorta. Antegrade flow is calculated at 140 mL/beat, retrograde flow is calculated at 40 mL/beat, and the regurgitant fraction is 33%.

CMR may be superior for these serial measurements. Quantification of AR with CMR showed significant associations with outcome, particularly when combined with CMR-derived LV volumes, including for patients who developed asymptomatic LV dilation or dysfunction.[54] Studies found a better predictive value of AR severity after TAVR when quantified by CMR compared with early echocardiography.[55] Using serial short-axis slices of the LV, it is possible to calculate LV volumes, mass, and EF very accurately. Several studies have shown that CMR is an excellent technique to monitor LV volumes and EF with a high degree of interobserver reproducibility. Using contrast agents (e.g., gadolinium-DTPA) and different magnetic resonance angiography sequences or 3D whole-chest SSFP sequences (without contrast), aortic root and ascending aortic anatomy and diameters can be determined.

CMR is a useful technique to obtain a global evaluation of patients with AR, to determine the evolution of the regurgitation and its impact on LV volume and function, and to decide the optimal time for AVR.

Cardiac computed tomography. The utility of 64-slice multidetector CT has been studied in patients with AR. CT is used in clinical practice if the ascending aorta is not well imaged by TTE or to check the aortic diameter when approaching a surgical threshold. It may be better to use CT when considering referral for AVR because it can also detect calcium in the ascending aorta and identify porcelain aorta as an indication for a transcatheter procedure instead of conventional surgery. Aortic root and LV parameters measured by CT correlate well with corresponding measurements by transthoracic echocardiography.[56] Direct planimetry of the aortic valve anatomic regurgitant orifice accurately detects and quantifies AR.[57] CT coronary angiography is also useful for the detection of coronary artery disease in patients with AR[58] particularly in those at no more than moderate coronary risk (e.g., younger patients with a bicuspid aortic valve), CT can produce in one evaluation an assessment of the aorta and coronary arteries before surgical treatment.

Radionuclide angiography. Radionuclide ventriculograms can provide accurate measurements of LV volumes and function and can be used as an alternative technique to echocardiography in patients with suboptimal echocardiograms or in patients showing discrepancies between clinical and echocardiographic data.[59]

Exercise Testing

Exercise stress testing is useful for assessing functional capacity and symptomatic responses in patients with equivocal symptoms. It is also useful in patients with AR before participation in athletic activities. Several investigators have suggested that exercise testing, with or without concurrent imaging, may help to identify patients with early systolic LV dysfunction. On exercise electrocardiography, the finding of at least 1.0 mm of ST-segment depression is associated with a lower resting and exercise EF, a higher wall stress, and a greater end-systolic dimension compared with those with no ST-segment changes with exercise.[60] Reduced maximal oxygen consumption and aerobic threshold also predict moderate to severe LV dysfunction, suggesting that cardiopulmonary stress testing may be useful in some patients.[61]

Exercise echocardiography can be used to measure the incremental change in LV dimensions and EF with exercise in patients with AR. Contractile reserve may be more predictive of clinical outcome than resting EF.[62,63] An increase in radionuclide EF with exercise of at least 5% correlates with preserved LV systolic function, whereas any decrease or increase of less than 5 units indicates an elevated end-systolic wall stress, increased end-systolic dimension, and impaired systolic function.[59] However, one study reported that in asymptomatic AR, resting LV strain, resting right ventricular (RV) strain, and exercise tricuspid annular plane systolic excursion (TAPSE) were independently associated with the need for earlier AVR but no other exercise parameters.[64]

The role of exercise testing must be individualized. It may be helpful when there is a discrepancy between the clinical presentation and the resting echocardiographic findings. However, clinical decisions should not be based solely on changes in EF with exercise or on data from stress echocardiography because these indices have not been adequately validated.

Beyond assessment of LV volumes and EF, there is a need for early identification of systolic dysfunction for indicating surgery before the onset of permanent LV dysfunction. Biomarkers such as brain natriuretic peptide (BNP) provide independent markers for asymptomatic patients with normal LV systolic function for subsequent symptoms and/or LV dysfunction, even after adjustment for LV volumes.[65]

Disease Stages
Pathophysiology

The LV responds to the volume load of chronic AR with a series of compensatory mechanisms, including an increase in end-diastolic volume, an increase in chamber compliance that accommodates the increased volume without an increase in filling pressures, and a combination of eccentric and concentric hypertrophy. The central hemodynamic feature of chronic AR is combined volume and pressure overload of the LV.[66,67] Because total LV stroke volume equals forward plus regurgitant stroke volume, normal cardiac output is maintained by an increase in total stroke volume corresponding to the severity of regurgitation. This increase in total stroke volume is achieved by progressive ventricular dilatation, with increased end-diastolic and end-systolic volumes. The greater diastolic volume permits the ventricle to eject a large total stroke volume, keeping forward stroke volume in the normal range.

Despite an increase in end-systolic dimension and pressure early in the course of the disease, end-systolic wall stress is maintained in the normal range by a compensatory increase in wall thickness. Patients with compensated chronic AR have substantial increases in LV mass and LV volumes, and the EF tends to be normal. As the disease progresses, recruitment of preload reserve and compensatory hypertrophy permit the LV to maintain normal ejection performance despite the elevated afterload. Most patients remain asymptomatic during this compensated phase, which may last for decades. During the compensated phase, ejection phase indices of LV systolic function at rest are normal. In a large subset of patients, however, the balance among afterload excess, preload reserve, and hypertrophy cannot be maintained indefinitely. Preload reserve may be exhausted or the hypertrophic response may be inadequate so that further increases in afterload result in a reduction in EF, first into the low-normal range and then below normal. Impaired contractility may also contribute to this process.

LV systolic dysfunction (i.e., EF below normal at rest) is initially a reversible phenomenon related predominantly to afterload excess, and full recovery of LV size and function is possible with AVR. With time, during which the LV develops progressive chamber enlargement and a more spherical geometry, depressed myocardial contractility predominates over excessive loading as the cause of progressive dysfunction. This can progress to the extent that the full benefit of surgical correction of the regurgitant lesion in terms of recovery of LV function and improved survival can no longer be achieved. Several studies have identified LV systolic function and end-systolic size as the most important determinants of survival and postoperative recovery of LV function in patients undergoing AVR for chronic AR.[45,68-84]

Aortic Regurgitation Progression

There is little information in the literature regarding the progression from mild to moderate and severe AR. It has been postulated that decreased aortic distensibility with age contributes to progressive AR due to the increase in LV afterload.[85] Doppler measures of jet width and

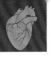

regurgitant orifice area suggest that there is progressive enlargement of the regurgitant orifice over time.[86] One echocardiographic study showed that the severity of AR increased in 30% of patients with at least two echocardiographic studies, with associated increases in severity of LV dilation; the greatest increases in LV volumes and mass were observed in those with severe AR.[87]

Normal left ventricular systolic function. The data regarding the natural history of asymptomatic patients with severe AR with normal LV systolic function derive from nine published series involving a total of 593 such patients[19–21,23,28,88–92] (Table 10.4).

These studies consistently show that patients can remain asymptomatic and with preserved LV function for a long time. The rate of progression to symptoms or LV dysfunction, or both, averaged 4.3% per year, development of asymptomatic LV dysfunction was 1.2% per year, and sudden death was 0.2% per year. It should be emphasized that more than one fourth of patients in these series did so before the onset of warning symptoms.

In the serial evaluation of patients, quantitative assessment of LV function is indispensable. LV size measured by echocardiography has

TABLE 10.4 Natural History of Asymptomatic Aortic Regurgitation.

Study	No. of Patients	Mean Follow-Up (Years)	Progression to Symptoms, Death, or LV Dysfunction (Rate/Year)	PROGRESSION TO ASYMPTOMATIC LV DYSFUNCTION		No. of Patient Deaths	Comments
				N	Rate/Year		
Bonow et al, 1983, 1991[19,23]	104	8.0	3.8%	4	0.5%	2	Outcome predicted by LV ESD, EDD, change in EF with exercise, and rate of change in ESD and EF at rest with time
Scognamiglio et al,[a] 1986[88]	30	4.7	2.1%	3	2.1%	0	3 patients developing asymptomatic LV dysfunction initially had lower PAP/ESV ratios and trend toward higher LV ESD and EDD and lower FS
Siemienczuk et al, 1989[89]	50	3.7	4.0%	1	0.5%	0	Patients included those receiving placebo and medical dropouts in a randomized drug trial; included some patients with NYHA FC II symptoms; outcome predicted by LV ESV, EDV, change in EF with exercise, and end-systolic wall stress
Scognamiglio et al,[a] 1994[90]	74	6.0	5.7%	15	3.4%	0	All patients received digoxin as part of a randomized trial
Tornos et al, 1995[20]	101	4.6	3.0%	6	1.3%	0	Outcome predicted by pulse pressure, LV ESD, EDD, and EF at rest
Ishii et al, 1996[21]	27	14.2	3.6%	—	—	0	Development of symptoms predicted by systolic BP, LV ESD, EDD, mass index, and wall thickness. LV function not reported in all patients
Borer et al, 1998[91]	104	7.3	6.2%	7	0.9%	4	20% of patients in NYHA FC II; outcome predicted by initial FC II symptoms, change in LV EF with exercise, LV ESD, and LV FS
Tarasoutchi et al, 2003[92]	72	10	4.7%	1	0.1%	0	Development of symptoms predicted by LV ESD and EDD. LV function not reported in all patients
Evangelista et al, 2005[28]	31	7	3.6%	—	—	1	Placebo control group in 7-year vasodilator clinical trial
Average	593	6.6	4.3%	37	1.2%	(0.18%/yr)	

[a]Two studies by same authors involved separate patient groups.

BP, Blood pressure; *EDD*, end-diastolic dimension; *EDV*, end-diastolic volume; *EF*, ejection fraction; *ESD*, end-systolic dimension; *ESV*, end-systolic volume; *FC*, functional class; *FS*, fractional shortening; *LV*, left ventricular; *NYHA*, New York Heart Association; *PAP*, pulmonary artery pressure.

a major predictive value. Patients with an end-systolic diameter greater than 50 mm had a likelihood of death, symptoms, or LV dysfunction of 19% per year. For those with end-systolic dimensions of 40 to 50 mm, the likelihood was 6% per year, and when the dimensions were less than 40 mm, it was zero.

In later studies, severe AR defined by quantitative methods, regurgitant volume, or regurgitant fraction using Doppler echocardiography[93] or CMR[52] were stronger predictors of outcome than LVEF or any of the LV dilation measurements. Although these parameters may enable identification of early LV dysfunction, their role in surgical indication requires confirmation.

Left ventricular systolic dysfunction. Despite very limited data for asymptomatic patients with depressed LV function, it has been estimated that the average rate of symptom onset in these patients is greater than 25% per year.[72] Symptoms caused by AR are a strong predictor of clinical outcome.[73] The data developed in the presurgical era indicate that patients with dyspnea, angina, or overt heart failure have a poor outcome with medical therapy, with mortality rates of greater than 10% for those with angina and 20% for those with heart failure.[72]

Medical Management

The aim of medical management of patients with significant AR is to carefully follow the clinical course to identify the best timing for surgical intervention and prevent complications.

Vasodilator Therapy

Vasodilator therapy has been designed to reduce regurgitant volume overload, LV volumes, and wall stress. Theoretically, these effects can be beneficial in AR by preserving LV function and reducing LV mass. Vasodilators are useful in patients with severe AR and symptoms or LV dysfunction who are considered poor candidates for AVR because of severe comorbidities. Vasodilators are also useful for improving the hemodynamic profile in patients with severe heart failure symptoms before AVR.

The most controversial effect of vasodilators is their use to alter the natural history of asymptomatic patients with preserved LV systolic function and prolong the compensated phase of the disease. If vasodilator therapy successfully delays decompensation of the LV, it would postpone the need for AVR. Several studies with small numbers of patients and short-term follow-up periods found different beneficial effects of vasodilators on hemodynamic and echocardiographic parameters of LV function.[94–101]

Regarding long-term effects, only one study reported that long-acting nifedipine therapy produced a reduction in LV dimensions and an increase in EF,[90] and two studies demonstrated improvement in hemodynamic parameters with enalapril and quinapril, particularly when accompanied by a drop in blood pressure.[95,101] A subsequent clinical trial using nifedipine, enalapril, or no treatment in asymptomatic patients with severe AR and normal LV function failed to demonstrate any significant benefit of such therapy. Vasodilators did not delay the need for AVR after an extended follow-up period and did not result in a reduction in regurgitant volume or beneficial effect on LV size or function.[28]

Guidelines[102,103] recommend treatment of hypertension (systolic blood pressure >140 mmHg) in patients with chronic AR (stages B and C), preferably with dihydropyridine calcium channel blockers or angiotensin-converting enzyme (ACE) inhibitors or angiotensin-receptor blockers (ARBs). Medical therapy with ACE inhibitors or ARBs and β-blockers is reasonable in patients with severe AR who have symptoms and/or LV dysfunction (stages C2

and D) when surgery is not performed because of comorbidities (Table 10.5).

Historically, β-blocker therapy has been discouraged for patients with severe AR because a reduction in heart rate can prolong diastole, increasing the aortic regurgitant volume. Nevertheless, an observational study indicated that β-blocker therapy was associated with better survival of patients with severe AR, mainly in the subgroup with higher heart rates.[104] A published trial showed that 6 months of treatment with metoprolol was associated with a decrease in heart rate (i.e., mean of 8 beats/min) and a mild increase in LVEF, but there was no effect on regurgitant fraction or LV volumes quantified by CMR and no effect on exercise capacity and peak oxygen consumption.[105]

The data are not sufficient to recommend β-adrenergic blockers for patients with AR. Further study is needed to determine whether these agents will be valuable for patients with significant AR and concomitant conditions, such as ascending aorta dilation, hypertension, arrhythmias, or coronary artery disease.[106]

Endocarditis Prevention

Patients with AR should be instructed about the importance of good oral hygiene and regular dental cleaning and examinations. Patients should also be instructed on early reporting of unexplained fever lasting for more than 1 week and on the importance of refraining from self-medication with antibiotics in the case of fever.

According to the 2007 American Heart Association guidelines on endocarditis prevention, antibiotic prophylaxis before dental work or other invasive procedures is no longer recommended for patients with AR or other forms of native valve disease. Antibiotic prophylaxis is recommended only for patients with AR who have a prior history of endocarditis.[107]

Serial Evaluations

The aims of serial evaluation of asymptomatic patients with chronic AR are to detect the onset of clinical symptoms and to objectively assess changes in LV function and size that can occur in the absence of symptoms to determine the optimal time for AVR. All asymptomatic patients with severe AR and normal LV function should have clinical evaluations at least every year. In patients with a new diagnosis of AR or in those in whom LV diameter and/or EF show significant changes or are approaching the thresholds for surgery, follow-up evaluations should be more frequent (i.e., intervals of 3 to 6 months). In inconclusive cases, the use of stress echocardiography or BNP, or both, may be helpful because elevation during follow-up has been related to deterioration of LV function.[108,109]

CMR or radionuclide angiography can be used in the serial assessment as an alternative to echocardiography, particularly in patients with technically suboptimal echocardiograms. Patients with mild to moderate AR can be reviewed on a yearly basis, and echocardiography can be performed every 2 years.

In patients with aortic root dilation, serial echocardiograms should include accurate measurements of the aorta. Indexing for body surface area can be recommended, especially for patients of small body size and for women. If the ascending aorta is dilated (>40 mm or 21 mm/m²), CT or CMR should be performed.[110] Depending on the agreement among imaging techniques, follow-up should be performed by echocardiography or by CMR or CT angiography. Any increase greater than 3 mm defined by echocardiography should be validated by CT angiography or CMR.

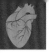

TABLE 10.5   Stages of Chronic Aortic Regurgitation.

Stage	Definition	Valve Anatomy	Valve Hemodynamics	Hemodynamic Consequences	Symptoms
A	At risk of AR	Bicuspid aortic valve (or other congenital valve anomaly) Aortic valve sclerosis Diseases of the aortic sinuses or ascending aorta History of rheumatic fever or known rheumatic heart disease IE	AR severity: none or trace	None	None
B	Progressive AR	Mild-to-moderate calcification of a trileaflet valve bicuspid aortic valve (or other congenital valve anomaly) Dilated aortic sinuses Rheumatic valve changes Previous IE	Mild AR: Jet width <25% of LVOT Vena contracta <0.3 cm RVol <30 mL/beat RF <30% ERO <0.10 cm^2 Angiography grade 1+ Moderate AR: Jet width 25%–64% of LVOT Vena contracta 0.3–0.6 cm RVol 30–59 mL/beat RF 30%–49% ERO 0.10–0.29 cm^2 Angiography grade 2+	Normal LV systolic function Normal LV volume or mild LV dilation	None
C	Asymptomatic severe AR	Calcific aortic valve disease Bicuspid valve (or other congenital abnormality) Dilated aortic sinuses or ascending aorta Rheumatic valve changes IE with abnormal leaflet closure or perforation	Severe AR: Jet width ≥65% of LVOT Vena contracta >0.6 cm Holodiastolic flow reversal in the proximal abdominal aorta RVol ≥60 mL/beat RF ≥50% ERO ≥0.3 cm^2 Angiography grade 3+ to 4+ Diagnosis of chronic severe AR also requires evidence of LV dilation	C1: normal LVEF (≥50%) and mild to moderate LV dilation (LVESD ≤50 mm) C2: abnormal LV systolic function with depressed LVEF (<50%) or severe LV dilation (LVESD >50 mm or indexed LVESD >25 mm/m^2)	None; exercise testing is reasonable to confirm symptom status
D	Symptomatic severe AR	Calcific valve disease Bicuspid valve (or other congenital abnormality) Dilated aortic sinuses or ascending aorta Rheumatic valve changes Previous IE with abnormal leaflet closure or perforation	Severe AR: Doppler jet width ≥ 65% of LVOT Vena contracta >0.6 cm Holodiastolic flow reversal in the proximal abdominal aorta RVol ≥60 mL/beat RF ≥50% ERO ≥0.3 cm^2 Angiography grade 3+ to 4+ Diagnosis of chronic severe AR also requires evidence of LV dilation	Sysmptomatic severe AR may occur with normal systolic function (LVEF ≥50%), mild to moderate LV dysfunction (LVEF 40%–50%), or severe LV dysfunction (LVEF <40%) Moderate to severe LV dilation is present	Exertional dyspnea or angina or more severe HF symptoms

AR, Aortic regurgitation; *ERO*, effective regurgitant orifice; *HF*, heart failure; *IE*, infective endocarditis; *LV*, left ventricular; *LVEF*, left ventricular ejection fraction; *LVESD*, left ventricular end-systolic dimension; *LVOT*, left ventricular outflow tract; *RF*, regurgitant fraction; *RVol*, regurgitant volume.
From Nishimura RA, Otto CM, Bonow RO, et al. 2014 AHA/ACC guideline for the management of patients with valvular heart disease: a report of the American College of Cardiology/American Heart Association Task Force on Practice Guidelines. Circulation. 2014;129:e521-e643.

Indications for Surgery
Aortic Valve Replacement or Repair

The surgical management of AR usually requires AVR. However, in selected patients and in surgical centers of excellence, there is increasing experience in aortic valve repair.[111,112] In younger patients, the pulmonic autograft procedure (i.e., Ross procedure) is an option if performed by surgical teams experienced in this more technically challenging operation.[113] The indications for surgery on the aortic valve are the same irrespective of the surgical technique used.

The goals of operation are to improve outcome, to diminish symptoms, to prevent the development of postoperative heart failure and cardiac death, and to avoid aortic complications in patients who have aortic aneurysms. Several investigators[32,44,68–85] have identified preoperative predictors of patient outcome and LV function after AVR for chronic AR. The most consistent measures are the functional class, EF, and end-systolic dimension. On the basis of robust observational evidence, the recommended indications for surgical intervention for severe AR are similar in the American College of Cardiology/American Heart Association (ACC/AHA) and the European guidelines[102,103] (Fig. 10.10).

Symptom onset is an indication for AVR, irrespective of LV function. When the LV systolic function is normal and the patient experiences symptoms, every effort should be made to clearly relate the symptoms to AR. Especially when the symptoms are mild, such as New York Heart Association (NYHA) functional class II dyspnea, clinical judgment is necessary, and in this setting, the role of exercise testing is valuable. However, for patients with LV dilation and progressive enlargement in chamber size or decline in EF on serial studies, the onset of mild symptoms is a clear indication for AVR.

For symptomatic patients with decreased LV systolic function (i.e., subnormal EF), AVR is clearly indicated. Several studies have shown that the long-term outcome is excellent when these patients undergo AVR when asymptomatic or only mildly symptomatic or with mild degrees of LV dysfunction.[44,55,68] Every effort should be made to refer patients to

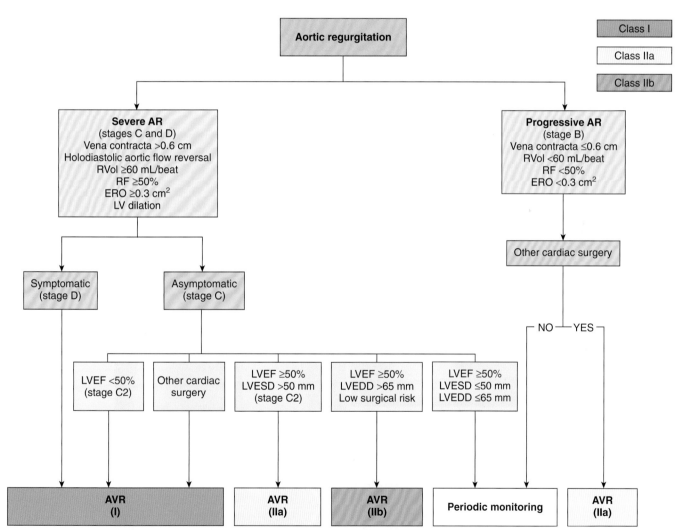

Fig. 10.10 Indications for Aortic Valve Replacement *(AVR)* for Chronic Aortic Regurgitation *(AR)*. Instead of AVR, valve repair may be appropriate in selected patients. *ERO*, Effective regurgitant orifice; *LV*, left ventricular; *LVEDD*, left ventricular end-diastolic dimension; *LVEF*, left ventricular ejection fraction; *LVESD*, left ventricular end-systolic dimension; *RF*, regurgitant fraction; *RVol*, regurgitant volume. (From Nishimura RA, Otto CM, Bonow RO, et al. 2014 AHA/ACC guideline for the management of patients with valvular heart disease: a report of the American College of Cardiology/American Heart Association Task Force on Practice Guidelines. Circulation 2014;129:e521-e643.)

surgery at this stage. Postoperative survival and the likelihood of recovery of systolic function is worse for patients with preoperative NYHA functional class IV symptoms or with extremely enlarged ventricles (>55 mm at end-systole) and those with very depressed EFs (<30%).[68,84,114,115] However, even for very ill patients, AVR and subsequent medical treatment is a better alternative than long-term medical therapy alone or cardiac transplantation. Surgical series demonstrating an improvement in postoperative survival for patients with AR and severe preoperative LV dysfunction reinforce this opinion.[116]

AVR should also be considered for asymptomatic patients with severe AR and impaired LV function at rest (resting EF < 50%) or extreme degrees of LV dilation (LV end-systolic diameter [LVESD] >50 mm or indexed LVESD >25 mm/m²). In these patients, the likelihood that symptoms will develop in the short term is high but perioperative mortality is very low, and the postoperative long-term results are excellent. Other studies have suggested that end-systolic volume index is a more sensitive predictor of cardiac events than end-systolic dimension for asymptomatic patients, but values of end-systolic volume index identifying high-risk patients have varied between 35 and 45 mL/m². More data are needed to determine threshold values of the end-systolic volume index with which to make recommendations for AVR in asymptomatic patients.

LV end-diastolic dimension is indicative of the severity of LV volume overload in patients with chronic AR. It is significantly associated with development of symptoms and LV systolic dysfunction in asymptomatic patients but less so than the LV end-systolic dimension. However, especially in young patients with severe AR, progressive increases in the end-diastolic dimension are associated with a subsequent need for surgery.

AVR may be considered for asymptomatic patients with severe AR and normal LV systolic function at rest but with progressive severe LV dilation (LV end-diastolic dimension >65 mm) if surgical risk is low. Some studies have pointed out that the natural history of many patients may not be as benign as reported in earlier studies in which patients were meticulously followed. Detaint and colleagues[93] reported a 10-year survival rate of 78% (suggesting an annual mortality rate of 2.2%/yr) in contrast to the annual mortality rate of 0.2% reported in earlier studies.

A retrospective study[117] of 1417 asymptomatic patients with chronic severe AR and preserved LV EF undergoing AVR reported long-term survival rates similar to those of age- and sex-matched individuals without valvular heart disease. However, the risk of death increased when the indexed LVESD exceeded 2.0 cm/m², a threshold lower than the currently recommended value of 2.5 cm/m².

For patients with AR undergoing other cardiac operations, such as coronary bypass surgery or mitral valve surgery, the decision to replace the aortic valve should be individualized according to the severity of AR, age, and overall clinical situation. If the AR is moderate or severe, AVR is almost always indicated, whereas AVR can be postponed when the AR is mild.

Concomitant Disease of the Ascending Aorta and Aortic Root

Dilation of the ascending aorta is one of the most common causes of isolated AR (Fig. 10.11). In these cases, AR is often not severe, and the decisions for surgical intervention are based more on the severity of ascending aorta dilation than on the severity of AR. Patients include those with Marfan syndrome, bicuspid aortic valves, annulo-aortic ectasia, or degenerative aortic aneurysms. When AR is mild or moderate, management should focus on treating the underlying aortic and aortic root disease. In some patients, AR may be severe, in which case decision making should consider both conditions.

In patients with Marfan syndrome, β-blockers may slow the progression of aortic dilation.[118] The efficacy of losartan, an angiotensin II receptor 1 blocker, was evaluated in the COMPARE clinical trial,[119] which reported that losartan reduced the rate of aortic dilation in patients with Marfan syndrome. The Pediatric Heart Network trial using echocardiography[120] and the LOAT trial using CMR showed that either atenolol or losartan was effective in reducing the rate of aortic dilation.[121] However, the Marfan Sartan randomized clinical trial

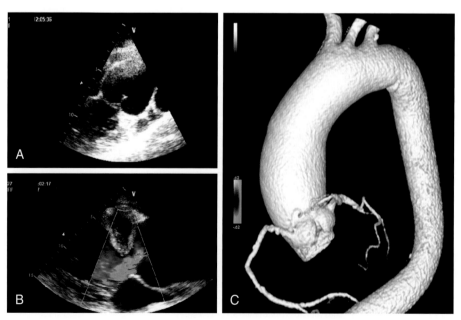

Fig. 10.11 Ascending Aortic Aneurysms. (A) Annulo-aortic ectasia shown in the parasternal long-axis view. The aortic annulus (28 mm) and aortic root (46 mm) were dilated. (B) Aortic root and ascending aorta aneurysms in a patient with severe atherosclerosis. Aortic regurgitation is severe and functional due to aorta dilation. (C) Volume-rendered image from an electrocardiographically gated thoracic computed tomographic aortogram in the presurgical study of a patient with ascending aortic aneurysm.

reported that losartan lowered blood pressure but had no effect on progression of aortic dilation.[122] All patients with known or suspected Marfan syndrome and aortic root dilation should receive medical therapy with adequate doses of β-blockers or possibly ARBs. The available evidence is less clear for patients with Marfan syndrome without aortic dilation.

Whether the same beneficial effect of β-blockers or other drugs occurs in patients with bicuspid aortic valves and aortic dilation is unknown. In patients with hypertension, blood pressure control with any effective antihypertensive medication is warranted. β-blockers and ARB have conceptual advantages for reduction of the progression rate, but these advantages have not been demonstrated in clinical studies.

Aortic root dilation greater than 55 mm should be considered a surgical indication regardless of the degree and cause of AR. In patients with bicuspid aortic valve, surgery is recommended at a lower degree of aortic dilation (>50 mm) only if there is a family history of aortic dissection or rapid progression (3–5 mm/yr).[102,103,123] The risk of progressive aortic dilation and dissection after AVR in patients with bicuspid aortic valves has been the subject of several studies, although definitive data are lacking.

For patients who have reached the recommended indications for surgery based on symptoms or AR severity, a lower threshold can be used for combining surgery on the ascending aorta. In patients with bicuspid aortic valves undergoing AVR because of severe aortic stenosis or AR, replacement of the ascending aorta is reasonable when the aortic diameter is greater than 4.5 cm. In borderline cases, the decision to replace the ascending aorta also relies on perioperative surgical findings such as aortic valve thickness and the status of the rest of the aorta.

REFERENCES

1. Singh JP, Evans JC, Levy D, et al. Prevalence and clinical determinants of mitral, tricuspid, and aortic regurgitation (the Framingham Heart Study). Am J Cardiol 1999;83(6):897-902.
2. Lebowitz NE, Bella JN, Roman MJ, et al. Prevalence and correlates of aortic regurgitation in American Indians: the Strong Heart Study. J Am Coll Cardiol 2000;36(2):461-467.
3. Roberts WC, KO JM, Moore TR, Jones WH. Causes of pure aortic regurgitation in patients having isolated aortic valve replacement in a single US tertiary hospital (1993-2005). Circulation 2006;114:422-429.
4. Baszyk H, Witkiewicz AJ, Edwards WD. Acute aortic regurgitation due to pontaneous rupture of a fenestrated cusp: report in a 65 year old man and review of seven additional cases. Cardiovasc Pathol 1999;8:213-216.
5. Sinning JM, Vasa-Nicotera M, Chin D, et al. Evaluation and management of paravalvular aortic regurgitation after transcatheter aortic valve replacement. J Am Coll Cardiol 2013;62(1):11-20.
6. Sadaniantz A, Malhotra R, Korr KS. Transient acute severe aortic regurgitation complicating balloon aortic valvuloplasty. Cath Cardiovasc Diagnosis 1989;17:186-189.
7. Aggarwal A, Raghuvir R, Eryazici P, et al. The development of aortic insufficiency in continuous-flow left ventricular assist device-supported patients. Ann Thorac Surg 2013;95(2):493-498.
8. Iung B, Baron G, Butchart EG et al. A prospective survey of patients with valvular heart disease in Europe: the Euro Heart Survey on Valvular Heart Disease. Eur Heart J 2003;24:1231-1243.
9. Hamirani YS, Dietl CA, Voyles W, et al. Acute aortic regurgitation. Circulation 2012;126:1121-1126.
10. Evangelista A, Carro A, Sergio M, et al. Imaging modalities for the early diagnosis of acute aortic syndrome. Nature Rev Cardiol 2013;10:477-486.
11. Mith MD, Cassidy JM, Souther S, et al. Transesophageal echocardiography in the diagnosis of traumatic rupture of the aorta. N Engl J Med 1995; 332:356-362.
12. Movsowitz HD, Levine RA, Hilgenberg AD, Isselbacher EM. Transesophageal echocardiographic description of the mechanisms of aortic regurgitation in

13. Dervan J, Goldberg S. Acute aortic regurgitation: pathophysiology and management. Cardiovasc Clin 1986;16:281-288.
14. Lerakis S, Hayek SS, Douglas PS. Paravalvular aortic leak after transcatheter aortic valve replacement: current knowledge. Circulation 2013;127: 397-407.
15. Graeter TP, Langer F, Nikoloudakis N, et al. Valve-preserving operations in acute aortic dissection type A. Ann Thorac Surg 2000;70:1460-1465.
16. Kallenbach K, Oelze T, Salcher R, et al. Evolving strategies for treatment of acute aortic dissection type A. Circulation 2004;110(Suppl II): II-243-II-249.
17. Cabell CH, Abrutyn E, Fowler VG, et al. Use of surgery in patients with native valve endocarditis: results from the international collaboration on endocarditis merged database. Am Heart J 2005;150:1092-1098.
18. Aksoy O, Sexton DJ, Wang A et al. Early surgery in patients with infective endocarditis: a propensity score analysis. Clin Infect Dis 2007;44:364-372.
19. Bonow RO, Rosing DR, McIntosh CL, et al. The natural history of asymptomatic patients with aortic regurgitation and normal left ventricular function. Circulation 1983;68:509-515.
20. Tornos MP, Olona M, Permanyer-Miralda G, et al. Clinical outcome of severe asymptomatic chronic aortic regurgitation: a long term prospective follow up study. Am Heart J 1995;130:333-339.
21. Ishii K, Hirota Y, Suwa M, et al. Natural history and left ventricular response in chronic aortic regurgitation. Am J Cardiol 1996;78: 357-361.
22. Nitenberg A, Foult JM, Blanchet F, Rahali M. Coronary flow and resistance reserve in patients with chronic aortic regurgitation, angina pectoris and normal coronary arteries. J Am Coll Cardiol 1988;11:478-486.
23. Bonow RO, Lakatos E, Maron BJ, Epstein SE. Serial long-term assessment of the natural history of asymptomatic patients with chronic aortic regurgitation and normal left ventricular systolic function. Circulation 1991; 84:1625-1635.
24. Grayburn PA, Smith MD, Handshoe R, et al. Detection of aortic insufficiency by standard echocardiography, pulsed Doppler echocardiography and auscultation: a comparison of accuracies. Ann Intern Med 186;104:599-605.
25. Aronow WS, Krozon I. Correlation of prevalence and severity of aortic regurgitation detected by pulsed Doppler echocardiography with the murmur of aortic regurgitation in elderly patients in a long term health facility. Am J Cardiol 1989;63:128-129.
26. Desjardin VA, Enriquez Sarano M, Tajik AJ, et al. Intensity of murmurs correlates with severity of valvular regurgitation. Am J Med 1996; 100:149-156..
27. Emi S, Fukuda N, Oki T, et al. Genesis of the Austin Flint murmur: relation to mitral flow and aortic regurgitant flow dynamics. J Am Coll Cardiol 1993;21:1399-1405.
28. Evangelista A, Tornos P, Sambola A, et al. Long-term vasodilator therapy in patients with severe aortic regurgitation. N Engl J Med 2005;353: 1342-1349.
29. Chen J, Okin PM, Roman MJ, et al. Combined rest and exercise electrocardiographic repolarization findings in relation to structural and functional abnormalities in symptomatic aortic regurgitation. Am Heart J 1996;132:343-347.
30. Reichek N, Deverex RB. Left ventricular hypertrophy: relationship of anatomic, echocardiographic and electrocardiographic findings. Circulation 1981;63:1391-1398.
31. Martinez Useros C, Tornos P, Montoyo J, et al. Ventricular arrhythmias in aortic valve disease: a further marker of impaired ventricular function. Int J Cardiol 1992;34:49-56.
32. Tribouilloy CM, Enriquez-Serrano M, Bailey KR, et al. Assessment of severity of aortic regurgitation using the width of the vena contracta: a clinical color Doppler imaging study. Circulation 2000;102(5):558-564.
32a. Zoghbi WA, Adams D, Bonow RO, et al. Recommendations for non-invasive evaluation of native valvular regurgitation. A report from the American Society of Echocardiography developed in collaboration with the Society for Cardiovascular Magnetic Resonance. J Am Soc Echocardiogr 2017;30: 303-371.

acute type A aortic dissection: implications for aortic valve repair. J Am Coll Cardiol 2000;36:884-890.

34. Panaro A, Moral S, Huguet M, et al. Descending aorta diastolic retrograde flow assessment for aortic regurgitation quantification. Rev Argent Cardiol 2016;84:336-341.

35. Bech-Hanssen O, Polte CL, Svensson F, et al. Pulsed-wave Doppler recordings in the proximal descending aorta in patients with chronic aortic regurgitation: insights from cardiovascular magnetic resonance. J Am Soc Echocardiogr 2018;31(3):304-313.

36. Evangelista A, del Castillo HG, Calvo F, et al. Strategy for optimal aortic regurgitation quantification by Doppler echocardiography: agreement among different methods. Am Heart J 2000;139(5):773-781.

37. Gao SA, Polte CL, Lagerstrand KM, et al. Evaluation of the integrative algorithm for grading chronic aortic and mitral regurgitation severity using the current American Society of Echocardiography recommendations: to discriminate severe from moderate regurgitation. J Am Soc Echocardiogr 2018 May 31. pii: S0894-7317(18)30181-0. doi: 10.1016/j.echo.2018.04.002.

38. Tribouilloy CM, Enriquez-Serrano M, Fett SL, et al. Application of the proximal flow convergence method to calculate the effective regurgitant orifice area in aortic regurgitation. J Am Coll Cardiol 1998;32(4):1032-1039.

39. Pouleur AC, de Waroux JB, Goffinet C, et al. Accuracy of the flow convergence method for quantification of aortic regurgitation in patients with central versus eccentric jets. Am J Cardiol 2008;102(4):475-480.

40. Lancellotti P, Tribouilloy C, Hagendorff A, et al. Recommendations for the echocardiographic assessment of native valvular regurgitation: an executive summary from the European Association of Cardiovascular Imaging. Eur Heart J Cardiovasc Imaging 2013;14:611-644.

41. Le Polain de Waroux JB, Pouleur AC, Goffinet C, et al. Functional anatomy of aortic regurgitation. Accuracy, prediction of surgical reparability and outcome implications of transesophageal echocardiography. Circulation 2007;116(Suppl):I 264-269.

42. Khoury El, Glineur D, Rubay J, et al: Functional classification of aortic root/valve abnormalities and their correlation with etiologies and surgical procedures. Curr Opin Cardiol 2005;20(2):115-121.

43. Lancellotti P, Tribouilloy C, Hagendorff A, et al. Recommendations for the echocardiographic assessment of native valvular regurgitation: an executive summary from the European Association of Cardiovascular Imaging. Eur Heart J Cardiovasc Imaging 2013;14:611-644.

44. Perez de Isla L, Zamorano J, Fernandez-Golfin C, et al. 3D color-Doppler echocardiography and chronic aortic regurgitation: a novel approach for severity assessment. Int J Cardiol 2013;166(3):640-645.

45. Klodas E, Enriquez-Sarano M, Tajik AJ, et al. Optimizing timing of surgical correction in patients with severe aortic regurgitation: role of symptoms. J Am Coll Cardiol 1997;30:746-752.

46. Sambola A, Tornos P, Ferreira I, Evangelista A. Prognostic value of preoperative indexed end-systolic left ventricular diameter in the outcome after surgery in patients with chronic aortic regurgitation. Am Heart J 2008; 155:1114-1120.

47. Olsen NT, Sogaard P, Larsson HB, et al. Speckle-tracking echocardiography for predicting outcome in chronic aortic regurgitation during conservative management and after surgery. JACC Cardiovasc Imaging 2011; 4(3):223-230.

48. Kaneko A, Tanaka H, Onishi T, et al. Subendocardial dysfunction in patients with chronic severe aortic regurgitation and preserved ejection fraction detected with speckle-tracking strain imaging and transmural myocardial strain profile. Eur Heart J Cardiovasc Imaging 2013;14:399-346.

49. Ewe S-H, Haeck MLA, Ng ACT, et al. Detection of subtle left ventricular systolic dysfunction in patients with significant aortic regurgitation and preserved left ventricular ejection fraction: speckle tracking echocardiographic analysis. Eur Heart J Cardiovasc Imaging 2015;16:992-999.

50. Lee JKT, Franzone A, Lanz J, et al. Early detection of subclinical myocardial damage in chronic aortic regurgitation and strategies for timely treatment of asymptomatic patients. Circulation 2018;137(2):184-196

51. Rodríguez-Palomares JF, Teixidó-Tura G, Galuppo V, et al. Multimodality assessment of ascending aortic diameters: comparison of different measurement methods. J Am Soc Echocardiogr 2016;29(9):819-826

52. Goffinet C, Kersten V, Pouleur AC, et al. Comprehensive assessment of the severity and mechanism of aortic regurgitation using multidetector CT and MR. Eur Radiol 2010;20(2):326-336.

53. Cawley PJ, Hamilton-Craig C, Owens DS, et al. Prospective comparison of valve regurgitation quantitation by cardiac magnetic resonance imaging and transthoracic echocardiography. Circ Cardiovasc Imaging 2013;6:48-57.

54. Myerson SG, d'Arcy J, Mohiaddin R, et al. Aortic regurgitation quantification using cardiovascular magnetic resonance association with clinical outcome. Circulation 2012;126:1452-1460.

55. Ribeiro HB, Orwat S, Hayek SS, et al. Cardiovascular magnetic resonance to evaluate aortic regurgitation after transcatheter aortic valve replacement. J Am Coll Cardiol 2016;68(6):577-585.

56. Alkadhi H, Desbioller L, Husmann L, et al. Aortic regurgitation: assessment with 64 section CT. Radiology 2007;245:111-121.

57. Jassae DS, Shapiro MD, Neilan Th, et al. 64-slice multidetector computed tomography (MDTC) for detection of aortic regurgitation and quantification of severity. Invest Radiol 2007;42:507-512.

58. Scheffeld H, Leschkas S, Plass A, et al. Accuracy of 64-slice computed tomography for the preoperative detection of coronary artery disease in patients with chronic aortic regurgitation. Am J Cardiol 2007;100:701-706.

59. Iskandrian AS, Heo J. Radionuclide angiographic evaluation of left ventricular performance at rest and exercise response in aortic regurgitation. Am J Cardiol 1985;55:428-431.

60. Misra M, Thakur R, Bhandari K, Puri VK. Value of treadmill exercise test in asymptomatic and minimally symptomatic patients with chronic severe aortic regurgitation. Int J Cardiol 1987;15:309-316.

61. Scriven AJ, Lipkin DP, Fox KM, Poole Wilson PA. Maximal oxygen uptake in severe aortic regurgitation: a different view of left ventricular function. Am Heart J 1990;120:902-909.

62. Wahi S, Haluska B, Pasquet A, et al. Exercise echocardiography predicts development of left ventricular dysfunction in medically and surgically treated patients with asymptomatic aortic regurgitation. Heart 2000;84: 606-614.

63. Park SJ, Enriquez-Sarano M, Song JE, et al. Contractile reserve determined on exercise echocardiography in patients with severe aortic regurgitation. Circ J 2013;77(9):2390-2398.

64. Kusunose K, Agarwal S, Marwick TH, et al. Decision making in asymptomatic aortic regurgitation in the era of guidelines: incremental values of resting and exercise cardiac dysfunction. Circ Cardiovasc Imaging 2014; 7(2):352-362

65. Pizarro R, Bazzino OO, Oberti PF, et al. Prospective validation of the prognostic usefulness of B-type natriuretic peptide in asymptomatic patients with chronic severe aortic regurgitation. J Am Coll Cardiol 2011;58(16):1705-1714

66. Carabello BA. Aortic regurgitation. a lesion with similarities to both aortic stenosis and mitral regurgitation. Circulation 1990;82:1051-1053.

67. Borow KM. Surgical outcome in chronic aortic regurgitation: a physiologic framework for assessing preoperative predictors. J Am Coll Cardiol 1987;10:1165-1170.

68. Cuhna CL, Giuliani ER, Fuster V, et al. Preoperative M mode echocardiography as predictor of surgical results in chronic aortic insufficiency. J Thorac Cardiovasc Surg 1980;79:256-265.

69. Forman R, Firth BG, Barnard MS. Prognostic significance of preoperative left ventricular ejection fraction and valve lesion in patients with aortic valve replacement. Am J Cardiol 1980;45:1120-1125.

70. Greves J, Rahimtoola SH, McAnulty JH, et al. Preoperative criteria predictive of late survival following valve replacement for severe aortic regurgitation. Am Heart J 1981;101:300-308.

71. Gaasch WH, Carroll JD, Levine H, Cristicello MG. Chronic aortic regurgitation: prognostic value of left ventricular end-systolic dimension and end-diastolic radius/thickness ratio. J Am Coll Cardiol 1983;1:775-782.

72. Bonow RO, Picone AL, McIntosh CL, et al. Survival and functional results after valve replacement for aortic regurgitation from 1976 to 1983: impact of preoperative left ventricular function. Circulation 1985;72: 1244-1256.

73. Carabello BA, Williams H, Gaasch AK, et al. Hemodynamic predictors of outcome in patients undergoing valve replacement. Circulation 1986; 72:1244-1256.

74. Michel PL, Iung B, Abou JS, et al. The effect of left ventricular systolic function on long term survival in mitral and aortic regurgitation. J Heart Valve Dis 1995;4(Suppl 2):S160-S168.

75. Henry WL, Bonow RO, Borer JS, et al. Observations on the optimum time for operative intervention for aortic regurgitation. I. Evaluation of the results of aortic valve replacement in symptomatic patients. Circulation 1980;61:471-483.

76. Kumpuris AG, Quinones MA, Waggoner AD, et al. Importance of preoperative hypertrophy, wall stress and end-systolic dimension as echocardiographic predictors of normalization of left ventricular dilatation after valve replacement in symptomatic patients. Am J Cardiol 1982;49:1091-1100.

77. Fioretti P, Roelandt J, Bos RJ, et al. Echocardiography in chronic aortic insufficiency: is valve replacement too late when left ventricular end systolic dimension reaches 55 mm? Circulation 1983;67:216-221.

78. Stone PH, Clark RD, Goldschlager N, et al. Determinants of prognosis of patients with aortic regurgitation who undergo aortic valve replacement. J Am Coll Cardiol 1984;3:1118-1126.

79. Daniel WG, Hood WP Jr, Siart A, et al. Chronic aortic regurgitation: reassessment of the prognostic value of preoperative left ventricular end systolic dimension and fractional shortening. Circulation 1985;7:669-680.

80. Cormier B, Vahanian A, Luxereaux P, et al. Should asymptomatic or mildly symptomatic aortic regurgitation be operated on? Z Kardiol 1986;75(Suppl 2):141-145.

81. Sheiban I, Trevi GP, Carassotto D, et al. Aortic valve replacement in patients with aortic incompetence: preoperative parameters influencing long term results. Z Kardiol 1986;75(suppl 2):146-154.

82. Klodas E, Enriquez-Sarano M, Tajik AJ, et al. Aortic regurgitation complicated by extreme left ventricular dilation: long-term outcome after surgical correction. J Am Coll Cardiol 1996;27:670-677.

83. Turina J, Milinic J, Seifert B, Turina M. Valve replacement in chronic aortic regurgitation: true predictors of survival after extended follow-up. Circulation 1998;98(Suppl II):II-100–II-106.

84. Tornos P, Sambola A, Permanyer-Miralda G, et al. Long term outcome of surgically treated aortic regurgitation: influence of guidelines adherence toward early surgery. J Am Coll Cardiol 2006;47:1012-1017.

85. Wilson RA, McDonald RW, Bristow JD, et al. Correlates of aortic distensibility in chronic aortic regurgitation and relation to progression to surgery. J Am Coll Cardiol 1992;19:259-265.

86. Rimold SC, Orav EJ, Come PC, et al. Progressive enlargement of the regurgitant orifice in patients with chronic aortic regurgitation. J Am Soc Echocardiogr 1998;11:259-265.

87. Padial LR, Oliver A, Vivaldi M, et al. Doppler echocardiographic assessment of progression of aortic regurgitation. Am J Cardiol 1997;80:306-314.

88. Scognamiglio R, Fasoli G, Dalla Volta S. Progression of myocardial dysfunction in asymptomatic patients with severe aortic insufficiency. Clin Cardiol 1986;9:151-156.

89. Siemienczuk D, Greenberg B, Morris C, et al. Chronic aortic insufficiency: factors associated with progression to aortic valve replacement. Ann Intern Med 1989;110:587-592.

90. Scognamiglio R, Rahimtoola SH, Fasoli G, et al. Nifedipine in asymptmatic paients with severe aortic regurgitation and normal left ventricular function. N Engl J Med 1994;331:689-694.

91. Borer JS, Hochreiter C, Herrold E, et al. Prediction of indications for valve replacement among asymptomatic or minimally symptomatic patients with chronic aortic regurgitation and normal left ventricular performance. Circulation 1998;97:525-534.

92. Tarasoutchi F, Grinberg M, Spina GS, et al. Ten year clinical laboratory follow up after application of a symptom-based therapeutic strategy to patients with severe aortic regurgitation of predominant rheumatic etiology. J Am Coll Cardiol 2003;41:1316-1324.

93. Detaint D, Messika-Zeitoun D, Maalouf J, et al. Quantitative echocardiographic determinants of clinical outcome in asymptomatic patients with aortic regurgitation: a prospective study. JACC Cardiovasc Imaging 2008:1:1-11.

94. Greenberg BH, Massie B, Bristow JD, et al. Long term vasodilator therapy of chronic aortic insufficiency: a randomized double-blinded, placebo controlled clinical trial. Circulation 1988;78:92-103.

95. Schon HR, Dorn R, Barthel P, Schomig A. Effects of 12 month quinapril therapy in asymptomatic patients with chronic aortic regurgitation. J Heart Valve Dis 1994;3:500-509.

96. Sondegaard L, Aldershvile J, Hildebrant P, et al. Vasodilatation with felodipine in chronic asymptomatic aortic regurgitation. Am Hear J 2000;139:667-674.

97. Greenberg BH, DeMots H, Murphy E, Rahimtoola SH. Mechanism for improved cardiac performance with arteriolar dilators in aortic insufficiency. Circulation 1981;63:263-268.

98. Greenberg BH, DeMots H, Murphy E, Rahimtoola SH. Beneficial effects of hydralazine on rest and exercise hemodynamics in patients with chronic severe aortic insufficiency. Circulation 1980;62:49-55.

99. Fioretti P, Benussi B, Scardi S, et al. Afterload reduction with nifedipine in aortic insufficiency. Am J Cardiol 1982;49:1728-1732.

100. Scognamiglio R, Fasoli G, Ponchia A, Dalla Volta S. Long term nifedipine unloading therapy in asymptomatic patients with chronic severe aortic regurgitation. J Am Coll Cardiol 1990;1:424-429.

101. Lin M, Chiang H, Lin S, et al. Vasodilator therapy in chronic asymptomatic aortic regurgitation: enalapril versus hydralazine therapy. J Am Coll Cardiol 1994;24:1046-1053.

102. Nishimura RA, Otto CM, Bonow RO, et al. 2014 AHA/ACC guideline for the management of patients with valvular heart disease: a report of the American College of Cardiology/American Heart Association Task Force on Practice Guidelines. Circulation 2014;129:e521-e643.

103. Baumgartner H, Falk V, Bax JJ, et al. 2017 ESC/EACTS guidelines for the management of valvular heart disease. The Task Force for the Management of Valvular Heart Disease of the European Society of Cardiology (ESC) and the European Association for Cardio-Thoracic Surgery (EACTS). Eur Heart J 2017;38:2739-2791.

104. Sampat U, Varadarajan P, Turk R, et al. Effect of beta-blocker therapy on survival in patients with severe aortic regurgitation: results from a cohort of 756 patients. J Am Coll Cardiol 2009;54:452-457.

105. Broch K, Urheim S, Lønnebakken MT, et al. Controlled release metoprolol for aortic regurgitation: a randomised clinical trial. Heart 2016;102(3):191-197.

106. Evangelista A. Medical treatment for chronic aortic regurgitation: β-blockers—maybe not bad, but good? Heart 2016;102:168-169.

107. Wilson W, Taubert KA, Gewitz M, et al. Prevention of infective endocarditis. A guideline from the American Heart Association Rheumatic Fever, Endocarditis, and Kawasaki Disease Committee, Council on Cardiovascular Disease in the Young, and the Council on Clinical Cardiology, Council on Cardiovascular Surgery and Anesthesia, and the Quality of Care and Outcomes Research Interdisciplinary Working Group. Circulation 2007;116:1736-1754.

108. Gabriel RS, Kerr AJ, Sharma V, et al. B-type natriuretic peptide and left ventricular dysfunction on exercise echocardiography in patients with chronic aortic regurgitation. Heart 2008;94:897-902.

109. Eimer MJ, Ekery DL, Rigolin VH, et al. Elevated B type natriuretic peptide in asymptomatic men with chronic aortic regurgitation and preserved left ventricular function. Am J Cardiol 2004;94:676-678.

110. Evangelista A. Diseases of the aorta: aneurysm of the ascending aorta. Heart 2010;96(12):979-985.

111. Sharma V, Suri RM, Dearani JA, et al. Expanding relevance of aortic valve repair-is earlier operation indicated? J Thorac Cardiovasc Surg 2014;147(1):100-107.

112. Boodhwani M, El Khoury G. Aortic valve repair: indications and outcomes. Curr Cardiol Rep 2014;16(6):490.

113. Hanke T, Stierle U, Boehm JO, et al. Autograft regurgitation and aortic root dimensions after the Ross procedure: the German Ross Registry experience. Circulation 2007;116(Suppl I):I-251–I-258.

114. Dujardin KS, Enriquez-Sarano M, Schaff HV, et al. Mortality and morbidity of aortic regurgitation in clinical practice: a long-term follow up study. Circulation 1999;99:1851-1857.

115. Bonow RO, Nikas D, Elefteriades JA. Valve replacement for regurgitant lesions of the aortic or mitral valve in advanced left ventricular dysfunction. Cardiol Clin 1995;13:73-83.

116. Kamath AR, Varadarajan P, Turk R, et al. Survival in patients with severe aortic regurgitation and severe left ventricular dysfunction is improved by aòrtic valve replacement: results from a cohort of 166 patients with an ejection fraction <35%. Circulation 2009;120(Suppl 1):S134-S138.

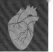

117. Mentias A, Feng K, Alashi A, et al. Long-term outcomes in patients with aortic regurgitation and preserved left ventricular ejection fraction. J Am Coll Cardiol 2016;68(20):2144-2153.

118. Shores J, Berger KR, Murphy EA, Pyeritz RE. Progression of aortic dilatation and the benefit of long term beta-adrenergic blockade in Marfan's syndrome. N Engl J Med 1994;330:1335-1341.

119. Groenink M, den Hartog AW, Franken R, et al. Losartan reduces aortic dilatation rate in adults with Marfan syndrome: a randomized controlled trial. Eur Heart J 2013;34(45):3491-3500.

120. Lacro RV, Dietz HC, Sleeper LA, et al. Atenolol versus losartan in children and young adults with Marfan's syndrome. N Engl J Med 2014;371(22):2061-2067.

121. Forteza A, Evangelista A, Sánchez V, et al. Efficacy of losartan vs. atenolol for the prevention of aortic dilation in Marfan syndrome: a randomized clinical trial. Eur Heart J 2016;37(12):978-985.

122. Milleron O, Arnoult F, Ropers J, et al. Marfan Sartan: a randomized, double-blind, placebo-controlled trial. Eur Heart J 2015;36(32): 2160-2166.

123. Hiratzka LF, Nishimura RA, Bonow RO, et al. Surgery for aortic dilatation in patients with bicuspid aortic valves. A statement of clarification from the American College of Cardiology/American Heart Association Task Force on Clinical Practice Guidelines. Circulation 2016; 133:680-686.

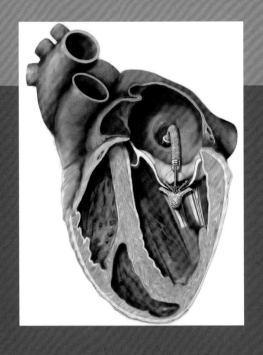

中文导读

第11章
二叶式主动脉瓣和相关的主动脉疾病

二叶式主动脉瓣是主动脉瓣的两个瓣叶在胎儿发育过程中融合，形成了双瓣，长期以来被认为是瓣膜性心脏病的一个重要原因，也是最常见的先天性心脏病之一，此种常染色体显性遗传可能伴随其他先天性心血管缺陷和疾病，包括主动脉夹层、特纳综合征、升主动脉和（或）主动脉根部的扩张等。二叶式主动脉瓣除自身作为独立的心血管疾病外，也可能作为其他系统性疾病的众多表现之一。遗传学和信号通路的发现、临床影像学的进步、主动脉和瓣膜介入手术及外科手术的改进，提高了我们对二叶式主动脉瓣及其相关并发症的认识和管理。

本章内容从二叶式主动脉瓣的可能致病基因、遗传倾向、临床解剖结构、临床表现与各种不同筛查诊断工具（包括经胸超声心动图、经食管超声心动图、心脏MRI或心脏CT诊断中的影像特征）等方面进行详实描述，并围绕二叶式主动脉瓣造成的影响、可能的并发症、各种治疗的手段选择及最合适的干预时机展开讨论，针对临床中不同情况（包括围手术期、远期并发症，影响预后的危险因素或诱因）进行分析探讨。最后，本章总结了二叶式主动脉瓣患者的完整临床治疗路径建议，包括早期筛查、确诊后、干预后近远期随访监测指标，以及该患病人群的生活运动建议，最后也对孕产妇高危人群提出了具体建议，以利于心脏团队对此部分患者进行全面的终生治疗管理。

丁　诚

The Bicuspid Aortic Valve and Associated Aortic Disease

Alan C. Braverman, Andrew Cheng

CHAPTER OUTLINE

KEY POINTS

- The bicuspid aortic valve (BAV) is the most common congenital heart condition, affecting approximately 1% of the population.
- Familial BAV occurs in 9% to 10% of first-degree relatives. Familial aortic aneurysm with or without BAV may occur in certain families; it is inherited as an autosomal dominant condition with incomplete penetrance and inconsistent expression.
- BAV may accompany other congenital cardiovascular defects and conditions, including coarctation of the aorta and Turner syndrome.
- When transthoracic echocardiography is not diagnostic, transesophageal echocardiography, cardiac magnetic resonance imaging, or cardiac computed tomography may be useful in diagnosing BAV disease.
- Aortic dilation, involving the ascending aorta and/or aortic root, occurs frequently in individuals with BAV disease, even in the absence of aortic stenosis or aortic regurgitation, and may occur late after aortic valve replacement.

- Abnormal aortic systolic flow patterns through the BAV lead to abnormal regional aortic wall stress and contribute to the aortopathy in this disorder.
- The aortopathy of BAV disease is associated with cystic medial degeneration, alterations in signaling pathways and matrix metalloproteinase activity, and apoptosis, all of which place the patient with BAV at increased risk for aortic aneurysm and aortic dissection.
- The BAV may be part of certain syndromic and nonsyndromic thoracic aortic aneurysm disorders.
- Most patients with BAV will require surgical therapy on the valve and/or aorta during their lifetime.
- After BAV replacement, the patient remains at risk for late ascending aortic aneurysm formation and aortic dissection. These complications may be related to the prior valve lesion and aortopathy phenotype, and they are more common with regurgitant than with stenotic valves, especially with the root phenotype. Surveillance of the aorta late after BAV replacement is important.

Bicuspid aortic valve (BAV) is an inherited form of heart disease in which two of the leaflets of the aortic valve fuse during fetal development, resulting in a two-leaflet valve. It is the most common congenital heart disorder and has long been recognized as an important cause of valvular heart disease.[1]

Leonardo da Vinci sketched the bicuspid variant of the aortic valve more than 400 years ago.[1] The clinical and valvular sequelae of the BAV were realized more than 150 years ago. Osler emphasized endocarditis as a complication in 1886. The association of congenital BAV with diseases of the aorta was first recorded by Abbott in 1927.[1]

TABLE 11.1 Prevalence of Bicuspid Aortic Valve in Autopsy Studies.

Study Authors	Year	Study Population *(N)*	BAV Prevalence (%)
Olsery	1886	800	1.2
Lewis and Grant	1923	215	1.39
Wauchope	1928	9,966	0.5
Grant et al	1928	1,350	0.89
Gross	1937	5,000	0.56
Roberts	1970	1,440	0.9
Larson and Edwards	1984	21,417	1.37
Datta et al	1988	8,800	0.59
Pauperio et al	1999	2,000	0.65

BAV, Bicuspid aortic valve.
Adapted from Basso C, Boschello M, Perrone C, et al. An echocardiographic survey of primary school children for bicuspid aortic valve. Am J Cardiol 2004;93:661-663.

In 1984, the relationship between BAV and aortic dissection risk was emphasized, observing a ninefold greater risk of aortic dissection among BAV patients.[1] Discoveries in genetics and signaling pathways, advances in imaging, and improvements in aortic and valve surgery have improved the understanding and management of BAV and its associated complications.

PREVALENCE

The prevalence of BAV is approximately 1% of the population, with a 2:1 to 3:1 male-to-female ratio (Table 11.1).[1] In the largest reported autopsy series, involving 21,417 consecutive cases, the prevalence of BAV was 1.37%.[1] In a study of 1075 neonates, the prevalence of BAV was 4.6 per 1000 live births.[2] Among 20,946 military recruits, the prevalence of BAV was 0.8%.[3] Certain groups of patients have a much higher prevalence of BAV than the general population; the rates are approximately 30% to 50% for patients with coarctation of the aorta (CoA) and 30% for Turner syndrome (TS) females.[1]

ETIOLOGY

Embryology

The semilunar valves originate from the mesenchymal outgrowths along the ventricular outflow tract of the primary heart tube. Several molecular signaling pathways have been implicated in its development, including transforming growth factor-β (TGF-β), RAS, WNT/β-catenin, vascular endothelial growth factor (VEGF), and NOTCH signaling.[4,5] Anomalous behavior of cells derived from the neural crest has been implicated as a possible cause of BAV because BAV is often associated with congenital malformations of the aortic arch and other neural crest–derived systems.[1,6–8] A primary molecular abnormality of the extracellular matrix may trigger abnormal valvulogenesis.[9] Endothelial nitric oxide (eNOS) signaling may also be important in the pathogenesis of BAV and aortic disease.[5–8]

Different pathways were shown to be responsible for BAV leaflet orientation in animal models: one that relies on a nitric oxide–dependent epithelial-to-mesenchymal transformation and another

that results from the distorted behavior of neural crest cells.[6] *GATA5* gene expression is restricted to endocardial cushions, and targeted inactivation of *GATA5* in mice leads to development of BAV, involving several signaling pathways, including that of *NOTCH*.[10] The ubiquitin fusion degradation 1–like gene *(UFD1L)*, which is expressed in the embryonic outflow tract, is downregulated in BAV tissue.[11] *NOTCH1* encodes for a transmembrane protein that is important in cardiac embryogenesis, including the aortic and pulmonary valves and aorta. *NOTCH1* mutations (9q34.3) are found in a small number of families with BAV and ascending aortic aneurysms.[5,8] Animal models propose deficient signal exchanges among the endocardial cushions, second heart field, and neural crest cells (with different embryologic origins of the outflow tract and aortic segmental anatomy) as a link between BAV and aortic wall abnormalities[12,13] (Fig. 11.1).

Genetics

Family studies report the prevalence of BAV among first-degree relatives of an individual with a BAV is 9% to 10%.[14,15] The inheritance of BAV is consistent with an autosomal dominant pattern with reduced penetrance.[14] Monozygotic twins do not necessarily both have BAV, highlighting the incomplete penetrance of this disorder.[16]

Although BAV is a heritable trait, the genetic causes remain elusive. In most patients, no specific genetic variant has been discovered. Mutations in *NOTCH1* are associated with familial and nonfamilial BAV and may result in aortic aneurysms and early aortic calcification.[1] Mutations in other single genes such as *GATA5*, *GATA6*, and *NKX2-5* have been associated with BAV; *ACTA2*, *TGFB2*, *LOX*, *SMAD6*, and other genes have been associated with BAV and thoracic aortic aneurysm[17] (Table 11.2). Polymorphisms in other genes may be associated with BAV risk.[18] BAV is also associated with genetic conditions such as DiGeorge syndrome, Loeys-Dietz syndrome, Anderson syndrome (i.e., *KCNJ2* mutation), and complex congenital heart conditions such as

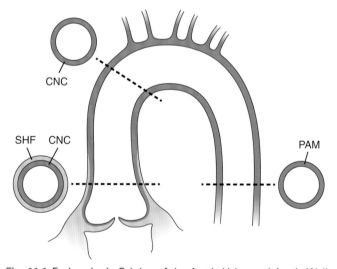

Fig. 11.1 Embryologic Origins of the Aortic Valve and Aortic Wall. The aortic valve is derived predominantly from the second heart field *(yellow)* and the cardiac neural crest cells *(blue)*. The embryologic origin of the aortic root also consists predominantly of the second heart field and neural crest cells, whereas the ascending aorta and aortic arch originate mainly from neural crest cells alone. The descending aorta distal to the subclavian artery originates from paraxial mesoderm cells *(green)*. The shared embryologic derivation suggests a link between bicuspid aortic valve and aortic wall abnormalities. *CNC*, Cardiac neural crest; *PAM*, paraxial mesoderm; *SHF*, second heart field. (From Yassine NM, Shahram JT, Body SC. Pathogenic mechanisms of bicuspid aortic valve aortopathy. Front Physiol 2017;8:687.)

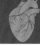

TABLE 11.2 Gene Mutations Associated With Bicuspid Aortic Valve With or Without Familial Thoracic Aortic Aneurysm.

Mutated Gene	Genetic Defect and Phenotype
ACTA2	FTAA with premature CAD, CVD, livedo reticularis; BAV in 3%
ELN	BAV may occur with cutis laxa
FBN1	Marfan syndrome or nonsyndromic FTAA; reported increased frequency of BAV
FLNA	BAV may occur with X-linked cardiac valve dysplasia
GATA5	Rarely associated with familial BAV
GATA6	Loss-of-function mutation associated with BAV
KCNJ2	Anderson syndrome; associated with BAV
LOX	FTAA; associated with BAV
MAT2A	FTAA and BAV
MYH11	FTAA; BAV may occur
NKX2-5	Rarely associated with familial BAV
NOTCH1	Isolated BAV with AS, familial BAV or FTAA
SMAD3	Syndromic FTAA (LDS type 3, aneurysm-osteoarthritis syndrome); may have BAV
SMAD6	Rarely associated with BAV, AS, and CoA
TGFB2	Syndromic FTAA (LDS type 4); may have BAV
TGFB3	Syndromic FTAA (LDS type 5); may have BAV
TGFBR1 TGFBR2	Syndromic (LDS) or nonsyndromic FTAA; BAV in 2%–17%

AS, Aortic stenosis; *BAV*, bicuspid aortic valve; *CAD*, coronary artery disease; *CoA*, coarctation of the aorta; *CVD*, cerebrovascular disease; *FTAA*, familial thoracic aortic aneurysm disorder; *LDS*, Loeys-Dietz syndrome; *TAA*, thoracic aortic aneurysm.

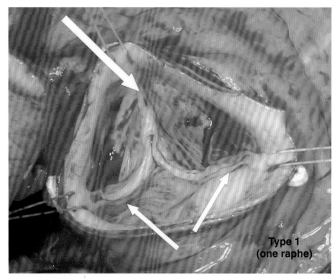

Fig. 11.2 Intraoperative Picture of a Bicuspid Aortic Valve. Bicuspid aortic valve type 1 (i.e., right-left coronary cusp fusion) with one completely developed noncoronary cusp, two completely developed commissures *(small arrows)*, and one raphe between the underdeveloped left and right coronary cusps extending to the corresponding malformed commissures *(large arrow)* cause hemodynamic signs of insufficiency due to prolapse of the conjoint cusps. (From Sievers HH, Schmidtke C. A classification system for the bicuspid aortic valve from 304 surgical specimens. J Thorac Cardiovasc Surg 2007;133:1226-1233.)

Shone complex and hypoplastic left heart syndrome. One cross-sectional exome-wide association study found no association signals for BAV with or without thoracic aortic aneurysm,[17] but whole-genome sequencing may provide more comprehensive understanding of the genetics of BAV.[5,19]

CLINICAL PHENOTYPE

Valve Anatomy

BAV anatomy typically includes unequal cusp size due to fusion of two cusps, leading to one larger cusp (Fig. 11.2). Fusion most commonly occurs between the right and left coronary leaflets (70%–86%). There may also be fusion between the right and noncoronary leaflets (12%) or between the left and noncoronary leaflets (3%).[1,20] Several classification systems have been used to describe BAVs based on the fused cusp orientation (i.e., right-left, right-noncoronary, or left-noncoronary) and the presence or absence of a raphe (Fig. 11.3). The raphe (89% of cases) is the site of fusion of the conjoined cusps.[20] The presence of a raphe is associated with a higher prevalence of valve dysfunction.[21]

Associated Cardiovascular Lesions

In most instances, BAV is an isolated cardiovascular finding. However, BAV may coexist with other congenital cardiovascular defects or syndromes.

Coarctation of the Aorta

BAV is associated with CoA in 30% to 50% of patients with CoA, whereas CoA has been found in 6% of patients with BAV.[1,22] Interrupted aortic arch is also frequently associated with BAV. Coexistence of BAV and CoA is predominantly associated with right-left coronary cusp fusion (85%). During infancy and adolescence, valvular dysfunction in patients with BAV and CoA tends to occur at the same rate as in those with isolated BAV.[22] However, during adulthood, valvular complications from BAV, such as aortic stenosis (AS) or aortic regurgitation (AR), are more prevalent among people with both CoA and BAV.

Pediatric patients with CoA and BAV may have smaller aortic dimensions than those with isolated BAV.[22] However, individuals with CoA and BAV have larger aortas than those with a CoA alone, and even those with CoA alone have been found to have aortic dimensions similar to those of the normal tricuspid aortic valve (TAV) population.[23] BAV is an important predictor of subsequent aortic wall complications (i.e., aortic aneurysm, aortic dissection, and aortic rupture) in patients with CoA.[24,25]

Among patients with BAV and CoA, the aortic abnormalities are not confined to the ascending aorta, suggesting a more diffuse process.[24] Hypertension and intrinsic aortic wall disease may be important in the pathogenesis of aortic dissection related to CoA.[1] Among CoA patients, BAV is a major risk factor for death or future cardiovascular events.[26] Individuals with BAV require long-term follow-up of the coarctation repair, the BAV, and the ascending aorta.[24–27]

Turner Syndrome

TS, which is caused by complete or partial absence of one X chromosome, is associated with cardiovascular defects in up to 75% of cases.[28] BAV is the most common defect, occurring in up to 30% of cases; other associated defects include ascending aortic dilation, CoA, pseudocoarctation, elongated aortic arch, and hypoplastic left heart syndrome.[28]

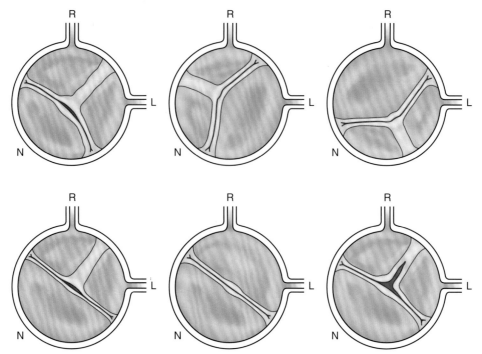

Fig. 11.3 Schematic of Bicuspid Aortic Valve (BAV) Phenotypes as Seen by Transthoracic Echocardiography. The schematic represents the parasternal short-axis echocardiographic view. Bicuspid valves are classified as type 1 (i.e., right cusp *[R]*–left coronary cusp *[L]* fusion), type 2 (i.e., R-noncoronary *[N]* cusp fusion), and type 3 (i.e., L-N cusp fusion). BAV phenotypes are shown. *Top left*, type 1 BAV (commissures at 10 and 5 o'clock) with complete raphe, asymmetric (the nonfused cusp [noncoronary] is smaller than the conjoined anterior cusp). *Top middle*, type 2 BAV (commissures at 1 and 7 o'clock) with complete raphe and asymmetric (the nonfused cusp [left] is larger than the conjoined cusp). *Top right*, type 3 BAV (shown with commissures at 2 and 8 o'clock but could be 1 and 7 o'clock) with complete raphe, asymmetric (the nonfused cusp [right] is larger than the conjoined one). *Bottom left*, symmetric type 1 BAV with complete raphe. *Bottom middle*, symmetric type 1 BAV without raphe (true BAV). *Bottom right*, type 1 BAV with incomplete raphe, partially fused. (From Michelena HI, Prakash SK, Della Corte A, et al. Bicuspid aortic valve: identifying knowledge gaps and rising to the challenge from the International Bicuspid Aortic Valve Consortium (BAVCon). Circulation 2014;129:2691-2704.)

Identification of a left-sided outflow tract lesion in a female infant should prompt evaluation for TS.

The finding of BAV in TS is associated with larger aortic dimensions at the annulus, sinuses, sinotubular junction, and ascending aorta.[29] Because TS patients have short stature, ascending aortic dimensions may be significantly dilated relative to body surface area (BSA), and absolute measurement of the aortic root or ascending aortic diameter may not predict the risk of aortic dissection. Prophylactic aortic surgery is recommended for these patients at smaller aortic dimensions, and the aortic size should be indexed to BSA.[29,30]

Coronary Artery Anomalies

Congenital coronary anomalies have been described in patients with BAV, including a short left main coronary artery and increased frequency of left-dominant circulation (24%–57%).[1] Isolated congenital coronary artery anomalies, particularly with a separate ostia for the left anterior descending and circumflex arteries, are associated with BAV and are related to fusion of the left and right coronary cusps.[31] High take-off coronary arteries are more common in BAV with associated congenital heart disease.[32] Coronary artery ectasia is also reported in BAV patients.[33]

Other Congenital Heart Malformations

Other congenital heart diseases and syndromes commonly associated with BAV are listed in Table 11.3.[1,22]

Aortopathy

BAV is associated with disorders of the thoracic aorta, including aortic aneurysm, CoA, and aortic dissection.[1,34–36] Patients with BAVs have larger aortic roots and/or ascending aortic diameters than controls after accounting for age, valvular lesions, and hypertension.[1,37] Aortic dilation is greater in those with regurgitant rather than stenotic or functionally normal BAV.[1,37] However, dilation of the aorta (which can involve the root to the arch) frequently accompanies BAV (50%), even in the absence of AS or AR.[1,35] Few patients with TAV disease have aortic dilation, whereas BAV is frequently associated with a dilated proximal aorta. Compared with TAV patients with severe AS, those with BAV have significantly larger aortic roots and ascending aortic diameters[34] (Fig. 11.4).

Pathophysiology

Several mechanisms are responsible for the aortopathy of BAV disease, including intrinsic (genetic) aortic wall defects and abnormal valve-related hemodynamic stress.[38,39] Developmental defects in neural crest cells affecting the aortic valve and proximal aorta are hypothesized to contribute to the genetic underpinnings.[35] In support of the genetic hypothesis, aortopathy has been reported in some studies of first-degree relatives of patients with BAV.[40,41] Among families with BAV and aneurysm, there are individuals with ascending aneurysm alone,

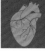

TABLE 11.3 Bicuspid Aortic Valve and Associated Cardiovascular Conditions.

Condition	Incidence of BAV	Comments
Coarctation of the aorta	30%–50%	BAV confers increased risk of aortic complications
Interrupted aortic arch	36%	BAV frequently associated
Turner syndrome	30%	Most frequent cardiac abnormality; CoA and TAA may be present
Supravalvular aortic stenosis	30%	Usually part of William syndrome
Hypoplastic left heart syndrome	25%	Frequently associated
Subvalvular aortic stenosis	10%–20%	May result in significant AR
Patent ductus arteriosus	2%	Usually diagnosed in infancy or childhood
Sinus of Valsalva aneurysm	15%–20%	Most commonly involves right coronary sinus
Ventricular septal defect	4%–30%	May result in significant AR
Shone complex	60%–85%	Series of left-sided obstructive lesions (supravalvular mitral ring, parachute mitral valve, subaortic stenosis, CoA)
Ascending aortic dilation	Common	BAV commonly associates with a dilated ascending aorta
Aortic aneurysm syndromes		
Loeys-Dietz syndrome	2.5%–17%	*TGFBR1* or *TGFBR2* mutations
ACTA2-related FTAA syndrome	3%	*ACTA2* mutations
NOTCH1	?	AS and TAA
Others: *TGFBR1, TGFBR2, SMAD3, TGFB2, TGFB3, MAT2A, LOX, SMAD6*	?	Syndromic and nonsyndromic FTAAs that may involve BAV

AR, Aortic regurgitation; *AS*, aortic stenosis; *BAV*, bicuspid aortic valve; *CoA*, coarctation of the aorta; *FTAA*, familial thoracic aortic aneurysm; *TAA*, thoracic aortic aneurysm.

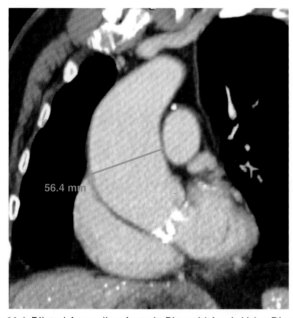

56.4 mm

Fig. 11.4 Dilated Ascending Aorta in Bicuspid Aortic Valve Disease. A CT angiogram shows a 5.6-cm ascending aortic aneurysm complicating a calcified bicuspid aortic valve.

suggesting that BAV and ascending aortic aneurysm are manifestations of a genetic defect with variable expression. Abnormalities of regulation of the endothelial/epithelial-mesenchymal transition during embryogenesis of the aortic valve and ascending aorta in BAV disease may contribute to aortopathy.[12]

A genetic trigger may underlie some cases of BAV-related thoracic aortic aneurysm, but in most cases, a specific underlying genetic disorder is not recognized. Some patients with BAV have syndromic or nonsyndromic genetic disorders related to specific mutations[5,19] (see Table 11.2). Potential mutations of loci at 5q, 13q, 15q, and 18q are reported for BAV and aortic aneurysm.[5,42] Rare copy number variants have been identified in patients with BAV and early-onset thoracic aortic aneurysm disease, suggesting that these variants may alter gene expression and affect aortopathy.[19,43]

A wide spectrum of rare genetic variants has been reported for many patients with BAV root phenotype.[44] Although the root phenotype is associated with a genetic underpinning, any aortopathy phenotype may be present in a patient with familial BAV and aneurysm disease.[42,45,46] Thorough evaluation of the aortic valve and ascending aorta is important for first-degree relatives of patients with BAV and ascending aortic aneurysm.[42,47]

BAV may also occur with syndromes associated with aortic or vascular disease.[5,8,46] BAV is reported in 2.5% to 17% of patients with Loeys-Dietz syndrome[46] and in approximately 3% of familial thoracic aortic aneurysm (FTAA) disorders due to *ACTA2* mutations.[48] Other FTAA disorders, some syndromic and others nonsyndromic, may be associated with an increased prevalence of BAV (see Table 11.2).

Genetic heterogeneity, complexity of the trait, noncoding sequence variants, and epigenetic factors may explain the absence of a unifying genetic pathogenesis of BAV aneurysm disease.[49] The patient with BAV and aneurysm should undergo a careful family history, evaluation for a phenotype suggesting an aneurysm syndrome and mutation analysis when appropriate.

Expanding the phenotype of BAV aortopathy is the recognition of an increased frequency (7.7%–9.8%) of intracranial aneurysms among BAV patients.[50,51] The rate was 5.7% for those without and 12.9% for those with CoA in a nonrandomized population from a tertiary referral center,[51] and an association was found between BAV and cervicocephalic arterial dissection.[1]

Hemodynamic factors are likely predominant in the aortic pathology in most BAV patients.[38,39,52–55] The BAV exhibits abnormal leaflet

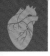

folding and wrinkling and increased leaflet doming, resulting in turbulence even in the absence of valve stenosis.[38,39] Markedly abnormal helical flow is demonstrated in the ascending aorta of BAV patients, including those without aortic aneurysm or AS.[52,54] Increased mid-ascending aortic wall shear stress related to asymmetric and higher flow velocity are identified in BAV models compared with TAVs.[54]

Leaflet orientation also influences areas of maximum aortic wall stress.[54,55] In BAV models, the orientation of the BAV with respect to the plane of aortic curvature results in different jet shapes and distribution of wall stress on the aorta.[53,54] The BAV cusp opening angle correlates with aortic growth rate, as do the angle between the left ventricular outflow tract and aortic root and the degree of aortic enlargement.[56] Patients with BAV have increased aortic wall stress compared with TAV patients matched for aortic diameter size.[57]

Abnormal systolic flow patterns and distribution of wall stress may underlie vascular remodeling and aneurysm formation in BAV patients.[8,38,39,52-54,58,59] Wall shear stress affects mechanotransduction pathways associated with vascular remodeling.[60] In patients with BAV and aneurysm, sites of greater wall shear stress demonstrate more cystic medial degeneration (CMD), elevated matrix metalloproteinase activity, increased TGF-β expression, and decreased fibrillin 1 content compared with sites of lower wall shear stress[55,61] (Fig. 11.5). An asymmetric pattern of elastic fiber degeneration and apoptosis are evident in the convexity compared with the concavity of the dilated ascending aorta in BAV patients.[7,39,62,63]

Regional variation in wall shear stress in BAV aortopathy is related to valve fusion type and aortic diameter[58,59,63,64] (Fig. 11.6). Pure BAVs (with no raphes) have more laminar flow than BAVs with right-left leaflet fusion and a raphe.[65] BAV leaflet morphology may also affect the aortic dilation pattern.[66,67] The asymmetric opening of the BAV alters flow, resulting in uneven wall stress on the aorta.[7,59] The right-left leaflet fusion is associated with a right anterior jet, whereas right-noncoronary leaflet fusion is associated with an eccentric left posterior jet. Right-left leaflet fusion results in aortic dilation at the convexity (i.e., outer curvature), whereas right-noncoronary leaflet fusion is associated with a tubular aortic enlargement extending into the arch.[7,59]

Among BAV patients with AS, flow patterns predict medial changes in the aortic wall.[68] Localized ascending aortic dilation occurs with stenotic BAV, and a more extensive aortopathy occurs among young patients with regurgitant BAV. This suggests that hemodynamics plays a greater role in stenotic BAV and genetics in regurgitant BAV.[20]

Histopathology

The histopathology underlying aortic root and/or ascending aortic complications in BAV is CMD, which may occur in the aortic wall with BAV, even in the absence of aneurysm formation (see Fig. 11.5).[1,9,55,58,69] The type of valve lesion (AS vs. AR) predicts the severity of CMD.[69] A higher degree of CMD occurs in BAV AR compared with BAV AS. The CMD is more diffuse when associated with AR, whereas in AS, medial changes are more focal at the site of the jet lesion.[69,70] Among patients with BAV undergoing aortic valve replacement (AVR) and aortic aneurysm resection, almost one half of those with AR had CMD, whereas only a minority of those with AS had these changes.[69]

Matrix architecture and aortic remodeling are different in BAV and TAV disease.[71] Compared with TAV aneurysm disease, the aortic wall in BAV aneurysm disease is characterized by less differentiated vascular smooth muscle cells, a lower expression of lamin A/C, decreased FBN1 expression, and marked elastic fiber thinning.[72] Compared with

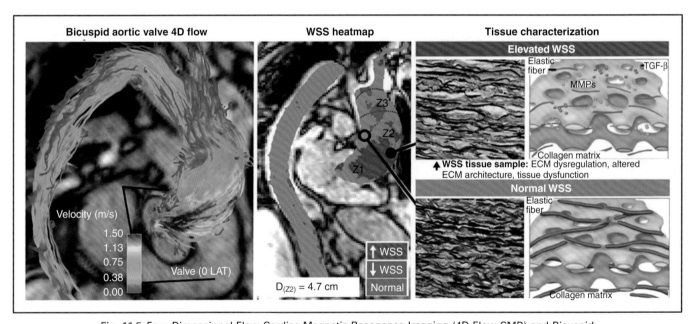

Fig. 11.5 Four-Dimensional Flow Cardiac Magnetic Resonance Imaging (4D Flow CMR) and Bicuspid Aortic Valve (BAV) Aortopathy. Using 4D flow CMR, the relationship between wall shear stress (WSS) and regional aortic tissue remodeling in BAV patients was assessed. Elevated aortic WSS generated by aberrant flow from cusp fusion corresponded to more severe extracellular matrix (ECM) dysregulation than adjacent regions of normal WSS in the same patient's aorta. Characteristic medial degeneration was observed throughout the aorta, but elastic fiber degeneration was more severe in regions of elevated WSS (i.e., less elastin, thinner fibers, and greater distances between laminae), where higher concentrations of mediators of ECM dysregulation (i.e., matrix metalloproteinase [MMP] and transforming growth factor-β [TGF-β]) are also observed. These data implicate valve-related hemodynamics as a contributing factor to BAV aortopathy. (From Guzzardi DG, Barker AJ, van Ooij P, et al. Valve-related hemodynamics mediate human bicuspid aortopathy: insights from wall shear stress mapping. J Am Coll Cardiol 2015;66:892-900.)

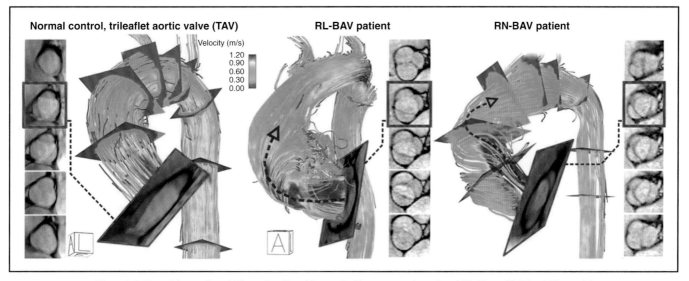

Fig. 11.6 Four-Dimensional Flow Cardiac Magnetic Resonance Imaging (4D Flow CMR) of Bicuspid Aortic Valve *(BAV)*–Mediated Hemodynamics. Images show the control patient, a BAV patient with a right-left *(RL)* fusion pattern, and a BAV patient with a right-noncoronary *(RN)* fusion pattern. The RL-BAV resulted in a marked eccentric aortic outflow jet (but not higher velocity *[arrow]*) impinging on the aortic wall compared with the trileaflet aortic valve. The BAV phenotype (RL vs. RN) strongly impacts aortic outflow and aortic regions exposed to elevated wall shear stress. (From Fedak PW, Barker AJ, Verma S. Year in review: bicuspid aortopathy. Curr Opin Cardiol 2016;31:132-138.)

TAV aortic aneurysm, BAV aortic aneurysm demonstrates increased apoptosis, more severe elastic fiber fragmentation, higher levels of matrix metalloproteinases (MMP2 and MMP9), and lower levels of tissue inhibitors of MMP (TIMP1).[55,73,74] The imbalance between MMP and TIMP1 levels may be influenced by BAV leaflet orientation and may affect aortopathy.[73,74] Elevated circulating MMP levels occur in BAV aneurysm disease.[58,75] Alterations in matrix fiber orientation in the aortic media vary depending on BAV leaflet orientation.[76] As in Marfan syndrome, fibrillin 1 content is reduced in BAV aortas (and pulmonary arteries) compared with that in TAV aortas and is related to the valve and aortopathy phenotype.[1,55]

In BAV aneurysms, as in Marfan and Loeys-Dietz syndromes, increased TGF-β levels and increased TGF-β signaling are demonstrated in the aortic wall.[77] There is upregulation of TGF-β signaling proteins in BAV compared with TAV aneurysm tissue.[78] Defective TGF-β splicing of fibronectin mRNA is seen in BAV patients, and it potentially contributes to defective vascular repair of BAV aortopathy.[79]

Ascending Aortic Dilation

Distinct patterns of aortic enlargement may be seen in patients with BAV[8,35,80] (Fig. 11.7). In contrast to the aortic sinus enlargement seen in Marfan syndrome, the enlargement in BAV may arise in the sinuses or the ascending aorta, or both, and may extend to the arch.[34,35,70,80] Most commonly, the mid-ascending aorta is dilated. The root phenotype is identified in 10% of cases; it is associated with an increased risk of late aortic events and is the phenotype most associated with genetic disease (Fig. 11.8).[35,44]

The prevalence of aortic dilation among BAV patients ranges from 20% to 84%, depending on the definition of dilation and patient-specific characteristics (e.g., age, valve lesion).[35,81] Children with BAV have larger aortic dimensions than controls, independent of any functional abnormality of the BAV.[1,80,82] Among children and young adults with BAV, the aortic root was dilated (Z-score > 2) in 22%, and more marked dilation (Z-score > 4) occurred in 5%, whereas the ascending aorta was dilated (Z-score > 2) in 49%, and 16% had Z-scores greater than 4.[82]

BAV leaflet orientation may influence the aortic root shape and phenotype.[20,65,82,83] Right-left cusp fusion is associated with larger aortic root diameter compared with right-noncoronary fusion, and right-noncoronary cusp fusion is associated with a larger ascending aorta and/or aortic arch diameter.[82,84] This may reflect the different eccentric flow jets of cusp fusion phenotypes, causing differential flow patterns, aortic wall shear stress, and medial changes.[55,83] However, other investigators have not reported a relationship between cusp orientation and aortic size[80] or pattern of aortic dilation.[85]

Reduced aortic wall elasticity and distensibility is reported for patients with nonstenotic BAV.[86] Aortic wall strain, aortic wall distention, and recoil are different in patients compared with those with TAV.[87] The elastic tissue properties of the BAV aorta may be related to cusp orientation.[88]

CLINICAL PRESENTATION AND DIAGNOSIS

Physical Examination

Most young patients with isolated BAV are asymptomatic and are diagnosed incidentally when a systolic ejection sound or murmur is heard or by echocardiography. However, routine clinical examination detects only about 50% of BAV patients.[15]

A functionally normal BAV has an ejection sound or click that is often followed by a systolic flow murmur.[1] In the setting of progressive AS, the ejection murmur becomes harsher and peaks later. The ejection sound diminishes as the valve cusps become more immobile. In the setting of AR, the examination findings vary with severity. An ejection sound is present with mild to moderate AR and absent with severe AR.[1] With significant AR, an early diastolic decrescendo murmur is best heard at the left lower sternal border. If the murmur of AR is heard loudest at the right midsternal border, concern should arise for the presence of a dilated ascending aorta. BAV may accompany other cardiovascular lesions, and the examination should assess for CoA and other lesions.

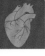

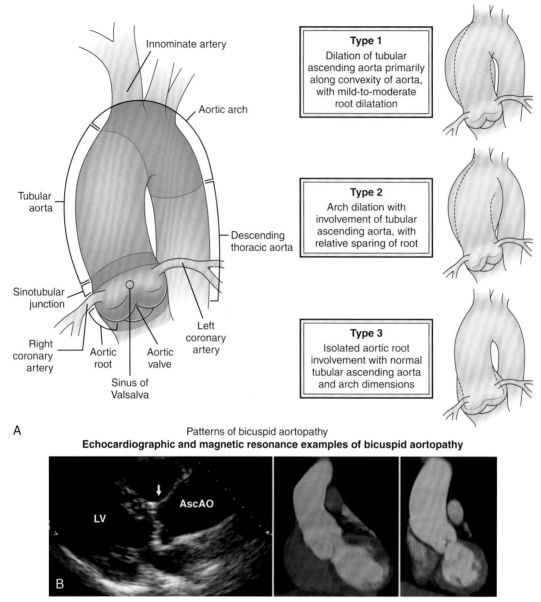

Fig. 11.7 Patterns of Bicuspid Aortopathy With Representative Findings on Echocardiography and Computed Tomography (CT). (A) Biologic features of the aorta and the three types of bicuspid aortopathy. (B) The transthoracic echocardiogram *(left)* shows normal dimensions of the sinuses of Valsalva *(arrow)* and a dilated ascending aorta. The CT images *(middle* and *right)* show dilation of the aortic root and dilation of the ascending aorta and proximal arch, respectively. *AscAO,* Proximal ascending aorta; *LV,* left ventricle. (From Verma S, Siu SC. Aortic dilation in patients with bicuspid aortic valve. New Engl J Med 2014;370:1920-1929.)

Transthoracic Echocardiography

Transthoracic echocardiography (TTE) reveals several distinct features of the BAV (Box 11.1).[1] The valve must be assessed in systole and diastole. In patients with a prominent raphe, the valve may appear to be trileaflet in diastole, but the distinct elliptical or football-shaped orifice can be visualized in systole, indicating that the raphe is not a functional commissure (Fig. 11.9A, B; Video 11.9A ▶).

The leaflets of a BAV are often thickened and calcified out of proportion to the patient's age. Prominent systolic doming of the leaflets and eccentric valve closure are often observed (see Fig. 11.9C; Video 11.9B ▶). Up to 25% of BAVs may not demonstrate eccentric closure, and conversely, TAVs may infrequently have eccentric closure. Leaflet redundancy should suggest a BAV. Unexplained eccentric jets of AR may also suggest an underlying BAV.

Valvular calcification is a function of age, increasing significantly after 40 years of age. Significant calcification may limit the degree of systolic doming and may give the appearance of a stenotic trileaflet valve on short-axis views. The BAV tends to open from the center and to separate at the commissures in a curvilinear manner (Video 11.9A ▶), whereas TAV leaflets maintain a straighter shape in diastole, pivoting from their point of annular insertion.[1]

In the diagnosis of BAV, TTE has a sensitivity of 78% to 92% and a specificity of 96%, but the accuracy depends on image quality, valve calcification, existence of aneurysm disease, and experience of the interpreter.[1,89] Both false-negative and false-positive results occur. Heavy calcification limits the ability to discern leaflet number accurately. A prominent raphe may often give the appearance of a third

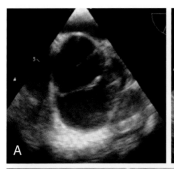
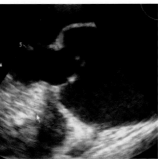
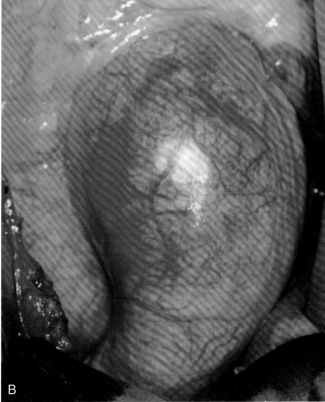

Fig. 11.8 The root phenotype is associated with an increased risk of late aortic events and is most often associated with genetic disease. transthoracic echocardiography (A) and intraoperative findings (B) in the bicuspid aortic valve root phenotype. (From Girdauskas E, Borger MA. Bicuspid aortic valve and associated aortopathy: an update. Semin Thorac Cardiovasc Surg 2013;25:310-316.)

BOX 11.1 Echocardiographic Features of the Bicuspid Aortic Valve

- Systolic doming
- Eccentric valve closure
- Leaflet redundancy
- Raphe (often calcified)
- Elliptical (football-shaped) systolic orifice
- Distinct opening pattern: opens from the center and separates at the commissures in a curvilinear fashion
- Eccentric jets of aortic regurgitation
- Premature calcification
- Dilated aortic root and/or ascending aorta

---

coaptation line, suggesting a trileaflet valve. Conversely, the aortic valve may appear bicuspid when one of the cusps is diminutive.[1]

Ascending aortic enlargement should trigger a careful evaluation for a BAV (see Fig. 11.9D).[34] So-called incomplete BAVs with very small raphes may be underappreciated and should be sought out, especially in cases of aortic dilation.[90] Because aortic dilation is frequently largest in the ascending aorta, the entire aspect of the aortic root and proximal ascending aorta should be visualized (see Fig. 11.9D; Video 11.9C ▶).[1,34,47]

TTE for BAV disease should include a formal assessment of valvular complications. Because BAV patients often have larger left ventricular outflow tracts, use of the continuity equation may yield larger calculated valve areas, potentially underestimating the hemodynamic severity. The use of serial gradients and velocity-time integral (VTI) ratios may more accurately reflect the hemodynamic burden.[91] AR may be the main clinical manifestation of BAV in adolescents or young adults. The jets of BAV AR may be highly eccentric (Video 11.9D ▶), making severity more difficult to assess.

With improved imaging technology, the routine use of three-dimensional (3D) TTE is becoming more common. With the ability to display an *en face* view of the aortic valve, 3D TTE provides an additional modality with which to assess BAV structure and function.[92] TTE examination of BAV should include a routine evaluation of coexisting cardiovascular lesions (see Table 11.3).

Transesophageal Echocardiography

For a subset of patients, the morphology of the aortic valve cannot be accurately determined by TTE. When aortic valve morphology is inadequately visualized, two-dimensional (2D) and 3D forms of transesophageal echocardiography (TEE) are useful for the diagnosis of BAV (Fig. 11.10). The sensitivity of TEE approaches 100% if little valvular calcification is present, but it is lower with moderate to severe valvular calcification,[93] and 3D TEE may help provide assessment of aortic valve area.[94]

TEE provides details about coexisting disease, including aortic abnormalities (e.g., ascending aortic aneurysm and dissection, sinus of Valsalva aneurysm, supravalvular stenosis), outflow tract defects (e.g., subvalvular stenosis, membranous ventricular septal defect), and valvular complications (e.g., AS, AR, endocarditis).

Other Tomographic Imaging

Cardiac magnetic resonance (CMR) imaging and coronary computed tomographic angiography (CCTA) can provide helpful information for the diagnosis and management of BAV. Multidetector cardiac computed tomography (MDCT) has a high sensitivity (94%) and specificity (100%) for detecting BAV (Fig. 11.11).[95] CMR is also highly accurate in diagnosing BAV, with a reported sensitivity of 100% and specificity of 95%.[96,97] MDCT may more accurately identify BAV and assess aortic valve area than CMR, TEE, or TTE. CMR can accurately assess BAV leaflet orientation and raphes and correlates well with TTE and invasive techniques for the evaluation of AS and AR.[98]

CCTA and CMR can assess associated vascular complications and congenital lesions, many of which are suboptimally visualized and defined by TTE, and they can assist in planning transcatheter aortic valve replacement (TAVR).[99,100] Magnetic resonance angiography (MRA) or CT follow-up is warranted in the setting of ascending aortic aneurysm and CoA.

OVERALL DISEASE COURSE

The natural history of BAV is defined by the occurrence of specific complications, including valvular disease, endocarditis, aortic aneurysm, aortic dissection, and coexisting congenital cardiovascular abnormalities

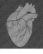
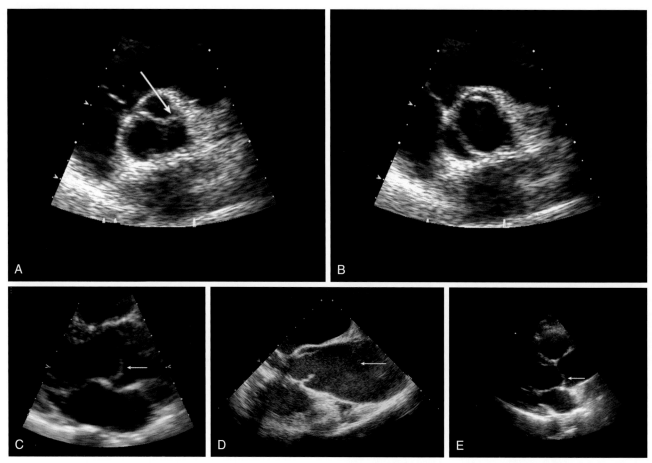

Fig. 11.9 Transthoracic Echocardiogram of Bicuspid Aortic Valve. (A) Short-axis view of the bicuspid aortic valve (BAV) in diastole demonstrates fusion of the right and left coronary cups and a raphe *(arrow)* (Video 11.9A ▶). (B) BAV in systole with elliptical opening pattern. (C) Parasternal long-axis view of a BAV demonstrates mild valve thickening and prominent systolic doming of the aortic valve leaflets *(arrow)* (Video 11.9B ▶). (D) Dilated ascending aorta (5.3 cm) complicates a BAV *(arrow)* (Video 11.9C ▶). (E) Color Doppler denotes a highly eccentric jet of aortic regurgitation *(arrow)* (Video 11.9D ▶).

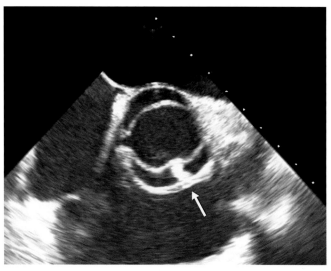

Fig. 11.10 Transesophageal echocardiography (TEE) is useful for the diagnosis of bicuspid aortic valve (BAV). TEE of a BAV with a raphe *(arrow)* (Video 11.10 ▶).

(Table 11.4). In some patients, the BAV may remain asymptomatic for a lifetime, whereas in others, a valve disorder or aortic complication may occur early in life. It has been estimated that most BAV patients will develop a complication during their lifetime.[1,81,101]

In natural history studies, aortic valve surgery for complications of BAV (more due to AS than AR) was required in 21% to 53% of patients followed for 21 to 25 years (see Table 11.4). In a series of 218 patients (mean age, 55 years; range, 21–89 years) with congenitally malformed aortic valves studied at autopsy, 87% had a BAV.[102] AS was identified in 65%, pure AR in 1%, endocarditis (native and prosthetic) in 14%, and a normally functioning BAV in 25%. Of the 218 patients, 65% died of their valvular disease (*n* = 124) or ascending aortic dissection (*n* = 17).[102] Although there is a 3:1 male predominance, men with BAV more frequently have significant AR at presentation, whereas women more often have AS.[21]

Minimally symptomatic or asymptomatic BAV patients treated at tertiary referral centers have a life expectancy no different from that of controls.[81,101] In a cohort study, 212 patients with asymptomatic and minimally dysfunctional BAV (mean age, 32 ± 20 years) were followed for 15 ± 6 years.[81] The survival rates were 97% ± 1% at 10 years and 90% ± 3% at 20 years after diagnosis, which were identical to the expected survival rates of the age-matched population

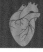

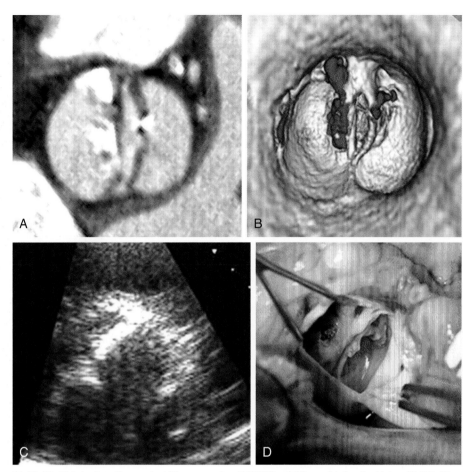

Fig. 11.11 Multidetector Computed Tomography (MDCT) of Bicuspid Aortic Valve (BAV) Stenosis. (A) Multiplanar reformatted image obtained by MDCT depicts calcified BAV with severe stenosis. (B) Virtual endoscopic image (cranial view) obtained by MDCT shows the BAV leaflets are almost the same size and show dense calcifications. (C) Transthoracic echocardiography is not able to depict the type of valve due to acoustic shadow from a densely calcified leaflet. (D) Densely calcified BAV was confirmed at the time of surgery. (From Tanaka R, Yoshioka K, Niinuma H, et al. Diagnostic value of cardiac CT in the evaluation of bicuspid aortic stenosis: comparison with echocardiography and operative findings. AJR Am J Roentgenol 2010;195:895-899. Reprinted with permission from the American Journal of Roentgenology.)

(see Table 11.4). The incidence of cardiovascular events (i.e., cardiac death, heart failure, new symptoms, endocarditis, or stroke) was 33% ± 5% at 20 years after diagnosis. At 20 years, the incidence of aortic valve surgery was 24% ± 4%, the incidence of aortic surgery for ascending aortic aneurysm was 5% ± 2%, and the combined incidence for both types of surgical events was 27% ± 4%. The rate of any medical or surgical cardiovascular event is 42%.[81]

In a study of 642 adults (mean age, 35 ± 16 years) with BAV, the survival rates over a 9-year follow-up period were not different from those of the general population.[101] Age and severity of valvular dysfunction predicted future events in BAV patients (Fig. 11.12).[101] Similar conclusions were drawn in a study of adults with BAV followed for up to 40 years.[103] Independent predictors for a BAV-related intervention included age older than 30 years, hyperlipidemia, hypertension, and moderate or severe AS or AR.[103] Findings in multiple large studies outlining BAV outcomes are summarized in Table 11.4.

Surgical interventions are common in subjects with BAV. In a cohort study of 1890 BAV patients (mean age, 50 years; 75% men), 49% of patients required surgery by 8 years of follow-up.[104] Of those, 36% underwent AVR alone, 42% underwent AVR and aortic grafting, and

3% required aortic grafting alone. Surgery related to BAV (as a time-dependent covariate) was related to significantly fewer events, and the rate of freedom from primary end point was similar to that of the normal age-matched U.S. population.[104]

VALVULAR COMPLICATIONS

Aortic Stenosis

AS is the most common complication of BAV. Calcific aortic valve disease is a result of ectopic mineralization and fibrosis.[7] Abnormal leaflet architecture is evident in infants with BAV disease with an increased volume of matrix substance, which may impact subsequent valvular calcification (Fig. 11.13).[7] Calcium deposition and fibrosis of the BAV increases with age.[1] This process in BAV patients is similar to that in people with TAVs, but it occurs at an accelerated rate and includes lipid deposition, neoangiogenesis, and inflammatory cell infiltration.[1] BAVs demonstrate folding and doming of the leaflets and increased turbulence, even when the leaflets are not stenotic.[38] These factors may increase susceptibility to BAV degeneration.

TABLE 11.4 Clinical Outcomes Studies of Bicuspid Aortic Valve Disease.

Study Parameters	Michelena et al, 2008[81] (N = 212)	Tzemos et al, 2008[101] (N = 642)	Michelena et al, 2011[118] (N = 416)	Davies et al, 2007[116] (N = 70)	Russo et al, 2002[125] (N = 50)	Borger et al, 2004[130] (N = 201)	McKellar et al, 2010[132] (N = 1286)	Girdauskas et al, 2012[134] (N = 153)	Girdauskas et al, 2015[45] (N = 56)	Masri et al, 2015[104] (N = 1890)	Rodrigues et al, 2016[103] (N = 227)
Setting	Community, population based	Tertiary referral center	Community, population based	Tertiary referral center	Tertiary referral center	Tertiary referral center	Tertiary referral center	Tertiary referral center	Tertiary referral center	Tertiary referral center	Tertiary referral center
Inclusion characteristics	Minimal BAV dysfunction	Any BAV dysfunction	Any BAV dysfunction	Any BAV dysfunction with ascending aortic aneurysm (mean diameter = 46 mm)	Status after AVR	Status after AVR	Status after AVR	Status after isolated AVR for AS with aortic diameter = 40–50 mm (mean diameter = 46 mm)	Status after isolated AVR for AR with root phenotype, aortic diameter = 40–50 mm (mean diameter = 45 mm)	Any BAV dysfunction, no prior AVR or aneurysm surgery; 21% with aortic diameter > 45 mm	Any BAV dysfunction
Age (years, mean ± SD)	32 ± 20	35 ± 16	35 ± 21	49	51 ± 12	56 ± 15	58 ± 14	54 ± 11	47 ± 11	50 ± 14	28 ± 14
Follow-up (years ± SD)	15 ± 6	9 ± 5	16 ± 7	5	20 ± 2	10 ± 4	12 ± 7	12 ± 3	11 ± 4	8 ± 2	13 ± 9
Survival[a]	90% at 20 yr	96% at 10 yr	80% at 25 yr	91% at 5 yr	40% at 15 yr	67% at 15 yr	52% at 15 yr	78% at 15 yr	90% at 10 yr 78% at 15 yr	95% at 7 yr[b] 88% at 7 yr[c]	96% at 10 yr 94% at 20 yr
Aortic valve surgery	24% at 20 yr	21%	53% at 25 yr	68%	—	—	—	100%	100%	47%	35% at 20 yr
Indication for aortic valve surgery	AS 67% AR 15%	AS 61% AR 27%	AS 61% AR 29%	—	—	—	—	AS 100%	AS 100%	AR > moderate in 40%	AS 64% AR 28%
Endocarditis	2%	2%	2%	—	4%	2%	—	—	—	1%	5%
Ascending aortic aneurysm formation (size)	39% (>40 mm)	45% (>35 mm)	26% at 25 yr (≥45 mm)	—	—	9% (≥50 mm)	10% (≥50 mm)	3% (≥50 mm)	13% (≥50 mm)	—	12% (>45 mm)
Aortic surgery (for aneurysm)	5% at 20 yr	7%	9%	73%	6%	9%	1%	3%	5%	25%	10%
Aortic dissection	0% at 20 yr	1%	0.5% at 20 yr	9%	10% at 20 yr	0.5%	1% at 15 yr	0%	4%	0.2%	1%

aSurvival rates in the studies led by Michelena,[81] Tzemos,[101] Michelena,[48] and Masri[104] was not different from survival rates for the general population. The survival rate in the study led by McKellar[132] was inferior to that of the general population. The other studies listing survival rates were not compared with survival rates for the general population.

bSurvival rate at 7 years for patients undergoing aortic valve and/or aortic surgery was 95%.

csurvival rate at 7 years was 88% for patients not undergoing cardiac surgery.

AR, Aortic regurgitation; AS, aortic stenosis; AVR, aortic valve replacement; BAV, bicuspid aortic valve.

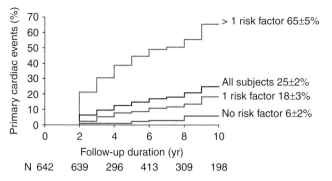

N 642   639   296   413   309   198

Fig. 11.12 Frequency of Adverse Cardiac Events in Adults With Bicuspid Aortic Valve Disease Stratified According to Risk Profile. Risk factors included: age > 30 years, moderate or severe aortic regurgitation, and moderate or severe aortic stenosis. (From Tzemos N, Therrien J, Yip J, et al. Outcomes in adults with bicuspid aortic valves. J Am Med Assoc 2008;300: 1317-1325 (original content); Siu SA, Silversides CK. Bicuspid aortic valve disease. J Am Coll Cardiol 2010;55:2789-2800.)

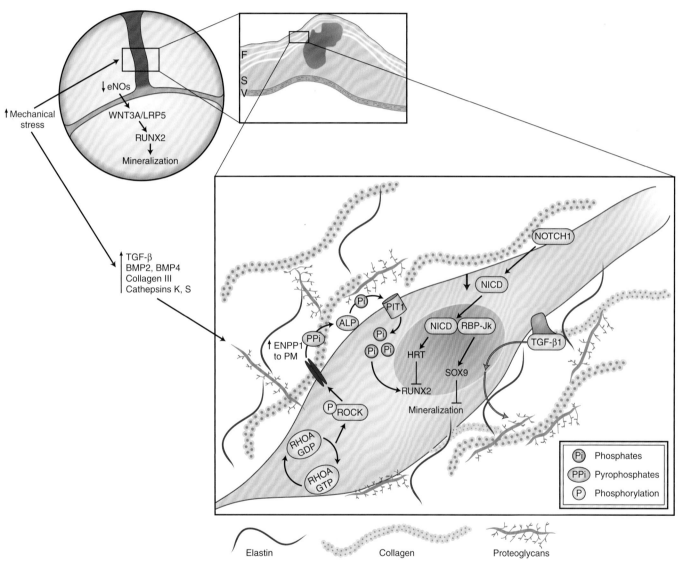

Fig. 11.13 Schematic of Pathophysiologic Mechanisms Involved in Bicuspid Aortic Valve (BAV). Dysregulation of nitric oxide signaling is suspected to play a role in the osteogenic transition of valvular interstitial cells through the WNT pathway. Increased content of prostaglandins and glycosaminoglycans and disorganized tissue architecture also can promote lipid retention and increase the bioavailability of transforming growth factor-β1 (TGF-β1). Elevated mechanical strain promotes the production of bone morphogenetic proteins (BMPs) 2 and 4, collagen type III, and cathepsins K and S, which participate in tissue remodeling in the BAV. ALP, Alkaline phosphatase; eNOS, endothelial nitric oxide synthase; ENPP1, ectonucleotide pyrophosphatase/phosphodiesterase 1; HRT, hairy-related family of transcription factors; LRP5, low-density lipoprotein receptor-related protein 5; NICD, NOTCH1 intracellular domain; RBP-jk, recombination signal binding protein for immunoglobulin kappa J region; ROCK, RHO-associated protein kinase; RUNX2, RUNT-related transcription factor 2. (From Mathieu P, Bosse Y, Huggins GS, et al. The pathology and pathobiology of bicuspid aortic valve: state of the art and novel research perspectives. J Pathol Clin Res 2015;1:195-206.)

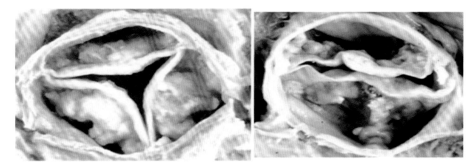

Fig. 11.14 Calcific aortic valve disease is a result of ectopic mineralization and fibrosis. Stenotic mineralized tricuspid *(left)* and bicuspid *(right)* aortic valves are shown. (From Mathieu P, Bosse Y, Huggins GS, et al. The pathology and pathobiology of bicuspid aortic valve: state of the art and novel research perspectives. J Pathol Clin Res 2015;1:195-206.)

Patients with BAV undergo surgery for AS 5 to 10 years earlier than those with TAV.[1] Approximately 25% of BAV patients without significant AS will have undergone AVR at 20-year follow-up.[81,103]

The reported incidence of AS complicating BAV in autopsy series is 15% to 75%.[1,102] Surgical pathology series have assessed the incidence of AS complicating BAV at 5% to 50% (Fig. 11.14).[1,105,106] Among adults with nonrheumatic AS, the incidence of BAV leading to AVR depends on the patient's age. Among those 50 years of age or younger, two thirds had a BAV (one third had a unicuspid aortic valve); among patients 50 to 70 years old, two thirds had a BAV, and one third had a TAV; and among patients older than 70 years of age, 40% had a BAV.[107] Among octogenarians and nonagenarians undergoing AVR, 22% and 18%, respectively, had a BAV.[106]

Progression of BAV stenosis is age related, with fibrosis beginning in the second decade and calcification progressing after the fourth decade.[1] Valve orientation may predict subsequent valvular pathology. In children, fusion of the right and noncoronary cusps correlates with both AS and AR, whereas fusion of the right and left cusps correlates with CoA.[82] In adults, investigations of valve morphology as a predictor of valve dysfunction have yielded varied results. Early studies suggested that right-left coronary fusion leads to more rapid progression of AS;[1,8] however, a larger, more contemporary study found that significant AS is more strongly associated with right-noncoronary cusp BAV.[84] Two population studies did not find any effect on BAV valve leaflet orientation and valve degeneration.[81,101]

BAV stenosis requires surgery on average 5 to 10 years earlier than expected for TAV stenosis.[107] In a population study from Toronto, Canada, of BAV patients with baseline age 35 ± 16 years, 22% had at least moderate AS at study entry.[101] Over a 9 ± 5-year follow-up period, 21% required valve surgery. Most of the patients undergoing valve surgery had symptomatic AS (63%) or progressive left ventricular dysfunction (28%).

Aortic Regurgitation

Isolated AR in BAV patients is less common than isolated AS, affecting 2% to 10% of patients.[1] In adults, AR may coexist with AS but is often only mild to moderate in severity. The prevalence of any AR in BAV disease is 47% to 64%, and that of moderate to severe AR is 13% to 32%.[108] There has been no consistent association between BAV valve morphology and AR, but pure AR is more common in younger patients and in the male population, and it is often associated with aortic root enlargement.[1,84] BAV is the most frequent cause of primary AR in the developed world.[81]

Multiple mechanisms may lead to AR in patients with BAV disease (Box 11.2). It may result from leaflet fibrosis with retraction of the

commissural margins of the leaflets, cusp prolapse, aneurysmal root enlargement, aortic dissection, or valvular destruction from endocarditis. A ventricular septal defect, subaortic membrane, or sinus of Valsalva aneurysm also may result in AR. Prior balloon aortic valvuloplasty for childhood BAV AS may lead to AR. Endocarditis accounts for up to 60% of cases of severe BAV AR and may be the presenting symptom for previously undiagnosed BAV.[1,109]

AVR due to BAV AR occurs much earlier in life (typically, 20–50 years of age) compared with AVR due to BAV AS. Population studies report AVR for AR in 3% to 7% of BAV patients.[81,101,103] Among patients undergoing AVR for AR, 15% to 20% of cases are related to BAV disease.[1] In BAV patients with the root phenotype pattern of dilation, AR is common and an underlying genetic defect may be present.[45]

Infective Endocarditis

The BAV, whether related to abnormal leaflet structure and function or turbulent flow across the leaflets, is at risk for infective endocarditis (IE). *Staphylococcus* and *Streptococcus* are the most common pathogenic microorganisms. Older pathologic studies reported that more than one third of aortic valve specimens with IE were BAVs.[1] Contemporary estimates place the BAV population risk for IE closer to 2% to 5%[81,101,103,105,109] (see Table 11.4). The incidence of IE (definite and possible) among patients with BAV was reported to be 9.9 cases per 10,000 patient-years, resulting in an age-adjusted relative risk of IE for those with BAV of 16.9 compared with that of the general population, and the 25-year risk of IE was 5% ± 2%.[110]

Acute IE may be the initial diagnosis of BAV for previously asymptomatic patients.[109] Endocarditis accounts for up to 60% of the cases of severe AR in BAV patients, most commonly due to cusp perforation.[1] BAV IE has a high complication rate, requiring surgery in 54% to 85% of cases,[103,109] and there is a higher rate of perivalvular abscess compared with TAV IE.[109,111] The lifetime risk of developing IE by patients with congenital AS has been estimated at 271 cases per 100,000 patient-years, whereas the risk for the general population is 5 cases per 100,000 patient-years.[112]

BAV is not included in the most recent guidelines for antibiotic prophylaxis. However, some investigators have suggested that because of the risk of IE and a higher risk of severe complications, BAV patients may be considered for antibiotic prophylaxis therapy, making the case for shared decision making.[111,113]

AORTIC COMPLICATIONS

Progressive Aortic Dilation

The rate of aortic dilation among patients with BAV varies, ranging from 0.2 to 2.3 mm/yr.[1,35,114] A small percentage of patients demonstrate more rapid growth rates.[114] Age, underlying valve disease (AR vs. AS), location of the dilation, baseline aortic diameter, family history of aortic valve or aortic disease, and other factors affect the rate of growth.[35,46,114] In children with BAV, the mean rate of ascending aortic growth was 1.2 mm/yr, but this must be correlated with age, BSA, and linear growth rate.[115] Among pediatric BAV patients, the ascending aortic diameter Z-score showed minimal changes during a 6-year follow-up. More rapid aortic dilation occurred among right-noncoronary leaflet fusion BAV compared with left-right leaflet fusion.[82] Thoracic aortic aneurysms associated with a BAV grow faster than aneurysms associated with TAV.[116,117]

Among 416 adults with BAV (55 ± 17 years old), 7.7% of patients had an ascending aortic aneurysm at baseline (mean size, 48 ± 6 mm).[118] Among patients without an aneurysm (aortic size < 45 mm) at the time of BAV diagnosis, 13% developed an aneurysm at 14 ± 6 years after diagnosis, and the 25-year risk of aneurysm was 26%.[118] Of 304 BAV operations, 90 patients (30%) had an ascending aortic aneurysm of at least 5 cm.[119] A tertiary center reported that repair of a dilated aorta (≥4.5 cm) encompassed 20% of all operations on BAV patients.[83]

Risk of Aortic Dissection

In autopsy and clinical series of aortic dissection, BAV was identified in 7% of cases (5%–15% of cases with ascending aortic dissections).[1,120] In the International Registry of Aortic Dissection (IRAD), a BAV was found in 9% of dissection patients younger than 40 years of age but in only 1% of those older than 40 years.[121] The average size of the ascending aorta at the time of dissection in the BAV group was 5.4 ± 1.8 cm.[121] Aortic dissection occurs at a younger age in patients with BAVs than in those with TAVs.[1,120,122] In a series of 460 type A dissections, 8.4% had underlying BAV.[120] BAV patients were younger (48 ± 13 years) than those with TAV (62 ± 12 years); they had larger aortic diameters (available in 37% of cases) at the time of dissection (62 vs. 53 mm), and they were more likely to have underlying CMD.

The incidence of aortic dissection in BAV populations is unclear and depends on the study population. Pooled estimation of cases associated with BAV has been reported as approximately 4%[11] (see Table 11.4). However, the absolute lifetime risk of aortic dissection for the BAV patient followed with routine imaging surveillance is very low and depends on many factors, most significantly the size of the aorta and the patient's age.[81,101,117,118] Among BAV patients (age at diagnosis of 35 ± 12 years) followed for a mean of 16 years, only 2 patients suffered aortic dissection, for an incidence of 3.1 cases per 10,000 patient-years and an age-adjusted relative risk of 8.4 compared with the general population.[118] Higher rates of dissection were observed for patients older than 50 years of age at baseline (17.4 cases per 10,000 patient-years) and for those with aortic diameters greater than 4.5 cm at baseline (44.9 cases per 10,000 patient-years, compared with an age-matched population risk of 0.31 cases per 10,000 person-years).

Outcomes of 1181 BAV patients with aortic diameters greater than 4.7 cm at the aortic root or ascending aorta were reported in one

series.[123] In 801 of the patients, aneurysm repair was performed (68% with aortic valve surgery). The 380 patients not undergoing surgery were observed for a median of 3 years (range, 0–17 years), during which 175 had aortic surgery. Ten (2.6%) of the 380 patients had a type A dissection. The risk-adjusted probability of dissection increased when the aortic diameter was greater than 5 cm in the aortic sinuses or greater than 5.3 cm in the ascending aorta. The risk of dissection was 3.8% for an ascending aortic diameter of 5.3 cm and 10% for a diameter greater than 6 cm.[123]

Late Aortic Complications After Aortic Valve Replacement

The rate of aortic root and ascending aorta dilation after isolated valve surgery for BAV is controversial and has varied among studies.[1,124–126] Given the uncertainty of progressive aortic growth, physicians should continue to evaluate the aorta in BAV patients after valve surgery. After valve-sparing root replacement for BAV aortopathy, wall shear stress differs along aortic segments depending on the BAV leaflet orientation.[65] However, late aortic events are uncommon in BAV patients who have normal or mildly enlarged aortic diameters at the time of AVR.[127,128] Of 1449 BAV patients who underwent AVR, only 3 patients had late aortic events when aortic diameters were less than 4.5 cm at the time of valve surgery.[129]

Borger and colleagues reported the 10-year follow-up results for 201 patients who underwent AVR for BAV without ascending aortic aneurysm replacement.[130] Ascending aortic size was less than 4.0 cm in 57%; 4.0 to 4.4 cm in 32%; and 4.5 to 4.9 cm in 11% of patients. During the follow-up period, 9% required late ascending aortic replacement due to a mean aortic diameter of 58 ± 9 mm. Freedom from ascending aortic complications (i.e., aneurysm repair, dissection, or sudden death) was 78% ± 6%; 81% ± 6%; and 43% ± 15% in the three increasing size groups, respectively[130] (Fig. 11.15). Others have reported a much lower risk of aortic complications after AVR for BAV disease.[131,132]

Of the 1286 BAV patients who underwent isolated AVR followed for a median of 12 years (range, 0–38 years), there were 13 aortic dissections (1%), 11 ascending aortic replacements (1%), and 127 cases (10%) of progressive ascending aortic dilation (>5 cm or >10 mm from the time of AVR).[132] The 15-year freedom from aortic complications rate was 89% for this population. Of the 323 patients for whom aortic dimensions were available, 75 had aortic dilation greater than 40 mm at the time of AVR. In this group with aortic dilation, 3 patients (4%) had aortic dissection,

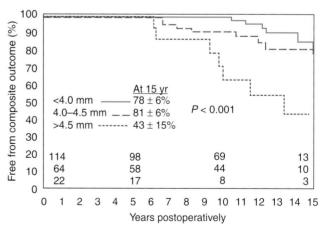

Fig. 11.15 Kaplan-Meier Curves for Freedom From Ascending Aortic Complications According Ascending Aortic Diameter in Patients With Bicuspid Aortic Valve Replacement Surgery. Patients with an ascending aortic diameter of 4.5 cm or greater had a significantly increased risk of future aortic complications (i.e., aneurysm, dissection, or sudden death) (P < 0.001). (From: Borger MA, Preston M, Ivanov J, et al. Should the ascending aorta be replaced more frequently in patients with bicuspid aortic valve disease? J Thorac Cardiovasc Surg 2004;128:677-683.)

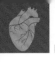

7 (9.3%) underwent aortic aneurysm resection, and 12 (16%) had aortic growth greater than 10 mm during follow-up.[132] Iagaki and coworkers reported late aortic event rates similar to those of a control population and lower than in those with Marfan syndrome.[133]

The BAV lesion requiring AVR may predict late aortic events (see Table 11.4). Late follow-up after BAV AVR revealed more aortic growth in patients with prior AR compared with those with AS.[124] Among 153 BAV patients with BAV AS and ascending aortic dilation (40–50 mm) who underwent isolated AVR and were followed for a mean of 12 ± 3 years, ascending aortic aneurysm surgery was required in only 3%.[134] No late aortic dissections occurred, and rates of freedom from aortic events at 10 and 15 years postoperatively were 95% and 93%, respectively. However 24% of BAV patients with predominant aortic root dilation (mean diameter, 45 mm) who underwent AVR for AR had an adverse aortic event (i.e., aortic root replacement, aortic dissection, or sudden death) after a mean follow-up of 10.3 ± 4.6 years.[134] In a meta-analysis of late aortic dissection after isolated AVR for BAV disease, aortic dissection was 10 times more common when the valve lesion was AR rather than AS.[135]

RECOMMENDATIONS FOR TREATING BICUSPID AORTIC VALVE PATIENTS

There are important relationships between the BAV and its valvular lesions, and in some patients, aortopathy may lead to significant morbidity and mortality. Patients must be educated about the potential for valve dysfunction, the possibility of aortic aneurysm formation, and the risk of aortic dissection (when appropriate).

All patients with known or suspected BAV should have an initial TTE to determine valve morphology, severity of AS or AR, the size of the aortic root (at the sinus of Valsalva), and the size of the ascending aorta.[136] The person with a BAV should undergo serial clinical and imaging follow-up evaluations to detect valve or aortic complications and plan timely surgical intervention. The imaging frequency depends on the severity of AS or AR (see Chapters 9 and 10), aortic size, and clinical status and should be based on the lesion requiring greatest frequency of surveillance.[47,136,137] If the aortic root or ascending aorta diameter is greater than 4.5 cm or there is a rapid rate of change in aortic diameter or a family history of aortic dissection, reassessment of the aortic root and ascending aorta size should be performed at least yearly.[136] The examination interval is also determined by the degree and rate of progression of aortic dilation and by the family history, with less frequent imaging suggested if the aortic diameter remains stable.[136,138] CT or MRA is indicated for patients with BAV when the morphology of the aortic root or ascending aorta cannot be assessed accurately by echocardiography and to evaluate further the dilated aorta visualized by echocardiography.[34,47,136]

To lessen the risk of repeated radiation exposure, MRA is recommended for long-term follow-up. For patients with CoA, screening for intracerebral aneurysm is recommended.[138] The 2014 American College of Cardiology/American Heart Association (AHA/ACC) valvular heart disease guidelines state that echocardiographic screening of first-degree relatives is appropriate if the patient with a BAV has associated aortopathy or a family history of valvular disease or aortopathy.[136] Many valve experts and the 2018 American Association for Thoracic Surgery (AATS) Consensus Guidelines recommend echocardiographic screening of all first-degree relatives of patients with BAV,[137,138] but data are lacking on the impact of screening on clinical outcomes and cost-effectiveness. In some instances, genetic testing for mutations associated with thoracic aortic aneurysm disease may be useful in patients with BAV and aneurysm.[139] Table 11.5 provides the ACC/AHA, European Society of Cardiology (ESC), and AATS recommendations for imaging of patients with BAV. Fig. 11.16 provides a proposed flow diagram for treating the BAV patient.[36]

For patients with BAV who have AS, AR, and/or aortic root or ascending aortic aneurysms, there are no studies demonstrating benefit of medical therapy, including β-blockers, angiotensin-converting enzyme (ACE) inhibitors, and angiotensin receptor blockers (ARBs), to alter the natural history of BAV disease or associated aortopathy. Whereas the 2014 ESC guidelines consider β-blockade reasonable for those with BAV and ascending aortic dimensions greater than 4.0 cm, neither the 2014 ACC/AHA nor the 2018 AATS guidelines recommend pharmacologic treatment for BAV patients in the absence of hypertension[136,138] (see Table 11.5). In the setting of hypertension, patients with BAV should be treated with standard guideline-based medical therapy to control blood pressure. When the BAV patient has AR and hypertension, treatment of blood pressure with a dihydropyridine calcium channel blocker or an ACE inhibitor or ARB is recommended.[136]

Other traditional risk factors for atherosclerosis may play a role in the progression of AS in BAV patients.[1,81] Cigarette smoking and hypercholesterolemia are risk factors for progression to severe AS.[140] There are no studies demonstrating that pharmacologic therapy with statins alters the natural history of BAV AS. The ATRONOMER study, in which patients with AS were treated with statin therapy, failed to show any improvement in BAV or TAV AS,[141] and BAV therefore is not in itself an indication for statin therapy.

Although BAV is a risk factor for IE, current guidelines do not endorse antibiotic prophylaxis in the setting of isolated BAV.[137] However, patients with BAV should be counseled on maintaining optimal oral health because this is most effective intervention to prevent future valvular infection.[136] Because patients with BAV have a relatively high frequency of IE compared with the general population and because their clinical profile is similar to that of high-risk IE patients, some investigators have suggested that antibiotic prophylaxis for BAV patients should be reconsidered.[111,113]

Patients with BAV should be counseled about appropriate lifestyle modifications and about a safe approach to exercise, physical activity, and competitive athletics.[142] There are limited prospective data on the effects of exercise in patients with BAV, but available studies do not demonstrate adverse effects of exercise on aortic dilation, valvular hemodynamics, or left ventricular (LV) morphology or function.[143] The ACC/AHA provided guidelines regarding participation in competitive athletics for those of high school age or older. Competitive athletes with BAV can participate in all competitive athletics if the aortic root and ascending aorta are not dilated (i.e., Z-score < 2, < 2 standard deviations from the mean, or aortic diameter < 40 mm in adults).

The function of the BAV (whether stenotic or regurgitant) is also important in determining participation recommendations. Athletes with a BAV and aortic dimensions above the normal range (Z-score = 2–3 or aortic diameter of 40–42 mm in men or 36–39 mm in women) should undergo echocardiographic or MRA surveillance of the aorta every 12 months. Athletes with BAV and a mild to moderately dilated aorta (Z-score = 2–3.5 or aortic root or ascending aortic diameter of 40–42 mm in men or 36–39 mm in women) and no features of associated connective tissue disorder or familial thoracic aortic aneurysm syndrome may participate in low and moderate static and dynamic competitive sports (i.e., classes IA, IB, IC, IIA, IIB, and IIC according to the AHA/ACC eligibility and disqualification recommendations for competitive athletes with cardiovascular abnormalities) with a low likelihood of significant bodily collision. For these athletes, intense weight training should be avoided. Athletes with BAV and a dilated aorta measuring 43 to 45 mm may participate in low-intensity competitive sports (i.e., class IA) with a low likelihood of bodily collision.

Athletes with BAV and a markedly dilated aorta (Z-score > 3.5–4 or aortic diameter > 43 mm in men or > 40 mm in women) should not participate in any competitive sports that involve the potential for

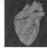

TABLE 11.5   Guidelines for the Management of Bicuspid Aortic Valve Disease.

ACC/AHA Guidelines	ESC Guidelines	AATS Guidelines	Class	Level
Imaging Recommendations				
Initial TTE is indicated to evaluate severity of valve disease, LV size and function, and dimensions and anatomy of ascending aorta and associated lesions.			I	C
If ascending aorta cannot be adequately evaluated by TTE, aortic CMR or CT angiography is recommended.			I	C
Interval evaluation of aortic root and ascending aorta by echocardiography, CMR, or CT angiography *when aorta >4.0 cm*; frequency based on aortic rate of growth or family history.	Interval evaluation of aortic root and ascending aorta by echocardiography, CMR, or CT angiography for *all BAV patients*; frequency based on aortic rate of growth or family history.	Interval evaluation of aortic root and ascending aorta by echocardiography, CMR, or CT angiography for *all BAV patients*. In patients with normal initial aortic diameters by TTE, the thoracic aorta should be reimaged every 3–5 yr.	I	C
If aortic sinus or ascending aorta > 4.5 cm, evaluation of aortic dimensions is recommended annually.		For patients with initial aortic dilation (root or tubular ascending aorta 4.0–4.9 cm), the thoracic aorta should be reimaged at 12 mo. If stability is confirmed, reimaging can be performed every 2 or 3 yr. For patients with more advanced initial aortic dilation (root or tubular ascending aorta 5.0–5.4 cm), the thoracic aorta should be reimaged yearly.	I	C
Athletes with BAV and aortic diameters of 40–42 mm (men) and 36–39 mm (women) or Z-score of 2–3, surveillance echocardiography or MRA should occur yearly, with more frequent imaging for increased aortic size.			I	C
Screening of first-degree relatives for BAV and thoracic aortic disease should be considered.			IIa	B
Pharmacologic Treatment				
In patients with hypertension, control of BP with any effective antihypertensive medication is warranted. β-Blockers and ARBs have conceptual advantages to reduce rate of progression but have not been beneficial in clinical studies.	β-Blockers may be considered for patients with BAV and a dilated aortic root > 4.0 cm.	β-Blockers and inhibitors of the renin-angiotensin system should be considered for BP control based on evidence extrapolated from connective tissue disease populations.	IIa	C
Surgical Treatment				
Repair/replace aortic sinus or ascending aorta in BAV patients with aortic dimensions ≥5.5 cm.			I	B-NR
Repair/replace aortic sinus or ascending aorta in BAV patients with aortic dimensions ≥5.0 cm and additional risk factors such as family history of dissection, aortic growth rate > 0.3 cm (ESC & AATS) or > 0.5 cm (ACC/AHA) per year			IIa	B-NR
Repair/replace aortic sinus or ascending aorta in BAV patients with aortic diameter ≥5.0 cm and surgical risk < 4% at an established surgical center for excellence.		Repair of the ascending aorta/root in patients with an aortic diameter ≥ 5.0 cm when surgical risk is low and when performed by an experienced aortic team in a center with established surgical results.	IIa (AHA/ ACC) IIb (AATS)	B-NR C
Repair/replace aortic sinus or ascending aorta in BAV patients with aortic diameter > 4.5 cm when aortic valve surgery is considered.			IIa	C (AHA/ ACC; ESC) B (AATS)
		Repair of the aortic arch is recommended in patients with an aortic arch diameter of ≥ 5.5 cm.	IIa	B
		Concomitant repair of the aortic arch should be performed in patients undergoing cardiac surgery with an aortic arch diameter of ≥ 5.0 cm, provided the surgical risk is low and when performed by an experienced aortic team.	IIb	C

Continued

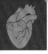

TABLE 11.5   Guidelines for the Management of Bicuspid Aortic Valve Disease.—cont'd

ACC/AHA Guidelines	ESC Guidelines	AATS Guidelines	Class	Level
		Concomitant repair of the aortic arch may be performed in patients undergoing cardiac surgery with an aortic arch diameter of ≥ 4.5 cm, provided surgical risk is low and when performed by an experienced aortic team with established surgical results.		C
Exercise Recommendations				
No competitive sports limitations in high school and older athletes with isolated BAV and normal aortic root and ascending aortic dimensions (Z-score <2.0 cm or < 4.0 cm in adults)			I	C
High school and older athletes with isolated BAV with an aortic diameter of				
40–42 mm (men), 36–39 mm (women), and Z-score 2–3.5;	Low and moderate competitive sports activities allowed with low likelihood of bodily collisions		I, II	A-C
>43 mm (men), >40 mm (women), Z-score 3.5–4	No competitive sports with potential for bodily collisions		III	C
High school and older athletes with BAV and an aorta > 4.5 cm should not participate in any competitive sports.	In patients with BAV and aorta >4.0 cm, isometric exercise with high static load is discouraged.	In patients with BAV and aorta >4.5 cm, avoid heavy lifting or competitive sports involving isometric exercise. Patients with BAV and dilated aorta should be precluded from private driving if the ascending aorta diameter is > 6.0 cm and restricted from commercial driving if the ascending thoracic aorta diameter is > 5.5 cm.	III	C

AATS, American Association for Thoracic Surgery; *ACC/AHA,* American College of Cardiology/American Heart Association; *ARB,* angiotensin receptor blocker; *BAV,* bicuspid aortic valve; *BP,* blood pressure; *CMR,* cardiac magnetic resonance imaging; *CT,* computed tomographic; *ESC,* European Society of Cardiology; *LV,* left ventricle; *MRA,* magnetic resonance angiography; *TEE,* transesophageal echocardiography; *TTE,* transthoracic echocardiography. Data from Nishimura RA, Otto CM, Bonow RO, et al. 2014 AHA/ACC guideline for the management of patients with valvular heart disease: executive summary: a report of the American College of Cardiology/American Heart Association Task Force on Practice Guidelines. J Am Coll Cardiol 2014;63:2438-2488; Hiratzka LF, Creager MA, Isselbacher EM, et al. Surgery for aortic dilatation in patients with bicuspid aortic valves: a statement of clarification from the American College of Cardiology (ACC)/American Heart Association (AHA) task force on clinical practice guidelines. J Am Coll Cardiol 2016;67:724-731; Braverman AC, Harris KM, Kovacs RJ, et al. Eligibility and disqualification recommendations for competitive athletes with cardiovascular abnormalities: Task Force 7: aortic diseases, including Marfan syndrome: a scientific statement from the American Heart Association and American College of Cardiology. J Am Coll Cardiol 2015;66:2398-2405; Erbel R, Aboyans V, Boileau C, et al. 2014 ESC guidelines on the diagnosis and treatment of aortic diseases: document covering acute and chronic aortic diseases of the thoracic and abdominal aorta of the adult. The Task Force for the Diagnosis and Treatment of Aortic Diseases of the European Society of Cardiology (ESC). Eur Heart J 2014;35:2873-926; Borger MA, Fedak PWM, Stephens EH. et al. The American Association for Thoracic Surgery (AATS) consensus guidelines on bicuspid aortic valve-related aortopathy: executive summary. J Thorac Cardiovasc Surg 2018;156:473-480.

significant bodily collision[142] (see Table 11.5). The 2018 AATS Consensus Guidelines suggest that patients with BAV and a dilated aorta should be precluded from private driving if the ascending aorta is greater than 6.0 cm and restricted from commercial driving if the ascending aorta diameter is greater than 5.5 cm.[138]

For carefully followed individuals with BAV, the survival rates are not significantly different from those of the general population[81,101,118] (see Fig. 11.12). However, timely surgical treatment of valve lesions and aortic aneurysm are critical for the longevity of the BAV patient. Even after surgical replacement of the BAV, a subset of patients is at risk for future aortic dilation, aneurysm formation, and aortic dissection and must undergo long-term imaging surveillance. Radiologic imaging after surgery to establish a postrepair baseline is suggested.[138] Long-term surveillance depends on individual factors. It is reasonable to image the aorta by CT or CMR after aortic surgery to establish a

baseline and every 3 to 5 years after repair based on anatomic, clinical, and surgical factors or if there is residual aortic pathology.[138]

SURGICAL TREATMENT OF THE BICUSPID AORTIC VALVE AND ASCENDING AORTA

The surgical procedure for a patient with BAV disease depends on whether intervention is required for the aortic valve or aorta, or both. The indications for replacement or repair of a BAV with AS or AR are well established and consistent with standard AHA/ACC, AATS, and ESC valvular guidelines. Aortic valve intervention depends on the severity of the valvular lesion, existence of cardiovascular symptoms, degree of LV function, and for AR, progression of LV dilation (see Chapter 9).[136] However, patients undergoing AVR for BAV are often young, making the decision to implant a mechanical or bioprosthetic valve more complex.[1,136]

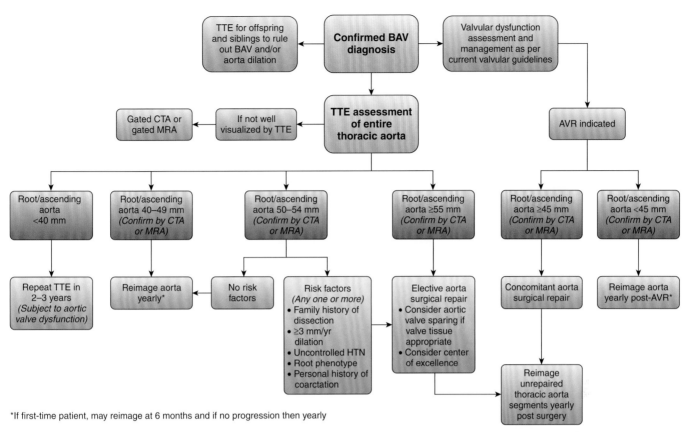

Fig. 11.16 Bicuspid Aortic Valve *(BAV)* Aortopathy Management Algorithm. An aortic root or ascending tubular aorta ≥ 55 mm with no risk factors or ≥ 50 mm with any one or more risk factors should prompt referral for elective surgical aortic repair regardless of aortic valve function. If the aortic valve does not have degeneration features (e.g., no calcium deposits, good mobility, no significant thickening), a valve-sparing aortic repair may be considered, and patient referral to a center of excellence may be warranted. Patients undergoing primary aortic valve replacement *(AVR)* for valvular dysfunction should have their root and/or ascending tubular aorta concomitantly repaired if they measure ≥ 45 mm. Patients who undergo isolated AVR without aortic repair should be followed with yearly thoracic aorta diameter assessments. *CTA,* Computed tomographic angiography; *MRA,* magnetic resonance angiography; *TTE,* transthoracic echocardiography. (From Michelena HI, Della Corte A, Prakash SK, et al. Bicuspid aortic valve aortopathy in adults: incidence, etiology, and clinical significance. Int J Cardiol 2015;201:400-407.)

Valve repair for the regurgitant BAV is performed in selected cases in centers of excellence, providing good short- and mid-term outcomes, but long-term durability of the repair is uncertain.[138,144] Of 728 patients who underwent BAV repair, 50% had at least moderate AR 5 years after repair, and 22% underwent AVR by 10 years' follow-up.[145] Among 85 patients undergoing valve-sparing root replacement for BAV aneurysm disease, 99% were free of more than moderate AR at 8 years.[146] Of 40 patients with BAV and aneurysm disease who underwent valve-sparing root replacement, the 5-year freedom from more than mild AR or reoperation rate was 100%.[147] Among 265 patients undergoing combined aortic valve repair and root surgery for significant AR and root disease, there was a cumulative incidence of reoperation of 22% at 15 years.[148]

The timing of prophylactic aortic root or ascending aortic surgery in the setting of BAV aneurysm disease is complex, and the optimal aortic diameter threshold requires individual decision making[46,129,138,149–152] (Fig. 11.17). Surveys of cardiac surgeons have reported marked variations in practice patterns.[153] The surgical risk must be weighed against that of aortic complications.[150] Most natural history studies have included patients for whom aortic aneurysm surgery was performed at various (and unpublished) size thresholds, and they reported a less than

1% per year risk of aortic dissection when the aortic diameter was less than 50 mm.[117,149,154]

For isolated BAV aneurysm, guidelines recommend elective surgery at thresholds of aortic diameter ranging from 5.0 to 5.5 cm (see Table 11.5).[46,136,138,155] The 2016 ACC/AHA updated guidelines recommend prophylactic aortic repair for asymptomatic BAV without high risk features at an aortic aneurysm diameter of 5.5 cm or greater, the same threshold recommended for those with a TAV.[30] However, if an additional risk factor (i.e., family history of aortic dissection or aortic growth rate ≥ 0.5 cm/yr) for dissection exists or the BAV patient is at low surgical risk (<4%) and the procedure is performed by an experienced aortic team in a center of excellence, surgery to replace or repair the aortic root or ascending aorta, or both, may be considered at a diameter 5.0 cm or greater.[30]

Gender and BSA may also be important factors in the timing of ascending aortic surgery. Some surgeons advocate use of an aortic cross-sectional area/height ratio greater than 10 cm/m^2 to inform decision making before surgery.[30,46,156]

Aortic diameter is the primary but not the only factor affecting timing of aortic repair.[152] Other factors include valve dysfunction (i.e., AS or AR), rate of aortic growth, age, BSA, family history, associated conditions

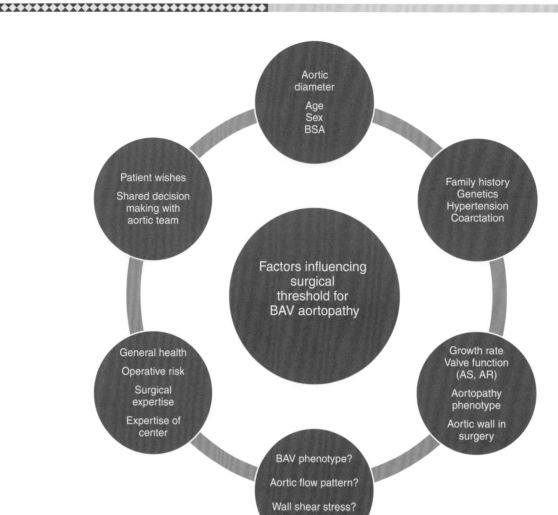

Fig. 11.17 Factors Influencing Surgical Threshold in Bicuspid Aortic Valve *(BAV)* Aneurysm. Many factors other than aortic diameter affect the surgical threshold for BAV aortopathy. *AS,* Aortic stenosis; *AR,* aortic regurgitation; *BSA,* body surface area. (From Braverman AC. Aortic replacement for bicuspid aortic valve aortopathy: when and why? J Thorac Cardiovasc Surg 2019;157:520-525.)

(e.g., hypertension, CoA), operative risk, and overall prognosis (see Fig. 11.17).[46,138,152] The pattern of aortic dilation is important, with the root phenotype associated with more growth and worse outcomes if not repaired.[45,157–159] Aortic imaging techniques incorporating regional hemodynamic stress, measurements of localized matrix proteolytic activity, and biomarker levels may help predict aortic repair outcomes.[73,152]

Although experienced centers report a very low operative risk,[129] the risk is greater with aortic root and ascending aortic replacement compared with isolated AVR.[150] Guidelines recommend surgery to replace the aortic root or ascending aorta, or both, at the time of valve surgery for appropriate BAV patients if the aortic aneurysm exceeds 4.5 cm.[30,130,138] Concomitant aortic arch repair is recommended if the arch diameter is 50 mm or greater and may be considered at an aortic diameter of 45 mm or greater if the patient is at low surgical risk and the operation is performed by an experienced aortic surgeon at a center with established surgical results.[138]

Individual decision making about BAV aneurysm disease is relevant for determining the surgical threshold.[46,152,157,160,161] The underlying valve lesion may predict later aortic events (more are reported for regurgitant BAVs).[135] Stenotic BAVs with mild to moderate aortic dilation present relatively low risk of aortic complications after AVR

alone,[134,162] whereas patients with root phenotype BAV and AR have a higher risk of late aortic events after AVR.[45,128,159]

For patients requiring simultaneous valve surgery and ascending aortic replacement for BAV, operations are tailored to specific characteristics of the patient, valve, and aorta.[1,129,151] Surgical options include the following:

- Valve replacement (or repair) and supracoronary graft replacement of the ascending aorta, leaving the sinuses intact
- Aortic valve and root replacement with a composite valve-graft conduit and coronary reimplantation (i.e., modified Bentall procedure)
- Valve-sparing root replacement using the David (reimplantation) or Yacoub (remodeling) technique
- Reduction aortoplasty

When the aortic sinuses are not significantly dilated, separate AVR and ascending aortic grafting leads to satisfactory long-term outcome and low risk of significant late sinus dilation.[163] Aortoplasty is controversial because of concerns about the risk of recurrent dilation, but it has been used successfully by some.[151]

The Ross procedure is an alternative to prosthetic valve replacement in BAV disease.[164] Initial reports of late autograft dilation raised concerns about this procedure for adult patients, especially in the setting of significant annular or aortic dilation.[1,165] The pulmonary autograft dilates in some patients with BAV who have a dilated aortic root before performance of the Ross procedure,[1,166] and concerns have been raised about the appropriateness of this procedure for patients with BAV disease and ascending aortic enlargement.[164–166] A dilated aortic annulus, mismatch in annular diameters, and AR are all associated with late pulmonary autograft failure.[167] However, for a carefully selected population of 129 patients (mean age, 35 years) with pure AR due to BAV, a 20-year freedom from reoperation rate of 85% was realized.[168]

BAV has been considered an exclusion criterion in pivotal trials of TAVR for severe AS due to concerns about risks of paravalvular regurgitation, poor valve seating, and aortic characteristics. Aortic root dilation or angulation, elliptical annulus, and heavy calcification, including a calcified raphe, may have contributed to paravalvular AR in early-generation devices.[169] TAVR in selected BAV patients has demonstrated acceptable outcomes.[170–172] Studies of TAVR for BAV AS have reported similar 1-year mortality rates for these patients compared with TAV patients.[172] Although no significant difference in post-TAVR paravalvular AR was reported in a meta-analysis of BAV compared with TAV patients (26% vs. 20%, respectively),[172] AR remains a significant concern after TAVR.[169]

CT-based valve sizing may lessen the incidence of post-TAVR paravalvular leak,[169] and imaging classification schemes have been proposed to improve outcomes.[100] Studies of next-generation TAVR devices for BAV AS reported no more than mild paravalvular AR[173,174] and 30-day and 1-year mortality rates of 4.3% and 14.4%, respectively[174] (Fig. 11.18). For BAV patients receiving new-generation devices, the procedural results were comparable across different prostheses, and the cumulative all-cause 2-year mortality rates were comparable for BAV AS and TAV AS (17.2% vs. 19.4%; P = 0.28).[175] Early-generation devices resulted in more frequent aortic root injury compared with new-generation devices (4.5% vs. 0%).[175]

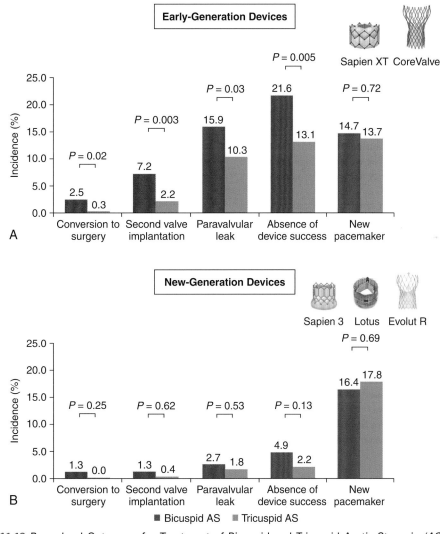

Fig. 11.18 Procedural Outcomes for Treatment of Bicuspid and Tricuspid Aortic Stenosis *(AS)* With Early- and New-Generation Transcatheter Aortic Valve Replacement (TAVR) Devices. Rates of conversion to surgery, second valve implantation, moderate or severe paravalvular leak, absence of device success, and new permanent pacemaker insertion after TAVR using (A) early-generation devices (i.e., Sapien XT or CoreValve) and (B) new-generation devices (i.e., Sapien 3, Lotus, or Evolut R). (From Yoon, S.H. Bleiziffer S, De Backer O, et al. Transcatheter aortic valve replacement for bicuspid versus tricuspid aortic valve stenosis. J Am Coll Cardiol 2017;69:2579-2589.)

PREGNANCY IN PATIENTS WITH A BICUSPID AORTIC VALVE

The most common valve lesion associated with AS during pregnancy is BAV.[176] Women with mild to moderate AS or class I/II symptoms with AR typically tolerate pregnancy well, whereas severe AS (especially if symptomatic) and AS with ventricular dysfunction are risk factors for increased maternal and fetal risk.[176,177] In older studies of pregnancy and AS, maternal mortality rates ranged from 11% to 20%, but in recent series, cardiac event rates were lower and death was rare.[176] Examination of pregnancy-related complications in congenital AS shows that maternal arrhythmias occurred in 2.4%, heart failure in 7%, and combined myocardial infarction, stroke, and cardiovascular death in 2.5% of cases.[178]

The multinational Registry on Pregnancy and Cardiac Disease (ROPAC) reported outcomes of pregnancy for women with moderate or severe AS.[176] Cardiovascular complications requiring hospitalization occurred in 20% of women (i.e., 13% of those with moderate AS, 35% of those with severe AS, and 42% of those with severe symptomatic AS), and there were no maternal deaths. Heart failure occurred in 7% of asymptomatic and 26% of symptomatic patients but was medically managed successfully except in one case that required balloon valvotomy.[176] Preterm birth and low birth weight occurred in one third of women with severe AS. In symptomatic severe AS during pregnancy, conservative therapy may be effective.[176,177] Because fetal congenital heart disease may occur in women with congenital AS, fetal echocardiography is recommended.[177]

Despite the moderate complication rate during pregnancy, many mothers with severe AS require surgical intervention during short-term follow-up. Clinical deterioration during pregnancy is associated with increased maternal and fetal risk. For women at high risk (severe AS or class III/IV symptoms), pregnancy should be proscribed until after surgical correction.[177]

Pregnancy may be associated with aortic complications due to hormone-induced histologic changes in the aortic wall coupled with the hemodynamic stress of pregnancy. BAV with aortic aneurysm increases the risk of aortic dissection during pregnancy.[1] For TS patients using assisted reproductive technology, there is an increased risk of aortic dissection during pregnancy, especially in the setting of BAV, aortic dilation, CoA, or hypertension.[179] Although BAV with aortic aneurysm is a risk factor for aortic dissection in pregnancy, the absolute risk of aortic dissection for women with BAV is very low.[180,181]

Women with BAV and aortic diameters greater than 4.5 cm should be counseled about the risk of pregnancy.[11,137] For women at increased risk (i.e., aortic diameter > 4.5 cm or increase in aortic root size during pregnancy), close monitoring is recommended during and up to 3 months after delivery. Cesarean section may be warranted for women with a significantly dilated aorta.[47] CoA may further increase peripartum risk of dissection.[182] Surgery before pregnancy is recommended when the aortic diameter is greater than 5 cm.[137]

REFERENCES

1. Braverman AC, Guven H, Beardslee MA, et al. The bicuspid aortic valve. Curr Probl Cardiol 2005;30:470-522.
2. Tutar E, Ekici F, Atalay S, Nacar N. The prevalence of bicuspid aortic valve in newborns by echocardiographic screening. Am Heart J 2005;150: 513-515.
3. Nistri S, Basso C, Marzari C, et al. Frequency of bicuspid aortic valve in young male conscripts by echocardiogram. Am J Cardiol 2005;96: 718-721.
4. Markwald RR, Norris RA, Moreno-Rodriguez R, Levine RA. Developmental basis of adult cardiovascular diseases: valvular heart diseases. Ann N Y Acad Sci 2010;1188:177-183.
5. Prakash SK, Bosse Y, Muehlschlegel JD, et al. A roadmap to investigate the genetic basis of bicuspid aortic valve and its complications: insights from the International BAVCon (Bicuspid Aortic Valve Consortium). J Am Coll Cardiol 2014;64(8):832-839.
6. Fernandez B, Duran AC, Fernandez-Gallego T, et al. Bicuspid aortic valves with different spatial orientations of the leaflets are distinct etiological entities. J Am Coll Cardiol 2009;54(24):2312-2318.
7. Mathieu P, Bosse Y, Huggins GS, et al. The pathology and pathobiology of bicuspid aortic valve: state of the art and novel research perspectives. J Pathol Clin Res 2015;1(4):195-206.
8. Michelena HI, Prakash SK, Della Corte A, et al. Bicuspid aortic valve: identifying knowledge gaps and rising to the challenge from the International Bicuspid Aortic Valve Consortium (BAVCon). Circulation 2014;129(25):2691-2704.
9. Fedak PW, Verma S, David TE, et al. Clinical and pathophysiological implications of a bicuspid aortic valve. Circulation 2002;106(8): 900-904.
10. Laforest B, Andelfinger G, Nemer M. Loss of Gata5 in mice leads to bicuspid aortic valve. J Clin Invest 2011;121(7):2876-2887.
11. Siu SC, Silversides CK. Bicuspid aortic valve disease. J Am Coll Cardiol 2010;55(25):2789-2800.
12. Maleki S, Kjellqvist S, Paloschi V, et al. Mesenchymal state of intimal cells may explain higher propensity to ascending aortic aneurysm in bicuspid aortic valves. Sci Rep 2016;6:35712.
13. Yassine NM, Shahram JT, Body SC. Pathogenic mechanisms of bicuspid aortic valve aortopathy. Front Physiol 2017;8:687.
14. Cripe L, Andelfinger G, Martin LJ, et al. Bicuspid aortic valve is heritable. J Am Coll Cardiol 2004;44(1):138-143.
15. Hales AR, Mahle WT. Echocardiography screening of siblings of children with bicuspid aortic valve. Pediatrics 2014;133(5):e1212-e1217.
16. Hui DS, Bonow RO, Stolker JM, et al. Discordant aortic valve morphology in monozygotic twins: a clinical case series. JAMA Cardiol 2016;1(9): 1043-1047
17. Gago-Diaz M, Brion M, Gallego P, et al. The genetic component of bicuspid aortic valve and aortic dilation. An exome-wide association study. J Mol Cell Cardiol 2017;102:3-9.
18. Dargis N, Lamontagne M, Gaudreault N, et al. Identification of gender-specific genetic variants in patients with bicuspid aortic valve. Am J Cardiol 2016;117(3):420-426.
19. Andreassi MG, Della Corte A. Genetics of bicuspid aortic valve aortopathy. Curr Opin Cardiol 2016;31(6):585-592.
20. Sievers HH, Stierle U, Hachmann RM, Charitos EI. New insights in the association between bicuspid aortic valve phenotype, aortic configuration and valve haemodynamics. Eur J Cardiothorac Surg 2016;49(2):439-446.
21. Kong WK, Delgado V, Poh KK, et al. Prognostic implications of raphe in bicuspid aortic valve anatomy. JAMA Cardiol 2017;2(3):285-292.
22. Niaz T, Poterucha JT, Johnson JN, et al. Incidence, morphology, and progression of bicuspid aortic valve in pediatric and young adult subjects with coexisting congenital heart defects. Congenit Heart Dis 2017;12(3):261-269.
23. Frandsen EL, Burchill LJ, Khan AM, Broberg CS. Ascending aortic size in aortic coarctation depends on aortic valve morphology: understanding the bicuspid valve phenotype. Int J Cardiol 2018;250:106-109.
24. Oliver JM, Gallego P, Gonzalez A, et al. Risk factors for aortic complications in adults with coarctation of the aorta. J Am Coll Cardiol 2004; 44(8):1641-1647.
25. Oliver JM, Alonso-Gonzalez R, Gonzalez AE, et al. Risk of aortic root or ascending aorta complications in patients with bicuspid aortic valve with and without coarctation of the aorta. Am J Cardiol 2009;104(7): 1001-1006.
26. Bambul Heck P, Pabst von Ohain J, et al. Survival and cardiovascular events after coarctation-repair in long-term follow-up (COAFU): predictive value of clinical variables. Int J Cardiol 2016;228:347-351.
27. Vonder Muhll IF, Sehgal T, Paterson DI. The adult with repaired coarctation: need for lifelong surveillance. Can J Cardiol 2016;32(8): 1038.e11-5.

28. Mortensen KH, Young L, De Backer J, et al. Cardiovascular imaging in Turner syndrome: state-of-the-art practice across the lifespan. Heart 2018 Sep 18. pii: heartjnl-2017-312658. doi: 10.1136/heartjnl-2017-312658.

29. Quezada E, Lapidus J, Shaughnessy R, et al. Aortic dimensions in Turner syndrome. Am J Med Genet A 2015;167A(11):2527-2532.

30. Hiratzka LF, Creager MA, Isselbacher EM, et al. Surgery for aortic dilatation in patients with bicuspid aortic valves: a statement of clarification from the American College of Cardiology/American Heart Association Task Force on Clinical Practice Guidelines. J Am Coll Cardiol 2016; 67(6):724-731.

31. Koenraadt WM, Tokmaji G, DeRuiter MC, et al. Coronary anatomy as related to bicuspid aortic valve morphology. Heart 2016;102(12):943-949.

32. Koenraadt WMC, Bartelings MM, Bokenkamp R, et al. Coronary anatomy in children with bicuspid aortic valves and associated congenital heart disease. Heart 2018;104(5):385-393.

33. Meindl C, Achatz B, Huber D, et al. Coronary artery ectasia are frequently observed in patients with bicuspid aortic valves with and without dilatation of the ascending aorta. Circ Cardiovasc Interv 2016;9(10).

34. Braverman AC. Aortic involvement in patients with a bicuspid aortic valve. Heart 2011;97(6):506-513.

35. Verma S, Siu SC. Aortic dilatation in patients with bicuspid aortic valve. N Engl J Med 2014;370(20):1920-1929.

36. Michelena HI, Della Corte A, Prakash SK, et al. Bicuspid aortic valve aortopathy in adults: incidence, etiology, and clinical significance. Int J Cardiol 2015;201:400-407.

37. Cecconi M, Manfrin M, Moraca A, et al. Aortic dimensions in patients with bicuspid aortic valve without significant valve dysfunction. Am J Cardiol 2005;95(2):292-294.

38. Robicsek F, Thubrikar MJ, Cook JW, Fowler B. The congenitally bicuspid aortic valve: how does it function? Why does it fail? Ann Thorac Surg 2004;77(1):177-185.

39. Girdauskas E, Borger MA, Secknus MA, et al. Is aortopathy in bicuspid aortic valve disease a congenital defect or a result of abnormal hemodynamics? A critical reappraisal of a one-sided argument. Eur J Cardiothorac Surg 2011;39(6):809-814.

40. Biner S, Rafique AM, Ray I, et al. Aortopathy is prevalent in relatives of bicuspid aortic valve patients. J Am Coll Cardiol 2009;53(24): 2288-2295.

41. Bissell MM, Biasiolli L, Oswal A, et al. Inherited aortopathy assessment in relatives of patients with a bicuspid aortic valve. J Am Coll Cardiol 2017;69(7):904-906.

42. Loscalzo ML, Goh DL, Loeys B, et al. Familial thoracic aortic dilation and bicommissural aortic valve: a prospective analysis of natural history and inheritance. Am J Med Genet A 2007;143A(17):1960-1967.

43. Prakash S, Kuang SQ, Gen TACRI, et al. Recurrent rare genomic copy number variants and bicuspid aortic valve are enriched in early onset thoracic aortic aneurysms and dissections. PLoS One 2016;11(4): e0153543.

44. Girdauskas E, Geist L, Disha K, et al. Genetic abnormalities in bicuspid aortic valve root phenotype: preliminary results. Eur J Cardiothorac Surg 2017;52(1):156-162.

45. Girdauskas E, Disha K, Rouman M, et al. Aortic events after isolated aortic valve replacement for bicuspid aortic valve root phenotype: echocardiographic follow-up study. Eur J Cardiothorac Surg 2015;48(4): e71-e76.

46. Adamo L, Braverman AC. Surgical threshold for bicuspid aortic valve aneurysm: a case for individual decision-making. Heart 2015;101(17): 1361-1367.

47. Hiratzka LF, Bakris GL, Beckman JA, et al. 2010 ACCF/AHA/AATS/ACR/ ASA/SCA/SCAI/SIR/STS/SVM Guidelines for the diagnosis and management of patients with thoracic aortic disease. A report of the American College of Cardiology Foundation/American Heart Association Task Force on Practice Guidelines, American Association for Thoracic Surgery, American College of Radiology, American Stroke Association, Society of Cardiovascular Anesthesiologists, Society for Cardiovascular Angiography and Interventions, Society of Interventional Radiology, Society of Thoracic Surgeons, and Society for Vascular Medicine. J Am Coll Cardiol 2010;55(14):e27-e129.

48. Guo DC, Pannu H, Tran-Fadulu V, et al. Mutations in smooth muscle alpha-actin (ACTA2) lead to thoracic aortic aneurysms and dissections. Nat Genet 2007;39(12):1488-1493.

49. Andelfinger G, Loeys B, Dietz H. A decade of discovery in the genetic understanding of thoracic aortic disease. Can J Cardiol 2016;32(1):13-25.

50. Schievink WI, Raissi SS, Maya MM, Velebir A. Screening for intracranial aneurysms in patients with bicuspid aortic valve. Neurology 2010; 74(18):1430-1433.

51. Egbe AC, Padang R, Brown RD, et al. Prevalence and predictors of intra-cranial aneurysms in patients with bicuspid aortic valve. Heart 2017; 103(19):1508-1514.

52. Hope MD, Hope TA, Meadows AK, et al. Bicuspid aortic valve: four-dimensional MR evaluation of ascending aortic systolic flow patterns. Radiology 2010;255(1):53-61.

53. Viscardi F, Vergara C, Antiga L, et al. Comparative finite element model analysis of ascending aortic flow in bicuspid and tricuspid aortic valve. Artif Organs 2010;34(12):1114-1120.

54. Vergara C, Viscardi F, Antiga L, Luciani GB. Influence of bicuspid valve geometry on ascending aortic fluid dynamics: a parametric study. Artif Organs 2012;36(4):368-378.

55. Guzzardi DG, Barker AJ, van Ooij P, et al. Valve-related hemodynamics mediate human bicuspid aortopathy: insights from wall shear stress mapping. J Am Coll Cardiol 2015;66(8):892-900.

56. Girdauskas E, Rouman M, Disha K, et al. Functional aortic root parame-ters and expression of aortopathy in bicuspid versus tricuspid aortic valve stenosis. J Am Coll Cardiol 2016;67(15):1786-1796.

57. Nathan DP, Xu C, Plappert T, et al. Increased ascending aortic wall stress in patients with bicuspid aortic valves. Ann Thorac Surg 2011;92(4):1384-1389.

58. Fedak PW, Barker AJ, Verma S. Year in review: bicuspid aortopathy. Curr Opin Cardiol 2016;31(2):132-138.

59. Mahadevia R, Barker AJ, Schnell S, et al. Bicuspid aortic cusp fusion mor-phology alters aortic three-dimensional outflow patterns, wall shear stress, and expression of aortopathy. Circulation 2014;129(6):673-682.

60. Garcia J, Barker AJ, Murphy I, et al. Four-dimensional flow magnetic resonance imaging-based characterization of aortic morphometry and haemodynamics: impact of age, aortic diameter, and valve morphology. Eur Heart J Cardiovasc Imaging 2016;17(8):877-884.

61. Wisneski AD, Mookhoek A, Chitsaz S, et al. Bicuspid aortic valve-associated ascending thoracic aortic aneurysm: patient-specific finite element analysis. J Heart Valve Dis 2015;24(6):714-721.

62. Cotrufo M, Della Corte A. The association of bicuspid aortic valve disease with asymmetric dilatation of the tubular ascending aorta: identification of a definite syndrome. J Cardiovasc Med (Hagerstown) 2009;10(4):291-297.

63. Barker AJ, Markl M, Burk J, et al. Bicuspid aortic valve is associated with altered wall shear stress in the ascending aorta. Circ Cardiovasc Imaging 2012;5(4):457-466.

64. Rodriguez-Palomares JF, Dux-Santoy L, Guala A, et al. Aortic flow pat-terns and wall shear stress maps by 4D-flow cardiovascular magnetic resonance in the assessment of aortic dilatation in bicuspid aortic valve disease. J Cardiovasc Magn Reson 2018;20(1):28.

65. Stephens EH, Hope TA, Kari FA, et al. Greater asymmetric wall shear stress in Sievers' type 1/LR compared with 0/LAT bicuspid aortic valves after valve-sparing aortic root replacement. J Thorac Cardiovasc Surg 2015;150(1):59-68.

66. Kang JW, Song HG, Yang DH, et al. Association between bicuspid aortic valve phenotype and patterns of valvular dysfunction and bicuspid aor-topathy: comprehensive evaluation using MDCT and echocardiography JACC Cardiovasc Imaging 2013;6(2):150-161.

67. Longobardo L, Jain R, Carerj S, et al. Bicuspid aortic valve: unlocking the morphogenetic puzzle. Am J Med 2016;129(8):796-805.

68. Girdauskas E, Rouman M, Disha K, et al. Correlation between systolic trans-valvular flow and proximal aortic wall changes in bicuspid aortic valve ste-nosis. Eur J Cardiothorac Surg 2014;46(2):234-239; discussion 239.

69. Roberts WC, Vowels TJ, Ko JM, et al. Comparison of the structure of the aortic valve and ascending aorta in adults having aortic valve replacement for aortic stenosis versus for pure aortic regurgitation and resection of the ascending aorta for aneurysm. Circulation 2011;123(8):896-903.

70. Girdauskas E, Rouman M, Disha K, et al. Morphologic and functional markers of aortopathy in patients with bicuspid aortic valve insufficiency versus stenosis. Ann Thorac Surg 2017;103(1):49-57.

71. Phillippi JA, Green BR, Eskay MA, et al. Mechanism of aortic medial matrix remodeling is distinct in patients with bicuspid aortic valve. J Thorac Cardiovasc Surg 2014;147(3):1056-1064.

72. Grewal N, Gittenberger-de Groot AC. Pathogenesis of aortic wall complications in Marfan syndrome. Cardiovasc Pathol 2018;33:62-69.

73. Spinale FG, Bolger AF. Fate versus flow: wall shear stress in the aortopathy associated with bicuspid aortic valves. J Am Coll Cardiol 2015; 66(8):901-904.

74. Ikonomidis JS, Ruddy JM, Benton SM, Jr., et al. Aortic dilatation with bicuspid aortic valves: cusp fusion correlates to matrix metalloproteinases and inhibitors. Ann Thorac Surg 2012;93(2):457-463.

75. Wang Y, Wu B, Dong L, et al. Circulating matrix metalloproteinase patterns in association with aortic dilatation in bicuspid aortic valve patients with isolated severe aortic stenosis. Heart Vessels. 2016;31(2): 189-197.

76. Tsamis A, Phillippi JA, Koch RG, et al. Extracellular matrix fiber microarchitecture is region-specific in bicuspid aortic valve-associated ascending aortopathy. J Thorac Cardiovasc Surg. 2016;151(6):1718-1728 e1715.

77. Lindsay ME, Dietz HC. Lessons on the pathogenesis of aneurysm from heritable conditions. Nature 2011;473(7347):308-316.

78. Rocchiccioli S, Cecchettini A, Panesi P, et al. Hypothesis-free secretome analysis of thoracic aortic aneurysm reinforces the central role of TGF-beta cascade in patients with bicuspid aortic valve. J Cardiol 2017; 69(3):570-576.

79. Maleki S, Bjorck HM, Paloschi V, et al. Aneurysm development in patients with bicuspid aortic valve (BAV): possible connection to repair deficiency? Aorta (Stamford) 2013;1(1):13-22.

80. Kari FA, Fazel SS, Mitchell RS, et al. Bicuspid aortic valve configuration and aortopathy pattern might represent different pathophysiologic substrates. J Thorac Cardiovasc Surg 2012;144(2):516-517.

81. Michelena HI, Desjardins VA, Avierinos JF, et al. Natural history of asymptomatic patients with normally functioning or minimally dysfunctional bicuspid aortic valve in the community. Circulation 2008;117(21):2776-2784.

82. Fernandes S, Khairy P, Graham DA, et al. Bicuspid aortic valve and associated aortic dilation in the young. Heart 2012;98(13):1014-1019.

83. Schaefer BM, Lewin MB, Stout KK, et al. The bicuspid aortic valve: an integrated phenotypic classification of leaflet morphology and aortic root shape. Heart 2008;94(12):1634-1638.

84. Evangelista A, Gallego P, Calvo-Iglesias F, et al. Anatomical and clinical predictors of valve dysfunction and aortic dilation in bicuspid aortic valve disease. Heart 2018;104(7):566-573.

85. Della Corte A, Bancone C, Quarto C, et al. Predictors of ascending aortic dilatation with bicuspid aortic valve: a wide spectrum of disease expression. Eur J Cardiothorac Surg 2007;31(3):397-404; discussion 404-395.

86. Grotenhuis HB, Ottenkamp J, Westenberg JJ, et al. Reduced aortic elasticity and dilatation are associated with aortic regurgitation and left ventricular hypertrophy in nonstenotic bicuspid aortic valve patients. J Am Coll Cardiol 2007;49(15):1660-1665.

87. Donato Aquaro G, Ait-Ali L, Basso ML, et al. Elastic properties of aortic wall in patients with bicuspid aortic valve by magnetic resonance imaging. Am J Cardiol 2011;108(1):81-87.

88. Schaefer BM, Lewin MB, Stout KK, et al. Usefulness of bicuspid aortic valve phenotype to predict elastic properties of the ascending aorta. Am J Cardiol 2007;99(5):686-690.

89. Hillebrand M, Koschyk D, Ter Hark P, et al. Diagnostic accuracy study of routine echocardiography for bicuspid aortic valve: a retrospective study and meta-analysis. Cardiovasc Diagn Ther 2017;7(4):367-379.

90. Sperling JS, Lubat E. Forme fruste or 'Incomplete' bicuspid aortic valves with very small raphes: the prevalence of bicuspid valve and its significance may be underestimated. Int J Cardiol 2015;184:1-5.

91. Ahmed S, Honos GN, Walling AD, et al. Clinical outcome and echocardiographic predictors of aortic valve replacement in patients with bicuspid aortic valve. J Am Soc Echocardiogr 2007;20(8):998-1003.

92. Sadron Blaye-Felice MA, Seguela PE, Arnaudis B, et al. Usefulness of three-dimensional transthoracic echocardiography for the classification of congenital bicuspid aortic valve in children. Eur Heart J Cardiovasc Imaging 2012;13(12):1047-1052.

93. Takeda H, Muro T, Saito T, et al. Diagnostic accuracy of transthoracic and transesophageal echocardiography for the diagnosis of bicuspid aortic valve: comparison with operative findings. Osaka City Med J 2013; 59(2):69-78.

94. Machida T, Izumo M, Suzuki K, et al. Value of anatomical aortic valve area using real-time three-dimensional transoesophageal echocardiography in patients with aortic stenosis: a comparison between tricuspid and bicuspid aortic valves. Eur Heart J Cardiovasc Imaging 2015;16(10): 1120-1128.

95. Tanaka R, Yoshioka K, Niinuma H, et al. Diagnostic value of cardiac CT in the evaluation of bicuspid aortic stenosis: comparison with echocardiography and operative findings. AJR Am J Roentgenol 2010;195(4):895-899.

96. Gleeson TG, Mwangi I, Horgan SJ, et al. Steady-state free-precession (SSFP) cine MRI in distinguishing normal and bicuspid aortic valves. J Magn Reson Imaging 2008;28(4):873-878.

97. Lee SC, Ko SM, Song MG, et al. Morphological assessment of the aortic valve using coronary computed tomography angiography, cardiovascular magnetic resonance, and transthoracic echocardiography: comparison with intraoperative findings. Int J Cardiovasc Imaging 2012;28(Suppl 1): 33-44.

98. Buchner S, Hulsmann M, Poschenrieder F, et al. Variable phenotypes of bicuspid aortic valve disease: classification by cardiovascular magnetic resonance. Heart 2010;96(15):1233-1240.

99. Al-Najafi S, Sanchez F, Lerakis S. The Crucial role of cardiac imaging in transcatheter aortic valve replacement (TAVR): pre- and post-procedural assessment. Curr Treat Options Cardiovasc Med 2016;18(12):70.

100. Jilaihawi H, Chen M, Webb J, et al. A bicuspid aortic valve imaging classification for the TAVR era. JACC Cardiovasc Imaging 2016; 9(10):1145-1158.

101. Tzemos N, Therrien J, Yip J, et al. Outcomes in adults with bicuspid aortic valves. JAMA 2008;300(11):1317-1325.

102. Roberts WC, Vowels TJ, Ko JM. Natural history of adults with congenitally malformed aortic valves (unicuspid or bicuspid). Medicine (Baltimore) 2012;91(6):287-308.

103. Rodrigues I, Agapito AF, de Sousa L, et al. Bicuspid aortic valve outcomes. Cardiol Young 2016:1-12.

104. Masri A, Kalahasti V, Alkharabsheh S, et al. Characteristics and long-term outcomes of contemporary patients with bicuspid aortic valves. J Thorac Cardiovasc Surg 2016;151(6):1650-1659 e1651.

105. Lewin MB, Otto CM. The bicuspid aortic valve: adverse outcomes from infancy to old age. Circulation 2005;111(7):832-834.

106. Roberts WC, Janning KG, Ko JM, et al. Frequency of congenitally bicuspid aortic valves in patients ≥80 years of age undergoing aortic valve replacement for aortic stenosis (with or without aortic regurgitation) and implications for transcatheter aortic valve implantation. Am J Cardiol 2012;109(11):1632-1636.

107. Roberts WC, Ko JM. Frequency by decades of unicuspid, bicuspid, and tricuspid aortic valves in adults having isolated aortic valve replacement for aortic stenosis, with or without associated aortic regurgitation. Circulation 2005;111(7):920-925.

108. Masri A, Svensson LG, Griffin BP, Desai MY. Contemporary natural history of bicuspid aortic valve disease: a systematic review. Heart 2017; 103(17):1323-1330.

109. Tribouilloy C, Rusinaru D, Sorel C, et al. Clinical characteristics and outcome of infective endocarditis in adults with bicuspid aortic valves: a multicentre observational study. Heart 2010;96(21): 1723-1729.

110. Michelena HI, Katan O, Suri RM, et al. Incidence of infective endocarditis in patients with bicuspid aortic valves in the community. Mayo Clin Proc 2016;91(1):122-123.

111. Kiyota Y, Della Corte A, Montiero Vieira V, et al. Risk and outcomes of aortic valve endocarditis among patients with bicuspid and tricuspid aortic valves. Open Heart 2017;4(1):e000545.

112. Wilson W, Taubert KA, Gewitz M, et al. Prevention of infective endocarditis: guidelines from the American Heart Association: a guideline from the American Heart Association Rheumatic Fever, Endocarditis, and Kawasaki Disease Committee, Council on Cardiovascular Disease in the Young, and the Council on Clinical Cardiology, Council on Cardiovascular Surgery and Anesthesia, and the Quality of Care and Outcomes Research Interdisciplinary Working Group. Circulation 2007;116(15):1736-1754.

113. Zegri-Reiriz I, de Alarcon A, Munoz P, et al. Infective endocarditis in patients with bicuspid aortic valve or mitral valve prolapse. J Am Coll Cardiol 2018;71(24):2731-2740.

114. Avadhani SA, Martin-Doyle W, Shaikh AY, Pape LA. Predictors of ascending aortic dilation in bicuspid aortic valve disease: a five-year prospective study. Am J Med 2015;128(6):647-652.

115. Holmes KW, Lehmann CU, Dalal D, et al. Progressive dilation of the ascending aorta in children with isolated bicuspid aortic valve. Am J Cardiol 2007;99(7):978-983.

116. Davies RR, Kaple RK, Mandapati D, et al. Natural history of ascending aortic aneurysms in the setting of an unreplaced bicuspid aortic valve. Ann Thorac Surg 2007;83(4):1338-1344.

117. Kim JB, Spotnitz M, Lindsay ME, et al. Risk of aortic dissection in the moderately dilated ascending aorta. J Am Coll Cardiol 2016;68(11):1209-1219.

118. Michelena HI, Khanna AD, Mahoney D, et al. Incidence of aortic complications in patients with bicuspid aortic valves. JAMA 2011;306(10):1104-1112.

119. Sievers HH, Schmidtke C. A classification system for the bicuspid aortic valve from 304 surgical specimens. J Thorac Cardiovasc Surg 2007;133(5):1226-1233.

120. Etz CD, von Aspern K, Hoyer A, et al. Acute type A aortic dissection: characteristics and outcomes comparing patients with bicuspid versus tricuspid aortic valve. Eur J Cardiothorac Surg 2015;48(1):142-150.

121. Januzzi JL, Isselbacher EM, Fattori R, et al. Characterizing the young patient with aortic dissection: results from the International Registry of Aortic Dissection (IRAD). J Am Coll Cardiol 2004;43(4):665-669.

122. Roberts CS, Roberts WC. Dissection of the aorta associated with congenital malformation of the aortic valve. J Am Coll Cardiol 1991;17(3):712-716.

123. Wojnarski CM, Svensson LG, Roselli EE, et al. Aortic dissection in patients with bicuspid aortic valve-associated aneurysms. Ann Thorac Surg 2015;100(5):1666-1673; discussion 1673-1664.

124. Wang Y, Wu B, Li J, et al. Impact of aortic insufficiency on ascending aortic dilatation and adverse aortic events after isolated aortic valve replacement in patients with a bicuspid aortic valve. Ann Thorac Surg 2016;101(5):1707-1714.

125. Russo CF, Mazzetti S, Garatti A, et al. Aortic complications after bicuspid aortic valve replacement: long-term results. Ann Thorac Surg 2002;74(5):S1773-S1776; discussion S1792-S1779.

126. Regeer MV, Versteegh MI, Klautz RJ, et al. Effect of aortic valve replacement on aortic root dilatation rate in patients with bicuspid and tricuspid aortic valves. Ann Thorac Surg 2016;102(6):1981-1987.

127. Disha K, Rouman M, Secknus MA, et al. Are normal-sized ascending aortas at risk of late aortic events after aortic valve replacement for bicuspid aortic valve disease? Interact Cardiovasc Thorac Surg 2016;22(4):465-471.

128. Girdauskas E, Disha K, Borger MA, Kuntze T. Long-term prognosis of ascending aortic aneurysm after aortic valve replacement for bicuspid versus tricuspid aortic valve stenosis. J Thorac Cardiovasc Surg 2014;147(1):276-282.

129. Svensson LG, Kim KH, Blackstone EH, et al. Bicuspid aortic valve surgery with proactive ascending aorta repair. J Thorac Cardiovasc Surg 2011;142(3):622-629, 629. e621-623.

130. Borger MA, Preston M, Ivanov J, et al. Should the ascending aorta be replaced more frequently in patients with bicuspid aortic valve disease? J Thorac Cardiovasc Surg 2004;128(5):677-683.

131. Roberts WC. Prophylactic replacement of a dilated ascending aorta at the time of aortic valve replacement of a dysfunctioning congenitally unicuspid or bicuspid aortic valve. Am J Cardiol 2011;108(9):1371-1372.

132. McKellar SH, Michelena HI, Li Z, et al. Long-term risk of aortic events following aortic valve replacement in patients with bicuspid aortic valves. Am J Cardiol 2010;106(11):1626-1633.

133. Itagaki S, Chikwe JP, Chiang YP, et al. Long-term risk for aortic complications after aortic valve replacement in patients with bicuspid aortic valve versus Marfan syndrome. J Am Coll Cardiol 2015;65(22):2363-2369.

134. Girdauskas E, Disha K, Raisin HH, et al. Risk of late aortic events after an isolated aortic valve replacement for bicuspid aortic valve stenosis with concomitant ascending aortic dilation. Eur J Cardiothorac Surg 2012;42(5):832-837; discussion 837-838.

135. Girdauskas E, Rouman M, Disha K, et al. Aortic dissection after previous aortic valve replacement for bicuspid aortic valve disease. J Am Coll Cardiol 2015;66(12):1409-1411.

136. Nishimura RA, Otto CM, Bonow RO, et al. 2014 AHA/ACC guideline for the management of patients with valvular heart disease: executive summary: a report of the American College of Cardiology/American Heart Association Task Force on Practice Guidelines. J Am Coll Cardiol 2014;63(22):2438-2488.

137. Warnes CA, Williams RG, Bashore TM, et al. ACC/AHA 2008 guidelines for the management of adults with congenital heart disease: a report of the American College of Cardiology/American Heart Association Task Force on Practice Guidelines (Writing Committee to Develop Guidelines on the Management of Adults With Congenital Heart Disease). Developed in collaboration with the American Society of Echocardiography, Heart Rhythm Society, International Society for Adult Congenital Heart Disease, Society for Cardiovascular Angiography and Interventions, and Society of Thoracic Surgeons. J Am Coll Cardiol 2008;52(23):e143-e263.

138. Borger MA, Fedak PW, Stephens EH, et al. The American Association for Thoracic Surgery consensus guidelines on bicuspid aortic valve-related aortopathy: executive summary. J Thorac Cardiovasc Surg 2018;146(2);473-480.

139. Freeze SL, Landis BJ, Ware SM, Helm BM. Bicuspid aortic valve: a review with recommendations for genetic counseling. J Genet Couns 2016;25(6):1171-1178.

140. Chan KL, Ghani M, Woodend K, Burwash IG. Case-controlled study to assess risk factors for aortic stenosis in congenitally bicuspid aortic valve. Am J Cardiol 2001;88(6):690-693.

141. Chan KL, Teo K, Dumesnil JG, et al. Effect of lipid lowering with rosuvastatin on progression of aortic stenosis: results of the Aortic Stenosis Progression Observation: Measuring Effects of Rosuvastatin (ASTRONOMER) trial. Circulation 2010;121(2):306-314.

142. Braverman AC, Harris KM, Kovacs RJ, Maron BJ. eligibility and disqualification recommendations for competitive athletes with cardiovascular abnormalities: Task Force 7: aortic diseases, including Marfan syndrome: a scientific statement from the American Heart Association and American College of Cardiology. J Am Coll Cardiol 2015;66(21):2398-2405.

143. Stefani L, Galanti G, Innocenti G, et al. Exercise training in athletes with bicuspid aortic valve does not result in increased dimensions and impaired performance of the left ventricle. Cardiol Res Pract 2014;2014:238694.

144. Kari FA, Siepe M, Sievers HH, Beyersdorf F. Repair of the regurgitant bicuspid or tricuspid aortic valve: background, principles, and outcomes. Circulation 2013;128(8):854-863.

145. Svensson LG, Al Kindi AH, Vivacqua A, et al. Long-term durability of bicuspid aortic valve repair. Ann Thorac Surg 2014;97(5):1539-1547; discussion 1548.

146. Kari FA, Kvitting JP, Stephens EH, et al. Tirone David procedure for bicuspid aortic valve disease: impact of root geometry and valve type on mid-term outcomes. Interact Cardiovasc Thorac Surg 2014;19(3):375-381; discussion 381.

147. Bavaria JE, Desai N, Szeto WY, et al. Valve-sparing root reimplantation and leaflet repair in a bicuspid aortic valve: comparison with the 3-cusp David procedure. J Thorac Cardiovasc Surg 2015;149(2 Suppl):S22-S28.

148. Schneider U, Feldner SK, Hofmann C, et al. Two decades of experience with root remodeling and valve repair for bicuspid aortic valves. J Thorac Cardiovasc Surg 2017;153(4):S65-S71.

149. Hardikar AA, Marwick TH. Surgical thresholds for bicuspid aortic valve associated aortopathy. JACC Cardiovasc Imaging 2013;6(12):1311-1320.

150. Sundt TM. Aortic replacement in the setting of bicuspid aortic valve: how big? How much? J Thorac Cardiovasc Surg 2015;149(2 Suppl):S6-S9.

151. Sievers HH, Stierle U, Mohamed SA, et al. Toward individualized management of the ascending aorta in bicuspid aortic valve surgery: the role of valve phenotype in 1362 patients. J Thorac Cardiovasc Surg 2014; 148(5):2072-2080.

152. Braverman AC. Aortic replacement for bicuspid aortic valve aortopathy: when and why? J Thorac Cardiovasc Surg 2019;157:520–525.

153. Verma S, Yanagawa B, Kalra S, et al. Knowledge, attitudes, and practice patterns in surgical management of bicuspid aortopathy: a survey of 100 cardiac surgeons. J Thorac Cardiovasc Surg 2013;146(5):1033-1040 e1034.

154. Girdauskas E, Disha K, Borger MA, Kuntze T. Risk of proximal aortic dissection in patients with bicuspid aortic valve: how to address this controversy? Interact Cardiovasc Thorac Surg 2014;18(3):355-359.

155. Braverman AC. Guidelines for management of bicuspid aortic valve aneurysms: what's the clinician to do? Curr Opin Cardiol 2014;29(6):489-491.

156. Masri A, Kalahasti V, Svensson LG, et al. Aortic cross-sectional area/height ratio and outcomes in patients with bicuspid aortic valve and a dilated ascending aorta. Circ Cardiovasc Imaging 2017;10(6):e006249.

157. Della Corte A, Bancone C, Dialetto G, et al. Towards an individualized approach to bicuspid aortopathy: different valve types have unique determinants of aortic dilatation. Eur J Cardiothorac Surg 2014;45(4):e118-e124; discussion e124.

158. Della Corte A, Bancone C, Dialetto G, et al. The ascending aorta with bicuspid aortic valve: a phenotypic classification with potential prognostic significance. Eur J Cardiothorac Surg 2014;46(2):240-247; discussion 247.

159. Girdauskas E, Disha K, Secknus M, et al. Increased risk of late aortic events after isolated aortic valve replacement in patients with bicuspid aortic valve insufficiency versus stenosis. J Cardiovasc Surg (Torino) 2013;54(5):653-659.

160. Sievers HH. Everybody is different: a plea for individualizing treatment of aortopathy. J Thorac Cardiovasc Surg 2018;156(2):481-482.

161. David TE. Bicuspid aortic valve with aortic aneurysms. J Thorac Cardiovasc Surg 2018;156(2):467-468.

162. Girdauskas E, Rouman M, Disha K, et al. The fate of mild-to-moderate proximal aortic dilatation after isolated aortic valve replacement for bicuspid aortic valve stenosis: a magnetic resonance imaging follow-up study. Eur J Cardiothorac Surg 2016;49(4):e80-e86; discussion e86-e87.

163. Park CB, Greason KL, Suri RM, et al. 3rd. Fate of nonreplaced sinuses of Valsalva in bicuspid aortic valve disease. J Thorac Cardiovasc Surg 2011;142(2):278-284.

164. Zimmermann CA, Weber R, Greutmann M, et al. Dilatation and dysfunction of the neo-aortic root and in 76 patients after the Ross procedure. Pediatr Cardiol 2016;37(6):1175-1183.

165. Hanke T, Charitos EI, Stierle U, et al. The Ross operation - a feasible and safe option in the setting of a bicuspid aortic valve? Eur J Cardiothorac Surg 2010;38(3):333-339.

166. Myers MR, Magruder JT, Crawford TC, et al. Surgical repair of aortic dissection 16 years post-Ross procedure. J Surg Case Rep 2016;2016(4).

167. David TE, David C, Woo A, Manlhiot C. The Ross procedure: outcomes at 20 years. J Thorac Cardiovasc Surg 2014;147(1):85-93.

168. Poh CL, Buratto E, Larobina M, et al. The Ross procedure in adults presenting with bicuspid aortic valve and pure aortic regurgitation: 85% freedom from reoperation at 20 years. Eur J Cardiothorac Surg 2018;54(3):420-426.

169. Mylotte D, Lefevre T, Sondergaard L, et al. Transcatheter aortic valve replacement in bicuspid aortic valve disease. J Am Coll Cardiol 2014;64(22):2330-2339.

170. Bauer T, Linke A, Sievert H, et al. Comparison of the effectiveness of transcatheter aortic valve implantation in patients with stenotic bicuspid versus tricuspid aortic valves (from the German TAVI Registry). Am J Cardiol 2014;113(3):518-521.

171. Hayashida K, Bouvier E, Lefevre T, et al. Transcatheter aortic valve implantation for patients with severe bicuspid aortic valve stenosis. Circ Cardiovasc Interv 2013;6(3):284-291.

172. Phan K, Wong S, Phan S, et al. Transcatheter aortic valve implantation (TAVI) in patients with bicuspid aortic valve stenosis—systematic review and meta-analysis. Heart Lung Circ 2015;24(7):649-659.

173. Perlman GY, Blanke P, Dvir D, et al. Bicuspid aortic valve stenosis: favorable early outcomes with a next-generation transcatheter heart valve in a multicenter study. JACC Cardiovasc Interv 2016;9(8):817-824.

174. Yoon SH, Lefevre T, Ahn JM, et al. Transcatheter aortic valve replacement with early- and new-generation devices in bicuspid aortic valve stenosis. J Am Coll Cardiol 2016;68(11):1195-1205.

175. Yoon SH, Bleiziffer S, De Backer O, et al. Outcomes in transcatheter aortic valve replacement for bicuspid versus tricuspid aortic valve stenosis. J Am Coll Cardiol 2017;69:2579-2589.

176. Orwat S, Diller GP, van Hagen IM, et al. Risk of pregnancy in moderate and severe aortic stenosis: from the multinational ROPAC Registry. J Am Coll Cardiol 2016;68(16):1727-1737.

177. Pessel C, Bonanno C. Valve disease in pregnancy. Semin Perinatol. 2014;38(5):273-284.

178. Drenthen W, Pieper PG, Roos-Hesselink JW, et al. Outcome of pregnancy in women with congenital heart disease: a literature review. J Am Coll Cardiol 2007;49(24):2303-2311.

179. Bons LR, Roos-Hesselink JW. Aortic disease and pregnancy. Curr Opin Cardiol 2016;31(6):611-617.

180. Immer FF, Bansi AG, Immer-Bansi AS, et al. Aortic dissection in pregnancy: analysis of risk factors and outcome. Ann Thorac Surg 2003;76(1):309-314.

181. McKellar SH, MacDonald RJ, Michelena HI, et al. Frequency of cardiovascular events in women with a congenitally bicuspid aortic valve in a single community and effect of pregnancy on events. Am J Cardiol 2011;107(1):96-99.

182. Vriend JW, Drenthen W, Pieper PG, et al. Outcome of pregnancy in patients after repair of aortic coarctation. Eur Heart J 2005;26(20):2173-2178.

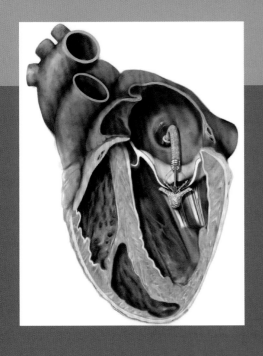

第12章
经导管主动脉瓣置换术：
适应证、手术操作和结局

　　本章主要介绍了经导管主动脉瓣置换术的适应证、手术操作和结局。有症状的重度主动脉瓣狭窄患者药物治疗预后差，其中外科手术高风险患者的1年死亡率高达51%，2年死亡率达68%。目前最常使用的经导管心脏瓣膜包括安装在网状支架上的球囊扩张式和自膨胀式生物瓣膜。更多新瓣膜正在研发和临床研究中。不论外科手术进行瓣膜置换的风险，与药物治疗相比，经导管主动脉瓣置换术均可改善患者的1年和2年无事件生存率。筛选适合经导管主动脉瓣置换术的患者需要多学科团队合作，包括有经验的结构性心脏病介入专家，心血管外科医师，麻醉医师，影像评估专家和专科护士。对患者的评估应识别出可显著改善生存率和生活质量的患者，包括神经认知功能评价、虚弱状态、功能状态和社会支持在内的综合评估非常重要。经导管主动脉瓣置换术在术前需行经胸和经食管超声心动图、心脏CT和心血管造影检查以进行手术操作相关的解剖评价。经导管主动脉瓣置换术成功率、术后30天生存率均＞95%，可明显改善生活质量，并发症发生率较低（如操作相关卒中＜2%，血管入路并发症＜5%，永久起搏器植入率约5%）。对于所有外科手术风险等级的患者，经导管主动脉瓣置换术均可作为外科主动脉瓣置换术的等效或优效替代治疗。低流速低压差主动脉瓣狭窄、二叶式主动脉瓣、伴左心室收缩功能下降的中度主动脉瓣狭窄和无症状的重度主动脉瓣狭窄行经导管主动脉瓣置换术是目前研究的热点。经导管主动脉瓣置换术的替代治疗包括外科主动脉瓣置换术和主动脉瓣球囊成形术。

张洪亮

Transcatheter Aortic Valve Replacement: Indications, Procedure, and Outcomes

Amisha Patel, Susheel Kodali

CHAPTER OUTLINE

KEY POINTS

- The prognosis for patients with symptoms due to severe valvular aortic stenosis treated medically is poor, with death rates as high as 51% at 1 year and 68% at 2 years for a series of patients at very high risk for surgical invention.
- Balloon-expandable and self-expanding bioprosthetic valves mounted in a mesh frame are the most commonly used transcatheter heart valves. Many new valve technologies are in development and undergoing clinical investigation.
- Data from multiple randomized trials indicate that transcatheter aortic valve replacement (TAVR) results in higher 1- and 2-year event-free survival rates than medical therapy, regardless of estimated surgical risk.
- Evaluation of potential TAVR candidates requires a collaborative, multidisciplinary approach by a heart valve team that includes interventional cardiologists with expertise in structural heart disease, cardiac and vascular surgeons, anesthesiologists, imaging specialists, and specialized nurses.
- Evaluation of patients should identify those for whom significant improvement in survival and quality of life is likely. Comprehensive evaluation, including neurocognitive assessment, frailty, functional status, and social support, is important.
- Transthoracic and transesophageal echocardiography, cardiac computed tomography, and invasive angiography are used to perform anatomic evaluations necessary for procedural planning before TAVR.
- Randomized trials and large registries of TAVR indicate procedural success rates of more than 95%, 30-day survival rates of more than 95%, meaningful improvement in quality of life, and acceptable complication rates (e.g., procedure-related stroke < 2%, vascular access site complications < 5%, permanent pacemaker rates ≈ 5%). TAVR has been validated as an equal or superior alternative to surgical aortic valve replacement across the spectrum of surgical risk.
- Expanding uses for TAVR in patients with low-flow, low-gradient aortic stenosis, bicuspid aortic valves, moderate aortic stenosis with left ventricular systolic dysfunction, and asymptomatic severe aortic stenosis are areas of active investigation.
- More than 300,000 TAVR procedures have been performed. Alternatives to TAVR include surgical aortic valve replacement and balloon aortic valvuloplasty.

Patients with symptomatic valvular aortic stenosis (AS) have a poor prognosis without intervention. In one series, these individuals, when treated with medical therapy alone (including balloon aortic valvuloplasty [BAV]), had death rates of 51% at 1 year and 68% at 2 years.[1] Treatment entails valve replacement by open surgical aortic valve replacement (SAVR) or transcatheter aortic valve replacement (TAVR). SAVR for severe AS has been the gold standard for decades and offers excellent long-term results.[2] However, during the past decade, TAVR has emerged as an effective and minimally invasive treatment for aortic valve disease. Although percutaneous TAVR was initially reserved for patients at excessive risk for traditional surgery,[3,4] it is now commonly used for patients at low, intermediate, and high risk for surgery and has outcomes that are similar or superior to those of the traditional surgery.[5,6]

BAV can be used as a temporizing measure for the treatment of severe AS, but it does not provide a definitive solution. Initial results were disappointing, with neither hemodynamic nor clinical improvement over the long term.[7] BAV is recommended as a palliative therapy or as a bridge to SAVR or TAVR in patients with severe symptomatic AS.[8]

TAVR started with the work of Andersen and colleagues in pigs in 1992 and was followed by the work of a number of other groups.[9] Cribier and associates reported the first implantation of a transcatheter aortic valve in humans in 2002.[10] In 2006, Webb and coworkers first described delivery of a transcatheter aortic valve by a retrograde approach through the femoral artery, a technique that has become the predominant approach today.[11] From these initial advances, the field rapidly evolved as a result of groundbreaking technologic advances and robust clinical research.

TAVR has become a safe and common procedure used widely across the developed world. Since its U.S. Food and Drug Administration (FDA) approval in the United States in 2011, more than 150,000 TAVR procedures (commercial and research) have been performed.[12,13] TAVR is approved for the treatment of native calcific AS, and its use as a treatment for expanding indications, including native aortic regurgitation (AR), bicuspid aortic valve disease, and degenerated bioprosthetic valves, continues to provide areas of active clinical research.

This chapter presents available valve designs, summarizes outcome data from TAVR randomized trials and registries, and discusses issues related to patient selection in adults with AS, and describes future directions of the field.

PERCUTANEOUS AORTIC VALVE DESIGNS

Two types of aortic valves for percutaneous implantation are most commonly used and commercially available: balloon-expandable valves and self-expanding valves (Fig. 12.1).

Balloon-Expandable Valves

Balloon-expandable prostheses for human implantation include the first-generation Cribier-Edwards valve, the modified second-generation Sapien (i.e., Sapien and Sapien XT) series of valves, and the third-generation Sapien 3 valve (all from Edwards Lifesciences Corp., Irvine, CA).

The Edwards Sapien 3 transcatheter heart valve comprises a balloon-expandable cobalt-chromium alloy tubular frame, within which are sewn bovine pericardium leaflets. It has a low delivery profile (14 Fr for 20-, 23-, and 26-mm valves and 16 Fr for the 29-mm valve) and an outer skirt that is designed to minimize paravalvular leaks (PVLs) (see Fig. 12.1). For transarterial implantation, the transcatheter valve is crimped onto a Commander delivery catheter (Edwards Lifesciences) and introduced through a sheath placed in the femoral artery. When transfemoral access is not feasible, multiple alternative access sites have been described, including the subclavian artery, carotid artery, transcaval access using the inferior vena cava to obtain access to the abdominal

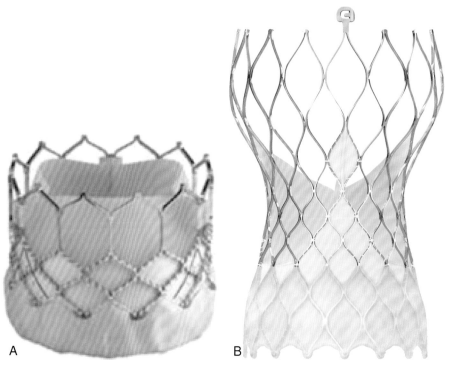

A   B

Fig. 12.1 Available Transcatheter Valves. (A) The Edwards Sapien 3 balloon-expandable valve (Edwards Lifesciences Corp., Irvine, CA) incorporates a cobalt-chromium alloy frame and bovine pericardial leaflets. It is delivered by lower-profile delivery catheters. (B) The Medtronic CoreValve Evolut R (Medtronic, Inc., Minneapolis, MN) incorporates a self-expandable nitinol frame, porcine pericardial leaflets, and an extended scalloped sealing skirt.

aorta, suprasternal access, direct aortic access, and transapical access (through the left ventricular [LV] apex).

The Sapien 3 valve is balloon expanded within the diseased native valve under rapid ventricular pacing, displacing the diseased native leaflets and anchoring in the calcium of the native aortic annulus. Whereas the Sapien 3 valve is delivered by a 14- or 16-Fr sheath, the older-generation Sapien XT/NovaFlex transfemoral system used a 16- or 19-Fr sheath. The earliest-generation devices used in the Placement of Aortic Transcatheter Valve (PARTNER) trial (discussed later) required the use of larger-diameter (22–24 Fr) sheaths.

Self-Expanding Valves

The self-expanding valve with the longest history and the most published data is the CoreValve system (Medtronic, Minneapolis, MN). The iteration of the CoreValve with the most contemporary data is the Evolut R (see Fig. 12.1), a supra-annular valve made from porcine pericardium that features a self-expanding nitinol frame and an extended scalloped sealing skirt that conforms and seals to the native aortic annulus to minimize paravalvular regurgitation. The Evolut-R system can be recaptured to optimize positioning before final valve deployment and does not require rapid ventricular pacing at the time of deployment.

The CoreValve Evolut R is compressed within an EnVeo R delivery system catheter (Medtronic) and introduced into the femoral or subclavian artery through a 14-Fr–equivalent system for the 23-, 26-, and 29-mm valves or a 16-Fr–equivalent system for the 34-mm valves. After the valve is positioned correctly within the diseased native valve, the delivery catheter is withdrawn, releasing the valve. The multistage frame is anchored within the aortic annulus, but because of its length, it also extends superiorly to anchor in the aorta above the coronaries. The latest iteration of this valve is the Evolut Pro valve, which has an external pericardial wrap designed to reduce paravalvular regurgitation.[14] This system requires adequate vascular access to allow for a delivery system that is 2-Fr larger than the comparable Evolut R valve.

Other Valve Systems

Other well-studied valve systems are displayed in Fig. 12.2. The Lotus valve (Boston Scientific, Natick, MA) (Fig. 12.2D) has a braided nitinol frame with bovine pericardial leaflets that is deployed by controlled mechanical expansion within the annulus. It is fully repositionable before release and has an adaptive seal on the outside of the valve to improve sealing and reduce paravalvular regurgitation. The latest iteration, Lotus Edge, features technology that aims to minimize the depth of deployment and interaction in the left ventricular outflow tract, potentially lowering the need for permanent pacemaker placement. It has been approved for commercial use in patients at high surgical risk and is under active investigation for those at intermediate surgical risk.[15]

The Portico transcatheter aortic heart valve (St. Jude Medical, St. Paul, MN) (see Fig. 12.2C) is a self-expanding, nitinol-based valve that is made of bovine pericardium, delivered transfemorally, and fully repositionable and retrievable. Similar to the CoreValve, it extends from the annulus to the supracoronary aorta to assist in coaxial alignment and fixation. In contrast to the CoreValve leaflets, which are supra-annular, the leaflets with the Portico device are intra-annular.

The Acurate neo valve (Symetis/Boston, Ecublens, Switzerland) (see Fig. 12.2A) is a transfemoral aortic bioprosthesis composed of a porcine pericardial tissue valve sutured within a self-expanding nitinol stent covered by a pericardial skirt on the inner and outer surface of the stent body to improve sealing and reduce PVL. The valve is supra-annular but is designed to have a smaller footprint in the ascending aorta and therefore provide easier access to the coronaries. Transfemoral and transapical delivery systems are available.

The JenaValve (JenaValve Technology, Irvine, CA) (see Fig. 12.2B) is an aortic porcine root valve mounted on a nitinol, self-expanding stent that can be delivered by a transfemoral or transapical approach. The frame design is unique in that it anchors by clipping onto the native leaflets rather than by radial force in the left ventricular outflow tract. It is currently the only transcatheter aortic valve that has been approved for the treatment of AS and AR. The mechanism of anchoring may also help protect against important complications such as coronary obstruction by holding the native leaflets away from the coronary ostium.

The Edwards Sapien, Medtronic CoreValve, and Boston Scientific Lotus systems are approved for commercial use by the FDA in the United States. The other platforms are commercially available in Europe. Clinical trials are ongoing in the United States for evaluation of the Lotus and Portico valve systems.

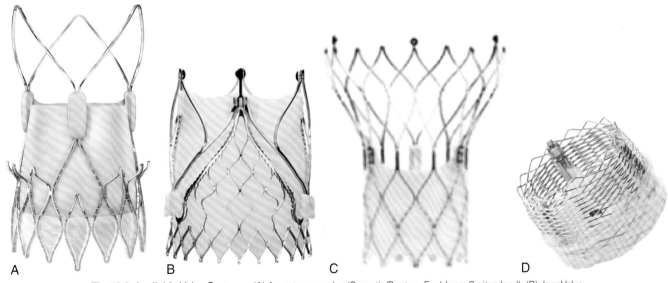

Fig. 12.2 Available Valve Systems. (A) Acurate neo valve (Symetis/Boston, Ecublens, Switzerland). (B) JenaValve (JenaValve Technology, Irvine, CA). (C) Portico transcatheter aortic heart valve (Portico is a trademark of Abbott and its related companies. Reproduced with permission of Abbott, 2019. All rights reserved.). (D) Lotus Edge valve (Boston Scientific Inc., Natick, MA).

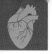

RANDOMIZED TAVR TRIALS

PARTNER

The primary results of the PARTNER trial at 1 and 5 years are presented in Table 12.1.[1,3,4,16] This trial used early-generation TAVR systems (i.e., Sapien 23-mm and 26-mm valves with 22-Fr and 24-Fr femoral delivery catheters) in centers with limited operator experience with TAVR.

Cohort B of the PARTNER trial compared transfemoral TAVR with standard therapy (including BAV). The mean operative mortality risk identified by the Society of Thoracic Surgeons (STS) score of patients enrolled in this trial was 11.6%. At 1-year follow-up, the rates of death were 50.7% for the standard therapy group and 30.7% for the TAVR group. Based on these results, only five patients needed to be treated with TAVR to prevent one death at 1 year (i.e., number needed to treat = 5) (Fig. 12.3). TAVR was associated with a significant reduction in symptoms at 1 year as assessed by New York Heart Association (NYHA) functional class (74.8% of surviving patients who had undergone TAVR were in NYHA class II or lower vs. 42.0% of those treated with standard therapy) and by Kansas City Cardiomyopathy Questionnaire (KCCQ) scores. The rate of major stroke was numerically higher with TAVR but not statistically significant, whereas the rates of vascular complications and major bleeding were significantly higher (see Table 12.1).

The 5-year follow-up of PARTNER Cohort B showed that the mortality rate remained lower for the TAVR group compared with that for the standard therapy group (71.8% vs. 93.6%, hazard ratio [HR]= 0.50, 95% confidence interval [CI]: 0.39–0.65, $P < 0.0001$).[17]

Echocardiography after TAVR showed durable hemodynamic benefit (aortic valve area of 1.52 cm[2] and mean gradient of 10.6 mmHg at 5 years), with no evidence of structural valve deterioration. TAVR did not improve the mortality rate for patients with an STS risk score higher than 14.9% on entry into the trial.[1]

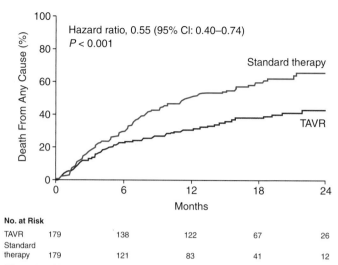

Fig. 12.3 Time-To-Event Curve for Death From Any Cause in the PARTNER Trial, Cohort B. (From Leon MB, Smith CR, Mack M, et al. Transcatheter aortic-valve implantation for aortic stenosis in patients who cannot undergo surgery. N Engl J Med 2010;363:1597-1607.)

Cohort A of the PARTNER trial compared transfemoral and transapical TAVR with SAVR.[4] One-year data showed the noninferiority of TAVR (i.e., death from all causes of 24.2% with TAVR vs. 26.8% with standard surgery) (Fig. 12.4). Rates of major strokes were numerically but not significantly higher in the TAVR group compared with the surgical group (3.8% vs. 2.1%, respectively, at 30 days; $P = 0.20$). Major vascular complications were significantly more frequent with transcatheter replacement (11.0% vs. 3.2%, $P < 0.01$), whereas adverse

TABLE 12.1 Randomized Clinical Trials of Transcatheter Aortic Valve Replacement.

TRIAL	Risk Category	Mean Age (yr)	% Male	Mean STS Score (%)	No. of Patients	Device Studied and Comparator	Primary End Point	Rate of Primary End Point (%)
PARTNER	High	83	46	11.8	699	Sapien vs. SAVR	Death at 1 yr	TAVR: 24.2 SAVR: 26.8
CoreValve U.S. Pivotal	High	83	53	7.4	747	CoreValve vs. SAVR	Death at 1 yr	TAVR: 14.2 SAVR: 9.1
PARTNER 2	Intermediate	82	54	5.8	2032	Sapien XT vs. SAVR	Death or disabling stroke at 2 yr	TAVR: 19.3 SAVR: 21.1
SURTAVI	Intermediate	80	56	4.5	1660	CoreValve/Evolut R vs. SAVR	Death or disabling stroke at 2 yr	TAVR: 12.6 SAVR: 14.0
PARTNER 3	Low	73	69	1.9	1000	Sapien 3 vs. SAVR	Death, stroke, rehospitalization at 1 yr	TAVR: 8.5 SAVR: 15.1
Evolut Low Risk Trial	Low	74	65	1.9	1468	CoreValve/Evolut R/ Evolut Pro vs. SAVR	Death or disabling stroke at 2 yr	TAVR: 5.3 SAVR: 6.7
CHOICE	High	81	36	5.9	121	CoreValve vs. Sapien XT	Device success	Sapien XT: 95.9 CoreValve: 77.5
REPRISE III	High	83	49	6.8	912	Lotus vs. CoreValve/ Evolut-R	Death, disabling stroke, and moderate or great PVL at 1 yr	Lotus: 15.4 CoreValve: 25.5
NOTION	Low	79	53	3.0	280	CoreValve vs. SAVR	Death at 1 yr	TAVR: 4.9 SAVR: 7.5

PVL, Paravalvular leak; *SAVR,* surgical aortic valve replacement; *STS,* Society of Thoracic Surgeons; *TAVR,* transcatheter aortic valve replacement.

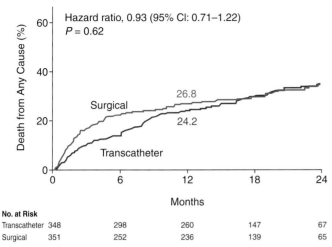

Death From Any Cause, All Patients

Hazard ratio, 0.93 (95% CI: 0.71–1.22)
$P = 0.62$

No. at Risk

Transcatheter	348	298	260	147	67
Surgical	351	252	236	139	65

Fig. 12.4 Time-To-Event Curve for Death From Any Cause in the PARTNER Trial, Cohort A. (From Smith CR, Leon MB, Mack MJ, et al. Transcatheter versus surgical aortic-valve replacement in high-risk patients. N Engl J Med 2011;364:2187-2198.)

events that were more frequent after SAVR included major bleeding and new-onset atrial fibrillation.

The 5-year follow-up of PARTNER Cohort A showed similar rates of death for the TAVR group and the surgical group (67.8% vs. 62.4%, respectively, HR = 1.04, 95% CI: 0.86–1.24, $P = 0.76$).[16] There was no structural valve deterioration requiring SAVR in either group. Moderate or severe AR occurred more often in the TAVR group (14% vs. 1%, $P < 0.01$) and was associated with an increased 5-year risk of death (72.4% for moderate or severe AR vs. 56.6% for mild AR or less, $P = 0.003$).

CoreValve U.S. Pivotal Trial

Self-expanding valves have been associated with higher rates of survival at 1 year compared with surgical valve replacement in patients at high operative risk. In the CoreValve U.S. pivotal trial, patients with severe symptomatic AS at high operative risk were randomized to TAVR with the CoreValve self-expanding bioprosthesis or to SAVR. The results are summarized in Table 12.1. The mean STS score was 7.4%. The rate of the primary end point of death from any cause at 1 year was lower for the TAVR group compared with the surgical group (14.2% vs. 19.1%, $P < 0.01$ for noninferiority). The rate of major adverse cardiovascular and cerebrovascular events at 1 year was significantly lower for the TAVR group than the surgical group (20.4% vs. 27.3%, $P = 0.03$). The rates of any stroke were lower in the TAVR group compared with the surgical group (4.9% vs. 6.2% and $P = 0.46$ at 30 days; 8.8% vs. 12.6% and $P = 0.10$ at 1 year). Major vascular complications and permanent pacemaker implantations were significantly more frequent in the TAVR group than in the surgical group, whereas bleeding, acute kidney injury, and new-onset or worsening atrial fibrillation were significantly more common in the surgical group. The rates of paravalvular regurgitation were higher in the TAVR group than in the surgical group at all time points after the procedure.[18]

PARTNER 2

The PARTNER 2 trial randomized intermediate-risk patients to TAVR with a Sapien XT valve or to SAVR.[5] The results are summarized in Table 12.1. The mean STS score for each group was 5.8%. The trial showed that TAVR was noninferior to SAVR with respect to the

primary end point of death (16.7% after TAVR and 18.0% after surgery, $P = 0.001$) or disabling stroke (6.2% after TAVR and 6.4% after surgery, $P = 0.001$) at 2 years. In the transfemoral-access cohort, TAVR resulted in a lower rate of death or disabling stroke than surgery (HR = 0.79, 95% CI: 0.62–1.00, $P = 0.05$), whereas in the transthoracic-access cohort, outcomes were similar between the two groups. TAVR also resulted in lower rates of acute kidney injury, severe bleeding, and new-onset atrial fibrillation, whereas surgery resulted in fewer major vascular complications and less paravalvular aortic regurgitation.[5]

Sapien 3 Intermediate-Risk Registry

Additional data from observational studies demonstrated that TAVR may be superior to SAVR in intermediate-risk patients. In the Sapien 3 intermediate-risk registry, 1077 patients with a mean STS score of 5.2% and an average age of 81 years were assigned to receive the Sapien 3 valve (88% by transfemoral access through 14-Fr and 16-Fr delivery systems) at more than 50 sites in the United States and Canada.[19,20] One-year outcomes of these patients, including all-cause mortality and incidence of strokes, reintervention, and aortic valve regurgitation were then compared with outcomes of intermediate-risk patients treated with SAVR in the PARTNER 2A trial using propensity-matching analysis (see Table 12.1). This study was conducted in the same centers as the randomized PARTNER 2A study. The clinical events committee and the echocardiography and CT core laboratories were the same for this registry as for the PARTNER 2A study. At 30 days, the mortality rate was 1.1% after TAVR compared with 4.0% for the surgical arm of PARTNER 2A. Stroke rates were also significantly lower after TAVR compared with SAVR in this intermediate-risk population (disabling strokes: 1.0% vs. 4.4%). Although rates of paravalvular regurgitation were higher with TAVR than with SAVR, other important complications, including bleeding, atrial fibrillation, and acute kidney injury, were lower with TAVR.

The reduction in early complications translated to improved late outcomes. For the primary composite end point of death, stroke, and moderate or severe AR at 1 year, TAVR was superior to SAVR (−9.2%, 95% CI: −13.0 to −5.4, $P < 0.0001$). Based on this analysis, the study authors concluded that TAVR should be a treatment alternative to SAVR for intermediate-risk patients.

SURTAVI

The Surgical Replacement and Transcatheter Aortic Valve Implantation (SURTAVI) trial randomized 1746 intermediate-risk patients with severe symptomatic AS to TAVR using of a self-expanding prosthesis or to SAVR.[21] Clinical outcomes of these patients at 30 days, 12 months, and 24 months are shown in Table 12.1. The mean STS score was 4.5%. At 24 months, the estimated incidence of the primary end point of death from any cause or disabling stroke was 12.6% for the TAVR group and 14.0% for the surgery group (95% CI: −5.2% to 2.3%; posterior probability of noninferiority > 0.999).

As in the PARTNER 2 trial, surgery was associated with higher rates of acute kidney injury, atrial fibrillation, and transfusion requirements, whereas TAVR led to higher rates of residual AR and need for pacemaker implantation. TAVR resulted in lower mean gradients and larger aortic valve areas than SAVR. Structural valve deterioration at 24 months did not occur in either group. Based on these data, TAVR with a self-expanding valve was considered a noninferior alternative to surgery in patients with severe AS at intermediate surgical risk.

REPRISE III

The REPRISE III study is the largest randomized comparison of two transcatheter heart valves.[22] It randomized 912 patients with severe aortic stenosis at high risk for surgery 2:1 to Lotus or CoreValve. The results are shown in Table 12.1. There was no difference in the composite prior safety end point between the two devices at 30 days or 1 year. However, the requirement for implantation of a new permanent pacemaker was significantly higher for the Lotus valve (35.5% vs. 19.6%, $P < 0.001$). For the primary efficacy end point, which was a composite of death, disabling stroke, and moderate or greater PVL at 1 year, the Lotus valve performed significantly better than CoreValve (16.4% vs. 28.6%). This was primarily driven by the significantly lower rates of moderate or greater PVL in the Lotus arm (2.0% vs. 11.1%, $P < 0.001$).

One of the strengths of the Lotus platform is that exceptionally low rates of PVL were seen across all of the studies. Whether these differences in short-term outcomes will translate to improved long-term outcomes remains to be seen.

PORTICO

The PORTICO study evaluated the safety and effectiveness of the St. Jude Medical Portico valve in a randomized trial against commercially approved transcatheter heart valves in patients at high surgical risk. The study had a primary effectiveness end point of composite all-cause death or disabling stroke at 1 year and a primary safety end point of composite all-cause death, disabling stroke, life-threatening bleeding, acute kidney injury, or major vascular complications at 30 days.

Although early feasibility results of the Portico valve were promising, this trial was halted due to an unexpected finding of reduced prosthesis leaflet motion on CT in a patient who had a stroke after TAVR.[23] This finding suggested subclinical valve thrombosis requiring further investigation.[23,24] The trial was resumed after FDA approval because reduced leaflet motion is not unique to the Portico valve and typically is not associated with adverse outcomes.[12] The results of the trial are shown in Table 12.1.[25] The study authors concluded that TAVR with the Portico valve in patients who are at increased surgical risk is associated with low 1-year death and stroke rates, and favorable hemodynamic results at 1 year were observed with low transvalvular pressure gradients and PVLs.

TAVR in Patients at Low Surgical Risk

Data have emerged comparing TAVR with conventional surgery in populations at low surgical risk.[26,27] In the PARTNER 3 trial, patients with severe AS at low surgical risk were randomly assigned to undergo TAVR with transfemoral placement of a balloon-expandable valve or conventional surgery. TAVR was shown to be superior to SAVR, with a significantly lower rate of death, stroke, or rehospitalization at 1 year.[26] Similarly, when patients at low surgical risk were randomized to TAVR with a self-expanding valve or to SAVR with a composite end point of death or disabling stroke at 24 months, TAVR was found to be noninferior to SAVR[27] (Figs. 12.5 and 12.6).

Overall, meta-analyses comparing TAVR with SAVR in low-risk patients revealed a significant reduction in death and disabling stroke. TAVR was also associated with improved quality of life, reduced bleeding, and lower rates of atrial fibrillation when compared with SAVR in this population.[29] These benefits initially came at the cost of increased rates of PVL and permanent pacemaker implantation in those who received TAVR. Although the rate of pacemaker placement remains a concern, particularly with self-expanding prostheses, the rate of PVL in more contemporary trials is not significantly different between TAVR and SAVR, largely due to improvement in valve design and the almost universal use of CT-guided valve-sizing techniques.

FINDINGS FROM TAVR REGISTRIES

In addition to the randomized, controlled trial data mentioned previously, several TAVR registries have been established in different countries to represent the real-world experience with this new technology. This

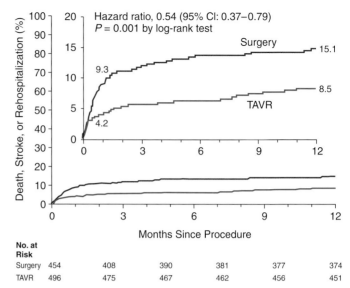

No. at Risk

Surgery	454	408	390	381	377	374
TAVR	496	475	467	462	456	451

Fig. 12.5 Time-To-Event Curve for Composite of Death, Stroke, or Rehospitalization in the PARTNER 3 Trial. (From Mack MJ, Leon MB, Thourani VH, et al. Transcatheter aortic-valve replacement with a balloon-expandable valve in low-risk patients. N Engl J Med 2019;380:1695-1705.)

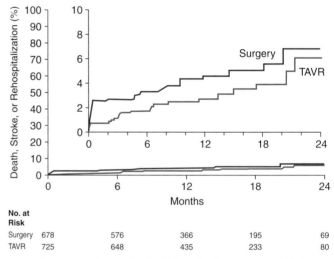

No. at Risk

Surgery	678	576	366	195	69
TAVR	725	648	435	233	80

Fig. 12.6 Transcatheter Aortic Valve Replacement (TAVR) Versus Surgical Aortic Valve Replacement (SAVR) for Patients at Low Surgical Risk. (From Popma JJ, Deeb GM, Yakubov SJ, et al. Transcatheter aortic-valve replacement with a self-expanding valve in low-risk patients. N Engl J Med 2019;380:1706-1715.)

section presents results from the United Kingdom Transcatheter Aortic Valve Implantation (U.K. TAVI) registry and the United States Transcatheter Valve Therapy (U.S. TVT) registry.

U.K. TAVI Registry

The U.K. TAVI registry includes 3980 TAVR procedures performed at 33 centers in the United Kingdom from 2007 through 2012.[30,31] The patients, who account for all TAVR cases performed in the country, received the Sapien/Sapien XT (Edwards Lifesciences; $n = 2036$) or the CoreValve (Medtronic; $n = 1897$) device. A minority of patients received a Portico (St. Jude; $n = 35$), Direct Flow (Direct Flow Medical, Santa Rosa, CA; $n = 3$), or JenaValve (JenaValve; $n = 3$) device. Most cases (71.2%) were performed through femoral access.

Predictors of 2-year mortality were atrial fibrillation, chronic obstructive pulmonary disease, and renal insufficiency (creatinine > 2.26 mg/dL). Patients who could be treated by the femoral route had a lower mortality rate than those for whom an alternative route was needed. Unadjusted survival for the direct aortic approach and the transapical approach were similar at 1 and 2 years. Postprocedural AR (moderate or severe) was associated with lower long-term survival rates on multivariate analysis at 1 and 2 years. There was no difference in survival at any point between Sapien and CoreValve devices; however, CoreValve was associated with a higher incidence of post-TAVR AR ($P < 0.001$) and need for pacemaker implantation ($P < 0.001$). The rate of pacemaker implantation decreased markedly with CoreValve, from 29% to 15% in the more recent years ($P < 0.001$). The 4-year survival rate was 55% for those treated in 2009 and 65% for those treated in 2011.

U.S. TVT Registry

The U.S. TVT Registry is a collaboration between the STS and the American College of Cardiology (ACC). It was initiated shortly after the commercial approval of first transcatheter heart valve (Edwards Sapien) in 2011. Since then, all commercial (nonresearch) cases must be entered into the TVT registry to meet the Center for Medicare and Medicaid Services (CMS) requirements for coverage as outlined in the national coverage decision.

One of the first publications from this registry included 12,182 patients (median age, 84 years; 52% female) undergoing TAVR using the Sapien valve between November 2011 and June 2013 at 299 U.S. hospitals.[30] Most cases (56.4%) were performed through femoral access, and the median STS score was 7.1%, with 30.8% of patients falling in the 8% to 15% range and 11.9% with a risk greater than 15%. The rate of comorbidities was high, and approximately 40% of patients had a slow gait suggesting frailty. Rates of death and stroke at 1 year were 23.7% and 4.1%, respectively. The 1-year composite outcome of incidence of death or stroke was 26%. On multivariate analysis, advanced age, male sex, renal failure, severe lung disease, preoperative atrial fibrillation, STS score greater than 15, and nontransfemoral access were among the factors associated with greater 1-year mortality rates.[30] These outcomes were similar to those seen in the carefully controlled, randomized trials that led to FDA approval, demonstrating a rational and controlled dispersion of this new technology.

The 2017 publication from TVT included 54,782 patients who underwent TAVR through 2015.[13] The data demonstrated a drop in the STS risk score of the patients between 2012 and 2015 (from 7% to 6%; $P < 0.0001$). Outcomes also improved during this time frame, with the in-hospital mortality rate decreasing from 5.7% to 2.9% and 1-year mortality rate decreasing from 25.8% to 21.6% (Table 12.2).

TABLE 12.2   Transcatheter Aortic Valve Replacement Outcomes in the Transcatheter Valve Therapy Registry.

Outcome Information	Overall (N = 54,782)	2012 (N = 4627)	2013 (N = 9052)	2014 (N = 16,295)	2015 (N = 24,808)	P Value
In-hospital death						<0.0001
Missing	10 (0.0)[a]	1 (0.0)	4 (0.0)	0 (0.0)	5 (0.0)	
Yes	2111 (3.9)	266 (5.7)	469 (5.2)	665 (4.1)	711 (2.9)	
30-day death						<0.0001
Missing	0 (0.0)	0 (0.0)	0 (0.0)	0 (0.0)	0 (0.0)	
Yes	2814 (5.7)	315 (7.5)	585 (7.1)	911 (6.0)	1003 (4.6)	
In-hospital stroke						0.2402
Missing	0 (0.0)	0 (0.0)	0 (0.0)	0 (0.0)	0 (0.0)	
Yes	1136 (2.1)	102 (2.2)	187 (2.1)	355 (2.2)	492 (2.0)	
30-day any strokes						0.0264
Missing	829 (1.9)	72 (2.2)	100 (1.5)	230 (1.8)	427 (2.1)	
Yes	917 (2.1)	75 (2.3)	156 (2.3)	292 (2.2)	394 (1.9)	
30-day pacemaker						0.0362
Missing	633 (1.8)	—	31 (1.8)	203 (1.5)	399 (2.0)	
Yes	4159 (11.8)	—	151 (8.8)	1,560 (11.9)	2,448 (12.0)	
New requirement for dialysis						<0.0001
Missing	0 (0.0)	0 (0.0)	0 (0.0)	0 (0.0)	0 (0.0)	
Yes	746 (1.4)	80 (1.7)	177 (2.0)	255 (1.6)	234 (0.9)	
Acute kidney injury						<0.0001
Missing	709 (1.3)	77 (1.7)	169 (1.9)	179 (1.1)	284 (1.1)	
Stage 3	2578 (4.7)	277 (6.0)	503 (5.6)	788 (4.8)	1010 (4.1)	
VARC degree of bleedings						<0.0001
Missing	0 (0.0)	0 (0.0)	0 (0.0)	0 (0.0)	0 (0.0)	
No threatening bleeding event	49,448 (91.6)	3927 (87.1)	7903 (89.0)	14,823 (92.0)	22,795 (93.1)	

Continued

TABLE 12.2   Transcatheter Aortic Valve Replacement Outcomes in the Transcatheter Valve Therapy Registry.—cont'd

Outcome Information	Overall (N = 54,782)	2012 (N = 4627)	2013 (N = 9052)	2014 (N = 16,295)	2015 (N = 24,808)	P Value
Major bleeding event	2337 (4.3)	271 (6.0)	446 (5.0)	674 (4.2)	946 (3.9)	
Life-threatening bleeding event	2200 (4.1)	309 (6.9)	535 (6.0)	618 (3.8)	738 (3.0)	
Transfusion of RBC/whole blood						<0.0001
Missing	210 (0.4)	46 (1.0)	29 (0.3)	55 (0.3)	80 (0.3)	
Yes	16,515 (30.1)	2069 (44.7)	4000 (44.2)	4990 (30.6)	5456 (22.0)	
Major vascular access site complication (VARC)						0.9874
Missing	0 (0.0)	0 (0.0)	0 (0.0)	0 (0.0)	0 (0.0)	
Yes	551 (1.3)	—	36 (1.6)	196 (1.2)	319 (1.3)	
Aortic regurgitation (most recent at discharge or 30 days)						<0.0001
Missing	0 (0.0)	0 (0.0)	0 (0.0)	0 (0.0)	0 (0.0)	
None/trace	31,686 (64.1)	2106 (54.3)	5003 (64.7)	9328 (63.0)	15,249 (66.2)	
Mild	14,339 (29.0)	1350 (34.8)	2226 (28.8)	4398 (29.7)	6365 (27.6)	
Moderate/severe	3428 (6.9)	419 (10.8)	509 (6.6)	1077 (7.3)	1423 (6.2)	
AV gradient (most recent at discharge or 30 days)						<0.0001
Missing	0 (0.0)	0 (0.0)	0 (0.0)	0 (0.0)	0 (0.0)	
<10 mmHg	27,644 (56.9)	1746 (46.5)	3862 (51.4)	8985 (61.7)	13,051 (57.3)	
10 and <20 mmHg	18,085 (37.2)	1721 (45.8)	3161 (42.0)	4902 (33.7)	8301 (36.4)	
≤20 mmHg	2886 (5.9)	288 (7.7)	495 (6.6)	674 (4.6)	1429 (6.3)	
30-Day AV reintervention						0.6271
Missing	859 (2.0)	74 (2.3)	102 (1.5)	233 (1.8)	450 (2.2)	
Yes	116 (0.3)	12 (0.4)	12 (0.2)	35 (0.3)	57 (0.3)	

[a]All trial data given as number of patients and percentage (%) of total.
AV, Aortic valve; *RBC,* red blood cells; *VARC,* Valve Academic Research Consortium.
From Grover FL, Vemulapalli S, Carroll JD, et al. 2016 Annual report of the Society of Thoracic Surgeons/American College of Cardiology Transcatheter Valve Therapy Registry. J Am Coll Cardiol 2017;69:1215-1230.

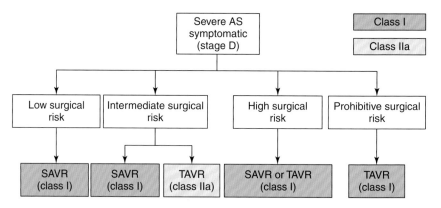

Fig. 12.7 Transcatheter Aortic Valve Replacement *(TAVR)* Versus Surgical Aortic Valve Replacement *(SAVR)* for Patients With Severe Symptomatic Aortic Stenosis *(AS).* (From Nishimura RA, Otto CM, Bonow RO, et al. 2017 AHA/ACC focused update of the 2014 AHA/ACC guideline for the management of patients with valvular heart disease: a report of the American College of Cardiology/American Heart Association Task Force on Clinical Practice Guidelines. Circulation 2017;135:e1159-e1195.)

TAVR GUIDELINES

Based on available clinical data, TAVR has been accepted by the American Heart Association (AHA)/ACC and European Society of Cardiology (ESC) guidelines as a class I indication in patients with severe symptomatic AS who are not candidates for SAVR or are at high risk and as a class IIa indication for patients with severely symptomatic AS who are at intermediate risk for death and complications after SAVR[8] (Figs. 12.7 through 12.9). A balanced interpretation of the literature and the prevailing sentiment from experts worldwide indicate that TAVR is the preferred therapy and the standard of care for patients with severe symptomatic AS who are at elevated risk for surgery or elderly.[32]

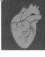

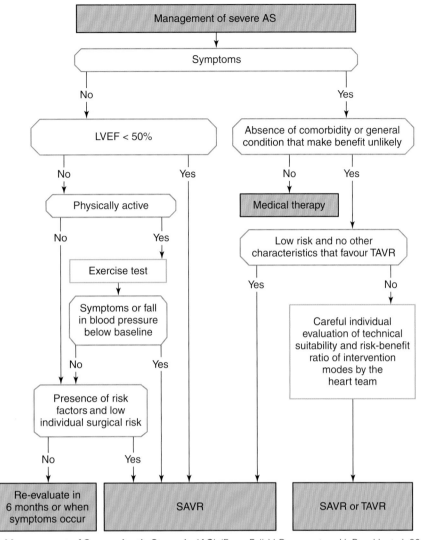

Fig. 12.8 Management of Severe Aortic Stenosis *(AS)*. (From Falk V, Baumgartner H, Bax JJ, et al. 2017 ESC/EACTS guidelines for the management of valvular heart disease. Eur J Cardiothorac Surg 2017;52:616-664.)

Aortic valve interventions should only be performed in centers with both departments of cardiology and cardiac surgery on site and with structured collaboration between the two, including a heart team (heart valve centers).	I	C
The choice for intervention must be based on careful individual evaluation of technical suitability and weighing of risks and benefits of each modality. Local expertise and outcomes data for the given intervention must be taken into account.	I	C
SAVR is recommended in patients at low surgical risk (STS or EuroSCORE II < 4% or logistic EuroSCORE I < 10% and no other risk factors not included in these scores, such as frailty, porcelain aorta, sequelae of chest irradiation).	I	B
TAVI is recommended in patients who are not suitable for SAVR as assessed by the heart team.	I	B
In patients who are at increased surgical risk (STS or EuroSCORE II ≥ 4% or logistic EuroSCORE I ≥ 10% or other risk factors not included in these scores such as frailty, porcelain aorta, sequelae of chest irradiation), the decision between SAVR and TAVI should be made by the heart team according to the individual patient characteristics, with TAVI being favored in elderly patients suitable for transfemoral access.	I	B
Balloon aortic valvotomy may be considered as a bridge to SAVR or TAVI in hemodynamically unstable patients or in patients with symptomatic severe aortic stenosis who require urgent major noncardiac surgery.	IIb	C
Balloon aortic valvotomy may be considered as a diagnostic means in patients with severe aortic stenosis or other potential causes for symptoms (i.e., lung disease) and in patients with severe myocardial dysfunction, prerenal insufficiency, or other organ dysfunction that may be reversible with balloon aortic valvotomy when performed in centers that can escalate to TAVI.	IIb	C

Fig. 12.9 Intervention for Severe Symptomatic Aortic Stenosis *(AS)*. (From Falk V, Baumgartner H, Bax JJ, et al. 2017 ESC/EACTS guidelines for the management of valvular heart disease. Eur J Cardiothorac Surg 2017;52:616-664.)

TABLE 12.3   Factors Favoring Surgical Aortic Valve Replacement, Transcatheter Valve Replacement, or Palliation Instead of Aortic Valve Intervention.

Decision-Making Factors	Favoring SAVR	Favoring TAVR	Favoring Palliation
Age and life expectancy[a]	Younger age/longer life expectancy	Older age/fewer expected remaining years of life	Limited life expectancy
Valve anatomy	Bicuspid aortic valve Rheumatic valve disease Small or large aortic annulus[b]	Calcific AS of a trileaflet valve	—
Prosthetic valve preference	Mechanical or surgical bioprosthetic valve preferred Concern for patient-prosthesis mismatch	Bioprosthetic valve preferred Favorable ratio of life expectancy to valve durability	—
Concurrent cardiac conditions	Aortic dilation[c] Severe primary MR Severe CAD requiring bypass grafting Septal hypertrophy requiring myectomy Atrial fibrillation	Severe calcification of the ascending aorta (porcelain aorta)	Irreversible severe LV systolic dysfunction Severe MR due to annular calcification
Noncardiac conditions	—	Severe lung, liver, or renal disease Mobility issues (high risk for sternotomy)	Symptoms likely due to noncardiac conditions Severe dementia Involvement of two or more other organ systems
Frailty	Not frail or few frailty measures	Frailty likely to improve after TAVR	Severe frailty unlikely to improve after TAVR
Estimated risk of SAVR or TAVR	SAVR risk low to high *or* TAVR risk high	TAVR risk low to medium *and* SAVR risk low to prohibitive (<15%)	Prohibitive SAVR risk (>15%) or post-TAVR life expectancy < 1 yr
Procedure-specific impediments	Valve anatomy, annular size, or coronary ostial height precludes TAVR Vascular access does not allow transfemoral TAVR	Previous cardiac surgery with at-risk coronary grafts Previous chest irradiation	Valve anatomy, annular size, or coronary ostial height precludes TAVR Vascular access does not allow transfemoral TAVR
Goals of care and patient preferences and values	Less uncertainty about valve durability Avoid repeat intervention Lower risk of permanent pacer Life prolongation Symptom relief Improved exercise capacity and QOL Avoids vascular complications Accepts longer hospital stay, pain in recovery period	Accepts uncertainty about valve durability and possible repeat intervention Higher risk of permanent pacer Life prolongation Symptom relief Improved exercise capacity and QOL Prefers shorter hospital stay, less postprocedure pain	Life prolongation not an important goal Avoid futile or unnecessary diagnostic or therapeutic procedures Avoid procedural stroke risk Avoid possibility of cardiac pacer

[a]Expected remaining years of life can be estimated based on U.S. actuarial life expectancy tables. The balance between expected patient longevity and valve durability varies across the age range, with more durable valves preferred for patients with a longer life expectancy. Bioprosthetic valve durability is finite (with shorter durability for younger patients), whereas mechanical valves are very durable but require lifelong anticoagulation. Long-term (20-year) data on outcomes with surgical bioprosthetic valves are available; robust data on transcatheter bioprosthetic valves extend only to 5 years, leading to uncertainty about longer-term outcomes. The decision about valve type should be individualized based on patient-specific factors that can affect expected longevity.

[b]A large aortic annulus may not be suitable for current transcatheter valve sizes. With a small aortic annulus or aorta, a surgical annular enlarging procedure may be needed to allow placement of a larger prosthesis and avoid patient-prosthesis mismatch.

[c]Dilation of the aortic sinuses or ascending aorta may require concurrent surgical replacement, particularly in younger patients with a bicuspid aortic valve.

AS, Aortic stenosis; *CAD*, coronary artery disease; *LV*, left ventricular; *MR*, mitral regurgitation; *QOL*, quality of life; *SAVR*, surgical aortic valve replacement; *TAVR*, transcatheter aortic valve replacement.

From Burke CR, Kirkpatrick IN, Otto CM. Goals of care in patients with severe aortic stenosis. Eur Heart J 2019 Aug 21, pii: ehz567. doi: 10.1093/eurheartj/ehz567 [Epub ahead of print].

Patient Selection

Evaluation of patients deemed suitable for TAVR is directed at identifying those for whom a significant improvement in quality and duration of life is likely and avoiding unnecessary intervention in patients for whom the procedure can be performed but benefit is unlikely (Table 12.3). Assessment of neurocognitive functioning, frailty, functional status, mobility, and social support is recognized as important in patient selection.[33]

Although each patient should be evaluated individually and there are no strict cutoffs for TAVR candidacy, trial data have shown that patients with very high STS scores (>15%) do not benefit from TAVR compared with standard therapy.[3] Registry data have shown that NYHA functional class III or IV symptoms, use of a transapical approach, and periprosthetic regurgitation grade 2 or higher (scale of 0 to 4) are independent predictors of death after TAVR.[34] Multivariate predictors of higher mortality rates for the TAVR group in the PARTNER 1A trial included a lower body mass index, lower preprocedure transvalvular gradient, reduced renal function, and prior vascular surgery or stent.[35] These factors should be considered before proceeding with TAVR in this patient population. TAVR-specific risk scores have been developed but need further validation.[36,37.]

The logistic EuroSCORE and the STS score incorporate many comorbidities. Before a patient is offered TAVR, these scores should be calculated and considered along with NYHA functional class, the preprocedural transvalvular gradient, renal function, prior vascular surgery or stent, adequacy of transfemoral vascular access, prior stroke, and pulmonary disease requiring supplemental oxygen. These important comorbidities may attenuate the benefit of TAVR in certain patient populations. Patients with anatomic considerations increasing the risk of SAVR, such as porcelain aorta or so-called hostile chest, may likely receive greater benefit from TAVR because the procedural risks are lower.

The 2017 ACC Expert Consensus Decision Pathway on TAVR for Adults with Aortic Stenosis outlines pre-TAVR selection and evaluation, pre-TAVR planning, TAVR imaging and assessment, and post-TAVR clinical management[38] (Fig. 12.10). Each patient considered for TAVR

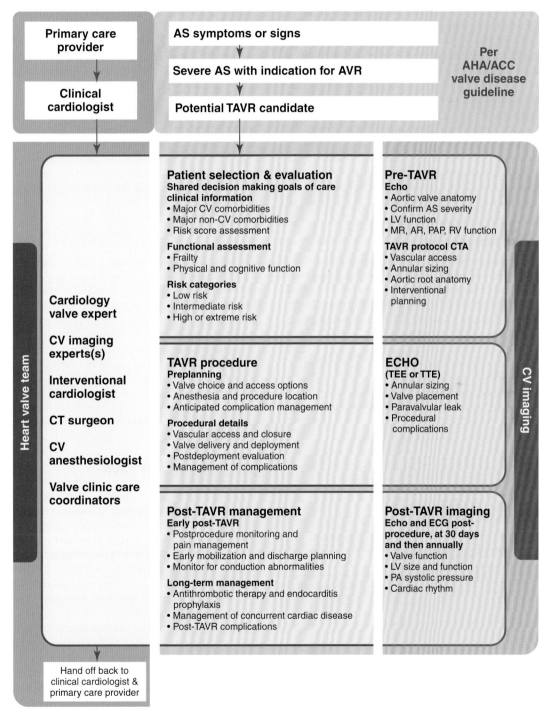

Fig. 12.10 TAVR Decision Pathway. (From Otto CM, Kumbhani DJ, Alexander KP, et al. 2017 ACC Expert Consensus decision pathway for transcatheter aortic valve replacement in the management of adults with aortic stenosis: a report of the American College of Cardiology Task Force on Clinical Expert Consensus Documents. J Am Coll Cardiol 2017;69:1313-1346.)

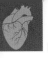

should be evaluated by a multidisciplinary and collaborative heart valve team composed of cardiologists with expertise in valvular heart disease, structural interventional cardiologists, imaging specialists, cardiovascular surgeons, cardiovascular anesthesiologists, and cardiovascular nursing professionals. Management relies on shared decision making and education of the patient, his or her family, and the referring physician, with realistic expectations about anticipated improvement in symptoms or survival (Fig. 12.11).

Transthoracic echocardiography (TTE), transesophageal echocardiography (TEE), multidetector computed tomography (MDCT), and invasive angiography are used to perform preprocedural anatomic evaluations specific to TAVR, with particular attention to aortic valve morphology and function, LV geometry, annular sizing, and aortic root measurements.[38–41] TTE, TEE, or MDCT (the gold standard) is commonly used to measure the dimensions of the aortic annulus, which determines valve size. It is imperative that some form of three-dimensional assessment of the valvar complex be performed as part of the screening process.

Assessment should include measurements of annular size and evaluate for high-risk anatomy for complications, such as annular or aortic root injury or coronary obstruction. These findings may influence the decision about whether to proceed with TAVR or the type of prosthesis (balloon expandable or self-expanding) to use.[42] Arterial access is typically assessed with invasive angiography or contrast MDCT[42,43] (Fig. 12.12).

Complications and Management

Intraprocedural complications from TAVR are usually the result of difficult vascular access, complex aortic annular and coronary anatomy, embolization, or technical intraprocedural aspects of the procedure itself. Complications include vascular injury and bleeding, stroke, valve embolization, coronary occlusion, aortic rupture, conduction disturbance, and paravalvular or central aortic regurgitation.

Postprocedural Care

Immediate postprocedural management of patients after TAVR should include postanesthesia monitoring with close attention paid to mental status as patients wake up from conscious sedation or general anesthesia. Patients should be monitored on telemetry for any signs of developing conduction disturbances. In the recovery area, the procedural access site should be checked frequently for signs of bleeding or pain. Early mobilization is critical to prevent deconditioning. Patients should be evaluated by physical or occupational therapists, or both, if necessary. A postprocedural echocardiogram should be done to check valve position and gradients, and a daily electrocardiogram should be obtained to monitor for heart block.

For pharmacologic therapy after TAVR, current guidelines recommend empiric dual antiplatelet therapy (DAPT) consisting of aspirin and clopidogrel for 6 months.[8] However, multiple studies and meta-analyses have shown that the use of aspirin monotherapy after TAVR is associated with lower rates of major bleeding compared with DAPT, with no significant difference in the rates of death, stroke, or vascular complications.[44–46]

Concern about subclinical leaflet thrombosis or hypo-attenuating leaflet thickening (HALT), often an incidental finding characterized by a thin layer of thrombus covering the aortic side of one or more leaflets, further raises the question about the need for anticoagulation after TAVR. Although anticoagulation may be a rational treatment option, few data exist on the safety and efficacy of this treatment. This is particularly important considering that TAVR patients also have a higher bleeding risk than the standard population.[47] The 2017 focused update of the AHA/ACC granted a level IIb recommendation to the use of vitamin K antagonists within the first 3 months after TAVR for patients without a high risk of bleeding.[8]

TAVR patients should be evaluated by the TAVR team 30 days after the procedure, and an echocardiogram should be done at that time to assess valve function, with a focus on increasing gradients, which may signal leaflet thrombosis. At that visit, patients should also be assessed for symptoms of heart failure, and the vascular access site should be checked. They should be advised about the importance of antibiotic prophylaxis before dental procedures. Because TAVR patients are often elderly and have multiple comorbidities, management of their other cardiac problems and promotion of a healthy lifestyle with risk factor reduction and an emphasis on physical activity should be stressed.

STATE-OF-THE-ART TAVR

More than 300,000 TAVR procedures have been performed at more than 1000 centers in more than 65 countries in the developed world. Some 55,000 of these procedures have been performed in the United States.[12.] Even so, TAVR remains a procedure in constant evolution. Multiple new TAVR devices have been developed to minimize complication rates and to simplify the procedure and patient recovery. In parallel with technology enhancements, patients have also benefited from increased operator experience, more refined case selection, and improved procedural methods.[32]

The cumulative impact of these favorable changes has resulted in a significant improvement in clinical outcomes. Comparison of mortality rates and stroke outcomes from the earliest PARTNER randomized trials (which began enrollment in 2007) with the most recent results from the Sapien 3 studies (reported in 2015 for similar-risk cohorts) indicates a reduction in 30-day mortality from 6.3% to 2.2% and a reduction in strokes from 6.7% to 2.6%.[32]

The identification of patients being considered for TAVR requires a noncompetitive and multidisciplinary team approach, as described

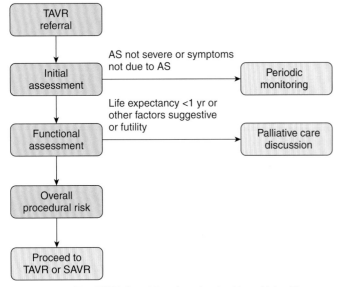

Fig. 12.11 Pre-TAVR Considerations by the Heart Valve Team.

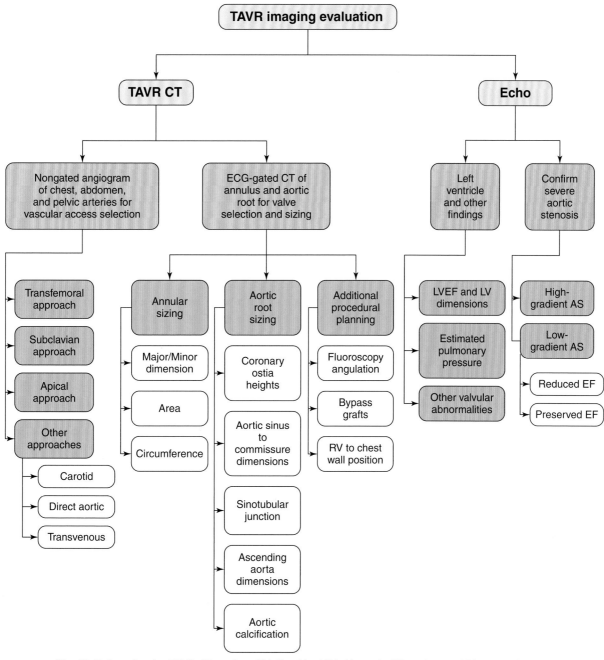

Fig. 12.12 Imaging for TAVR. (From Otto CM, Kumbhani DJ, Alexander KP, et al. 2017 ACC Expert Consensus decision pathway for transcatheter aortic valve replacement in the management of adults with aortic stenosis: a report of the American College of Cardiology Task Force on Clinical Expert Consensus Documents. J Am Coll Cardiol 2017;69:1313-1346.)

earlier. The routine use of a heart valve team approach is recommended for TAVR and is a class I indication in the AHA/ACC and the ESC guidelines.[8,48]

Looking forward, a progressive attitude to encourage optimal clinical outcomes after TAVR would favor the application of quality benchmarks. For example, an optimal quality TAVR center in the future should be able to achieve the following outcomes for high-risk AS patients: (1) all-cause mortality of approximately 1% to 3% at 30 days, depending on the patient risk profile; (2) significant strokes at 30 days in fewer than 2% of patients; (3) major vascular complications in 2% to 3%; (4) new permanent pacemakers in fewer than 10%; and (5) moderate or severe paravalvular regurgitation in fewer than 3%.

ANCILLARY DEVICES USED IN TAVR

As the TAVR procedure continues to evolve and indications expand to patients with lower-risk profiles, multiple ancillary devices have been developed to minimize procedural complications and improve outcomes.

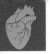
Cerebral Embolic Protection

Stroke remains a concerning complication of TAVR. Cerebral ischemic events are an independent predictor of morbidity and mortality.[49,50] The risk of thromboembolic events is highest during valve implantation.[51,52]

Several embolic protection devices have been developed to reduce the risk of neurologic events during TAVR. The only device approved in the United States is the Sentinel Cerebral Protection System (Boston Scientific), which consists of two independent filters placed in the innominate and the left carotid arteries through the right radial artery. The randomized CLaret Embolic Protection ANd TAVI - Trial (CLEAN-TAVI) study demonstrated a reduction in new cerebral lesion number and volume on diffusion-weighted magnetic resonance imaging at 2 and 7 days after TAVR with the Medtronic CoreValve when using the Sentinel Extrusion Protection Sensor (EPS).[53] Subsequently, a larger randomized, multicenter, international trial using multiple valve types (i.e., Edwards Sapien XT, Edwards Sapien 3, Medtronic CoreValve, and Medtronic Evolut) failed to demonstrate a significant reduction in new lesion volume on 30-day diffusion-weighted magnetic resonance imaging despite a 42% reduction in number of lesions. However, histopathologic analysis of the filters demonstrated debris capture in 99% of the patients. Secondary analysis showed a 63% reduction ($P = 0.05$) in stroke at 72 hours.

Based on this data set, the FDA approved the Sentinel EPS for commercial use in 2017.[54,55] Since then, the use of cerebral embolic protection devices that position filters in the carotid and innominate arteries has become more widespread during TAVR. The TriGuard 3 device (Keystone Heart, Tampa, FL) is a mesh device that is placed in the ascending aorta to deflect debris from the cerebral circulation rather than capturing it. The initial randomized trial of the TriGuard 3 demonstrated that the device was safe but did not show a significant reduction in neurologic events, although the patient sample was small (85 patients).[56] A larger multicenter, international, randomized trial is ongoing.

Although no randomized trial has demonstrated a significant reduction in stroke at 30 days as the primary end point, meta-analyses have shown that use of cerebral embolic protection devices in TAVR is associated with a lower risk of stroke, death, and major or life-threatening bleeding at 30 days.[57] Many other embolic protection devices in development aim to provide better coverage of all the cerebral vessels and have minimal interference with the TAVR delivery system.

Vascular Closure Devices

Vascular and bleeding complications remain a significant cause of morbidity and mortality after TAVR. During the early years of this procedure, surgical cutdown and open surgical closure were performed to close the large-bore access site used for valve entry. Currently, various vascular closure devices are used to achieve hemostasis after femoral artery puncture.

The Perclose ProGlide device (Abbott Vascular Devices, Redwood City, CA) is suture based and is commonly used for the preclose technique, in which two ProGlide preformed knots are advanced with the pusher and tightened to the arteriotomy to ensure adequate hemostasis.[58]

An alternative is the Manta vascular closure device (Teleflex, Morrisville, NC), which has an intraarterial footplate and an extraarterial absorbable collagen plug secured proximally by a nonabsorbable stainless steel clip that can be used to close an arteriotomy up to a 25-Fr outer diameter.[59] In the pivotal trial studying its use in patients undergoing TAVR, endovascular abdominal aortic aneurysm repair, and/or thoracic endovascular aortic aneurysm repair, the device was shown to

be safe and effective.[60] Although Manta and ProGlide have not been compared head to head, retrospective analyses have shown that Manta resulted in a significantly lower complication rate, especially for bleeding, than did ProGlide.[61]

EXPANDING CLINICAL INDICATIONS

Valve-in-Valve Procedures

The frequency of implantation of aortic and mitral bioprostheses now exceeds that of mechanical prostheses.[62] Structural deterioration of bioprosthetic valves results in hemodynamic failure (i.e., stenosis, regurgitation, or both), typically within 10 to 15 years after implantation. The novel use of transcatheter valves within failed bioprostheses (i.e., valve-in-valve procedures) has been studied[63] and is described in more detail in Chapter 27.

Bicuspid Aortic Valve Disease

Bicuspid valves account for about 20% of SAVR procedures.[64] There has been hesitancy to treat stenotic bicuspid valves with TAVR because of concerns that a more oval annulus shape, unequal leaflet size, heavy and uneven calcification of the leaflets, and calcified raphes might interfere with optimal TAVR deployment or lead to suboptimal hemodynamics with increased paravalvular regurgitation.[63,65]

Bicuspid aortic valves are often diagnosed in younger patients, raising the issue of valve durability requirements. Data from a TAVR bicuspid valve registry that included 139 patients from 12 centers in Europe supported a preliminary finding that TAVR is safe in these patients, with mortality rates of 5% at 30 days and 17.5% at 1 year.[66] However, there was a high incidence (28.4%) of postimplantation AR. Moving forward, clinical trials enrolling patients with bicuspid AS using next-generation TAVR devices will be helpful in determining the most appropriate clinical indications for this population.

Low-Flow Aortic Stenosis

Classically, patients with severe AS have a high transvalvular gradient and velocity. However, a sizeable subset of these patients has severe AS despite a low gradient and velocity because of concurrent LV systolic dysfunction (LVEF < 50%) or a low transaortic stroke volume with preserved left ventricular systolic function, or paradoxical low-flow, low-gradient (LFLG) AS.[8,67] The literature demonstrates that in classic LFLG AS with reduced LVEF it is crucial to rule out a pseudosevere AS because reduced LVEF may result in incomplete opening of the valve and lower velocities. Evaluation can be done by low-dose dobutamine stress echocardiography (Fig. 12.13). Patients with contractile reserve as demonstrated by increased stroke volume on dobutamine echocardiography and severe AS can benefit from TAVR and should undergo treatment. Patients with pseudosevere AS should be continued on medical therapy.

Data on paradoxical LFLG AS is limited, but the literature has shown that these patients have a mortality rate as high as twice that of patients with high-flow AS.[68] However, studies have demonstrated that these patients still benefit from treatment compared with medical therapy.[69] Patients with paradoxical LFLG AS are often underdiagnosed and mistakenly thought to have moderate AS because the gradients are not elevated.

The clinical approach and decision making in LFLG AS rely on integration of data from multiple sources, including hemodynamic data, echocardiography, and CT.[70] Aortic valve morphology, body surface area, and stroke volume index are parameters that can be used to determine clinical significance for patients with LFLG AS.

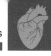

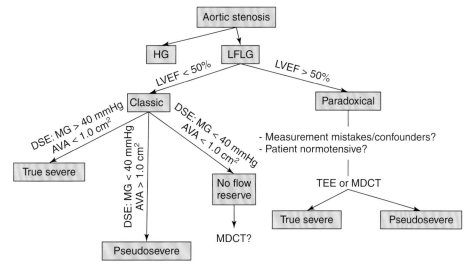

Fig. 12.13 Algorithm for the Diagnosis of Low-Flow, Low-Gradient Aortic Stenosis (AS). (From Vogelgesang A, Hasenfuss G, Jacobshagen C. Low-flow/low-gradient aortic stenosis—still a diagnostic and therapeutic challenge. Clin Cardiol 2017;40:654-659.)

Moderate Aortic Stenosis With Left Ventricular Dysfunction

Moderate AS and reduced LV ejection fraction (LVEF) constitute a clinical entity that has been proposed as a therapeutic target for TAVR. It is defined by a mean transaortic gradient between 20 and 40 mmHg and an aortic valve area between 1.0 and 1.5 cm² in patients with LVEF lower than 50%. In this population, the reduction in LVEF is not thought to be secondary to AS but rather to myocardial damage caused by ischemic conditions or nonischemic, nonvalvular cardiomyopathies.[71]

Because moderate AS may contribute significantly to increased overall LV afterload in these cases, TAVR has been considered as a treatment option to unload the LV and improve symptoms.[71] This is being investigated in the Transcatheter Aortic Valve Replacement to UNload the Left Ventricle in Patients with ADvanced Heart Failure (TAVR UNLOAD) trial (NCT02661451), which is an international, multicenter, randomized, open-label, clinical trial comparing TAVR using the Edwards Sapien 3 valve in addition to optimal heart failure therapy with optimal heart failure therapy alone in patients with moderate AS and reduced LVEF.[72]

Asymptomatic Severe Aortic Stenosis

Although current guidelines recommend SAVR or TAVR for patients with severe symptomatic AS as a class I indication,[8] as many as 50% of patients with severe AS report no symptoms at the time of diagnosis.[73] The optimal timing of intervention in these patients is unclear and somewhat controversial. A strategy of watchful waiting can be problematic because of the often vague nature of symptoms in elderly, sedentary patients and the sometimes variable and unpredictable nature of AS progression. The 1% to 1.5% risk of sudden cardiac death of patients with severe AS is also worrisome.

Exercise stress testing may be used as an adjunct to determine exercise-induced symptoms or an abnormal blood pressure response in the setting of severe AS.[74] Retrospective data suggest that the strategy of early aortic valve replacement is associated with improved survival in asymptomatic patients.[75,76] However, there are no randomized trial data evaluating watchful waiting versus aortic valve replacement. This is an area of active investigation, including the Evaluation of Transcatheter Aortic Valve Replacement Compared to SurveilLance for

Patients with AsYmptomatic Severe Aortic Stenosis (EARLY TAVR) trial (NCT03042104).

ALTERNATIVES TO TAVR

Surgical Aortic Valve Replacement

SAVR should be considered for all patients regardless of age. Survival rates at 1, 2, and 5 years among selected patients older than 80 years of age undergoing SAVR have been reported as 87%, 78%, and 68%, respectively.[77] It is recommended that the assessment of all patients being considered for TAVR include a multidisciplinary team approach that includes cardiac surgery consultation to ensure that SAVR is one of the options considered.

Balloon Aortic Valvuloplasty

Historically, indications for BAV have included hemodynamically significant AS and any of the following: as a bridge to SAVR in hemodynamically unstable patients; increased perioperative risk (STS score > 15); age in the late 80s or 90s and patient preference for an aortic valvuloplasty over SAVR; severe comorbidities (e.g., porcelain aorta, severe lung disease) for which the surgeon prefers not to operate; and severe neuromuscular or arthritic conditions that would limit the patient's ability to undergo postoperative rehabilitation.[78] TAVR can now be performed in most of the patients with these conditions.

BAV may be undertaken to assess the therapeutic response of a reduction in aortic gradient in borderline patients, often with multiple comorbidities, to assess symptomatic improvement before consideration of definitive TAVR intervention.[79] BAV can be used in patients with symptomatic severe AS who require urgent noncardiac surgery. BAV is typically reserved for hemodynamically unstable patients as a bridge to a more definitive treatment of AS, for patients with a predicted survival time from noncardiac causes measured in weeks to months, and for patients who have a contraindication to TAVR, for whom relief of the aortic obstruction will improve quality of life.

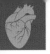
CONCLUSIONS

Aortic valve replacement by TAVR or SAVR in patients with severe AS undoubtedly improves symptoms and survival. Over the past decade, TAVR has emerged as a safe, effective, and well-tolerated alternative to SAVR in patients at all levels of surgical risk. TAVR has become widely recognized as equivalent or superior to open surgery. Newer iterations of TAVR devices, lower-profile delivery systems, and increased operator experience have substantially reduced complications pertaining to vascular access, stroke, paravalvular regurgitation, and need for permanent pacemaker placement.

As TAVR devices and technologies continue to evolve, clinical research in this area has become focused on novel applications of this technology to treat a variety of expanding indications. Ongoing investigation promises to further knowledge about the utility, safety, and efficacy of TAVR, with the hope of reducing risk and improving quality of life for patients with aortic valve disease.

REFERENCES

1. Makkar RR, Fontana GP, Jilaihawi H, et al. Transcatheter aortic-valve replacement for inoperable severe aortic stenosis. N Engl J Med 2012; 366:1696-1704.
2. Villablanca PA, Mathew V, Thourani VH, et al. A meta-analysis and meta-regression of long-term outcomes of transcatheter versus surgical aortic valve replacement for severe aortic stenosis. Int J Cardiol 2016;225: 234-243.
3. Leon MB, Smith CR, Mack M, et al. Transcatheter aortic-valve implantation for aortic stenosis in patients who cannot undergo surgery. N Engl J Med 2010;363:1597-1607.
4. Smith CR, Leon MB, Mack MJ, et al. Transcatheter versus surgical aortic-valve replacement in high-risk patients. N Engl J Med 2011;364: 2187-2198.
5. Leon MB, Smith CR, Mack MJ, et al. Transcatheter or surgical aortic-valve replacement in intermediate-risk patients. N Engl J Med 2016;374: 1609-1620.
6. Thourani VH, Kodali S, Makkar RR, et al. Transcatheter aortic valve replacement versus surgical valve replacement in intermediate-risk patients: a propensity score analysis. Lancet 2016;387:2218-2225.
7. Otto CM, Mickel MC, Kennedy JW, et al. Three-year outcome after balloon aortic valvuloplasty. Insights into prognosis of valvular aortic stenosis. Circulation 1994;89:642-650.
8. Nishimura RA, Otto CM, Bonow RO, et al. 2017 AHA/ACC focused update of the 2014 AHA/ACC guideline for the management of patients with valvular heart disease: a report of the American College of Cardiology/American Heart Association Task Force on Clinical Practice Guidelines. Circulation 2017;135:e1159–e1195.
9. Andersen HR, Knudsen LL, Hasenkam JM. Transluminal implantation of artificial heart valves. Description of a new expandable aortic valve and initial results with implantation by catheter technique in closed chest pigs. Eur Heart J 1992;13:704-708.
10. Cribier A, Eltchaninoff H, Bash A, et al. Percutaneous transcatheter implantation of an aortic valve prosthesis for calcific aortic stenosis: first human case description. Circulation 2002;106:3006-3008.
11. Webb JG, Chandavimol M, Thompson CR, et al. Percutaneous aortic valve implantation retrograde from the femoral artery. Circulation 2006;113:842-850.
12. Eleid MF, Holmes DRJ. Transcatheter aortic valve replacement: state of the art and future directions. Annu Rev Med 2017;68:15-28.
13. Grover FL, Vemulapalli S, Carroll JD, et al. 2016 annual report of the Society of Thoracic Surgeons/American College of Cardiology Transcatheter Valve Therapy registry. J Am Coll Cardiol 2017;69:1215-1230.
14. Mahtta D, Elgendy IY, Bavry AA. From CoreValve to Evolut Pro: reviewing the journey of self-expanding transcatheter aortic valves. Cardiol Ther 2017;6:183-192.
15. Reardon MJ, Feldman TE, Meduri CU, et al. Two-year outcomes after transcatheter aortic valve replacement with mechanical vs self-expanding valves: the REPRISE III randomized clinical trial. JAMA Cardiol 2019;4:223-229.
16. Mack MJ, Leon MB, Smith CR, et al. 5-year outcomes of transcatheter aortic valve replacement or surgical aortic valve replacement for high surgical risk patients with aortic stenosis (PARTNER 1): a randomised controlled trial. Lancet 2015;385:2477-2484.
17. Kapadia SR, Leon MB, Makkar RR, et al. 5-year outcomes of transcatheter aortic valve replacement compared with standard treatment for patients with inoperable aortic stenosis (PARTNER 1): a randomised controlled trial. Lancet 2015;385:2485-2491.
18. Adams DH, Popma JJ, Reardon MJ, et al. Transcatheter aortic-valve replacement with a self-expanding prosthesis. N Engl J Med 2014;370: 1790-1798.
19. Thourani VH, Kodali S, Makkar RR, et al. Transcatheter aortic valve replacement versus surgical valve replacement in intermediate-risk patients: a propensity score analysis. Lancet 2016;387:2218-2225.
20. Kodali S, Thourani VH, White J, et al. Early clinical and echocardiographic outcomes after SAPIEN 3 transcatheter aortic valve replacement in inoperable, high-risk and intermediate-risk patients with aortic stenosis. Eur Heart J 2016;37:2252-2262.
21. Reardon MJ, Van Mieghem NM, Popma JJ, et al. Surgical or transcatheter aortic-valve replacement in intermediate-risk patients. N Engl J Med 2017;376:1321-1331.
22. Feldman TE, Reardon MJ, Rajagopal V, et al. Effect of mechanically expanded vs self-expanding transcatheter aortic valve replacement on mortality and major adverse clinical events in high-risk patients with aortic stenosis: the REPRISE III randomized clinical trial. JAMA 2018; 319:27-37.
23. Makkar RR, Fontana G, Jilaihawi H, et al. Possible subclinical leaflet thrombosis in bioprosthetic aortic valves. N Engl J Med 2015;373: 2015-2024.
24. Marwan M, Mekkhala N, Goller M, et al. Leaflet thrombosis following transcatheter aortic valve implantation. J Cardiovasc Comput Tomogr 2018;12(1):8-13.
25. Sondergaard L, Rodes-Cabau J, Hans-Peter Linke A, et al. Transcatheter aortic valve replacement with a repositionable self-expanding prosthesis: the PORTICO-I trial 1-year outcomes. J Am Coll Cardiol 2018;72: 2859-2867.
26. Mack MJ, Leon MB, Thourani VH, et al. Transcatheter aortic-valve replacement with a balloon-expandable valve in low-risk patients. N Engl J Med 2019;380:1695-1705.
27. Popma JJ, Deeb GM, Yakubov SJ, et al. Transcatheter aortic-valve replacement with a self-expanding valve in low-risk patients. N Engl J Med 2019; 380:1706-1715.
28. Reference deleted in review.
29. Kheiri B, Osman M, Bakhit A, et al. Meta-analysis of transcatheter aortic valve replacement in low-risk patients. Am J Med 2020;133(2): e38-e41.
30. Suradi HS, Hijazi ZM. TAVR update: contemporary data from the UK TAVI and US TVT registries. Glob Cardiol Sci Pract 2015; 2015:21.
31. Ludman PF, Moat N, de Belder MA, et al. Transcatheter aortic valve implantation in the United Kingdom: temporal trends, predictors of outcome, and 6-year follow-up: a report from the UK Transcatheter Aortic Valve Implantation (TAVI) Registry, 2007 to 2012. Circulation 2015;131:1181-1190.
32. Vahl TP, Kodali SK, Leon MB. Transcatheter Aortic valve replacement 2016: a modern-day "Through the Looking-Glass" adventure. J Am Coll Cardiol 2016;67:1472-1487.
33. Green P, Woglom AE, Genereux P, et al. The impact of frailty status on survival after transcatheter aortic valve replacement in older adults with severe aortic stenosis: a single-center experience. JACC Cardiovasc Interv 2012;5:974-981.
34. Gilard M, Eltchaninoff H, Iung B, et al. Registry of transcatheter aortic-valve implantation in high-risk patients. N Engl J Med 2012;366: 1705-1715.

35. Kodali SK, Williams MR, Smith CR, et al. Two-year outcomes after transcatheter or surgical aortic-valve replacement. N Engl J Med 2012;366: 1686-1695.
36. Arsalan M, Weferling M, Hecker F, et al. TAVI risk scoring using established versus new scoring systems: role of the new STS/ACC model. EuroIntervention 2018;13(13):1520-1526.
37. Grossman Y, Barbash IM, Fefer P, et al. Addition of albumin to traditional risk score improved prediction of mortality in individuals undergoing transcatheter aortic valve replacement. J Am Geriatr Soc 2017;65:2413-2417.
38. Otto CM, Kumbhani DJ, Alexander KP, et al. 2017 ACC Expert Consensus decision pathway for transcatheter aortic valve replacement in the management of adults with aortic stenosis: a report of the American College of Cardiology Task Force on Clinical Expert Consensus Documents. J Am Coll Cardiol 2017;69:1313-1346.
39. Moss RR, Ivens E, Pasupati S, et al. Role of echocardiography in percutaneous aortic valve implantation. JACC Cardiovasc Imaging 2008;1:15-24.
40. Hahn RT. Use of imaging for procedural guidance during transcatheter aortic valve replacement. Curr Opin Cardiol 2013;28:512-517.
41. Nguyen G, Leipsic J. Cardiac computed tomography and computed tomography angiography in the evaluation of patients prior to transcatheter aortic valve implantation. Curr Opin Cardiol 2013;28:497-504.
42. Webb JG, Wood DA. Current status of transcatheter aortic valve replacement. J Am Coll Cardiol 2012;60:483-492.
43. Litmanovich DE, Ghersin E, Burke DA, et al. Imaging in Transcatheter Aortic Valve Replacement (TAVR): role of the radiologist. Insights Imaging 2014;5:123-145.
44. Stabile E, Pucciarelli A, Cota L, et al. SAT-TAVI (single antiplatelet therapy for TAVI) study: a pilot randomized study comparing double to single antiplatelet therapy for transcatheter aortic valve implantation. Int J Cardiol 2014;174:624-627.
45. Rodes-Cabau J, Masson J-B, Welsh RC, et al. Aspirin versus aspirin plus clopidogrel as antithrombotic treatment following transcatheter aortic valve replacement with a balloon-expandable valve: the ARTE (Aspirin Versus Aspirin + Clopidogrel Following Transcatheter Aortic Valve Implantation) randomized clinical trial. JACC Cardiovasc Interv 2017; 10:1357-1365.
46. Alrifai A, Soud M, Kabach A, et al. Dual antiplatelet therapy versus single antiplatelet therapy after transaortic valve replacement: meta-analysis. Cardiovasc Revasc Med 2018;19:47-52.
47. Rashid HN, Brown AJ, McCormick LM, et al. Subclinical leaflet thrombosis in transcatheter aortic valve replacement detected by multidetector computed tomography—a review of current evidence. Circ J 2018;82: 1735-1742.
48. Falk V, Baumgartner H, Bax JJ, et al. 2017 ESC/EACTS Guidelines for the management of valvular heart disease. Eur J Cardiothorac Surg 2017;52: 616-664.
49. Eggebrecht H, Schmermund A, Voigtlander T, et al. Risk of stroke after transcatheter aortic valve implantation (TAVI): a meta-analysis of 10,037 published patients. EuroIntervention 2012;8:129-138.
50. Tchetche D, Farah B, Misuraca L, et al. Cerebrovascular events post-transcatheter aortic valve replacement in a large cohort of patients: a FRANCE-2 registry substudy. JACC Cardiovasc Interv 2014;7: 1138-1145.
51. Van Belle E, Hengstenberg C, Lefevre T, et al. Cerebral embolism during transcatheter aortic valve replacement: the BRAVO-3 MRI study. J Am Coll Cardiol 2016;68:589-599.
52. Kapadia S, Agarwal S, Miller DC, et al. Insights into timing, risk factors, and outcomes of stroke and transient ischemic attack after transcatheter aortic valve replacement in the PARTNER Trial (Placement of Aortic Transcatheter Valves). Circ Cardiovasc Interv 2016;9.
53. Haussig S, Mangner N, Dwyer MG, et al. Effect of a cerebral protection device on brain lesions following transcatheter aortic valve implantation in patients with severe aortic stenosis: the CLEAN-TAVI randomized clinical trial. JAMA 2016;316:592-601.
54. Kapadia SR, Kodali S, Makkar R, et al. Protection against cerebral embolism during transcatheter aortic valve replacement. J Am Coll Cardiol 2017;69:367-377.
55. Seeger J, Gonska B, Otto M, et al. Cerebral embolic protection during transcatheter aortic valve replacement significantly reduces death and stroke compared with unprotected procedures. JACC Cardiovasc Interv 2017;10:2297-2303.
56. Lansky AJ, Schofer J, Tchetche D, et al. A prospective randomized evaluation of the TriGuard HDH embolic DEFLECTion device during transcatheter aortic valve implantation: results from the DEFLECT III trial. Eur Heart J 2015;36:2070-2078.
57. Ndunda PM, Vindhyal MR, Muutu TM, Fanari Z. Clinical outcomes of sentinel cerebral protection system use during transcatheter aortic valve replacement: a systematic review and meta-analysis. Cardiovasc Revasc Med 2019 Apr 25. pii: S1553-8389(19)30257-X. doi: 10.1016/j.carrev.2019.04.023. [Epub ahead of print]
58. Maniotis C, Andreou C, Karalis I, et al. A systematic review on the safety of Prostar XL versus ProGlide after TAVR and EVAR. Cardiovasc Revasc Med 2017;18:145-150.
59. De Palma R, Settergren M, Ruck A, et al. Impact of percutaneous femoral arteriotomy closure using the MANTA(TM) device on vascular and bleeding complications after transcatheter aortic valve replacement. Catheter Cardiovasc Interv 2018;92:954-961.
60. Wood DA, Krajcer Z, Sathananthan J, et al. Pivotal clinical study to evaluate the safety and effectiveness of the MANTA percutaneous vascular closure device. Circ Cardiovasc Interv 2019;12:e007258.
61. Moriyama N, Lindstrom L, Laine M. Propensity-matched comparison of vascular closure devices after transcatheter aortic valve replacement using MANTA versus ProGlide. EuroIntervention 2019;14:e1558–e1565.
62. Brennan JM, Edwards FH, Zhao Y, et al. Long-term safety and effectiveness of mechanical versus biologic aortic valve prostheses in older patients: results from the Society of Thoracic Surgeons Adult Cardiac Surgery National Database. Circulation 2013;127:1647-1655.
63. Gurvitch R, Cheung A, Ye J, et al. Transcatheter valve-in-valve implantation for failed surgical bioprosthetic valves. J Am Coll Cardiol 2011;58: 2196-2209.
64. Roberts WC, Ko JM. Frequency by decades of unicuspid, bicuspid, and tricuspid aortic valves in adults having isolated aortic valve replacement for aortic stenosis, with or without associated aortic regurgitation. Circulation 2005;111:920-925.
65. Patel A, Leon MB. Transcatheter aortic valve replacement in patients with bicuspid aortic valves. J Thorac Dis 2018;10:S3568–S3572.
66. Mylotte D, Lefevre T, Sondergaard L, et al. Transcatheter aortic valve replacement in bicuspid aortic valve disease. J Am Coll Cardiol 2014;64: 2330-2339.
67. Vogelgesang A, Hasenfuss G, Jacobshagen C. Low-flow/low-gradient aortic stenosis—still a diagnostic and therapeutic challenge. Clin Cardiol 2017; 40:654-659.
68. Fischer-Rasokat U, Renker M, Liebetrau C, et al. 1-Year survival after TAVR of patients with low-flow, low-gradient and high-gradient aortic valve stenosis in matched study populations. JACC Cardiovasc Interv 2019;12: 752-763.
69. Herrmann HC, Pibarot P, Hueter I, et al. Predictors of mortality and outcomes of therapy in low-flow severe aortic stenosis: a Placement of Aortic Transcatheter Valves (PARTNER) trial analysis. Circulation 2013;127: 2316-2326.
70. Magne J, Mohty D. Paradoxical low-flow, low-gradient severe aortic stenosis: a distinct disease entity. Heart 2015;101:993-995.
71. Spitzer E, Ren B, Kroon H, et al. Moderate aortic stenosis and reduced left ventricular ejection fraction: current evidence and challenges ahead. Front Cardiovasc Med 2018;5:111.
72. Spitzer E, Van Mieghem NM, Pibarot P, et al. Rationale and design of the Transcatheter Aortic Valve Replacement to UNload the Left ventricle in patients with ADvanced heart failure (TAVR UNLOAD) trial. Am Heart J 2016;182:80-88.
73. Genereux P, Stone GW, O'Gara PT, et al. Natural history, diagnostic approaches, and therapeutic strategies for patients with asymptomatic severe aortic stenosis. J Am Coll Cardiol 2016;67:2263-2288.
74. Rafique AM, Biner S, Ray I, et al. Meta-analysis of prognostic value of stress testing in patients with asymptomatic severe aortic stenosis. Am J Cardiol 2009;104:972-977.

75. Campo J, Tsoris A, Kruse J, et al. Prognosis of Severe asymptomatic aortic stenosis with and without surgery. Ann Thorac Surg 2019;108:74-79.

76. Lindman BR, Dweck MR, Lancellotti P, et al. Management of asymptomatic severe aortic stenosis: evolving concepts in timing of valve replacement. JACC Cardiovasc Imaging 2019.

77. Varadarajan P, Kapoor N, Bansal RC, Pai RG. Survival in elderly patients with severe aortic stenosis is dramatically improved by aortic valve replacement: results from a cohort of 277 patients aged > or =80 years. Eur J Cardiothorac Surg 2006;30:722-727.

78. Hara H, Pedersen WR, Ladich E, et al. Percutaneous balloon aortic valvuloplasty revisited: time for a renaissance? Circulation 2007;115:e344-e338.

79. Keeble TR, Khokhar A, Akhtar MM, et al. Percutaneous balloon aortic valvuloplasty in the era of transcatheter aortic valve implantation: a narrative review. Open Heart 2016;3:e000421.

80. Abdel-Wahab M, Mehilli, J, Frerker, C, et al. Comparison of balloon-expandable vs self-expandable valves in patients undergoing transcatheter aortic valve replacement: the CHOICE randomized clinical trial. JAMA 2014;311(15):1503-1514.

81. Thyregod HGH, Steinbruchel, DA, Ihlemann N, et al. Transcatheter versus surgical aortic valve replacement in patients with severe aortic valve stenosis: 1-year results from the all-comers NOTION randomized clinical trial. J Amer Coll Cardiol 2015;65(20):2184-2194.

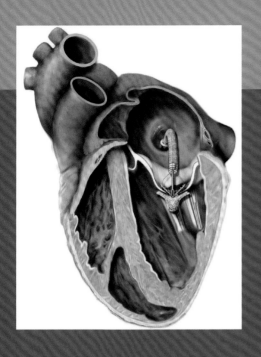

第13章
经导管主动脉瓣置换术的影像评估

　　经导管主动脉瓣置换术是治疗主动脉瓣重度狭窄患者的新兴介入技术，自2002年法国医师Cribier成功实施第一例经导管主动脉瓣置换术以来，这种基于微创介入技术的瓣膜置换术在全球蓬勃发展，目前已有超过10万例主动脉瓣重度狭窄患者因此受益。有别于传统外科瓣膜置换术，经导管主动脉瓣置换术因其"非直视"的手术特点，术前影像学评估对于筛选患者、了解主动脉根部解剖毗邻、人工瓣环型号的选择及规划入路极为重要。有效而准确的术前影像学评估可减低术中并发症发生率、提高手术成功率，是保证经导管主动脉瓣置换术顺利完成的关键。在本章中，作者首先对经导管主动脉瓣置换术的主要影像学评估方法，包括超声心动图、CT及MRI的各自优势、评估重点进行了总结，引导临床医师学会挑选合适的"武器"对患者进行综合且全面的评估；而后作者详细阐述了经导管主动脉瓣置换术的术前影像评估重点和操作流程，主要围绕主动脉瓣环与主动脉根部评估和血管入路评估；最后作者简要点明了围手术期和术后影像学方面所需关注的重点，为经导管主动脉瓣置换术保驾护航。整个章节全面细致、深入浅出、贴合临床实际操作，为经导管主动脉瓣置换术影像评估初学者搭建了一条高效学习的快车道。

王墨扬　赵庆豪

Imaging Assessment for Transcatheter Aortic Valve Replacement

James Lee, Paul Schoenhagen, Milind Desai

CHAPTER OUTLINE

KEY POINTS

- Accurate annular sizing is critical for valve selection and minimizing complications during the performance of transcatheter aortic valve replacement (TAVR).
- Electrocardiogram (ECG)-gated computed tomographic (CT) angiography before TAVR is an integral part of the preprocedural evaluation of the aortoannular complex for valve sizing and mitigation of complications.
- CT angiography before TAVR plays an important role in the evaluation of vascular access, potential vascular access complications, and nonstandard implantation routes.
- When CT angiography is not possible, alternative imaging options exist but should be performed at imaging centers of excellence that have an understanding of the specific needs of the structural heart disease proceduralist.

- Periprocedural guidance of TAVR replies primarily on fluoroscopy and echocardiography to assist with device delivery for the assessment of immediate catastrophic complications.
- Longitudinal postprocedural monitoring of TAVR focuses on an echocardiographic evaluation of paravalvular aortic regurgitation, valve migration, and valve degeneration, although increasingly ECG-gated CT angiography is used for evaluation of valve thrombosis.
- The unknown long-term durability of current-generation TAVR valves is an area of interest as implantation expands to lower-risk cohorts, and the ideal frequency of imaging surveillance is unclear.
- Dedicated imagers with expertise and training in structural heart disease interventions should perform the preprocedural imaging assessment of TAVR.

Since its inception, transcatheter aortic valve replacement (TAVR) has been at the forefront of technologic innovation. Its development and widespread adoption has relied on advances in interventional cardiology and cardiac imaging. From the first clinical TAVR implantation in humans by Criber and colleagues in 2002 as a bailout procedure for a patient with a bicuspid aortic valve and low-flow, low-gradient (LFLG) severe aortic stenosis (AS),[1] TAVR has pushed the limits of cardiology and its imaging techniques. Although TAVR is still performed on an urgent or emergent basis, the field has moved dramatically forward, and at many centers, it is widely accepted and routinely performed in the outpatient setting with a minimal hospital stay.[2] Currently, less than 10% of cases are done on an urgent or emergent basis, and registry data suggest outcomes are worse when TAVR is performed under duress.[3]

The successful move toward scheduled outpatient procedures has been facilitated by thoughtful and deliberate preprocedural planning. Central to this process is good-quality imaging, and what initially began as a small cottage industry of imaging specialists has now blossomed into the new field of multimodality structural and interventional imaging. This has been made possible by refinements in transcatheter technologies and the maturation of modern imaging techniques such as three-dimensional (3D) echocardiography, ECG-gated multidetector computed tomography (MDCT), and cardiac magnetic resonance imaging (CMR). The integration of these specialists into the multidisciplinary heart team has been critical for the growth and success of transcatheter therapies such as TAVR and has highlighted the importance of a collaborative approach to the complex decision making and problem solving often required for these cases.

PREPROCEDURAL CARDIAC IMAGING

General Principles

Many large, randomized clinical trials have been performed for TAVR therapy, and their outcomes are discussed in detail in Chapter 12. Relevant highlights of some of the major trials and their imaging implications are discussed in this chapter.

The first major multicenter trial for TAVR with a surgical comparison was the Placement of Aortic Transcatheter Valves (PARTNER I) trial, which studied an early-generation balloon-expandable transcatheter bioprosthetic valve.[4] At the time of the study, valve sizing was based on the transthoracic echocardiography (TTE) assessment of the aortic annulus. In this trial, although TAVR compared favorably with surgical aortic valve replacement (SAVR), the overall mortality rate was high, with many of the adverse events driven by paravalvular aortic regurgitation and vascular access complications.[5] As seen in Fig. 13.1, at 2 years after the procedure, paravalvular aortic regurgitation was proportionally related to increased mortality.[6] These adverse outcomes identified specific targets for improvement and have become a major focus of innovation for new TAVR related technologies. It is notable then, that the parallel CoreValve US Pivotal trial, which evaluated a self-expanding nitinol bioprosthetic TAVR valve, incorporated the routine use of MDCT to visualize the aortic annulus, thoracic vasculature, and iliofemoral vasculature. Perhaps due to large early-generation delivery

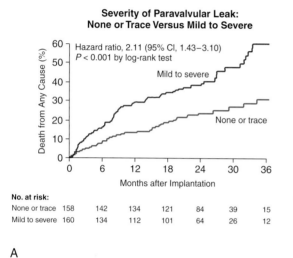

A

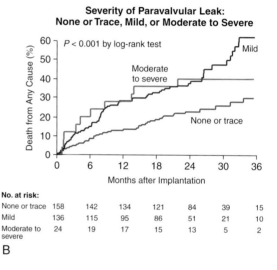

B

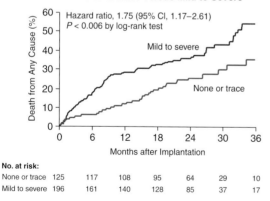

C

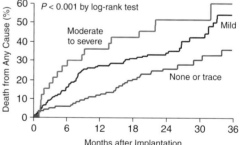

D

Fig. 13.1 Relationship of Aortic Regurgitation and All-Cause Mortality in the Placement of Aortic Transcatheter Valves (PARTNER I) Trial. In the 2-year follow-up of the PARTNER I trial, any paravalvular or total aortic regurgitation after TAVR was associated with an increase in late mortality (hazard ratio = 2.11, 95% CI: 1.43–3.10, $P < 0.001$). (A) Death from any cause for mild or greater PVL. (B) Death from any cause with PVL stratified by none or trace, mild, or moderate to severe. (C) Death from any cause for mild or greater total aortic regurgitation. (D) Death from any cause with total aortic regurgitation stratified by none or trace, mild, or moderate to severe. These data have spurred innovation for newer-generation devices and improved imaging for determination of device sizing. (From Kodali SK, Williams MR, Smith CR, et al. Two-year outcomes after transcatheter or surgical aortic-valve replacement. N Engl J Med 2012;366:1686-1695.)

sheaths, vascular access complications were still high. However, rates of moderate or severe paravalvular regurgitation were only 6.1% compared with the 12.2% seen PARTNER I,[7] which may potentially be attributed to the integrative use of MDCT for annular measurements. Due to clinical trial data and increasing evidence of the value of accurate annular sizing, all modern TAVR trials primarily use routine aortic annulus sizing performed with MDCT, although transesophageal echocardiography (TEE) or CMR is sometimes used in selected cases.

Despite improvements in TAVR, the importance of addressing paravalvular aortic regurgitation continues to be important. Data from an intermediate-risk TAVR cohort (Fig. 13.2) showed that although rates of moderate to severe paravalvular regurgitation were overall lower at only 3.7%, mortality rates continue to be driven by larger amounts of aortic regurgitation.[8] Given the continued importance of reducing paravalvular aortic regurgitation, technology continues to advance, with some of the newest-generation TAVR valves under

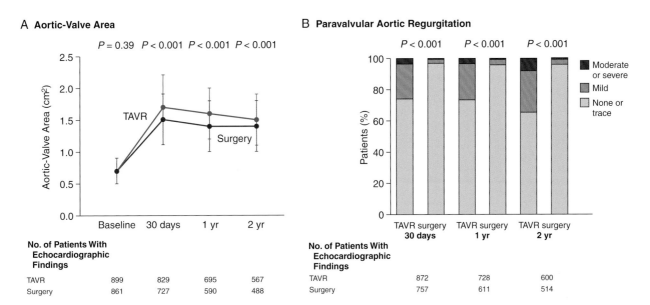

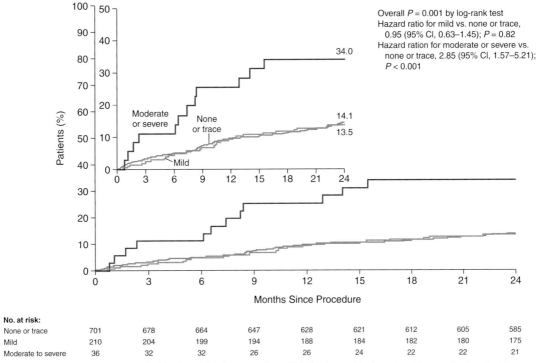

Fig. 13.2 Echocardiographic Findings for Intermediate-Risk Patients Undergoing Transcatheter Aortic Valve Replacement *(TAVR).* (A) Larger effective aortic valve area calculated by echocardiography in patients undergoing transcatheter aortic valve replacement (TAVR) vs. surgical aortic valve replacement (SAVR). (B) Presence and degree of paravalvular aortic regurgitation is greater in TAVR vs. SAVR at 30 days, 1 year, and 2 years. (C) In the intermediate risk TAVR population, moderate or greater PVL was associated with worse outcomes at 2 years (hazard ratio= 2.85, 95% CI: 1.57–5.21, *P* < 0.001). (From Leon MB, Smith CR, Mack MJ, et al. Transcatheter or surgical aortic-valve replacement in intermediate-risk patients. N Engl J Med 2016;374:1609-1620.)

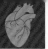

TABLE 13.1 Imaging Techniques Used for Preprocedural Planning of Transcatheter Aortic Valve Replacement.

Imaging Technique	Advantages	Limitations
3D transesophageal echocardiography	Portability No ionizing radiation Excellent temporal resolution Ability to perform live imaging	Semi-invasive Operator dependent Limited by available acoustic windows
Electrocardiogram-gated computed tomography	Rapid acquisition High spatial resolution Ability to perform 4D cine images Large field of view imaged in a single acquisition (e.g., heart, peripheral vasculature) Relatively operator independent	Nephrotoxic iodinated contrast Ionizing radiation exposure Relatively low temporal resolution Inability to do live imaging
Cardiovascular magnetic resonance imaging	No ionizing radiation High spatial resolution High temporal resolution	Time-intensive acquisition and processing Operator-dependent image aquisition Contraindications related to pacemakers, defibrillators Risk of nephrogenic systemic fibrosis in renal failure Suboptimal for assessment of calcific atherosclerosis Limited ability for live imaging

investigation reporting less than 1% rates of moderate or greater paravalvular regurgitation.[9,10] Although outcomes from TAVR are improving due to better operator experience and better imaging and technology, complications arising during TAVR are swift and frequently catastrophic.[11] This underlies the need for comprehensive preprocedural planning for TAVR using an integrative, multimodality imaging approach that uses the unique advantages of each imaging modality (Table 13.1).

Echocardiography

Echocardiography is the foundation of imaging for valvular heart disease. It is widely available, is cost-effective, and has years of validation regarding its use for diagnosis, staging, and prognostication.[12,13] Its high temporal resolution and tightly integrated use of Doppler echocardiography often makes echocardiography the ideal tool to evaluate valvular pathology. For the complex patients who are often referred for TAVR, the optimal use of echocardiography requires a nuanced understanding of the guideline-based evaluation of AS.[14-16] Echocardiography also provides interrogation of physiologic parameters such as diastolic function and right ventricular function, which may be helpful for patient selection and prognostication.[17,18] Beyond a standard evaluation, echocardiography continues to drive innovation with continually improving image quality and innovative technologies such as strain and 3D echocardiography, which continue to improve our understanding of valve physiology and pathology.

However, the minimally invasive approach of TAVR lacks the exposure and visualization of a traditional operative field; and echocardiography by itself often is insufficient for comprehensive preprocedural planning.[4-6,19] As clinical experience with TAVR has increased and transcatheter procedures have become more complex, it has become clear that inadequate planning before TAVR can increase complications such as suboptimal valve deployment, coronary obstruction, aortic injury, heart block, and embolization of the valve prosthesis.[20] Many of these complications (Table 13.2) can be predicted and mitigated by the use of supplemental imaging for patient selection, preprocedural planning, and periprocedural decision making.[21,22]

Computed Tomography

A multimodality approach to imaging is used for TAVR (Fig. 13.3). Integration of MDCT into TAVR clinical trials vastly increased understanding of the aortoannular complex, specific preprocedural planning needs, and potential surgical complications. Table 13.3 shows the checklist of imaging components that are routinely evaluated before TAVR. The standardized imaging pathway, which highlights integration of MDCT, was made possible by technologic advances in image acquisition and postprocessing that were initially developed for coronary computed tomographic angiography but then adapted to the planning of transcatheter therapies for structural heart disease therapies.

Most modern MDCT scanners have the required capabilities of ECG-synchronized acquisition and high spatial resolution that

TABLE 13.2 Transcatheter Aortic Valve Replacement Complications Mitigated by Imaging.

Risk Characteristics	Specific Issue	Complications
Valve deployment	High deployment Deep deployment	Valve embolization Heart block
Valve sizing	Valve undersized Valve oversized	Valve embolization Heart block Annular rupture Coronary occlusion
Annular characteristics	Long leaflets Low coronary ostia Highly eccentric annulus Eccentric calcifications	Coronary occlusion Coronary occlusion Misclassification of aortic stenosis severity Annular rupture Heart block Paravalvular leak Coronary occlusion
Vascular characteristics	Tortuosity Stenosis Calcification Dissection	Difficulty advancing prosthesis, dissection, vessel rupture

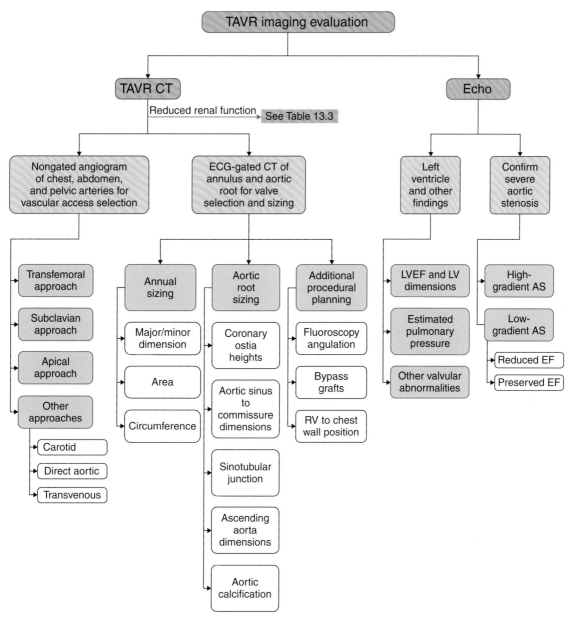

Fig. 13.3 Imaging Evaluation Before Transcatheter Aortic Valve Replacement *(TAVR)*. Imaging for the preprocedural planning for transcatheter aortic valve replacement starts with an initial evaluation with echo-cardiography to confirm the severity of aortic stenosis and assess elements of myocardial function and structure. Most patients who can receive iodinated contrast should undergo computed tomography *(CT)* angiography. Although protocols vary by vendor, this typically includes an electrocardiogram *(ECG)*-gated scan of the heart and aortic root and a nongated scan of the peripheral vasculature of the chest, abdomen, and pelvis. Alternative strategies can be employed for patients who cannot receive iodinated contrast by physicians who have expertise in other imaging modalities such as magnetic resonance imaging *(MRI)*. *AS,* Aortic stenosis; *EF,* ejection fraction; *LV,* left ventricular; (From Otto CM, Kumbhani DJ, Alexander KP, et al. 2017 ACC expert consensus decision pathway for transcatheter aortic valve replacement in the management of adults with aortic stenosis: a report of the American College of Cardiology Task Force on Clinical Expert Consensus Documents. J Am Coll Cardiol 2017;69:1313-1346.)

allow images to be reconstructed in any plane with sharp delinea-tion of various cardiac structures throughout the cardiac cycle. Fig. 13.4 demonstrates the technique of ECG gating and some of the anatomic and functional information that can extracted from the data sets, such as assessments of wall motion, ejection fraction, and valve motion. Additional MDCT tools include unique post-processing or rendering techniques that can be used to improve

understanding of complex valve disease. Fig. 13.5 highlights how these tools are valuable for making an accurate diagnosis and assist in quickly and effectively communicating unusual aspects of cardiac and valve pathology to the heart team to aid in a successful procedure.

Application of these new technologies and techniques to the pre-procedural planning of TAVR have given a new appreciation of the complex and dynamic nature of the aortoannular complex, vascular atherosclerotic burden, and characteristics of the thoracoabdominal aorta and iliofemoral branches.[23] All of the measurements routinely made with MDCT are shown in Table 13.4. Integration of MDCT improves the accuracy of TAVR prosthesis sizing, and paravalvular aortic regurgitation has decreased from approximately 75.3% to 55%,

and mild or more severe paravalvular regurgitation has decreased from approximately 20.5% to 7.5%.[24-27]

The accumulating body of evidence for the use of MDCT in the planning of TAVR is compelling. In most large-volume centers, MDCT is the foundation of the standard imaging pathway for TAVR preprocedural planning.[21,28]

TABLE 13.3   Imaging Assessment Checklist for Transcatheter Aortic Valve Replacement.
Preprocedure, Vascular Access, Periprocedure, Long-Term Postprocedure

Region of Interest	Recommended Approach and Key Measurements	Additional Comments
Preprocedure		
Aortic valve morphology	TTE[a] • Trileaflet, bicuspid, or unicuspid • Valve calcification • Leaflet motion • Annular size and shape	TEE if can be safely performed, particularly useful for subaortic membranes Cardiac MRI if echocardiography is nondiagnostic ECG-gated thoracic CTA if MRI contraindicated
Aortic valve function	TTE • Maximum aortic velocity • Mean aortic valve gradient • AVA • Stroke volume index • Presence and severity of AR	Additional parameters • Dimensionless index • AVA by planimetry (echocardiography, CT, MRI) • Dobutamine stress echocardiography for LFLG AS– reduced EF • Aortic valve calcium score if LFLG AS diagnosis in question
LV geometry and other cardiac findings	TTE • LVEF, regional wall motion • Hypertrophy, diastolic function • Pulmonary pressure estimate • Mitral valve (MR, MS, MAC) • Aortic sinus anatomy and size	CMR: identification of cardiomyopathies Myocardial ischemia and scar: CMR, PET, DSE, thallium CMR imaging for myocardial fibrosis and scar
Annular sizing	TAVR CTA-gated, contrast-enhanced CT thorax with multi-phasic acquisition; for annulus, typically reconstructed in systole between 30% and 40% of the R-R window	Major/minor annulus dimension Major/minor average Annular area Circumference/perimeter
Aortic root measurements	TAVR CTA: for aortic root, typically reconstructed in diastole at 60%–80%	Coronary ostia heights Mid-sinus of Valsalva (sinus to commissure, sinus to sinus) Sinotubular junction Ascending aorta (40 cm above valve plane, widest dimension, at level of PA) Aortic root and ascending aorta calcification
Coronary disease and thoracic anatomy	Coronary angiography Nongated thoracic CTA	Coronary artery disease severity Bypass grafts: number/location RV to chest wall distance Aorta to chest wall relationship
Noncardiac imaging	Carotid ultrasound Cerebrovascular MRI	May be considered, depending on clinical history
Renal Function	**Recommended Approach**	**Key Parameters**
Vascular Access (Imaging Depends on Renal Function)		
Normal renal function (GFR > 60) or ESRD not expected to recover	TAVR CTA[b]	Aorta, great vessel, and abdominal aorta dissection, atheroma, stenosis, calcification Iliac/subclavian/femoral luminal dimensions, calcification, and tortuosity
Borderline renal function	Contrast MRA Direct femoral angiography (low contrast)	Institutional-dependent protocols Luminal dimensions and tortuosity of peripheral vasculature
Acute kidney injury or ESRD with expected recovery	Noncontrast CT of chest, abdomen, and pelvis Noncontrast MRA Can consider TEE if balancing risk/benefits	Degree of calcification and tortuosity of peripheral vasculature

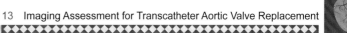

TABLE 13.3	Imaging Assessment Checklist for Transcatheter Aortic Valve Replacement.—cont'd	

Preprocedure, Vascular Access, Periprocedure, Long-Term Postprocedure

Imaging Goals	Recommended Approach	Additional Details
Periprocedure		
Interventional planning	TAVR CTA (preprocedural)	Predict optimal fluoroscopy angles for valve deployment
Confirmation of annular sizing	TAVR CTA (preprocedural)	Consider contrast aortic root injection if needed 3D TEE to confirm annular size
Valve placement	Fluoroscopy under general anesthesia	TEE (if using general anesthesia)
Paravalvular AR	Direct aortic root angiography	TEE (if using general anesthesia)
Procedural complications	TTE TEE (if using general anesthesia) Intracardiac echo (alternative)	See Table 13.2
Long-Term Postprocedure		
Evaluate valve function	TTE	Key elements of echocardiography • Maximum aortic velocity • Mean aortic valve gradient • Aortic valve area • Paravalvular and valvular AR
LV geometry and other cardiac findings	TTE • LVEF, regional wall motion • Hypertrophy, diastolic function • Pulmonary pressure estimate • Mitral valve (MR, MS, MAC)	—

[a]Given the use of CT, the role in annular sizing before TAVR with TEE is limited. Periprocedural use of TEE is limited to cases performed with general anesthesia.

[b]Unless otherwise noted, TAVR CTA refers to a CT angiogram of the chest, abdomen, and pelvis. Typically, the thorax is acquired using ECG-gated multiphase acquisition. At a minimum, acquisition and reconstruction should include end-systole, usually between 30% and 40% of the R-R window.

AR, Aortic regurgitation; *AS*, aortic stenosis; *AVA*, aortic valve area; *CMR*, cardiovascular magnetic resonance imaging; *CT*, computed tomography; *CTA*, computed tomography angiography; *DSE*, dobutamine stress echocardiography; *ECG*, electrocardiogram; *EF*, ejection fraction; *ESRD*, end-stage renal disease; *GFR*, glomerular filtration rate; *LFLG*, low flow, low gradient; *LVEF*, left ventricular ejection fraction; *MAC*, mitral annular calcification; *MR*, mitral regurgitation; *MRA*, magnetic resonance angiogram; *MRI*, magnetic resonance imaging; *MS*, mitral stenosis; *PA*, pulmonary artery; *PET*, positron emission tomography; *TAVR*, transcatheter aortic valve replacement.

From Otto CM, Kumbhani DJ, Alexander KP, et al. 2017 ACC expert consensus decision pathway for transcatheter aortic valve replacement in the management of adults with aortic stenosis: a report of the American College of Cardiology Task Force on Clinical Expert Consensus Documents. J Am Coll Cardiol 2017;69:1313-1346.

Magnetic Resonance Imaging

CMR and magnetic resonance angiography (MRA) can provide an alternative comprehensive assessment of the aortic valve, annulus, aortic root, thoracoabdominal aorta, and luminal caliber of the iliofemoral branches with good correlation with MDCT.[29-32] CMR also provides for interrogation of myocardial function and mechanisms of valve pathology. If quantification of hemodynamics is desired, a stack of cine images in a short-axis orientation can be used to quantify left ventricular (LV) volumes. This information can be used to calculate cardiac stroke volumes, which can be internally confirmed using velocity-encoded flow imaging. These techniques are useful for establishing the diagnosis of valve disease when the results of echocardiography are unclear.

The unique tissue characterization abilities of CMR are likely to play a growing role in patient selection. Evidence indicates that cardiac amyloid may be more prevalent in patients with AS,[33-35] and identification of cardiac amyloid or other coexisting cardiomyopathies may constrain post-TAVR outcomes and thereby inform patient-centered discussions about undergoing the procedure.

A checklist of the anatomic structures that can be evaluated with these techniques is shown in Table 13.5. However, image quality with CMR and MRA greatly depends on image pulse sequence selection, skill of the operator in proper image acquisition, and patient cooperation, including the ability to lie flat and perform breath holds. For valvular and structural heart disease, successful planning with CMR and MRA requires attention to detail and meticulous care in image acquisition and postprocessing of the images. CMR and MRA for valvular heart disease should be performed only at an imaging center of excellence, where dedicated and experienced imagers are facile with the nuances of CMR and understand the specific needs of the structural heart team.

Annular and Aortic Root Assessment

Correct assessment and sizing of the aortic annulus can be challenging because it is an elliptical, virtual ring formed by the basal attachments of the aortic valve leaflets. It is a dynamic structure that undergoes conformational pulsatile changes throughout the cardiac cycle, with an average relative difference between the maximum and minimum cross-sectional areas of 18.2 ± 6.1%.[36] Fig. 13.6 illustrates this change and shows that the predominance of the conformational change is driven by an increase in size of the minimum cross-sectional dimension, leading to a larger and more circular shape during systole (typically 30%–40% of the RR interval of the cardiac cycle).[37] The aortic

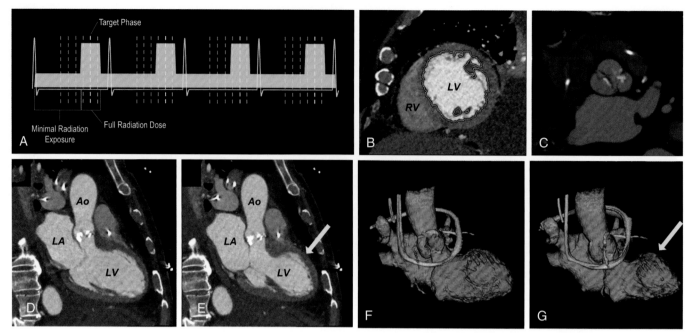

Fig. 13.4 Utility of ECG-Gated Computed Tomography (CT) Angiography for Structural Heart Disease. (A) ECG-gating of CT images allows freezing of cardiac motion and generation of full 3D data sets throughout the cardiac cycle. Radiation can be reduced or dose modulated during parts of the cardiac cycle of less clinical interest. For cine generation, wider windows that encompass systole should be included. (B) ECG-gated short-axis slice of the heart with automated endocardial segmentation. This can be done throughout the cardiac cycle to calculate ejection fractions and stroke volumes in challenging cases such as in low-flow, low-gradient aortic stenosis. (C) ECG-gated image of an aortic valve in systole shows the open leaflets and allows clear identification of structure and assessment of anatomic valve area by planimetry in challenging cases (Video 13.4C ▶). (D–E) Frozen frames in diastole (D; Video 13.4D ▶) and systole (E) of a reconstruction of a three-chamber long-axis view of a heart. *Arrow* identifies a region of segmental hypokinesis. (F–G) Corresponding volume-rendered images can be used for 3D visualization of cardiac function. *Arrow* identifies a region of segmental hypokinesis.

annulus is typically measured at peak systole to avoid undersizing of the TAVR prosthesis[36,38] because valve undersizing can lead to increased rates of paravalvular aortic regurgitation, valve migration, or valve embolization.[36,39–42]

Recommendations for valve selection and sizing vary by vendor, and these tasks have historically been performed using multiple measurement techniques, including minimum and maximum cross-sectional dimensions, circumference-derived area, and direct planimetry of the annular area.[28] To account for distortion and compliance of the annular tissue caused by valve deployment, oversizing of the valve (10%–15%) has traditionally been recommended,[28] although specifics depend on manufacture recommendations. Greater degrees of oversizing should be avoided because they increase the risk of complications such as coronary obstruction, heart block,[43,44] and annular rupture.[22,28,45] Complications such as heart block may be variable between vendors.[16] Whether these variations reflect differences in valve sizing methodology or intrinsic differences in risk between valve technologies is unknown, but the accuracy of valve sizing is likely to play a role because left bundle branch block (LBBB) prevalence during or after TAVR is high, and preexisting right bundle branch block (RBBB) is associated with sudden cardiac death and progression to complete heart block.

Due to the importance of the aortic annulus for TAVR, annular sizing should be performed carefully, particularly when using multiple imaging modalities. It is essential that the imaging provider understand the bias and comparative effectiveness and measurement biases for each imaging modality.

Computed Tomography

3D MDCT data sets are easily manipulated using dedicated workstations to visualize cardiac structures in any plane. The freedom to fully manipulate data allows ideal imaging of the aortic annulus (Fig. 13.7).

Because the aortic annulus is not a physical structure, but rather the virtual plane prescribed by the insertion points of each of the three coronary cusps, measurement reproducibility can be a challenge for an inexperienced operator. When performed by experienced operators, aortic annulus measurements have an excellent correlation (r values between 0.94 and 0.96).[46] However, even experienced operators using a single method of annulus measurement for valve sizing (e.g., dimensions, perimeter, area) can yield a difference in prosthesis sizing of 6% to 11% between observers.[46] If multiple measurement parameters are used for internal validation of prosthesis selection, differences in TAVR valve size selection occur in only 3% to 4% of patients.[46] This small but clinically significant variation highlights the critical importance of experience, training, and continual quality assessment to achieve accurate and reproducible valve sizing.

Beyond annular sizing, MDCT enables analysis of the degree and complexity of calcification of the aortic annulus and LV outflow tract. Extensive or eccentric calcifications may increase the risk of annular rupture, paravalvular aortic regurgitation, or coronary obstruction.

Coronary obstruction is a catastrophic complication of TAVR that can happen at the time of TAVR valve deployment or in a delayed fashion, in which case it most frequently occurs in the first 7 days after implantation.[47] Most data for this are provided by retrospective registry analysis, and the rarity of occurrence due to early identification of

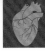

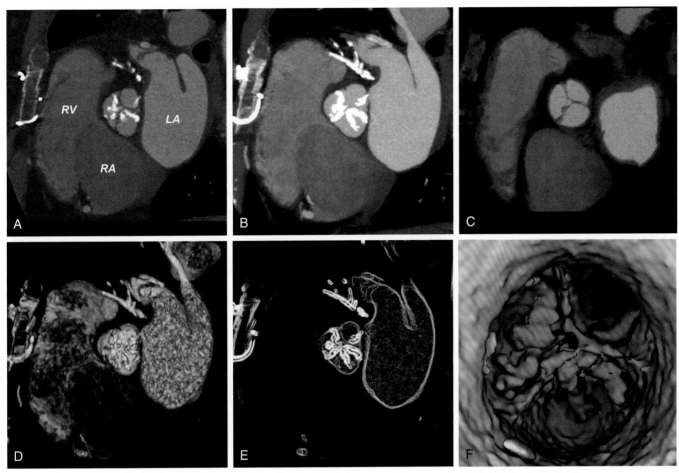

Fig. 13.5 Different Aortic Valve Visualizations With Computed Tomography (CT). (A) Standard thin-slice double-oblique reconstruction of the aortic valve with gated CT angiography. (B) A more complete visualization of the calcifications can be seen when using multiple stacked slices and a maximum-intensity projection (MIP) projection. (C) Minimum-intensity projections can be used to reduce calcium blooming (partial-volume effect) and more clearly see the aortic valve commissures. This view is particularly helpful in evaluation of regurgitant orifice areas and stenotic valve areas. (D) Volume-rendered image, which is helpful for spatial orientation of other cardiac and vascular structures. (E) Alternative volume-rendered image uses edge enhancements and transparency effects to demonstrate the nature and extent of valve calcifications. (F) Fly-through image of the aortic valve from the aorta can give an appreciation of the 3D nature of the calcifications and the orientation on the aortic valve. This view can help to evaluate abnormal valve motion. *LA,* Left atrium. *RA,* right atrium. *RV,* right ventricle.

TABLE 13.4 Computed Tomography–Specific Measurements for Transcatheter Aortic Valve Replacement.

Region of Interest	Specific Measurements	Measurement Technique	Additional Comments
Valve Size and Type			
Aortic valve morphology and function	Aortic valve	If cine images obtained, qualitative evaluation of valve opening Planimetry of aortic valve area in rare cases Calcium score with Agatston technique or a volumetric technique to quantify calcification of aortic valve	Most useful in cases of LFLG severe AS when diagnosis is otherwise unclear; may be helpful in defining number of valve cusps.
LV geometry and other cardiac findings	Left ventricular outflow tract	Measured with a double-oblique plane at most narrow portion of the left ventricular outflow tract Perimeter Area Qualitative assessment of calcification	Quantification of calcification not standardized Large eccentric calcium may predispose to paravalvular regurgitation and annular rupture during valve deployment

Continued

TABLE 13.4 Computed Tomography–Specific Measurements for Transcatheter Aortic Valve Replacement.—cont'd

Region of Interest	Specific Measurements	Measurement Technique	Additional Comments
Annular sizing	Aortic annulus	Defined as double-oblique plane at insertion point of all three coronary cusps Major/minor diameter Perimeter Area	Periprocedural TEE and/or balloon sizing can confirm dimensions during case
Aortic root measurements	Sinus of Valsalva	Height from annulus to superior aspect of each coronary cusp Diameter of each coronary cusp to the opposite commissure Circumference around largest dimension Area of the largest dimension	
Coronary and thoracic anatomy	Coronary arteries	Height from annulus to inferior margin of left main coronary artery and the inferior margin of the right coronary artery	Short coronary artery height increases risk of procedure Evaluation of coronary artery and bypass graft stenosis on selected studies Estimate risk of coronary occlusion during valve deployment
	Aortic root angulation	Angle of root to left ventricle Three-cusp angulation to predict best fluoroscopy angle	Reduce procedure time and contrast load by reducing number of periprocedural root injections
Vascular Access Planning			
Vascular access	Aorta	Major/minor diameters of the following: • Aorta at sinotubular junction • Ascending aorta in widest dimension • Ascending aorta before brachiocephalic artery • Mid-aortic arch • Descending aorta at isthmus • Descending aorta at level of pulmonary artery • Descending aorta at level of diaphragm • Abdominal aorta at level of renal arteries • Abdominal aorta at the iliac bifurcation	Measurements must be perpendicular to aorta in two orthogonal planes. Identify aortopathies. Evaluate burden of atherosclerosis. Identify dissection or aneurysms.
	Primary peripheral vasculature	Major/minor dimensions, tortuosity, calcification of the following: • Carotid arteries • Subclavian arteries • Brachiocephalic artery • Vertebral arteries • Bilateral subclavian arteries • Great vessels • Iliac arteries • Femoral arteries	No well-defined cutoff or definition of tortuosity or calcification has been established.
	Ancillary vasculature	Stenosis of the following: • Celiac artery • Superior mesenteric artery • Both renal arteries	—
	Relationship of femoral bifurcation and femoral head	Distance from inferior margin of femoral head to femoral bifurcation	—

AS, Aortic stenosis; *CT*, computed tomography; *LFLG*, low flow, low gradient; *TAVR*, transcatheter aortic valve repair.
From Otto CM, Kumbhani DJ, Alexander KP, et al. 2017 ACC expert consensus decision pathway for transcatheter aortic valve replacement in the management of adults with aortic stenosis: a report of the American College of Cardiology Task Force on Clinical Expert Consensus Documents. J Am Coll Cardiol 2017;69:1313-1346.

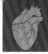

TABLE 13.5 Cardiovascular Magnetic Resonance Imaging Measurements for Transcatheter Aortic Valve Replacement.

Region of Interest	Specific Measurement	Purpose	Measurement Technique
Valve Size and Type			
Aortic valve morphology and function	Aortic valve	Confirmation of valve morphology if needed	SSFP cine images of aortic valve morphology Flow imaging can quantify degree of aortic regurgitation if not clear by echocardiography
LV geometry and other cardiac findings	Left ventricle	Evaluate systolic function	Quantitative assessment of myocardial systolic function by planimetry of the endocardial borders
		Myocardial mass	Quantitation of left ventricular mass
	LV outflow tract	Exclude subaortic membrane and dynamic outflow tract obstruction	SSFP cine images of LV outflow tract In-plane velocity encoded images of the LV outflow tract
Annular sizing	Aortic annulus	Valve sizing and selection	SSFP cine images of the aortic annulus Noncontrast gated angiography
Aortic root measurements	Sinus of Valsalva	Valve sizing and selection	Noncontrast ECG and respiratory gated angiography • Height from annulus to superior aspect of each coronary cusp • Diameter of each coronary cusp to the opposite commissure • Area of the largest dimension
Coronary and thoracic anatomy	Coronary arteries	Valve sizing and selection Estimate risk of coronary occlusion during valve deployment	Height from annulus to inferior margin of left main coronary artery and the inferior margin of the right coronary artery
Vascular Access Planning			
Vascular Access	Aorta	Vascular access planning Identify aortopathies Identify dissection or aneurysms	Typically gadolinium-based contrast angiography Noncontrast options based on local expertise Major/minor dimensions of the following: • Aorta at sinotubular junction • Ascending aorta in widest dimension • Ascending aorta before brachiocephalic artery • Mid-aortic arch • Descending aorta at isthmus • Descending aorta at level of pulmonary artery • Descending aorta at level of diaphragm • Abdominal aorta at level of renal arteries • Abdominal aorta at the iliac bifurcation
	Primary peripheral vasculature	Vascular access planning	Major/minor dimensions and tortuosity of the following: • Carotid arteries • Subclavian arteries • Brachiocephalic artery • Vertebral arteries • Bilateral subclavian arteries • Iliac arteries • Femoral arteries
	Ancillary vasculature	Vascular access planning	Stenosis of the following: • Celiac artery • Superior mesenteric artery • Both renal arteries

SSFP, Steady-state free progression (in this context, intrinsic bright blood cine images); *TAVR*, transcatheter aortic valve replacement.

the potential problem has limited the data for the specific metrics provided by MDCT to prevent immediate or delayed coronary obstruction. Practically, if coronary heights are greater than the valve struts at the predicted landing zone of the TAVR valve, the risk of coronary obstruction should be minimized. This risk is theoretically reduced if there is sufficient distance between predicted implantation distance of the TAVR valve and the coronary ostia.

The risk of coronary obstruction during TAVR increases with the placement of a valve-in-valve (VIV) TAVR, in which a transcatheter aortic valve is placed in a preexisting surgical aortic valve.[48] VIV TAVR is feasible and increasing in frequency, and understanding the imaging nuances of the procedure is important.[49] In addition to a higher risk of coronary obstruction, patients undergoing VIV TAVR are at higher risk for patient-prosthesis mismatch, which is associated with worse

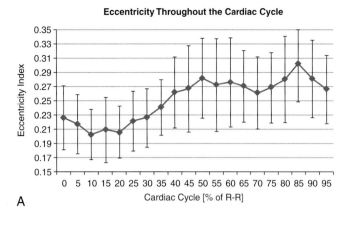

A

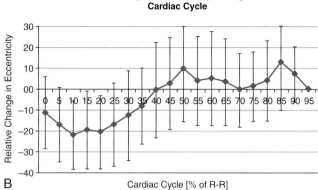

B

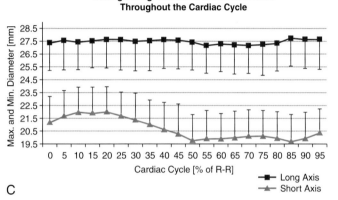

C

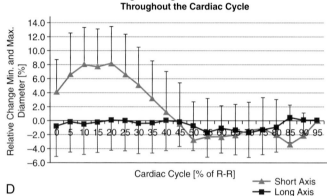

D

Fig. 13.6 Aortic Annular Conformational Changes Throughout the Cardiac Cycle. Aortic annular sizing is ideally performed during systole, when the annulus is at its largest, to prevent undersizing of the transcatheter aortic valve prosthesis. (A) Eccentricity of the aortic annulus throughout the cardiac cycle using an eccentricity index derived from the major and minor dimensions. (B) Decreased relative change in eccentricity of the aortic annulus consistent with a more circular shape during systole. (C) Decrease in eccentricity is driven largely by an increase in the minimum diameter during systole. (D) Relative change in minimum and maximum aortic annulus diameter throughout the cardiac cycle. (From Blanke P, Russe M, Leipsic J, et al. Conformational pulsatile changes of the aortic annulus: impact on prosthesis sizing by computed tomography for transcatheter aortic valve replacement. JACC Cardiovasc Interv 2012;5:984-994.)

outcomes.[50] To reduce the rate of patient-prosthesis mismatch, some groups have demonstrated that valve fracture with a balloon valvuloplasty before TAVR is feasible and can provide improved hemodynamics.[51,52] Preprocedural analysis with CTA is likely to improve the safety of VIV TAVR, particularly when facilitated by valve fracture. If preprocedural imaging suggests that a patient may be at high risk for coronary obstruction, transcatheter electrocautery for the intentional perforation and laceration of the high-risk leaflets before TAVR is technically feasible.[53]

MDCT holds promise for improving the diagnosis of AS in patients when echocardiographic parameters may be unclear. In diseases such as LFLG severe AS, aortic valve calcium scoring can improve the diagnosis. MDCT cine imaging of the stenotic valve with direct planimetry of the anatomic aortic valve area can help establish the severity of AS and determine whether the patient may benefit from treatment with TAVR. Other applications of MDCT for LFLG severe AS include using the improved visualization of the aortic annulus as part of the continuity equation for calculation of the aortic valve area. Compared with echocardiography, the MDCT-derived annulus is systematically larger, and it has been suggested an aortic valve area determined by MDCT of less than 1.2 cm² calculated with the continuity equation is comparable to the aortic valve area

calculated with echocardiography of less than 1.0 cm².[54] Fig. 13.8 shows a case in which these principles were helpful in clinical decision making.

MDCT should be avoided for some TAVR patients, most commonly those with acute kidney injury or significant chronic kidney disease not yet requiring dialysis. In these cases, iodinated contrast should be avoided if possible. Iodinated contrast is also best avoided for patients with severe anaphylaxis in response to iodinated contrast, even with prophylactic premedication protocols.

As the experience with transcatheter therapies increases, lower risk[8] and younger patients previously excluded from clinical trials, such as those with bicuspid aortic valves[55] and complex congenital heart diseases, are undergoing TAVR. This means that patients will begin undergoing serial evaluations with MDCT and exposure to fluoroscopy at younger ages. Although the effects of ionizing radiation at the doses administered for medical imaging are likely negligible for many of the high-risk elderly patients with severe AS being treated with TAVR, cumulative radiation exposure is an important consideration for the younger patients being considered in the future for transcatheter therapies.[56] These patients will create a need for using alternative imaging techniques such as CMR,[30] leveraging advances in 3D TEE, and creating novel fusion imaging techniques.

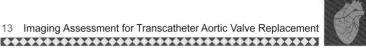

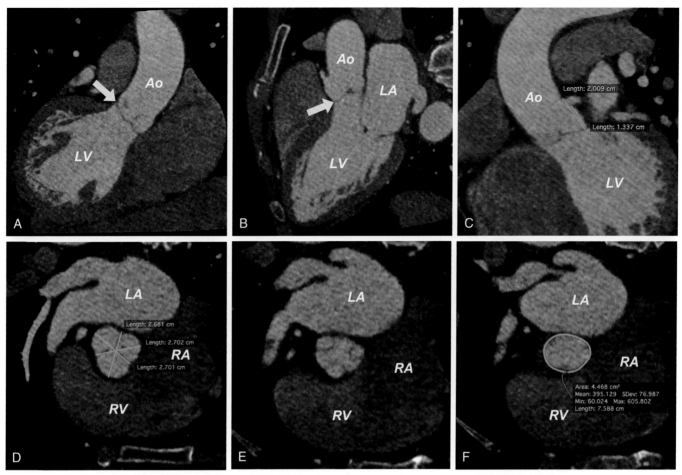

Fig. 13.7 Measurements of the Aortoannular Complex With Gated Computed Tomography (CT). (A and B) The left ventricular outflow tract (LVOT) and virtual aortic annulus *(arrows)* are demonstrated in two 90-degree, double-oblique views. (C) Distance from the aortic annulus to the superior and inferior aspects of the left main coronary artery. Shorter coronary heights and longer valve leaflets have been associated with coronary occlusion during valve deployment. (D) Double-oblique reconstruction of the aortic annulus at the widest point of the sinuses of Valsalva. (E) Transition point from the sinuses of Valsalva to their insertion points in the LVOT that define the virtual aortic annulus. (F) Aortic annulus as defined by CT. This is frequently measured in terms of its area, major and minor dimensions, and circumference. *Ao,* Aorta.

Echocardiography

Although echocardiography will continue to play a role in TAVR, its use in annular assessment can be problematic because standard two-dimensional (2D) TTE imaging most easily visualizes the short axis of an oval annulus.[26,57] Increasing availability of 3D TTE probes allow integration of newer techniques such as biplane guidance, and use of full-volume 3D acquisitions may offer improved delineation of valve and annular morphology. Full-volume 3D TTE data sets are similar to MDCT in that they allow for post hoc image processing. However, 3D TTE data sets are often limited in spatial and temporal resolution and require specific experience and training for efficient and reproducible postprocessing. Despite the technical hurdles, image quality of 3D imaging probes continues to improve and may become more reliable for routine use for direct preprocedural planning of TAVR.

Echocardiographic imaging with TEE plays a role in the preprocedural and periprocedural guidance of structural heart disease interventions.[26,31,39,58] TEE, especially with 3D imaging techniques, can provide reasonable anatomic delineation of the aortic annulus (Fig. 13.9). The annulus can be measured during an ongoing TEE study, but more commonly, it is acquired as a 3D data set to be manipulated and measured later.

TEE studies performed before the procedure are helpful in that multiple acquisitions can be made without concern for nephrotoxic iodinated contrast administration or ionizing radiation exposure. Annular measurements are a prime example of the importance of comparative imaging studies because direct planimetry of the aortic annulus on 3D TEE compared with MDCT shows systemic underestimation of the echocardiographically derived annular sizes.[58] This has important clinical implications and may lead to discrepant TAVR valve sizes in up to 50% of patients.[55] Fig. 13.10 shows that these types of sizing discrepancies can lead to increases in paravalvular aortic regurgitation.[59]

Another major drawback of performing preprocedural TEE for TAVR planning is that it adds a second procedure with incremental risks for a sick and frail population. These risks are somewhat mitigated if the TEE is performed immediately before TAVR as part of the procedure itself. However, when done in this fashion, there are often time constraints that do not allow thoughtful integration of the data a

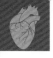
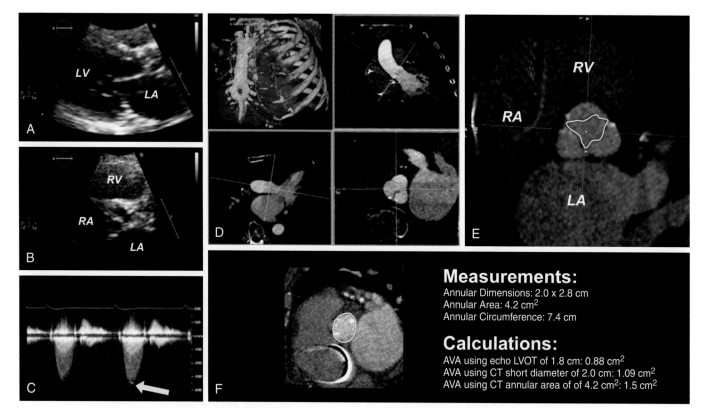

Measurements:
Annular Dimensions: 2.0 x 2.8 cm
Annular Area: 4.2 cm^2
Annular Circumference: 7.4 cm

Calculations:
AVA using echo LVOT of 1.8 cm: 0.88 cm^2
AVA using CT short diameter of 2.0 cm: 1.09 cm^2
AVA using CT annular area of of 4.2 cm^2: 1.5 cm^2

Fig. 13.8 Gated Computed Tomography (CT) in Low-Flow, Low-Gradient Aortic Stenosis. A patient with severe obesity and poor acoustic windows on transthoracic echocardiography (TTE) was suspected to have symptomatic low-flow, low-gradient severe aortic stenosis and was referred for transcatheter aortic valve replacement. (A–C) TTE images show a peak velocity of 3.5 m/s *(yellow arrow)*, mean gradient of 25 mmHg, aortic valve area (AVA) of 0.9 cm^2 by the continuity equation, stroke volume of 66 mL, and stroke volume index of 26 mL/m^2. (D) CT angiography image shows the aortic valve oriented in a double-oblique fashion. (E) Aortic valve on CT is well visualized during systole and has an anatomic valve area by planimetry of 1.9 cm^2. (F) Aortic annulus measured on CT was very eccentric, with the short axis on CT matching the annular dimension measured on TTE. Calculation of the continuity equation using different annular measurements has a significant effect on the AVA.

priori. Unusual situations, such as very small or large annuli, may also halt the procedure if an appropriately sized prosthesis is not on hand.

Large calcifications, which may predispose to paravalvular aortic regurgitation, are easily seen on MDCT but may be more difficult to assess by TEE due to acoustic shadowing. Many aspects of the MDCT planning process, such as coronary heights, are not as easily or reliably identified with TEE. If a hard stop is identified only by TEE at the time of the planned intervention, unnecessary procedures such as central vascular access may have been obtained, and the overall laboratory workflow may be disrupted.

Magnetic Resonance Imaging

CMR is most frequently used for physiologic assessment and clarification of many cardiovascular diagnoses (Fig. 13.11A,B). Particularly in highly calcified valves, it can be helpful in establishing the presence of a bicuspid or dysplastic aortic valve. Occasionally when MDCT or 3D echocardiography is not feasible, CMR with intrinsic bright blood cine imaging can be used to provide a detailed assessment of the aortic valve, aortic root, aortic annulus, and coronary ostia.

When available, a free-breathing, noncontrast, navigator-gated, whole-heart 3D acquisition can be helpful for annular measurements (Fig. 13.12).[31] Unlike standard 2D bright blood cine images, these fully 3D data sets allow accurate measurements and reconstructions of the aortic annulus and vasculature structures after the primary

acquisition period. However, unlike MDCT, the gated-MRA images typically are obtained only at a single phase of the cardiac cycle and are not adept at detecting the conformational changes of the aortic annulus.

The dual ECG and respiratory gating required for these studies can be fairly prolonged, proportionate to the spatial resolution desired, which may be problematic for elderly, frail patients. In some centers, gadolinium contrast–based MRA images can be used for the aortic annulus, but the ECG-gated sequences required for annular sizing are not widely available and probably offers little benefit over MDCT.

Novel Techniques

If all other avenues are exhausted and annular sizing remains unclear, confirmation of aortic annulus size can be performed invasively with a balloon at the time of the procedure. As procedures become more complex, novel techniques such as 3D printing have garnered significant interest and may be helpful in planning these challenging cases.[60] Beyond actual printing of 3D models, computer-aided modeling techniques with virtual valve implantation may also provide insights and planning information before TAVR.[61]

When alternatives to CT are used, many studies have demonstrated differences exist in measurements between techniques.[62] Caution and experience are important to understand the strengths and limits of each technology.

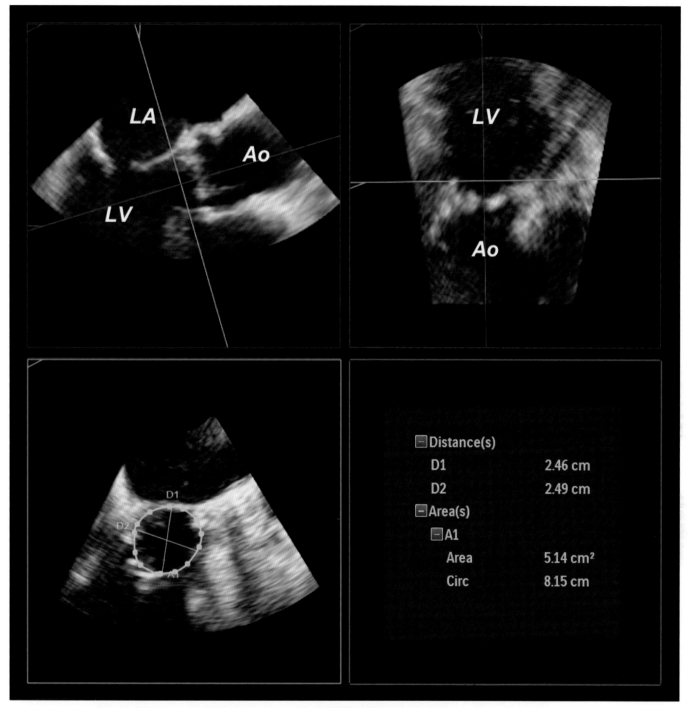

Fig. 13.9 Measurement of Aortic Annulus on 3D TEE. Most modern TEE systems permit 3D acquisitions. The 3D data sets can be manipulated in double-oblique planes similar to computed tomography (CT). The 3D images may allow more accurate annular evaluation and valve sizing than 2D images alone. *Ao*, Aorta.

Peripheral and Central Vascular Access

Because of the still relatively large diameter of the delivery sheaths, appropriate sizing and planning of vascular access area is critical for TAVR. As shown in Fig. 13.13, it is important to evaluate the entire thoracoabdominal aorta; the major thoracic peripheral arterial vasculature, including great vessels of the aorta; and the iliofemoral vasculature.

The central vasculature includes the aortic root, aortic arch, descending thoracic aorta, and abdominal aorta. The most proximal portion of the aortic root is the region from the aortic annulus to the sinotubular junction and encompasses the aortic valve leaflets.

Imaging of this region includes assessment of aortic valve morphology, which is discussed in more detail in Chapter 8. More distally, the extent of atherosclerotic plaque in the ascending aorta and aortic arch have been associated with worse outcomes after cardiac surgery and increased rates of complications after TAVR.[63] Full assessment of the central aortic vasculature includes evaluating for aneurysm, ectasia, calcification, mobile plaque, mural thrombus, dissection, intramural hematoma, and penetrating aortic ulcers. Aneurysms in the aortic root may increase risk of perforation, particularly at increased delivery angles of the valve landing zone.

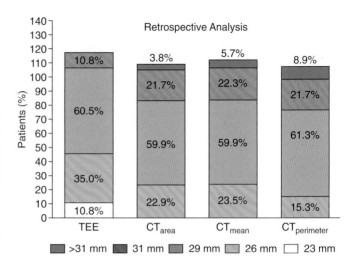

Fig. 13.10 Variation in Valve Sizing by Imaging Technique. Transcatheter aortic valves were sized using 2D transesophageal echocardiography (TEE) in patients who also had corresponding computed tomography (CT) images that were retrospectively evaluated. In general, valve sizes predicted by CT were often discordant and somewhat larger than the actual valves used based on 2D TEE sizing. This highlights the importance of knowing variations between imaging modalities and likely the benefits of 3D imaging of the complex annular structure (From Mylotte D, Dorfmeister M, Elhmidi Y, et al. Erroneous measurement of the aortic annular diameter using 2-dimensional echocardiography resulting in inappropriate CoreValve size selection: a retrospective comparison with multislice computed tomography. JACC Cardiovasc Interv 2014;7:652-661.).

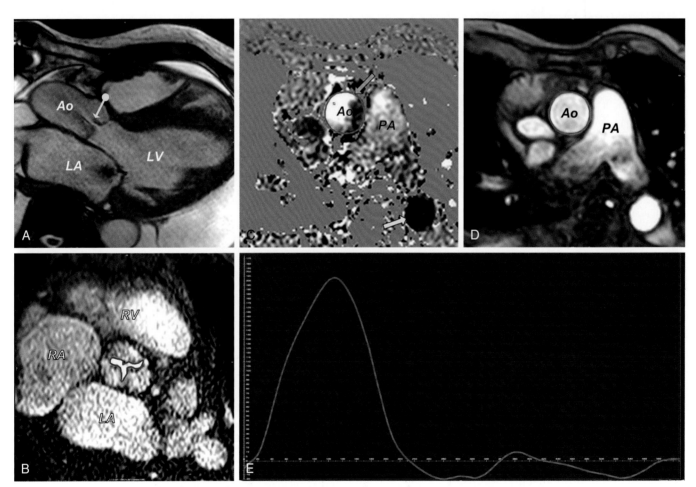

Fig. 13.11 Cardiovascular Magnetic Resonance Imaging Techniques for Evaluation of Aortic Valve Disease. (A) Intrinsic bright blood cardiac magnetic resonance (CMR) cine image of the three-chamber long-axis view at peak systole shows poor aortic valve leaflet excursion with a central jet of high-velocity turbulent flow as demonstrated by proton dephasing *(yellow arrow).* (B) Intrinsic bright blood CMR imaging of the aortic valve in cross section shows an anatomic valve area of 1.2 cm². (C) Velocity-encoded flow image shows forward flow through the aorta in white *(blue arrow).* Flow through the descending aorta is seen in *black (yellow arrow).* (D) Corresponding cine still frame image assists with drawing accurate regions of interest for flow quantification. (E) Quantitative flow through the aorta plotted over time is particularly useful for quantification of aortic regurgitation. *Ao,* Aorta; *PA,* pulmonary artery.

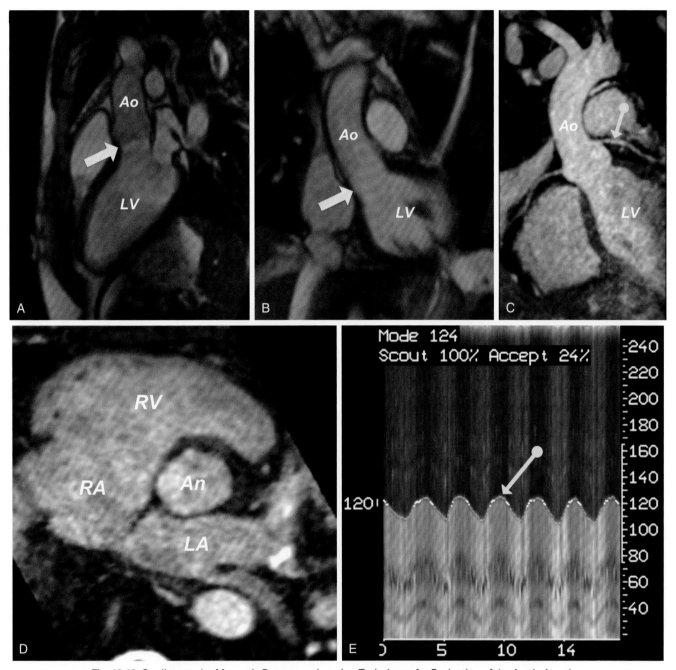

Fig. 13.12 **Cardiovascular Magnetic Resonance Imaging Techniques for Evaluation of the Aortic Annulus.** (A and B) Intrinsic bright blood cardiovascular magnetic resonance (CMR) image of the left ventricular outflow tract (LVOT) and virtual aortic annulus *(arrows)* is demonstrated in two 90-degree, double-oblique views. These images can be used to plan a cross-sectional cine of the aortic annulus itself, but this can be challenging to acquire due to the dynamic motion of the annulus (Video 13.12A ▶ and B ▶). (C) Noncontrast, ECG-gated magnetic resonance angiography (MRA) image of the aortoannular complex and proximal coronary arteries. Although not universally available, electrocardiogram (ECG)-gated MRA images are an excellent alternative to computed tomography (Video 13.12C ▶). (D) Same noncontrast ECG-gated MRA as in C has been lined up in a double-oblique orientation at the aortic annulus. (E) ECG-gated MRA images are often also gated to respirations using a pencil-thin navigator on the diaphragm that allows data to be acquired at end-expiration only *(arrow)*. *An,* Aortic annulus; *Ao,* aorta.

The peripheral vasculature in the thorax includes the great vessels off of the aorta inclusive of the brachiocephalic artery, carotid arteries, subclavian arteries, and more distally, the axillary arteries. In the pelvis, the main peripheral vessels evaluated include the iliofemoral vasculature, most notably the common iliac arteries, external iliac arteries, and common femoral arteries. Each of the peripheral vessels is carefully evaluated in terms of minimal luminal diameter, tortuosity, and degree or morphology of calcification. Circumferential calcification, horseshoe calcifications, and severe tortuosity are particularly common in the iliofemoral vasculature in patients undergoing TAVR, and they increase the risk of access site complications.[64]

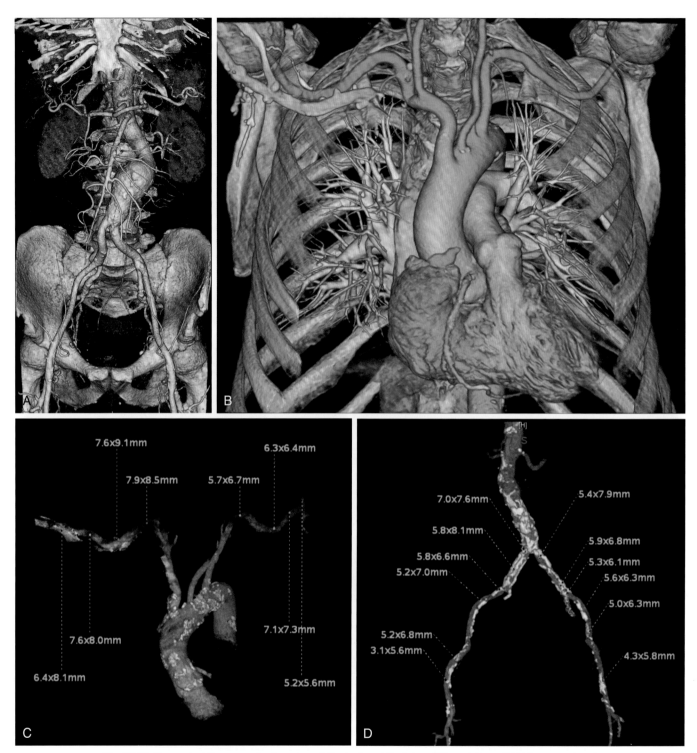

Fig. 13.13 Computed Tomography Imaging of Central and Peripheral Vasculature. (A) Volume-rendered image shows an abdominal aortic aneurysm, which has implications for the vascular access site for TAVR. (B) Volume-rendered image of the thoracic vasculature enables improved understanding of the spatial orientation of the cardiac and vascular structures (Video 13.13B ▶). (C and D) Volume-rendered images of the thoracic and iliofemoral vasculature demonstrate tortuosity, calcification, and vascular sizing. These images are often displayed as a roadmap for fluoroscopy during the procedure.

Evaluation of the remainder of the central and peripheral aortic vasculature plays a primary roll in selecting the route of access. The standard method is femoral artery access, but alternative access routes include apical, transcarotid,[65,66] transcaval,[67,68] subclavian, and direct aortic approaches.[69]

Computed Tomography

MDCT is widely available and enables measurements beyond that of the aortic annulus. It excels in evaluating the size of the sinuses of Valsalva, coronary ostia distance from the annulus, size of the aorta at the sinotubular junction, diameter of the aorta above the annulus, and extent and location of aortic calcifications.[70] MDCT is also excellent for evaluating the remainder of the thoracoabdominal vasculature for stenosis, tortuosity, and calcifications.

Other risks that can be assessed with MDCT include aortic or vascular dissections, intramural hematomas, aortic ulcerations, and extensive atheromas. In cases with challenging arterial access, imaging with MDCT can identify the feasibility of alternative access approaches. The primary challenge with MDCT for peripheral vasculature is that highly calcified vessels may exhibit a calcium blooming artifact, which can make smaller vessels more difficult to evaluate.

Despite its importance, MDCT is limited for patients with acute kidney injury or severe chronic renal injury. Some innovative solutions to this have been tried. Advances in MDCT technology such as iterative reconstruction techniques are now commonly used over the traditional reconstruction techniques of filtered back projection. Iterative reconstruction allows low tube voltage (kVp) scanning that reduces the radiation dose while maintaining image quality. Lower tube voltages (80–100 kVp) are also closer to the K-edge energies of iodine (33 keV) and have increased enhancement for a given amount of iodinated contrast. Combining these benefits allows reductions in contrast volume without loss in image quality. Some centers have taken advantage of this to use diluted mixtures of contrast to obtain excellent image quality with only 20 mL of contrast for pre-TAVR MDCT scans.[71] Others have employed an approach in which a femoral sheath is left in place after cardiac catheterization and used to perform a pelvic MDCT angiogram with the injection of contrast directly through the sheath into the pelvic arterial vasculature. This approach has been successful in evaluating the infrarenal abdominal aorta with very low doses (≈15 mL) of iodinated contrast.[72]

If absolutely no iodinated contrast administration is tenable, a noncontrast MDCT scan can be considered for the assessment of overall vessel size, calcification, and tortuosity. Often due to surrounding fat, the size of the outer lumen of the vessel can be estimated on noncontrast scans, which can potentially detect larger aneurysms. However, no information regarding actual vessel lumen is obtained, and this approach requires an alternative method to evaluate actual luminal stenosis, occlusion, dissection, or other arterial pathology.

Magnetic Resonance Imaging

Gadolinium-based contrast MRA serves as the most readily available alternative to MDCT for evaluation of the central and peripheral vasculature. Most commercial MRA pulse sequences are not ECG gated and are most useful for noncardiac structures such as the central aorta and peripheral vasculature. CMR or MRA sequences do not easily visualize calcium, which can be problematic, but in highly calcified vessels, the lack of the partial-volume calcium blooming artifacts can sometimes be an advantage over MDCT. On MRA, calcium typically generates a signal void that allows easier visualization of the true degree of stenosis.

Novel Techniques

For patients with poor renal function, there is interest in and growth of the use of fusion imaging. The scope of the potential is broad and limited by technologic innovations and local expertise. One example of fusion imaging for evaluation of the peripheral vasculature is the approach seen in Fig. 13.14, in which MRA is combined with noncontrast CT.[73] This may hold promise for patients with renal disease who cannot receive iodinated contrast. Other vendors are starting to integrate MDCT overlays on top of fluoroscopy images to aid in TAVR valve deployment. TEE fusion onto the fluoroscopy screen is used in certain institutions to gain improved understanding of the spatial orientation of cardiac structures relative to the fluoroscopy images.

Additional Case Planning

Before TAVR, it is important to plan and anticipate different aspects and potential outcomes of the procedure. Evaluation can include using MDCT to predict what the optimal valve delivery angle will be on fluoroscopy, plan for the use of cerebroembolic protection devices, understand potential complications, make decisions about concomitant procedures such as percutaneous coronary intervention (PCI), decide on the safety and route of surgical before bailout options, and identify other high risk features such as left atrial appendage thrombi.

Prediction of Delivery Angles

Knowledge about the correct delivery angle is helpful for TAVR valve deployment. Precise coaxial alignment of the stent-based valve along the centerline of the native aortic valve and aortic root is important

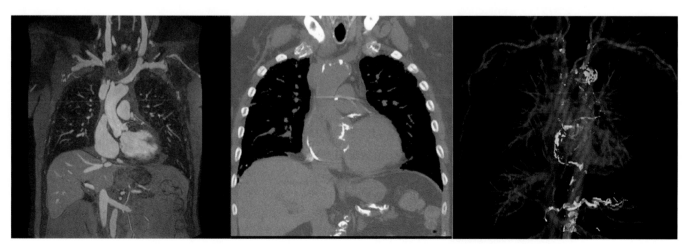

Fig. 13.14 Fusion Imaging for Preprocedural Planning in Challenging Cases. When computed tomography cannot be used for preprocedural planning because iodinated contrast is contraindicated, alternative imaging often relies on local expertise and creativity. Some centers are even venturing into fusion imaging in which magnetic resonance angiography is fused with calcifications from noncontrast computed tomography. (From Yoshida T, Han F, Zhou Z, et al. Ferumoxytol MRA and non-contrast CT fusion in TAVR candidates with renal failure. J Cardiovasc Magn Reson 2016;18[Suppl 1]:Q59.)

during TAVR valve positioning to avoid procedural complications.[20] Historically, this was done with root injections during invasive angiography in multiple imaging planes.[74,75] With routine MDCT use, the delivery angles of fluoroscopy can be accurately predicted ahead of time.[74,76] This can be done using double-oblique, multiplanar MDCT images or with volume-rendered images (Fig. 13.15A).

Preprocedural prediction of the aortic root angle is helpful in saving time and contrast by potentially decreasing the number of aortograms required during the procedure. Newer scanning systems that allow for C-arm CT at the time of the procedure can also be used and have shown excellent correlation with MDCT.[77]

Embolic Protection Planning

Because cerebrovascular events are a major cause of adverse outcomes in TAVR, there has been interest in developing techniques and devices to reduce the risk.[78] The definitive role and techniques for cerebrovascular embolic protection techniques vary, but one commercially available solution uses percutaneous basket filters placed in the brachiocephalic and left common carotid arteries.[79] MDCT is important for patient selection for this device to determine the size, tortuosity, and calcifications of the great vessels. As other solutions become commercially available, imaging will play a role in identifying appropriate patients and device sizing.

Coronary Artery and Bypass Graft Analysis

Cardiac computed tomography angiography (CCTA) is a rapid and accurate technique for evaluation of coronary artery stenosis. ECG gating and many of the postprocessing tools used in the evaluation of structural heart disease with MDCT were initially developed for CCTA applications, and due to similarities in image acquisition, most of the gated MDCT images used for pre-TAVR planning are timed in a fashion that allows coronary artery analysis. Fig. 13.15B–E shows some of the techniques that are particularly useful in pre-TAVR planning.

A few issues challenge the routine MDCT-based evaluation of coronary arteries in patients who are undergoing a standard pre-TAVR MDCT scan. First, the current temporal resolution of most MDCT scanners requires β-blockade to slow the heart rate enough so that

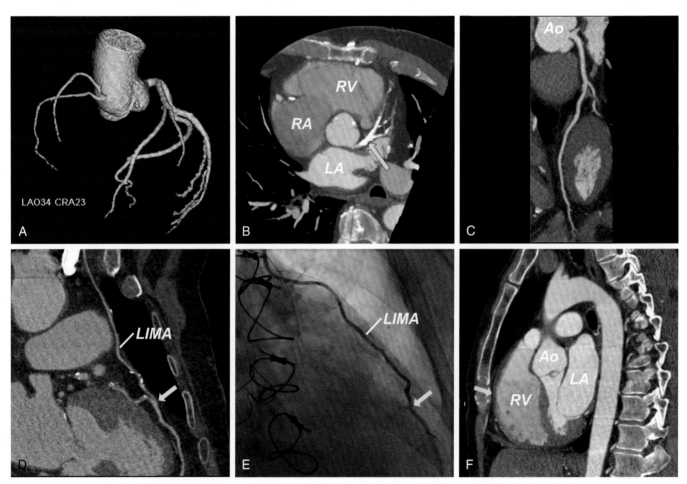

Fig. 13.15 Coronary Computed Tomographic Angiography Techniques for Transcatheter Aortic Valve Replacement Planning. (A) Volume-rendered image of the aortic root and coronary arteries allows planning of optimal transcatheter aortic valve replacement (TAVR) delivery angles on fluoroscopy. (B) Coronary computed tomography angiography (CCTA) image with a maximum-intensity projection demonstrates a highly calcified left main coronary artery *(arrow)* in an elderly patient. (C) CCTA is often technically difficult in patients undergoing TAVR due calcified vasculature and the typical need to avoid β-blockers and sublingual nitroglycerin. When images are of good quality (as shown), they can be of use in excluding significant coronary artery stenosis and avoiding invasive coronary angiography before TAVR. (D and E) CCTA and corresponding invasive angiography of a coronary artery bypass graft. Touchdown of a left internal mammary artery *(LIMA)* to the native left anterior descending artery is shown *(arrows)*. In addition to patency, the relationship of bypass grafts to the sternum is important for bailout surgical planning. (F) Proximity of the right ventricular free wall to the sternum *(arrow)* is also important for bailout surgical planning. *Ao,* Aorta.

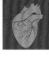

coronary motion can be frozen on the images (typically < 60 beats/min), and many of the patients undergoing TAVR are ill and cannot tolerate this aggressive regimen. Second, the sublingual nitrates typically used to dilate and improve coronary artery visualization are ill advised for most patients with severe AS.

Third, many of the patients undergoing evaluation for TAVR are elderly with preexisting complex and highly calcified coronary arteries that are particularly difficult to evaluate for significant coronary artery stenosis. Given the risks of repeat sternotomy, TAVR is increasingly performed in patients with prior coronary artery bypass grafts.[80,81] Coronary artery bypass grafts are typically well seen on CCTA, but the graft lumen may be obscured if excessive staples are used, and the native diseased coronary artery is often quite challenging to evaluate.

Fourth, coronary artery stents are often found in patients presenting for TAVR. Current CT imaging technology is most effective only for the largest stents, typically those greater than 3 mm, and requires processing with a sharp reconstruction kernel and higher radiation level to reduce the metallic artifacts. Even using most modern MDCT scanners, complete coronary assessment with CCTA is often limited in the elderly population undergoing evaluation for TAVR. However, in some cases, the coronary arteries can be seen well, and significant coronary artery disease can be excluded, allowing avoidance of coronary angiography before TAVR.

In an Italian cohort of 491 patients undergoing TAVR, 116 underwent both CCTA and invasive coronary angiography. Overall, 65 (56%) of 116 of these patients were thought to have significant lesions on CCTA and 31 (47.7%) were thought to have hemodynamically significant lesions on invasive coronary angiography. Using a combined CCTA and an invasive approach, the rate of periprocedural myocardial infarction was only 1.2%.[82] These data are compelling and suggest that although coronary artery analysis for TAVR patients may be more challenging and have reduced specificity, its routine and broad use can be implemented into the regular TAVR workflow to exclude significant coronary artery disease with very few adverse periprocedural outcomes.

Emergency Surgical Planning

MDCT is helpful in planning for possible surgical approaches if complications occur during TAVR valve delivery.[83,84] Its primary use is to evaluate the relationship of cardiovascular structures with the sternum (see Fig. 13.15F). Other structures of particular importance in relation to the sternum include the right ventricle (RV) free wall, ascending aorta, brachiocephalic vessels, and pericardium. The sternum should be evaluated for deformities and adhesions from prior surgeries. It is important to assess the relationship of coronary bypass grafts with the sternum, particularly for internal mammary bypass grafts.

Assessment of the burden of atherosclerotic calcification of the ascending aorta is helpful because a high degree of calcification may increase the risk of stroke in the cannulation of the aorta for cardiopulmonary bypass. In cases with a porcelain aorta, alternative vascular access sites should be considered for cannulation.

Left Atrial Appendage Thrombus

There is evidence for high rates of atrial fibrillation and particularly of left atrial appendage thrombus among patients being evaluated for TAVR. Prevalence ranges from 3.8% to 11% of patients undergoing evaluation for TAVR who have left atrial thrombus on the preprocedural planning MDCT study.[85,86] This additional finding may help risk stratify patients for TAVR and avoid certain access routes for which there is a risk of an interventional wire to potentially dislodge the thrombus.

TECHNICAL CONSIDERATIONS

Computed Tomography

In the context TAVR, MDCT systems with at least 64 detectors and a spatial resolution of 0.5 to 0.6 mm are recommended. Processing should be performed on a dedicated workstation that at minimum has the ability to manipulate double-oblique planes of a 3D data set. Many modern workstations use a semi-automated workflow with dedicated TAVR analysis packages to create a reproducible and efficient clinical workflow.[87–91]

Although scanning protocols vary by vendor, typical protocols involve two main components. The first is an ECG-gated acquisition of the aortic annulus and aortic root. ECG-synchronized imaging reduces motion artifact and allows reconstruction at any acquired phase of the cardiac cycle. These images serve a primary goal of valve sizing, and they provide detailed information on the relationships of the coronary arteries, leaflet morphology, calcification, and identification of other challenging anatomic features. Most facilities use a full retrospective ECG-gated acquisition, which increases radiation exposure but allows assessment of all cardiac structures throughout the entire cardiac cycle. The second step is a full chest, abdominal, and pelvic angiogram that typically does not require ECG gating to delineate the arterial vasculature.

Although quick and robust, MDCT does expose patients to potentially nephrotoxic iodinated contrast agents. Because a standard bolus of 80 to 120 mL of low-osmolar iodinated contrast is needed, the benefits and risks of iodinated contrast need to be carefully weighed, especially for the elderly patients.[92] For patients for whom iodinated contrast is absolutely contraindicated, alternative imaging is not standardized, depends highly on local expertise, and will likely require multimodality integration. The threshold for the safe performance of CT is highly individualized and depends in part on provider preferences and institutional protocols.

Magnetic Resonance Imaging

The mainstay of CMR imaging is intrinsic bright blood cine imaging (without contrast) with 2D ECG-gated noncontrast cine CMR sequences called balanced steady-state free precession (SSFP). SSFP images are typically acquired at a 6- to 10-mm slice thickness with or without a small gap between slices. The main drawback of SSFP imaging is that although it provides intrinsic bright blood imaging and high signal-to-noise ratios, the images are acquired over several heart beats and require an 8- to 12-second breath hold and the absence or irregular heart beats or rhythms. Typical SSFP images are acquired as 2D image sequences, and the precise imaging planes must be correctly lined up at the time of primary image acquisition because they cannot be manipulated after acquisition.

For noncontrast angiography, intrinsic bright blood MRA sequences are available, but acquisition times are too long to be acquired with a single breath hold. These images can instead by obtained using free-breathing, navigator-gated, 3D, whole-heart acquisition (typically at mid-diastole, voxel size of approximately 1.2 × 1.2 × 1.8 mm^3), similar to the volumetric acquisition of a MDCT image. These images are also often obtained only at a single phase of the R-R interval due to the prohibitive time required to obtain a fully dynamic data set. Noncontrast angiography sequences are not widely available, and gadolinium-based sequences often are required.

Gadolinium chelate is most often used for MRA studies. Although not directly nephrotoxic, it has been associated with nephrogenic systemic fibrosis in patients with impaired renal function with a glomerular filtration rate less than 30, acute renal failure, and in particular, end-stage renal disease requiring hemodialysis. This leaves a small

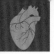

window of abnormal renal function for which these agents may have a role rather than using iodinated contrast, and they are typically used only in selected cases.

CMR for valvular heart disease is particularly enhanced by the use of velocity-encoded imaging, which is analogous to Doppler echocardiography. In-plane flow quantification can be performed to visualize the direction of flow through stenotic or regurgitant valve lesions.[93] Alternatively, through-plane flow imaging can be useful for quantifying aortic regurgitation (see Fig. 13.11C–E). Through-plane flows can be positioned to estimate a peak velocity of a stenotic aortic valve, but this systematically underestimates peak velocities compared with echocardiography. Newer 4D flow sequences are becoming more widely available, but this technology is limited by long acquisition times and lack of wide availability. Nonetheless, 4D flow has the potential to change how CMR is used to evaluate valvular heart disease.

PREPROCEDURAL NONCARDIOVASCULAR IMAGING

Because of the high prevalence of dementia and atherosclerosis among the elderly patient population, a preprocedural workup, including carotid ultrasound and cerebrovascular MRI, may be considered before recommending these patients for TAVR. However, further research is necessary before making conclusive recommendations. This type of evaluation is particularly relevant given the increased rates of cerebrovascular events among patients with TAVR compared with SAVR.

PERIPROCEDURAL EVALUATION

Immediate Preprocedural Evaluation

Fluoroscopy and TEE are the primary imaging modalities used at the time of the TAVR procedure. The aortic annulus can be evaluated with TEE immediately before the procedure, but using the standard imaging pathway with MDCT, this imaging should ideally be only confirmatory of the preprocedure planning. Isolated valve sizing with TEE should be reserved for urgent cases for which there is insufficient time for careful preplanning.[94]

If questions remain about the correct annular measurements, a sizing balloon can be inflated in the aortic annulus with subsequent aortic root angiography to evaluate for aortic regurgitation. The TAVR deployment angles obtained before the procedure with MDCT are also confirmed during this period with an aortic root injection. Fluoroscopic C-arm CT is becoming more widely available and may find a future periprocedural role, particularly for urgently performed procedures.

Periprocedural Guidance Considerations

When the decision is made to proceed with TAVR, real-time 3D imaging with TEE has improved in image quality and temporal resolution enough to provide full imaging guidance of an entire procedure.[62] 3D TEE tools such as biplane imaging and fusion imaging with fluoroscopy can be of particular value in this setting.

As with other imaging modalities, interventional TEE requires specific training and practice to achieve competence, particularly when performed under the pressure of an active intervention. However, what constitutes adequate training for these modalities is an evolving process. The future roll of TEE specifically for TAVR may also decrease in the future as many centers move toward standard use of monitored anesthesia care during TAVR cases.[95,96] Early data suggest that this shift away from the use of TEE has produced no significant change in outcomes.[97] However, dedicated skills with interventional TEE will remain important for guiding the most complex and highest-risk cases.[53]

Immediate Postprocedural Evaluation

The role of imaging in the immediate post-TAVR period employs simultaneous evaluation of the valve with fluoroscopy (often with a root injection of iodinated contrast) and assessment by TEE. The primary goals of evaluation include (1) assessing valve positioning and whether an ideal deployment occurred with minimal migration from the expected position; (2) evaluating immediate catastrophic complications; and (3) assessing the immediate degree of paravalvular aortic regurgitation.

Complications that can be seen on initial imaging include annular rupture from a large calcification in the LV outflow tract, and wall motion abnormalities from coronary artery occlusion from displacement of the native aortic valve leaflets by the prosthetic valve. If the degree of paravalvular aortic regurgitation is unacceptable, many solutions have been described depending on the reason for leak, the valve technology used, and whether the valve can be recaptured or repositioned. As many centers gain expertise with TAVR and monitored anesthesia care, particularly in the intermediate-risk population, TEE may be supplanted by a focused immediate postprocedural TTE or no immediate echocardiographic imaging.

POSTPROCEDURAL MONITORING

Postprocedural Valve Assessment

The definitive time frame for valve imaging after TAVR has not been determined. Most follow-up is performed using TTE with monitoring of valve gradients and velocities with Doppler echocardiography. Many centers obtain a TTE at regular intervals, such as before discharge and at 1 month, 6 months, and 1 year. However, these schedules often are driven by protocols from clinical trials and are discordant with current valve guidelines for SAVR, for which up until 10 years after implantation, only an initial follow-up study is recommended for baseline hemodynamics.[14] Whether these guidelines are relevant to TAVR remains an open question because the durability of TAVR valves compared with SAVR valves needs to be established.

MDCT has continued to play a role in the postprocedural evaluation of TAVR. It can be used to evaluate prosthesis implantation height, valve geometry, and better visualize complications such as chamber rupture.[98] MDCT can also be used to study the impact of TAVR on the geometry of the aortoannular complex. As the round valve is placed into the oval annulus, the annulus typically becomes more circular. Noncircular valve deployment can be quantified by eccentricity greater than 10%,[99] and highly eccentric valves are theorized to distort prosthetic valve geometry after expansion and may contribute to early valve degeneration.[100] For balloon-expandable valves up to 2.5 years after deployment, the finding of highly eccentric valves is rare and suggests that valve geometry is reasonably stable after implantation.[101]

Quantification of paravalvular aortic regurgitation by echocardiography is not fully standardized. In challenging cases with poor visualization, postprocedural assessment of residual aortic insufficiency by quantitative MRI may have a role in monitoring post-TAVR patients.[102]

Replacement Valve Durability

The issue of valve durability is coming under increasing scrutiny as TAVR becomes more widespread, particularly as it expands to younger and lower-risk cohorts.[8,103] Case reports of early valve failure show that the primary reported causes are endocarditis, structural valve failure, and valve thrombosis.[104] This is discordant from the 5-year outcomes reported in the PARTNER I trial, in which no structural valve degeneration was seen in the TAVR or SAVR groups.[19]

Individual sites have shown signs of moderate prosthetic valve failure in 3.4% of patients who received a balloon-expandable TAVR valve.[105] Similar results were reported for the 5-year experience with a self-expanding prosthesis, with late prosthesis failure occurring in 1.4% of cases and 2.8% showing late mild stenosis.[106] Worsening dyspnea and an increasing TAVR valve gradient have been associated with valve thrombosis in 0.61% of patients, occurring mostly within 2 years of implantation. Treatment with anticoagulation appears to be effective, even when the thrombosis is not clearly seen on echocardiography.[107]

Due to the available acquisition windows with TTE, it is often difficult to obtain a detailed assessment of prosthetic valve leaflet motion, and subclinical leaflet thrombosis may be underestimated. Using MDCT cine images, valve motion can often be visualized more readily. The use of this technique was reported in a study by Makkar and colleagues, which raised concern about possible subclinical leaflet thrombosis in a variety of transcatheter and surgically placed bioprosthetic aortic valves.[108]

The clinical impact of early leaflet thrombosis after TAVR is a significant concern and remains an area of active research. Some early observational evidence suggests that this is not associated with increased mortality or stroke rates in the intermediate term.[109] However the impact on long-term valve durability is unknown and of significant interest as TAVR becomes more widespread among lower-risk cohorts.

Postprocedural Evaluation for Cerebrovascular Events

As a result of antecedent balloon valvuloplasty and subsequent TAVR valve placement, there is an increased risk of dislodgement of microdebris from an arch atheroma or from the TAVR valve itself, producing embolic stroke. This complication has been seen in various studies, which reported a higher incidence of stroke after TAVR.[4,5]

In a study using intraprocedural transcranial Doppler during TAVR, cerebral microemboli were observed in all patients, especially during balloon valvuloplasty and delivery of the prosthetic valve.[110] Multiple studies using cerebral diffusion-weighted MRI have demonstrated a very high incidence (>70%) of new cerebral embolic foci after TAVR.[111–114] In short-term follow-up, these foci were not associated with apparent neurologic events or measurable deterioration of neurocognitive function. However, the high incidence of such foci may portend greater clinical significance when patients are followed for longer periods and when younger patients start to undergo TAVR. Future research should study the timing and frequency of assessing for these embolic foci, their long-term clinical impact, and techniques to reduce such embolic events.

FUTURE DIRECTIONS

The growth of TAVR has pushed current imaging technology forward, and integration of MDCT with the standard evaluation and preprocedural planning of TAVR has expanded knowledge of the aortoannular complex. Accurate annular sizing is critical for TAVR valve selection and for minimizing complications during the procedure, solidifying the importance of multimodality imaging by dedicated imaging specialists before TAVR.[94]

Incorporation of new imaging technologies with TAVR has set the stage for integrative imaging in the rapidly growing world of structural heart disease interventions, and techniques such as ECG-gated MDCT continue to play a greater role in more complex interventions such as transcatheter mitral valve replacement.[115] Fusion imaging techniques are an exciting outgrowth of structural heart disease imaging, and innovations such as the integration of live TEE images with fluoroscopy may change how complex structural heart disease interventions are performed.[116]

As the scope of transcatheter interventions expand, the experience with TAVR has shown the importance of meticulous planning and periprocedural imaging guidance. The continued growth of transcatheter procedures will require training of more specialty structural imagers who are knowledgeable about all cardiac imaging modalities and how they fit into the planning and performance of these challenging procedures. Given the complexity of structural imaging, the most complex of procedures should be performed in structural imaging centers of excellence, where dedicated experts are able to use an integrative multimodality imaging approach for the best outcomes.

REFERENCES

1. Cribier A, Eltchaninoff H, Bash A, et al. Percutaneous transcatheter implantation of an aortic valve prosthesis for calcific aortic stenosis: first human case description. Circulation 2002;106(24):3006-3008.
2. Kamioka N, Wells J, Keegan P, et al. Predictors and clinical outcomes of next-day discharge after minimalist transfemoral transcatheter aortic valve replacement. JACC Cardiovasc Interv 2018;11(2):107-115.
3. Kolte D, Khera S, Vemulapalli S, et al. Outcomes following urgent/emergent transcatheter aortic valve replacement: insights from the STS/ACC TVT Registry. JACC Cardiovasc Interv 2018;11(12):1175-1185.
4. Leon MB, Smith CR, Mack M, et al. Transcatheter aortic-valve implantation for aortic stenosis in patients who cannot undergo surgery. N Engl J Med 2010;363(17):1597-1607.
5. Smith CR, Leon MB, Mack MJ, et al. Transcatheter versus surgical aortic-valve replacement in high-risk patients. N Engl J Med 2011;364(23):2187-2198.
6. Kodali SK, Williams MR, Smith CR, et al. Two-year outcomes after transcatheter or surgical aortic-valve replacement. N Engl J Med 2012;366(18):1686-1695.
7. Adams DH, Popma JJ, Reardon MJ, et al. Transcatheter aortic-valve replacement with a self-expanding prosthesis. N Engl J Med 2014;370(19):1790-1798.
8. Leon MB, Smith CR, Mack MJ, et al. Transcatheter or surgical aortic-valve replacement in intermediate-risk patients. N Engl J Med 2016;374(17):1609-1620.
9. Feldman TE, Reardon MJ, Rajagopal V, et al. Effect of mechanically expanded vs self-expanding transcatheter aortic valve replacement on mortality and major adverse clinical events in high-risk patients with aortic stenosis: the REPRISE III Randomized Clinical Trial. JAMA 2018;319(1):27-37.
10. Reichenspurner H, Schaefer A, Schafer U, et al. Self-expanding transcatheter aortic valve system for symptomatic high-risk patients with severe aortic stenosis. J Am Coll Cardiol 2017;70(25):3127-3136.
11. Eggebrecht H, Vaquerizo B, Moris C, et al. Incidence and outcomes of emergent cardiac surgery during transfemoral transcatheter aortic valve implantation (TAVI): insights from the European Registry on Emergent Cardiac Surgery during TAVI (EuRECS-TAVI). Eur Heart J 2018;39(8):676-684.
12. Otto CM, Burwash IG, Legget ME, et al. Prospective study of asymptomatic valvular aortic stenosis. Clinical, echocardiographic, and exercise predictors of outcome. Circulation 1997;95(9):2262-2270.
13. Rosenhek R, Zilberszac R, Schemper M, et al. Natural history of very severe aortic stenosis. Circulation 2010;121(1):151-156.
14. Nishimura RA, Otto CM, Bonow RO, et al. 2014 AHA/ACC guideline for the management of patients with valvular heart disease: executive summary: a report of the American College of Cardiology/American Heart Association Task Force on Practice Guidelines Circulation 2014;129(23):2440-2492.
15. Baumgartner H, Hung J, Bermejo J, et al. Echocardiographic assessment of valve stenosis: EAE/ASE recommendations for clinical practice. J Am Soc Echocardiogr 2009;22(1):1-23.
16. Siontis GC, Juni P, Pilgrim T, et al. Predictors of permanent pacemaker implantation in patients with severe aortic stenosis undergoing TAVR: a meta-analysis. J Am Coll Cardiol 2014;64(2):129-140.
17. Asami M, Lanz J, Stortecky S, et al. The impact of left ventricular diastolic dysfunction on clinical outcomes after transcatheter aortic valve replacement. JACC Cardiovasc Interv 2018;11(6):593-601.

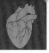
18. Asami M, Stortecky S, Praz F, et al. Prognostic value of right ventricular dysfunction on clinical outcomes after transcatheter aortic valve replacement. JACC Cardiovasc Imaging 2018.

19. Mack MJ, Leon MB, Smith CR, et al. 5-year outcomes of transcatheter aortic valve replacement or surgical aortic valve replacement for high surgical risk patients with aortic stenosis (PARTNER 1): a randomised controlled trial. Lancet 2015;385(9986):2477-2484.

20. Al Ali AM, Altwegg L, Horlick EM, et al. Prevention and management of transcatheter balloon-expandable aortic valve malposition. Catheter Cardiovasc Interv 2008;72(4):573-578.

21. Schoenhagen P, Tuzcu EM, Kapadia SR, et al. Three-dimensional imaging of the aortic valve and aortic root with computed tomography: new standards in an era of transcatheter valve repair/implantation. Eur Heart J 2009;30(17):2079-2086.

22. Bloomfield GS, Gillam LD, Hahn RT, et al. A practical guide to multimodality imaging of transcatheter aortic valve replacement. JACC Cardiovasc Imaging 2012;5(4):441-455.

23. Piazza N, de Jaegere P, Schultz C, et al. Anatomy of the aortic valvar complex and its implications for transcatheter implantation of the aortic valve. Circ Cardiovasc Interv 2008;1(1):74-81.

24. Binder RK, Webb JG, Willson AB, et al. The impact of integration of a multidetector computed tomography annulus area sizing algorithm on outcomes of transcatheter aortic valve replacement: a prospective, multicenter, controlled trial. J Am Coll Cardiol 2013;62(5):431-438.

25. Toggweiler S, Gurvitch R, Leipsic J, et al. Percutaneous aortic valve replacement: vascular outcomes with a fully percutaneous procedure. J Am Coll Cardiol 2012;59(2):113-118.

26. Kempfert J, Van Linden A, Lehmkuhl L, et al. Aortic annulus sizing: echocardiographic versus computed tomography derived measurements in comparison with direct surgical sizing. Eur J Cardiothorac Surg 2012;42(4):627-633.

27. Jilaihawi H, Kashif M, Fontana G, et al. Cross-sectional computed tomographic assessment improves accuracy of aortic annular sizing for transcatheter aortic valve replacement and reduces the incidence of paravalvular aortic regurgitation. J Am Coll Cardiol 2012;59(14):1275-1286.

28. Achenbach S, Delgado V, Hausleiter J, et al. SCCT expert consensus document on computed tomography imaging before transcatheter aortic valve implantation (TAVI)/transcatheter aortic valve replacement (TAVR). J Cardiovasc Comput Tomogr 2012;6(6):366-380.

29. Quail MA, Nordmeyer J, Schievano S, et al. Use of cardiovascular magnetic resonance imaging for TAVR assessment in patients with bioprosthetic aortic valves: comparison with computed tomography. Eur J Radiol 2012;81(12):3912-3917.

30. Cavalcante JL, Lalude OO, Schoenhagen P, Lerakis S. Cardiovascular magnetic resonance imaging for structural and valvular heart disease interventions. JACC Cardiovasc Interv 2016;9(5):399-425.

31. Koos R, Altiok E, Mahnken AH, et al. Evaluation of aortic root for definition of prosthesis size by magnetic resonance imaging and cardiac computed tomography: implications for transcatheter aortic valve implantation. Int J Cardiol 2012;158(3):353-358.

32. Jabbour A, Ismail TF, Moat N, et al. Multimodality imaging in transcatheter aortic valve implantation and post-procedural aortic regurgitation comparison among cardiovascular magnetic resonance, cardiac computed tomography, and echocardiography. J Am Coll Cardiol 2011;58(21):2165-2173.

33. Scully PR, Treibel TA, Fontana M, et al. Prevalence of cardiac amyloidosis in patients referred for transcatheter aortic valve replacement. J Am Coll Cardiol 2018;71(4):463-464.

34. Cavalcante JL, Rijal S, Abdelkarim I, et al. Cardiac amyloidosis is prevalent in older patients with aortic stenosis and carries worse prognosis. J Cardiovasc Magn Reson 2017;19(1):98.

35. Castano A, Narotsky DL, Hamid N, et al. Unveiling transthyretin cardiac amyloidosis and its predictors among elderly patients with severe aortic stenosis undergoing transcatheter aortic valve replacement. Eur Heart J 2017;38(38):2879-2887.

36. Blanke P, Russe M, Leipsic J, et al. Conformational pulsatile changes of the aortic annulus: impact on prosthesis sizing by computed tomography for transcatheter aortic valve replacement. JACC Cardiovasc Interv 2012;5:984–994.

37. Murphy DT, Blanke P, Alaamri S, et al. Dynamism of the aortic annulus: effect of diastolic versus systolic CT annular measurements on device selection in transcatheter aortic valve replacement (TAVR). J Cardiovasc Comput Tomogr 2016;10(1):37-43.

38. Sucha D, Tuncay V, Prakken NH, et al. Does the aortic annulus undergo conformational change throughout the cardiac cycle? A systematic review. Eur Heart J Cardiovasc Imaging 2015;16(12):1307-1317.

39. Messika-Zeitoun D, Serfaty JM, et al. Multimodal assessment of the aortic annulus diameter: implications for transcatheter aortic valve implantation. J Am Coll Cardiol 2010;55(3):186-194.

40. Akhtar M, Tuzcu EM, Kapadia SR, et al. Aortic root morphology in patients undergoing percutaneous aortic valve replacement: evidence of aortic root remodeling. J Thorac Cardiovasc Surg 2009;137(4):950-956.

41. Tops LF, Wood DA, Delgado V, et al. Noninvasive evaluation of the aortic root with multislice computed tomography implications for transcatheter aortic valve replacement. JACC Cardiovasc Imaging 2008;1(3):321-330.

42. O'Brien B, Schoenhagen P, Kapadia SR, et al. Integration of 3D imaging data in the assessment of aortic stenosis: impact on classification of disease severity. Circ Cardiovasc Imaging 2011;4(5):566-573.

43. Nazif TM, Dizon JM, Hahn RT, et al. Predictors and clinical outcomes of permanent pacemaker implantation after transcatheter aortic valve replacement: the PARTNER (Placement of AoRtic TraNscathetER Valves) trial and registry. JACC Cardiovasc Interv 2015;8(1 Pt A):60-69.

44. Piazza N, Onuma Y, Jesserun E, et al. Early and persistent intraventricular conduction abnormalities and requirements for pacemaking after percutaneous replacement of the aortic valve. JACC Cardiovasc Interv 2008;1(3):310-316.

45. Blanke P, Reinohl J, Schlensak C, et al. Prosthesis oversizing in balloon-expandable transcatheter aortic valve implantation is associated with contained rupture of the aortic root. Circ Cardiovasc Interv 2012;5(4):540-548.

46. Schmidkonz C, Marwan M, Klinghammer L, et al. Interobserver variability of CT angiography for evaluation of aortic annulus dimensions prior to transcatheter aortic valve implantation (TAVI). Eur J Radiol 2014;83(9):1672-1678.

47. Jabbour RJ, Tanaka A, Finkelstein A, et al. Delayed coronary obstruction after transcatheter aortic valve replacement. J Am Coll Cardiol 2018;71(14):1513-1524.

48. Ribeiro HB, Webb JG, Makkar RR, et al. Predictive factors, management, and clinical outcomes of coronary obstruction following transcatheter aortic valve implantation: insights from a large multicenter registry. J Am Coll Cardiol 2013;62(17):1552-1562.

49. Tuzcu EM, Kapadia SR, Vemulapalli S, et al. Transcatheter aortic valve replacement of failed surgically implanted bioprostheses: the STS/ACC Registry. J Am Coll Cardiol 2018;72(4):370-382.

50. Pibarot P, Simonato M, Barbanti M, et al. Impact of pre-existing prosthesis-patient mismatch on survival following aortic valve-in-valve procedures. JACC Cardiovasc Interv 2018;11(2):133-141.

51. Chhatriwalla AK, Allen KB, Saxon JT, et al. Bioprosthetic valve fracture improves the hemodynamic results of valve-in-valve transcatheter aortic valve replacement. Circ Cardiovasc Interv 2017;10(7).

52. Saxon JT, Allen KB, Cohen DJ, Chhatriwalla AK. Bioprosthetic valve fracture during valve-in-valve TAVR: bench to bedside. Interv Cardiol 2018;13(1):20-26.

53. Khan JM, Dvir D, Greenbaum AB, et al. Transcatheter laceration of aortic leaflets to prevent coronary obstruction during transcatheter aortic valve replacement: concept to first-in-human. JACC Cardiovasc Interv 2018;11(7):677-689.

54. Clavel MA, Malouf J, Messika-Zeitoun D, Araoz PA, Michelena HI, Enriquez-Sarano M. Aortic valve area calculation in aortic stenosis by CT and Doppler echocardiography. JACC Cardiovasc Imaging 2015;8(3):248-257.

55. Mylotte D, Lefevre T, Sondergaard L, et al. Transcatheter aortic valve replacement in bicuspid aortic valve disease. J Am Coll Cardiol 2014;64(22):2330-2339.

56. Einstein AJ, Henzlova MJ, Rajagopalan S. Estimating risk of cancer associated with radiation exposure from 64-slice computed tomography coronary angiography. JAMA 2007;298(3):317-323.

57. Tzikas A, Schultz CJ, Piazza N, et al. Assessment of the aortic annulus by multislice computed tomography, contrast aortography, and transthoracic echocardiography in patients referred for transcatheter aortic valve implantation. Catheter Cardiovasc Interv 2011;77(6):868-875.

58. Ng AC, Delgado V, van der Kley F, et al. Comparison of aortic root dimensions and geometries before and after transcatheter aortic valve implantation by 2- and 3-dimensional transesophageal echocardiography and multislice computed tomography. Circ Cardiovasc Imaging 2010;3(1):94-102.

59. Mylotte D, Dorfmeister M, Elhmidi Y, et al. Erroneous measurement of the aortic annular diameter using 2-dimensional echocardiography resulting in inappropriate CoreValve size selection: a retrospective comparison with multislice computed tomography. JACC Cardiovasc Interv 2014;7:652–661.

60. O'Neill B, Wang DD, Pantelic M, et al. Transcatheter caval valve implantation using multimodality imaging: roles of TEE, CT, and 3D printing. JACC Cardiovasc Imaging 2015;8(2):221-225.

61. Qian Z, Wang K, Liu S, et al. Quantitative prediction of paravalvular leak in transcatheter aortic valve replacement based on tissue-mimicking 3D printing. JACC Cardiovasc Imaging 2017;10(7):719-731.

62. Janosi RA, Kahlert P, Plicht B, et al. Measurement of the aortic annulus size by real-time three-dimensional transesophageal echocardiography. Minim Invasive Ther Allied Technol 2011;20(2):85-94.

63. Kurra V, Lieber ML, Sola S, et al. Extent of thoracic aortic atheroma burden and long-term mortality after cardiothoracic surgery: a computed tomography study. JACC Cardiovasc Imaging 2010;3(10):1020-1029.

64. Kurra V, Schoenhagen P, Roselli EE, et al. Prevalence of significant peripheral artery disease in patients evaluated for percutaneous aortic valve insertion: preprocedural assessment with multidetector computed tomography. J Thorac Cardiovasc Surg 2009;137(5):1258-1264.

65. Mylotte D, Sudre A, Teiger E, et al. Transcarotid transcatheter aortic valve replacement: feasibility and safety. JACC Cardiovasc Interv 2016;9(5):472-480.

66. Debry N, Delhaye C, Azmoun A, et al. Transcarotid transcatheter aortic valve replacement: general or local anesthesia. JACC Cardiovasc Interv 2016;9(20):2113-2120.

67. Martinez-Clark PO, Singh V, Cadena JA, et al. Transcaval retrograde transcatheter aortic valve replacement for patients with no other access: first-in-man experience with CoreValve. JACC Cardiovasc Interv 2014;7(9):1075-1077.

68. Greenbaum AB, Babaliaros VC, Chen MY, et al. Transcaval access and closure for transcatheter aortic valve replacement: a prospective investigation. J Am Coll Cardiol 2017;69(5):511-521.

69. Bapat V, Thomas M, Hancock J, Wilson K. First successful trans-catheter aortic valve implantation through ascending aorta using Edwards SAPIEN THV system. Eur J Cardiothorac Surg 2010;38(6):811-813.

70. Delgado V, Ewe SH, Ng AC, et al. Multimodality imaging in transcatheter aortic valve implantation: key steps to assess procedural feasibility. EuroIntervention 2010;6(5):643-652.

71. Azzalini L, Abbara S, Ghoshhajra BB. Ultra-low contrast computed tomographic angiography (CTA) with 20-mL total dose for transcatheter aortic valve implantation (TAVI) planning. J Comput Assist Tomogr 2014;38(1):105-109.

72. Joshi SB, Mendoza DD, Steinberg DH, et al. Ultra-low-dose intra-arterial contrast injection for iliofemoral computed tomographic angiography. JACC Cardiovasc Imaging 2009;2(12):1404-1411.

73. Yoshida T, Han F, Zhou Z, et al. Ferumoxytol MRA and non-contrast CT fusion in TAVR candidates with renal failure. J Cardiovasc Magn Reson 2016;18(Suppl 1):Q59.

74. Gurvitch R, Wood DA, Leipsic J, et al. Multislice computed tomography for prediction of optimal angiographic deployment projections during transcatheter aortic valve implantation. JACC Cardiovasc Interv 2010;3(11):1157-1165.

75. Kurra V, Kapadia SR, Tuzcu EM, et al. Pre-procedural imaging of aortic root orientation and dimensions: comparison between X-ray angiographic planar imaging and 3-dimensional multidetector row computed tomography. JACC Cardiovasc Interv 2010;3(1):105-113.

76. Samim M, Stella PR, Agostoni P, et al. Automated 3D analysis of pre-procedural MDCT to predict annulus plane angulation and C-arm positioning: benefit on procedural outcome in patients referred for TAVR. JACC Cardiovasc Imaging 2013;6(2):238-248.

77. Binder RK, Leipsic J, Wood D, et al. Prediction of optimal deployment projection for transcatheter aortic valve replacement: angiographic 3-dimensional reconstruction of the aortic root versus multidetector computed tomography. Circ Cardiovasc Interv 2012;5(2):247-252.

78. Testa L, Latib A, Casenghi M, et al. Cerebral protection during transcatheter aortic valve implantation: an updated systematic review and meta-analysis. J Am Heart Assoc 2018;7(10):e008463.

79. Kapadia SR, Kodali S, Makkar R, et al. Cerebral embolic protection during transcatheter aortic valve replacement. J Am Coll Cardiol 2016;69(4):367-377.

80. Ibrahim H, Welt FGP. Surgical versus transcatheter aortic valve replacement in patients with prior coronary bypass surgery: tie goes to the runner. Circ Cardiovasc Interv 2018;11(4):e006593.

81. Gupta T, Khera S, Kolte D, et al. Transcatheter versus surgical aortic valve replacement in patients with prior coronary artery bypass grafting: trends in utilization and propensity-matched analysis of in-hospital outcomes. Circ Cardiovasc Interv 2018;11(4):e006179.

82. Chieffo A, Giustino G, Spagnolo P, et al. Routine screening of coronary artery disease with computed tomographic coronary angiography in place of invasive coronary angiography in patients undergoing transcatheter aortic valve replacement. Circ Cardiovasc Interv 2015;8(7):e002025.

83. Feuchtner G, Goetti R, Plass A, et al. Dual-step prospective ECG-triggered 128-slice dual-source CT for evaluation of coronary arteries and cardiac function without heart rate control: a technical note. Eur Radiol 2010;20(9):2092-2099.

84. Rajiah P, Schoenhagen P. The role of computed tomography in pre-procedural planning of cardiovascular surgery and intervention. Insights Imaging 2013;4(5):671-689.

85. Palmer S, Child N, de Belder MA, et al. Left atrial appendage thrombus in transcatheter aortic valve replacement: incidence, clinical impact, and the role of cardiac computed tomography. JACC Cardiovasc Interv 2017;10(2):176-184.

86. Salemi A, De Micheli A, Aftab A, et al. Transcatheter aortic valve replacement in the setting of left atrial appendage thrombus. Interact Cardiovasc Thorac Surg 2018;27(6):842-849.

87. Van Linden A, Kempfert J, Blumenstein J, et al. Manual versus automatic detection of aortic annulus plane in a computed tomography scan for transcatheter aortic valve implantation screening. Eur J Cardiothorac Surg 2014;46(2):207-212; discussion 212.

88. Entezari P, Kino A, Honarmand AR, et al. Analysis of the thoracic aorta using a semi-automated post processing tool. Eur J Radiol 2013;82(9):1558-1564.

89. Swee JK, Grbic S. Advanced transcatheter aortic valve implantation (TAVI) planning from CT with ShapeForest. Med Image Comput Comput Assist Interv 2014;17(Pt 2):17-24.

90. Lou J, Obuchowski NA, Krishnaswamy A, et al. Manual, semiautomated, and fully automated measurement of the aortic annulus for planning of transcatheter aortic valve replacement (TAVR/TAVI): analysis of interchangeability. J Cardiovasc Comput Tomogr 2015;9(1):42-49.

91. Watanabe Y, Morice MC, Bouvier E, et al. Automated 3-dimensional aortic annular assessment by multidetector computed tomography in transcatheter aortic valve implantation. JACC Cardiovasc Imaging 2013;6(9):955-964.

92. Bagur R, Webb JG, Nietlispach F, et al. Acute kidney injury following transcatheter aortic valve implantation: predictive factors, prognostic value, and comparison with surgical aortic valve replacement. Eur Heart J 2010;31(7):865-874.

93. Krieger EV, Lee J, Branch KR, Hamilton-Craig C. Quantitation of mitral regurgitation with cardiac magnetic resonance imaging: a systematic review. Heart 2016;102(23):1864-1870.

94. Otto CM, Kumbhani DJ, Alexander KP, et al. 2017 ACC Expert Consensus decision pathway for transcatheter aortic valve replacement in the management of adults with aortic stenosis: a report of the American College of Cardiology task force on clinical expert consensus documents. J Am Coll Cardiol 2017;69:1313–1346.

95. Durand E, Borz B, Godin M, et al. Transfemoral aortic valve replacement with the Edwards SAPIEN and Edwards SAPIEN XT prosthesis using exclusively local anesthesia and fluoroscopic guidance: feasibility and 30-day outcomes. JACC Cardiovasc Interv 2012;5(5):461-467.

96. Babaliaros V, Devireddy C, Lerakis S, et al. Comparison of transfemoral transcatheter aortic valve replacement performed in the catheterization laboratory (minimalist approach) versus hybrid operating room (standard approach): outcomes and cost analysis. JACC Cardiovasc Interv 2014;7(8):898-904.

97. Bhatnagar UB, Gedela M, Sethi P, et al. Outcomes and safety of transcatheter aortic valve implantation with and without routine use of transesophageal echocardiography. Am J Cardiol 2018;122(7):1210-1214

98. Delgado V, Ng AC, van de Veire NR, et al. Transcatheter aortic valve implantation: role of multi-detector row computed tomography to evaluate prosthesis positioning and deployment in relation to valve function. Eur Heart J 2010;31(9):1114-1123.

99. Willson AB, Webb JG, Labounty TM, et al. 3-dimensional aortic annular assessment by multidetector computed tomography predicts moderate or severe paravalvular regurgitation after transcatheter aortic valve replacement: a multicenter retrospective analysis. J Am Coll Cardiol 2012;59(14):1287-1294.

100. Schultz CJ, Weustink A, Piazza N, et al. Geometry and degree of apposition of the CoreValve ReValving system with multislice computed tomography after implantation in patients with aortic stenosis. J Am Coll Cardiol 2009;54(10):911-918.

101. Willson AB, Webb JG, Gurvitch R, et al. Structural integrity of balloon-expandable stents after transcatheter aortic valve replacement: assessment by multidetector computed tomography. JACC Cardiovasc Interv 2012;5(5):525-532.

102. Sherif MA, Abdel-Wahab M, Beurich HW, et al. Haemodynamic evaluation of aortic regurgitation after transcatheter aortic valve implantation using cardiovascular magnetic resonance. EuroIntervention 2011;7(1):57-63.

103. Sedrakyan A, Dhruva SS, Sun T, et al. Trends in use of transcatheter aortic valve replacement by age. JAMA 2018;320(6):598-600.

104. Mylotte D, Andalib A, Theriault-Lauzier P, et al. Transcatheter heart valve failure: a systematic review. Eur Heart J 2015;36(21):1306-1327.

105. Toggweiler S, Humphries KH, Lee M, et al. 5-year outcome after transcatheter aortic valve implantation. J Am Coll Cardiol 2013;61(4):413-419.

106. Barbanti M, Petronio AS, Ettori F, et al. 5-Year outcomes after transcatheter aortic valve implantation with corevalve prosthesis. JACC Cardiovasc Interv 2015;8(8):1084-1091.

107. Latib A, Naganuma T, Abdel-Wahab M, et al. Treatment and clinical outcomes of transcatheter heart valve thrombosis. Circ Cardiovasc Interv 2015;8(4):e001779.

108. Makkar RR, Fontana G, Jilaihawi H, et al. Possible subclinical leaflet thrombosis in bioprosthetic aortic valves. N Engl J Med 2015;373(21):2015-2024.

109. Ruile P, Minners J, Breitbart P, et al. Medium-term follow-up of early leaflet thrombosis after transcatheter aortic valve replacement. JACC: Cardiovasc Interv 2018;11(12):1164-1171.

110. Drews T, Pasic M, Buz S, et al. Transcranial Doppler sound detection of cerebral microembolism during transapical aortic valve implantation. Thorac Cardiovasc Surg 2011;59(4):237-242.

111. Kahlert P, Knipp SC, Schlamann M, et al. Silent and apparent cerebral ischemia after percutaneous transfemoral aortic valve implantation: a diffusion-weighted magnetic resonance imaging study. Circulation 2010;121(7):870-878.

112. Astarci P, Glineur D, Kefer J, et al. Magnetic resonance imaging evaluation of cerebral embolization during percutaneous aortic valve implantation: comparison of transfemoral and trans-apical approaches using Edwards Sapiens valve. Eur J Cardiothorac Surg 2011;40(2):475-479.

113. Ghanem A, Muller A, Nahle CP, et al. Risk and fate of cerebral embolism after transfemoral aortic valve implantation: a prospective pilot study with diffusion-weighted magnetic resonance imaging. J Am Coll Cardiol 2010;55(14):1427-1432.

114. Fairbairn TA, Mather AN, Bijsterveld P, et al. Diffusion-weighted MRI determined cerebral embolic infarction following transcatheter aortic valve implantation: assessment of predictive risk factors and the relationship to subsequent health status. Heart 2012;98(1):18-23.

115. Wang DD, Eng M, Greenbaum A, et al. Predicting LVOT obstruction after TMVR. JACC Cardiovasc Imaging 2016;9(11):1349-1352.

116. Biaggi P, Fernandez-Golfin C, Hahn R, Corti R. Hybrid imaging during transcatheter structural heart interventions. Curr Cardiovasc Imaging Rep 2015;8(9):33.

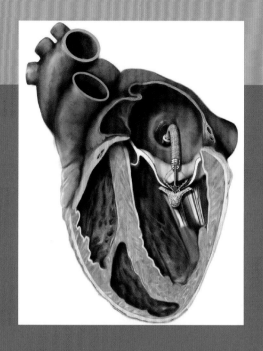

中文导读

第14章
主动脉瓣和主动脉根部疾病的外科手术策略

主动脉瓣和主动脉根部疾病，由于解剖毗邻，二者可依据具体病情个体化处理，或同期联合手术治疗。

手术入路首选经典胸骨正中切口。在主动脉瓣置换术中，瓣膜选择至关重要，本章详述了常见生物瓣和机械瓣的瓣膜工艺特征，相应的术式特点；并基于大量临床研究及指南，介绍两类瓣膜的优缺点，有助于患者和医师做出最佳选择。瓣膜修复部分介绍了可修复瓣膜的特征，修复手术相对瓣膜置换的优劣点及具体瓣膜修复的手术技巧。在瓣膜手术风险方面，依据患者术前风险评估，近期最新的研究及既往经典的研究结果，对长期及围手术期风险结局进行讲解。

主动脉根部疾病章节讲述了升主动脉疾病病因构成及风险，并对相应的手术指征、手术时机进行了详细介绍；针对不同的疾病，介绍了不同手术术式的具体流程和注意事项；对是否联合瓣膜手术，以及不同情况下需要进行的瓣膜联合主动脉根部手术方案进行讨论。

本章还对一些特殊疾病情况的处理进行讲解，如升主动脉夹层合并主动脉瓣反流、冠状动脉旁路移植术后的瓣膜置换、瓣膜置换术后二次手术、升主动脉根部二次手术、磁化主动脉手术策略等。

最后，本章讲述了主动脉瓣瓣膜材质工艺的改进，以及新型抗凝药物的临床应用可能为今后瓣膜病的治疗提供新的契机。

王彬成

Surgical Approach to Diseases of the Aortic Valve and Aortic Root

S. Chris Malaisrie, Patrick M. McCarthy

CHAPTER OUTLINE

KEY POINTS

- Aortic valve replacement (AVR) has become increasingly safe even though an older population of patients is now being treated, with the best outcomes achieved at high-volume centers.
- Complete primary median sternotomy is the standard approach for aortic valve and aortic root replacement, but minimally invasive approaches, including upper hemisternotomy and right anterior thoracotomy, can be performed with equivalent safety and improved outcomes.
- More stented bioprosthetic valves are being used than mechanical valves, homografts, and pulmonary autografts combined, reflecting advances in valve technology and changing patient preferences.
- Sutureless and rapid-deployment valves combine the advantages of surgical AVR procedure (e.g., control of aortic atheroemboli, resection of diseased native valve) with those of transcatheter technology (e.g., decreased procedure time, improved valve hemodynamics).

- Aortic root replacement with a composite valve-graft (i.e., Bentall procedure) is the gold standard operation for aortic root aneurysm; however, valve-sparing aortic root replacement (i.e., David or Yacoub procedure) is a good option for patients who want to avoid the long-term oral anticoagulation that is required with mechanical valves and the structural valve deterioration associated with bioprosthetic valves.
- Aortic regurgitation from acute type A aortic dissections is life-threatening and is commonly managed by valve repair, reserving aortic root replacement for patients with intrinsic root pathology.
- Repeat aortic valve and aortic root surgery can be performed safely with the use of preoperative imaging, advanced techniques for myocardial protection, and safe management of existing bypass grafts, but the transcatheter valve-in-valve procedure is an increasingly attractive option in selected patients.

Since the placement of the first ball-in-cage mechanical valve more than 50 years ago, advances in surgical technique and valve technology have revolutionized the approach to aortic valve and aortic root disease. Surgical techniques encompass valve replacement for aortic stenosis (AS) and valve repair for aortic regurgitation (AR) and infective endocarditis. Replacement of the entire aortic root has become a safe and commonplace procedure in cases of aortic root aneurysm, and it is lifesaving in cases of aortic dissection.

Minimally invasive procedures through incisions other than a median sternotomy have been facilitated by technologic advances in

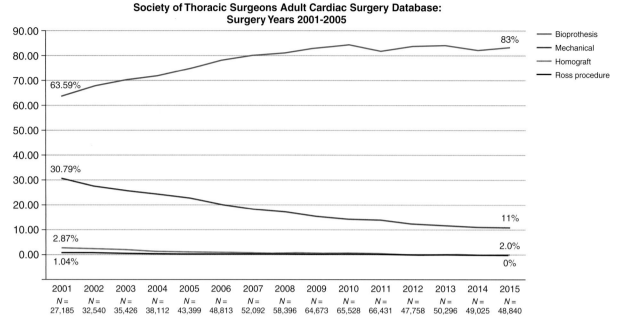

Society of Thoracic Surgeons Adult Cardiac Surgery Database:
Surgery Years 2001-2005

Fig. 14.1 Trends in Valve Choice for Aortic Valve Replacement. Bioprosthetic valves are the type most commonly implanted in the current era. Mechanical valves, homografts, and pulmonary autografts have declined in use over time.

surgical instruments and valve design, perhaps most significantly the advent of transcatheter heart valve procedures. During the past decade, transcatheter aortic valve implantation (TAVI) was developed and tested, leading to U.S. Food and Drug Administration (FDA) approval of a new treatment option for patients with AS that previously would have been managed by medical therapy and for patients who are at elevated risk (Society of Thoracic Surgeons [STS] score ≥ 3%) during conventional aortic valve replacement (AVR).[1–4] Additional testing is ongoing in randomized clinical trials to determine the proper use of TAVI in patients with low surgical risk.[5,6]

The field has been influenced by new valve guidelines that emphasize the patient's role in decision making. These developments have led to the most dramatic change in the clinical practice of aortic valve surgery in decades. Fig. 14.1 demonstrates by year the changing pattern of valve replacement choices. There has been a striking shift in the choice of prosthesis. In 2001, 63.6% of AVRs were bioprosthetic valves, a percentage that steadily rose to 83% in 2015. Mechanical valve use dropped by almost two thirds, from 30.8% to 11%. Homograft replacement fell from 2.9% to 2.0%, and use of the Ross procedure dropped from 1.0% to almost none in 2015.

This chapter explores the data that led to the change in valve prosthesis choice and reviews the advances in surgical techniques and valve technology that are relevant in clinical settings.

APPROACHES TO THE AORTIC VALVE AND ROOT

Median Sternotomy

The median sternotomy is the standard and most common approach for aortic valve and root procedures. The skin incision is vertical and directly overlies the sternum, which is divided from the sternal notch superiorly to the xyphoid process inferiorly. Complete exposure of the aorta and heart allows concomitant procedures such as coronary artery bypass grafting (CABG), multiple-valve procedures, surgical ablation of atrial fibrillation, and left atrial appendage closure. Rigid closure of the

divided sternum at the completion of the case with steel wire cerclage is generally well tolerated, although temporary upper-body weight restrictions (i.e., sternal precautions) are required during convalescence.

Minimally Invasive Approaches

Minimally invasive approaches to AVR include any incision that does not involve a complete median sternotomy, most commonly the upper hemisternotomy and the right anterior thoracotomy. Cosmesis has been the driving factor associated with the development of minimally invasive approaches, and these approaches have not been shown to compromise safety despite longer periods of cardiopulmonary bypass.[7–10] Potential benefits of a minimally invasive approach include reduction in postoperative bleeding, intensive care unit stay, and hospital length of stay.[7]

Upper Hemisternotomy

The upper hemisternotomy is performed through a vertical skin incision 5 to 8 cm below the angle of Louis (Fig. 14.2). The sternotomy is extended into the right third or fourth interspace as a J-shaped incision. Alternatively, the sternum can be divided transversely with a T-shaped incision. Cannulation for cardiopulmonary bypass and cardioplegic arrest can be performed through the incision or through peripheral sites. Exposure of the aortic valve and root is uncompromised, and conduct of the operation is unchanged compared with the median sternotomy approach.[11]

Right Anterior Thoracotomy

The right anterior thoracotomy is performed through a horizontal skin incision 4 to 7 cm lateral to the sternum (Fig. 14.3). The chest cavity is entered in the second or third interspace, often with division of the right internal thoracic vessels. The lower rib is disconnected from the sternal edge to improve exposure. Cannulation for cardiopulmonary bypass and cardioplegic arrest is performed peripherally. The aortic valve is well visualized, but long-handled instruments are required to complete the valve replacement. No sternal precautions are required for the minithoracotomy approach.[11]

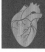

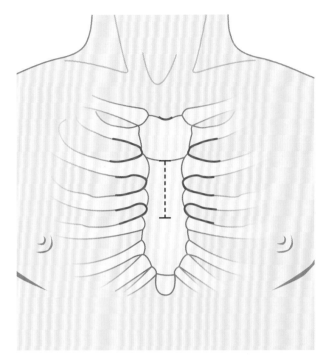

Fig. 14.2 Upper Hemisternotomy. Through a vertical skin incision, the upper sternotomy is divided and extended into the third or the fourth interspace, typically to the right.

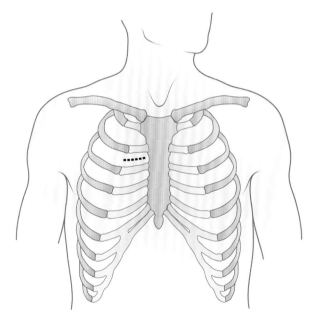

Fig. 14.3 Right Anterior Thoracotomy. By means of a horizontal skin incision, the right pleural cavity is entered through the second or third interspace, directly lateral to the sternal border.

AORTIC VALVE REPLACEMENT

Bioprosthetic Valves: Stented

The valve most commonly used to replace the aortic valve is a stented bioprosthetic valve constructed of bovine pericardium (Fig. 14.4A) or an actual porcine valve (see Fig. 14.4B). These valves have several

advantages: (1) ease of implantation and the rare occurrence of clinically significant patient-prosthesis mismatch (PPM) due to improving valve hemodynamics; (2) no need for lifelong oral anticoagulation (unless the patient requires it for a different reason); (3) a relatively straightforward future reoperation, if one is necessary; and (4) the potential for a valve-in-valve (VIV) procedure using a transcatheter heart valve for bioprosthetic valve failure. The most important disadvantage to tissue valves is the occurrence of structural valve deterioration (SVD), which is primarily age dependent.

The technical aspects of AVR with a stented bioprosthetic valve are straightforward. The aortic valve can be exposed through a variety of aortotomy incisions (i.e., hockey stick, transverse, or oblique). The aortic valve is excised, and the annulus is completely debrided of calcific plaques, with care taken in the area of the conduction system (below the commissure between the noncoronary and right coronary cusps). Calcific extensions on the aortic root, left ventricular outflow tract, and anterior leaflet of the mitral valve are removed. With adequate debridement of annular calcification, paravalvular leak is rare,[12] and with current-generation bioprostheses, clinically significant PPM is uncommon.[13]

Sutureless Valves

The most recent advance in bioprosthetic valve technology is the sutureless or rapid-deployment valve (see Fig. 14.4C and D, respectively). First implanted in humans in 2005,[14] sutureless valves have a metallic stent frame similar to those seen in transcatheter heart valves. The frames extend beyond the aortic annulus into the left ventricular outflow tract and achieve a seal without the need for complete suturing. Unlike the case with transcatheter valves, complete excision of the native aortic valve is required.

Two valves have been approved for commercial use in the United States and Europe and have shown safety and efficacy (Table 14.1).[15–17] Benefits include shorter aortic cross-clamp and cardiopulmonary bypass times, which may facilitate minimally invasive approaches[18] and cases of difficult full-sternotomy AVR involving reoperation, delicate aortic wall, concomitant procedures, or small aortic root.[19] A symmetric bicuspid aortic valve (BAV) with two commissures and no raphes (i.e., Sievers type 0)[20] and annular destruction due to complex infectious endocarditis are contraindications for this class of valves.[18,19]

Use of sutureless and rapid-deployment valves has reduced early postoperative complications, potentially translating into reduced resource consumption such as length of stay and hospital costs.[21] As with all new valve technology, the long-term durability of sutureless valves has not been proved, and equipoise remains regarding the durability in younger patients.

Bioprosthetic Valves: Stentless

Stentless bioprosthetic valves made from porcine aortic valves became available in the 1990s (see Fig. 14.4E) and were followed by stentless bovine pericardial valves (see Fig. 14.4F). The advantages of this type of valve are (1) improved hemodynamics compared with stented biologic and mechanical valves[22–24] and (2) the option to replace the entire aortic root, including the aortic valve, for combined valve and aortic disease (using the stentless porcine root). The disadvantages of stentless valves are (1) a more complex operation requiring a full root technique with reimplantation of the coronary ostia (Fig. 14.5), a root inclusion technique, or a subcoronary technique and (2) recent concerns regarding freedom from SVD.[25] The full root technique requires resection of the aortic root in addition to the aortic valve (described later). In the subcoronary and root inclusion techniques, only the aortic valve is excised, and the stentless valve is implanted within the native aortic root. Of these two, the subcoronary technique is more commonly performed (Fig. 14.6).

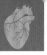

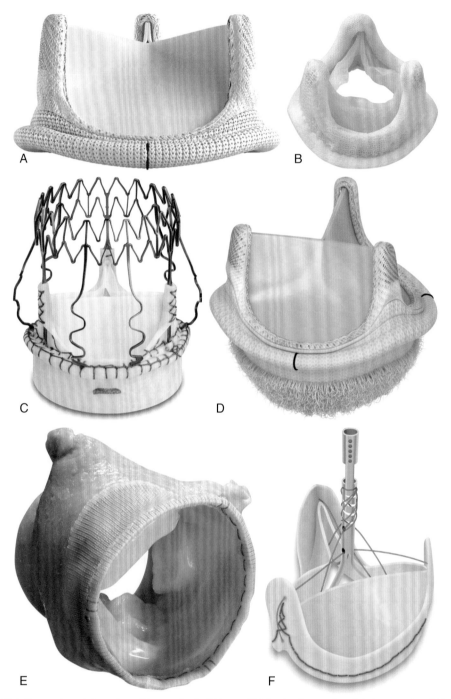

Fig. 14.4 Stented and Stentless Bioprosthetic Valves. (A) The bovine pericardial tissue valve (Edwards Magna Ease, Edwards Lifesciences, Irvine, CA) is attached to the supporting frame with an incorporated sewing ring. (B) The leaflets of the stented porcine valve (Medtronic Mosaic Ultra, Medtronic, Minneapolis, MN) are attached to the supporting frame with an incorporated sewing ring. (C). The Perceval sutureless aortic heart valve incorporates bovine pericardial leaflets on a nitinol, self-expanding frame. (D) The rapid-deployment valve (Edwards Intuity Elite, Edwards Lifesciences) incorporates bovine pericardial leaflets on a stainless steel, balloon-expandable frame. (E) The stentless porcine valve (Medtronic Freestyle, Medtronic). (F) The Solo Smart stentless bovine pericardial aortic heart valve. (B and F, Reproduced with permission of Medtronic, Inc., Minneapolis, MN. C. Reproduced with permission of LivaNova, London, England.)

Typically, two suture lines are required for the stentless porcine valve. The proximal line is a circular suture line at the level of the annulus, and the distal line follows the scallop-shaped leaflet insertion line below the level of the coronary arteries. In some stentless bovine pericardial valves, only a single distal line is required for implantation.[26]

Mechanical Valves

Mechanical valves have the advantages of long-term durability and a long track record with designs that have been durable for decades. The major disadvantages are (1) the need for lifelong anticoagulation (i.e., warfarin), (2) a higher risk for thromboembolism compared with

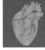

TABLE 14.1 Sutureless and Rapid-Deployment Aortic Valves.

Feature	LivaNova Sorin Perceval S	Edwards Intuity Elite
Leaflet material	Bovine pericardium	Bovine pericardium
Metal frame	Nitinol stent	Cobalt-chromium stent
	Nitinol skirt	Stainless steel skirt
Sizes (mm)	21, 23, 25, 27	19, 21, 23, 25, 27
Trial name	CAVALIER[16,17]	TRANSFORM[15]
Patients (N)	658	839
Age (yr)/STS predicted risk (%)	78/7.2	74/2.5
Minimally invasive approach (%)	33	41
Cross-clamp time (minutes)	32–38	49–63
30-Day mortality rate (%)	3.7	0.8
PPM implantation (%) at index procedure	11.6	11.9
Mean gradient (mmHg) at 1 yr	9.2	10.3
Perivalvular regurgitation (%) mild or greater at 1 yr	3.3	8.5
CE mark obtained	2011	2012
U.S. FDA approval obtained	2016	2016

CE mark, Conformité Européene (European Conformity) certification required for manufacturers seeking access to markets in the European Union; *FDA*, Food and Drug Administration; *PPM*, patient-prosthesis mismatch; *STS*, Society of Thoracic Surgeons.

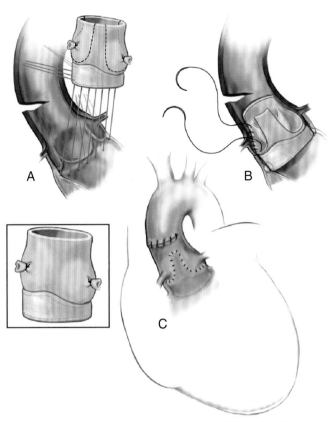

Fig. 14.6 Stentless Porcine Root Replacement Using a Modified Sub-Coronary Technique. (A) Proximal interrupted suture line in a circular plane at or below the annulus. (B) Distal, continuous polypropylene suture line attaches the residual aortic wall to the native aortic wall running below the coronary ostia and preserves the porcine noncoronary sinus. (C) Aortotomy closed, showing relation of the distal suture line to coronary ostia.

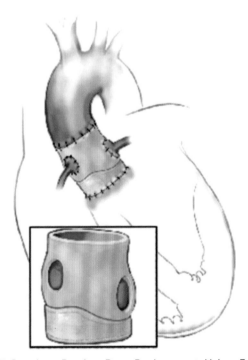

Fig. 14.5 Stentless Porcine Root Replacement Using Full Root Technique. The porcine root completely replaces the native aortic root, and the coronaries are reimplanted.

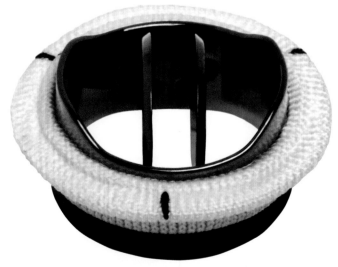

Fig. 14.7 Mechanical Valve. The On-X heart valve (Cryolife Inc., Austin, TX) is a bileaflet mechanical valve constructed with pyrolytic carbon.

bioprosthetic valves, and (3) audible clicking of the normally functioning mechanical valve, which may be troubling to some patients.

The On-X mechanical valve (Cryolife Inc., Austin, TX) was first implanted in 1996 (Fig. 14.7). It has a low rate of adverse clinical events per patient-year, including 0.6% for thromboembolism, 0.4% for bleeding, and 0% for thrombosis when the valve is used in the aortic position.[27]

A randomized clinical trial using the On-X aortic valve, completed in 2014, demonstrated the safety of lower doses of warfarin in AVR patients.[28] The valve was subsequently approved by the U.S. FDA for expanded labeling that allows patients, starting 3 months after AVR, to be maintained at an international normalized ratio (INR) clotting score of 1.5 to 2.0. This approval is reflected in guideline recommendations for the On-X valve (class IIb), rather than the standard target INR of 2.5 recommended for all other mechanical valves (class I).[29]

Aortic Homografts

The first successful orthotopic placement of an aortic homograft was performed in 1962 by Donald Ross.[30] The operation is more complex than the straightforward implantation of a stented tissue valve because a full root technique may be performed (Fig. 14.8) or the valve may be sewn in the subcoronary position (as with stentless bioprosthetic valves).

Perceived advantages of the homograft are (1) freedom from anticoagulation and a low risk of thromboembolic events similar to that of native aortic valves and (2) greater resistance to reinfection, making it the valve of choice in complex infective endocarditis cases. The disadvantages of a homograft are (1) the increased complexity of implantation, (2) difficulty of reoperation in many patients due to calcification that develops in the wall,[15] and (3) greater incidence of SVD than was originally hoped.[31,32]

Ross Procedure

Donald Ross developed the Ross procedure using the pulmonic root autograft for AVR and homograft replacement of the patient's pulmonic valve (Fig. 14.9).[33] The perceived advantages of this technique are freedom from anticoagulation and decreased risk for stroke. In children, the tissue continues to grow with the child, unlike homografts and bioprosthetic valves. The disadvantages are (1) a much more

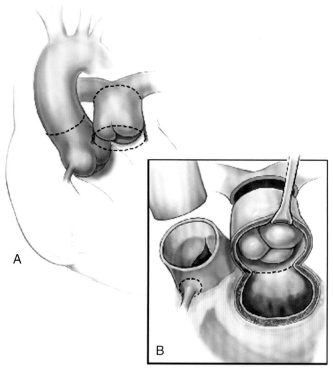

Fig. 14.9 Ross Procedure. (A) Incision lines are illustrated for the aortic (transverse and distal) and pulmonary roots. (B) The distal pulmonary incision is made first to allow inspection of the valve and accurate placement of the proximal incision below the annulus.

complex operation than other procedures that simply replace the pathologic aortic valve, (2) the potential for dysfunction of two valves (i.e., pulmonic homograft and autograft), (3) development of late aneurysms requiring reoperation, and (4) potential for injury to the first septal perforator during mobilization of the pulmonary autograft.

Guidelines for Valve Choice

Valve choice according to age is controversial. European guidelines[34] recommend mechanical valves for patients younger than 60 years of age, whereas the upper limit recommended in American guidelines[29,35] when only age is considered is 50 years (Table 14.2). The European guidelines include a class I recommendation for mechanical valves in patients younger than 40 years of age. Bioprosthetic valves are preferred in older patients (>65 years in European and >70 years in American guidelines).

Both guidelines acknowledge that the most important factor in valve choice is patient preference. Shared decision making between the clinician and the patient after informed consent should balance the

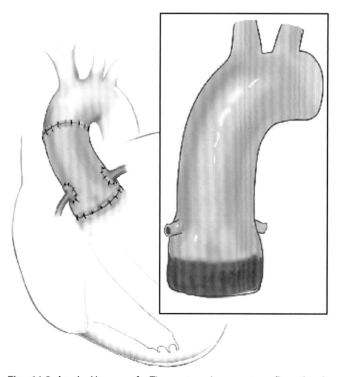

Fig. 14.8 Aortic Homograft. The root replacement configuration is shown. The cryopreserved aortic homograft is used with reimplantation of the coronary ostia.

TABLE 14.2 Age Thresholds for Valve Choice.

Valve Type	ACC/AHA 2017	ESC/EACTS 2017
Mechanical valve	<50 years (Class IIa, B)[a]	<60 years (Class IIa, C)
		<40 years (Class I, C)
Bioprosthetic valve	>70 years (Class IIa, B)	>65 years (Class IIa, C)

[a]Class of recommendation and level of evidence are shown in parentheses.
ACC/AHA, American College of Cardiology/American Heart Association; *ESC/EACTS,* European Society of Cardiology/European Association for Cardio-Thoracic Surgery.

risk of long-term anticoagulation required for mechanical valves and the risk of SVD requiring reintervention associated with bioprosthetic valves. Other factors favoring the use of mechanical valves are listed in Table 14.3, and factors favoring the use of bioprosthetic valves are listed in Table 14.4.

Several large series have shown good durability (>15 years) with long-term follow-up of commonly used stented bioprosthetic valves in the aortic position (Table 14.5). Overall, the rate of freedom from SVD for stented bovine pericardial valves has been 48.5% at 20 years for the Carpentier-Edwards Perimount valve[36] (Edwards Lifesciences, Irvine, CA) and 62.3% at 20 years for the Sorin Mitroflow valve[37] (LivaNova, London, England). For stented porcine valves, the rate for freedom from SVD was 63.4% at 20 years for the Medtronic Hancock II valve[38] (Medtronic, Inc., Minneapolis, MN), and freedom from reoperation for SVD was 61.1% for the Biocor valve[39] (St. Jude Medical, Inc., St. Paul, MN). In the largest reported series of 12,569 patients receiving

TABLE 14.3 Factors Favoring Mechanical Valves.

Factor	ACC/AHA 2017	ESC/EACTS 2017
Patient preference	Class I, C[a]	Class I, C
Accelerated risk of SVD (age <40 yr, hyperparathyroidism)	None	Class I, C
Already on anticoagulation for mechanical prosthesis in another position	[b]	Class IIa, C
Already on anticoagulation due to high risk of thromboembolism (AF, VTE, thrombophilia, severe LV dysfunction)	[b]	Class IIb, C
Reasonable life expectancy (>10 yr) and high risk for future repeat AVR	[b]	Class IIa, C
Small aortic root precluding future valve-in-valve procedure	[b]	None

[a]Class of recommendation and level of evidence are shown.
[b]Factor acknowledged but with no graded recommendations.
ACC/AHA, American College of Cardiology/American Heart Association; *AF,* atrial fibrillation; *AVR,* aortic valve replacement; *ESC/EACTS,* European Society of Cardiology/European Association for Cardio-Thoracic Surgery; *LV,* left ventricular; *SVD,* structural valve deterioration; *VTE,* venous thromboembolism.

TABLE 14.4 Factors Favoring Bioprosthetic Valves.

Factor	ACC/AHA 2017	ESC/EACTS 2017
Patient preference	Class I, C[a]	Class I, C
Anticoagulation contraindicated	Class I, C	Class I, C
Reoperation of mechanical valve thrombosis despite good long-term anticoagulation	None	Class I, C
Woman of child-bearing age contemplating pregnancy	None	Class IIa, C
Low risk for future repeat AVR	[b]	Class IIa, C

[a]Class of recommendation and level of evidence are shown.
[b]Factor acknowledged but with no graded recommendations.
ACC/AHA, American College of Cardiology/American Heart Association; *ESC/EACTS,* European Society of Cardiology/European Association for Cardio-Thoracic Surgery; *AVR,* aortic valve replacement.

TABLE 14.5 Freedom From Structural Valve Deterioration in Stented Bioprosthetic Valves Used for Aortic Valve Replacement.

Study	Mean Follow-Up	No. of Valves	Time of SVD Estimate (yr)	Age (yr)	Actuarial Freedom From Reoperation for SVD (%)	Valve Type
Yankah et al, 2008	—	1513	20	>65	71.8 ± 6.0	Mitroflow pericardial valve
				>70	84.8 ± 0.7	
Mykén et al, 2009	6.0 ± 4.5	1518	20	≤50	37.7 ± 8.6	St. Jude Medical Biocor porcine bioprothesis
				51–60	60.7 ± 10.3	
				61–70	81.0 ± 5.1	
				71–80	97.8 ± 1.2	
				>80	100	
David et al, 2010	12.2	1134	20	<60	32.6 ± 6.2	Hancock II bioprosthesis in the aortic position
				60–70	89.8 ± 3.2	
				>70	100	
Bourgignon et al, 2015	6.7 ± 4.8	2659	20	<60	38.1 ± 5.6	Carpentier-Edwards pericardial aortic valve bioprosthesis
				60–70	59.6 ± 7.6	
				>70	98.1 ± 0.8	

SVD, Structural valve deterioration.
From Yankah CA, Pasic M, Musci M, et al. Aortic valve replacement with the Mitroflow pericardial bioprosthesis: durability results up to 21 years. J Thorac Cardiovasc Surg 2008;136:688-696; Myken PS, Bech-Hansen O. A 20-year experience of 1712 patients with the Biocor porcine bioprosthesis. J Thorac Cardiovasc Surg 2009;137:76-81; David TE, Armstrong S, Maganti M. Hancock II bioprosthesis for aortic valve replacement: the gold standard of bioprosthetic valves durability? Ann Thorac Surg 2010;90:775-781; Bourgignon T, Bourquiaux-Stablo AL, Candolfi P, et al. Very long-term outcomes of the Carpentier-Edwards Perimount valve in aortic position. Ann Thorac Surg 2015;99:831-837.

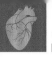

TABLE 14.6   Freedom From Valve-Related Complications in Mechanical Valves Used for Aortic Valve Replacement.

Study	N and Mean Age	Mean Follow-Up	Time (yr)	Freedom from Valve-Related Mortality (%)	Thromboembolism, Cumulative Incidence (%)	Bleeding, Cumulative Incidence (%)	Reoperation, Cumulative Incidence (%)	Valve Type
Emery et al, 2005	2982 65 yr	7 ± 5 yr	5	95	7.2	12.4	1.0	St. Jude Medical, St. Paul, MN
			10	90	11.3	17.5	1.4	
			15	85	14.7	20.7	1.6	
			20	76	16.6	22.5	1.9	
Bouchard et al, 2014	2242 56 yr	7 ± 5 yr	5	97	3.1	2.7	2.9	CarboMedics, Inc., Austin, TX
			10	93	4.9	6.1	4.9	
			15	88	7.4	9.5	6.2	
			20	78	8.4	10.5	10.8	

From Emery RW, Krogh CC, Arom KV, et al. The St. Jude Medical cardiac valve prosthesis: a 25-year experience with single valve replacement. Ann Thorac Surg 2005;79:776-782; discussion 782-773; Bouchard D, Mazine A, Stevens LM, et al. Twenty-year experience with the CarboMedics mechanical valve prosthesis. Ann Thorac Surg 2014;97:816-823.

a Carpentier-Edwards Perimount valve (mean age, 71 years), the rate of freedom from reoperation for SVD was 85% at 20 years.[40] Patient age is the most important determinant of durability, and most series have shown almost 100% freedom from reoperation for SVD in patients older than 70 years, making a bioprosthetic valve the valve of choice in this age group.

Durability remains the hallmark of mechanical valves, and many centers have shown a 0% incidence of SVD.[41,42] Valve thrombosis and prosthetic valve endocarditis are also uncommon (<3% and <2%, respectively, through 20 years).[41,42] However, valve-related morbidity and mortality rates, driven mostly by thromboembolism or anticoagulation-related bleeding, are higher among patients receiving a mechanical valve.[43] Two of the largest series of commonly used bileaflet mechanical valves demonstrated a risk of approximately 25% for valve-related mortality through 20 years (Table 14.6). Whether newer-generation mechanical valves (described earlier) can mitigate these complications remains to be seen.

Very limited comparative data exist to inform younger patients who should receive a mechanical valve but prefer a bioprosthetic valve. Two major randomized clinical trials were not consistent regarding difference in long-term survival between bioprosthetic and mechanical valves.[44,45] Both trials compared first-generation porcine valves and single-tilting disc Bjork-Shiley valves, neither of which is currently in use. The Veterans Affairs Cooperative Study[45] showed improved 15-year survival for mechanical valves compared with bioprosthetic valves, whereas the Edinburgh Heart Valve Trial[44] showed no difference in 20-year survival. Although 20-year durability is decidedly worse among younger patients who receive a bioprosthetic valve, many young patients can expect to achieve reasonable 10-year durability: 85% freedom from SVD among 45-year-old patients[46] and 85.8% freedom from all valve-related complications among 25-year-old patients.[47] For young patients who eventually develop SVD, reintervention can be performed as an open surgical procedure or a transcatheter procedure (i.e., VIV). The safety of reoperative AVR is discussed in later sections.

TAVI is approved for high-risk patients with failing bioprosthetic valves in the aortic position. An international registry[48] of 202 patients demonstrated a 30-day mortality rate after VIV of 8.4% and a 1-year survival rate of 85.8%. Procedural concerns included coronary ostial obstruction (in 3.5%) and relatively high mean gradients (15.9 ± 8.6 mmHg).

Registry data from the PARTNER 2 trial (365 patients)[49] and the CoreValve U.S. Expanded Use trial (233 patients)[50] demonstrated improved rates of mortality at 30 days (2.7% and 2.2%, respectively) and survival at 1 year (87.6% and 85.4%, respectively) after VIV with newer devices. The rate of coronary obstruction decreased to less than 1% in both trials, but the average mean gradient remained higher than after TAVI for native AS (17 mmHg for both valve types). The availability of a future VIV procedure nevertheless makes AVR with a bioprosthetic valve more attractive to younger patients.

Ultimately, valve choice is based on patient preference and shared decision making between the physician and the patient. The risk of SVD in bioprosthetic valves is weighed against the risk of thromboembolism and anticoagulation-related bleeding in mechanical valves. The future role of the VIV procedure for failed bioprosthetic valves and the possibility of non-warfarin options for mechanical valves (e.g., novel oral anticoagulants, dual antiplatelet therapy) should be considered.

AORTIC VALVE REPAIR

Aortic valve repair can be performed in patients with AR. However, valve repair for patients with AS involving leaflet decalcification is not a feasible treatment option and has been associated with early postoperative AR due to leaflet scarring and late restenosis due to recalcification.[51] The benefit of aortic valve repair compared with AVR is avoidance of prosthetic valve-related complications such as thromboembolism and infective endocarditis. Data on aortic valve repair durability are limited to experienced centers, but the 10-year freedom from reoperation rate can be as high as 93% for trileaflet aortic valves.[52–54] BAV repair is less durable than repair of tricuspid aortic valves, and repair in patients with BAV remains controversial. No professional society–driven guidelines exist for the role of aortic valve repair.

Repair of a regurgitant tricuspid aortic valve uses a combination of cusp repair and annuloplasty. Typically, one or more cusps are redundant, which causes cusp prolapse. Central free margin plication at the nodulus of Arantius effectively shortens the cusp, resulting in a higher zone of coaptation with the other cusps (Fig. 14.10).[55]

An alternative method of cusp shortening is free margin resuspension with a continuous over-and-over suture from commissure to

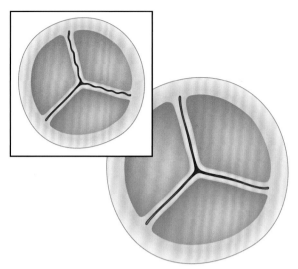

Fig. 14.10 Free Margin Plication. After identification of the prolapsing leaflets, the free margin is plicated at the nodulus of Arantius with a simple, interrupted 5-0 polypropylene stitch. By shortening the free margin, this procedure brings the leaflet coaptation surface higher in the aortic root.

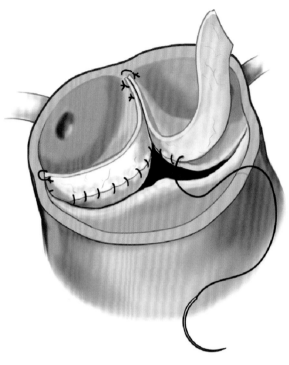

Fig. 14.12 Leaflet Extension. When the aortic valve leaflet is retracted or shortened, the cusp can be extended with the use of pericardium. The pericardium is sewn from commissure to commissure, along the free margin of the leaflet, thereby increasing the coaptation surface.

commissure (Fig. 14.11). This technique is also useful for closing cusp fenestrations, which are typically located near the commissures where cusp stress is highest. The least common technique of cusp repair is cusp extension with pericardium in cases of inadequate cusp tissue (Fig. 14.12). Occasionally, leaflet perforations (e.g., after healed endocarditis) can be repaired with a pericardial patch (Fig. 14.13). A reduction annuloplasty may also be required in cases of annuloaortic ectasia.

The simplest technique is commissural plication (Fig. 14.14). This technique achieves narrowing of the interleaflet triangle below the commissure and reduces the diameter of the aortic root, thereby increasing coaptation of the cusp surfaces. Alternatively, the aortic annulus may be stabilized by suture annuloplasty, which can be placed internal[56] or external[57] to the aortic root. The concept of ring annuloplasty has been applied to the aortic valve, first with the use of available material such as Dacron graft[58] and currently with manufactured aortic valve rings (Fig. 14.15) that can be placed internally (i.e., HAART ring, BioStable Science and Engineering, Austin, TX)[59] or externally (i.e., Extra-Aortic Ring, Coroneo Inc., Montreal, Quebec).[60]

Repair of the BAV can be performed with similar techniques of cusp repair and reduction annuloplasty. The goal of BAV repair is to restore a competent BAV rather than to create a tricuspid aortic valve. In cases with equal-size cusps and commissure oriented at 180 degrees to each other, repair can be performed readily, as with a tricuspid aortic valve. However, in the more common type of BAV involving a conjoint (fused) cusp (Fig. 14.16), the raphe may be sclerosed and immobile, necessitating additional techniques. In these cases, a triangular resection of the raphe can be performed with reapproximation of the edges to create a shortened and pliable cusp (Fig. 14.17). If tissue is inadequate in the conjoint cusp, the raphe can be released from the commissure and shaved to improve cusp mobility. Judgment must be

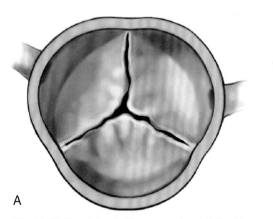

A

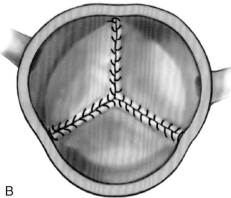

B

Fig. 14.11 Free Margin Resuspension. (A) Continuous over-and-over suturing from commissure to commissure is one method for shortening leaflets. (B) 6-0 Gore-Tex is suggested for this maneuver, with the knots placed outside the aorta.

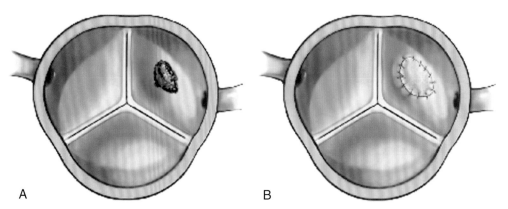

Fig. 14.13 Leaflet Patch. A simple leaflet perforation (A) can be repaired with an autologous pericardial patch (B).

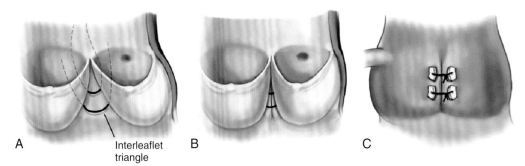

Fig. 14.14 Commissural Plication. The wide interleaflet triangle (A) is narrowed with sutures that plicate this area (B) to increase coaptation. (C) Completed repair.

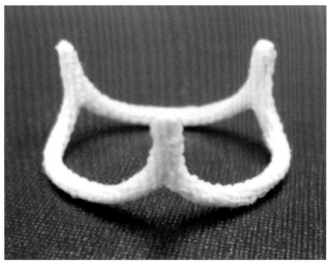

Fig. 14.15 Aortic Valve Ring. HAART 300 aortic annuloplasty device (BioStable Science & Engineering, Austin, TX).

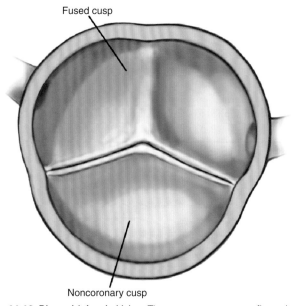

Fig. 14.16 Bicuspid Aortic Valve. The most common configuration of a bicuspid aortic valve is a fusion of two leaflets (usually the right and left coronary leaflets) with a rudimentary commissure of raphe where the normal commissure would be.

used in cases with severely sclerosed valves because the durability of a diseased BAV may be less than even that of a bioprosthetic valve.

Complete leaflet reconstruction has undergone a revival since it was first described in 1964.[61] Several techniques for leaflet reconstruction have been described, mostly using glutaraldehyde-fixed autologous pericardium (Fig. 14.18).[62–64] The entire aortic valve leaflet is resected, and new leaflets are constructed from a sizing template and then sewn into the aortic root. The benefits of leaflet reconstruction with autologous pericardium are the complete avoidance of prosthetic material and the ability to treat all types of aortic valve disease (i.e., AS,

AR, and endocarditis) and all valve morphologies (i.e., unicuspid, bicuspid, tricuspid, and quadricuspid). Whether these benefits translate into improved outcomes in terms of reduced valve-related complications, improved valve gradients, and long-term durability is unclear[65]; however, excellent mid-term results with newer, standardized techniques are rapidly emerging.[66]

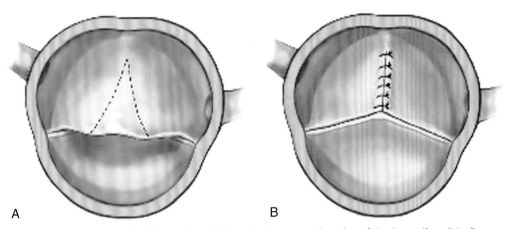

Fig. 14.17 Raphe Resection. The raphe and the redundant central portion of the larger (fused) leaflet are resected and closed primarily (A) to restore normal coaptation level (B).

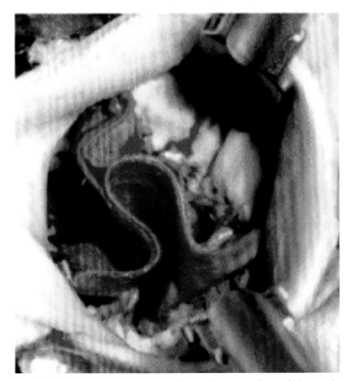

Fig. 14.18 Leaflet Replacement. The individual leaflets of the aortic valve are replaced with glutaraldehyde-fixed, autologous pericardium.

RISKS OF AORTIC VALVE SURGERY

The risks of aortic valve surgery can be objectively determined with the use of several risk models, including the STS Predicted Risk of Mortality (STS PROM),[67] the European System for Cardiac Operative Risk Evaluation (EuroSCORE) II,[68] and the Ambler scores.[69] In addition to operative mortality, the STS PROM provides an estimate of important complications such as prolonged hospitalization, stroke, respiratory failure, mediastinitis, renal failure, and reoperation. These risk models are important for surgical decision making and require informed consent before the planned operation.

Data from the STS National Database indicate that the operative mortality rate for patients 70 years of age or older who underwent isolated AVR or AVR with CABG fell from 10% in 1994 to less than 6% in 2003.[70] An STS analysis of 108,687 patients who underwent isolated

AVR between 1997 and 2006 (mean age, 68 years) reported an in-hospital mortality rate in 2006 of 2.6%; the observed stroke rate was 1.3%, and the average length of hospital stay was 7.8 days.[71] Among patients 80 to 85 years of age, the 30-day mortality rate was 4.9%, and the observed stroke rate was 2.0%.[71]

Experience at centers of excellence has demonstrated significantly improved operative mortality rates (<1% after isolated AVR).[72–76] The incidence of perioperative stroke in those series ranged from 0% to 1.9%, and the median length of stay was as low as 5 days.[73] Di Eusanio and colleagues reported a 3-year patient survival rate, comparable to the life expectancy of an age- and gender-matched 2006 population (82% vs. 81%, $P = 0.157$).[75] Overall, the reported survival in these series was 94% to 97% at 1 year and 88% to 94% at 3 years.

In the prospective, randomized, multicenter Placement of Aortic Transcatheter Valves (PARTNER) trial comparing high-risk patients (mean STS score, 11.8%) receiving TAVI versus AVR for severe, symptomatic AS, outcomes for both procedures were excellent.[2] Patients undergoing AVR ($n = 351$; mean age, 85 years) had a 30-day mortality rate of 6.5%.[2] As reported in the SURTAVI trial that enrolled an intermediate-risk cohort (mean STS score of 4.5%), patients undergoing AVR ($n = 796$; mean age, 80 years) had a 30-day mortality rate of only 1.7%.[77] Both trials set a new benchmark for operative outcomes for patients treated at centers of excellence.

AORTIC ROOT SURGERY

Indications

Indications for aortic root replacement include aneurysms of the ascending aorta, aortic valve endocarditis with annular abscess, and acute type A aortic dissection. The most common indication is aneurysms of the aortic root or ascending aorta. The size threshold for aneurysm repair depends on whether the aneurysm is the primary indication for surgery or coexists in a patient who already requires cardiac surgery.

Primary aneurysms of the aortic root result from genetically mediated disorders or acquired disorders. The acquired disorders include degenerative thoracic aortic aneurysm, chronic aortic dissection, intramural hematoma, penetrating atherosclerotic ulcer, mycotic aneurysm, and pseudoaneurysm. The size threshold for surgical repair in this group of patients is 5.5 cm for both the aortic root and the ascending aorta according to class I recommendations by the 2010 Guidelines for Thoracic Aortic Disease.[78]

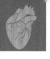

The genetically mediated disorders include Marfan syndrome, vascular Ehlers-Danlos syndrome, Turner syndrome, familial thoracic aortic aneurysm and dissection, and Loeys-Dietz syndrome. These disorders, particularly Loeys-Dietz syndrome, are associated with a greater risk of rupture, dissection, and death. The size threshold for operative intervention in this group of patients is 5.0 cm; patients with Loeys-Dietz syndrome may be considered for surgical repair with aortic diameters as low as 4.2 cm, depending on imaging modality.[78]

Previous recommendations for early repair of aneurysms associated with BAV have become less aggressive.[29,79] The current recommendation is a threshold of 5.0 cm in patients who have additional risk factors for dissection or who are at low operative risk when the surgery is performed at an experienced center (class IIa).[80]

When aortic root aneurysm or aneurysm of the ascending aorta exist in a patient who already requires cardiac surgery, the threshold for concomitant aortic replacement is an aortic diameter of 4.5 cm (class I in the Thoracic Aortic Disease guidelines).[78] In the most common clinical scenario of patients with BAV requiring aortic valve surgery, the size threshold is similarly 4.5 cm (class IIa).[80] The rationale for prophylactic repair at a smaller size is to prevent future aneurysmal degeneration requiring later reoperative cardiac surgery.[81]

These guidelines are predicated on an operative risk for aortic root replacement of less than 5%. Although no risk model is available to predict the risk of operative mortality for aortic root replacement, results from two national registries demonstrate that elective aortic root replacement is associated with an operative mortality rate of 4.5% to 5.8%.[82,83] The U.K. registry (1962 patients undergoing any first-time aortic root replacement between 1986 and 2004) identified concomitant CABG (odds ratio [OR] = 3.38), nonelective surgery (OR = 3.20), left ventricular ejection fraction of less than 50% (OR = 2.63), valve size less than 23 mm (OR = 1.97), hospital volume of eight or fewer cases per year (OR = 1.53), and age greater than 70 years (OR = 1.20) as independent risk factors for early mortality.[83] The STS National Database includes 13,358 patients undergoing either elective aortic root replacement or an AVR/ascending aortic procedure between 2004 and 2007; the records demonstrated 58% lower operative mortality in high- versus low-volume centers, with the most pronounced difference in centers performing fewer than 30 cases per year ($P = 0.001$).[82] Moreover, when complicating factors such as reoperative cardiac surgery, emergency operation for aortic dissections, and complex infective endocarditis are involved, outcome differences in high- versus low-volume centers may be even more pronounced.

Aortic Root Replacement With Composite Valve-Graft: Modified Bentall Procedure

Replacement of the entire aortic root, including the aortic wall and the aortic valve, was first described in 1968 by Bentall and De Bono.[84] In this procedure, a mechanical valve was attached to the end of a Dacron tube graft to construct a composite valve-graft (CVG). The CVG was then implanted inside the native aortic root at the level of the aortic annulus. Holes were made in the side of the Dacron graft, and the two coronary ostia were reattached to the graft by sewing the graft to the aortic wall around the ostia. The distal end of the graft was sewn inside the distal aorta, and the native aortic wall was completely closed over the Dacron graft. The classic Bentall procedure was performed to control bleeding from the coronary artery suture lines and porous graft material used in that era; however, long-term follow-up showed that this procedure was prone to pseudoaneurysm formation. This classic procedure is no longer performed in modern practice.

The current technique of aortic root replacement with CVG is a modification of the Bentall procedure (Fig. 14.19).[85] The CVG is implanted at

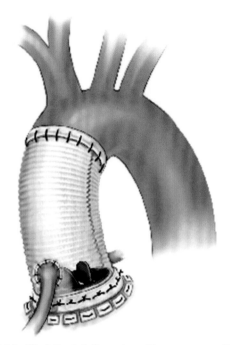

Fig. 14.19 Modified Bentall Procedure. The current configuration of freestanding complete aortic root replacement with a mechanical valved conduit is shown with coronary buttons reimplanted into the conduit.

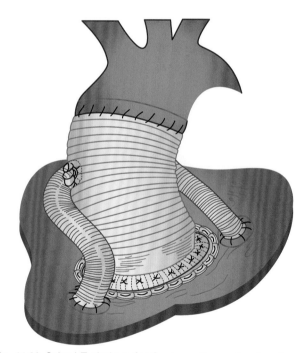

Fig. 14.20 Cabrol Technique for Coronary Reconstruction. In cases in which the coronary arteries cannot be safely mobilized for reimplantation in the conduit, coronary reconstruction can be accomplished by sewing a Dacron tube graft from coronary os to os, followed by a side-to-side anastomosis to the conduit.

the aortic annulus in a similar fashion, but coronary reconstruction is performed by reattaching the coronary ostia as buttons rather than using the classic inclusion technique. Other, less common techniques of coronary reconstruction include creation of a Dacron bypass graft to the coronary ostia (i.e., Cabrol technique [Fig. 14.20]),[86] interposition of a saphenous vein graft to the coronary ostia (i.e., Kay-Zubiate technique

[Fig. 14.21]),[87] and traditional CABG to the epicardial arteries. These advanced techniques for coronary reconstruction are typically used during reoperative aortic root surgery in which the coronary arteries are frozen and cannot be mobilized from the surrounding scar tissue.

The modified Bentall procedure using a mechanical valve has been extensively used in young patients with Marfan syndrome. In 2002, the Johns Hopkins group reported 24 years of experience with this operation in 271 Marfan patients.[88] The results showed an operative mortality rate of 0%, with an 84% overall survival rate at 24 years. Actuarial 20-year freedom from thromboembolism, endocarditis, and reoperation rates were 93%, 90%, and 74%, respectively.

Similarly, the modified Bentall procedure using a bioprosthetic valve (Fig. 14.22) was shown to have excellent outcomes. In 2007, the Mount Sinai group reported 12 years of experience with 275 patients.[89] The results showed an operative mortality rate of 6.2%, with 75% overall survival at 5 years. The rates of stroke and significant hemorrhage were 0.85% and 0.3% per 100 patient-years, respectively. Only one patient required a reoperation. Because impregnated Dacron grafts cannot be stored with bioprosthetic valves, CVGs are not typically premanufactured. Construction of the CVG at the time of operation allows greater versatility in bioprosthetic valve type and size while adding little time to the operation (see Fig. 14.20).

Overall, the modified Bentall procedure with replacement of the ascending aorta and aortic valve is the gold standard operation for aortic root replacement. The technique is reproducible and safe. Proven durability for greater than 20 years is the benchmark for the many alternative techniques.

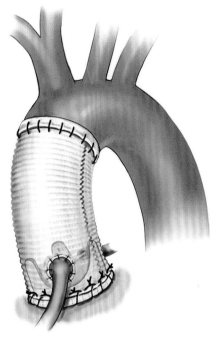

Fig. 14.22 Biological Bentall Procedure. The biological valve is first attached to the conduit, and the composite then is attached to the aortic root. Coronary arteries are reimplanted into the graft.

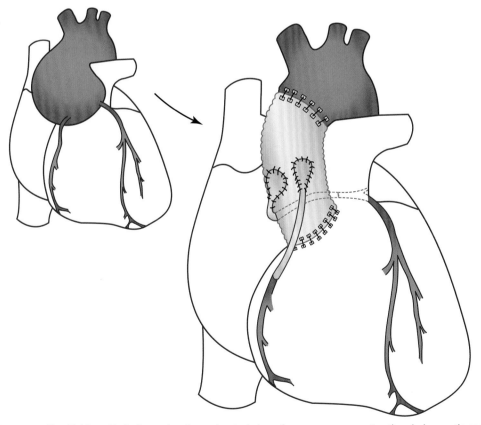

Fig. 14.21 Kay-Zubiate Technique. An alternative technique for coronary reconstruction during aortic root replacement is performed using saphenous vein to create interposition grafts between the aortic graft and native origins of the coronary arteries.

Valve-Sparing Aortic Root Replacement: David and Yacoub Procedures

Aortic root replacement with preservation of the native aortic valve was first described in the early 1990s by Sir Magdi Yacoub and Tirone David. The remodeling technique (i.e., Yacoub procedure) and the reimplantation technique (i.e., David procedure) have the advantage of sparing the native aortic valve, eliminating the need for a prosthetic valve, and preserving the flow characteristics of a normal aortic valve. Theoretical disadvantages of valve-sparing aortic root replacement include abnormal eddy currents within the neoroot, which can increase stress during leaflet closure and contribute to abnormal coronary flow reserve.[90] The possibility of leaflet trauma on the Dacron graft may be mitigated by recreation of pseudosinuses with the Dacron graft.[91]

Successful preservation of the native aortic valve is more likely in patients with normal or near-normal leaflets. Thinning of the cusps due to severely enlarged roots can cause stress fenestrations toward the commissures. When more than one cusp is involved, repair is not advised.[92] Valves with AR, which typically results from cusp prolapse, can be repaired using techniques described earlier. Prevention of leaflet prolapse during the procedure can improve durability.[52]

Results of valve-sparing aortic root replacement have been reported for both procedures, and long-term follow-up has shown that reintervention rates are lower with the David procedure than with the Yacoub procedure.[93]

Yacoub Procedure

The remodeling technique for valve-sparing aortic root replacement (i.e., Yacoub procedure) involves resection of the sinus tissue and construction of neosinuses using a tailored Dacron graft (Fig. 14.23). The coronary arteries are reimplanted in their corresponding neosinuses as buttons, similar to the modified Bentall procedure. Because the aortic annulus is not supported by the Dacron graft in the Yacoub procedure, it is best suited for patients without annular dilation or a predisposition to future annular dilation.

David Procedure

The reimplantation technique for valve-sparing aortic root replacement (i.e., David technique) involves resection of the sinus tissue and reimplantation of the native aortic valve within a Dacron graft (Fig. 14.24). The coronary arteries are reconstructed as coronary buttons to the corresponding neosinus. Because the annulus is enclosed with the Dacron graft, the size of the annulus can be reduced and further dilation prevented. Several modifications of the David procedure have been described; newer modifications attempt to construct bulging neosinuses to mimic the natural aortic root.[94,95]

Aortic Root Enlargement

The aortic root can be enlarged by dividing the annulus and augmenting the root with a patch. The most common technique involves enlarging the posterior annulus of the aortic root at the noncoronary cusp, as described by Nicks and associates[96] (Fig. 14.25). The division of the aortic root can be extended through the aortic annulus into the anterior leaflet of the mitral valve, as described by Manougian and coworkers.[97] Both procedures require repair of the defect with a patch of bovine pericardium, autologous pericardium, or synthetic graft, which effectively enlarges the aortic annulus. The Manougian procedure allows for placement of a larger patch but also requires repair of the dome of the left atrium and the anterior leaflet of the mitral valve.[97]

Anterior annulus enlargement (i.e., Konno procedure)[98] is more commonly used in the pediatric population when the left ventricular outflow tract requires enlargement for subvalvular stenosis. This technique enlarges the anterior aortic annulus just to the left of the right coronary os, through the ventricular septum, and into the right ventricular outflow tract. The resulting defect is closed with a pericardial or synthetic patch. Posterior and anterior aortic root enlargement techniques allow implantation of a larger aortic prosthesis.

The indication for a root enlargement procedure is a small aortic annulus that would accommodate an aortic prosthesis that is too small relative to patient size, resulting in patient-prosthesis mismatch (PPM).

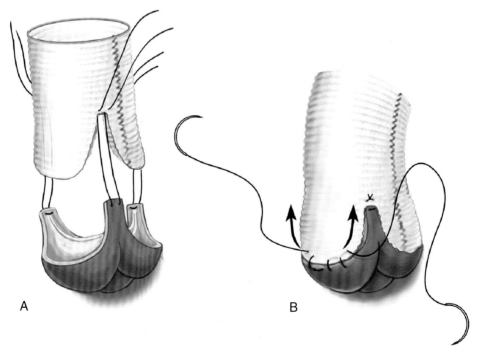

Fig. 14.23 Yacoub Procedure. (A) The sinuses are cut out, and the commissures are carefully suspended to maintain root height. (B) The sinuses are effectively replaced with tailored tongues of vascular graft, with the longest parts of the graft placed at the depth of each sinus.

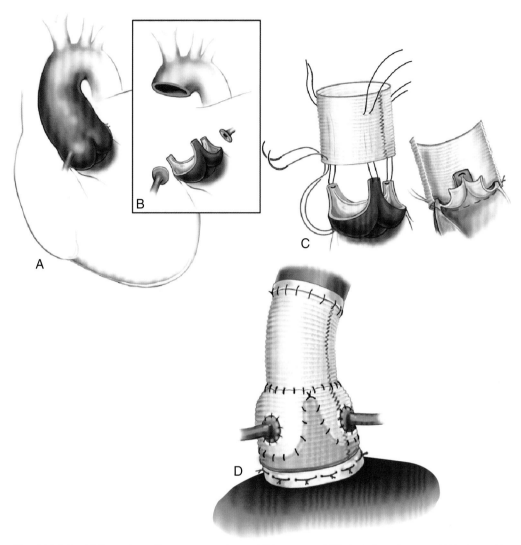

Fig. 14.24 David Procedure. The aneurysmal root (A) is resected (B), including sinuses of Valsalva, with coronary buttons mobilized away. (C) Six to eight subannular sutures are placed. Commissural posts are drawn up inside the valve, and the annular sutures are passed through the proximal end of the graft. (D) Annular sutures are tied gently. The valve then is reimplanted with continuous 5-0 polypropylene suture inside the graft. Aortic continuity is reestablished with another graft of a size appropriate to the desired sinotubular junction and proximal arch.

The concept of PPM can be quantified using the indexed effective orifice area (EOAi). Guidelines published by the American Society of Echocardiography define PPM as absent, moderate, or severe if EOAi is greater than or equal to 0.85 cm^2/m^2, between 0.60 and 0.85 cm^2/m^2, or equal to or less than 0.6 cm^2/m^2, respectively.[99] The guidelines also suggest that PPM should not be considered unless corroborated by additional echocardiographic evidence such as aortic jet velocity greater than 3 m/s, acceleration time less than 100 ms, and dimensionless velocity index less than 0.25.

The significance of PPM remains controversial in terms of incidence and clinical relevance. Pibarot and Dumesnil reported PPM in up to 70% of aortic valve replacements,[100] whereas other studies have reported a prevalence of less than 1% for severe PPM.[101] Several large studies have provided evidence that PPM has a significant negative impact on postoperative survival, [102–105] but others have suggested that PPM has no impact on short-term or long-term mortality rates.[13,106,107]

Prevention of PPM by means of aortic root enlargement during AVR has declined as a result of improved hemodynamics of mechanical and bioprosthetic valves. An alternative strategy to prevent PPM is aortic root replacement (described earlier). The possibility of a VIV procedure for a failed bioprosthesis is another consideration when performing AVR in a small aortic root. Patients with small bioprosthetic valves (e.g., 19 or 21 mm) may not be candidates for future VIV procedures because the rigid stent of the bioprosthetic valve limits the size of the intended transcatheter heart valve.

SPECIAL CHALLENGES

Aortic Dissection

Significant AR affects approximately one half of patients with acute type A aortic dissections, and it is typically caused by prolapse of detached commissures from the aortic wall.[108] Intraoperative transesophageal echocardiography (TEE) is mandatory in the evaluation of the aortic root to assist the surgeon with aortic root management. Correction of the AR can be performed by resuspension of the aortic valve by suture fixation of the commissure to the aortic adventitia

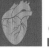

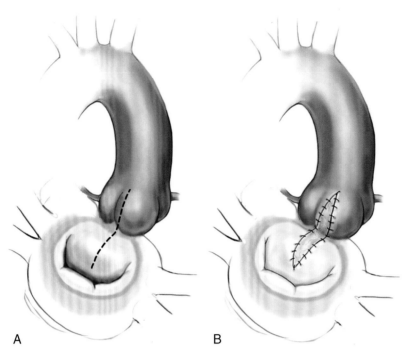

Fig. 14.25 Root Enlargement. Incision in the noncoronary sinus (A) is carried down into the anterior mitral leaflet. A patch of pericardium (B) is used to expand the leaflet, annulus, and aortic wall to allow implantation of a larger aortic valve.

(Fig. 14.26). Reattachment of the dissected layers can be supplemented with biological glue, felt, or fabric graft reinforcement. Valve resuspension is expeditious and effectively addresses acute AR during an emergent operation, but patients undergoing valve resuspension have a 20% to 25% risk of late aortic root enlargement or significant AR requiring reoperation.[109]

Alternatively, an aortic root replacement with CVG or using a valve-sparing technique can be employed. Patients with intrinsic root abnormality (e.g., Marfan syndrome, preexisting annuloaortic ectasia prone to future root enlargement, progression of AR) are ideal candidates for aortic root replacement. To avoid future aortic root surgery, some centers favor an aggressive approach to aortic root replacement for acute type A aortic dissections.[110]

In patients with normal aortic sinuses, AVR can be performed when the aortic valve has intrinsic pathology such as sclerosis, calcifications, or stenosis. The technique of AVR with a separate supracoronary graft has limited utility in acute type A aortic dissections because of the combined disadvantage of retaining abnormal aortic sinus tissue and exposing the patient to the risks of a prosthetic valve.

Aortic Valve Replacement After Previous Coronary Artery Bypass Graft

AS and coronary artery disease frequently coexist due to common pathophysiology.[111] A significant subset of patients with AS requiring AVR has undergone previous CABG.[2] Often, AS is recognized at the time of the index CABG, and guidelines recommend AVR at the time of CABG in patients with AS that is severe (class I) or moderate (class IIa).[35] Similarly, AVR is indicated in patients with AR who are undergoing cardiac surgery for another indication if the AR is severe (class I) or moderate (class IIa). Addressing aortic valve pathology at the time of index CABG can prevent the need for later reoperative surgery for the aortic valve.

Reoperative cardiac surgery can be complicated by injury to cardiovascular structures during sternal reentry, particularly injury to patent

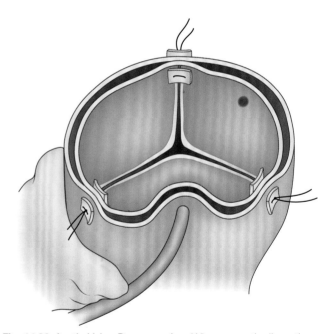

Fig. 14.26 Aortic Valve Resuspension. When an aortic dissection extends into the aortic root, the valve competency can be restored by resuspending the commissures to the aortic adventitia using Teflon felt pledgeted sutures. The dissected layers can then by reapproximated with surgical adhesives or fabrics.

bypass grafts in patients after previous CABG. AVR after prior CABG was previously associated with an operative mortality rate as high as 14%.[112] However, later series showed that the operative mortality rate is approximately 3.8% even for patients with patent bypass grafts.[113] Reoperative cardiac surgery has therefore become safer with appropriate perioperative planning and is not a contraindication to AVR.

Management of a patient's internal mammary artery (IMA) graft during AVR after CABG requires attention to preoperative planning and operative technique. Some surgeons consider a patent IMA graft crossing the midline and directly adherent to the sternum to be a high-risk factor because injury to the IMA graft during reoperation is associated with an increased operative mortality rate.

Routine preoperative high-resolution cardiac computed tomography is indispensable in identifying patients with cardiovascular structures at risk for injury during sternal reentry.[114] Exposure of peripheral vessels (axillary or femoral) for cardiopulmonary bypass and institution of cardiopulmonary bypass before sternal reentry are useful strategies when injury to underlying structures is imminent.[115] Nevertheless, injury to the IMA graft has been associated in large series with operative mortality rates of 12% to 17.9%.[114,115]

Myocardial protection in patients with a patent left IMA (LIMA) graft to the left anterior descending artery poses another challenge during AVR. The traditional strategy of clamping the LIMA graft during cardioplegic arrest of the heart can risk injury to the LIMA graft during the initial identification and exposure. The alternative strategy of leaving the LIMA graft unclamped can safely be performed by including moderate systemic hypothermia and delivery of retrograde cardioplegia during cardioplegic arrest. This alternative strategy has been associated with comparable operative mortality rates and avoids the risk of injury to the graft.[116,117]

Aortic Valve Replacement After Previous Aortic Valve Replacement

SVD of bioprosthetic valves is the most common indication for repeat AVR. Other indications include prosthetic valve endocarditis, pannus formation, and valve thrombosis with bioprosthetic or mechanical valves. Increasing use of bioprosthetic valves in younger populations may lead to the need for interventions due to SVD. Fortunately, repeat AVR remains a safe procedure, with an operative mortality rate of 5%.[118]

A special concern about repeat AVR is the management of new ascending aortic aneurysms after a previous AVR. Preoperatively, the use of contrast-enhanced imaging to determine the relation of the aneurysm to the sternum can significantly change the operative technique. For patients with an aneurysm adherent to the sternum, cardiopulmonary bypass by peripheral cannulation should be instituted before sternal reentry. Use of the axillary rather than the femoral artery for arterial cannulation is preferred in these cases because of the reduced risk of stroke and operative mortality.[119] This technique can allow temporary decompression of the aneurysm by inducing low pump flows to permit safe division of the sternum. Rapid institution of cardiopulmonary bypass with hypothermia can avert major neurologic injury if catastrophic arterial injury to the aneurysm occurs during reentry.

Patent saphenous vein bypass grafts arising from a new ascending aortic aneurysm are managed according to the amount of disease affecting the graft. For vein grafts with no significant atherosclerotic disease, a patch of aorta containing the proximal anastomoses can be reimplanted on the Dacron graft (Fig. 14.27). Alternatively, a new saphenous vein graft can be used to replace part or all of the old diseased graft with construction of a separate proximal anastomosis.

Failed Aortic Root Replacement

Patients who have had previous aortic root replacements, particularly younger patients, may require reoperation for SVD leading to AS, AR, or aneurysm of the ascending aorta (i.e., aneurysm of the unresected native aorta or pseudoaneurysm of the replaced root at the anastomotic lines). Common clinical scenarios include failed pulmonary autografts (i.e., Ross procedure) and failed aortic homografts. The outcomes after reoperative aortic root replacement are understandably less favorable than those after primary aortic root replacement but are acceptable. The largest series of repeat aortic root replacement demonstrated an operative mortality rate of 7%.[120]

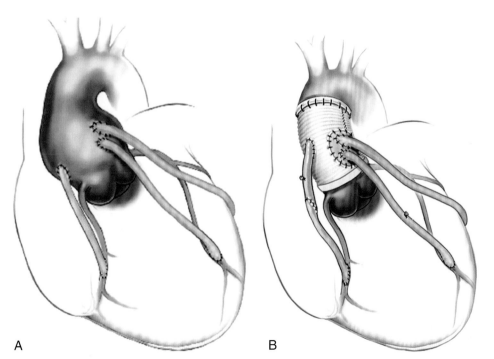

Fig. 14.27 Aneurysm After Bypass Grafting. (A) Patent grafts arise from a new ascending aneurysm. (B) The right coronary graft is extended with a new segment of saphenous vein. The left-sided grafts are reimplanted as a single island of native aorta.

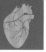

The challenge in reoperative aortic root replacements is management of the native coronary arteries as they arise from the replaced root. Unlike in primary operations, the coronary arteries can be difficult to mobilize from the surrounding scar tissue, which can result in the inability to fashion a reliable coronary button for reimplantation (i.e., frozen button). Alternative techniques to manage frozen buttons include construction of a Dacron tube connecting the ostia of both coronary arteries (see Fig. 14.20) and construction of an interposition vein graft (see Fig. 14.21), as described earlier.[86,87] If the coronary arteries cannot be reconstructed, ligation with standard CABG is a less desirable but viable option.

In some circumstances after failed aortic root replacement, only the aortic valve requires replacement. This option is attractive because the coronary arteries can be left in place without the need for complex reconstruction.

Porcelain Aorta

The term *porcelain aorta* refers to concentric calcification of the entire ascending aorta (Fig. 14.28). During standard AVR, the ascending aorta is typically cannulated and cross-clamped. A porcelain aorta prevents standard approaches to AVR. Alternative sites of cannulation for cardiopulmonary procedures can easily be performed; the most common peripheral site is the right axillary artery.

Because the porcelain aorta cannot be clamped, hypothermic circulatory arrest (HCA) must be used to open the ascending aorta in a bloodless fashion. During HCA, three procedures can be performed. The first procedure is opening the aorta (without cross-clamping) and completing the entire valve replacement. The second is performing an aortic endarterectomy, clamping the decalcified ascending aorta, resuming cardiopulmonary bypass, and performing the valve replacement in the standard fashion. The third is replacing the ascending aorta with a synthetic graft (typically Dacron), clamping the synthetic graft, resuming cardiopulmonary bypass, and completing the valve replacement in standard fashion. Results of these approaches are shown in Table 14.7.

TABLE 14.7   Results of Hypothermic Circulatory Arrest for Patients With Porcelain Aorta.

Study	Method (n)	Stroke Rate (%)	Mortality Rate (%)
Gillinov et al, 2000	AVR, HCA (n = 24)	17	12
	AVR, aortic endarterectomy, HCA (n = 16)	12	19
	AVR, aortic replacement, HCA (n = 12)	0	25
Aranki et al, 2005	AVR, HCA (n = 13)	15	0
	AVR, aortic endarterectomy, HCA (n = 13)	7.6	0
	AVR, aortic replacement, HCA (n = 44)	11.3	6.8

AVR, Aortic valve replacement; *HCA*, hypothermic circulatory arrest. From Gillinov AM, Lytle BW, Hoang V, et al. The atherosclerotic aorta at aortic valve replacement: surgical strategies and results. J Thorac Cardiovasc Surg 2000;120:957-963; Aranki SF, Nathan M, Shekar P, et al. Hypothermic circulatory arrest enables aortic valve replacement in patients with unclampable aorta. Ann Thorac Surg 2005;80:1679-1686.

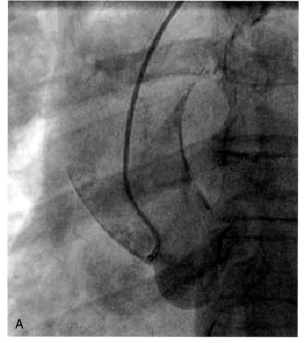
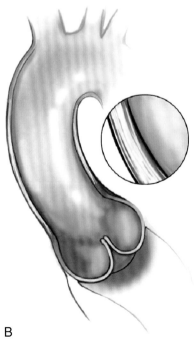

Fig. 14.28 Porcelain Aorta. (A) Radiographic appearance of calcified aortic wall at catheterization. A dense strip of calcification is seen in the greater and lesser curvatures in this left anterior oblique aortogram. (B) Artist's conception of the calcified wall seen in cutaway view with close-up inset.

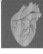

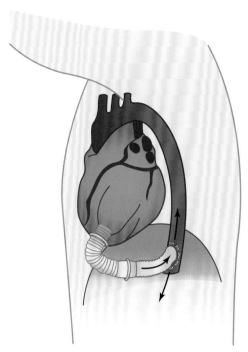

Fig. 14.29 Apico-Aortic Conduit. A valved conduit is attached to the left ventricular apex and the descending thoracic aorta through a left thoracotomy.

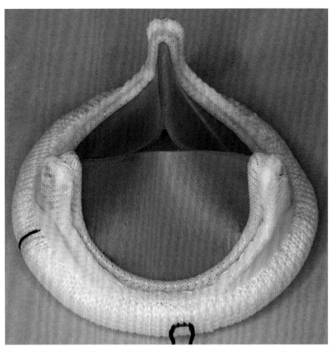

Fig. 14.30 New Tissue Technology. Bovine pericardium is treated with glycerolization, allowing the bioprosthetic valve (Edwards Lifesciences, Irvine, CA) to be dry-stored.

Another surgical approach to porcelain aorta is the apico-aortic conduit (i.e., aortic valve bypass).[121] In this approach, a left thoracotomy is performed, and the ascending aorta is avoided altogether. A valved conduit is then constructed from the left ventricular apex to the descending thoracic aorta (Fig. 14.29). The stenosed native aortic valve is left in place, and blood is bypassed extra-anatomically through the valved conduit. Outcomes of the apico-aortic conduit are limited, but a 13% perioperative mortality was demonstrated for a high-risk cohort (average age, 81 years; 16% with porcelain aorta).[122] Disadvantages of this procedure are that it cannot be performed in patients who have significant AR or a severely calcified descending aorta.

FUTURE PERSPECTIVES

New Bioprosthetic Leaflet Technology

Dystrophic calcification is the major factor contributing to SVD of bioprosthetic valves.[123] Ongoing development of anticalcification treatment for bioprosthetic valves seeks to reduce the incidence of SVD. Treatments are proprietary and include Thermafix tissue preparation (Edwards Lifesciences), AOA anticalcification tissue treatment (Medtronic), Linx anticalcification technology (St. Jude Medical), and phospholipid reduction treatment (PRT, LivaNova) in FDA-approved valves. Other tissue treatments of bovine pericardium are available for patches but not as valves; they include ADAPT (Admedus, Egan, MN) and Photofix (Cryolife).

Tissue treatment with glycerolization (Resilia, Edwards Lifesciences) has reduced calcification in an ovine model[124] and currently has the CE mark and FDA approval for an aortic bioprosthetic valve that can be dry-stored (Fig. 14.30) rather than being stored in glutaraldehyde. These tissue treatments aim to improve the durability of bioprosthetic valves and increase their applicability among younger patients.

Non-Warfarin Therapy for Mechanical Valves

Lifelong warfarin therapy for mechanical valves exposes patients to the competitive risks of thromboembolism and bleeding. FDA-approved anticoagulant alternatives include dabigatran, rivaroxaban, apixaban, and edoxaban. Dabigatran, which is a direct thrombin inhibitor, is inferior to warfarin in patients with mechanical valves.[125] The others are factor X inhibitors, which have not been studied in newer-generation mechanical valves. Dual antiplatelet therapy without an anticoagulant was only recently studied (PROACT trial, NCT #00291525). The use of non-warfarin therapy may increase the applicability of mechanical valves for older patients.

CONCLUSIONS

Surgery of the aortic valve can be accomplished with increased safety and efficacy in most patients. In those with higher operative risks, TAVI is already a proven acceptable alternative to AVR. The choice of valve prosthesis is guided by patient preference, life expectancy, and comorbidities relevant to SVD and anticoagulation.

Aortic valve repair in the young patient with AR avoids the risks associated with valve prostheses. Aortic root surgery similarly can be performed with replacement of the aortic valve and aortic wall, but valve-sparing techniques may offer the advantage of durability equivalent to normal native aortic valves along with avoidance of prosthetic valve–related complications. Reoperative aortic valve and aortic root surgery, like isolated AVR, can be performed safely, with the best outcomes achieved at high-volume centers.

REFERENCES

1. Leon MB, Smith CR, Mack M, et al. Transcatheter aortic-valve implantation for aortic stenosis in patients who cannot undergo surgery. N Engl J Med 2010;363(17):1597-1607.

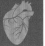
2. Smith CR, Leon MB, Mack MJ, et al. Transcatheter versus surgical aortic-valve replacement in high-risk patients. N Engl J Med 2011;364(23): 2187-2198.

3. Leon MB, Smith CR, Mack MJ, et al. Transcatheter or surgical aortic-valve replacement in intermediate-risk patients. N Engl J Med 2016;374(17): 1609-1620.

4. Popma JJ, Adams DH, Reardon MJ, et al. Transcatheter aortic valve replacement using a self-expanding bioprosthesis in patients with severe aortic stenosis at extreme risk for surgery. J Am Coll Cardiol 2014;63(19):1972-1981.

5. The PARTNER 3 Trial The Safety and Effectiveness of the SAPIEN 3 Transcatheter Heart Valve in Low Risk Patients with Aortic Stenosis (P3). ClinicalTrials.gov. Identifier: NCT02675114. Available at https://clinicaltrials. gov/ct2/show/NCT02675114.

6. Medtronic Transcatheter Aortic Valve Replacement in Low Risk Patients ClinicalTrials.gov. Identifier: NCT02701283. Available at https://clinicaltrials. gov/ct2/show/NCT02701283.

7. Kirmani BH, Jones SG, Malaisrie SC, et al. Limited versus full sternotomy for aortic valve replacement. Cochrane Database Syst Rev 2017;4:CD011793.

8. Brown ML, McKellar SH, Sundt TM, Schaff HV. Ministernotomy versus conventional sternotomy for aortic valve replacement: a systematic review and meta-analysis. J Thorac Cardiovasc Surg 2009;137(3):670-679. e675.

9. Khoshbin E, Prayaga S, Kinsella J, Sutherland FW. Mini-sternotomy for aortic valve replacement reduces the length of stay in the cardiac intensive care unit: meta-analysis of randomised controlled trials. BMJ Open 2011;1(2):e000266.

10. Phan K, Xie A, Di Eusanio M, Yan TD. A meta-analysis of minimally invasive versus conventional sternotomy for aortic valve replacement. Ann Thorac Surg 2014;98(4):1499-1511.

11. Malaisrie SC, Barnhart GR, Farivar RS, et al. Current era minimally invasive aortic valve replacement: techniques and practice. J Thorac Cardiovasc Surg 2014;147(1):6-14.

12. Duncan BF, McCarthy PM, Kruse J, et al. Paravalvular regurgitation after conventional aortic and mitral valve replacement: a benchmark for alternative approaches. J Thorac Cardiovasc Surg 2015;150(4):860-868. e861.

13. Chacko SJ, Ansari AH, McCarthy PM, et al. Prosthesis-patient mismatch in bovine pericardial aortic valves: evaluation using 3 different modalities and associated medium-term outcomes. Circ Cardiovasc Imaging 2013;6(5):776-783.

14. Sadowski J, Kapelak B, Pfitzner R, Bartus K. Sutureless aortic valve bioprothesis '3F/ATS Enable'—4.5 years of a single-centre experience. Kardiol Pol 2009;67(8A):956-963.

15. Barnhart GR, Accola KD, Grossi EA, et al. TRANSFORM (Multicenter Experience With Rapid Deployment Edwards INTUITY Valve System for Aortic Valve Replacement) US clinical trial: performance of a rapid deployment aortic valve. J Thorac Cardiovasc Surg 2017;153(2):241-251. e242.

16. Fischlein T, Meuris B, Hakim-Meibodi K, et al. The sutureless aortic valve at 1 year: a large multicenter cohort study. J Thorac Cardiovasc Surg 2016;151(6):1617-1626. e1614.

17. Laborde F, Fischlein T, Hakim-Meibodi K, et al. Clinical and haemodynamic outcomes in 658 patients receiving the Perceval sutureless aortic valve: early results from a prospective European multicentre study (the Cavalier Trial). Eur J Cardiothorac Surg 2016;49(3):978-986.

18. Glauber M, Moten SC, Quaini E, et al. International expert consensus on sutureless and rapid deployment valves in aortic valve replacement using minimally invasive approaches. Innovations (Phila) 2016;11(3):165-173.

19. Gersak B, Fischlein T, Folliguet TA, et al. Sutureless, rapid deployment valves and stented bioprosthesis in aortic valve replacement: recommendations of an international expert consensus panel. Eur J Cardiothorac Surg 2016;49(3):709-718.

20. Sievers HH, Schmidtke C. A classification system for the bicuspid aortic valve from 304 surgical specimens. J Thorac Cardiovasc Surg 2007;133(5): 1226-1233.

21. Pollari F, Santarpino G, Dell'Aquila AM, et al. Better short-term outcome by using sutureless valves: a propensity-matched score analysis. Ann Thorac Surg 2014;98(2):611-616; discussion 616-617.

22. Ali A, Halstead JC, Cafferty F, et al. Early clinical and hemodynamic outcomes after stented and stentless aortic valve replacement: results from a randomized controlled trial. Ann Thorac Surg 2007;83(6):2162-2168.

23. Cohen G, Christakis GT, Joyner CD, et al. Are stentless valves hemodynamically superior to stented valves? A prospective randomized trial. Ann Thorac Surg 2002;73(3):767-775; discussion 775-768.

24. Cohen G, Zagorski B, Christakis GT, et al. Are stentless valves hemodynamically superior to stented valves? Long-term follow-up of a randomized trial comparing Carpentier-Edwards pericardial valve with the Toronto Stentless Porcine Valve. J Thorac Cardiovasc Surg 2010;139(4):848-859.

25. Desai ND, Merin O, Cohen GN, et al. Long-term results of aortic valve replacement with the St. Jude Toronto stentless porcine valve. Ann Thorac Surg 2004;78(6):2076-2083; discussion 2076-2083.

26. Repossini A, Kotelnikov I, Bouchikhi R, et al. Single-suture line placement of a pericardial stentless valve. J Thorac Cardiovasc Surg 2005;130(5): 1265-1269.

27. Chambers JB, Pomar JL, Mestres CA, Palatianos GM. Clinical event rates with the On-X bileaflet mechanical heart valve: a multicenter experience with follow-up to 12 years. J Thorac Cardiovasc Surg 2013;145(2):420-424.

28. Puskas J, Gerdisch M, Nichols D, et al. Reduced anticoagulation after mechanical aortic valve replacement: interim results from the Prospective Randomized On-X Valve Anticoagulation Clinical Trial randomized Food and Drug Administration investigational device exemption trial. J Thorac Cardiovasc Surg 2014;147(4):1202-1211. e1202.

29. Nishimura RA, Otto CM, Bonow RO, et al. 2017 AHA/ACC focused update of the 2014 AHA/ACC guideline for the management of patients with valvular heart disease: a report of the American College of Cardiology/American Heart Association Task Force on Clinical Practice Guidelines. J Am Coll Cardiol 2017;70(2):252-289.

30. Ross DN. Homograft replacement of the aortic valve. Lancet.1962;2(7254):487.

31. Sales VL, McCarthy PM, Carr JC, et al. Near-complete obstruction of an aortic homograft. Circulation 2012;125(8):e392-394.

32. Nowicki ER, Pettersson GB, Smedira NG, et al. Aortic allograft valve reoperation: surgical challenges and patient risks. Ann Thorac Surg 2008;86(3): 761-768. e762.

33. Ross D. The Ross operation. J Card Surg 2002;17(3):188-193.

34. Falk V, Baumgartner H, Bax JJ, et al. Corrigendum to '2017 ESC/EACTS Guidelines for the management of valvular heart disease' [Eur J Cardiothorac Surg 2017;52:616-664]. Eur J Cardiothorac Surg 2017;52(4):832.

35. Nishimura RA, Otto CM, Bonow RO, et al. 2014 AHA/ACC guideline for the management of patients with valvular heart disease: a report of the American College of Cardiology/American Heart Association Task Force on Practice Guidelines. J Am Coll Cardiol 2014;63:e57-e185.

36. Bourguignon T, Bouquiaux-Stablo AL, Candolfi P, et al. Very long-term outcomes of the Carpentier-Edwards Perimount valve in aortic position. Ann Thorac Surg 2015;99(3):831-837.

37. Yankah CA, Pasic M, Musci M, et al. Aortic valve replacement with the Mitroflow pericardial bioprosthesis: durability results up to 21 years. J Thorac Cardiovasc Surg 2008;136(3):688-696.

38. David TE, Armstrong S, Maganti M. Hancock II bioprosthesis for aortic valve replacement: the gold standard of bioprosthetic valves durability? Ann Thorac Surg 2010;90(3):775-781.

39. Myken PS, Bech-Hansen O. A 20-year experience of 1712 patients with the Biocor porcine bioprosthesis. J Thorac Cardiovasc Surg 2009;137(1): 76-81.

40. Johnston DR, Soltesz EG, Vakil N, et al. Long-term durability of bioprosthetic aortic valves: implications from 12,569 implants. Ann Thorac Surg 2015;99(4):1239-1247.

41. Bouchard D, Mazine A, Stevens LM, et al. Twenty-year experience with the CarboMedics mechanical valve prosthesis. Ann Thorac Surg 2014;97(3):816-823.

42. Emery RW, Krogh CC, Arom KV, et al. The St. Jude Medical cardiac valve prosthesis: a 25-year experience with single valve replacement. Ann Thorac Surg 2005;79(3):776-782; discussion 782-773.

43. El Oakley R, Kleine P, Bach DS. Choice of prosthetic heart valve in today's practice. Circulation 2008;117(2):253-256.

44. Oxenham H, Bloomfield P, Wheatley DJ, et al. Twenty year comparison of a Bjork-Shiley mechanical heart valve with porcine bioprostheses. Heart 2003;89(7):715-721.

45. Hammermeister K, Sethi GK, Henderson WG, et al. Outcomes 15 years after valve replacement with a mechanical versus a bioprosthetic

valve: final report of the Veterans Affairs randomized trial. J Am Coll Cardiol 2000;36(4):1152-1158.

46. Banbury MK, Cosgrove DM, 3rd, White JA, et al. Age and valve size effect on the long-term durability of the Carpentier-Edwards aortic pericardial bioprosthesis. Ann Thorac Surg 2001;72(3):753-757.

47. Berrebi AJ, Carpentier SM, Phan KP, et al. Results of up to 9 years of high-temperature-fixed valvular bioprostheses in a young population. Ann Thorac Surg 2001;71(5 Suppl):S353-S355

48. Dvir D, Webb J, Brecker S, et al. Transcatheter aortic valve replacement for degenerative bioprosthetic surgical valves: results from the global valve-in-valve registry. Circulation 2012;126(19):2335-2344.

49. Webb JG, Mack MJ, White JM, et al. Transcatheter aortic valve implantation within degenerated aortic surgical bioprostheses: PARTNER 2 Valve-in-Valve Registry. J Am Coll Cardiol 2017;69(18):2253-2262.

50. Deeb GM, Chetcuti SJ, Reardon MJ, et al. 1-Year results in patients undergoing transcatheter aortic valve replacement with failed surgical bioprostheses. JACC Cardiovasc Interv 2017;10(10):1034-1044.

51. Enright LP, Hancock EW, Shumway NE. Aortic debridement—long-term follow-up. Circulation 1971;43(5 Suppl):I68-I72.

52. Aicher D, Fries R, Rodionycheva S, et al. Aortic valve repair leads to a low incidence of valve-related complications. Eur J Cardiothorac Surg 2010;37(1):127-132.

53. El Khoury G, Vanoverschelde JL, Glineur D, et al. Repair of aortic valve prolapse: experience with 44 patients. Eur J Cardiothorac Surg 2004; 26(3):628-633.

54. El Khoury G, de Kerchove L. Principles of aortic valve repair. J Thorac Cardiovasc Surg 2013;145(3 Suppl):S26-S29.

55. Schafers HJ, Langer F, Glombitza P, et al. Aortic valve reconstruction in myxomatous degeneration of aortic valves: are fenestrations a risk factor for repair failure? J Thorac Cardiovasc Surg 2010;139(3):660-664.

56. Taylor WJ, Thrower WB, Black H, Harken DE. The surgical correction of aortic insufficiency by circumclusion. J Thorac Surg 1958;35(2):192-205 passim.

57. Schneider U, Aicher D, Miura Y, Schafers HJ. Suture annuloplasty in aortic valve repair. Ann Thorac Surg 2016;101(2):783-785.

58. Lansac E, Di Centa I, Varnous S, et al. External aortic annuloplasty ring for valve-sparing procedures. Ann Thorac Surg 2005;79(1):356-358.

59. Rankin JS. An intra-annular 'hemispherical' annuloplasty frame for aortic valve repair. J Heart Valve Dis 2010;19(1):97-103.

60. Lansac E, Di Centa I, Raoux F, et al. An expansible aortic ring for a physiological approach to conservative aortic valve surgery. J Thorac Cardiovasc Surg 2009;138(3):718-724.

61. Bjoerk VO, Hultquist G. Teflon and pericardial aortic valve prostheses. J Thorac Cardiovasc Surg 1964;47:693-701.

62. Rankin JS, Nobauer C, Crooke PS, et al. Techniques of autologous pericardial leaflet replacement for aortic valve reconstruction. Ann Thorac Surg 2014;98(2):743-745.

63. Ozaki S, Kawase I, Yamashita H, et al. Aortic valve reconstruction using self-developed aortic valve plasty system in aortic valve disease. Interact Cardiovasc Thorac Surg 2011;12(4):550-553.

64. Duran CM, Gallo R, Kumar N. Aortic valve replacement with autologous pericardium: surgical technique. J Card Surg 1995;10(1):1-9.

65. Al Halees Z, Al Shahid M, Al Sanei A, et al. Up to 16 years follow-up of aortic valve reconstruction with pericardium: a stentless readily available cheap valve? Eur J Cardiothorac Surg 2005;28(2):200-205; discussion 205.

66. Ozaki S, Kawase I, Yamashita H, et al. A total of 404 cases of aortic valve reconstruction with glutaraldehyde-treated autologous pericardium. J Thorac Cardiovasc Surg 2014;147(1):301-306.

67. Shroyer AL, Coombs LP, Peterson ED, et al. The Society of Thoracic Surgeons: 30-day operative mortality and morbidity risk models. Ann Thorac Surg 2003;75(6):1856-1864; discussion 1864-1855.

68. Nashef SA, Roques F, Sharples LD, et al. EuroSCORE II. Eur J Cardiothorac Surg 2012;41(4):734-745.

69. Ambler G, Omar RZ, Royston P, et al. Generic, simple risk stratification model for heart valve surgery. Circulation 2005;112(2):224-231.

70. Rankin JS, Hammill BG, Ferguson TB, Jr., et al. Determinants of operative mortality in valvular heart surgery. J Thorac Cardiovasc Surg 2006;131(3): 547-557.

71. Brown JM, O'Brien SM, Wu C, et al. Isolated aortic valve replacement in North America comprising 108,687 patients in 10 years: changes in risks, valve types, and outcomes in the Society of Thoracic Surgeons National Database. J Thorac Cardiovasc Surg 2009;137(1):82-90.

72. Filsoufi F, Rahmanian PB, Castillo JG, et al. Excellent early and late outcomes of aortic valve replacement in people aged 80 and older. J Am Geriatr Soc 2008;56(2):255-261.

73. Malaisrie SC, McCarthy PM, McGee EC, et al. Contemporary perioperative results of isolated aortic valve replacement for aortic stenosis. Ann Thorac Surg 2010;89(3):751-756.

74. Bakaeen FG, Chu D, Huh J, Carabello BA. Is an age of 80 years or greater an important predictor of short-term outcomes of isolated aortic valve replacement in veterans? Ann Thorac Surg 2010;90(3):769-774.

75. Di Eusanio M, Fortuna D, De Palma R, et al. Aortic valve replacement: results and predictors of mortality from a contemporary series of 2256 patients. J Thorac Cardiovasc Surg 2011 Apr;141(4):940-947.

76. Thourani VH, Myung R, Kilgo P, et al. Long-term outcomes after isolated aortic valve replacement in octogenarians: a modern perspective. Ann Thorac Surg 2008;86(5):1458-1464; discussion 1464-1455.

77. Reardon MJ, Van Mieghem NM, Popma JJ, et al. Surgical or transcatheter aortic-valve replacement in intermediate-risk patients. N Engl J Med 2017;376(14):1321-1331.

78. Hiratzka LF, Bakris GL, Beckman JA, et al. 2010 ACCF/AHA/AATS/ACR/ASA/SCA/SCAI/SIR/STS/SVM guidelines for the diagnosis and management of patients with thoracic aortic disease: a report of the American College of Cardiology Foundation/American Heart Association Task Force on Practice Guidelines, American Association for Thoracic Surgery, American College of Radiology, American Stroke Association, Society of Cardiovascular Anesthesiologists, Society for Cardiovascular Angiography and Interventions, Society of Interventional Radiology, Society of Thoracic Surgeons, and Society for Vascular Medicine. Circulation 2010;121(13):e266-e369.

79. Bonow RO, Carabello BA, Kanu C, et al. ACC/AHA 2006 guidelines for the management of patients with valvular heart disease: a report of the American College of Cardiology/American Heart Association Task Force on Practice Guidelines (writing committee to revise the 1998 Guidelines for the Management of Patients With Valvular Heart Disease): developed in collaboration with the Society of Cardiovascular Anesthesiologists: endorsed by the Society for Cardiovascular Angiography and Interventions and the Society of Thoracic Surgeons. Circulation 2006;114(5):e84-e231.

80. Hiratzka LF, Creager MA, Isselbacher EM, et al. Surgery for aortic dilatation in patients with bicuspid aortic valves: a statement of clarification from the American College of Cardiology/American Heart Association Task Force on Clinical Practice Guidelines. J Am Coll Cardiol 2016;67(6): 724-731.

81. Borger MA, Preston M, Ivanov J, et al. Should the ascending aorta be replaced more frequently in patients with bicuspid aortic valve disease? J Thorac Cardiovasc Surg 2004;128(5):677-683.

82. Hughes GC, Zhao Y, Rankin JS, et al. Effects of institutional volumes on operative outcomes for aortic root replacement in North America. J Thorac Cardiovasc Surg 2013;145(1):166-170.

83. Kalkat MS, Edwards MB, Taylor KM, Bonser RS. Composite aortic valve graft replacement: mortality outcomes in a national registry. Circulation 2007;116(11 Suppl):I301-I306.

84. Bentall H, De Bono A. A technique for complete replacement of the ascending aorta. Thorax 1968;23(4):338-339.

85. Kouchoukos NT, Karp RB. Resection of ascending aortic aneurysm and replacement of aortic valve. J Thorac Cardiovasc Surg 1981;81(1): 142-143.

86. Cabrol C, Pavie A, Gandjbakhch I, et al. Complete replacement of the ascending aorta with reimplantation of the coronary arteries: new surgical approach. J Thorac Cardiovasc Surg 1981;81(2):309-315.

87. Zubiate P, Kay JH. Surgical treatment of aneurysm of the ascending aorta with aortic insufficiency and marked displacement of the coronary ostia. J Thorac Cardiovasc Surg 1976;71(3):415-421.

88. Gott VL, Cameron DE, Alejo DE, et al. Aortic root replacement in 271 Marfan patients: a 24-year experience. Ann Thorac Surg 2002;73(2): 438-443.

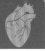
89. Etz CD, Homann TM, Rane N, et al. Aortic root reconstruction with a bioprosthetic valved conduit: a consecutive series of 275 procedures. J Thorac Cardiovasc Surg 2007;133(6):1455-1463.

90. Kvitting JP, Kari FA, Fischbein MP, et al. David valve-sparing aortic root replacement: equivalent mid-term outcome for different valve types with or without connective tissue disorder. J Thorac Cardiovasc Surg 2013;145(1):117-126, 137.e1-5; discussion 126-127.

91. De Paulis R, Scaffa R, Nardella S, et al. Use of the Valsalva graft and long-term follow-up. J Thorac Cardiovasc Surg 2010;140(6 Suppl):S23-S27; discussion S45-S51.

92. David TE, Armstrong S, Maganti M, et al. Long-term results of aortic valve-sparing operations in patients with Marfan syndrome. J Thorac Cardiovasc Surg 2009;138(4):859-864; discussion 863-854.

93. Benedetto U, Melina G, Takkenberg JJ, et al. Surgical management of aortic root disease in Marfan syndrome: a systematic review and meta-analysis. Heart 2011;97(12):955-958.

94. Demers P, Miller DC. Simple modification of "T. David-V" valve-sparing aortic root replacement to create graft pseudosinuses. Ann Thorac Surg 2004;78(4):1479-1481.

95. De Paulis R, De Matteis GM, Nardi P, et al. One-year appraisal of a new aortic root conduit with sinuses of Valsalva. J Thorac Cardiovasc Surg 2002;123(1):33-39.

96. Nicks R, Cartmill T, Bernstein L. Hypoplasia of the aortic root. The problem of aortic valve replacement. Thorax 1970;25(3):339-346.

97. Manouguian S, Seybold-Epting W. Patch enlargement of the aortic valve ring by extending the aortic incision into the anterior mitral leaflet: new operative technique. J Thorac Cardiovasc Surg 1979;78(3):402-412.

98. Konno S, Imai Y, Iida Y, et al. A new method for prosthetic valve replacement in congenital aortic stenosis associated with hypoplasia of the aortic valve ring. J Thorac Cardiovasc Surg 1975;70(5):909-917.

99. Zoghbi WA, Chambers JB, Dumesnil JG, et al. Recommendations for evaluation of prosthetic valves with echocardiography and doppler ultrasound: a report from the American Society of Echocardiography's Guidelines and Standards Committee and the Task Force on Prosthetic Valves, developed in conjunction with the American College of Cardiology Cardiovascular Imaging Committee, Cardiac Imaging Committee of the American Heart Association, the European Association of Echocardiography, a registered branch of the European Society of Cardiology, the Japanese Society of Echocardiography and the Canadian Society of Echocardiography, endorsed by the American College of Cardiology Foundation, American Heart Association, European Association of Echocardiography, a registered branch of the European Society of Cardiology, the Japanese Society of Echocardiography, and Canadian Society of Echocardiography. J Am Soc Echocardiogr 2009; 22(9):975-1014; quiz 1082-1014.

100. Pibarot P, Dumesnil JG. Prosthesis-patient mismatch: definition, clinical impact, and prevention. Heart 2006;92(8):1022-1029.

101. Flameng W, Meuris B, Herijgers P, Herregods MC. Prosthesis-patient mismatch is not clinically relevant in aortic valve replacement using the Carpentier-Edwards Perimount valve. Ann Thorac Surg 2006;82(2):530-536.

102. Blackstone EH, Cosgrove DM, Jamieson WR, et al. Prosthesis size and long-term survival after aortic valve replacement. J Thorac Cardiovasc Surg 2003;126(3):783-796.

103. Blais C, Dumesnil JG, Baillot R, et al. Impact of valve prosthesis-patient mismatch on short-term mortality after aortic valve replacement. Circulation 2003;108(8):983-988.

104. Hanayama N, Christakis GT, Mallidi HR, et al. Patient prosthesis mismatch is rare after aortic valve replacement: valve size may be irrelevant. Ann Thorac Surg 2002;73(6):1822-1829; discussion 1829.

105. Rao V, Jamieson WR, Ivanov J, et al. Prosthesis-patient mismatch affects survival after aortic valve replacement. Circulation 2000;102 (19 Suppl 3):III5-III9.

106. Howell NJ, Keogh BE, Ray D, et al. Patient-prosthesis mismatch in patients with aortic stenosis undergoing isolated aortic valve replacement does not affect survival. Ann Thorac Surg 2010;89(1):60-64.

107. Mascherbauer J, Rosenhek R, Fuchs C, et al. Moderate patient-prosthesis mismatch after valve replacement for severe aortic stenosis has no impact on short-term and long-term mortality. Heart 2008;94(12): 1639-1645.

108. Movsowitz HD, Levine RA, Hilgenberg AD, Isselbacher EM. Transesophageal echocardiographic description of the mechanisms of aortic regurgitation in acute type A aortic dissection: implications for aortic valve repair. J Am Coll Cardiol 2000;36(3):884-890.

109. Bonser RS, Ranasinghe AM, Loubani M, et al. Evidence, lack of evidence, controversy, and debate in the provision and performance of the surgery of acute type A aortic dissection. J Am Coll Cardiol 2011;58(24):2455-2474.

110. Halstead JC, Spielvogel D, Meier DM, et al. Composite aortic root replacement in acute type A dissection: time to rethink the indications? Eur J Cardiothorac Surg 2005;27(4):626-632; discussion 632-623.

111. Stewart BF, Siscovick D, Lind BK, et al. Clinical factors associated with calcific aortic valve disease. Cardiovascular Health Study. J Am Coll Cardiol 1997;29(3):630-634.

112. Fighali SF, Avendano A, Elayda MA, et al. Early and late mortality of patients undergoing aortic valve replacement after previous coronary artery bypass graft surgery. Circulation 1995;92(9 Suppl):II163-II168.

113. Dobrilovic N, Fingleton JG, Maslow A, et al. Midterm outcomes of patients undergoing aortic valve replacement after previous coronary artery bypass grafting. Eur J Cardiothorac Surg 2012;42(5):819-825.

114. Park CB, Suri RM, Burkhart HM, et al. Identifying patients at particular risk of injury during repeat sternotomy: analysis of 2555 cardiac reoperations. J Thorac Cardiovasc Surg 2010;140(5):1028-1035.

115. Roselli EE, Pettersson GB, Blackstone EH, et al. Adverse events during reoperative cardiac surgery: frequency, characterization, and rescue. J Thorac Cardiovasc Surg 2008;135(2):316-323, 323.e1-6.

116. Park CB, Suri RM, Burkhart HM, et al. What is the optimal myocardial preservation strategy at re-operation for aortic valve replacement in the presence of a patent internal thoracic artery? Eur J Cardiothorac Surg 2011;39(6):861-865.

117. Smith RL, Ellman PI, Thompson PW, et al. Do you need to clamp a patent left internal thoracic artery-left anterior descending graft in reoperative cardiac surgery? Ann Thorac Surg 2009;87(3):742-747.

118. Potter DD, Sundt TM, 3rd, Zehr KJ, et al. Operative risk of reoperative aortic valve replacement. J Thorac Cardiovasc Surg 2005;129(1):94-103.

119. Svensson LG, Blackstone EH, Rajeswaran J, et al. Does the arterial cannulation site for circulatory arrest influence stroke risk? Ann Thorac Surg 2004;78(4):1274-1284; discussion 1274-1284.

120. Etz CD, Plestis KA, Homann TM, et al. Reoperative aortic root and transverse arch procedures: a comparison with contemporary primary operations. J Thorac Cardiovasc Surg 2008;136(4):860-867, 867.e1-3.

121. Gammie JS, Brown JW, Brown JM, et al. Aortic valve bypass for the high-risk patient with aortic stenosis. Ann Thorac Surg 2006;81(5): 1605-1610.

122. Gammie JS, Krowsoski LS, Brown JM, et al. Aortic valve bypass surgery: midterm clinical outcomes in a high-risk aortic stenosis population. Circulation 2008;118(14):1460-1466.

123. Schoen FJ, Levy RJ. Calcification of tissue heart valve substitutes: progress toward understanding and prevention. Ann Thorac Surg 2005;79(3): 1072-1080.

124. Flameng W, Hermans H, Verbeken E, Meuris B. A randomized assessment of an advanced tissue preservation technology in the juvenile sheep model. J Thorac Cardiovasc Surg 2015;149(1):340-345.

125. Eikelboom JW, Connolly SJ, Brueckmann M, et al. Dabigatran versus warfarin in patients with mechanical heart valves. N Engl J Med 2013;369(13):1206-1214.

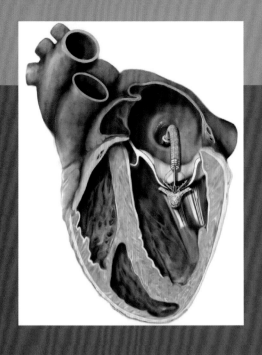

第15章
二尖瓣反流的诊断评估

　　经胸超声心动图可准确判断大多数患者二尖瓣反流的原因，但在干预瓣膜时通常需要三维经食管超声心动图进一步补充。原发性二尖瓣反流由小叶或腱索疾病引起，最常见的是二尖瓣脱垂、风湿性心脏病或感染性心内膜炎。继发性二尖瓣反流可能由局部或整体左心室扩张和收缩功能障碍相关的缺血性或非缺血性原因引起。指南对原发性和继发性二尖瓣反流严重程度使用相同的定量标准，但需考虑患者的症状、左心室大小和功能、左心房大小、肺循环压力和二尖瓣反流严重程度。了解二尖瓣反流束的起源和方向有助于确定二尖瓣反流的确切机制和决定具体干预措施。二尖瓣反流严重程度的评估基于许多定性和定量参数的综合评估（如缩流颈宽度），如果可能的话，建议测量反流容积和反流孔面积。二尖瓣反流严重程度评估需考虑动态变化，尤其在前、后负荷和左心室收缩性变化时。左心室大小、形状和收缩功能的成像是评估二尖瓣反流患者的关键因素。继发性二尖瓣反流经导管治疗的研究为了解左心室大小和功能与二尖瓣反流严重程度之间的复杂相互作用提供了见解。除经胸超声心动图和经食管超声心动图外，心脏MRI、CT和有创性左心室血管造影对二尖瓣反流测量提供一定帮助。

赵振燕

Diagnostic Evaluation of Mitral Regurgitation

Akhil Narang, Jyothy Puthumana, James D. Thomas

CHAPTER OUTLINE

KEY POINTS

- Transthoracic echocardiography (TTE) provides an accurate diagnosis of the cause of mitral regurgitation (MR) in most patients, although three-dimensional transesophageal imaging (TEE) often is needed for decisions about timing and type of intervention.
- Primary MR is caused by disease of the leaflets or chords, most often mitral valve prolapse (MVP), rheumatic heart disease, or infective endocarditis. Secondary MR may be caused by ischemic or nonischemic conditions associated with regional or global left ventricular (LV) dilation and systolic dysfunction.
- Guidelines use similar quantitative measures of MR severity for primary and secondary MR. Consideration is given to the patient's symptoms, LV size and function, left atrial size, pulmonary pressures, and MR severity.
- It is helpful to know the origin and direction of the MR jet when determining the exact mechanism of regurgitation and deciding on specific interventions to reduce MR severity.
- Evaluation of MR severity is based on integration of many qualitative and quantitative parameters (e.g., vena contracta width), and

measurement of regurgitant volume and regurgitant orifice area is recommended when possible.
- A simple, practical approach to quantitation of MR severity is measurement of the proximal isovelocity surface area (PISA) radius on color-flow Doppler imaging with the aliasing velocity set at 40 cm/s. The estimated effective regurgitation orifice area (EROA) is one half of the square of the PISA radius ($r^2/2$); a radius of approximately 1.0 cm indicates severe MR (EROA > 0.4 cm²).
- Evaluation of MR should take into account the dynamic changes in severity that can occur with changes in preload, afterload, and LV contractility.
- Imaging of LV size, geometry, and systolic function is a key element in the evaluation of patients with MR. Studies on transcatheter therapy for secondary MR offer insights into the complex interaction between LV size and function and MR severity.
- In addition to TTE and TEE, cardiac magnetic resonance imaging, computed tomographic imaging, and invasive LV angiography may be helpful for selected patients.

IMAGING MITRAL VALVE ANATOMY

The first step in imaging a patient with mitral valve (MV) disease is to diagnose the underlying disease process leading to valve dysfunction. Worldwide, mitral stenosis is most often caused by rheumatic valve disease. In developed countries, severe mitral annular calcification extending onto the valve leaflets is emerging as a cause of

mitral stenosis in elderly patients. Mitral stenosis is discussed in Chapter 16. This chapter focuses on imaging of patients with mitral regurgitation (MR).

The most common causes of MR include myxomatous MV disease (i.e., mitral valve prolapse [MVP] and ruptured or flail mitral chordae), rheumatic heart disease, infective endocarditis, hypertrophic cardiomyopathy, mitral annular calcification, dilated cardiomyopathy, and ischemic heart disease. Less common causes of MR include connective tissue disorders (e.g., Marfan syndrome, Loeys-Dietz syndrome), trauma, hypereosinophilic syndrome, metastatic carcinoid tumors, and exposure to certain drugs.

The causes of MR are categorized as primary (i.e., organic or degenerative) MR, which result from abnormalities of the MV apparatus itself, or secondary (i.e., functional) MR, which is associated with pathology of the left ventricle (LV), left atrium (LA), or mitral annulus but with relatively normal valve leaflets and chords. Ischemic MR is a subset of secondary MR that results from myocardial infarction with subsequent LV dysfunction and remodeling. Primary and secondary forms of MR are two distinct disease states with distinct pathologies, outcomes, and management considerations (see Chapters 17 and 18).

The next step in imaging the patient with MR is to determine the specific mechanism of MR. Abnormalities in the MV leaflets, chordae tendineae, papillary muscles, mitral annulus, LA, or LV can result in MR (Figs. 15.1 and 15.2).[1] One useful approach to categorizing the mechanism of MR is based on the pattern of leaflet motion: normal (type I), excessive (type II), or restricted (type IIIa, restricted opening; type IIIb, restricted closure) (see Fig. 19.3 in Chapter 19). This classification system is useful in considering potential surgical or transcatheter interventions for reducing MR severity. Types II and IIIa usually are caused by primary disorders of the valve leaflets, whereas in types I and IIIb, the leaflets are relatively normal but leaflet motion is distorted by LV, LA, and/or annular remodeling causing secondary MR.

Valve Leaflets

Transthoracic echocardiography (TTE) is adequate for routine evaluation of the anatomy and motion of the valve leaflets, but transesophageal echocardiography (TEE) often is necessary for optimal visualization of valve anatomy and quantitation of regurgitant severity, particularly when surgical or transcatheter intervention is being considered.

Myxomatous disease occurs on a spectrum according to the relative degree of leaflet thickening and redundancy versus weakness in the mitral chords. On one end of the spectrum is Barlow syndrome (Fig. 15.3), which is characterized by significant leaflet thickening and redundancy, prolapse of multiple scallops, and severe regurgitation arising from multiple points along the valve closure line. At the other end of the spectrum is fibroelastic deficiency, in which the leaflets are relatively thin; at presentation, there is isolated prolapse or flail of a single scallop with regurgitation originating from a single focus. Intermediate forms lie between these two extremes.[2]

Infective endocarditis causes MR by destruction of valve leaflets, which results in inadequate coaptation, or by frank leaflet perforation. Vegetations on the MV can prevent complete leaflet closure. Even after effective treatment of endocarditis, valvular retraction and calcification can lead to persistent or worsening MR.

In the developing world, rheumatic heart disease remains a common cause of MR. In contrast to mitral stenosis, rheumatic MR is more frequent in men than in women. It is a consequence of shortening, rigidity, deformity, and retraction of one or both MV cusps and is associated with shortening and fusion of the chordae tendineae and papillary muscles.

MR can occur with exposure to drugs that cause fibrotic changes in the valve leaflets.[3] Among drugs associated with MR are the ergot alkaloids methysergide and ergotamine, the anorexigens (dex)fenfluramine and benfluorex, the dopamine agonists pergolide and cabergoline, and MDMA (Ecstacy). The thickened, rigid leaflets are similar to those usually seen in patients with carcinoid and suggest a common pathophysiologic cause: overstimulation of the serotonin 2B receptor. In carcinoid limited to the gastrointestinal tract, the excess serotonin is metabolized in the lungs, and mitral involvement is not seen. However, with lung metastases or right-to-left shunting, mitral and aortic thickening and regurgitation may develop as a result of exposure to serotonin.

Mitral Annulus
Dilation

The normal mitral annulus in an adult has a circumference of approximately 10 cm. The annulus is soft and flexible, with systolic annular constriction caused by contraction of the surrounding LV muscle that contributes importantly to valve closure.[4] Smooth muscle cells within the annulus and mitral leaflets may also exert a sphincter action on the valve.[5] MR due to dilation of the mitral annulus can occur in any form of heart disease characterized by dilation of the LV or LA, especially in dilated cardiomyopathy and long-standing atrial fibrillation.[6,7]

Aneurysm of the basal inferoposterior LV wall (i.e., submitral aneurysm) has been reported as a cause of annular MR in sub-Saharan Africa. It appears to result from a congenital defect in the posterior aspect of the annulus. Primary diseases of the leaflets, such as myxomatous disease, are associated with annular dilation and abnormal annular motion, which may worsen the severity of MR.[8,9]

Calcification

Idiopathic (degenerative) calcification of the mitral annulus or leaflets is commonly found at autopsy and is usually of little functional consequence. However, if severe annular or leaflet calcification develops (Fig. 15.4), it can cause MR and even significant mitral stenosis. Mitral annular calcification shares common risk factors with atherosclerosis, including hypertension, dyslipidemia, and diabetes, and it is associated with coronary and carotid atherosclerosis and aortic valve calcification. Patients with significant annular or leaflet calcification are at higher risk for cardiovascular morbidity and mortality. Annular calcification may be accelerated by an intrinsic defect in the fibrous skeleton of the heart, as in patients with Marfan and Hurler syndromes, in which annular dilation further contributes to MR. The

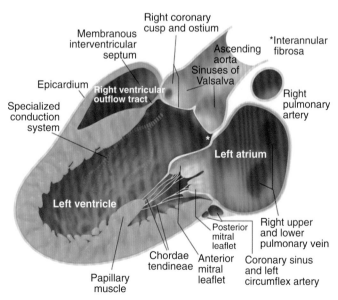

Fig. 15.1 Normal Mitral Valve Anatomy. An anatomic illustration oriented similar to an echocardiographic parasternal long-axis view in diastole shows normal mitral valve anatomy, including the mitral annulus, anterior and posterior mitral leaflets, mitral chords, and papillary muscles. The medial papillary muscle is shown for reference, although slight medial angulation typically is needed to visualize this structure in the long-axis view.

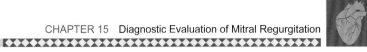

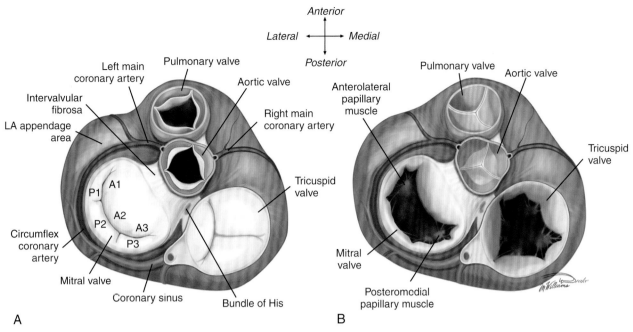

Anterior

Lateral ← → Medial

Posterior

Left main coronary artery
Pulmonary valve
Aortic valve
Intervalvular fibrosa
Right main coronary artery
LA appendage area
A1
P1
A2
P2
A3
P3
Circumflex coronary artery
Tricuspid valve
Mitral valve
Coronary sinus
Bundle of His

A

Pulmonary valve
Aortic valve
Anterolateral papillary muscle
Tricuspid valve
Mitral valve
Posteromedial papillary muscle

B

Fig. 15.2 Anatomic Relationships of the Mitral Valve. The base of the heart is shown in an anatomic orientation from the left atrial aspect. The relationship of the mitral valve and adjacent cardiac structures is demonstrated. (A) Systole. The posterior leaflet of the mitral valve has two natural clefts. The clefts divide the posterior leaflet into three segments that (using the Carpentier nomenclature) are called P1, P2, and P3. Although there are no natural clefts in the anterior leaflet, its corresponding segments are called A1, A2, and A3. For purposes of echocardiographic orientation, it is useful to observe that P1 is adjacent to the left atrial appendage and P3 is adjacent to the tricuspid valve. (B) Diastole. The anterolateral and posteromedial papillary muscles support the anterior and posterior leaflets symmetrically. The anterolateral muscle supports A1/P1 and the anterolateral half of A2/P2; the posteromedial muscle supports A3/P3 and the posteromedial half of A2/P2. (From Drake DH, Zimmerman KG, Sidebotham DA. Transesophageal echocardiography for surgical repair of mitral regurgitation. In: Otto C, editor. The practice of clinical echocardiography. 5th ed. Philadelphia: Elsevier; 2017. p. 343-373.)

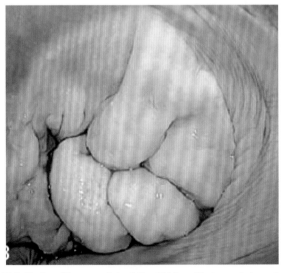

Fig. 15.3 Barlow Disease of the Mitral Valve. Photograph from the left atrial perspective with the anterior leaflet at the top and the posterior leaflet at the bottom shows significant leaflet thickening and redundancy. Multiscallop prolapse has resulted in significant mitral regurgitation.

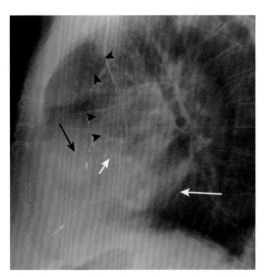

Fig. 15.4 Calcification of the Heart. Chest radiograph shows aortic stenosis calcification (*short white arrow*), mitral annular calcification (*long white arrow*), anterior ascending aortic wall calcification (*black arrowheads*), and calcified density crossing the aortic root along the left anterior descending coronary artery (*black arrow*).

incidence of mitral annular calcification is increased in patients who have chronic renal failure with secondary hyperparathyroidism and in those with rheumatic involvement.

Chordae Tendineae

Abnormalities of the chordae tendineae are important causes of MR (Fig. 15.5).[10] Lengthening and rupture of the chordae tendineae are cardinal features of the MVP syndrome (Fig. 15.6), particularly in cases of fibroelastic deficiency. The chordae may be congenitally abnormal; rupture may be spontaneous (primary), or it may occur as a consequence of infective endocarditis, trauma, rheumatic fever, or, rarely, osteogenesis imperfecta or relapsing polychondritis.

In most patients, no cause for chordal rupture is apparent other than increased mechanical strain on thin, myxomatous chords. Chords to the posterior leaflet rupture more frequently than those to the anterior leaflet. Depending on the number of chords involved in rupture and the rate at which rupture occurs, the resultant MR may be mild, moderate, or severe and acute, subacute, or chronic. Chordal rupture also has been reported as a result of trauma from percutaneous circulatory support devices.[11]

Papillary Muscles

The LV papillary muscles are perfused by the terminal portion of the coronary vascular bed, making them particularly vulnerable to ischemia, and any disturbance in coronary perfusion may result in papillary muscle dysfunction. Transient ischemia causes temporary papillary muscle dysfunction and transient episodes of MR that are sometimes associated with attacks of angina pectoris or pulmonary edema. If papillary muscle ischemia is severe and prolonged, papillary muscle dysfunction and scarring lead to chronic MR. MR occurs in approximately 20% of patients after acute myocardial infarction, and even when mild, it is associated with a higher risk of adverse outcomes.[12–14]

The posterior papillary muscle, which is supplied by the posterior descending branch of the right coronary artery, becomes ischemic and infarcted more frequently than the anterolateral papillary muscle. The latter is often dually supplied by diagonal branches of the left anterior descending coronary artery and marginal branches from the left circumflex artery. Ischemia of the papillary muscles usually is caused by coronary atherosclerosis but also may occur in patients with severe anemia, shock, coronary arteritis of any cause, or an anomalous left coronary artery.

With remote myocardial infarction, MR may result from regional myocardial tissue at the base of a papillary muscle, most commonly due to right coronary or left circumflex coronary disease, which results in tethering of the mitral leaflets and incomplete leaflet coaptation.[13,15] Necrosis of a papillary muscle can complicate myocardial infarction, but frank rupture of the full papillary muscle is rarely diagnosed premortem because it usually causes severe or fatal acute MR. However, rupture of one or two of the apical heads of a papillary muscle can result in a flail leaflet (Fig. 15.7) with a lesser degree of MR (although still usually severe). Survival is possible, usually with prompt surgical therapy,[16,17] although percutaneous repairs have also been reported.[18]

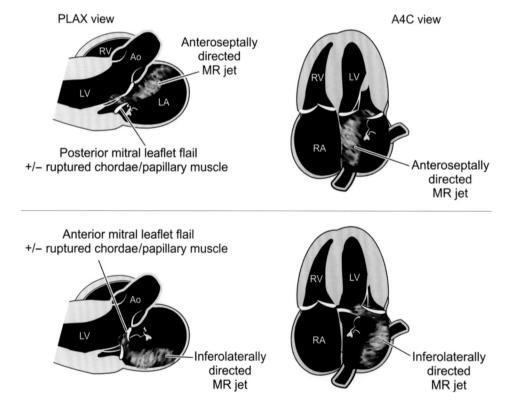

Fig. 15.5 Acute Mitral Regurgitation. Schematic diagrams show the jet directions resulting from acute mitral regurgitation caused by posterior mitral leaflet flail *(top)* and by anterior mitral leaflet flail *(bottom)*. (From Solomon D, Wu JC, Gillam L. Echocardiography. In: Zipes DP, Libby P, Bonow RO, et al, editors. Braunwald's heart disease: a textbook of cardiovascular medicine. 11th ed. Philadelphia: Elsevier; 2018. p. 174-251.)

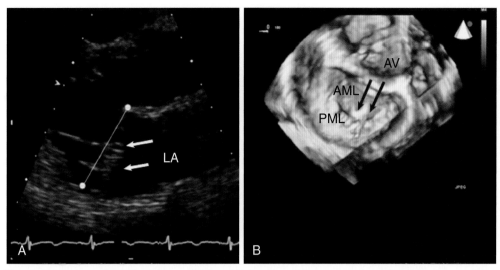

Fig. 15.6 Degenerative Mitral Regurgitation. (A) Parasternal long-axis echocardiographic image shows bileaflet prolapse demonstrating billowing of both leaflets *(arrows)* above the annular plane *(white line)*. (B) Three-dimensional transesophageal image shows anterior mitral leaflet flail segments *(arrows)*. *AML,* Anterior mitral leaflet; *AV,* aortic valve; *LA,* left atrium; *PML,* posterior mitral leaflet.

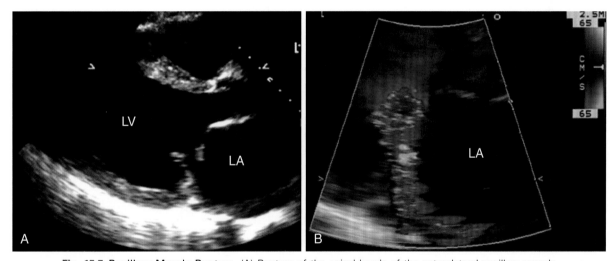

Fig. 15.7 Papillary Muscle Rupture. (A) Rupture of the apical heads of the anterolateral papillary muscle results in flail anterior mitral valve leaflet, as shown in a parasternal long-axis view. This results in posterior mitral regurgitation on color Doppler flow imaging (B). *LA,* Left atrium; *LV,* left ventricle.

Various other disorders of the papillary muscles may be responsible for the development of MR. They include congenital malposition of the papillary muscles, absence of one papillary muscle (leading to the parachute MV syndrome), and involvement or infiltration of the papillary muscles by a variety of processes such as abscesses, granulomas, neoplasms, amyloidosis, and sarcoidosis.

Left Ventricular Dysfunction

Ischemic LV dysfunction and dilated cardiomyopathy are contributors to the development of MR and represent the second leading cause of MR (after MVP) in the United States.[13] LV dilation of any cause, including ischemia, can alter the spatial relationships between the papillary muscles and chordae tendineae and thereby result in

secondary MR (Fig. 15.8). For a given amount of LV dilation, MR is greater when there is asymmetric tethering of the MV caused by inferior and inferolateral ventricular scarring rather than symmetric dilation as in dilated cardiomyopathy (Fig. 15.9).[17]

Some degree of MR is found in approximately 30% of patients with coronary artery disease who are referred for coronary artery bypass grafting (CABG). In most of these patients, MR develops from tethering of the posterior leaflet because of regional LV dysfunction. Other pathologic changes may include additional ischemic damage to the papillary muscles, dilation of the MV ring, and loss of systolic annular contraction contributing further to MR. The incidence and severity of regurgitation vary inversely with LV ejection fraction and directly with LV end-systolic volume (ESV).

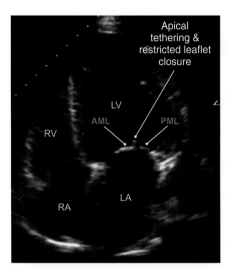
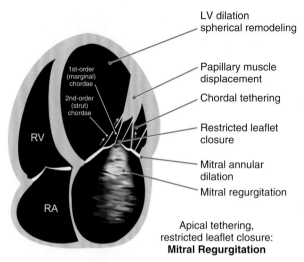

Fig. 15.8 Mechanisms of Secondary Mitral Regurgitation. Secondary (including ischemic) mitral regurgitation develops as a consequence of annular dilation and papillary muscle traction, both caused by LV remodeling. This leads to apical displacement of leaflet coaptation. *AML,* Anterior mitral leaflet; *PML,* posterior mitral leaflet. (From Solomon D, Wu JC, Gillam L. Echocardiography. In: Zipes DP, Libby P, Bonow RO, et al, editors. Braunwald's heart disease: a textbook of cardiovascular medicine. 11th ed. Philadelphia: Elsevier; 2018. p. 174-251.)

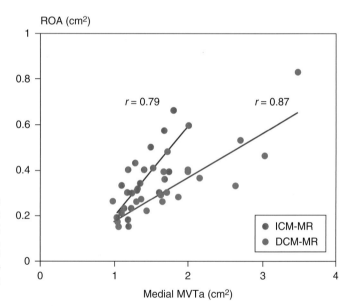

Fig. 15.9 Mitral Leaflet Tenting Area. Correlation between mitral valve tenting area *(MVTa)* and regurgitation orifice area *(ROA)* in patients with ischemic or dilated mitral regurgitation. *DCM,* Dilated cardiomyopathy; *ICM,* ischemic cardiomyopathy; *MR,* mitral regurgitation. (From Kwan J, Shiota T, Agler DA, et al. Geometric differences of the mitral apparatus between ischemic and dilated cardiomyopathy with significant mitral regurgitation: real-time three-dimensional echocardiography study. Circulation 2003;107:1135-1140.)

ECHOCARDIOGRAPHIC EVALUATION OF MITRAL REGURGITATION

Echocardiography plays a central role in quantifying MR severity. An integral part of evaluating MR severity is consideration of the degree of LA and LV enlargement and assessment of LV systolic function[19–22] (Tables 15.1 through 15.3). Doppler echocardiography characteristically reveals a high-velocity signal in the regurgitant orifice with flow from the LV to the LA during systole.[19] Qualitative assessment of the color Doppler regurgitant jet size in the LA correlates reasonably well with quantitative methods in estimating MR severity. However, color-flow jet areas are significantly influenced by the driving pressure (i.e., LV-LA gradient), jet eccentricity, and a host of instrument factors such as transmission power and frequency, receiver gain, Nyquist limit, and wall filter, limiting the accuracy of this approach (Table 15.4).

Quantitative methods to measure regurgitant fraction, regurgitant volume, and regurgitant orifice area have greater accuracy when done carefully[23–26] (Figs. 15.10 through 15.12). An integrative approach with consideration of multiple parameters of MR severity is strongly recommended (Fig. 15.13).

TEE imaging with three-dimensional (3D) visualization provides better assessment of mitral anatomy and leaflet motion, identification of the exact mechanism and origin of the regurgitant jet, and quantitation of regurgitant severity. MR assessment, with LV volumes routinely available, and surface rendering of the valve directly demonstrate the pathology. Multiplane imaging allows the valve to be interrogated in a structured fashion to optimally localize the pathology (Fig. 15.14; see Fig. 15.7). 3D Doppler imaging[4,9,27] helps elucidate the mechanism of MR (Fig. 15.15).

(Text Continued on Page 303)

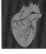

TABLE 15.1 American College of Cardiology/American Heart Association Stages of Primary MR.

Grade	Definition	Valve Anatomy	Valve Hemodynamics*	Hemodynamic Consequences	Symptoms
A	At risk of MR	• Mild mitral valve prolapse with normal coaptation • Mild valve thickening and leaflet restriction	• No MR jet or small central jet area < 20% LA on Doppler • Small vena contracta < 0.3 cm	• None	• None
B	Progressive MR	• Severe mitral valve prolapse with normal coaptation • Rheumatic valve changes with leaflet restriction and loss of central coaptation • Prior IE	• Central jet MR 20%–40% LA or late systolic eccentric jet MR • Vena contracta < 0.7 cm • Regurgitant volume < 60 mL • Regurgitant fraction < 50% • ERO < 0.40 cm² • Angiographic grade 1–2+	• Mild LA enlargement • No LV enlargement • Normal pulmonary pressure	• None
C	Asymptomatic severe MR	• Severe mitral valve prolapse with loss of coaptation or flail leaflet • Rheumatic valve changes with leaflet restriction and loss of central coaptation • Prior IE • Thickening of leaflets with radiation heart disease	• Central jet MR > 40% LA or holosystolic eccentric jet MR • Vena contracta ≥ 0.7 cm • Regurgitant volume ≥ 60 mL • Regurgitant fraction ≥ 50% • ERO ≥ 0.40 cm² • Angiographic grade 3–4+	• Moderate or severe LA enlargement • LV enlargement • Pulmonary hypertension may be present at rest or with exercise • **C1:** LVEF > 60% and LVESD < 40 mm • **C2:** LVEF ≤ 60% and LVESD ≤ 40 mm	• None
D	Symptomatic severe MR	• Severe mitral valve prolapse with loss of coaptation or flail leaflet • Rheumatic valve changes with leaflet restriction and loss of central coaptation • Prior IE • Thickening of leaflets with radiation heart disease	• Central jet MR > 40% LA or holosystolic eccentric jet MR • Vena contracta ≥ 0.7 cm • Regurgitant volume ≥ 60 mL • Regurgitant fraction ≥ 50% • ERO ≥ 0.40 cm² • Angiographic grade 3–4+	• Moderate or severe LA enlargement • LV enlargement • Pulmonary hypertension present	• Decreased exercise tolerance • Exertional dyspnea

*Several valve hemodynamic criteria are provided for assessment of MR severity, but not all criteria for each category will exist in each patient. Categorization of MR severity as mild, moderate, or severe depends on data quality and integration of these parameters in conjunction with other clinical evidence.

ERO, Effective regurgitant orifice; *IE*, infective endocarditis; *LA*, left atrium/atrial; *LV*, left ventricular; *LVEF*, left ventricular ejection fraction; *LVESD*; left ventricular end-systolic dimension; *MR*, mitral regurgitation.

From Nishimura RA, Otto CM, Bonow RO, et al. 2017 AHA/ACC focused update of the 2014 AHA/ACC guideline for the management of patients with valvular heart disease: a report of the American College of Cardiology/American Heart Association Task Force on Clinical Practice Guidelines. J Am Coll Cardiol 2017;70:252-289.

TABLE 15.2 American College of Cardiology/American Heart Association Stages of Secondary MR.

Grade	Definition	Valve Anatomy	Valve Hemodynamics*	Associated Cardiac Findings	Symptoms
A	At risk of MR	• Normal valve leaflets, chords, and annulus in a patient with coronary disease or cardiomyopathy	• No MR jet or small central jet area < 20% LA on Doppler • Small vena contracta < 0.30 cm	• Normal or mildly dilated LV size with fixed (infarction) or inducible (ischemia) regional wall motion abnormalities • Primary myocardial disease with LV dilation and systolic dysfunction	• Symptoms due to coronary ischemia or HF may be present that respond to revascularization and appropriate medical therapy
B	Progressive MR	• Regional wall motion abnormalities with mild tethering of mitral leaflet • Annular dilation with mild loss of central coaptation of the mitral leaflets	• ERO < 0.40 $cm^{2\dagger}$ • Regurgitant volume < 60 mL • Regurgitant fraction < 50%	• Regional wall motion abnormalities with reduced LV systolic function • LV dilation and systolic dysfunction due to primary myocardial disease	• Symptoms due to coronary ischemia or HF may be present that respond to revascularization and appropriate medical therapy
C	Asymptomatic severe MR	• Regional wall motion abnormalities and/or LV dilation with severe tethering of mitral leaflet • Annular dilation with severe loss of central coaptation of the mitral leaflets	• ERO ≥ 0.40 $cm^{2\dagger}$ • Regurgitant volume ≥ 60 mL • Regurgitant fraction ≥ 50%	• Regional wall motion abnormalities with reduced LV systolic function • LV dilation and systolic dysfunction due to primary myocardial disease	• Symptoms due to coronary ischemia or HF may be present that respond to revascularization and appropriate medical therapy
D	Symptomatic severe MR	• Regional wall motion abnormalities and/or LV dilation with severe tethering of mitral leaflet • Annular dilation with severe loss of central coaptation of the mitral leaflets	• ERO ≥ 0.40 $cm^{2\dagger}$ • Regurgitant volume ≥ 60 mL • Regurgitant fraction ≥ 50%	• Regional wall motion abnormalities with reduced LV systolic function • LV dilation and systolic dysfunction due to primary myocardial disease	• HF symptoms due to MR persist even after revascularization and optimization of medical therapy • Decreased exercise tolerance • Exertional dyspnea

*Several valve hemodynamic criteria are provided for assessment of MR severity, but not all criteria for each category will exist in each patient. Categorization of MR severity as mild, moderate, or severe depends on data quality and integration of these parameters in conjunction with other clinical evidence.

†Measurement of the proximal isovelocity surface area by 2D TTE in patients with secondary MR underestimates the true ERO because of the crescentic shape of the proximal convergence.

2D, Two-dimensional; *ERO*, effective regurgitant orifice; *HF*, heart failure; *LA*, left atrium; *LV*, left ventricular; *MR*, mitral regurgitation; *TTE*, transthoracic echocardiogram.

From Nishimura RA, Otto CM, Bonow RO, et al. 2017 AHA/ACC focused update of the 2014 AHA/ACC guideline for the management of patients with valvular heart disease: a report of the American College of Cardiology/American Heart Association Task Force on Clinical Practice Guidelines. J Am Coll Cardiol 2017;70:252-289.

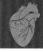

TABLE 15.3 Mitral Valve Apparatus, Cardiac Remodeling, and Jet Characteristics in Primary and Secondary Mitral Regurgitation.

Parameter	Primary MR[a]	SECONDARY MR Regional LV Dysfunction	Global LV Dysfunction
Cause	Myxomatous or calcific leaflet degeneration	Inferior myocardial infarction	Nonischemic cardiomyopathy, large anterior or multiple myocardial infarctions
LV remodeling	Global if severe chronic MR	Primarily inferior wall	Global dilation with increased sphericity
LA remodeling	Moderate to severe if chronic MR	Varies	Usually severe
Annulus	Dilated, preserved dynamic function	Mild to no dilation, less dynamic	Dilated, flattened, nondynamic
Leaflet morphology			
Thickening	Yes/moderate, severe	No/mild	No/mild
Prolapse or flail	Usually present	No	No
Calcification	Varies	No/mild	No/mild
Tethering pattern	None	Asymmetric	Symmetric
Systolic tenting	None	Increased	Markedly increased
Papillary muscle distance	Normal	Increased posterior papillary-intervalvular fibrosa distance	Increased interpapillary muscle distance
MR jet direction	Eccentric or central	Posterior	Usually central
CWD	May be late systolic (if MVP) or uniform if flail or with calcific degeneration	Density usually uniform throughout systole	Biphasic pattern, with increased density in early- and late-systolic flow and midsystolic dropout
PISA	Often hemispheric	Often not hemispheric	Often not hemispheric; may be biphasic

[a]Primary and secondary MR may coexist.
CWD, Continuous-wave Doppler; *LV*, left ventricle; *MR*, mitral regurgitation; *MVP*, mitral valve prolapse; *PISA*, proximal isovelocity surface area.
From Zoghbi WA, Adams D, Bonow RO, et al. Recommendations for noninvasive evaluation of native valvular regurgitation: a report from the American Society of Echocardiography Developed in collaboration with the Society for Cardiovascular Magnetic Resonance. J Am Soc Echocardiogr 2017;30:303-371.

TABLE 15.4 Doppler Echocardiography in Evaluating the Severity of Mitral Regurgitation.

Modality	Optimization	Example	Advantages	Pitfalls
Color-Flow Doppler Proximal flow convergence	Align direction of flow with insonation beam to avoid distortion of hemisphere from noncoaxial imaging Zoomed view Variance off Change baseline of Nyquist limit in the direction of the jet Adjust lower Nyquist limit to obtain the most hemispheric flow convergence (typically 30–40 cm/s) Measure the radius from the point of color aliasing to the VC		Rapid qualitative assessment Absence of proximal flow convergence usually a sign of mild MR	Multiple jets Eccentric jets Constrained jet (LV wall) Nonhemispheric shape, particularly functional MR Overestimation when MR not holosystolic
VCW	Parasternal long-axis view Zoomed view Imaging plane for optimal VC Best measured when proximal flow convergence, VC, and MR jet aligned in same plane		Surrogate for regurgitant orifice size Independent of flow rate and driving pressure for a fixed orifice Can be applied to eccentric jets Depends less on technical factors Good at separating mild (<0.3 cm) from severe MR (≥0.7 cm)	Problematic in the setting of multiple jets Convergence zone needs to be visualized for adequate measurement Overestimation when MR not holosystolic

Continued

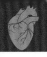

TABLE 15.4   Doppler Echocardiography in Evaluating the Severity of Mitral Regurgitation.—cont'd

Modality	Optimization	Example	Advantages	Pitfalls
Jet area or jet area/LA area ratio	Apical view Zoom view Measure largest jet alone or as ratio to LA area in same view		Easy to measure	Shown to be imprecise in multiple studies, particularly in eccentric, wall-impinging jets Depends on hemodynamic (especially LV systolic pressure) and technical variables Overestimation when MR not holosystolic
3D VCA	Color-flow sector should be as narrow as possible to improve volume rates and line density Align orthogonal cropping planes along the axis of the jet Planimeter the high velocity aliased signal of VC, avoiding low velocity (dark color) signals		Multiple jets of different directions may be measured Can identify severe functional MR in some cases when PISA underestimates EROA (arrow)	Subject to color Doppler blooming Limited temporal and spatial resolution Overestimation when MR not holosystolic Multiple jets may be in different planes, must be analyzed separately and then added Cumbersome; often requires offline analysis
Pulse-Wave Doppler Mitral inflow velocity	Align insonation beam with the flow across the MV at leaflet tips in apical four-chamber view		E velocity ≥ 1.2 m/s is a supportive sign of severe MR (volume load) Dominant A-wave inflow pattern virtually excludes severe MR Can be obtained with TTE and TEE	Depends on LV relaxation and filling pressures High E velocity not specific for severe MR in secondary MR, atrial fibrillation, and mitral inflow stenosis
Pulmonary vein flow pattern	Use small sample volume (3–5 mm) placed 1 cm into the pulmonary vein		Systolic flow reversal in more than one pulmonary vein is specific for severe MR Normal pulmonary vein pattern suggests low LA pressure and non-severe MR	Eccentric MR of mild or moderate severity directed into a pulmonary vein alters flow pattern Systolic blunting is not specific for significant MR (common in secondary MR and present in elevated LA pressure, atrial fibrillation)
Continuous-Wave Doppler Density and contour of regurgitant jet	Align insonation beam with the flow		Simple Density is proportional to the number of red blood cells reflecting the signal Faint or incomplete jet is compatible with mild MR A triangular contour (early MR peak velocity; arrow) denotes a large regurgitant pressure wave and hemodynamic significance	Qualitative Perfectly central jets may appear denser than eccentric jets of higher severity Density is gain dependent A contour with an early peak velocity is not sensitive for severe MR

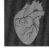

TABLE 15.4 Doppler Echocardiography in Evaluating the Severity of Mitral Regurgitation.—cont'd

Modality	Optimization	Example	Advantages	Pitfalls
Quantitative Doppler: EROA, RVol, and Fraction				
Flow convergence method (PISA) 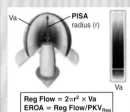	Align insonation beam with the flow, usually in apical views; zoomed view Lower the color Doppler baseline in the direction of the jet Look for the hemispheric shape to guide the best low Nyquist limit Look for need for angle correction if flow convergence zone is nonplanar Measure PISA radius at roughly the same time as CW jet peak velocity	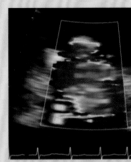 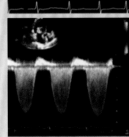	Rapid quantitative assessment of lesion severity (EROA) and volume overload (RVol) Shown to predict outcomes in degenerative and functional MR	May not be accurate in multiple jets Less accurate in eccentric jets or markedly crescent-shaped orifices Small errors in radius measurement can lead to substantial errors in EROA due to squaring of error; this is less likely to misclassify patients at very large ($\geq$1.0 cm) or very small radii ($\leq$0.4 cm)
SV method 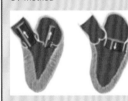 $RVol = SV_{MV} - SV_{LVO}$	LVOT diameter measured at the annulus in systole and pulsed Doppler from apical views at same site Mitral annulus measured at mid-diastole; pulse-wave Doppler at the annulus level in diastole Total LVSV can be measured by pulsed Doppler technique at mitral annulus or by the difference between LV end-diastolic volume and end-systolic volume LV volumes are best measured by 3D; contrast may be needed to better trace endocardial borders; if 3D not feasible, use 2D method of disks	Mitral annulus  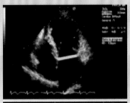 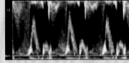 LVOT 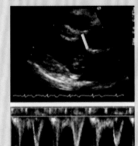	Quantitative, valid with multiple jets and eccentric jets Provides lesion severity (EROA, RF) and volume overload (RVol) Validated against CMR in isolated MR	Not valid for combined MR and AR unless pulmonic site is used Cumbersome, needs training; small errors in each different measurement can combine to magnify error in final results Pulse-wave Doppler method (mitral SV) and LV volume method may give different results

CMR, Cardiac magnetic resonance imaging; *EROA*, effective regurgitant orifice area; *LA*, left atrium/atrial; *LV*, left ventricular/ventricle; *LVOT*, left ventricular outflow tract; *MR*, mitral regurgitation; *MV*, mitral valve; *PISA*, proximal isovelocity surface area method; *RF*, regurgitant fraction; *Rvol*, regurgitant volume; *SV*, stoke volume; *VC*, vena contracta; *VCW*, vena contracta width.

From Zoghbi WA, Adams D, Bonow RO, et al. Recommendations for noninvasive evaluation of native valvular regurgitation: a report from the American Society of Echocardiography developed in collaboration with the Society for Cardiovascular Magnetic Resonance. J Am Soc Echocardiogr 2017;30:303-371.

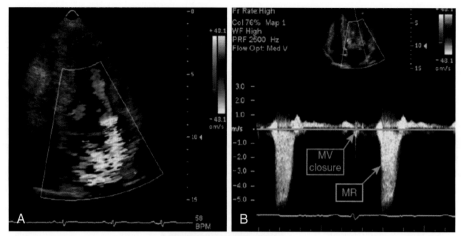

Fig. 15.10 Late Systolic Mitral Regurgitation. A limitation of the proximal isovelocity surface area (PISA) method when mitral regurgitation *(MR)* is not holosystolic is shown here. Despite a large proximal convergence zone (A) with an effective regurgitant orifice area (EROA) of 0.6 cm^2, the CW Doppler (CWD) pattern (B) shows that the regurgitation begins in the second half of systole. This is commonly seen in mitral valve prolapse. The actual regurgitation is less severe than a single frame showing the largest jet, vena contracta, or convergence zone would suggest. When calculating the regurgitant volume, one should multiply EROA by the velocity-time integral (VTI) from the dense part of the CWD signal, not including the faint, early systolic portion of the MR flow, which is relatively mild compared with the later portion. *MV*, Mitral valve.

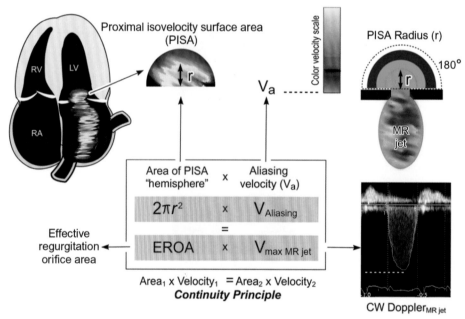

Fig. 15.11 PISA Quantification of Mitral Regurgitant Orifice Area for Mitral Regurgitation. To optimize the proximal isovelocity surface area (PISA) shell, a baseline shift in the direction of the jet is needed. The effective mitral regurgitant orifice area (EROA) is computed as follows: EROA = 2(πr^2)($V_{aliasing}$/V_{MaxMR}). Regurgitant volume = EROA × VTI$_{MR}$, where VTI$_{MR}$ is the velocity-time integral of the MR spectrum. (From Solomon D, Wu JC, Gillam L. Echocardiography. In: Zipes DP, Libby P, Bonow RO, et al, editors. Braunwald's heart disease: a textbook of cardiovascular medicine. 11th ed. Philadelphia: Elsevier; 2018. p. 174-251.)

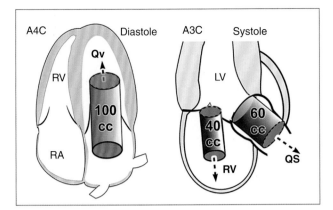

Fig. 15.12 Quantitative Doppler Technique to Assess Mitral Regurgitation Severity. Regurgitant volume is calculated as the difference between total transmitral flow, or Qv, and antegrade flow across the left ventricular outflow tract (LVOT), or Qs. Qv and Qs are determined using the continuity approach (CSA × VTI). Alternatively, Qv, which is identical to LVSV in the absence of a ventricular shunt of significant aortic regurgitation, may be calculated as LVEDV − LVESV. *CSA,* Cross-sectional area; *LVEDV,* left ventricular end-diastolic volume; *LVESV,* left ventricular end-systolic volume; *LVSV,* total volume of blood ejected from the left ventricle; *SV,* stroke volume; *VTI,* velocity-time integral. (From Solomon D, Wu JC, Gillam L. Echocardiography. In: Zipes DP, Libby P, Bonow RO, et al, editors. Braunwald's heart disease: a textbook of cardiovascular medicine. 11th ed. Philadelphia: Elsevier; 2018. p. 174-251.)

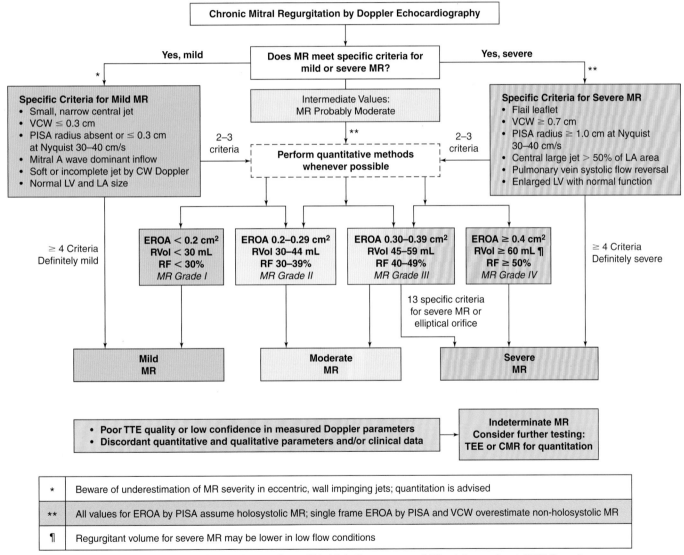

Fig. 15.13 Algorithm for the Integration of Multiple Parameters of Mitral Regurgitant *(MR)* Severity. Good-quality echocardiographic imaging and complete data acquisition are assumed. If imaging is technically difficult, consider TEE or cardiac magnetic resonance imaging *(CMR)*. MR severity may be indeterminate due to poor image quality, technical issues with data, internal inconsistency among echocardiographic findings, or discordance with clinical findings. *CW,* Continuous-wave; *EROA,* effective mitral regurgitant area; *LA,* left atrium; *LV,* left ventricle; *PISA,* proximal isovelocity surface area; *RF,* regurgitant fraction; *RVol,* regurgitant volume; *TTE,* transthoracic echocardiography; *VCW,* vena contracta width. (From Zoghbi WA, Adams D, Bonow RO, et al. Recommendations for noninvasive evaluation of native valvular regurgitation: a report from the American Society of Echocardiography developed in collaboration with the Society for Cardiovascular Magnetic Resonance. J Am Soc Echocardiogr 2017;30:303-371.)

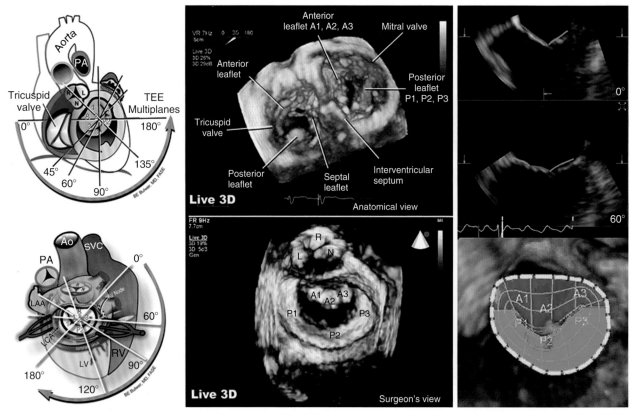

Fig. 15.14 Anatomy of the Mitral Valve From Transesophageal Echocardiography. The panels on the *left* represent the position of the TEE probe and omni plane orientation, sweeping across the entire mitral valve. The middle panels show the mitral valve on a 3D echocardiogram with adjacent cardiac structures *(middle, top)* and leaflet scallops *(middle, bottom)*. The panels on the *right* show 2D still images of the mitral valve leaflets at 0 degrees (i.e., four-chamber view) *(right, top)* and 60 degrees *(right, middle)*. The panel at *bottom right* depicts 3D analysis of the mitral valve. (From Solomon D, Wu JC, Gillam L. Echocardiography. In: Zipes DP, Libby P, Bonow RO, et al, editors. Braunwald's heart disease: a textbook of cardiovascular medicine. 11th ed. Philadelphia: Elsevier; 2018. p. 174-251.)

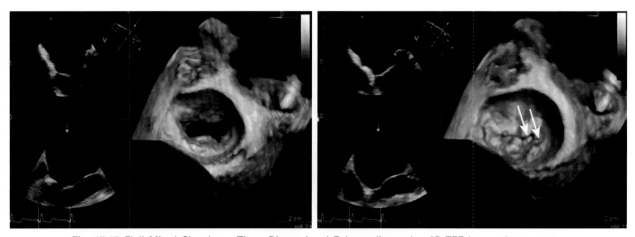

Fig. 15.15 Flail Mitral Chords on Three-Dimensional Echocardiography. 3D TEE image demonstrates pathology of the mitral valve (P2, P3 flail chordae) *(arrows)* as observed during systole *(right)*. The corresponding diastolic image is shown on the *left*.

Jet Origin and Direction

In interrogating the MV, it is important to localize the origin and direction of the regurgitant jet. In patients with myxomatous MV disease, jet direction typically is opposite the affected leaflet. For example, posterior leaflet prolapse results in an anteriorly directed jet, whereas anterior leaflet dysfunction results in a posteriorly directed regurgitation. This rule breaks down in functional MR, for which the typical cause is overriding of a tethered posterior leaflet by the anterior leaflet, which produces a posteriorly directed jet.

Visualizing the exact origin and number of regurgitant jets may impact clinical decision making. The parasternal and apical long-axis views identify pathology of the posterior and anterior leaflets and jet direction, whereas the often-neglected parasternal short-axis and apical two-chamber views can show where along the commissural closure line the dominant jet originates (Fig. 15.16).

Regurgitant Volume

Regurgitant volume (Rvol) is a theoretically simple concept but is challenging to measure in practice. In principle, stroke volume is measured in two places, one that includes the MR (i.e., forward flow across the mitral annulus or total LV stroke volume) and one that does not (i.e., forward flow though the LV outflow tract [if no aortic regurgitation exists] or right-sided stroke volume). However, each of these stroke volumes requires multiple measurements, and any error propagates throughout the calculation, compounded at the end by the need to subtract one large number from another. Nonetheless, this technique may be more helpful for patients who have very eccentric jets and those for whom it is challenging to obtain good vena contracta diameters or PISA measurements.

Vena Contracta

The vena contracta, which is the narrowest cross-sectional area of the regurgitant jet as mapped by color-flow Doppler echocardiography, can predict the severity of MR, but the measurement may suffer from color-blooming artifact and limitation of lateral resolution. The vena contracta diameter ideally should be measured in a parasternal long-axis or short-axis view. Alternatively, the apical views can be used if the parasternal windows are suboptimal.

The diameter (i.e., perpendicular to flow) should be measured at the neck between the flow convergence and the atrial color jet. Consideration should be given to techniques to optimize measurement, such as zoom mode and narrow color Doppler box width.

Proximal Isovelocity Surface Area Method

The proximal isovelocity surface area (PISA) method offers the most practical quantitative method for daily use. It exploits the predictable acceleration of flow leading into the MV, which forms roughly hemispheric isovelocity shells; this can be highlighted by shifting the aliasing velocity of the color display and identified where the color changes from blue to red.

If r is the radial distance from the vena contracta to the contour with velocity v, the flow rate Q will be given by $Q = 2\pi r^2 v$. From this calculation, the effective regurgitant orifice area (EROA) can be obtained by dividing Q by V_{max}, the maximal velocity through the orifice obtained by continuous-wave (CW) Doppler imaging. A handy simplification that works in most cases assumes a driving pressure of approximately 100 mmHg across the regurgitant orifice (leading by the Bernoulli equation to a 5 m/s maximal jet velocity). If the aliasing velocity is set to approximately 40 cm/s, the EROA becomes one half of the square of the PISA radius, or $EROA = r^2/2$.

An approximation to Rvol can be obtained by multiplying the EROA by the velocity-time integral (VTI) of the regurgitant CW signal (Fig. 15.17). The ideal PISA acquisition is taken from the apical four-chamber or long-axis view in a narrow sector width with zoom and with the aliasing velocity set to approximately 40 cm/s.

There are some important caveats for using the PISA equation, the most critical of which involves non-holosystolic jets. Fig. 15.10 shows a very large proximal convergence zone with an EROA of 0.6 cm^2, but CW Doppler demonstrates that this is a case of MVP in which the regurgitation does not begin until the latter half of systole. The regurgitation is much less severe than would be implied by a single frame showing the largest jet, the vena contracta, or the convergence zone.

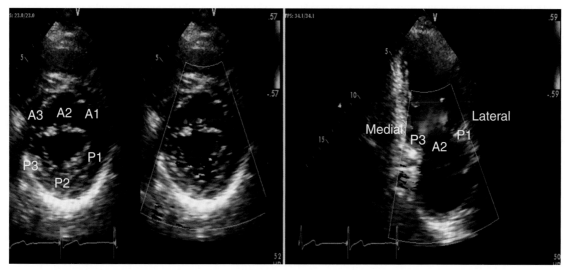

Fig. 15.16 Two-Dimensional Evaluation of Mitral Regurgitant Jet Origin. When examining the origin of mitral regurgitation in two dimensions, it is important to use all available views. The parasternal long-axis and apical long-axis views identify anterior versus posterior jet locations. The often-neglected parasternal short-axis and apical two-chamber views identify regurgitation along the commissural closure line and aid in determining medial versus lateral origination. *A1, A2, A3,* Anterior leaflet segments; *P1, P2, P3,* posterior leaflet segments.

- Assume LV-LA Δp is 100 mmHg
- Set aliasing velocity to (near) 40 cm/sec
- Then ROA = $r^2/2$

ROA = $9^2/2$ = 40 mm^2

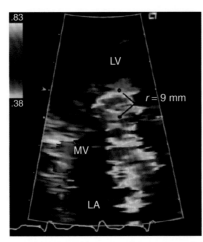

Fig. 15.17 Simplified Approach to Estimating the Regurgitant Orifice Area Using the Proximal Convergence Method. This method assumes that the systolic pressure difference (Δp) between the left ventricle *(LV)* and left atrium *(LA)* is approximately 100 mmHg (producing a 5 m/s regurgitant jet velocity) and sets the color aliasing velocity to approximately 40 cm/s. The radius *(r)* is then measured. The regurgitant orifice area (ROA) calculation can be simplified to the equation $r^2/2$, which has been validated against the complete formula. (From Pu M, Prior DL, Fan X, et al. Calculation of mitral regurgitant orifice area with use of a simplified proximal convergence method: initial clinical application. J Am Soc Echocardiogr 2001;14:180-185.)

When calculating Rvol, the EROA should be multiplied by the VTI from the dense part of the CW signal, not including the faint early systolic portion when regurgitation is mild. Non-holosystolic jets are common in MVP (without flail) and in cases of functional MR in which the MR is most prominent during early systole and isovolumic relaxation, with relatively little regurgitation in mid-systole, when the MV is firmly closed by LV pressure.

Additional pitfalls of the PISA method include slight flow underestimation (on the order of V/V_{max}) as contours flatten approaching the orifice, some overestimation as convergence zones are distorted by surrounding walls (a problem typically confined to already severe MR), and further underestimation when the regurgitant orifice is elongated, as is common in functional MR.

PISA can also be measured with the use of 3D echocardiography. Although the assumption of a hemisphere is integral to the PISA calculation, the observed LV geometry can vary considerably (depending on the cause of the MR) and can include circular, elliptical, and irregular slitlike orifices. Often, this better appreciated by 3D echocardiographic visualization of the PISA flow convergence. 3D PISA is feasible and potentially more accurate than 2D PISA, which can underestimate the severity of MR, especially in eccentric jets with flat convergence zones,[28] and overestimate it in patients with oval-shaped zones. When multiple MR jets exist, a combination of both PISA techniques is often needed to quantify the overall MR.

Supportive Evidence for Mitral Regurgitant Severity

Supportive evidence for MR severity can be found in pulmonary venous flow. A normal pattern, characterized by a systolic (S) wave greater than the diastolic (D) wave, indicates mild MR, and frank systolic reversal indicates severe MR, but the common blunted pattern (S < D) may be seen in all degrees of MR. However, pulmonary venous flow patterns may be abnormal in nonsinus rhythms, even when MR is not severe. A transmitral E wave (i.e., peak mitral inflow velocity during early diastole) greater than 1.2 m/s is supportive evidence of severe MR,

whereas a pattern in which the E wave is less than the A wave (i.e., peak mitral inflow velocity during late diastole at atrial contraction) virtually excludes severe MR.

Doppler echocardiography is an important tool to estimate the pulmonary artery systolic pressure, which typically is significantly elevated in patients with chronic severe MR.

CHALLENGING ISSUES IN EVALUATION OF MITRAL REGURGITATION

Dynamic Changes in Mitral Regurgitation Severity

Because the regurgitant mitral orifice is anatomically in parallel with the aortic valve, the impedance to LV emptying is reduced in patients with MR. MR enhances LV emptying, and a significant proportion of the regurgitant volume is ejected into the LA before the aortic valve opens and after it closes. The volume of MR flow depends on the instantaneous size of the regurgitant orifice and the (reverse) pressure gradient between the LV and LA,[29] both of which are labile and dynamic. LV systolic pressure and therefore the LV-LA gradient depend on systemic vascular resistance, and LA pressure may rise dramatically with severe MR, sometimes reducing the LV-LA gradient to zero by end-systole.

In patients whose mitral annulus has normal flexibility, its cross-sectional area may be altered by many interventions. Increases in preload and afterload and depression of contractility increase LV size and enlarge the mitral annulus, thereby enlarging the regurgitant orifice. When LV size is reduced by treatment with positive inotropic agents, diuretics, and particularly vasodilators, the regurgitant orifice size decreases and the volume of regurgitant flow declines, as reflected in the height of the *v* wave (i.e., LA filling against a closed mitral valve) in the LA pressure pulse and in the intensity and duration of the systolic murmur. Conversely, LV dilation, regardless of cause, may increase MR.

Role of Exercise Echocardiography

Exercise echocardiography can be helpful in determining the severity of MR and hemodynamic abnormalities (e.g., pulmonary hypertension) during exercise.[30–32] This is a useful, objective means to evaluate symptoms in patients who appear to have only mild MR at rest and to determine functional status and dynamic changes in hemodynamics in patients who otherwise appear stable and asymptomatic. Especially helpful is an observation that late-systolic MR becomes more holosystolic with exercise, particularly if the pulmonary artery pressure rises significantly.

When ordering a treadmill exercise echocardiogram, guidance should be provided to the sonographer about the priority for the various data sets to be obtained after exercise because it is often impossible to obtain diagnostic mitral and tricuspid imaging and wall motion assessment while the heart rate is still optimally high. If the focus is on the MV, rapid acquisition of mitral color images, mitral CW Doppler, and tricuspid CW Doppler is usually a priority. Comprehensive imaging can be obtained of all relevant parameters if the exercise is on a supine bicycle. Dobutamine echocardiography has little role in the assessment of organic MR but may be useful for ischemia or viability assessment in functional MR.

Quantitation of Secondary Mitral Regurgitation

For patients with secondary MR, echocardiography is important for identifying the degree of LV dilation and systolic dysfunction and the presence, severity, and mechanisms responsible for the MR.[4,13,33] MR develops as a result of annular dilation and tethering of the leaflets due to geometric displacement or traction of the papillary muscles; this tethering results in restricted leaflet closure with incomplete coaptation during systole, often with concomitant mitral annular dilation as

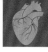

a consequence of an ischemic or nonischemic cardiomyopathy.[13] Most commonly, the posterior leaflet is more severely restricted in closure, allowing the anterior leaflet to override it. This produces a posteriorly directed jet of MR that may arise broadly along the commissural closure line. Because the magnitude of MR can vary widely with loading conditions and ischemia, evaluation with exercise echocardiography can be highly informative.[15]

The clinical stages of secondary MR (see Table 15.3)[34] are based on the same quantitative measurements of MR severity as for primary MR in current guidelines.[24] However, the optimal definitions of severity for secondary MR remain controversial. Numerous studies have shown that secondary MR identifies patients with heart failure who are at higher risk for hemodynamic deterioration and death than those without MR. Even mild degrees of MR that would be well tolerated for decades in patients with primary MR stemming from MVP are associated with increased mortality rates over 3 to 5 years.[12,14]

Because the mechanism of ischemic and nonischemic (or functional) MR is related to the magnitude of LV remodeling, patients with MR usually have lower ejection fractions and higher ESVs than those without MR, and MR of greater severity is associated with more severe LV dysfunction and remodeling. MR is therefore a marker of significant regional or global LV dysfunction. It is less clear whether secondary MR, once established, contributes to progression of LV dysfunction and plays a causative role in the observed worse outcomes or is more a marker for poor outcome even if the MR were not present. Whether secondary MR should be a target for surgical or device intervention remains uncertain (see Chapter 18).

IMAGING THE LEFT VENTRICLE

Pathophysiology

The LV initially compensates for the development of acute MR by emptying more completely and by increasing preload (i.e., according to the Frank-Starling principle). Because acute MR reduces late-systolic LV pressure and radius, LV wall tension declines markedly (and proportionately to a greater extent than LV pressure), permitting a reciprocal increase in the extent and velocity of myocardial fiber shortening, which leads to a reduced ESV (see Chapter 5). When MR, particularly severe MR, becomes chronic, the LV end-diastolic volume (EDV) increases and the ESV returns to normal.

The Laplace principle states that myocardial wall tension is related to the product of intraventricular pressure and radius divided by wall thickness. The increased LV EDV increases wall tension to normal or supranormal levels in the so-called chronic compensated stage of severe MR. As a result, LV EDV and mitral annular diameter increase. A vicious cycle may be created in which MR leads to more MR.

In patients with chronic MR, LV EDV and mass are increased, and typical volume overload (eccentric) hypertrophy develops. However, the degree of hypertrophy is often not proportional to the degree of LV dilation, and the ratio of LV mass to EDV may be less than normal, increasing wall stress. Nonetheless, the reduced afterload permits maintenance of ejection fraction in the normal to supranormal range, giving false reassurance; the effective ejection fraction (i.e., forward stroke volume divided by LV EDV) may be quite depressed and is often unmasked after mitral surgery.[35] The reduced LV afterload allows a greater proportion of the contractile energy of the myocardium to be expended in shortening than in tension development. This explains how the LV can adapt to the load imposed by MR.

The eccentric LV hypertrophy that accompanies the elevated EDV of chronic MR occurs because new sarcomeres are laid down in series.

A shift to the right (i.e., greater volume at any pressure) occurs in the LV diastolic pressure-volume curve in patients with chronic MR. With decompensation, chamber stiffness increases, raising the diastolic pressure at any given volume.

Many patients with severe primary MR maintain compensation for years, but in some patients, the prolonged hemodynamic overload ultimately leads to myocardial decompensation.[29] ESV, preload, and afterload all increase, whereas ejection fraction and stroke volume decline. These patients have evidence of neurohormonal activation and elevation of circulating proinflammatory cytokines. Plasma natriuretic peptide levels also increase in response to the volume load,[36] more so in patients with symptomatic decompensation.

Myocardial ischemia in the absence of coronary disease is rare in patients with primary MR. Coronary flow rates may be increased in patients with severe MR, but the increases in myocardial oxygen consumption (MVo_2) are relatively modest compared with those in patients with aortic stenosis or aortic regurgitation. Myocardial fiber shortening, which is elevated in patients with MR, is not one of the principal determinants of MVo_2. Mean LV wall tension is normal to reduced, whereas the other two determinants of MVo_2, contractility and heart rate, are not affected. The incidence of clinical manifestations of myocardial ischemia is lower among patients with MR and much higher among those with aortic stenosis or aortic regurgitation, conditions in which MVo_2 is greatly augmented.

Assessment of Myocardial Contractility

Because the ejection phase indices of myocardial contractility are inversely correlated with afterload, patients with early MR (i.e., reduced LV afterload) often exhibit elevations in these indices, including ejection fraction, fractional fiber shortening, and velocity of circumferential fiber shortening (VCF).[37] Many patients ultimately develop symptoms because of elevated LA and pulmonary venous pressures related to the regurgitant volume but have no change in ejection phase indices, which remain elevated. In other patients, major symptoms reflect serious contractile dysfunction, by which time ejection fraction, fractional shortening, and mean VCF have declined to low-normal or below-normal levels.

As MR persists, the reduction in afterload, which increases myocardial fiber shortening and ejection phase indices, is opposed by the impairment of myocardial function that is characteristic of severe chronic diastolic overload. However, even in patients with overt heart failure due to MR, the ejection fraction and fractional shortening may be only modestly reduced. Values in the low-normal range for the ejection phase indices of myocardial performance in patients with chronic MR may actually reflect impaired myocardial function, whereas moderately reduced values (e.g., ejection fraction of 40% to 50%) usually signify severe, often irreversible, impairment of contractility, identifying patients who may do poorly after surgical correction of the MR (see Chapter 17). In these patients, parameters of longitudinal shortening, such as global longitudinal strain, may better predict postoperative LV dysfunction than ejection fraction does.[33] An ejection fraction of less than 35% in patients with chronic severe organic MR usually represents advanced myocardial dysfunction, and these patients are at high operative risk and may not experience satisfactory improvement after MV replacement.

End-Systolic Volume

Preoperative myocardial contractility is an important determinant of the risk of operative death, perioperative cardiac failure, and postoperative LV function. It is not therefore surprising that the end-systolic pressure-volume (or stress-dimension) relationship has emerged as a useful index for evaluating LV function in patients with MR.

The measurement of ESV or end-systolic diameter (ESD) is a predictor of function and survival after MV surgery.[21,29] A preoperative LV ESD that exceeds 40 mm identifies a patient with a high likelihood of impaired LV systolic function after surgery.[25] Global longitudinal strain magnitude less than 19.3% (i.e., a normal value in the absence of severe MR) is more strongly predictive of postoperative LV dysfunction than traditional parameters such as ejection fraction and ESD.[37]

Left Atrial Compliance

Compliance of the LA and pulmonary venous bed is an important determinant of the hemodynamic and clinical picture in patients with severe MR. Three major subgroups of patients with severe MR based on LA compliance have been identified, and they correlate commonly with the chronicity of severe regurgitation.

When severe MR develops acutely (e.g., with rupture of the chordae tendineae, infarction of one of the heads of a papillary muscle, leaflet disruption from trauma or endocarditis), the LA is initially normal in size and compliance. The pressure-volume relationship of the relaxed atrium is curvilinear, and the sudden volume load from the MR forces it to operate on a steeper portion of that curve, with an exaggerated rise in pressure (*v* wave) for a given regurgitant volume. This marked elevation of mean LA pressure leads to pulmonary congestion as a prominent symptom. Sinus rhythm usually is present, at least initially.

Over time, the LA dilates, and its wall becomes hypertrophied to maintain contractile function. Chamber dilation shifts the pressure-volume curve to the right, increasing compliance at a given volume, whereas hypertrophy has the opposite effect, shifting the curve upward. The balance of these two remodeling processes determines the overall impact on mean LA pressure and the *v* wave.

As severe MR becomes chronic, dilation predominates, and the *v* wave may fall, leading to an increase in operating compliance. If symptoms are tolerated or nonexistent, this stage may last years with progressive LA enlargement, which increases the risk of atrial fibrillation. At the extremes, patients may present with massive atrial enlargement and markedly increased compliance but relatively modest LA pressure elevation. Atrial fibrillation is likely, and the atrial wall may largely be replaced by fibrous tissue.

EVALUATION OF MITRAL REGURGITATION IN PATIENTS UNDERGOING TRANSCATHETER INTERVENTIONS

Preprocedural Evaluation

The advent of transcatheter therapies (i.e., edge-to-edge repair) has revolutionized the treatment of primary MR, particularly in cases of MVP or flail chordae. This technology was evaluated in patients with functional MR in the MITRA-FR and COAPT trials.[38,39] Although the MITRA-FR trial showed no difference in clinical outcomes for patients treated with transcatheter MV repair versus medical therapy, the COAPT study demonstrated lower risks of death and hospitalization due to heart failure among patients who underwent transcatheter repair. A closer examination of the study populations revealed a new framework to understand functional MR.[40] When the LV progressively dilates, the degree of resultant MR due to malcoaptation of the MV leaflets may be proportionate to the LV EDV, as in MITRA-FR patients, or disproportionate (i.e., more severe), as in COAPT.

Perhaps not surprisingly, therapies to modify the MV (i.e., edge-to-edge repair) may not be as clinically beneficial in patients with severe MR who have proportionate LV dilation compared with those in whom the degree of LV dilation is disproportionate. Care should be taken to properly measure volumes through use of contrast with 2D echocardiography or, when available, through 3D echocardiography.[41]

Postprocedural Evaluation

Assessment of residual MR after percutaneous intervention is challenging. Although in many ways the echocardiographic evaluation is similar for native valve MR and surgical prosthetic MR, special considerations are given to patients treated with transcatheter options. There are four broad categories of transcatheter MV therapies: leaflet repair (i.e., edge-to-edge repair, artificial chord placement), transcatheter mitral valve replacement (TMVR), mitral annuloplasty devices, and paravalvular leak closure.[41]

Because most transcatheter MV therapies involve image guidance, the first evaluation of residual MR is made immediately after the procedure, using TEE. Accurate evaluation of residual MR is obtained based on general echocardiographic findings, color Doppler information, spectral Doppler information, quantitative parameters, and invasive hemodynamics (Fig. 15.18; Table 15.5).

A postprocedural decline in LV ejection fraction often reflects the hemodynamic changes that result in LV afterload mismatch after significant reduction in MR (in the absence of other causes). The appearance of spontaneous contrast in the LA or left atrial appendage often signifies improvement in MR. These two general echocardiographic findings are often immediately obvious after MR intervention.

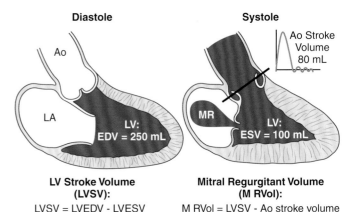

LV Stroke Volume (LVSV):
LVSV = LVEDV - LVESV
LVSV = 250 mL - 100 mL
LVSV = 150 mL

Mitral Regurgitant Volume (M RVol):
M RVol = LVSV - Ao stroke volume
M RVol = 150 mL - 80 mL
M RVol = 70 mL

Fig. 15.18 Use of the Cardiac Magnetic Resonance Imaging Method for Quantification of Magnetic Resonance (MR). The volume of the left ventricle (LV) is calculated during end-diastole (EDV) and during end-systole (ESV) by summation of the volume (area × thickness) of each short-axis slice. The total volume of blood ejected from the LV (LVSV) is computed as the difference between LVEDV and LVESV. In this example, LVSV is 150 mL. The volume of blood crossing the aortic valve is measured by a phase-contrast acquisition in the aorta (Ao); in this example, it is 80 mL. The mitral regurgitant volume (M RVol) is computed as the difference between LVSV and Ao forward stroke volume; in this example, it is 70 mL. (From Zoghbi WA, Adams D, Bonow RO, et al. Recommendations for noninvasive evaluation of native valvular regurgitation: a report from the American Society of Echocardiography developed in collaboration with the Society for Cardiovascular Magnetic Resonance. J Am Soc Echocardiogr 2017;30: 303-371.)

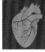

TABLE 15.5   Hemodynamics and TEE Parameters for Determining Residual Mitral Regurgitation Severity During Mitral Valve Interventions in the Catheterization Laboratory.

Method	Assessing Severity of Residual MR
Invasive hemodynamics	Decrease in regurgitant *v* wave, LA pressure, and pulmonary pressures are specific signs of reduction in MR severity; consider effects of general anesthesia on MR severity
General Echocardiographic Findings	
Spontaneous echo contrast in LA	Appearance of spontaneous contrast after MV intervention suggests significant reduction in MR severity
LVEF	Decline in LVEF after MV intervention suggests significant MR reduction in the absence of other causes (ischemia, pacemaker-related, etc.)
Color Doppler	
Color Doppler jet (size, number, location, eccentricity)	Easy to obtain with a comprehensive, systematic approach Difficult to assess multiple and eccentric jets Jet area affected by eccentricity, technical and hemodynamic factors (especially driving velocity)
Flow convergence	Large flow convergence denotes significant residual MR whereas a small or no flow convergence suggests mild MR Difficult to use in presence of multiple jets or very eccentric jets, or may be masked by the device
Vena contracta width	VCW ≥ 0.7 cm specific for severe MR Difficult to use in presence of multiple small jets or very eccentric jets for which orifice shape is not well delineated
Vena contracta area (3D planimetry)	Allows better delineation of eccentric orifice shape and possibly the addition of VCA of multiple jets Prone to blooming artifacts
Spectral Doppler	
Pulmonary vein flow pattern	Systolic flow reversal in >1 vein specific for severe MR Increase in forward systolic velocity after MV intervention helps confirm MR reduction
MR jet profile by CWD (contour, density, peak velocity)	Dense, triangular pattern suggests severe MR May be hard to line up CWD properly in flail leaflet or very eccentric jet after intervention
Mitral inflow pattern	In sinus rhythm, mitral A wave–dominant flow excludes severe MR Decrease in mitral E velocity and VTI suggests reduction in MR severity
Pulsed Doppler of LVOT (deep transgastric view)	Increase in LVOT velocity and VTI after procedure suggests MR reduction
Quantitative Parameters[a]	
EROA by PISA	Not recommended after edge-to-edge repair because assumption of hemispheric proximal flow convergence is violated by the device PISA often underestimates MR severity in the setting of multiple jets or markedly eccentric jets Not feasible in PVR of mechanical prosthetic MV or possibly TMVR (flow masking in LV by TEE)
Regurgitant volume	Difficult to perform volumetric RVol with pulsed Doppler by TEE

[a]In general, more difficult to perform; some procedure-specific limitations in quantitation.

CWD, Continuous-wave Doppler; *EROA*, effective regurgitant orifice area; *LA*, left atrium; *LVEF*, left ventricular ejection fraction; *LVOT*, left ventricular outflow tract; *MR*, mitral regurgitation; *MV*, mitral valve; *PISA*, proximal isovelocity surface area; *PVR*, paravalvular regurgitation; *TEE*, transesophageal echocardiography; *TMVR*, transcatheter mitral valve replacement; *VCA*, vena contracta area; *VCW*, vena contracta width; *VTI*, velocity-time integral.

From Zoghbi WA, Asch FM, Bruce C, et al. Guidelines for the evaluation of valvular regurgitation after percutaneous valve repair or replacement: a report from the American Society of Echocardiography Developed in collaboration with the Society for Cardiovascular Angiography and Interventions, Japanese Society of Echocardiography, and Society for Cardiovascular Magnetic Resonance. J Am Soc Echocardiogr 2019;32:431-475.

Color Doppler imaging provides critical insight into the evaluation of residual MR after transcatheter intervention. The residual color jets (i.e., number, size, location, and eccentricity) provide for visual inspection of the MR before and after intervention. Measurement of flow convergence zones, vena contracta width (2D), and vena contracta area (3D) also provides semiquantitative parameters to assess residual MR severity. Because acoustic shadowing from the specific

transcatheter intervention performed can lead to inaccurate assessment of MR, special care must be given to fully interrogate the MR using multiple conventional TEE angles (on and off axis) in addition to 3D echocardiography.

Spectral Doppler parameters are useful for determining the amount of residual MR. Specific indices reflecting improvement in MR include change in the pulmonary venous flow pattern (i.e., transition from

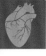
flow reversal or blunted systolic flow to systolic dominant flow), the MR jet profile (i.e., decreased density of jet with loss of triangular shape), presence of A-wave dominance, decrease in E velocity, and increase in LV outflow tract velocity.

Quantitative parameters such as PISA and regurgitant volumes are also useful after transcatheter MV intervention. These measurements must be performed with caution because the specific assumptions of the PISA formula may be violated after certain interventions (e.g., edge-to-edge repair).

OTHER IMAGING APPROACHES

Cardiac Magnetic Resonance

CMR provides accurate measurements of regurgitant flow that correlate well with quantitative Doppler imaging.[42] It also is the most accurate noninvasive technique for measuring LV EDV, LV ESV, and mass[43] and has been included in guidelines for imaging in valvular regurgitation[24] (Fig. 15.19). Although detailed visualization of MV structure and function is obtained more reliably with echocardiography, particularly TEE, CMR offers a promising approach for more accurate assessment of regurgitant severity and its impact on chamber size.[44,45] For patients with secondary MR, CMR is useful in assessing the severity of LV remodeling and contractile dysfunction and in evaluating the pattern of myocardial fibrosis as it relates to regional dysfunction and papillary muscle dysfunction.[24,46]

Cardiac Computed Tomography

Cardiac CT imaging can provide useful structural information about the regurgitant MV[47–50] and is particularly valuable in sizing the mitral annulus and quantifying the degree of annular calcification.[51] It appears to be especially useful in planning for percutaneous MV replacement[52] and

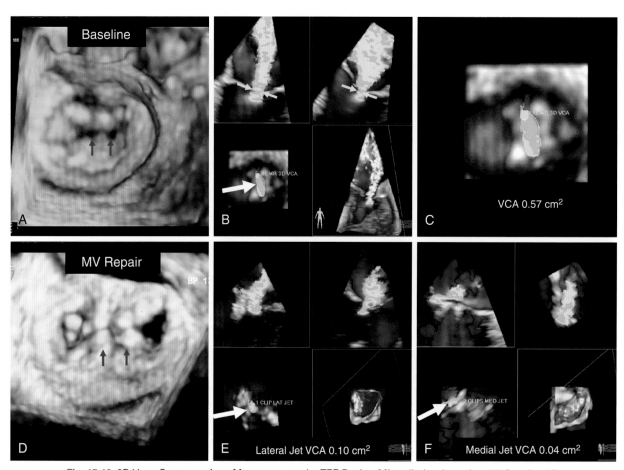

Fig. 15.19 3D Vena Contracta Area Measurements by TEE During Mitraclip Implantation. (A) Baseline 3D *en face* view from the left atrium. Both leaflets were restricted with coaptation defects *(arrows)*. (B) 3D quad images show vena contracta width *(yellow arrows)* that is wider in the bicommissural view *(top left)* than in the long-axis view *(top right)*. (C) The elliptical 3D vena contracta area *(VCA), bottom left,* is shown in a magnified view; it measures 0.57 cm². (D) 3D *en face* view from the left atrium after placement of two MitraClips *(arrows)*. (E) 3D vena contracta measurements after placement of two MitraClips orienting the cut planes to the lateral jet *(arrow)* with a VCA of 0.10 cm². (F) 3D vena contracta measurements orienting the cut planes to the medial jet *(arrow)* with a VCA of 0.04 cm². The combined VCA is 0.14 cm², consistent with mild mitral regurgitation. *MV,* Mitral valve. (From Zoghbi WA, Asch FM, Bruce C, et al. Guidelines for the evaluation of valvular regurgitation after percutaneous valve repair or replacement: a report from the American Society of Echocardiography developed in collaboration with the Society for Cardiovascular Angiography and Interventions, Japanese Society of Echocardiography, and Society for Cardiovascular Magnetic Resonance. J Am Soc Echocardiogr 2019;32:431-475.)

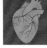

has been used in conjunction with 3D printing to ensure an adequate fit of the valve within the mitral apparatus.[53,54] Some have proposed CT imaging for quantification of the actual regurgitant severity, specifically the planimetered size of the EROA, but this approach will likely remain adjunctive given the availability of echocardiography and CMR.[55]

Left Ventricular Angiography

Because echocardiography and CMR are readily available, there is little reason to perform left ventriculography for the purpose of characterizing MR. The prompt appearance of contrast material in the LA after its injection into the LV indicates MR. The injection should be rapid enough to permit LV opacification but slow enough to avoid the development of premature ventricular contractions, which can induce spurious regurgitation.

The regurgitant volume can be determined from the difference between the total LV stroke volume, estimated by angiocardiography, and the effective forward stroke volume measured simultaneously by the Fick method. In patients with severe MR, the regurgitant volume may approach, or even exceed, the effective forward stroke volume. Qualitative but clinically useful estimates of the severity of MR may be made by cineangiographic observation of the degree of opacification of the LA and pulmonary veins after injection of contrast material into the LV.

REFERENCES

1. Drake DH, Zimmerman KG, Sidebotham DA. Transesophageal echocardiography for surgical repair of mitral regurgitation. In: Otto CM, ed. The practice of clinical echocardiography. 5th ed. Philadelphia: Elsevier; 2017. p. 343-373.
2. Adams DH, Rosenhek R, Falk V. Degenerative mitral valve regurgitation: best practice revolution. Eur Heart J 2010;31(16):1958-1966.
3. Cosyns B, Droogmans S, Rosenhek R, Lancellotti P. Drug-induced valvular heart disease. Heart 2013;99(1):7-12.
4. Tsang W, Freed BH, Lang RM. Three-dimensional anatomy of the aortic and mitral valves. In: Otto CM, Bonow RO, eds. Valvular heart disease: a companion to Braunwald's heart disease. 4th ed. Philadelphia: Saunders; 2013. p. 14-29.
5. Nordrum IS, Skallerud B. Smooth muscle in the human mitral valve: extent and implications for dynamic modelling. APMIS 2012;120(6):484-494.
6. Kilic A, Schwartzman DS, Subramaniam K, Zenati MA. Severe functional mitral regurgitation arising from isolated annular dilatation. Ann Thorac Surg 2010;90(4):1343-1345.
7. Gertz ZM, Raina A, Saghy L, et al. Evidence of atrial functional mitral regurgitation due to atrial fibrillation. J Am Coll Cardiol 2011;58(14):1474-1481.
8. Grewal J, Suri R, Mankad S, et al. Mitral annular dynamics in myxomatous valve disease: new insights with real-time 3-dimensional echocardiography. Circulation 2010;121(12):1423-1431.
9. Little SH, Ben Zekry S, Lawrie GM, Zoghbi WA. Dynamic annular geometry and function in patients with mitral regurgitation: insight from three-dimensional annular tracking. J Am Soc Echocardiogr 2010;23(8):872-879.
10. Solomon D, Wu JC, Gillam L. Echocardiography. In: Zipes DP, Libby P, Bonow RO, et al, eds. Braunwald's heart disease: a textbook of cardiovascular medicine. 11th ed. Philadelphia: Elsevier; 2018. p. 174-251.
11. Bhatia N, Richardson TD, Coffin ST, Keebler ME. Acute mitral regurgitation after removal of an impella device. Am J Cardiol 2017;119(8):1290-1291.
12. Deja MA, Grayburn PA, Sun B, et al. Influence of mitral regurgitation repair on survival in the surgical treatment for ischemic heart failure trial. Circulation 2012;125(21):2639-2648.
13. Foster E, Rao RK. Secondary mitral regurgitation. In: Otto CM, Bonow RO, eds. Valvular heart disease: a companion to Braunwald's heart disease. 4th ed. Philadelphia: Saunders; 2013. p. 295-309.
14. Rossi A, Dini FL, Faggiano P, et al. Independent prognostic value of functional mitral regurgitation in patients with heart failure. A quantitative analysis of 1256 patients with ischaemic and non-ischaemic dilated cardiomyopathy. Heart 2011;97(20):1675-1680.
15. Bertrand PB, Schwammenthal E, Levine RA, Vandervoort PM. Exercise dynamics in secondary mitral regurgitation: pathophysiology and therapeutic implications. Circulation 2017;135(3):297-314.
16. Bouma W, Wijdh-den Hamer IJ, Koene BM, et al. Long-term survival after mitral valve surgery for post-myocardial infarction papillary muscle rupture. J Cardiothorac Surg 2015;10:11.
17. Bouma W, Wijdh-den Hamer IJ, Koene BM, et al. Predictors of in-hospital mortality after mitral valve surgery for post-myocardial infarction papillary muscle rupture. J Cardiothorac Surg 2014;9:171.
18. Wolff R, Cohen G, Peterson C, et al. MitraClip for papillary muscle rupture in patient with cardiogenic shock. Can J Cardiol 2014;30(11):1461.e1413-1464.
19. Otto CM. Echocardiographic evaluation of valvular heart disease. In: Otto CM, Bonow RO, eds. Valvular heart disease: a companion to Braunwald's heart disease. 4th ed. Philadelphia: Saunders; 2013. p. 62-85.
20. Grayburn PA, Weissman NJ, Zamorano JL. Quantitation of mitral regurgitation. Circulation 2012;126(16):2005-2017.
21. Hung J. Mitral valve anatomy, quantification of mitral regurgitation, and timing of surgical intervention for mitral regurgitation. In: Otto CM, ed. The clinical practice of echocardiography. 4th ed. Philadelphia: Saunders; 2012. p. 330-350.
22. Thavendiranathan P, Phelan D, Collier P, et al. Quantitative assessment of mitral regurgitation: how best to do it. JACC Cardiovasc Imaging 2012;5(11):1161-1175.
23. Thavendiranathan P, Phelan D, Thomas JD, et al. Quantitative assessment of mitral regurgitation: validation of new methods. J Am Coll Cardiol 2012;60(16):1470-1483.
24. Zoghbi WA, Adams D, Bonow RO, et al. Recommendations for Noninvasive Evaluation of Native Valvular Regurgitation: A Report from the American Society of Echocardiography Developed in Collaboration with the Society for Cardiovascular Magnetic Resonance. J Am Soc Echocardiogr 2017;30(4):303-371.
25. Nishimura RA, Otto CM, Bonow RO, et al. 2014 AHA/ACC guideline for the management of patients with valvular heart disease: executive summary: a report of the American College of Cardiology/American Heart Association Task Force on Practice Guidelines. J Am Coll Cardiol 2014;63(22):2438-2488.
26. Lancellotti P, Moura L, Pierard LA, et al. European Association of Echocardiography recommendations for the assessment of valvular regurgitation. Part 2: mitral and tricuspid regurgitation (native valve disease). Eur J Echocardiogr 2010;11(4):307-332.
27. Tsang W, Lang RM. Three-dimensional echocardiography is essential for intraoperative assessment of mitral regurgitation. Circulation 2013;128(6):643-652.
28. Choi J, Heo R, Hong GR, et al. Differential effect of 3-dimensional color Doppler echocardiography for the quantification of mitral regurgitation according to the severity and characteristics. Circ Cardiovasc Imaging 2014;7(3):535-544.
29. Nishimura RA, Schaff HV. Mitral regurgitation: timing of surgery. In: Otto CM, Bonow RO, eds. Valvular heart disease: a companion to Braunwald's heart disease. 4th ed. Philadelphia: Saunders; 2013. p. 310-325.
30. Lancellotti P, Magne J. Stress testing for the evaluation of patients with mitral regurgitation. Curr Opin Cardiol 2012;27(5):492-498.
31. Magne J, Lancellotti P, Pierard LA. Stress echocardiography and mitral valvular heart disease. Cardiol Clin 2013;31(2):311-321.
32. Rosenhek R, Maurer G. Management of valvular mitral regurgitation: the importance of risk stratification. J Cardiol 2010;56(3):255-261.
33. Hung JW. Ischemic (functional) mitral regurgitation. Cardiol Clin 2013;31(2):231-236.
34. Nishimura RA, Otto CM, Bonow RO, et al. 2017 AHA/ACC Focused Update of the 2014 AHA/ACC Guideline for the Management of Patients With Valvular Heart Disease: A Report of the American College of Cardiology/American Heart Association Task Force on Clinical Practice Guidelines. J Am Coll Cardiol 2017;70(2):252-289.
35. Witkowski TG, Thomas JD, Debonnaire PJ, et al. Global longitudinal strain predicts left ventricular dysfunction after mitral valve repair. Eur Heart J Cardiovasc Imaging 2013;14(1):69-76.

36. Magne J, Mahjoub H, Pierard LA, et al. Prognostic importance of brain natriuretic peptide and left ventricular longitudinal function in asymptomatic degenerative mitral regurgitation. Heart 2012;98(7):584-591.

37. Witkowski TG, Thomas JD, Delgado V, et al. Changes in left ventricular function after mitral valve repair for severe organic mitral regurgitation. Ann Thorac Surg 2012;93(3):754-760.

38. Obadia JF, Messika-Zeitoun D, Leurent G, et al. Percutaneous repair or medical treatment for secondary mitral regurgitation. N Engl J Med 2018;379(24):2297-2306.

39. Stone GW, Lindenfeld J, Abraham WT, et al. Transcatheter mitral-valve repair in patients with heart failure. N Engl J Med 2018;379(24):2307-2318.

40. Grayburn PA, Sannino A, Packer M. Proportionate and disproportionate functional mitral regurgitation: a new conceptual framework that reconciles the results of the MITRA-FR and COAPT trials. JACC Cardiovasc Imaging 2019;12(2):353-362.

41. Zoghbi WA, Asch FM, Bruce C, et al. Guidelines for the evaluation of valvular regurgitation after percutaneous valve repair or replacement: a report from the american society of echocardiography developed in collaboration with the society for cardiovascular angiography and interventions, japanese society of echocardiography, and society for cardiovascular magnetic resonance. J Am Soc Echocardiogr 2019;32(4):431-475.

42. Cawley PJ, Hamilton-Craig C, Owens DS, et al. Prospective comparison of valve regurgitation quantitation by cardiac magnetic resonance imaging and transthoracic echocardiography. Circ Cardiovasc Imaging 2012;6(1):48-57.

43. Schiros CG, Dell'Italia LJ, Gladden JD, et al. Magnetic resonance imaging with 3-dimensional analysis of left ventricular remodeling in isolated mitral regurgitation: implications beyond dimensions. Circulation 2012;125(19):2334-2342.

44. Myerson SG, Francis JM, Neubauer S. Direct and indirect quantification of mitral regurgitation with cardiovascular magnetic resonance, and the effect of heart rate variability. MAGMA 2010;23(4):243-249.

45. Uretsky S, Gillam L, Lang R, et al. Discordance between echocardiography and MRI in the assessment of mitral regurgitation severity: a prospective multicenter trial. J Am Coll Cardiol 2015;65(11):1078-1088.

46. Chinitz JS, Chen D, Goyal P, et al. Mitral apparatus assessment by delayed enhancement CMR: relative impact of infarct distribution on mitral regurgitation. JACC Cardiovasc Imaging 2013;6(2):220-234.

47. Naoum C, Blanke P, Cavalcante JL, Leipsic J. Cardiac computed tomography and magnetic resonance imaging in the evaluation of mitral and tricuspid valve disease: implications for transcatheter interventions. Circ Cardiovasc Imaging 2017;10(3).

48. Koo HJ, Yang DH, Oh SY, et al. Demonstration of mitral valve prolapse with CT for planning of mitral valve repair. Radiographics 2014;34(6):1537-1552.

49. van Rosendael PJ, Katsanos S, Kamperidis V, et al. New insights on Carpentier I mitral regurgitation from multidetector row computed tomography. Am J Cardiol 2014;114(5):763-768.

50. Pontone G, Andreini D, Bertella E, et al. Pre-operative CT coronary angiography in patients with mitral valve prolapse referred for surgical repair: comparison of accuracy, radiation dose and cost versus invasive coronary angiography. Int J Cardiol 2013;167(6):2889-2894.

51. Mak GJ, Blanke P, Ong K, et al. Three-dimensional echocardiography compared with computed tomography to determine mitral annulus size before transcatheter mitral valve implantation. Circ Cardiovasc Imaging 2016;9(6).

52. Blanke P, Dvir D, Cheung A, et al. Mitral annular evaluation with CT in the context of transcatheter mitral valve replacement. JACC Cardiovasc Imaging 2015;8(5):612-615.

53. Vukicevic M, Mosadegh B, Min JK, Little SH. Cardiac 3D printing and its future directions. JACC Cardiovasc Imaging 2017;10(2):171-184.

54. Vukicevic M, Puperi DS, Jane Grande-Allen K, Little SH. 3D printed modeling of the mitral valve for catheter-based structural interventions. Ann Biomed Eng 2017;45(2):508-519.

55. Arnous S, Killeen RP, Martos R, et al. Quantification of mitral regurgitation on cardiac computed tomography: comparison with qualitative and quantitative echocardiographic parameters. J Comput Assist Tomogr 2011;35(5):625-630.

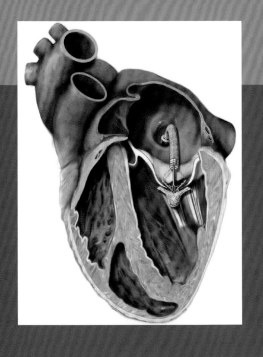

第16章
风湿性和钙化性
二尖瓣狭窄与二尖瓣分离术

尽管风湿性心脏病的发病率有所下降，但二尖瓣狭窄仍普遍存在，尤其在发展中国家非常常见且未得到充分诊断。

风湿性二尖瓣狭窄的主要机制是二尖瓣瓣膜连合部融合，评估风湿性二尖瓣狭窄的主要目的为明确干预的最佳时机和最佳方案——球囊二尖瓣分离术或外科手术。关于球囊二尖瓣分离术的大型长期随访系列报道提升了该干预决策的证据等级，其也与目前指南一致。二维超声心动图平面测量可获得风湿性二尖瓣狭窄患者二尖瓣面积，当二尖瓣瓣口面积<1.5 cm²时，对有症状患者应予以干预；无症状患者可考虑行球囊二尖瓣分离术，尤其是存在血栓栓塞高风险的患者。

钙化性二尖瓣狭窄是二尖瓣瓣环广泛钙化的结果，其患病率随年龄增长而显著增加。在钙化性二尖瓣狭窄患者中，决策时必须考虑手术难度和老年患者存在的高风险特征。经导管二尖瓣置换术为选定患者提供了一种外科开胸手术的替代方法，但因其手术操作复杂且与患者死亡率升高相关，并且缺乏长期的研究结果作为证据支持，需谨慎评估和使用。

本章详细介绍了风湿性和钙化性二尖瓣狭窄的评估及治疗策略，重点介绍了二尖瓣分离术的选择策略、并发症及预后等内容，相信读者一定能从中学有所得。

段振娅

Rheumatic and Calcific Mitral Stenosis and Mitral Commissurotomy

Bernard Iung, Alec Vahanian

CHAPTER OUTLINE

KEY POINTS

- Although the incidence of rheumatic heart diseases has decreased, mitral stenosis (MS) remains prevalent in developed countries. It is common and underdiagnosed in developing countries.
- Calcific MS is the consequence of extensive mitral annular calcification, the prevalence of which increases markedly with age.
- Clinical assessment is paramount to detect MS in asymptomatic patients and to evaluate symptoms.
- Planimetry using bidimensional echocardiography is the reference measurement for the mitral valve area (MVA) in patients with rheumatic MS.
- Intervention is needed in symptomatic patients who have rheumatic MS with an MVA smaller than 1.5 cm^2.

- Balloon mitral commissurotomy (BMC) can be considered for selected asymptomatic patients who have rheumatic MS with an MVA of less than 1.5 cm^2, particularly those who have a high risk of thromboembolism.
- The choice between BMC and surgery should be individualized and based on valve anatomy and other clinical and echocardiographic characteristics.
- Decision making for interventions is difficult for calcific MS because of the technical difficulties of surgery and the frequently high-risk profile of patients. Transcatheter mitral valve replacement may be an alternative for selected patients, but it carries significant early morbidity and mortality, and long-term results are lacking.

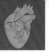

Mitral stenosis (MS) remains prevalent despite the decreased incidence of rheumatic heart disease. The main purpose of investigation of rheumatic MS is to determine the optimal timing of intervention and the most appropriate treatment: balloon mitral commissurotomy (BMC) or surgery. Large series reporting long-term follow-up after BMC have improved the level of evidence for interventional decision making, as attested by contemporary guidelines.

In patients with calcific mitral stenosis, decision making must also consider the technical difficulties of surgery and the frequently high-risk profile of elderly patients. Transcatheter mitral valve replacement offers an alternative for selected patients, but it carries significant early morbidity and mortality, and long-term results are lacking.

EPIDEMIOLOGY

MS is the least common left-sided native valve disease in developed countries, accounting for 9% of single, moderate or severe native valve diseases in Europe in 2001.[1] The overall prevalence of MS, without assessment of cause, was estimated at 0.1% in the only large population-based study on valvular diseases comprising systematic echocardiographic examinations.[2] Unlike other valvular diseases, the most frequent cause of MS remains rheumatic heart disease, which is now rare in developed countries.

Calcific MS is the consequence of mitral annular calcification (MAC) extending to the leaflets. MAC is diagnosed by cardiac computed tomography (CT) in approximately 10% of unselected patients. Its prevalence increases with age and is greater than 25% after the age of 75 years (MESA study).[3] In the Euro Heart Survey, the percentage of calcific causes increased progressively with age.[1] MAC is favored by cardiovascular risk factors and reduced renal function.[3,4] Although MAC is common, it seldom causes significant hemodynamic impairment. Mitral regurgitation (MR) is more common than MS, which is encountered in less than 10% of patients with MAC.[5,6]

In developing countries, the estimated prevalence of rheumatic heart disease is between 1 and 10 cases per 1000 of school-age children according to clinical screening and between 20 and 30 cases per 1000 of school-age children by systematic echocardiographic screening.[7–9] Most valvular disease is of rheumatic origin and involves mainly young adults (mean age, 30–40 years).[10,11] Pure MS accounts for 5% to 10% of valvular disease in patients between 20 and 50 years of age, and MS with MR accounts for 20% to 30%.[11]

Intermediate patterns are observed in emerging countries. In a 2009 Turkish survey, rheumatic heart disease accounted for 46% of all valve diseases, followed by calcific causes in 29%.[12]

PATHOPHYSIOLOGY

Mechanisms of Valve Obstruction

The main mechanism of rheumatic MS is commissural fusion (Fig. 16.1). Posterior leaflet thickening and restriction are almost constant features. Thickening and rigidity of the anterior leaflet or subvalvular apparatus can also contribute to stenosis.[13] Commissural fusion explains why the area of the mitral orifice is relatively constant in severe MS, whereas it may vary according to flow conditions after the commissures have been opened by BMC.[14]

Degenerative MAC results from an active remodeling process favored by cardiovascular risk factors, increased mitral valve stress, and disorders of calcium-phosphorus metabolism.[4,6] It is frequently associated with atherosclerosis and calcific aortic stenosis.[6,15] The main mechanism of calcific MS is reduced anterior leaflet mobility due to rigidity without commissural fusion.[6,16]

Other causes are rare. Congenital MS is mainly the consequence of abnormalities of the subvalvular apparatus. Inflammatory diseases (e.g., systemic lupus), infiltrative diseases, carcinoid heart disease, and drug-induced valve diseases are characterized by a predominance of leaflet thickening and restriction, but commissures are seldom fused.

Hemodynamic Consequences of Mitral Stenosis
Mitral Gradient
The increase in diastolic mitral pressure gradient depends on the mitral valve area (MVA) and on other factors such as transvalvular flow and heart rate. Severe MS may therefore be associated with a low gradient in patients with low cardiac output, particularly those who have chronic atrial fibrillation (AF).

Left Atrium
Chronic left atrial (LA) pressure overload due to mitral gradient leads to enlargement of the LA, with important interpatient variations. LA enlargement and wall fibrosis favor the occurrence of AF.[17]

The severity of blood stasis can be assessed with Doppler echocardiography from the intensity of LA spontaneous contrast and the

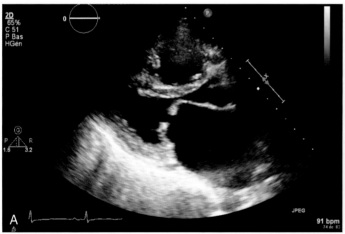
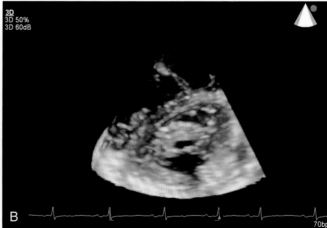

Fig. 16.1 Severe Mitral Stenosis. Transthoracic echocardiography: parasternal long-axis view (A) and short-axis 3D view from the left ventricle (B). Valve area is 0.5 cm². Leaflet tips are thickened, but the anterior leaflet is pliable. The short-axis view shows fusion of both commissures.

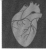

decrease of flow velocities in the LA appendage in patients in sinus rhythm. Blood stasis and LA appendage flow velocities are considerably impaired when AF occurs. The LA appendage is the most frequent location of LA thrombus.[18]

Pulmonary Circulation

Postcapillary pulmonary hypertension is the passive consequence of increased LA pressure. There may also be a component of precapillary pulmonary hypertension due to an increase in pulmonary vascular resistance, which determines a gradient of 7 mmHg or greater between diastolic pulmonary artery pressure (PAP) and pulmonary artery wedge pressure.[19]

Increased pulmonary vascular resistance involves endothelium-dependent vasoconstriction, which is reversible under inhaled nitric oxide, and structural changes of the pulmonary arterial wall.[20] Structural changes initially consist of intimal and medial thickening in muscular arteries and arterioles, which may be reversible with a decrease in PAP.[21] More severe lesions include fibrinoid necrosis and arteritis, loss of smooth muscle cell nuclei, fibrin deposition in the arterial wall, and inflammatory cells. Plexiform lesion is the hallmark of end-stage, irreversible pulmonary hypertension and accounts for persistently elevated PAP after intervention for MS. There is a wide range in PAP for any degree of MS because PAP depends on MVA and gradient and on left ventricular (LV) end-diastolic pressure, chronic pulmonary disease, and net atrioventricular compliance.[22,23]

Right Heart

Chronic pulmonary hypertension leads to right ventricular (RV) hypertrophy, dilation, and then reduced ejection fraction. This process may be exacerbated by significant tricuspid regurgitation from rheumatic involvement of the tricuspid valve or annular dilation due to RV enlargement. Although pulmonary hypertension presumably is the cause of right heart dysfunction, there is a poor correlation between pulmonary pressures and RV failure in patients with MS.

Left Ventricle

LV size is usually normal or moderately reduced in MS. The main consequence of MS on the LV is a prolongation of early diastolic filling and an increased contribution of LA contraction. AF further alters diastolic filling. LV filling may also be impaired by RV pressure or volume overload determining abnormal septal motion.

Although LV contractility typically is normal in isolated MS, forward stroke volume may be reduced due to low filling volumes across the stenotic mitral valve. LV ejection fraction is impaired in 5% to 10% of patients in the absence of other valve or coronary artery disease.[24] This does not seem to be explained by abnormal loading conditions because LV dysfunction typically persists after the relief of MS.

Exercise Physiology

Hemodynamic changes during exercise provide additional insights into the many factors interacting with the severity of the stenosis to determine its repercussions. The increase in transmitral gradient during exercise is the consequence of shortening of the diastolic filling period, and it determines an upstream increase in PAP. However, changes in mitral gradient and PAP vary greatly for a given degree of stenosis.[25] This heterogeneity may be explained by differences in the evolution of stroke volume during exercise and by differences in atrioventricular compliance, which depends mostly on LA compliance.[23,26] Besides valvular function, lung function, chronotropic incompetence, stroke volume reserve, and peripheral factors contribute to impaired exercise tolerance.[27]

Increased stroke volume during exercise is associated with an increase in MVA during exercise, which is observed in patients who have a moderate impairment of valve anatomy. In patients with severe impairment of valve anatomy, stroke volume does not increase or may even decrease during exercise. Besides valvular function, net atrioventricular compliance is a strong determinant of LA pressure and PAP at rest and during exercise.[23,26,28]

CLINICAL PRESENTATION

History

Dyspnea is the most frequent symptom of MS, and it has a prognostic value. It may be difficult to assess given the progressive course of the disease and in elderly patients with calcific MS. Paroxysmal dyspnea, cough, or hemoptysis should be looked for.

Patients sometimes complain more about fatigue than dyspnea, particularly elderly patients and those who have advanced heart disease with chronic AF. Asthenia and abdominal pain are suspicious for right heart failure.

Complications such as AF or embolic events may reveal MS in previously asymptomatic patients. Pregnancy is a common cause of decompensation of previously well-tolerated MS, because the increase in cardiac output and tachycardia causes a sharp increase in the mitral gradient and PAP during the second trimester.[29] The search for comorbidity is important in older patients, who account for a growing portion of patients with rheumatic or calcific MS in developed countries.[6,30,31]

Physical Examination

Auscultation reveals a loud first heart sound and an opening snap in early diastole just after the second heart sound, followed by a holodiastolic rumbling murmur that decreases in intensity with time and increases in end-diastole in patients in sinus rhythm (Fig. 16.2). Careful auscultation is needed because the murmur is often difficult to identify.

A loud murmur with a thrill suggests severe stenosis. However, a low-intensity murmur does not exclude severe stenosis in a patient with low cardiac output. The duration of the interval between the second aortic sound and the opening snap is shortened in severe stenosis. The intensity of the first sound and of the opening snap may be diminished in cases of extensive calcification that limits leaflet motion.

Auscultation should search for a holosystolic murmur at the apex, which suggests combined MR and MS. The holosystolic murmur of tricuspid regurgitation is usually located at the xiphoid or near the apex and increases with inspiration. It is important to pay attention even to a low-intensity mid-systolic murmur attesting to associated aortic stenosis, the severity of which tends to be underestimated when combined with MS. A diastolic murmur at the left sternal border is more likely to be the consequence of aortic than pulmonic regurgitation. The second pulmonary sound is louder in cases of pulmonary hypertension. Auscultation is also the first means of detecting arrhythmias, which should be confirmed by electrocardiography.

Clinical signs of left-sided heart failure are found in patients with severe symptoms. Signs of right heart failure are observed in patients with severe and often long-standing disease. Hepatomegaly may be expansive in cases of severe tricuspid regurgitation.

Chest Radiography and Electrocardiography

LA enlargement is characterized by LA double density and prominence of the LA appendage on chest radiograms. The pulmonary artery trunk and branches are often dilated. Heart size is initially normal but is enlarged in severe chronic MS with RV and right atrial enlargement. Interstitial edema is often seen even in patients without clinical signs of heart failure. Alveolar edema is a sign of acute hemodynamic decompensation. Transverse chest radiography is useful to detect RV enlargement, mild pleural effusion, and MAC.[4]

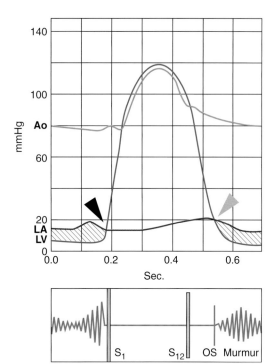

Fig. 16.2 Correspondence Between Hemodynamics and Auscultation of Mitral Stenosis. The diastolic rumbling murmur corresponds to the pressure gradient between the left atrium and left ventricle *(striped area)*. Murmur intensity decreases progressively and is reinforced in end-diastole with atrial contraction. The intensity of the first heart sound *(S₁)* is increased. The interval between the second heart sound *(S₂)* and the opening snap *(OS)* decreases as stenosis becomes more severe. The *black triangle* indicates mitral valve closure, and the *gray triangle* indicates mitral valve opening. *Ao*, Aortic pressure; *LA*, left atrial pressure; *LV*, left ventricular pressure.

LA enlargement is the only electrocardiographic abnormality at an early stage. RA and RV enlargement with right axis deviation and right bundle branch block are observed in more advanced disease. Electrocardiography plays a major role in the detection of atrial arrhythmias including frequent atrial premature beats, AF, and less frequently, atrial flutter or atrial tachycardia.

Echocardiography

Echocardiography is the cornerstone for confirming the diagnosis of MS, evaluating its cause, determining the severity and consequences of valve lesions, and assessing valve anatomy and associated diseases.[32]

Assessment of Severity

Planimetry using the parasternal short-axis view is the reference measurement of MVA because it directly measures the valve area independent of loading conditions and associated heart diseases.[33] Technical expertise is needed to scan the mitral valve apparatus to position the measurement plane on the leaflet tip. This may be facilitated with the use of three-dimensional (3D) echocardiography, which improves accuracy and reproducibility.[34,35] Planimetry is also useful during BMC to monitor the procedure and immediately after BMC, for which it is the most reliable technique.

Planimetry may be difficult or not feasible in cases of irregular orifice or severe calcification and in patients with poor echogenicity. Mitral orifice planimetry is particularly difficult to perform and lacks reliability in patients with degenerative MS due to the extent of calcification and the deformation of the mitral orifice. Limited data suggest that planimetry using 3D echocardiography has good concordance with the results obtained from use of the continuity equation.[33]

The parasternal short-axis view also assesses commissural fusion; accuracy is higher with 3D rather than two-dimensional (2D) echocardiography.[34] This is important for differentiating rheumatic from calcific MS and for determining the feasibility of BMC. Assessment of the commissural opening provides an additional indication of the efficacy of BMC during and after the procedure and during late follow-up.

The pressure half-time method is easier to perform and is therefore widely used, but it may be misleading in cases of aortic regurgitation, abnormal compliance of cardiac chambers, and immediately after BMC.[33] The validity of the pressure half-time method is questionable for patients with calcific MS because LV compliance is frequently impaired due to patient age and hypertension.[6]

Use of the continuity equation is not valid in cases of associated significant MR or aortic regurgitation. Its accuracy and reproducibility are limited due to the number of measurements involved.[33]

Assessment of the proximal isovelocity surface area is technically demanding.[36]

Mean mitral gradient, as assessed by pulsed or continuous-wave Doppler, depends greatly on flow conditions: cardiac output, heart rate, and associated MR. Its value should be consistent with the MVA, and it has prognostic value after BMC. Despite its flow dependence, the mean gradient is useful in patients with calcific MS because of limitations of the methods used to assess valve area. Severe MS is likely if the mean gradient is greater than 10 mmHg.[33]

The consistency of results obtained by planimetry, the pressure half-time method, and mitral gradient should always be checked, keeping in mind the limitations of the various measurements.[33,37–39] The continuity equation and proximal isovelocity surface area methods are not used routinely in rheumatic MS but may be useful when other methods lead to uncertain or discordant findings (Table 16.1). Given the limitations of planimetry and the pressure half-time method, the continuity equation is useful for assessment of calcific MS.[16]

When the MVA is greater than 1.5 cm², the hemodynamics are not affected at rest. Interventions for MS are considered when the MVA is smaller than 1.5 cm².[33,37,38] Mitral valve resistance has been proposed as a marker of severity but has no additional value compared with MVA.[33]

Assessment of Valve Morphology

Analysis of the morphology of the valve leaflets, mitral annulus, and subvalvular apparatus using 2D echocardiography is a key feature in the diagnosis of MS and its mechanism. It also has implications for the choice of the most appropriate intervention.[33]

Rheumatic MS is characterized by commissural fusion, restriction of posterior leaflet motion, and impairment of the subvalvular apparatus. Valve calcification may involve both leaflets but seldom affects the mitral annulus. Degenerative MS is characterized by extensive calcification of the mitral annulus, which appears as a dense band located between the posterior leaflet and the posterior wall with acoustic shadowing.[16] Calcification often extends to the base of the leaflets, but there is no commissural fusion, and the leaflet tips are less frequently involved.[6] Thickening and restriction of the motion of both leaflets is frequently observed when MAC causes severe MS.[6,16]

In rheumatic MS, echocardiographic evaluation assesses leaflet thickening (significant if ≥5 mm), leaflet mobility in the long-axis parasternal view, and calcification, which is best confirmed by fluoroscopic examination. The parasternal short-axis view is paramount for planimetry and for evaluating the homogeneity of the impairment of the mitral orifice, focusing on commissural areas (Fig. 16.3). The long-axis parasternal and apical views enable assessment of the subvalvular

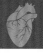

TABLE 16.1   Echocardiographic Assessment of the Severity of Mitral Stenosis and Alternative Methods.

Measurement	Method	Advantages	Disadvantages	Alternative Methods
Valve area (cm²)	Planimetry on 2D/3D parasternal short-axis view	Direct measurement, independent of flow conditions; reference method for rheumatic MS	Experience required; not feasible if there is severe valve deformity or a poor acoustic window	MSCT, CMR, Gorlin formula
	Pressure half-time using CW Doppler	Easy to obtain	Dependence on other factors (regurgitations, chamber compliance, diastolic function)	—
	Continuity equation	Independent of flow conditions; recommended for calcific MS	Errors of measurement (multiple variables); not valid in cases of significant regurgitation	—
	Proximal isovelocity surface	Independent of flow conditions	Technically difficult	—
Mean mitral gradient (mmHg)	CW Doppler on mitral flow	Easy to obtain	Depends on heart rate and flow conditions	Right + left catheterization
Pulmonary artery pressure (mmHg)	CW Doppler on tricuspid regurgitant flow	Easy to obtain in cases of tricuspid regurgitation	Arbitrary estimation of right atrial pressure; no estimation of pulmonary vascular resistance	Right catheterization (reference measurement)
Mean gradient and pulmonary artery pressure at exercise (mmHg)	CW Doppler of mitral and tricuspid regurgitant flow	Objective assessment of exercise tolerance	Lack of validation for decision making	—

CMR, Cardiac magnetic resonance; *MS*, mitral stenosis; *MSCT*, multislice computed tomography.

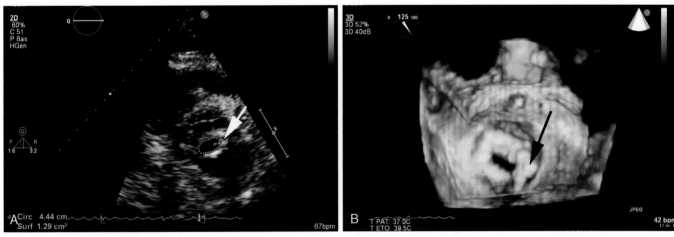

Fig. 16.3 Mitral Stenosis With Calcification of the Lateral Commissure. Transthoracic echocardiography: parasternal short-axis 2D view (A) and short-axis 3D view from the left atrium (B). Valve area is 1.3 cm². Both commissures are fused, and the lateral commissure is calcified *(arrows)*.

apparatus (i.e., thickening and/or shortening of chordae), although impairment tends to be underestimated compared with anatomic findings.

The severity of valvular and subvalvular involvement usually is described by a combined score in rheumatic MS. The Wilkins echocardiographic score grades each of the following components of the mitral apparatus from 1 to 4: leaflet mobility, thickness, calcification, and impairment of the subvalvular apparatus (Table 16.2).[40] Total scores range from 4 to 16. An alternative approach is to assess the whole mitral valve anatomy according to the best surgical alternative; three classifications are identified based on echocardiography and fluoroscopy (Table 16.3).[41]

These two scores share limitations related to the lack of a detailed location of calcification and leaflet thickening, particularly in relation to commissural areas, which are likely to influence the results of BMC.[42–45] They tend to underestimate the weight of subvalvular apparatus impairment.[46] Other scoring systems involve a more detailed approach, including quantitative approaches and analysis of commissural

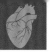

TABLE 16.2 Assessment of Mitral Valve Anatomy According to the Wilkins Score.

Grade[a]	Mobility	Thickening	Calcification	Subvalvular Thickening
1	Highly mobile valve with only leaflet tips restricted	Leaflets near normal in thickness (4–5 mm)	A single area of increased echocardiographic brightness	Minimal thickening just below the mitral leaflets
2	Leaflet middle and base portions have normal mobility	Mid-leaflets normal, considerable thickening of margins (5–8 mm)	Scattered areas of brightness confined to leaflet margins	Thickening of chordal structures extending to one of the chordal length
3	Valve continues to move forward in diastole, mainly from the base	Thickening extending through the entire leaflet (5–8 mm)	Brightness extending into the midportions of the leaflets	Thickening extended to distal third of the chords
4	No or minimal forward movement of the leaflets in diastole	Considerable thickening of all leaflet tissue (>8–10 mm)	Extensive brightness throughout much of the leaflet tissue	Extensive thickening and shortening of all chordal structures extending down to the papillary muscles

[a]Each component is graded separately, and the total score is the sum of the four items, ranging between 4 and 16.
From Wilkins GT, Weyman AE, Abascal VM, et al. Percutaneous balloon dilatation of the mitral valve: an analysis of echocardiographic variables related to outcome and the mechanism of dilatation. Br Heart J 1988;60:299-308.

TABLE 16.3 Assessment of Mitral Valve Anatomy According to the Cormier Score.

Echocardiographic Group	Mitral Valve Anatomy
Group 1	Pliable noncalcified anterior mitral leaflet and mild subvalvular disease (i.e., thin chordae ≥ 10 mm long)
Group 2	Pliable noncalcified anterior mitral leaflet and severe subvalvular disease (i.e., thickened chordae ≤ 10 mm long)
Group 3	Calcification of mitral valve of any extent as assessed by fluoroscopy, whatever the state of the subvalvular apparatus

From Vahanian A, Michel PL, Cormier B, et al. Results of percutaneous mitral commissurotomy in 200 patients. Am J Cardiol 1989;63:847-852.

areas.[33,47,48] Good prediction of the results of BMC has been shown for small numbers of patients, but validation in large series using multivariate analyses including other predictors is lacking. No comparative evaluation of scoring systems enables a particular one to be recommended.[39] It is unlikely that a single scoring system could combine reproducibility and accurate prediction of the results of BMC. Echocardiographers use a method with which they are familiar and that includes the assessment of valve morphology among other clinical and echocardiographic findings.

Consequences of Mitral Stenosis
Quantitation of LA enlargement with the use of time-motion measurement is the most widely used method but lacks accuracy. Estimation of LA area (or, better, LA volume) using 2D echocardiography is preferred and should include analysis of LA shape.[49,50]

Systolic PAP is estimated from the velocity of Doppler-indicated tricuspid flow. Diastolic and mean PAPs can be derived from pulmonary flow.[51]

Mitral Regurgitation
Quantitation of associated MR should combine different semiquantitative and quantitative measurements and check their consistency. An accurate evaluation using quantitative methods is of particular importance for moderate MR because it may have important implications for the choice of the type of intervention.[52] Quantitation of MR may be hampered in calcific MS because of acoustic shadowing of the LA.

Associated Lesions
Rheumatic aortic valve disease is frequently associated with MS, and calcific aortic disease can be associated with MAC.[15] Decreased stroke volume due to MS may lead to underestimation of aortic stenosis because of a low gradient. Valve area should be quantitated using the continuity equation or planimetry of the aortic valve, or both.

Secondary tricuspid regurgitation is caused by enlargement of right cavities due to pulmonary hypertension without rheumatic lesions of the valve. Quantitation of tricuspid regurgitation depends on loading conditions. Echocardiographic measurement of the tricuspid annulus is systematic given its prognostic implications for the persistence of severe tricuspid regurgitation after treatment of MS.[53] Assessment of RV size and function should be relevant but lacks standardization.[54] Rheumatic tricuspid disease is less common than secondary tricuspid regurgitation and is characterized by thickening and decreased leaflet mobility causing stenosis and regurgitation.

Thromboembolic Risk
Transesophageal echocardiography (TEE) has a much higher sensitivity than transthoracic echocardiography for detecting LA thrombus, particularly that located in the LA appendage (Fig. 16.4). TEE is therefore mandatory before BMC. TEE is also useful for assessing LA spontaneous contrast, which is a strong predictor of thromboembolic risk in patients with MS.

Stress Testing
Semisupine bicycle ergometry enables sequential assessment of hemodynamic changes with increasing workload, particularly mean mitral gradient and estimated systolic PAP (Fig. 16.5).[25] It is useful for patients whose symptoms are equivocal or discordant with the severity of MS. However, the thresholds of mitral gradient and PAP proposed for consideration of intervention in asymptomatic patients rely on low levels of evidence and are frequently achieved in practice.[33,55]

Dobutamine stress echocardiography, although less physiologic than exercise echocardiography, was shown to have a prognostic value in one study.[56]

Cardiac Computed Tomography
Cardiac CT is the reference study for the diagnosis of valvular or annular calcification because it has a higher specificity than echocardiography for differentiating calcification from dense fibrosis. Cardiac CT also ensures an accurate and reproducible location and quantitation of the extent of MAC, which requires electrocardiogram (ECG)–gated CT with intravenous contrast and 3D reconstruction. Cardiac CT plays

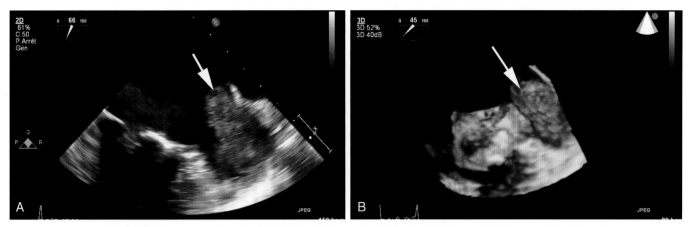

Fig. 16.4 Mitral Stenosis With Left Atrial Thrombus. TEE: 2D (A) and 3D (B) views show a large thrombus of the left atrial appendage *(arrow)*. The thrombus tip protrudes into the left atrial cavity. Dense left atrial spontaneous contrast is visible on the 2D view *(arrow)*.

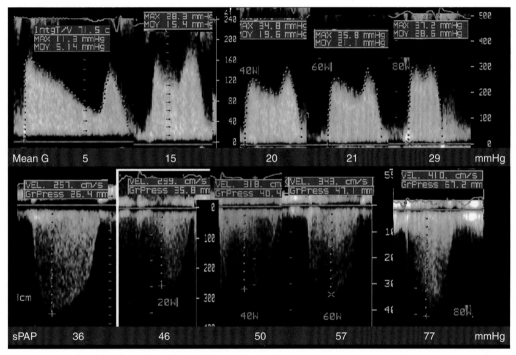

Fig. 16.5 Exercise Echocardiography in Mitral Stenosis. Monitoring of mitral gradient *(upper panels)* and pulmonary artery pressure *(lower panels)* with bicycle exercise in a semisupine position at rest and at 20, 40, 60, and 80 W *(left to right)*. *Mean G,* Mean mitral gradient; *sPAP,* systolic pulmonary artery pressure. (Courtesy Dr. Eric Brochet, Cardiology Department, Bichat Hospital, Paris, France.)

a role in the choice of the type of intervention in patients with calcific MS.[16] The usefulness of CT in the assessment of calcification has not been studied in rheumatic MS.

Cardiac CT and magnetic resonance imaging may be alternative techniques for planimetry of the mitral valve, and CT can be used to detect LA thrombus.[57,58]

Cardiac Catheterization

There is now little interest in the use of right and left heart cardiac catheterization to calculate MVA using the Gorlin formula which lacks reliability when cardiac output is decreased and immediately after BMC.[59] However, cardiac catheterization remains the reference method used to estimate PAP and the only technique for calculating

pulmonary vascular resistance, which is useful in patients with severe pulmonary hypertension.

In current practice, the main indication for invasive investigations is the assessment of associated coronary disease using coronary angiography. Monitoring the results of BMC now relies mainly on periprocedure echocardiography.

NATURAL HISTORY

Onset and Progression of Valvular Lesions

The development of MS takes many years after acute rheumatic fever. Severity of carditis, recurrences of acute rheumatic fever, and mother's low educational level are risk factors associated with progression of

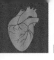

chronic rheumatic valve disease.[60] The course of the disease is rapid in countries where rheumatic fever is endemic, leading to severe MS in young adults, whereas in Western countries rheumatic MS frequently occurs after the age of 50 years.[61]

The progression of rheumatic MS has been evaluated in small, retrospective series, which reported an average decrease in valve area of 0.01 cm²/yr.[62–64] However, this reflects a mixture of patients: in one third to two thirds of patients, MVA remained stable, whereas patients experiencing progression had an annual decrease ranging from 0.1 to 0.3 cm². In another study, progression of calcific MS was observed in one half of the patients, who had a mean gradient increase of 2.0 mmHg/yr.[65]

Clinical Outcome Without Intervention

Studies of the natural history of rheumatic MS are frequently old, retrospective, and subject to inclusion bias. The prognosis of MS is poor after patients become symptomatic, with 10-year survival rates between 34% and 61% and 20-year rates between 14% and 21%.[66,67] One series reported a 44% survival rate at 5 years for patients refusing intervention.[68]

Survival is influenced by symptoms and AF. Asymptomatic patients have a 10-year survival rate greater than 80%, but approximately one half of them become symptomatic after 10 years.[66,69] The leading cause of death is heart failure, affecting about 60% of patients, followed by thromboembolic complications occurring in about 20%.[66] There are no specific data on the prognosis of degenerative MS, but MAC is an independent predictive factor of all-cause and cardiovascular mortality, regardless of its hemodynamic consequences.[6]

Complications

AF is frequently associated with rheumatic and calcific MS; it is largely related to LA enlargement and age.[17,30,70] One half of patients with MS in sinus rhythm have atrial arrhythmias according to Holter ECG monitoring, most often without symptoms.

AF impairs hemodynamics and may cause acute decompensation such as pulmonary edema. Because of blood stasis in the LA, AF further increases the thromboembolic risk.

The annual linearized risk of thromboembolism in AF without anticoagulant therapy is estimated to be 3.6% for patients with moderate rheumatic MS and 5.7% for those with severe MS. The corresponding figures for patients in sinus rhythm are 0.25% for moderate MS and 0.85% for severe MS.[68] Embolic events are cerebral in location in 60% to 70% of cases; they frequently have sequelae and are prone to recurrence. The risk of stroke is also increased among patients with MAC and is probably multifactorial.[4]

MEDICAL THERAPY

Prevention of Rheumatic Fever and Infective Endocarditis

Primary prevention of rheumatic fever relies on adapted antibiotic treatment of streptococcal pharyngitis. Secondary prevention is based on continuous antibiotic therapy, up to 40 years in cases of rheumatic carditis.[37,38] After rheumatic valve disease has occurred, no medical treatment has been shown to slow the progression of MS. Antibiotic prophylaxis is no longer advised for the prevention of infective endocarditis in MS, but dental and cutaneous hygiene measures should be applied.[71,72]

Treatment of Symptoms

Medical treatment of symptomatic MS relies on diuretics to relieve congestion and β-blockers to lengthen the diastolic filling period.

β-Blockers are particularly useful in pregnant women because they enable a dramatic decrease in the mean gradient and PAP in most cases. However, β-blockers do not seem to improve exercise tolerance in MS patients.[73,74]

In patients with MS and AF, restoration of sinus rhythm is superior to rate control in regard to indices of functional capacity and quality of life.[75] Amiodarone appears to be the most effective drug for maintaining sinus rhythm after cardioversion, but indications should be weighed against side effects, particularly in young patients.[17] When AF cannot be converted to sinus rhythm, rate control is obtained with the use of digitalis or β-blockers, or both. The respective indications of rhythm and rate control should be adapted to patient characteristics, taking into account the higher risk of recurrence of AF in MS.[17]

Prevention of Thromboembolism

Permanent or paroxysmal AF is a class I indication for oral anticoagulation, regardless of stenosis severity, as described in the American Heart Association (AHA)/American College of Cardiology (ACC) guidelines and the European Society of Cardiology (ESC)/European Association for Cardio-Thoracic Surgery (EACTS) guidelines.[37,38] In a retrospective study, oral anticoagulation decreased the annual risk of thromboembolism in patients with MS and AF from 5.7% to 1.0% for severe MS and from 3.6% to 0.9% for moderate MS.[68] Among patients with MS in sinus rhythm, the annual risk of thromboembolism decreased from 0.85% to 0.10% for severe MS and from 0.25% to 0.10% for moderate MS.[68] Given the risk of bleeding inherent associated with oral anticoagulation, risk-benefit analysis does not support systematic anticoagulant therapy in patients with MS in sinus rhythm.

Vitamin K antagonists are advised for selected patients with MS in sinus rhythm who are at high risk for thromboembolic events. Prior embolism and LA thrombus are class I indications for anticoagulation in the AHA/ACC and ESC/EACTS guidelines. Dense spontaneous echocardiographic contrast and enlargement of the LA are class IIa indications in the ESC/EACTS guidelines but not in the AHA/ACC guidelines. The target international normalized ratio is between 2.0 and 3.0.

Aspirin or other antiplatelet drugs alone are not valid alternatives to decrease thromboembolic risk in patients with MS. Direct inhibitors of factors II and X cannot be recommended because patients with MS were excluded from trials comparing these drugs with warfarin for the prevention of embolism in AF.[37,38]

Pharmacologic or electrical cardioversion should be attempted in patients with nonsevere MS who have persistent AF. For patients with severe MS, cardioversion should be postponed after the intervention on the mitral valve in most cases.[17,37]

Modalities of Follow-Up

Follow-up timing should be adapted to the severity of MS, symptoms, and potential complications. In asymptomatic patients with MS (MVA < 1.5 cm²) in whom intervention is not planned, systematic clinical and echocardiographic follow-up is performed yearly. Follow-up intervals can be longer for those with MS who have an MVA greater than 1.5 cm².

The patient should be educated to identify interim changes in symptoms, which should lead to a prompt visit. Women should be informed of the inherent risks of pregnancy, even if they are asymptomatic. Repeated monthly echocardiographic examinations are needed during the second and third trimesters of pregnancy to monitor the mean gradient and PAP.[76]

Follow-up after successful BMC is the same as for asymptomatic patients. Its periodicity can be adapted through use of a simple scoring system to estimate the probability of long-term, event-free survival according to baseline patient characteristics and the results of BMC.[77] Intervals should be shorter after restenosis occurs.

INTERVENTIONS FOR MITRAL STENOSIS

Surgical Commissurotomy

The initial surgical approach for relief of rheumatic MS, introduced in 1948, was closed commissurotomy (i.e., dilation of the stenotic valve through the LA without direct visualization of the valve). This procedure does not require cardiopulmonary bypass, but it carries the risks of embolic events caused by dislodged atrial thrombi, incomplete relief of MS, and induction of excessive MR due to leaflet tear. Closed mitral commissurotomy results in an increase in MVA and relief of symptoms with an operative mortality rate of 3% to 4%.[78–80] Long-term outcome is quite good, with 31% to 50% of patients requiring reoperation within 15 years after the initial procedure and 76% by 20 years.[78–80]

Multivariate predictors of the need for subsequent mitral valve replacement (MVR) are functional class, mitral valve calcification, subvalvular fusion, and the adequacy of the initial surgical procedure.[78,79] This operation is easily accessible and remains in use in developing countries.

Open mitral commissurotomy is usually performed through a median sternotomy under cardiopulmonary bypass. Fused commissures are dissected under direct vision, and this can be combined with release of fused chordae or correction of chordal shortening. If needed, an annuloplasty ring can be used to decrease the severity of coexisting MR.

The advantages of the open procedure are a more directed surgical repair and the possibility of detection and removal of LA thrombus. With appropriate patient selection and in experienced hands, open commissurotomy is feasible in 80% to 90% of referred patients, with an operative mortality rate of about 1%.[81] Long-term outcome after open surgical commissurotomy has been excellent, with survival rates of 80% to 90% at 10 years and approximately 40% at 20 years.[80,81]

Balloon Mitral Commissurotomy

Similar to surgical commissurotomy, BMC splits the closed commissures, and it is therefore applicable only to rheumatic MS.[82]

Patient Selection

The applicability of BMC depends on three major factors: the patient's clinical condition, the mitral valve anatomy, and the experience of the medical and surgical teams of the institution concerned.

Evaluation of the patient's clinical condition must take into account the degree of functional disability, any severe cardiothoracic deformity that may compromise BMC, and the alternative risk of surgery based on the underlying cardiac condition or comorbidities. Exercise testing is recommended to unmask symptoms in patients claiming to be asymptomatic and in those with doubtful symptoms.

The first step in the evaluation of valve anatomy is to establish the severity of MS. The performance of BMC is usually restricted to patients with an MVA smaller than 1.5 cm^2.[37,38] It is then critical to ensure that there are no anatomic contraindications to the technique. LA thrombosis must be excluded by systematic performance of TEE just before the procedure. Other contraindications are greater than moderate MR and the coexistence of another severe valve disease.

Echocardiographic assessment allows classification of patients into anatomic groups with a view toward predicting results. Most investigators use the Wilkins score, whereas others, such as Cormier and colleagues, use a more general assessment of valve anatomy.[33,39,83] Other

scores have been proposed to improve prediction of the results of BMC through the use of quantitative approaches or analysis of commissural areas, or both, but their validation remains limited, and they are seldom used in practice.[39,83]

The incidence of technical failures and complications is related to operator experience.[84] Experience also improves the selection of patients by means of clinical evaluation and echocardiographic assessment.[85–87] Complication rates have increased in the United States during the past decade due to increased patient age and more frequent comorbidities and because of decreased operator volume.[87] For this reason, BMC should be restricted to teams that have extensive experience with transseptal catheterization and are able to perform an adequate number of procedures. The interventionists who perform BMC must also be able to perform emergency pericardiocentesis. Immediate surgical backup does not seem to be compulsory.

Technique

The transvenous or antegrade approach with transseptal catheterization is the most widely used technique. The retrograde technique without transseptal catheterization is very seldom used.[88]

The Inoue technique (Fig. 16.6) is now almost exclusively used. The Inoue balloon is self-positioning, is pressure extensible, and has three distinct parts that can be inflated sequentially. Balloon size (24–30 mm) is chosen according to the patient's height and body surface area.[39,83,89] Use of a stepwise dilation technique under echocardiographic guidance is recommended (Fig. 16.7). The first inflation is performed to the minimum diameter of the balloon chosen. The balloon is then deflated and withdrawn into the LA. If MR has not increased and the MVA is insufficient, the balloon is readvanced across the mitral valve, and inflation is repeated with the balloon diameter increased by 1 to 2 mm.

The other techniques, such as use of the double balloons, multitrack balloons, and metallic commissurotome, are seldom employed, mainly in developing countries, where economic constraints lead to reuse of the devices.[90,91] The use of TEE or intracardiac echocardiography is limited to rare cases in which difficulty is encountered during the transseptal catheterization or in which high-risk circumstances, such as severe cardiothoracic deformity or pregnancy, are factors.[92]

Monitoring the Procedure and Assessing Immediate Results

Echocardiography during BMC provides essential information on the efficacy of the procedure and enables early detection of complications.[33,39] Evaluation of the results necessitates a combined analysis of the following: (1) the commissural opening, shown in the parasternal short-axis view by 2D transthoracic echocardiography or 3D real-time echocardiography; (2) the MVA, measured with planimetry because pressure half-time measurement is not adequate in the acute setting; (3) the mean gradient; and (4) the presence and degree of MR, as assessed in several views with special attention to MR originating in the commissural areas.

The following criteria have been proposed for the desired end point of the procedure: (1) MVA greater than 1 cm^2/m^2 of body surface area; (2) complete opening of at least one commissure; or (3) appearance or increment of regurgitation greater than grade 1/4 classification.[89] These criteria should be individualized. The expected final MVA is smaller in elderly patients, in cases of very tight MS or extensive valve and subvalvular disease, and in cases of calcification.

After the procedure, the most accurate evaluation of MVA is provided by planimetry using echocardiography, which also evaluates commissural opening.[33] Pressure half-time measurements should be interpreted with caution early after BMC. Despite its dependence on flow conditions and heart rate, the mean mitral gradient should be

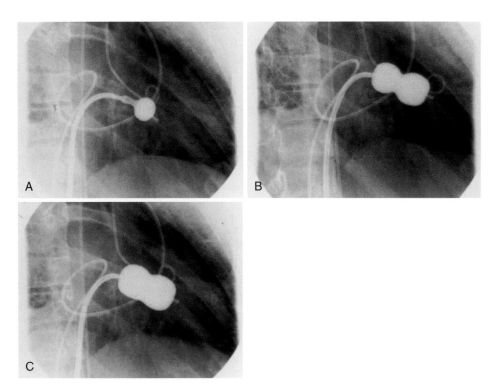

Fig. 16.6 Balloon Mitral Commissurotomy (BMC). Fluoroscopic images recorded during percutaneous BMC using an Inoue balloon. (A) The distal balloon has been inflated to secure the position at the valvular level. (B) The proximal segment also has been inflated. (C) The dilating segment is briefly inflated.

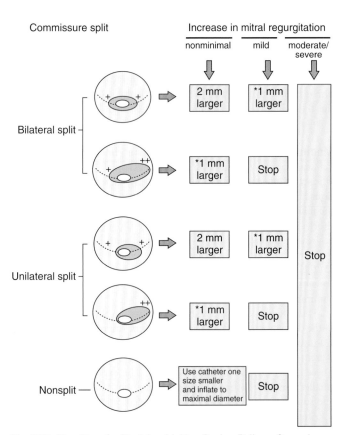

Fig. 16.7 Algorithm for Decision Making During Balloon Commissurotomy. The stepwise dilation technique using the Inoue balloon is modified according to echocardiographic findings after each balloon inflation. +, Incomplete split; ++, complete split; *, stop in cases of severely diseased valve or age > 65 years. (From Topol E. Textbook of interventional cardiology. 7th ed. Philadelphia: Elsevier; 2016.)

assessed because it has prognostic value (Fig. 16.8). Final assessment of the degree of regurgitation may be made with angiography or, more frequently, Doppler color-flow imaging. TEE is recommended in cases of severe MR to determine the mechanisms involved. The most sensitive method for the assessment of shunting is Doppler color-flow imaging, especially when TEE is used.

Immediate Results

Efficacy. BMC usually provides an increase of more than 100% in valve area (Table 16.4).[31,88,93–104] Overall good immediate results, defined by a final MVA greater than 1.5 cm^2 without an MR grade greater than 2/4, are observed in more than 80% of cases and in patients with diverse characteristics.[61] Gradual decreases in PAP and pulmonary vascular resistance are seen. High pulmonary vascular resistance continues to decrease in the absence of restenosis.[105]

BMC has a beneficial effect on exercise capacity.[106] Studies have shown that this technique also improves LA pump function and decreases LA stiffness.

Failures. The failure rates range from 1% to 17%.[31,84,88,93–101] Most failures occur in the early part of the investigators' experience and in low-volume centers. Others are the result of unfavorable anatomy.

Risks. Procedural mortality rates range from 0% to 3% (Table 16.5).[31,84,88,93–101] The main causes of death are LV perforation and poor general condition of the patient. The incidence of hemopericardium, mainly due to transseptal catheterization, varies from 0.5% to 12%. Embolism is typically encountered in less than 2% of cases.

The frequency of severe MR ranges from 2% to 19%. It is mostly related to noncommissural leaflet tearing, which can be associated with chordal rupture (Fig. 16.9).[86,98,107–111] The development of severe MR depends more on the distribution of the morphologic changes of the valve than on their severity, but it is largely unpredictable.[47] Severe acute MR is often poorly tolerated, and surgery is necessary. In most cases, MVR is required because of the severity of the underlying valve

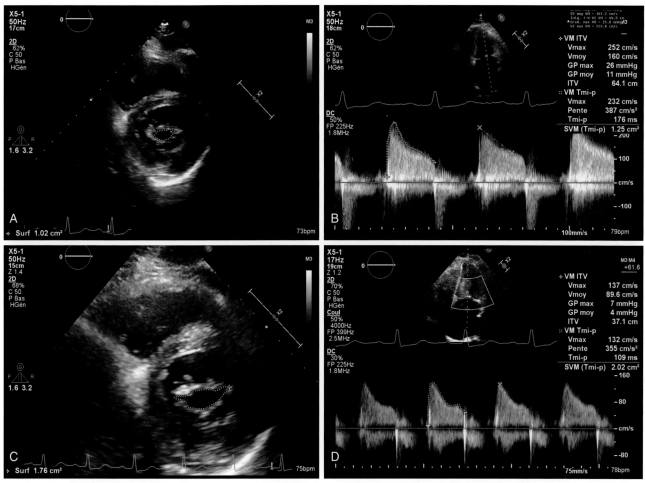

Fig. 16.8 Evaluation of the Immediate Result of Balloon Mitral Commissurotomy (BMC) by TTE. Before BMC *(upper panels)*: Parasternal short-axis view (A) shows severe MS with fusion of both commissures. Doppler imaging of transmitral flow (B) shows a mean mitral gradient of 11 mmHg. Mitral valve area is estimated to be 1.0 cm² by planimetry and 1.2 cm² by pressure half-time measurement. After BMC *(lower panels)*: Parasternal short-axis view (C) shows opening of both commissures. Doppler imaging of transmitral flow (D) shows a mean mitral gradient of 4 mmHg. Mitral valve area is estimated to be 1.8 cm² by planimetry and 2.0 cm² by pressure half-time measurement.

TABLE 16.4   Immediate Results of Balloon Mitral Commissurotomy: Increase in Mitral Valve Area.

| | | | MITRAL VALVE AREA (cm²) | | |
Study	Patients (N)	Age (yr)	Before BMC	After BMC	Technique
Arora et al.[93]	4850	27	0.7	1.9	Inoue, double-balloon or metallic commissurotome
Chen and Cheng[94]	4832	37	1.1	2.1	Inoue balloon
Iung et al.[31]	2773	47	1.0	1.9	Inoue, single-, or double-balloon
Meneguz-Moreno et al.[104]	1582	36	0.9	2.0	Inoue, double-balloon, metallic commissutrotome, multitrack
Neumayer et al.[95]	1123	57	1.1	1.8	Inoue balloon
Palacios et al.[96]	879	55	0.9	1.9	Inoue or double-balloon
Ben-Farhat et al.[97]	654	33	1.0	2.1	Inoue or double-balloon
Hernandez et al.[98]	561	53	1.0	1.8	Inoue balloon
Fawzy[99]	547	32	0.9	2.0	Inoue balloon
Meneveau et al.[100]	532	54	1.0	1.7	Double-balloon or Inoue balloon
Tomai et al.[101]	527	55	1.0	1.9	Inoue balloon
Eltchaninoff et al.[102]	500	34	0.9	2.1	Metallic commissurotome
Stefanadis et al.[88]	441	44	1.0	2.1	Modified single-, double-, or Inoue balloon (retrograde)
Lee et al.[103]	152	42	0.9	1.8	Inoue balloon
(randomized comparison)	150	40	0.9	1.9	Double-balloon

BMC, Balloon mitral commissurotomy.

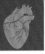

TABLE 16.5   Severe Complications of Balloon Mitral Commissurotomy.

Study	Patients (N)	Age (yr)	In-Hospital Deaths (%)	Tamponade (%)	Embolic Events (%)	Severe Mitral Regurgitation (%)
Arora et al.[93] (1987–2000)	4850	27	0.2	0.2	0.1	1.4
Chen and Cheng[94] (1985–1994)[a]	4832	37	0.1	0.8	0.5	1.4
Iung et al.[31] (1986–2001)	2773	47	0.4	0.2	0.4	4.1
Neumayer et al.[95] (1989–2000)	1123	57	0.4	0.9	0.9	6.0
Palacios et al.[96] (1986–2000)	879	55	0.6	1.0	1.8	9.4
NHLBI Registry[84] (1987–1989)[a]	738	54				
n < 25			2	6	4	4
25 ≤ n < 100			1	4	2	3
n ≥ 100			0.3	2	1	3
Ben-Farhat et al.[97] (1987–1998)	654	33	0.5	0.6	1.5	4.6
Hernandez et al.[98] (1989–1995)	620	53	0.5	0.6	—	4.0
Fawzy[99] (1989–2006)	578	32	0	0.9	0.5	1.6
Meneveau et al.[100] (1986–1996)	532	54	0.2	1.1	—	3.9
Tomai et al.[101] (1991–2010)	527	55	0.4	0.4	0.2	4.9
Stefanadis et al.[88] (1988–1996)[a]	441	44	0.2	0	0	3.4

[a]Multicenter series.
NHLBI, National Heart, Lung, and Blood Institute.

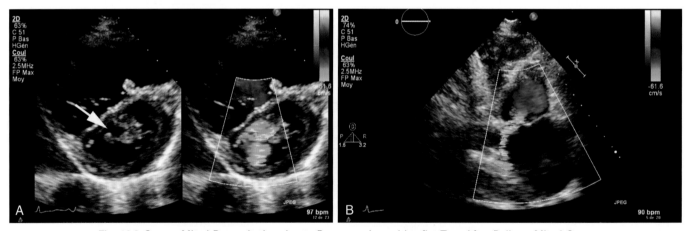

Fig. 16.9 Severe Mitral Regurgitation due to Paracommissural Leaflet Tear After Balloon Mitral Commissurotomy. TTE: (A) Parasternal short-axis 2D view shows mitral regurgitation originating from a paracommissural leaflet tear of the anterior leaflet *(arrow)*. (B) Apical four-chamber view shows eccentric jet of mitral regurgitation.

disease. Conservative surgery has been successfully performed in selected young patients with less severe valve deformity.[107]

Atrial septal defects after BMC are usually small and persist in less than 10% of patients after 6 months.[112] Emergency surgery (within 24 hours) is seldom needed. It is used primarily in cases of massive hemopericardium or severe MR with poor hemodynamic tolerance.[86,108–110]

Predictors of immediate results. The prediction of immediate results is multifactorial.[86,104,113–115] In addition to morphologic factors, whatever the score used, preoperative variables such as age, history of surgical commissurotomy, functional class, small MVA, presence of MR before BMC, AF, high PAP, severe tricuspid regurgitation, and procedural factors such as balloon type and size are independent predictors of the immediate results.

Two multivariate models derived from large series and validated for different populations showed that older age, higher New York Health Association (NYHA) class, impaired valve anatomy as assessed by echocardiography, and smaller MVA are the most important predictive factors of poor immediate results of BMC.[86,115] The sensitivity of predictive models is high, but the specificity is low.[86] Low specificity indicates insufficient prediction of poor immediate results, which is particularly true for the prediction of severe MR. This low specificity is related to the intrinsic limitations of the prediction of immediate results—that is, to the possibility of good results in patients who are at high risk for poor results.

Long-Term Results

Data from up to 20 years of follow-up can now be analyzed. In clinical terms, the overall long-term results of BMC are good (Table 16.6).[77,88,96–101,104,116–119] Late outcomes after BMC depend on patient characteristics and the quality of the immediate results (Figs. 16.10 and 16.11).

If the immediate results are unsatisfactory, patients experience only transient or no functional improvement, and delayed surgery is usually performed when the extracardiac conditions allow. Conversely, if BMC is initially successful, survival rates are excellent, functional improvement occurs in most cases, and secondary surgery is infrequently needed.

Two European series reported the longest follow-up data after initially successful BMC in 912 and 482 patients with a mean age of 49 and 55 years, respectively.[77,101] After 20 years, cardiovascular survival rates without intervention (i.e., repeat BMC or surgery) were 38%

± 2% and 36% ± 5%, and good functional results (NYHA class I–II) were observed in 33% ± 2% and 21% ± 5% of the patients, respectively.[77,101] The rate of long-term, event-free survival is higher (≥70% after 10–20 years) in series in which the most patients were young and had favorable anatomic conditions.[97,104]

Clinical deterioration occurs late and is mainly related to mitral restenosis. Restenosis has been defined as a loss of more than 50% of the initial gain, with the MVA becoming smaller than 1.5 cm². After a successful procedure, the incidence of restenosis ranges from 2% to 40% at time intervals of 3 to 9 years.[98,116,117] The possibility of repeat BMC in cases of recurrent MS is one of the advantages of this nonsurgical procedure, provided that the predominant mechanism of restenosis is commissural refusion.[120–125] Good immediate and midterm outcomes are obtained after repeat BMC in patients with favorable characteristics, particularly in those younger than 50 years of age.[125]

The degree of MR typically remains stable or slightly decreases during follow-up. Atrial septal defects are likely to close over time in most cases, and they very seldom require treatment on their own. BMC reduces markers of the risk of embolism such as intensity of LA echocardiographic contrast, size, and function.[126–131] Two nonrandomized comparative series suggested that BMC decreases the incidence of thromboembolic events in MS compared with medical management.[132,133] No direct evidence exists that BMC reduces the incidence of AF, but it has a favorable influence on predictors of AF, such as atrial size and degree of obstruction.[134–137] It is recommended that electric shock cardioversion be performed after successful BMC if AF is of recent onset and in the absence of severe LA enlargement.[75]

TABLE 16.6	Late Results After Balloon Mitral Commissurotomy (Follow-Up ≥5 years).				
Study	Patients (N)	Age (yr)	Maximum Follow-Up (yr)	Event-Free Survival (%)	Predictive Factors of Event-Free Survival
Meneguz-Moreno et al.[104a]	1582	36	23	76[b]	Age, NYHA class, post-BMC MVA
Bouleti et al.[77]	1024	49	20	30[c]	Age, sex, NYHA class, rhythm, anatomy, post-BMC MVA, post-BMC gradient
Palacios et al.[96]	879	55	12	33[c]	Age, NYHA IV, prior commissurotomy, anatomy, MR, post-BMC MR, post-BMC PAP
Ben-Farhat et al.[97]	654	34	10	72[c]	Anatomy, post-BMC LA pressure, post-BMC gradient, post-MR
Hernandez et al.[98]	561	53	7	69[c]	Post-BMC MVA, post-BMC MR
Fawzy[99a]	547	32	19	28[c]	Anatomy, rhythm
Meneveau et al.[100]	532	54	7.5	52[c]	Age, anatomy, CTI, post-BMC gradient, post-BMC PAP
Tomai et al.[101]	482	55	20	36[b]	Sex, AF, anatomy, post-BMC MVA
Stefanadis et al.[88]	441	44	9	75[c]	NYHA class, anatomy, post-BMC MVA
Song et al.[116]	402	44	9	90[b]	Age, post-BMC MVA, commissural opening, post-BMC MR
Wang et al.[117]	310	53	6	80	Age, anatomy, NYHA class, post-BMC gradient
Lee et al.[103]					Post-BMC MVA, post-BMC commissural MR
Inoue balloon	152	42	24	41[c]	
Double-balloon	150	40	24	43[c]	
Cohen et al.[118]	146	59	5	51[b]	Anatomy, post-BMC MVA, post-BMC LVED pressure
Orrange et al.[119]	132	44	7	65[b]	Post-BMC MVA, post-BMC capillary wedge pressure

[a]Patients with good immediate results.
[b]Survival without intervention.
[c]Survival without intervention and in NYHA class I or II.
AF, Atrial fibrillation; *BMC*, balloon mitral commissurotomy; *CTI*, cardiothoracic index; *LVED*, left ventricular end-diastolic diameter; *MVA*, mitral valve area; *MR*, mitral regurgitation; *NYHA*, New York Heart Association; *PAP*, pulmonary artery pressure.

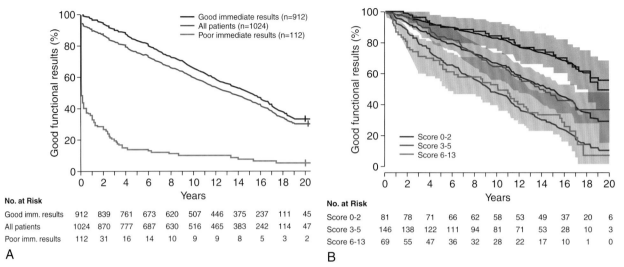

A

B

Fig. 16.10 Functional Results After Balloon Mitral Commissurotomy (BMC) for Rheumatic Mitral Stenosis. (A) Good functional results (i.e., survival considering cardiovascular-related deaths with no need for mitral surgery or repeat dilation and in NYHA functional class I or II) after BMC in 1024 patients. (B) Prediction of long-term success after BMC. Assessment of the performance of a 13-point score predicting good late functional results after percutaneous BMC. Observed rates *(colored lines)* with their 95% confidence intervals are shown along with the predicted rates *(black lines)*. (From Bouleti C, Iung B, Laouénan C, et al. Late results of percutaneous mitral commissurotomy up to 20 years: development and validation of a risk score predicting late functional results from a series of 912 patients. Circulation 2012;125:2119-2127.)

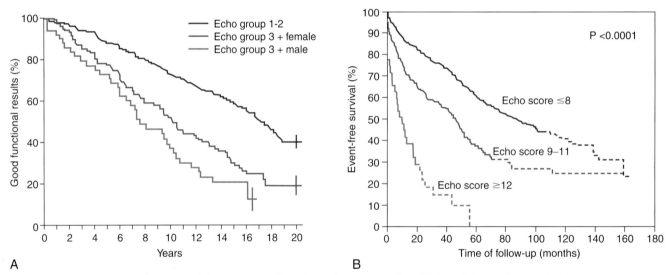

A

B

Fig. 16.11 Outcomes After Balloon Mitral Commissurotomy Stratified by Echocardiographic Morphology Score. (A) Influence of Cormier echocardiographic group. (B) Influence of Wilkins score. (From Bouleti C, Iung B, Laouénan C, et al. Late results of percutaneous mitral commissurotomy up to 20 years: development and validation of a risk score predicting late functional results from a series of 912 patients. Circulation 2012;125:2119-2127; Palacios IF, Sanchez PL, Harrell LC, et al. Which patients benefit from percutaneous mitral balloon valvuloplasty? Prevalvuloplasty and postvalvuloplasty variables that predict long-term outcome. Circulation 2002;105:1465-1471.)

Several randomized studies have compared surgical commissurotomy with BMC, mostly in young patients with favorable characteristics. They consistently showed that BMC is at least comparable to surgical commissurotomy in regard to short-term and midterm follow-up up to 15 years.[138–141] A nonrandomized series comparing BMC with mitral surgery showed no difference in overall survival but a better event-free survival rate for surgery in patients who had unfavorable valve anatomy or were in AF.[142]

Predictors of long-term results. Prediction of long-term results is multifactorial.[77,96,100,104,143] It is based on clinical variables such as age; valve anatomy as assessed by echocardiographic score or the presence of valve calcification; factors related to the evolutional stage of the disease

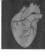

(i.e., a higher NYHA class before BMC); history of previous commissurotomy; severe tricuspid regurgitation; cardiomegaly; AF; high pulmonary vascular resistances; and the results of the procedure (see Table 16.6). Moderate MR after BMC does not consistently predict a poor late outcome.[144,145] However, postprocedural MVA and gradients are strong independent determinants of late functional results. The mitral gradient should be systematically taken into account in conjunction with MVA in the assessment of the results of BMC.[77]

Quality of the late results is considered to be independent of the technique used. Identification of the predictors provides important information for patient selection and is relevant to follow-up. Patients who have good immediate results but who are at high risk for further events must be carefully followed to detect deterioration and allow for timely intervention.

A 13-point score developed by Bouleti and colleagues combines seven variables and enables risk stratification to be easily performed. It is useful for patient information and for planning follow-up (Table 16.7; see Fig. 16.10B).[77]

Applications of Balloon Mitral Commissurotomy in Special Patient Groups

After surgical commissurotomy. In developed countries, recurrent MS is becoming more common than primary MS. BMC is feasible after surgical commissurotomy and significantly improves valve function.[146–148] Long-term outcome is less favorable than for native valves, with a 18% rate of good functional results 20 years after successful BMC for restenosis (Fig. 16.12).[148] However, the possibility of deferring

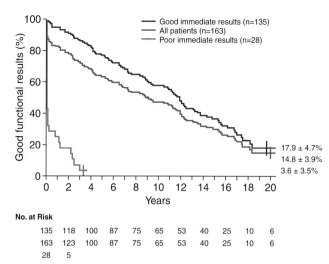

Fig. 16.12 Functional Result of Balloon Mitral Commissurotomy (BMC) for Restenosis. Good functional results (i.e., survival considering cardiovascular-related deaths with no need for mitral surgery or repeat dilatation and in NYHA functional class I or II) after BMC for mitral restenosis after previous commissurotomy in the whole population and according to immediate results. (From Bouleti C, Iung B, Himbert D, et al. Long-term efficacy of percutaneous mitral commissurotomy for restenosis after previous mitral commissurotomy. Heart 2013;99:1336-1341.)

TABLE 16.7 Predictive Factors of Poor Late Functional Results After Good Immediate Results of Balloon Mitral Commissurotomy[a]: Multivariable Analysis and Definition of a 13-Point Predictive Score.

Predictive Factor	Adjusted Hazard Ratio (95% CI)	P	Points for Score (Possible Total = 13)
Age (yr) and final MVA (cm²)			
<50 and MVA ≥ 2.00	1		0
<50 and MVA 1.50–2.00 Or 50–70 and MVA > 1.75	2.1 [1.6–2.9]	<0.0001	2
50–70 and MVA 1.50–1.75 Or ≥70 and MVA ≥1.50	5.1 [3.5–7.5]	<0.0001	5
Valve anatomy and gender			
No valve calcification	1	—	0
Valve calcification			
Female	1.2 [0.9–1.6]	0.18	0
Male	2.3 [1.6–3.2]	<0.0001	3
Rhythm and NYHA class			
Sinus rhythm Or AF and NYHA class I–II	1		0
AF and NYHA class III–IV	1.8 [1.4–2.3]	<0.0001	2
Final mean mitral gradient (mmHg)			
≤3	1		0
3–6	1.1 [1.0–1.8]	0.05	1
≥6	2.5 [1.8–3.5]	<0.0001	3

[a]Valve area ≥1.5 cm² with no regurgitation > 2/4.
AF, Atrial fibrillation; *CI,* confidence interval; *MVA,* mitral valve area; *NYHA,* New York Heart Association.
From Bouleti C, Iung B, Laouenan C, et al. Late results of percutaneous mitral commissurotomy up to 20 years: development and validation of a risk score predicting late functional results from a series of 912 patients. Circulation 2012;125:2119-2127.

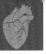

surgery by at least 10 years in one half of the patients enables prosthesis-related complications to be postponed. This is particularly attractive in young patients, who derive the greatest benefit from BMC for restenosis.[148]

Repeat BMC can also be performed for restenosis after a previous BMC in selected patients; the results are better for young patients with mild or no calcification.[125,147] Repeat BMC increases the average 20-year rate of cardiovascular survival without any mitral intervention (i.e., repeat BMC or surgery) after successful BMC from 38% to 46% when considering cardiovascular survival without surgery (Fig. 16.13).[124] The usefulness of repeat BMC is particularly marked in patients younger than 50 years of age, with a 20-year rate of survival without surgery of 57%. Echocardiographic examination must exclude any patients in whom restenosis is mainly caused by valve rigidity without significant commissural refusion (Fig. 16.14).

Patients for whom surgery poses a high risk. Preliminary series have suggested that BMC can be performed safely and effectively in patients with severe pulmonary hypertension.[149,150] In Western countries, patients with MS are older and may have concomitant noncardiac disease, which may also increase the risk of surgery.[31,83,151] BMC can be performed as a lifesaving procedure in critically ill patients[152] as the sole treatment when there is an absolute contraindication to surgery or as a bridge to surgery in other cases. In this context, dramatic improvement has been observed in young

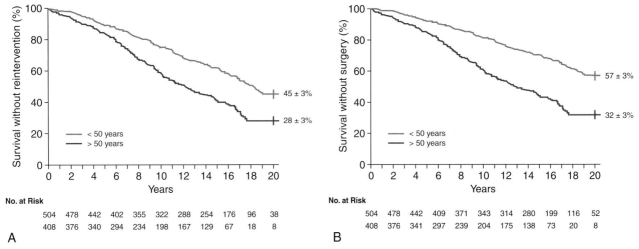

Fig. 16.13 Impact of Repeat Balloon Mitral Commissurotomy (BMC) on Survival Without Intervention. Survival considering cardiovascular-related deaths with no need for mitral intervention (i.e., surgery or repeat dilation) (A) and survival considering cardiovascular-related deaths with no need for mitral surgery (B) in 912 patients who had good immediate results after BMC (valve area ≥ 1.5 cm² and mitral regurgitation ≤ 2/4). (From Bouleti C, Iung B, Himbert D, et al. Reinterventions after percutaneous mitral commissurotomy during long-term follow-up, up to 20 years: the role of repeat percutaneous mitral commissurotomy. Eur Heart J 2013;34:1923-1930.)

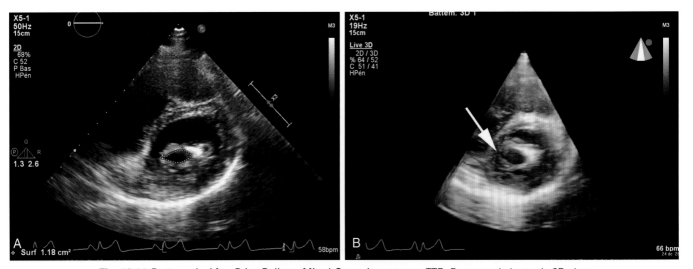

Fig. 16.14 Restenosis After Prior Balloon Mitral Commissurotomy. TTE: Parasternal short-axis 2D view (A) and short-axis 3D view from the left ventricle (B). Valve area is 1.2 cm². The lateral commissure is fused, but there is persistent opening of the medial commissure *(arrow)*.

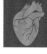

patients; however, the outcome is very poor in elderly patients with end-stage disease, who should probably be better treated conservatively.

In elderly patients, BMC results in moderate but significant improvement in valve function at an acceptable risk, although subsequent functional deterioration frequently occurs.[153–157] BMC is a valid, if only a palliative, treatment for these patients, particularly when the alternative of surgery carries a high risk. In elderly patients with calcified valves, MS of degenerative origin must be excluded before BMC is considered; this requires a thorough analysis of commissures and of the location of calcification.

During pregnancy, changes in cardiac output cause a marked increase in gradient and upstream pressures. Symptomatic MS carries a high risk of maternal and fetal complications in the absence of intervention.[158,159] Surgery under extracorporeal circulation is harmful for the fetus, with a mortality rate of 20% to 30%. BMC can be performed safely during pregnancy; the procedure is effective and results in normal delivery in most cases.[160] BMC should be performed by experienced teams in pregnant women who remain symptomatic despite medical therapy. It should preferably be performed after the 20th week of gestation and with abdominal protection using a shield.[76]

Surgical Mitral Valve Replacement

Surgical MVR is the only option when anatomic conditions preclude surgical commissurotomy or BMC, particularly because of extensive calcification or greater than moderate MR. The operative mortality rate for MVR ranges between 3% and 10% and correlates with age, functional class, pulmonary hypertension, and coronary artery disease.[161,162]

Long-term outcome after valve replacement for rheumatic MS depends on the durability, hemodynamics, and complications of the prosthetic valve; the risks of chronic anticoagulation; any residual anatomic or hemodynamic abnormalities due to MS, such as pulmonary hypertension, LA enlargement, AF, or RV enlargement and dysfunction; and involvement of other valves due to the rheumatic process.

MVR raises particular problems in calcific MS because patients are frequently old and have comorbidities and because of the extent of annular calcification.[4,6] MVR without annular calcium debridement carries a risk of paraprosthetic leak. Complete decalcification and reconstruction of the mitral annulus before placement of the prosthesis is challenging; it increases cardiopulmonary bypass duration and may cause ventricular wall hemorrhage or rupture due to atrioventricular groove disruption.[6,16] CT is useful to assess the extraannular extension of calcium into the myocardium, which increases the difficulty and the risks of surgical debridement.[16]

Nonanatomic implantation of the valve prosthesis has been described in patients with MAC and can include intraatrial implantation or an LA-to-LV apical conduit.[16] These surgical techniques require specific expertise, and it is not possible to compare their safety and effectiveness because of the small size of published series.[6]

Transcatheter Prosthesis Implantation

Transcatheter mitral valve replacement (TMVR) for calcific MS consists in the off-label use of a transcatheter aortic valve replacement prosthesis, which is implanted in the calcified mitral annulus. Experience in treating MAC with MS or MR is limited.[163] Most procedures have used a balloon-expandable prosthesis and a transapical or a transseptal approach. Surgical implantation of the prosthesis under direct vision has also been described.[164]

Preliminary experience shows that TMVR can improve valvular function and clinical status but is associated with substantial morbidity and mortality rates when performed in high-risk patients. In the

largest experience, from a registry of 116 patients with a mean Society of Thoracic Surgeons (STS) short-term risk calculator score of 15.3%, the all-cause mortality rate was 25% at 30 days and 54% at 1 year.[165] In a series of 27 patients with a mean European System for Cardiac Risk Evaluation score (EuroSCORE II) of 7.3%, the rate of all-cause mortality was 11% at 30 days, 42% at 1 year, and 58% at 2 years.[166] The most frequent procedural complication leading to early death was left ventricular outflow tract (LVOT) obstruction, followed by prosthesis migration and perforation.[165]

The feasibility of the procedure should be assessed by echocardiography and ECG-gated CT with intravenous contrast and 3D reconstruction (Fig. 16.15).[6,16] It is necessary to assess the annulus size, the circumferential extent of calcification, and the risk of LVOT obstruction according to aortomitral angle and LV size. LVOT obstruction is the consequence of protrusion of the prosthesis or displacement of the anterior mitral leaflet, or both. Other difficulties include prosthesis sizing and positioning to avoid migration and paraprosthetic leaks.

The transseptal approach has the advantage of being less invasive than the transapical approach but is technically challenging.[16] TMVR is an appealing treatment, but experience is currently limited, and several technical challenges remain to decrease the rates of early morbidity and mortality.

TREATMENT STRATEGY

Rheumatic Mitral Stenosis

In Europe in 2001, BMC was used in more than one third of patients with MS.[1] Other patients were treated by valve replacement, mostly with mechanical prostheses. Surgical commissurotomy was used in less than 5% of patients.

Intervention should be performed only in patients with an MVA smaller than 1.5 cm²; beyond that threshold, the risks probably outweigh the benefits.[37,38] The procedure may be offered to patients with slightly larger valve areas if they have a large stature, are symptomatic with elevated PAP at rest or with exercise, and have favorable presenting characteristics.

Surgery is the only alternative when BMC is contraindicated. The most important contraindication to BMC is LA thrombosis. Results of small series suggest that BMC can be performed under TEE guidance when the thrombus is located in the LA appendage, but there is no convincing evidence that this approach avoids the risk of embolism.[167,168] If the patient is clinically stable, BMC can be attempted if TEE shows that the thrombus has disappeared after 2 to 6 months of treatment with vitamin K antagonists.[169]

Other contraindications for BMC include the following (Table 16.8)[37,38]: (1) MR more than mild (but BMC can be considered in selected patients with moderate MR if the risk for surgery is high or even prohibitive); (2) severe calcification; (3) absence of commissural fusion; and (4) combined MS and severe aortic disease, when surgery is obviously indicated in the absence of contraindications.

BMC can be performed if MS is associated with moderate aortic valve disease to postpone multiple valve surgery. This is particularly the case if there is associated aortic regurgitation, which worsens slowly over time.[170] Combined severe tricuspid stenosis and tricuspid regurgitation with clinical signs of heart failure is an indication for surgery on both valves. The existence of tricuspid regurgitation is not a contraindication to the procedure even though it represents a negative prognostic factor.[171]

Less frequently, coronary disease may favor surgical therapy. In these patients, valve replacement is usually preferred, but open commissurotomy may be performed by experienced teams in young

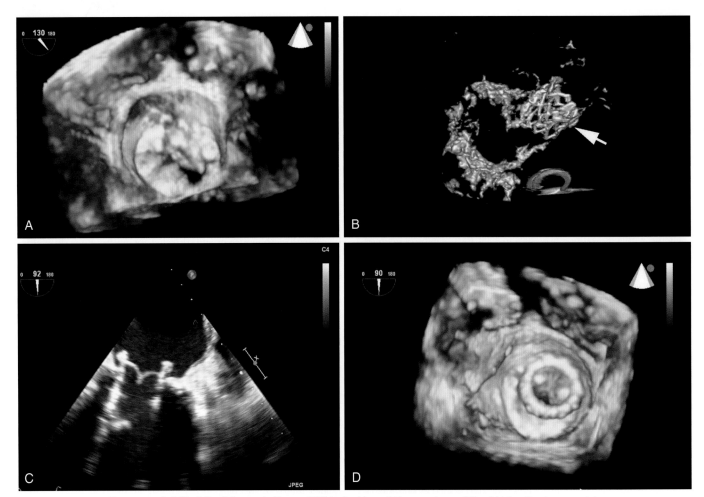

Fig. 16.15 Calcific Mitral Stenosis Treated With the Use of Transcatheter Mitral Valve Replacement in a Patient Who Had Undergone Prior Transcatheter Aortic Valve Replacement. (A) TEE 3D view from the left atrium shows extensive calcification of the mitral annulus. (B) CT 3D reconstruction shows extensive calcification of the mitral annulus and the prosthesis in aortic position (arrow). TEE 2D view (C) and 3D view from the left atrium (D) show a Sapien 3 prosthesis implanted in the stenotic mitral valve.

TABLE 16.8 Contraindications to Balloon Mitral Commissurotomy From ESC/EACTS Guidelines on the Management of Valvular Diseases.

- Mitral valve area > 1.5 cm^2
- Left atrial thrombus
- More than mild mitral regurgitation
- Severe or bicommissural calcification
- Absence of commissural fusion
- Severe concomitant aortic valve disease or severe combined tricuspid stenosis and regurgitation
- Concomitant coronary artery disease requiring bypass surgery

EACTS, European Association for Cardio-Thoracic Surgery; *ESC,* European Society of Cardiology.
From Baumgartner H, Falk V, Bax JJ, et al. 2017 ESC/EACTS guidelines for the management of valvular heart disease. the Task Force for the Management of Valvular Heart Disease of the European Society of Cardiology (ESC) and the European Association for Cardio-Thoracic Surgery (EACTS). Eur Heart J. 2017;38:2739-2791.

patients who are in sinus rhythm, have no or only mild calcification, and have mild to moderate MR.

BMC is the procedure of choice for symptomatic patients who have favorable characteristics such as young age and good anatomy (i.e., pliable valves and moderate subvalvular disease with an echocardiographic score ≤8). These patients are often seen in countries where rheumatic fever is endemic, and the results of BMC are generally excellent (Table 16.9; Figs. 16.16 and 16.17).[172–174] If restenosis occurs, patients treated by BMC often can undergo repeat BMC, avoiding the risk of iterative surgery. BMC is also preferable, at least as a first attempt, for patients for whom surgery carries increased risk, particularly those with severe pulmonary hypertension. BMC is favored as a lifesaving procedure in critically ill patients, in pregnant patients who remain symptomatic despite medical therapy, and in elderly patients as a palliative procedure.

Controversy remains regarding the performance of the procedure in asymptomatic patients and in those with unfavorable anatomy. The level of evidence for performing BMC in asymptomatic patients is low because no randomized comparison exists between the results of BMC and medical therapy for such patients. In these cases, the goal is not to prolong life or to decrease symptoms but rather to prevent

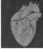

TABLE 16.9 Recommendations for Balloon Mitral Commissurotomy in Symptomatic Patients With Rheumatic Mitral Stenosis.

2014 AHA/ACC Guidelines	2017 ESC/EACTS Guidelines
PMBC is recommended for symptomatic patients with severe MS (MVA ≤ 1.5 cm², stage D) and favorable valve morphology in the absence of left atrial thrombus or moderate to severe mitral regurgitation (I, A)[a] PMBC may be considered for symptomatic patients with MVA > 1.5 cm² if there is evidence of hemodynamically significant MS based on pulmonary wedge pressure > 25 mmHg or mean mitral valve gradient > 15 mmHg during exercise (IIb, C) PMBC may be considered for severely symptomatic patients (NYHA class III to IV) with severe MS (MVA ≤ 1.5 cm², stage D) and a suboptimal valve anatomy who are not candidates for surgery or for whom surgery poses a high risk (IIb, C)	Patients with MS and MVA ≤ 1.5 cm²: • Symptomatic patients without unfavorable characteristics[b] for PMC (I, B) • Symptomatic patients with a contraindication or for whom surgery poses a high risk (I, C) • As initial treatment in symptomatic patients with suboptimal anatomy but no unfavorable clinical characteristics[b] for PMC (IIa, C)

[a]Numbers in parentheses indicate level of recommendation (I, IIa, or IIb) and level of evidence (A, B, or C).
[b]Unfavorable characteristics for PMC can be defined as follows. Clinical characteristics include old age, history of commissurotomy, NYHA class IV, permanent atrial fibrillation, and severe pulmonary hypertension. Anatomic characteristics include echocardiographic score > 8, Cormier score of 3 (calcification of mitral valve of any extent, as assessed by fluoroscopy), very small MVA, and severe tricuspid regurgitation.
ACC, American College of Cardiology; *AHA*, American Heart Association; *EACTS*, European Association for Cardio-Thoracic Surgery; *ESC*, European Society of Cardiology; *MR*, mitral regurgitation; *MS*, mitral stenosis; *MVA*, mitral valve area; *NYHA*, New York Heart Association; *PMC*, percutaneous mitral commissurotomy; *PMBC*, percutaneous mitral balloon commissurotomy.
Data from Baumgartner H, Falk V, Bax JJ, et al. 2017 ESC/EACTS Guidelines for the management of valvular heart disease. The Task Force for the Management of Valvular Heart Disease of the European Society of Cardiology (ESC) and the European Association for Cardio-Thoracic Surgery (EACTS). Eur Heart J. 2017;38:2739-2791; Nishimura RA, Otto CM, Bonow RO, et al. 2014 AHA/ACC guideline for the management of patients with valvular heart disease: a report of the American College of Cardiology/American Heart Association Task Force on Practice Guidelines. J Am Coll Cardiol 2014;63:e57-e185.

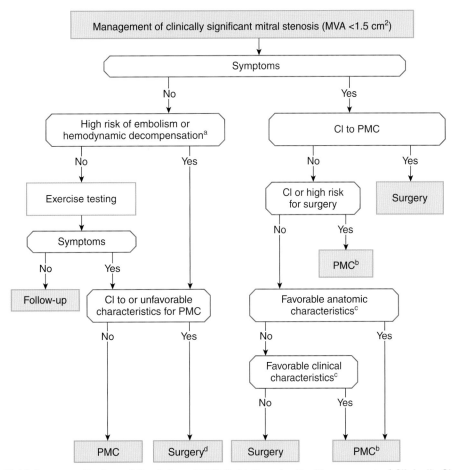

Fig. 16.16 European Society of Cardiology (ESC) Guidelines for the Management of Clinically Significant Mitral Stenosis. *a,* High thromboembolic risk is defined as a history of systemic embolism, dense spontaneous contrast in the left atrium, or new-onset atrial fibrillation. High risk of hemodynamic decompensation is defined as systolic pulmonary pressure greater than 50 mmHg at rest, need for major noncardiac surgery, or desire for pregnancy. *b,* Surgical commissurotomy may be considered by experienced surgical teams or in patients with contraindications to percutaneous mitral commissurotomy *(PMC). c,* Table 16.10 defines unfavorable characteristics. *d,* If symptoms occur with a low level of exercise and operative risk is low. *CI,* Contraindication; *MS,* mitral stenosis; *MVA,* mitral valve area. (From Baumgartner H, Falk V, Bax JJ, et al. 2017 ESC/EACTS Guidelines for the management of valvular heart disease. Eur Heart J 2017;38:2739-2791.)

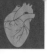

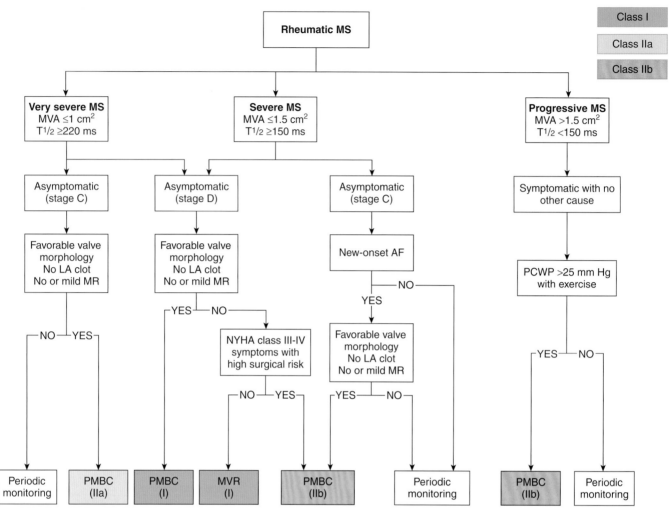

Fig. 16.17 American Heart Association/American College of Cardiology (AHA/ACC) Guidelines for Balloon Mitral Commissurotomy (BMC) in Patients With Mitral Stenosis. BMC is the procedure of choice for symptomatic patients who have favorable characteristics, such as young age and good anatomy (i.e., pliable valves and moderate subvalvular disease with an echocardiographic score ≤ 8). *AF*, Atrial fibrillation; *MR*, mitral regurgitation; *MS*, mitral stenosis; *MVA*, mitral valve area; *MVR*, mitral valve replacement; *NYHA*, New York Health Association; *PCWP*, pulmonary capillary wedge pressure; *PMBC*, percutaneous mitral balloon commissurotomy; *T½*, pressure half-time. (From Nishimura RA, Otto CM, Bonow RO, et al. 2014 AHA/ACC guideline for the management of patients with valvular heart disease: a report of the American College of Cardiology/American Heart Association Task Force on Practice Guidelines. J Am Coll Cardiol. 2014; 63:e57-e185.)

thromboembolism.[132,133] A prospective series reported higher rates of 11-year event-free survival among patients undergoing BMC with NYHA class I–II versus class III–IV designations.[175] The difference remained significant after propensity matching, with a particular benefit for patients at risk for thromboembolic events (i.e., with AF or previous embolic events).[175]

According to current guidelines, BMC should be considered in selected asymptomatic patients with favorable characteristics who are at high risk for thromboembolism (e.g., previous embolism, dense spontaneous contrast in the LA, recurrent atrial arrhythmias) or hemodynamic decompensation, particularly when the systolic PAP is greater than 50 mmHg at rest (Table 16.10; see Figs. 16.16 and 16.17).[37,38] BMC can also be considered for asymptomatic patients who require major extracardiac surgery or to allow for pregnancy.

Indications for BMC remain debated in regard to patients with unfavorable anatomy. For this group, some clinicians favor immediate surgery because of the less satisfying results of BMC, whereas others

prefer BMC as an initial treatment for selected candidates and reserve surgery for patients in whom BMC has failed. No randomized study has been performed examining this issue.

Indications for this subgroup of patients must take into account their heterogeneity with respect to anatomy and clinical status. An individualized approach is favored that allows for the multifactorial nature of prediction. Current opinion is that surgery can be considered the treatment of choice for patients with bicommissural or heavy calcification. However, BMC can be attempted as a first approach in patients with extensive lesions of the subvalvular apparatus or moderate or unicommissural calcification, the more so because their clinical status argues in favor of this. For patients with calcific rheumatic MS who are younger than 50 years of age, BMC provides good functional results with NYHA class I–II features in many cases (i.e., 57% at 10 years and 21% at 20 years) (Fig. 16.18).[176] Differences in long-term outcome with noncalcified valves are less marked when propensity-matched subgroups of patients are compared to account for

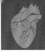

TABLE 16.10 Recommendations for Balloon Mitral Commissurotomy in Asymptomatic Patients With Rheumatic Mitral Stenosis.

2014 AHA/ACC Guidelines	2017 ESC/EACTS Guidelines
PMBC is reasonable for asymptomatic patients with very severe MS (MVA ≤ 1.0 cm², stage C) and favorable valve morphology in the absence of left atrial thrombus or moderate to severe mitral regurgitation (IIa, C)[a] PMBC may be considered for asymptomatic patients with severe MS (MVA ≤ 1.5 cm², stage C) and favorable valve morphology in the absence of left atrial thrombus or moderate to severe MR who have new onset of atrial fibrillation (IIb, C)	Asymptomatic patients with MS and MVA ≤ 1.5 cm² who are without unfavorable clinical and anatomic characteristics for PMC[b] and who have either or both of the following: • High thromboembolic risk (history of systemic embolism, dense spontaneous contrast in the left atrium, new-onset or paroxysmal atrial fibrillation) (IIa, C) • High risk of hemodynamic decompensation (systolic pulmonary pressure >50 mmHg at rest, need for major noncardiac surgery, desire for pregnancy) (IIa, C)

[a]Numbers in parentheses indicate level of recommendation (I, IIa, or IIb) and level of evidence (A, B, or C).
[b]Unfavorable characteristics for PMC can be defined as follows. Clinical characteristics include old age, history of commissurotomy, NYHA class IV, permanent atrial fibrillation, and severe pulmonary hypertension. Anatomic characteristics include echocardiographic score > 8, Cormier score of 3 (calcification of mitral valve of any extent, as assessed by fluoroscopy), very small MVA, and severe tricuspid regurgitation.
ACC, American College of Cardiology; *AHA*, American Heart Association; *EACTS*, European Association for CardioThoracic Surgery; *ESC*, European Society of Cardiology; *MR*, mitral regurgitation; *MS*, mitral stenosis; *MVA*, mitral valve area; *NYHA*, New York Heart Association; *PMC*, percutaneous mitral commissurotomy; *PMBC*, percutaneous mitral balloon commissurotomy.
Data from Baumgartner H, Falk V, Bax JJ, et al. 2017 ESC/EACTS Guidelines for the management of valvular heart disease. The Task Force for the Management of Valvular Heart Disease of the European Society of Cardiology (ESC) and the European Association for Cardio-Thoracic Surgery (EACTS). Eur Heart J. 2017;38:2739-2791; Nishimura RA, Otto CM, Bonow RO, et al. 2014 AHA/ACC guideline for the management of patients with valvular heart disease: a report of the American College of Cardiology/American Heart Association Task Force on Practice Guidelines. J Am Coll Cardiol. 2014;63:e57-e185.

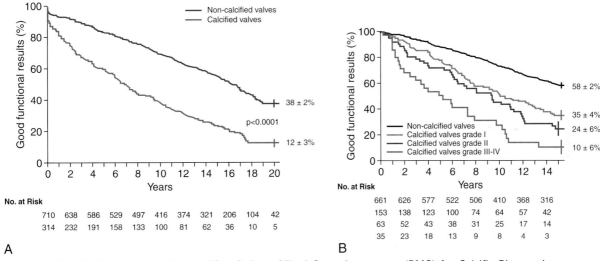

Fig. 16.18 Functional Results After Balloon Mitral Commissurotomy (BMC) for Calcific Rheumatic Mitral Stenosis. Good functional results (i.e., survival considering cardiovascular-related deaths with no need for mitral surgery or repeat dilatation and in NYHA functional class I or II) were obtained after BMC in patents with and without valve calcification (A) and according the extent of valve calcification (B). (From Bouleti C, Iung B, Himbert D, et al. Relationship between valve calcification and long-term results of percutaneous mitral commissurotomy for rheumatic mitral stenosis. Circ Cardiovasc Interv 2014;7:381-389.)

confounding factors.[176] BMC is therefore useful to postpone MVR in selected patients with rheumatic calcific MS. Conversely, there is a much lower likelihood of sustained improvement in older patients who have unfavorable mitral anatomy, tight stenosis, severe symptoms, and AF.[77,96]

AF ablation is more effective than antiarrhythmic drugs in maintaining sinus rhythm in patients with mitral disease requiring intervention. Indications should take into account age and consequences of MS, particularly LA enlargement, and the higher risk of AF recurrence

in MS. In patients with severe MS, ablation should not be considered without treatment of the MS.[17]

Calcific Mitral Stenosis

Medical therapy with the use of diuretics for heart rate control is the first-line treatment of calcific MS. Interventions should be discussed on a case-by-case basis only for patients who have severe symptoms despite medical therapy. Indications for interventions are much more restrictive for calcific MS than for rheumatic MS because both

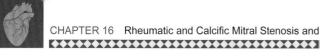

surgical MVR and TMVR are technically complex and associated with high rates of morbidity and mortality (especially because calcific MS most often occurs in elderly patients with comorbidities).[6]

Multimodality imaging is useful for determining the choice of technique. Deep extension of calcification into the myocardium, as assessed by CT, tends to discourage surgical calcium debridement. CT with accurate measurements is also mandatory to assess the feasibility of TMVR and to limit the risk of complications, particularly LVOT obstruction or prosthesis migration.

The potential benefits of surgical MVR and TMVR should be weighed against the risks of these procedures, taking into account the lack of long-term outcome data. No guidelines are available in this field, and these patients should be managed by specialized multidisciplinary teams with all interventional resources available.

The experience acquired with BMC supports a leading role in the treatment of rheumatic MS. BMC and MVR must be considered as complementary techniques. Calcific MS is the subject of growing attention due to the aging of the population and therapeutic innovations, but decision making remains particularly difficult, and continuing evaluation of interventions is needed.

REFERENCES

1. Iung B, Baron G, Butchart EG, et al. A prospective survey of patients with valvular heart disease in Europe: The Euro Heart Survey on Valvular Heart Disease. Eur Heart J 2003;24(13):1231-1243.
2. Nkomo VT, Gardin JM, Skelton TN, et al. Burden of valvular heart diseases: a population-based study. Lancet 2006;368(9540):1005-1011.
3. Kanjanauthai S, Nasir K, Katz R, et al. Relationships of mitral annular calcification to cardiovascular risk factors: the Multi-Ethnic Study of Atherosclerosis (MESA). Atherosclerosis 2010;213(2):558-562.
4. Abramowitz Y, Jilaihawi H, Chakravarty T, et al. Mitral annulus calcification. J Am Coll Cardiol 2015;66(17):1934-1941.
5. Labovitz AJ, Nelson JG, Windhorst DM, et al. Frequency of mitral valve dysfunction from mitral anular calcium as detected by Doppler echocardiography. Am J Cardiol 1985;55(1):133-137.
6. Sud K, Agarwal S, Parashar A, et al. Degenerative mitral stenosis: unmet need for percutaneous interventions. Circulation 2016;133(16):1594-1604.
7. Carapetis JR. Rheumatic heart disease in Asia. Circulation 2008;118(25):2748-2753.
8. Nkomo VT. Epidemiology and prevention of valvular heart diseases and infective endocarditis in Africa. Heart 2007;93(12):1510-1519.
9. Marijon E, Mirabel M, Celermajer DS, Jouven X. Rheumatic heart disease. Lancet 2012;379(9819):953-964.
10. Sliwa K, Carrington M, Mayosi BM, et al. Incidence and characteristics of newly diagnosed rheumatic heart disease in urban African adults: insights from the heart of Soweto study. Eur Heart J 2010;31(6):719-727.
11. Zühlke L, Engel M, Karthikeyan G, et al. Characteristics, complications, and gaps in evidence-based interventions in rheumatic heart disease: the Global Rheumatic Heart Disease Registry (the REMEDY study). Eur Heart J 2015;36(18):1115-1122a.
12. Demirbag R, Sade LE, Aydin M, et al. The Turkish registry of heart valve disease. Turk Kardiyol Dern Ars 2013;41(1):1-10.
13. Roberts WC, Virmani R. Aschoff bodies at necropsy in valvular heart disease. Evidence from an analysis of 543 patients over 14 years of age that rheumatic heart disease, at least anatomically, is a disease of the mitral valve. Circulation 1978;57(4):803-807.
14. Okay T, Deligonul U, Sancaktar O, Kozan O. Contribution of mitral valve reserve capacity to sustained symptomatic improvement after balloon valvulotomy in mitral stenosis: implications for restenosis. J Am Coll Cardiol 1993;22(6):1691-1696.
15. Mejean S, Bouvier E, Bataille V, et al. Mitral annular calcium and mitral stenosis determined by multidetector computed tomography in patients referred for aortic stenosis. Am J Cardiol 2016;118(8):1251-1257.
16. Eleid MF, Foley TA, Said SM, et al. Severe mitral annular calcification: multimodality imaging for therapeutic strategies and interventions. JACC Cardiovasc Imaging 2016;9(11):1318-1337.
17. Iung B, Leenhardt A, Extramiana F. Management of atrial fibrillation in patients with rheumatic mitral stenosis. Heart 2018;104(13):1062-1068.
18. Shaw TR, Northridge DB, Sutaria N. Mitral balloon valvotomy and left atrial thrombus. Heart 2005;91(8):1088-1089.
19. Galiè N, Humbert M, Vachiery J, et al. 2015 ESC/ERS Guidelines for the diagnosis and treatment of pulmonary hypertension: the Joint Task Force for the Diagnosis and Treatment of Pulmonary Hypertension of the European Society of Cardiology (ESC) and the European Respiratory Society (ERS): endorsed by: Association for European Paediatric and Congenital Cardiology (AEPC), International Society for Heart and Lung Transplantation (ISHLT). Eur Heart J 2016;37(1):67-119.
20. Fernandes JL, Sampaio RO, Brandao CM, et al. Comparison of inhaled nitric oxide versus oxygen on hemodynamics in patients with mitral stenosis and severe pulmonary hypertension after mitral valve surgery. Am J Cardiol 2011;107(7):1040-1045.
21. Remetz MS, Cleman MW, Cabin HS. Pulmonary and pleural complications of cardiac disease. Clin Chest Med 1989;10(4):545-592.
22. Otto CM, Davis KB, Reid CL, et al. Relation between pulmonary artery pressure and mitral stenosis severity in patients undergoing balloon mitral commissurotomy. Am J Cardiol 1993;71(10):874-878.
23. Nunes MC, Hung J, Barbosa MM, et al. Impact of net atrioventricular compliance on clinical outcome in mitral stenosis. Circ Cardiovasc Imaging 2013;6(6):1001-1008.
24. Gaasch WH, Folland ED. Left ventricular function in rheumatic mitral stenosis. Eur Heart J 1991;12(Suppl B):66-69.
25. Brochet E, Detaint D, Fondard O, et al. Early hemodynamic changes versus peak values: what is more useful to predict occurrence of dyspnea during stress echocardiography in patients with asymptomatic mitral stenosis? J Am Soc Echocardiogr 2011;24(4):392-398.
26. Schwammenthal E, Vered Z, Agranat O, et al. Impact of atrioventricular compliance on pulmonary artery pressure in mitral stenosis: an exercise echocardiographic study. Circulation 2000;102(19):2378-2384.
27. Laufer-Perl M, Gura Y, Shimiaie J, et al. Mechanisms of effort intolerance in patients with rheumatic mitral stenosis: combined echocardiography and cardiopulmonary stress protocol. JACC Cardiovasc Imaging 2017;10(6):622-633.
28. Li M, Dery JP, Dumesnil JG, et al. Usefulness of measuring net atrioventricular compliance by Doppler echocardiography in patients with mitral stenosis. Am J Cardiol 2005;96(3):432-435.
29. Samiei N, Amirsardari M, Rezaei Y, et al. Echocardiographic evaluation of hemodynamic changes in left-sided heart valves in pregnant women with valvular heart disease. Am J Cardiol 2016;118(7):1046-1052.
30. Shaw TR, Sutaria N, Prendergast B. Clinical and haemodynamic profiles of young, middle aged, and elderly patients with mitral stenosis undergoing mitral balloon valvotomy. Heart 2003;89(12):1430-1436.
31. Iung B, Nicoud-Houel A, Fondard O, et al. Temporal trends in percutaneous mitral commissurotomy over a 15-year period. Eur Heart J 2004;25(8):701-707.
32. Iung B, Vahanian A. Mitral stenosis: patient selection, hemodynamic results, complications and long-term outcome with balloon mitral commissurotomy. In: Otto CM, ed. The practice of clinical echocardiography. 5th ed. Philadelphia: Elsevier; 2017. p. 395-415.
33. Baumgartner H, Hung J, Bermejo J, et al. Echocardiographic assessment of valve stenosis: EAE/ASE recommendations for clinical practice. J Am Soc Echocardiogr 2009;22(1):1-23.
34. Messika-Zeitoun D, Brochet E, Holmin C, et al. Three-dimensional evaluation of the mitral valve area and commissural opening before and after percutaneous mitral commissurotomy in patients with mitral stenosis. Eur Heart J 2007;28(1):72-79.
35. Min SY, Song JM, Kim YJ, et al. Discrepancy between mitral valve areas measured by two-dimensional planimetry and three-dimensional transoesophageal echocardiography in patients with mitral stenosis. Heart 2013;99(4):253-258.
36. de Agustin J, Mejia H, Viliani D, et al. Proximal flow convergence method by three-dimensional color Doppler echocardiography for mitral valve

area assessment in rheumatic mitral stenosis. J Am Soc Echocardiogr 2014;27(8):838-845.

37. Baumgartner H, Falk V, Bax JJ, et al. 2017 ESC/EACTS Guidelines for the management of valvular heart disease. The Task Force for the Management of Valvular Heart Disease of the European Society of Cardiology (ESC) and the European Association for Cardio-Thoracic Surgery (EACTS). Eur Heart J 2017;38(36):2739-2791.

38. Nishimura RA, Otto CM, Bonow RO, et al. 2014 AHA/ACC guideline for the management of patients with valvular heart disease: a report of the American College of Cardiology/American Heart Association Task Force on Practice Guidelines. J Am Coll Cardiol 2014;63(22):e57-e185.

39. Wunderlich NC, Beigel R, Siegel RJ. Management of mitral stenosis using 2D and 3D echo-Doppler imaging. JACC Cardiovasc Imaging 2013;6(11):1191-1205.

40. Wilkins GT, Weyman AE, Abascal VM, et al. Percutaneous balloon dilatation of the mitral valve: an analysis of echocardiographic variables related to outcome and the mechanism of dilatation. Br Heart J 1988;60(4):299-308.

41. Vahanian A, Michel PL, Cormier B, et al. Results of percutaneous mitral commissurotomy in 200 patients. Am J Cardiol 1989;63(12):847-852.

42. Fatkin D, Roy P, Morgan JJ, Feneley MP. Percutaneous balloon mitral valvotomy with the Inoue single-balloon catheter: commissural morphology as a determinant of outcome. J Am Coll Cardiol 1993;21(2):390-397.

43. Cannan CR, Nishimura RA, Reeder GS, et al. Echocardiographic assessment of commissural calcium: a simple predictor of outcome after percutaneous mitral balloon valvotomy. J Am Coll Cardiol 1997;29(1):175-180.

44. Sutaria N, Shaw TR, Prendergast B, Northridge D. Transoesophageal echocardiographic assessment of mitral valve commissural morphology predicts outcome after balloon mitral valvotomy. Heart 2006;92(1):52-57.

45. Rifaie O, Esmat I, Abdel-Rahman M, Nammas W. Can a novel echocardiographic score better predict outcome after percutaneous balloon mitral valvuloplasty? Echocardiography 2009;26(2):119-127.

46. Bhalgat P, Karlekar S, Modani S, et al. Subvalvular apparatus and adverse outcome of balloon valvotomy in rheumatic mitral stenosis. Indian Heart J 2015;67(5):428-433.

47. Padial LR, Freitas N, Sagie A, Newell JB, et al. Echocardiography can predict which patients will develop severe mitral regurgitation after percutaneous mitral valvulotomy. J Am Coll Cardiol 1996;27(5):1225-1231.

48. Nunes MC, Tan TC, Elmariah S, et al. The echo score revisited: impact of incorporating commissural morphology and leaflet displacement to the prediction of outcome for patients undergoing percutaneous mitral valvuloplasty. Circulation 2014;129(8):886-895.

49. Keenan NG, Cueff C, Cimadevilla C, et al. Usefulness of left atrial volume versus diameter to assess thromboembolic risk in mitral stenosis. Am J Cardiol 2010;106(8):1152-1156.

50. Nunes MC, Handschumacher MD, Levine RA, et al. Role of LA shape in predicting embolic cerebrovascular events in mitral stenosis: mechanistic insights from 3D echocardiography. JACC Cardiovasc Imaging 2014;7(5):453-461.

51. Sohrabi B, Kazemi B, Mehryar A, et al. Correlation between pulmonary artery pressure measured by echocardiography and right heart catheterization in patients with rheumatic mitral valve stenosis (a prospective study). Echocardiography 2016;33(1):7-13.

52. Lancellotti P, Tribouilloy C, Hagendorff A, et al. Recommendations for the echocardiographic assessment of native valvular regurgitation: an executive summary from the European Association of Cardiovascular Imaging. Eur Heart J Cardiovasc Imaging 2013;14(7):611-644.

53. Dreyfus J, Durand-Viel G, Raffoul R, et al. Comparison of 2-dimensional, 3-dimensional, and surgical measurements of the tricuspid annulus size: clinical implications. Circ Cardiovasc Imaging 2015;8(7):e003241.

54. Lang R, Badano L, Mor-Avi V, et al. Recommendations for cardiac chamber quantification by echocardiography in adults: an update from the American Society of Echocardiography and the European Association of Cardiovascular Imaging. J Am Soc Echocardiogr 2015;28(1):1-39.e14.

55. Henri C, Pierard LA, Lancellotti P, et al. Exercise testing and stress imaging in valvular heart disease. Can J Cardiol 2014;30(9):1012-1026.

56. Reis G, Motta MS, Barbosa MM, et al. Dobutamine stress echocardiography for noninvasive assessment and risk stratification of patients with rheumatic mitral stenosis. J Am Coll Cardiol 2004;43(3):393-401.

57. Kim SS, Ko SM, Song MG, et al. Quantification of stenotic mitral valve area and diagnostic accuracy of mitral stenosis by dual-source computed tomography in patients with atrial fibrillation: comparison with cardiovascular magnetic resonance and transthoracic echocardiography. Int J Cardiovasc Imaging 2015;31(Suppl 1):203-214.

58. Choi BH, Ko SM, Hwang HK, et al. Detection of left atrial thrombus in patients with mitral stenosis and atrial fibrillation: retrospective comparison of two-phase computed tomography, transoesophageal echocardiography and surgical findings. Eur Radiol 2013;23(11):2944-2953.

59. Segal J, Lerner DJ, Miller DC, et al. When should Doppler-determined valve area be better than the Gorlin formula?: variation in hydraulic constants in low flow states. J Am Coll Cardiol 1987;9(6):1294-1305.

60. Meira ZM, Goulart EM, Colosimo EA, Mota CC. Long term follow up of rheumatic fever and predictors of severe rheumatic valvar disease in Brazilian children and adolescents. Heart 2005;91(8):1019-1022.

61. Marijon E, Iung B, Mocumbi AO, et al. What are the differences in presentation of candidates for percutaneous mitral commissurotomy across the world and do they influence the results of the procedure? Arch Cardiovasc Dis 2008;101(10):611-617.

62. Dubin AA, March HW, Cohn K, Selzer A. Longitudinal hemodynamic and clinical study of mitral stenosis. Circulation 1971;44(3):381-389.

63. Gordon SP, Douglas PS, Come PC, Manning WJ. Two-dimensional and Doppler echocardiographic determinants of the natural history of mitral valve narrowing in patients with rheumatic mitral stenosis: implications for follow-up. J Am Coll Cardiol 1992;19(5):968-973.

64. Sagie A, Freitas N, Padial LR, et al. Doppler echocardiographic assessment of long-term progression of mitral stenosis in 103 patients: valve area and right heart disease. J Am Coll Cardiol 1996;28(2):472-479.

65. Pressman GS, Agarwal A, Braitman LE, Muddassir SM. Mitral annular calcium causing mitral stenosis. Am J Cardiol 2010;105(3):389-391.

66. Rowe JC, Bland EF, Sprague HB, White PD. The course of mitral stenosis without surgery: ten- and twenty-year perspectives. Ann Intern Med 1960;52(741-749.

67. Olesen KH. The natural history of 271 patients with mitral stenosis under medical treatment. Br Heart J 1962;24:349-357.

68. Horstkotte D, Niehues R, Strauer BE. Pathomorphological aspects, aetiology and natural history of acquired mitral valve stenosis. Eur Heart J 1991;12(Suppl B):55-60.

69. Chandrashekhar Y, Westaby S, Narula J. Mitral stenosis. Lancet 2009;374(9697):1271-1283.

70. O'Neal W, Efird J, Nazarian S, et al. Mitral annular calcification and incident atrial fibrillation in the Multi-Ethnic Study of Atherosclerosis. Europace 2015;17(3):358-363.

71. Baddour LM, Wilson WR, Bayer AS, et al. Infective endocarditis in adults: diagnosis, antimicrobial therapy, and management of complications: a scientific statement for healthcare professionals from the American Heart Association. Circulation 2015;132(15):1435-1486.

72. Habib G, Lancellotti P, Antunes MJ, et al. 2015 ESC Guidelines for the management of infective endocarditis: the Task Force for the Management of Infective Endocarditis of the European Society of Cardiology (ESC). Endorsed by: European Association for Cardio-Thoracic Surgery (EACTS), the European Association of Nuclear Medicine (EANM). Eur Heart J 2015;36(44):3075-3128.

73. Patel JJ, Dyer RB, Mitha AS. Beta adrenergic blockade does not improve effort tolerance in patients with mitral stenosis in sinus rhythm. Eur Heart J 1995;16(9):1264-1268.

74. Stoll BC, Ashcom TL, Johns JP, et al. Effects of atenolol on rest and exercise hemodynamics in patients with mitral stenosis. Am J Cardiol 1995;75(7):482-484.

75. Hu CL, Jiang H, Tang QZ, et al. Comparison of rate control and rhythm control in patients with atrial fibrillation after percutaneous mitral balloon valvotomy: a randomised controlled study. Heart 2006;92(8):1096-1101.

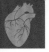
76. Regitz-Zagrosek V, Roos-Hesselink JW, Bauersachs J, et al; ESC Scientific Document Group. 2018 ESC Guidelines for the management of cardiovascular diseases during pregnancy. Eur Heart J 2018 Aug 25. doi: 10.1093/eurheartj/ehy340. [Epub ahead of print]

77. Bouleti C, Iung B, Laouenan C, et al. Late results of percutaneous mitral commissurotomy up to 20 years: development and validation of a risk score predicting late functional results from a series of 912 patients. Circulation 2012;125(17):2119-2127.

78. Rihal CS, Schaff HV, Frye RL, et al. Long-term follow-up of patients undergoing closed transventricular mitral commissurotomy: a useful surrogate for percutaneous balloon mitral valvuloplasty? J Am Coll Cardiol 1992;20(4):781-786.

79. Detter C, Fischlein T, Feldmeier C, et al. Mitral commissurotomy, a technique outdated? Long-term follow-up over a period of 35 years. Ann Thorac Surg 1999;68(6):2112-2118.

80. Reichart DT, Sodian R, Zenker R, et al. Long-term (</=50 years) results of patients after mitral valve commissurotomy-a single-center experience. J Thorac Cardiovasc Surg 2012;143(4 Suppl):S96-S98.

81. Smith WM, Neutze JM, Barratt-Boyes BG, Lowe JB. Open mitral valvotomy. Effect of preoperative factors on result. J Thorac Cardiovasc Surg 1981;82(5):738-751.

82. Inoue K, Owaki T, Nakamura T, et al. Clinical application of transvenous mitral commissurotomy by a new balloon catheter. J Thorac Cardiovasc Surg 1984;87(3):394-402.

83. Nunes M, Nascimento B, Lodi-Junqueira L, et al. Update on percutaneous mitral commissurotomy. Heart 2016;102(7):500-507.

84. Complications and mortality of percutaneous balloon mitral commissurotomy. A report from the National Heart, Lung, and Blood Institute Balloon Valvuloplasty Registry. Circulation 1992;85(6):2014-2024.

85. Tuzcu EM, Block PC, Palacios IF. Comparison of early versus late experience with percutaneous mitral balloon valvuloplasty. J Am Coll Cardiol 1991;17(5):1121-1124.

86. Iung B, Cormier B, Ducimetiere P, et al. Immediate results of percutaneous mitral commissurotomy. A predictive model on a series of 1514 patients. Circulation 1996;94(9):2124-2130.

87. Badheka AO, Shah N, Ghatak A, et al. Balloon mitral valvuloplasty in the United States: a 13-year perspective. Am J Med 2014;127(11):1126e1-1126e12.

88. Stefanadis CI, Stratos CG, Lambrou SG, et al. Retrograde nontransseptal balloon mitral valvuloplasty: immediate results and intermediate long-term outcome in 441 cases—a multicenter experience. J Am Coll Cardiol 1998;32(4):1009-1016.

89. Vahanian A, Himbert D, Brochet E, Iung B. Mitral valvuloplasty. In: Topol EJ, editor. Textbook of interventional cardiology. 7th ed. Philadelphia: Elsevier; 2016. p. 788-797.

90. Farman M, Khan N, Sial J, et al. Predictors of successful percutaneous transvenous mitral commissurotomy using the Bonhoeffer Multi-Track system in patients with moderate to severe mitral stenosis: can we see beyond the Wilkins score? Anatol J Cardiol 2015;15(5):173-179.

91. Cribier A, Eltchaninoff H, Koning R, et al. Percutaneous mechanical mitral commissurotomy with a newly designed metallic valvulotome: immediate results of the initial experience in 153 patients. Circulation 1999;99(6):793-799.

92. Liang KW, Fu YC, Lee WL, et al. Intra-cardiac echocardiography guided trans-septal puncture in patients with dilated left atrium undergoing percutaneous transvenous mitral commissurotomy. Int J Cardiol 2007;117(3):418-421.

93. Arora R, Kalra GS, Singh S, et al. Percutaneous transvenous mitral commissurotomy: immediate and long-term follow-up results. Catheter Cardiovasc Interv 2002;55(4):450-456.

94. Chen CR, Cheng TO. Percutaneous balloon mitral valvuloplasty by the Inoue technique: a multicenter study of 4832 patients in China. Am Heart J 1995;129(6):1197-1203.

95. Neumayer U, Schmidt HK, Fassbender D, et al. Early (three-month) results of percutaneous mitral valvotomy with the Inoue balloon in 1,123 consecutive patients comparing various age groups. Am J Cardiol 2002;90(2):190-193.

96. Palacios IF, Sanchez PL, Harrell LC, et al. Which patients benefit from percutaneous mitral balloon valvuloplasty? Prevalvuloplasty and postvalvuloplasty variables that predict long-term outcome. Circulation 2002;105(12):1465-1471.

97. Ben-Farhat M, Betbout F, Gamra H, et al. Predictors of long-term event-free survival and of freedom from restenosis after percutaneous balloon mitral commissurotomy. Am Heart J 2001;142(6):1072-1079.

98. Hernandez R, Banuelos C, Alfonso F, et al. Long-term clinical and echocardiographic follow-up after percutaneous mitral valvuloplasty with the Inoue balloon. Circulation 1999;99(12):1580-1586.

99. Fawzy ME. Long-term results up to 19 years of mitral balloon valvuloplasty. Asian Cardiovasc Thorac Ann 2009;17(6):627-633.

100. Meneveau N, Schiele F, Seronde MF, et al. Predictors of event-free survival after percutaneous mitral commissurotomy. Heart 1998;80(4):359-364.

101. Tomai F, Gaspardone A, Versaci F, et al. Twenty year follow-up after successful percutaneous balloon mitral valvuloplasty in a large contemporary series of patients with mitral stenosis. Int J Cardiol 2014;177(3):881-885.

102. Eltchaninoff H, Koning R, Derumeaux G, Cribier A. [Percutaneous mitral commissurotomy by metallic dilator. Multicenter experience with 500 patients]. Arch Mal Coeur Vaiss 2000;93(6):685-692.

103. Lee S, Kang DH, Kim DH, et al. Late outcome of percutaneous mitral commissurotomy: randomized comparison of Inoue versus double-balloon technique. Am Heart 2017;194(12):1-8.104.

104. Meneguz-Moreno RA, Costa JR Jr, Gomes NL, et al. Very long term follow-up after percutaneous balloon mitral valvuloplasty. JACC Cardiovasc Interv 2018 Jul 27. pii: S1936-8798(18)31204-4. doi: 10.1016/j.jcin.2018.05.039. [Epub ahead of print]

105. Krishnamoorthy KM, Dash PK, Radhakrishnan S, Shrivastava S. Response of different grades of pulmonary artery hypertension to balloon mitral valvuloplasty. Am J Cardiol 2002;90(10):1170-1173.

106. Tanabe Y, Oshima M, Suzuki M, Takahashi M. Determinants of delayed improvement in exercise capacity after percutaneous transvenous mitral commissurotomy. Am Heart J 2000;139(5):889-894.

107. Acar C, Jebara VA, Grare P, et al. Traumatic mitral insufficiency following percutaneous mitral dilation: anatomic lesions and surgical implications. Eur J Cardiothorac Surg 1992;6(12):660-663.

108. Choudhary SK, Talwar S, Venugopal P. Severe mitral regurgitation after percutaneous transmitral commissurotomy: underestimated subvalvular disease. J Thorac Cardiovasc Surg 2006;131(4):927; author reply 927-928.

109. Varma PK, Theodore S, Neema PK, et al. Emergency surgery after percutaneous transmitral commissurotomy: operative versus echocardiographic findings, mechanisms of complications, and outcomes. J Thorac Cardiovasc Surg 2005;130(3):772-776.

110. Zimmet AD, Almeida AA, Harper RW, et al. Predictors of surgery after percutaneous mitral valvuloplasty. Ann Thorac Surg 2006;82(3):828-833.

111. Nanjappa MC, Ananthakrishna R, Hemanna Setty S, et al. Acute severe mitral regurgitation following balloon mitral valvotomy: echocardiographic features, operative findings, and outcome in 50 surgical cases. Catheter Cardiovasc Interv 2013;81(4):603-608.

112. Manjunath CN, Panneerselvam A, Srinivasa KH, et al. Incidence and predictors of atrial septal defect after percutaneous transvenous mitral commissurotomy - a transesophageal echocardiographic study of 209 cases. Echocardiography 2013;30(2):127-130.

113. Herrmann HC, Ramaswamy K, Isner JM, et al. Factors influencing immediate results, complications, and short-term follow-up status after Inoue balloon mitral valvotomy: a North American multicenter study. Am Heart J 1992;124(1):160-166.

114. Feldman T, Carroll JD, Isner JM, et al. Effect of valve deformity on results and mitral regurgitation after Inoue balloon commissurotomy. Circulation 1992;85(1):180-187.

115. Cruz-Gonzalez I, Sanchez-Ledesma M, Sanchez PL, et al. Predicting success and long-term outcomes of percutaneous mitral valvuloplasty: a multifactorial score. Am J Med 2009;122(6):581 e511-589.

116. Song JK, Song JM, Kang DH, et al. Restenosis and adverse clinical events after successful percutaneous mitral valvuloplasty: immediate post-procedural mitral valve area as an important prognosticator. Eur Heart J 2009;30(10):1254-1262.

117. Wang A, Krasuski RA, Warner JJ, et al. Serial echocardiographic evaluation of restenosis after successful percutaneous mitral commissurotomy. J Am Coll Cardiol 2002;39(2):328-334.

118. Cohen DJ, Kuntz RE, Gordon SP, et al. Predictors of long-term outcome after percutaneous balloon mitral valvuloplasty. N Engl J Med 1992; 327(19):1329-1335.

119. Orrange SE, Kawanishi DT, Lopez BM, et al. Actuarial outcome after catheter balloon commissurotomy in patients with mitral stenosis. Circulation 1997;95(2):382-389.

120. Pathan AZ, Mahdi NA, Leon MN, et al. Is redo percutaneous mitral balloon valvuloplasty (PMV) indicated in patients with post-PMV mitral restenosis? J Am Coll Cardiol 1999;34(1):49-54.

121. Kim JB, Ha JW, Kim JS, et al. Comparison of long-term outcome after mitral valve replacement or repeated balloon mitral valvotomy in patients with restenosis after previous balloon valvotomy. Am J Cardiol 2007;99(11):1571-1574.

122. Turgeman Y, Atar S, Suleiman K, et al. Feasibility, safety, and morphologic predictors of outcome of repeat percutaneous balloon mitral commissurotomy. Am J Cardiol 2005;95(8):989-991.

123. Chmielak Z, Klopotowski M, Kruk M, et al. Repeat percutaneous mitral balloon valvuloplasty for patients with mitral valve restenosis. Catheter Cardiovasc Interv 2010;76(7):986-992.

124. Yazicioglu N, Arat Ozkan A, Orta Kilickesmez K, et al. Immediate and follow-up results of repeat percutaneous mitral balloon commissurotomy for restenosis after a succesful first procedure. Echocardiography 2010;27(7):765-769.

125. Bouleti C, Iung B, Himbert D, et al. Reinterventions after percutaneous mitral commissurotomy during long-term follow-up, up to 20 years: the role of repeat percutaneous mitral commissurotomy. Eur Heart J 2013;34(25):1923-1930.

126. Stefanadis C, Dernellis J, Stratos C, et al. Effects of balloon mitral valvuloplasty on left atrial function in mitral stenosis as assessed by pressure-area relation. J Am Coll Cardiol 1998;32(1):159-168.

127. Cormier B, Vahanian A, Iung B, et al. Influence of percutaneous mitral commissurotomy on left atrial spontaneous contrast of mitral stenosis. Am J Cardiol 1993;71(10):842-847.

128. Porte JM, Cormier B, Iung B, et al. Early assessment by transesophageal echocardiography of left atrial appendage function after percutaneous mitral commissurotomy. Am J Cardiol 1996;77(1):72-76.

129. Zaki A, Salama M, El Masry M, et al. Immediate effect of balloon valvuloplasty on hemostatic changes in mitral stenosis. Am J Cardiol 2000; 85(3):370-375.

130. Chen MC, Wu CJ, Chang HW, et al. Mechanism of reducing platelet activity by percutaneous transluminal mitral valvuloplasty in patients with rheumatic mitral stenosis. Chest 2004;125(5):1629-1634.

131. Vieira M, Silva M, Wagner C, et al. Left atrium reverse remodeling in patients with mitral valve stenosis after percutaneous valvuloplasty: a 2- and 3-dimensional echocardiographic study. Rev Esp Cardiol 2013; 66(1):17-23.

132. Chiang CW, Lo SK, Ko YS, et al. Predictors of systemic embolism in patients with mitral stenosis. A prospective study. Ann Intern Med 1998; 128(11):885-889.

133. Liu TJ, Lai HC, Lee WL, et al. Percutaneous balloon commissurotomy reduces incidence of ischemic cerebral stroke in patients with symptomatic rheumatic mitral stenosis. Int J Cardiol 2008;123(2):189-190.

134. Krasuski RA, Assar MD, Wang A, et al. Usefulness of percutaneous balloon mitral commissurotomy in preventing the development of atrial fibrillation in patients with mitral stenosis. Am J Cardiol 2004;93(7): 936-939.

135. Leon MN, Harrell LC, Simosa HF, et al. Mitral balloon valvotomy for patients with mitral stenosis in atrial fibrillation: immediate and long-term results. J Am Coll Cardiol 1999;34(4):1145-1152.

136. Fan K, Lee KL, Chow WH, et al. Internal cardioversion of chronic atrial fibrillation during percutaneous mitral commissurotomy: insight into reversal of chronic stretch-induced atrial remodeling. Circulation 2002;105(23):2746-2752.

137. Krittayaphong R, Chotinaiwatarakul C, Phankingthongkum R, et al. One-year outcome of cardioversion of atrial fibrillation in patients with

138. Turi ZG, Reyes VP, Raju BS, et al. Percutaneous balloon versus surgical closed commissurotomy for mitral stenosis. A prospective, randomized trial. Circulation 1991;83(4):1179-1185.

139. Reyes VP, Raju BS, Wynne J, et al. Percutaneous balloon valvuloplasty compared with open surgical commissurotomy for mitral stenosis. N Engl J Med 1994;331(15):961-967.

140. Ben Farhat M, Ayari M, Maatouk F, et al. Percutaneous balloon versus surgical closed and open mitral commissurotomy: seven-year follow-up results of a randomized trial. Circulation 1998;97(3):245-250.

141. Rifaie O, Abdel-Dayem MK, Ramzy A, et al. Percutaneous mitral valvotomy versus closed surgical commissurotomy. Up to 15 years of follow-up of a prospective randomized study. J Cardiol 2009;53(1):28-34.

142. Song JK, Kim MJ, Yun SC, et al. Long-term outcomes of percutaneous mitral balloon valvuloplasty versus open cardiac surgery. J Thorac Cardiovasc Surg 2010;139(1):103-110.

143. Langerveld J, Thijs Plokker HW, Ernst SM, et al. Predictors of clinical events or restenosis during follow-up after percutaneous mitral balloon valvotomy. Eur Heart J 1999;20(7):519-526.

144. Jneid H, Cruz-Gonzalez I, Sanchez-Ledesma M, et al. Impact of pre- and postprocedural mitral regurgitation on outcomes after percutaneous mitral valvuloplasty for mitral stenosis. Am J Cardiol 2009;104(8): 1122-1127.

145. Iung B, Garbarz E, Michaud P, et al. Late results of percutaneous mitral commissurotomy in a series of 1024 patients. Analysis of late clinical deterioration: frequency, anatomic findings, and predictive factors. Circulation 1999;99(25):3272-3278.

146. Jang IK, Block PC, Newell JB, et al. Percutaneous mitral balloon valvotomy for recurrent mitral stenosis after surgical commissurotomy. Am J Cardiol 1995;75(8):601-605.

147. Fawzy ME, Hassan W, Shoukri M, et al. Immediate and long-term results of mitral balloon valvotomy for restenosis following previous surgical or balloon commissurotomy. Am J Cardiol 2005;96(7):971-975.

148. Bouleti C, Iung B, Himbert D, et al. Long-term efficacy of percutaneous mitral commissurotomy for restenosis after previous mitral commissurotomy. Heart 2013;99(18):1336-1341.

149. Umesan CV, Kapoor A, Sinha N, et al. Effect of Inoue balloon mitral valvotomy on severe pulmonary arterial hypertension in 315 patients with rheumatic mitral stenosis: immediate and long-term results. J Heart Valve Dis 2000;9(5):609-615.

150. Maoqin S, Guoxiang H, Zhiyuan S, et al. The clinical and hemodynamic results of mitral balloon valvuloplasty for patients with mitral stenosis complicated by severe pulmonary hypertension. Eur J Intern Med 2005;16(6):413-418.

151. Iung B, Baron G, Tornos P, et al. Valvular heart disease in the community: a European experience. Curr Probl Cardiol 2007;32(11):609-661.

152. Goldman JH, Slade A, Clague J. Cardiogenic shock secondary to mitral stenosis treated by balloon mitral valvuloplasty. Cathet Cardiovasc Diagn 1998;43(2):195-197.

153. Tuzcu EM, Block PC, Griffin BP, et al. Immediate and long-term outcome of percutaneous mitral valvotomy in patients 65 years and older. Circulation 1992;85(3):963-971.

154. Iung B, Cormier B, Farah B, et al. Percutaneous mitral commissurotomy in the elderly. Eur Heart J 1995;16(8):1092-1099.

155. Hildick-Smith DJ, Taylor GJ, Shapiro LM. Inoue balloon mitral valvuloplasty: long-term clinical and echocardiographic follow-up of a predominantly unfavourable population. Eur Heart J 2000;21(20):1690-1697.

156. Sutaria N, Elder AT, Shaw TR. Long term outcome of percutaneous mitral balloon valvotomy in patients aged 70 and over. Heart 2000;83(4): 433-438.

157. Chmielak Z, Klopotowski M, Demkow M, et al. Percutaneous mitral balloon valvuloplasty beyond 65 years of age. Cardiol J 2013;20(1): 44-51.

158. Diao M, Kane A, Ndiaye MB, et al. Pregnancy in women with heart disease in sub-Saharan Africa. Arch Cardiovasc Dis 2011;104(6-7):370-374.

159. van Hagen IM, Thorne SA, Taha N, et al; ROPAC Investigators and EORP Team. Pregnancy outcomes in women with rheumatic mitral valve

disease: results from the registry of pregnancy and cardiac disease. Circulation 2018;137(8): 806-816.

160. Hameed AB, Mehra A, Rahimtoola SH. The role of catheter balloon commissurotomy for severe mitral stenosis in pregnancy. Obstet Gynecol 2009;114(6):1336-1340.

161. O'Brien SM, Shahian DM, Filardo G, et al. The Society of Thoracic Surgeons 2008 cardiac surgery risk models: part 2—isolated valve surgery. Ann Thorac Surg 2009;88(1 Suppl):S23-S42.

162. Rankin JS, Hammill BG, Ferguson TB, Jr., et al. Determinants of operative mortality in valvular heart surgery. J Thorac Cardiovasc Surg 2006;131(3):547-557.

163. Himbert D, Bouleti C, Iung B, et al. Transcatheter valve replacement in patients with severe mitral valve disease and annular calcification. J Am Coll Cardiol 2014;64(23):2557-2558.

164. Murashita T, Suri R, Daly R. Sapien XT transcatheter mitral valve replacement under direct vision in the setting of significant mitral annular calcification. Ann Thorac Surg 2016;101(3):1171-1174.

165. Guerrero M, Urena M, Himbert D, et al. 1-Year outcomes of transcatheter mitral valve replacement in patients with severe mitral annular calcification. J Am Coll Cardiol 2018;71(17):1841-1853.

166. Urena M, Brochet E, Lecomte M, et al. Clinical and haemodynamic outcomes of balloon-expandable transcatheter mitral valve implantation: a 7-year experience. Eur Heart 2018;39(28):2679-2689.

167. Chen WJ, Chen MF, Liau CS, et al. Safety of percutaneous transvenous balloon mitral commissurotomy in patients with mitral stenosis and thrombus in the left atrial appendage. Am J Cardiol 1992;70(1):117-119.

168. Liu Y, Guo GL, Wen B, et al. Feasibility and effectiveness of percutaneous balloon mitral valvuloplasty under echocardiographic guidance only.

Echocardiography 2018 Jun 19. doi: 10.1111/echo.14055. [Epub ahead of print]

169. Silaruks S, Thinkhamrop B, Kiatchoosakun S, et al. Resolution of left atrial thrombus after 6 months of anticoagulation in candidates for percutaneous transvenous mitral commissurotomy. Ann Intern Med 2004;140(2):101-105.

170. Vaturi M, Porter A, Adler Y, et al. The natural history of aortic valve disease after mitral valve surgery. J Am Coll Cardiol 1999;33(7): 2003-2008.

171. Song H, Kang DH, Kim JH, et al. Percutaneous mitral valvuloplasty versus surgical treatment in mitral stenosis with severe tricuspid regurgitation. Circulation 2007;116(11 Suppl):I246-I250.

172. Gamra H, Betbout F, Ben Hamda K, et al. Balloon mitral commissurotomy in juvenile rheumatic mitral stenosis: a ten-year clinical and echocardiographic actuarial results. Eur Heart J 2003;24(14):1349-1356.

173. Fawzy ME, Stefadouros MA, Hegazy H, et al. Long term clinical and echocardiographic results of mitral balloon valvotomy in children and adolescents. Heart 2005;91(6):743-748.

174. Kothari SS, Ramakrishnan S, Kumar CK, et al. Intermediate-term results of percutaneous transvenous mitral commissurotomy in children less than 12 years of age. Catheter Cardiovasc Interv 2005;64(4):487-490.

175. Kang DH, Lee CH, Kim DH, et al. Early percutaneous mitral commissurotomy vs. conventional management in asymptomatic moderate mitral stenosis. Eur Heart J 2012;33(12):1511-1517.

176. Bouleti C, Iung B, Himbert D, et al. Relationship between valve calcification and long-term results of percutaneous mitral commissurotomy for rheumatic mitral stenosis. Circ Cardiovasc Interv 2014;7(3): 381-389.

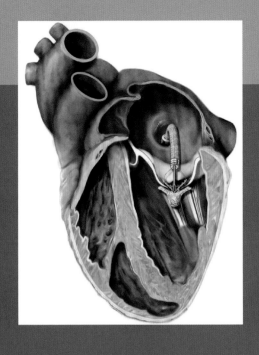

第17章
二尖瓣脱垂

　　二尖瓣脱垂是西方国家原发性二尖瓣反流的最常见病因，其人群患病率约为2.4%。二尖瓣脱垂是指由于腱索和（或）瓣膜延长导致的瓣叶延长，进而导致收缩期二尖瓣瓣叶活动度增大的瓣膜解剖学和功能学异常。一般情况下，超声心动图发现心脏收缩期瓣叶摆动幅度超过二尖瓣瓣环上≥2 mm则可诊断二尖瓣脱垂。多种疾病均可导致二尖瓣脱垂，包括纤维弹性缺陷症（可累及单一的瓣叶节段，以二尖瓣后叶P2区的局部脱垂较为常见）、广泛的黏液样变性疾病（如Balow氏病，弥漫累及两个瓣叶的多个节段，其解剖学异常以腱索延长、瓣叶增厚松软为主要表现）。有研究表明，二尖瓣脱垂具有家族聚集性。然而，黏液样变性相关的基因突变尚不十分明确。二尖瓣脱垂的解剖学改变主要与二尖瓣反流的程度、左心室和左心房的解剖学和功能学改变（如左室射血分数、左心室收缩末期内径、左房扩大、心房颤动）、肺动脉压增高等相关，但与预后的相关性较小。二尖瓣脱垂增加恶性心律失常和猝死风险，双瓣叶脱垂、黏液瘤样瓣叶增厚、瓣环撕裂可能与心肌纤维化密切相关，后者可诱发室性心律失常。若患者出现左心室扩大（如左心室收缩末期内径≥40～45 mm）、左心室功能异常（如左室射血分数≤60%）、心房颤动（即使是阵发性）的相关症状，则应尽快请外科医师评估有无手术指征。对于无症状的重度二尖瓣反流患者，应行运动负荷试验以进一步明确是否可诱发心力衰竭症状。对于左室射血分数保留且处于窦性心律的无症状性重度二尖瓣反流患者，是否应该干预仍存在争议。虽然缺乏随机对照试验证据，但越来越多的研究表明，早期手术能够使患者获益。对于外科手术低风险且二尖瓣解剖结构合适的患者，可考虑在有经验的瓣膜中心接受外科瓣膜手术治疗。

张而立

Mitral Valve Prolapse

David Messika-Zeitoun, Maurice Enriquez-Sarano

KEY POINTS

- The estimated prevalence of mitral valve prolapse (MVP) for the general population is 2.4%.
- The term *mitral valve prolapse* refers to leaflet prolapse resulting from an elongated chorda and/or leaflet. It is usually diagnosed with the use of echocardiography as excessive systolic movement of a leaflet (≥ 2 mm) beyond the level of the saddle-shaped annulus.
- Anatomic lesions encompass a wide spectrum of disease, from fibro-elastic deficiency (i.e., disease localized to an isolated segment lesion, usually the middle scallop of the posterior leaflet) to extensive myxomatous disease (i.e., Barlow disease) with diffuse disease in bileaflet segments that are thickened and floppy with elongated chordae.
- Familial clustering of MVP has been reported, but identification of mutations associated with myxomatous degeneration has remained elusive.
- Mitral valve anatomy has little impact on outcome, which correlates much more with mitral regurgitation severity (ideally assessed quantitatively) and its effects on the left ventricle (i.e., ejection fraction [EF] or end-systolic diameter), left atrium (i.e., enlargement and atrial fibrillation), pulmonary artery pressure, and functional impairment.

- MVP is associated with an increased risk of malignant arrhythmia and sudden death. Bileaflet prolapse, myxomatous mitral valve with thickened leaflet, and mitral annular disjunction may be responsible for localized myocardial fibrosis that can trigger ventricular arrhythmias.
- Patients with symptoms such as left ventricular enlargement (i.e., end-systolic diameter ≥ 40–45 mm) or dysfunction (i.e., EF $\leq 60\%$), systolic pulmonary hypertension (≥ 50 mmHg at rest), or atrial fibrillation (even if paroxysmal) should be promptly referred for surgery.
- An exercise stress test is recommended for allegedly asymptomatic patients to unveil symptoms.
- Indications for intervention in asymptomatic patients with preserved EF in sinus rhythm are disputed because of the absence of large randomized, controlled trials, but there is increasing evidence favoring early surgery. Surgery may be considered for those who have a low surgical risk and favorable anatomy when it can be performed in expert valve centers.

Mitral valve prolapse (MVP) is the leading cause of organic mitral regurgitation (MR) in Western countries and is associated with increased morbidity and mortality, especially when severe MR is left untreated and not appropriately and timely managed. MVP is a disease of the extracellular matrix with a possible genetic component, although this has not been completely elucidated. It can manifest with markedly different phenotypes, such as the extreme form called Barlow disease. This chapter describes MVP epidemiology, pathogenesis, clinical presentation, evaluation, and management, including intervention.

DEFINITION AND ANATOMY

The term *mitral valve prolapse* refers to leaflet prolapse resulting from an elongated chorda and/or leaflet. It is usually diagnosed with the use of echocardiography. The common definition is excessive systolic movement of a leaflet (≥ 2 mm) beyond the level of the saddle-shaped annulus (Fig. 17.1; Video 17.1A ▶). Flail leaflets are caused by rupture of the chordae and are defined as eversion and systolic movement of the leaflet tip into the left atrium (LA) with complete failure of leaflet cooptation (Video 17.1B ▶).

MVP corresponds to a type II mitral valve (MV) lesion, according to the classification of Carpentier. The importance of the prolapse and of a possible associated rupture of chordae determines the degree of systolic malcoaptation and therefore MR existence and severity. A flail leaflet is usually responsible for severe MR.

The term *degenerative mitral valve disease* is often used interchangeably with MVP. In contrast, *myxomatous disease* relates to the tissue characteristics of leaflet thickening and chordae and tissue

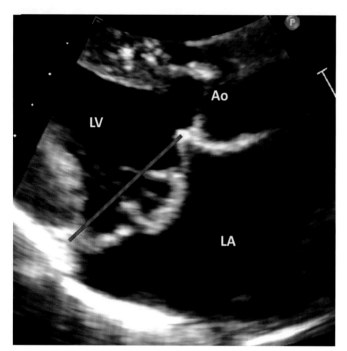

Fig. 17.1 Echocardiographic Diagnosis of Mitral Valve Prolapse. TTE parasternal long-axis view shows a displacement equal to or greater than 2 mm of the mitral valve leaflets beyond the plane of the mitral annulus *(red line)* (Videos 17.1A ⊙ and 17.1B ⊙). *Ao,* Aorta; *LA,* left atrium; *LV,* left ventricle.

predictability of mitral repair. However, the decision-making process mainly relies (in addition to functional status) on the assessment of MR severity and its effects on the left-sided chambers and pulmonary artery pressure (PAP).

The MV apparatus is composed of two leaflets attached through chordae to the anterolateral and posterolateral papillary muscles. Both leaflets are attached to the mitral annulus. The anterior valve is usually larger but is attached to only about one third of the annulus circumference, contiguous to the aortomitral curtain; the smaller posterior valve is attached to the remaining posterior two thirds of the annulus circumference. The MV annulus is nonplanar and saddle-shaped with posterior and anterior peaks.[1] Three-dimensional (3D) modeling studies have shown that the mitral annulus is a dynamic structure[2] and that this activity is profoundly abnormal in Barlow disease compared with fibroelastic deficiency.[3]

Each leaflet is usually divided into three segments (i.e., lateral, middle, and medial). For the posterior leaflet, this division relies on a true anatomic segmentation. Incisures or clefts of varied depth divide the leaflet into three individual scallops (i.e., P1, P2, and P3 from lateral to medial). There are no similar anatomic features for the anterior leaflet, which is usually a single structure. The segments directly facing P1, P2, and P3 are named A1, A2, and A3, respectively. The regions joining the two leaflets are the anterolateral and posteromedial commissures. According to the Carpentier classification, eight segments are individually identified (Fig. 17.3). However, wide variations exist, and especially in Barlow disease, segmentation may be more complex, with additional scallops exceeding the conventional nomenclature.

The surface of the anterior and posterior leaflets is significantly larger than the surface of the mitral annulus; therefore, coaptation between the two leaflets does not occur at the level of the edges of each leaflet but through 7 to 10 mm of their atrial side. This reserve of coaptation explains why an isolated annular dilation is usually insufficient to cause significant MR.[4] The anterolateral papillary muscle provides chordae to the lateral half of the anterior leaflet and the posterior leaflet, whereas the posterolateral papillary muscle provides chordae to the medial half of the anterior leaflet and the posterior leaflet. Three types of chordae can be individualized: primary chordae attached to the leaflets' edge, secondary chordae attached to the ventricular surface of the leaflets, and tertiary chordae arising from the ventricular trabeculae and inserting into the posterior annulus.

redundancy. The anatomic lesions encompass a wide disease spectrum, from fibroelastic deficiency (i.e., disease localized to an isolated segment lesion, usually the middle scallop of the posterior leaflet) to extensive myxomatous disease (i.e., Barlow disease) with diffuse disease in bileaflet segments that are thickened and floppy with elongated chordae. However, there is a continuum between these two conditions (Fig. 17.2). Barlow disease is also associated with a large annulus, suggesting involvement of the mitral annular tissue in the disease process.

A very large annulus in some patients may affect the surgical technique. The extent of disease may play a role in the management of MVP, especially in asymptomatic patients in regard to the

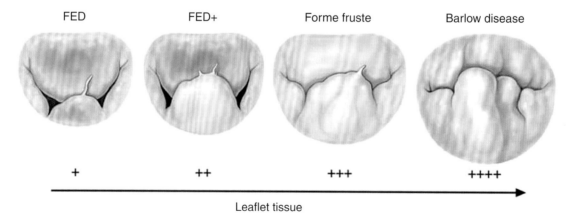

Fig. 17.2 Spectrum of Degenerative Mitral Disease. The spectrum of mitral valve prolapse ranges from fibroelastic deficiency *(FED),* in which disease is localized to an isolated segment lesion, to extensive myxomatous disease (i.e., Barlow disease) with diffuse disease in bileaflet segments that are thickened and floppy with elongated chordae, and to intermediate forms. (From Adams DH, Rosenhek R, Falk V. Degenerative mitral valve regurgitation: best practice revolution. Eur Heart J 2010;31:1958-1966.)

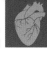

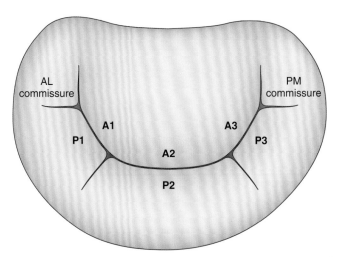

Fig. 17.3 Mitral Valve Segmentation. An *en-face* surgical view of the mitral valve from the left atrium. *A*, Anterior valve; *AL*, anterolateral; *P*, posterior valve; *PM*, posteromedial. (From Messika-Zeitoun D, Topilsky Y, Enriquez-Sarano M. The role of echocardiography in the management of patients with myxomatous disease. Cardiol Clin 2013;31:217-229.)

PATHOGENESIS

An important step in understanding MVP pathogenesis was the demonstration that the MV is not a passive element but an actor capable of biologic and consequently phenotypic changes (i.e., MV plasticity). The mitral leaflet is a complex structure with important 3D variations in components and biomechanical properties.

Each leaflet is composed of three layers: the atrialis, the spongiosa, and the fibrosa/ventricularis. They are covered on both sides with an endothelial layer (Fig. 17. 4).[5] Each layer has a different thickness and matrix composition, and these characteristics change radially from the basal part of the leaflet inserted on the annulus to the free edge. Quiescent noncontractile valvular interstitial cells exist in the deep subendocardial layers. These cells originate from endocardial cells and contribute to the homeostatic remodeling of the extracellular matrix. There is an important interplay between the biology and composition of the extracellular matrix and the biomechanical properties of the tissue. Myxomatous degeneration is caused by a default in the normal leaflets' extracellular matrix regeneration process, with an imbalance toward excessive catabolism and pathologic tissue remodeling. More details are provided in the works of Levine et al[6] and Delling and Vasan.[7]

Identification of mutations associated with myxomatous degeneration has remained elusive. Such identifications are crucial to better understand the pathogenesis of MVP and to elucidate pathways and targets that are potentially modifiable with the use of therapeutic agents.

MVP can occur in several inherited connective tissue disorders, including Marfan syndrome (i.e., syndromic MVP). Marfan syndrome results from a mutation in the fibrillin 1 gene *(FBN1)*, and these patients often have Barlow-like MV disease. Much evidence shows that Marfan syndrome is associated with increased transforming growth factor-β (TGF-β) activation and signaling.

A few other mutations, both X-linked (i.e., mutation in the filamin A *[FLNA]* gene) and autosomal, have been described.[8–14] Familial clustering of MVP has been reported, and MVP heritability may have been underestimated due to underrecognition and lack of systematic screening in families of probands with MVP.[15] However, penetrance may vary, and expression is influenced by environmental factors that need to be identified. More work needs to be done to ascertain whether fibroelastic deficiency and Barlow disease are different phenotypes of

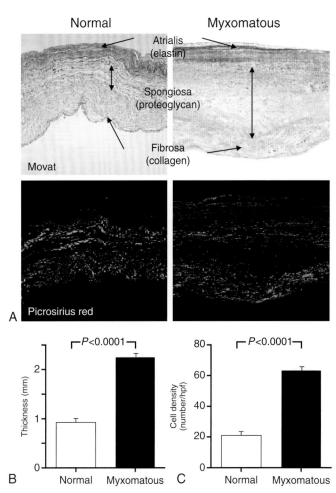

Fig. 17.4 Morphologic Features of Normal and Myxomatous Mitral Valves. (A) Normal mitral valves *(left)* and valves with myxomatous degeneration *(right)*. Myxomatous valves have an abnormal layered architecture: loose collagen in the fibrosa, an expanded spongiosa strongly positive for proteoglycans, and disrupted elastin in the atrialis. Normal and myxomatous mitral valves differ in both thickness (B) and cell density (C). (From Rabkin E, Aikawa M, Stone JR, et al. Activated interstitial myofibroblasts express catabolic enzymes and mediate matrix remodeling in myxomatous heart valves. Circulation 2001;104:2525-2532.)

the same disease sharing the same pathophysiology or represent two pathologies with different underlying mechanisms and pathways.

NATURAL HISTORY

Prevalence

The prevalence of MVP varies widely according to studies that used unclear and not strict definitions of MVP. Diagnosis of MVP should be made in parasternal long-axis view because of the saddle shape of the mitral annulus with at least 2 mm displacement of the leaflet into the LA beyond the annular hinge points. Other views may lead to a false diagnosis of MVP. The echocardiographic measurement of leaflet thickness proposed in several studies, usually between 2 and 3 mm, is challenging and poorly reproducible. Using this strict definition, the prevalence of MVP is estimated to be 2.4% in the general population based on Framingham data.[16]

In the Oxvalve study, a prospective cohort study conducted in Oxfordshire, United Kingdom, in which subjects 65 years of age and older without known valvular heart disease were screened using echocardiography,

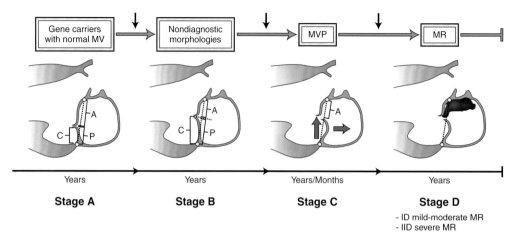

Fig. 17.5 Proposed Temporal Spectrum of Mitral Valve Prolapse *(MVP)* Progression. MVP can evolve over a period of 3 to 16 years. *A,* projection of anterior leaflets onto the mitral annulus. *C,* Mitral leaflet coaptation height; *MR,* mitral regurgitation; *MV,* mitral valve; *P,* projection of posterior leaflets onto the mitral annulus. (From Delling FN, Vasan RS. Epidemiology and pathophysiology of mitral valve prolapse: new insights into disease progression, genetics, and molecular basis. Circulation 2014;129:2158-2170.)

the prevalence of any degree of MR was 20.1% (including 2.3% with moderate to severe MR).[17] The cause of MR was not specifically reported, but MVP can be assumed to be the main cause in Western countries.

In a familial context, subtle MV abnormalities—so called nondiagnostic MVP morphologies—were found in carriers of the mutation linked to MVP.[12] These findings led to the hypothesis that the nondiagnostic MVP morphologies may represent a mild or early stage or expression of the disease. Two forms were reported. Individuals with less than 2 mm of leaflet displacement but a posterior (normal) coaptation were defined as having minimal systolic displacement, whereas individuals with anterior coaptation (>40%, similar to MVP) were said to have abnormal anterior coaptation.

Among individuals who participated in the fifth examination cycle of the Framingham Heart Study offspring cohort, patients with nondiagnostic MVP morphologies shared anatomic features of MVP with regard to annular size and leaflet thickness and a higher rate of MR compared with healthy controls.[18] The prevalence of these nondiagnostic MVP morphologies remains unclear, but in another study, the same investigators showed that MVP can evolve over a period of 3 to 16 years (Fig. 17.5).[19] However, sample size was relatively modest in this study, and the findings require confirmation. Progression was slow and uncertain. If nondiagnostic MVP morphologies need clinical (and research) attention, these limitations raise caution regarding information that should be given to patients.

Patients with MVP are significantly younger than those with aortic valve stenosis. Patients with fibroelastic deficiency are typically about 60 years of age at the time of surgery and often have abrupt MR onset. Patients with Barlow disease are usually younger, in their fourth or fifth decade at presentation, with a progressive evolution and a long history of a regurgitant murmur. MV lesions and MR worsen with time and possibly with aging, but prospective longitudinal studies are scarce, and disease progression and its determinants remain poorly understood.[19–21] For patients with moderate to severe MR, transthoracic echocardiography (TTE) should be repeated annually or semiannually for those approaching thresholds for intervention.

Prognosis for Mitral Valve Prolapse

There has been considerable debate concerning the prognosis associated with MVP. In the Framingham Heart Study, among 3491 individual participants, MVP was reported as a benign entity with a low occurrence of adverse sequelae.[16] These data, however, contradicted

those obtained from the community, such as the Olmsted County study. A Mayo Clinic study identified 833 Olmsted County residents first diagnosed with asymptomatic MVP.[22] Diagnosis was motivated by auscultatory findings in two thirds and was incidental in one third of the patients, and all cases were confirmed by echocardiography. At 10 years, rates of death, cardiovascular morbidity, and MVP-related events were 19%, 30%, and 20%, respectively.

An important result of this study was the identification of major and minor predictors of outcome. Major predictors were moderate or severe MR and depressed ejection fraction (EF); minor predictors were LA diameter 40 mm or greater, flail leaflet, atrial fibrillation, and age 50 years or older. Patients with none of these predictors did not experience excess mortality and morbidity rates beyond the expected levels; patients with two minor risk factors incurred an excess morbidity but no excess mortality; and patients with one major risk factor incurred both excess morbidity and excess mortality (Fig. 17.6).

Several reasons may explain the differences in outcome between the Framingham and Olmsted studies. First, in the Framingham study, the number of patients with MVP was relatively small, only 84 patients, and most of them had no or only mild MR. Second, the benign MVP feature in the Framingham study was reported on the basis of cross-sectional observations. In contrast, the community-based Olmsted County study[22] enrolled a large number of patients with MVP and demonstrated a considerable heterogeneity in outcomes according to phenotype.

In a later study from the Framingham cohort, it was shown that MVP progressed to significant MR in one fourth of the patients with MVP and was associated with increased mortality and morbidity rates, although statistical significance was not reached.[19] The literature indicates that MV anatomy has little impact on outcome, which is much more closely related to MR severity and its effects on the left-sided chambers, PAP, and functional impairment.

Mortality, Atrial Fibrillation, and Heart Failure Risks

Many studies have shown the increased mortality and morbidity associated with MR and have identified several important prognostic factors. Severely symptomatic patients incur excess morbidity and mortality compared with the expected rates. Patients with left ventricular (LV) systolic dysfunction assessed by EF (<60%) or by end-systolic diameter (>40 mm) also experience an excess mortality.

The rate of atrial fibrillation under conservative management is high among patients with severe MR initially in sinus rhythm (18% at

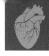

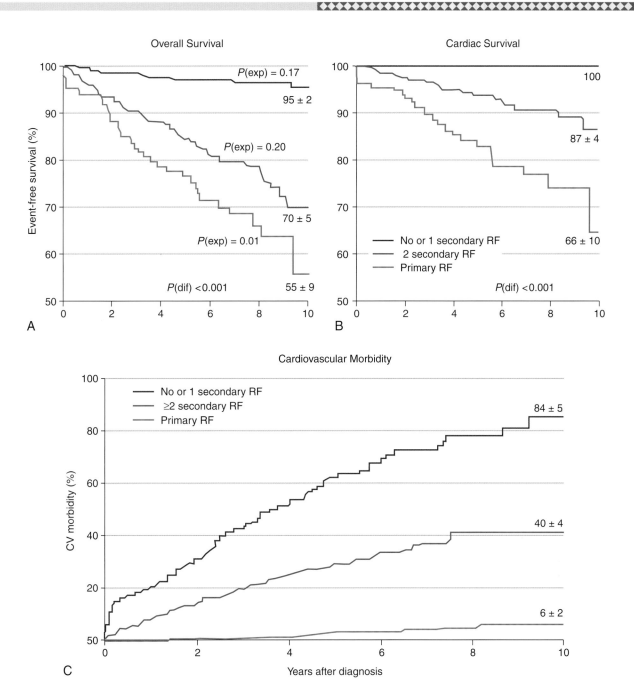

Fig. 17.6 Natural History of Asymptomatic Mitral Valve Prolapse in the Community. Overall survival (A), cardiovascular survival (B), and cardiovascular morbidity (C) according to the categories of baseline risk factors *(RFs)*: (1) no primary RFs and 0 or 1 secondary RFs; (2) no primary RFs but 2 or more secondary RFs, and (3) primary RFs. *P(dif)*, Difference in total mortality between subgroups; *P(exp)*, probabilities regarding the difference between observed and expected mortality within each subgroup. (From Avierinos JF, Gersh BJ, Melton LJ 3rd, et al. Natural history of asymptomatic mitral valve prolapse in the community. Circulation 2002;106:1355-1361.)

5 years; 48% at 10 years) and is predicted by the size of the LA. Occurrence of secondary atrial fibrillation is responsible for the excess mortality and morbidity rates. Among patients with flail leaflet, atrial fibrillation is associated with a 29% increased risk of death.[23] In the same population, annualized rates of atrial fibrillation, heart failure, all-cause mortality, and the composite end point of cardiac death, atrial fibrillation, and heart failure were 5.4%, 8%, 2.6%, and 12.4%, respectively.

Severe MR, quantitatively assessed, is a major prognostic factor, with a 62% event rate at 5 years among those with an effective regurgitant orifice of 40 mm² or greater. The adjusted hazard ratios for mortality for the regurgitant orifice (per 10-mm² increment) and regurgitant volume (per 10-mL increment) were 1.11 and 1.05, respectively, for a

large, unselected cohort of almost 4000 patients with isolated MVP.[24] Kaplan-Meier curves illustrating the prognostic value of these parameters are presented in Fig. 17.7. The cumulative effects of these parameters, as assessed by the Mitral Regurgitation International Database (MIDA) mortality risk score, have been shown for both medical and surgical management.[23]

Arrhythmias and Risk of Sudden Death

A potential association between MVP and malignant arrhythmia or sudden death has been recognized for decades but is still debated and controversial, with highly discordant data regarding prevalence of MVP in registries of sudden death ranging from 0% to 24%. One pitfall is the

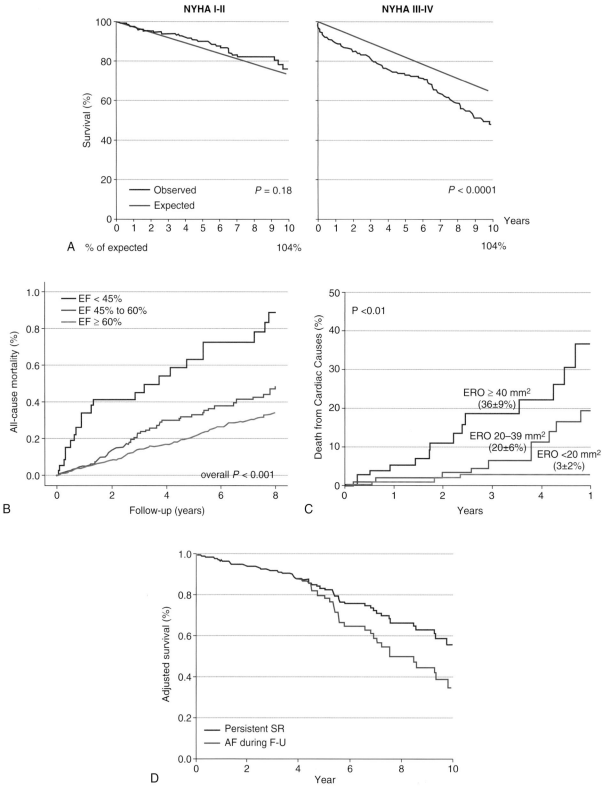

Fig. 17.7 Prognostic Factors for Patients With Mitral Valve Regurgitation. Kaplan-Meier curves illustrate the prognostic value of New York Heart Association *(NYHA)* functional class, (A), ejection fraction *(EF)* (B), atrial fibrillation *(AF)* (C), and mitral regurgitation severity (D). *ERO,* Effective regurgitant orifice; *F-U,* follow-up; *SR,* sinus rhythm. (Data from Enriquez-Sarano M, Avierinos JF, Messika-Zeitoun D, et al. Quantitative determinants of the outcome of asymptomatic mitral regurgitation. N Engl J Med 2005;352:875-883; Tribouilloy C, Rusinaru D, Grigioni F, et al. Long-term mortality associated with left ventricular dysfunction in mitral regurgitation due to flail leaflets: a multicenter analysis. Circ Cardiovasc Imaging 2014;7:363-370; Grigioni F, Avierinos JF, Ling LH, et al. Atrial fibrillation complicating the course of degenerative mitral regurgitation: determinants and long-term outcome. J Am Coll Cardiol 2002;40:84-92; Tribouilloy C, Enriquez-Sarano M, Schaff H, et al. Impact of preoperative symptoms on survival after surgical correction of organic mitral regurgitation: rationale for optimizing surgical indications. Circulation 1999;99:400-405.)

lack of differentiation between the role of MVP itself and the role of MR and its effects on left-sided chambers in the occurrence of sudden death.

An excess mortality rate due to sudden death has been reported for patients with significant MR.[25] The rate of sudden death for 348 patients with flail leaflets was 8.6% at 5 years and 18.8% at 10 years. Sudden death accounted for one fourth of all deaths. This study also highlighted important risk factors: severe symptoms (New York Heart Association [NYHA] class III/IV), depressed left ventricular ejection fraction (LVEF), and atrial fibrillation, which are all class I or IIa indications for surgery. A striking finding was that although the rate of sudden death was markedly increased in these subgroups, most of the sudden deaths occurred among patients in NYHA functional class I or II who had normal LV EF and sinus rhythm. This may represent an important incentive for early or preventive surgery, but these findings need confirmatory study.

The situation is completely different for patients with isolated MVP without MR. Life-threatening ventricular arrhythmias in patients with MVP have been reported, but their prevalence in registries has varied across series, from less than 1% to 7% of all sudden cardiac deaths.[26,27] The reality of this association remained uncertain and speculative in the absence of a pathophysiologic hypothesis. Among 650 young adults (≤40 years of age) who experienced a sudden death, Basso et al identified 43 individuals with MVP. The usual phenotype was a female with a click at auscultation, bileaflet involvement of the MV, T-wave abnormalities on inferior leads, and right bundle branch block–type or polymorphic arrhythmias on electrocardiograms.

The researchers identified a possible origin of malignant arrhythmia using pathology and magnetic resonance imaging (MRI). They noticed patchy fibrosis interspersed within surviving hypertrophic cardiomyocytes at the level of the papillary muscles and adjacent free wall and at the inferobasal basal wall (in keeping with the morphology of the ventricular arrhythmia).

The same group later refined the potential pathophysiology of malignant arrhythmia in MVP.[28] They reported a strong association for the mitral annular disjunction (i.e., separation between the LA wall at the level of the MV junction and the LV free wall; Fig. 17.8), systolic curling of the posterior MV leaflet, and ultimately myocardial fibrosis. The researchers hypothesized that the mitral annular disjunction was responsible for an annular hypermobility with systolic curling of the posterior MV leaflet and consequently an excessive mobility of the MV apparatus. The excessive mobility induced increased myocardial stress at the level of the papillary muscles and the LF inferobasal segment, resulting in myocardial fibrosis. Myocardial fibrosis served as the substrate of malignant arrhythmias induced by the mechanical stretch, which acted as the trigger.

Myocardial dispersion, a parameter of heterogeneous ventricular contraction that correlates with myocardial fibrosis, can be assessed with the use of speckle-tracking echocardiography and has been

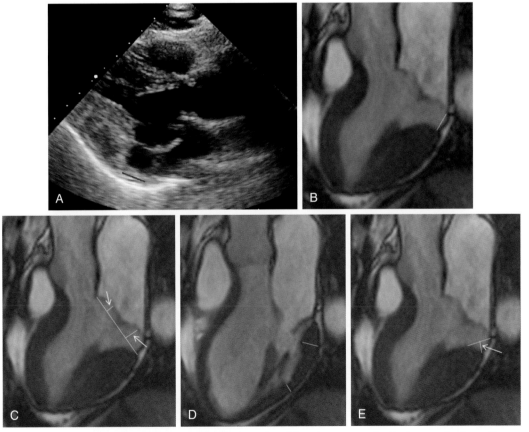

Fig. 17.8 Mitral Annulus Disjunction. (A) Mitral annulus disjunction assessed with the use of echocardiography (parasternal long-axis view) in a patient with trivial mitral regurgitation admitted for resuscitated out-of-hospital cardiac arrest (Video 17.8 ▶). (B) Mitral annulus disjunction is assessed with cardiac magnetic resonance imaging in the three-chamber, long-axis view. (C) The prolapsed distance is measured as the maximum distance of the leaflet beyond the mitral annulus (*white arrows*). (D) The LV thickness of basal and mid-segments of the inferolateral wall is measured in the same long-axis view on diastole. (E) The quantitative assessment of curling (*white arrow*) is provided by tracing a line between the top of LV inferobasal wall and the LA wall–posterior MV leaflet junction, and from this line, a perpendicular line to the lower limit of the mitral annulus during end systole. (From Perazzolo Marra M, Basso C, De Lazzari M, et al. Morphofunctional abnormalities of mitral annulus and arrhythmic mitral valve prolapse. Circ Cardiovasc Imaging 2016;9:e005030.)

associated with a higher prevalence of arrhythmic complications among patients with MVP. It may help to identify MVP patients who are at higher arrhythmic risk.[29] The role of severe myxomatous MVP disease (defined by the combination of bileaflet prolapse, myxomatous MV with thickened leaflet, and mitral annular disjunction) was also highlighted in a multicenter study gathering 42 patients who had survived a documented ventricular fibrillation with no detectable structural or electric cause other than MVP.[30]

Evaluation of the exact prevalence of sudden death and validation of the prognostic value of myocardial fibrosis could benefit from prospective registries of patients with MVP free of MR, but in the absence of such data, clinicians should pay special attention to patients with MVP and inferolateral electrocardiographic abnormalities, ventricular arrhythmias (especially right bundle branch block morphology), and a history of syncope or presyncope. MRI may help to stratify risk for such patients.

Infective Endocarditis

In regard to the marked simplification of antimicrobial preventive strategies for infective endocarditis (IE)[31] and their complete suppression by the United Kingdom's National Institute for Health and Care Excellence (NICE), it is important to evaluate IE rates in the population of patients with MVP. Estimation of IE rates has been hindered in several studies by nonspecific criteria for the diagnosis of MVP or by selection or recruitment bias.[32,33]

A community study reported a 1.1% IE rate at 15 years among 896 MVP patients in the Olmsted County population, an 8.1% increase in relative risk compared with the expected incidence.[34] Several points need to be emphasized. No age and gender or anatomic features were associated with an increased IE risk. The main determinant of the risk of IE occurrence was the presence and degree of MR (Fig. 17.9). Although the increased relative risk was high, the increased absolute risk was modest (1.1% vs. 0.2% in the population at 15 years, or 1 of every 1100 patients with MVP). Whether patients with MVP and a moderate or greater degree of MR should be considered to be at high risk for IE is therefore uncertain.

Antibiotic prophylaxis is recommended only for high-risk procedures, including dental procedures involving manipulation of the gingival or periapical region of the teeth or manipulation of the oral mucosa, and for patients with prosthetic valves (including transcatheter valves) or repairs using prosthetic material and those with previous episodes of IE.[31,35,36] However, the absence of antibiotic prophylaxis does not mean absence of prophylaxis, and strict dental hygiene and aseptic measures during any invasive procedures are required for patients with MVP.

ECHOCARDIOGRAPHIC EVALUATION

Echocardiography is the preferred method for evaluation of MVP and other MV disease. Echocardiography establishes the MVP diagnosis, characterizes its phenotype, and assesses and quantifies associated MR and its effects on the LV, LA, and systolic PAP. Based on this information, echocardiography plays a major role in the clinical management of MVP.

Computed tomography (CT) and MRI are useful adjuncts for the evaluation of MV disease and its effects. CT may identify lesions responsible for MR and possibly its severity.[37,38] MRI is considered the method of choice for quantification of LV size and function, and it has been used to assess MR severity.[39] However, both modalities represent second- or even third-line methods for the assessment of MV morphology and MR quantification. In this section, we focus on echocardiography.

Assessment of Regurgitant Severity

Accurate assessment of MR severity is of paramount importance because MR degree is the main determinant of outcome of patients with MVP. Assessment of MR severity (see Chapter 15) relies on the integration of semiquantitative and qualitative parameters in addition to the underlying MR mechanism.[40] The two main recommended techniques are the vena contracta method and the flow convergence method. There is a general consensus regarding avoidance of the use of color Doppler imaging for the assessment of MR severity.[41] Color Doppler should be used for the diagnosis but not for MR quantification. Nevertheless, tiny regurgitant jets strongly suggest mild MR, whereas large regurgitant jets with a large coaptation defect suggest severe MR.

The vena contracta is the narrowest neck of the regurgitant flow through the regurgitant orifice. It can be regarded as the diameter of the regurgitant orifice as measured by color flow. A value of 3 mm or less rules out severe MR, whereas a value of 7 mm or greater suggests severe MR with high sensitivity and high specificity. Between these two values, there is a gray and nonconclusive zone. The vena contracta should be measured perpendicular to the direction of the regurgitant flow (usually the parasternal long-axis view).

The proximal isovelocity surface area (PISA) measurement, also known as the flow convergence method, is based on the conservation of mass. The principle is presented elsewhere.[42] Two parameters can be derived from the PISA method: the effective regurgitant orifice (ERO), which reflects anatomic damage, and the regurgitant volume (RVol),

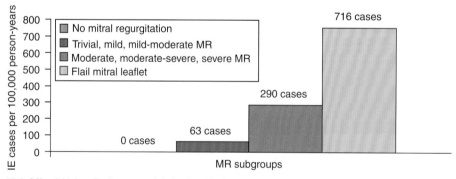

Fig. 17.9 Mitral Valve Prolapse and Infective Endocarditis. Incidence of infective endocarditis *(IE)* per 100,000 person-years according to presence and degree of mitral regurgitation *(MR)*. The expected IE incidence was 6 cases per 100,000 person-years. Patients with flail leaflet (also included in the group of moderate to severe MR) are individualized in the last bar graph. (From Katan O, Michelena HI, Avierinos JF, et al. Incidence and predictors of infective endocarditis in mitral valve prolapse: a population-based study. Mayo Clin Proc 2016;91:336-342.)

which reflects the volume overload. Simple technical rules need to be respected when using the PISA method:

- In contrast to the vena contracta measurement, the PISA measurement should be made parallel to the regurgitant flow (usually the four-chamber view).
- Use of the zoom is strongly recommended to avoid the translation of minimal errors in radius measurement into marked differences in ERO/RVol calculations.
- There is no unique aliasing velocity for all PISA studies, and the aliasing velocity should be chosen to obtain a nice hemispheric flow convergence shape. It should be adapted according to the estimated MR degree (i.e., smaller aliasing velocities in mild or moderate MR and higher velocities in severe MR).
- In MVP, the ERO increases throughout systole. To obtain an average systolic ERO, the radius of the flow convergence should be measured at the level of the T-wave, and the maximal MR peak velocity should be used.[42]

It is established that PISA is an accurate and reproducible method for quantification of MR severity. Nevertheless, some pitfalls and limitations should not be forgotten. In the setting of MVP, several specific situations also need to be underlined:

- Mid-late systolic MR is a common feature in MVP, especially in patients with Barlow disease. It has been demonstrated that PISA can still be used, but the ERO should be disregarded and only the RVol considered. Only the hemi-envelope of the MR jet should be traced; no extrapolation should be performed.[43]
- Multiple jets are common in bileaflet prolapse or Barlow disease. The PISA method may be used, but each jet has to be quantified separately, which may make the procedure lengthy and challenging. Other techniques, such as the debit method or the Simpson method, can be used in the absence of associated aortic regurgitation and very irregular rhythm. In the debit method, the regurgitant volume is calculated as the difference between the mitral inflow stroke volume (which requires measurement of the mitral annulus diameter and the mitral inflow) and the aortic inflow stroke volume.[44] Similarly, the Simpson method obtains regurgitant volume as the difference between LV stroke volume (i.e., end-diastolic minus end-systolic volume) and the aortic inflow stroke volume.
- A very eccentric jet may not fulfill the hemispheric assumption due to flow constraint. An angle correction might be used, but the debit or Simpson method may be the best option.

Severe MR is defined by an ERO of 40 mm^2 or greater or an RVol of 60 mL or greater, or both. The prognostic value of these measurements has been demonstrated and largely supersedes that of the semiquantitative measurements.[24,45]

Transesophageal echocardiography (TEE) is not recommended for routine evaluation and follow-up, but it is indicated when TTE provides nondiagnostic information about the MR mechanism or severity.[46] Use of 3D echocardiography has been proposed for MR quantification, and several methods have been evaluated. The 3D capability allows direct measurement, not of the diameter of the ERO but of the area and therefore the ERO.[47] It also allows acquisition of the 3D flow convergence, which may overcome the hemispheric assumption of the PISA method. With 3D MV modeling, the anatomic regurgitant orifice area can also be measured.[48] Temporal and spatial resolutions of 3D echocardiography remain suboptimal, and treatment afterward is lengthy and operator dependent, but these new modalities are very promising.

Assessment of Mitral Regurgitation Effects

In addition to symptomatic status, clinical decision making strongly depends on the effects of MR on the LV, the LA, and the systolic PAP. LV size

and function are major prognostic markers. These respective impacts and the most appropriate thresholds that should be considered in surgical indications have been refined based on data from the MIDA registry, a multicenter compilation of patients diagnosed with mitral flail as a surrogate marker for severe MR in six centers in Europe and the United States.[49] Although criticized because of the decrease in afterload, EF is a valuable parameter for assessing LV dysfunction in patients with MR. Spline analysis has shown that the threshold of 60% is a turning point in terms of risk; below that threshold, the risk increases gradually. Patients with an EF lower than 45% are at very high risk compared with those with an EF greater than 60%, and those with EF between 45% and 60% are at intermediate risk. These findings apply to conservative management and overall or when considering only the postoperative period. Nevertheless, despite incurring a higher surgical risk, patients with an EF of less than 45% and those between 45% and 60% markedly benefit from the surgery. With an EF greater than 60%, no further stratification can be performed.

An end-systolic LV diameter of 40 mm or greater is associated with an increased mortality rate, and patients with a diameter above this threshold who are operated on continue to incur excess risk, suggesting that surgery may be considered earlier when the LV end-systolic diameter is between 36 and 39 mm.[50] No adjusted threshold could be validated. Several studies have suggested that the global longitudinal strain assessed by speckle-tracking echocardiography, a method that is reputedly more sensitive in assessing LV myocardial contractility than EF, provides further prognostic information, but larger multicenter series are needed before this parameter can be definitively recommended in clinical practice.[51]

LA enlargement is a normal physiologic response to the volume overload induced by the regurgitation. Pioneering studies have shown that LA diameter is associated with increased risks of heart failure, atrial fibrillation, and death.[52-55] However, LA enlargement is often asymmetric and more accurately reflected by the evaluation of LA volume.[56] LA volume should be estimated using biplane methods, the biplane Simpson method or the biplane area-length method, which is our preference. Using the latter method, LA enlargement is defined by an LA volume greater than or equal to 40 mL/m^2 of body surface area, and severe enlargement is defined by an LA volume greater than or equal to 60 mL/m^2. The prognostic value of these thresholds has been validated[57] and incorporated in guidelines.[35]

Systolic PAP is the third main parameter to consider. Pulmonary hypertension, defined as a systolic PAP greater than 50 mmHg, is associated with increased mortality and morbidity rates. A study from the MIDA registry showed that pulmonary hypertension doubles the risk of death and heart failure after diagnosis.[58] Surgery incompletely abolishes the impact of pulmonary hypertension on outcome.

Morphologic Assessment of the Valve

A precise anatomic evaluation is essential to estimate the probability of successful repair, plan the intervention, and guide the surgeon. Morphologic assessment may also provide important complementary information about MR severity because a flail leaflet is in most cases responsible for severe MR. The evaluation relies on the assessment of MR mechanism and disease localization (i.e., identification of the diseased leaflets and segments or scallops). Because multiple lesions may coexist, a systematic and rigorous approach is recommended.

Usually, TTE allows identification and localization of the diseased segments. It requires some expertise and analysis of the MV from multiple angles. The parasternal short-axis view without and with color is often very informative. Inclination of the probe medially and laterally in the parasternal long-axis view, in combination with the apical two-chamber view, usually identifies medial or lateral prolapse. In difficult cases, TEE may produce the final answer. Compared with TTE, TEE provides a more precise anatomic assessment and detection of finer details. Although TEE

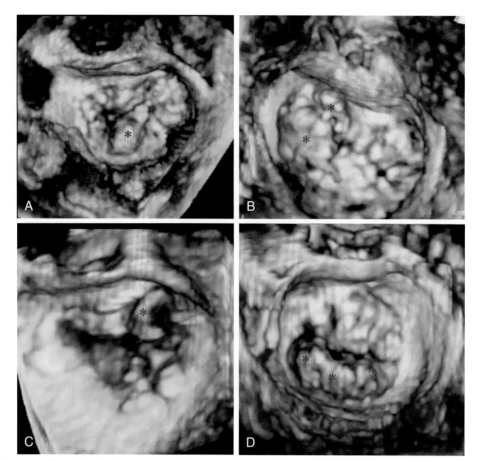

Fig. 17.10 Morphologic Assessment of Diseased Segments Using 3D TEE. Examples of prolapsed segments visualized by 3D TEE. *Red asterisks* indicate the identified leaflets. (A) P2 prolapse. Notice the rupture of chordae. (B) P1/A1 flail. (C) A3 prolapse. (D) Large, complete prolapse involving P1, P2, and P3. (From Messika-Zeitoun D, Topilsky Y, Enriquez-Sarano M. The role of echocardiography in the management of patients with myxomatous disease. Cardiol Clin 2013;31:217-229.)

is not required in many cases to provide an accurate analysis of valve lesions, it is mandatory in the operating room to provide a final assessment of the lesions and to monitor surgical results.

Similar to TTE, analysis of valve lesions by TEE requires the use of multiple views and angles. Real-time 3D echocardiography has considerably simplified this assessment, providing an immediate and intuitive assessment of the anatomy of the MV (Fig. 17.10). Real-time 3D echocardiography also helps the communication between echocardiographers and surgeons. 3D TEE remains much more precise and informative than 3D TTE, but the latter is expected to improve as technology progresses.

MANAGEMENT AND TIMING OF INTERVENTION

MVP alone does not require specific therapy, but treatment may be needed for patients with MVP and significant MR. No medical therapy can prevent MR progression or MR consequences, and MV surgery is the only approved treatment for patients with severe MR, although a transcatheter option (MitraClip, Abbott Laboratories, Chicago, IL) has emerged as a valuable alternative for patients considered to be at high surgical risk.[59,60]

Class I or IIa Indications for Intervention

Treatment of patients with symptoms who have LV enlargement (end-systolic diameter ≥ 40 mm) or dysfunction (EF ≤ 60%), systolic pulmonary hypertension (≥50 mmHg at rest), and/or atrial fibrillation

(even paroxysmal) is relatively simple, and they should be promptly referred for surgery (Table 17.1).[35,36]

The European guidelines consider an end-systolic threshold of 40 mm only when there is a high likelihood of durable repair for patients at low surgical risk who have flail leaflet or LA enlargement (≥60 mL/m²); a 45-mm threshold is recommended in other cases (see Table 17.1). Caution is warranted for patients with a very low EF (<30%), although registries have shown that this is rare.[49] Algorithms for the management of primary MR drawn from the American and European guidelines are presented in Fig. 17.11.

Evaluation of Asymptomatic Patients and Identification of High-Risk Subsets

Management of asymptomatic patients with severe MR and no class I or IIa indications for surgery is controversial. As with other valvular diseases, it is crucial to ensure that patients are really asymptomatic. Careful questioning of the patient and family members is important, as is exercise testing. Patients with degenerative MR are usually 15 years younger than those with aortic valve stenosis and usually are able to perform an exercise test. Exercise testing should not be performed by patients with class I or IIa indications for surgery.

Several types of exercise testing can be used. Because typically the information sought is whether the functional capacity is preserved or reduced, a simple exercise test may be sufficient. Cardiopulmonary exercise testing has the advantage of providing robust data regarding

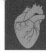

TABLE 17.1   Recommendations for Surgery in Primary Mitral Regurgitation According to 2017 AHA/ACC and ESC Guidelines for the Management of Patients With Valvular Heart Disease.

PATIENTS WITH CHRONIC SEVERE PRIMARY MR	CLASS and LOE	
	AHA/ACC	**ESC**
Mitral valve surgery is recommended for		
• Symptomatic patients (stage D) and LVEF > 30%	I B	I B
• Asymptomatic patients LV dysfunction (EF 30%–60% and/or LVESD 40 mm [AHA/ACC] or 45 mm [ESC] or greater [stage C2])	I B	I B
Mitral valve surgery is reasonable for		
• Asymptomatic patients with normal LV systolic function (EF > 60% and LVESD < 40 mm [AHA/ACC] or 40–44 mm [ESC]) if the likelihood of a durable repair without residual MR is > 95% with an expected surgical mortality < 1% when performed at a heart valve center of excellence	IIa B	IIa C
• Asymptomatic patients with normal LV systolic function (EF > 60% and LVESD < 40 mm) with a progressive increase in LV size or decrease in EF on serial imaging studies	IIa C	
• Asymptomatic patients with normal LV systolic function (EF > 60% and LVESD < 40 mm) if the likelihood of a durable repair when there is new onset of AF or a resting PA systolic pressure > 50 mmHg	IIa B	IIa B
• Patients with chronic moderate primary MR (stage B) when undergoing cardiac surgery for other indications	IIa C	
Mitral valve surgery may be considered for		
• Symptomatic patients with an LVEF < 30%	IIb C	IIb C
Transcatheter mitral valve repair may be considered for		
• Severe symptomatic patients (NYHA class III-IV) who have valve anatomy favorable for the repair procedure and a reasonable life expectancy but have a prohibitive surgical risk and remain severely symptomatic despite optional GDMT for heart failure	IIb B	IIb C
Mitral valve repair is recommended in preference to MVR when surgical treatment is indicated when		
• Prolapse is limited to the posterior leaflet or	I B	
• Prolapse involves the anterior leaflet or both leaflets when a successful and durable repair can be accomplished	I B	
• In all cases when results are expected to be durable		I C
Commitment mitral valve repair or MVR is indicated if undergoing cardiac surgery for other indications	I B	

ACC, American Collage of Cardiology; *AF,* atrial fibrillation; *AHA,* American Heart Association; *ESC,* European Society of Cardiology; *GDMT,* guideline-directed medical therapy; *LD,* limited data; *LOE,* Level of Evidence; *LV,* left ventricular; *LVEF,* left ventricular ejection fraction; *LVESD,* left vebtricular end-systolic dimension; *MR,* mitral regurgitaion; *MVR,* mitral valve replacement; *NYHA,* New York Heart Association; *PA,* pulmonary artery.
Data from Baumgartner H, Falk V, Bax JJ, et al. 2017 ESC/EACTS guidelines for the management of valvular heart disease: the Task Force for the Management of Valvular Heart Disease of the European Society of Cardiology (ESC) and the European Association for Cardio-Thoracic Surgery (EACTS). Eur Heart J 2017 21;38:2739-2791; Nishimura RA, Otto CM, Bonow RO, et al. 2017 AHA/ACC focused update of the 2014 AHA/ACC guideline for the management of patients with valvular heart disease: a report of the American College of Cardiology/American Heart Association Task Force on Clinical Practice Guidelines. Circulation 2017;135:e1159-e1195.

age- gender-, and weight-adjusted reference values; a peak oxygen uptake ($\dot{V}o_2$) value less than 84% of the expected value is considered functional impairment. Exercise testing usually unveils a functional impairment in 20% of patients with severe MR, and these patients incur an excess risk compared with those who have a normal functional capacity.[61] Patients with functional limitation should be considered symptomatic and therefore referred for surgery.

Exercise echocardiography has been proposed as an alternative to simple electrocardiographic exercise testing or cardiopulmonary exercise testing. In addition to assessing functional capacity, it can be used to determine systolic PAP, left myocardial contractile reserve, and right ventricular (RV) performance. PAP during exercise, defined as a systolic PAP of 60 mmHg or higher, was found to be an important prognostic marker of event-free survival for 78 patients with at least moderate MR.[62] It was also associated with an increased risk of cardiac events after MV surgery.[63] However, these studies suffered from small sample sizes, and patients with pulmonary artery hypertension at rest were also included. Pulmonary artery hypertension at peak exercise is not specific and may be observed in healthy controls, especially those older than 60 years of age.[64,65] These findings need to be validated by other centers and ideally in multicenter studies.

Contractile reserve can be evaluated during exercise testing. Several studies have shown that preoperative LV contractile reserve predicts postoperative EF, exercise capacity, and outcome.[66–68] Global longitudinal strain seems to be more sensitive than EF,[69] but these findings need further validation before being applied to the clinical management of

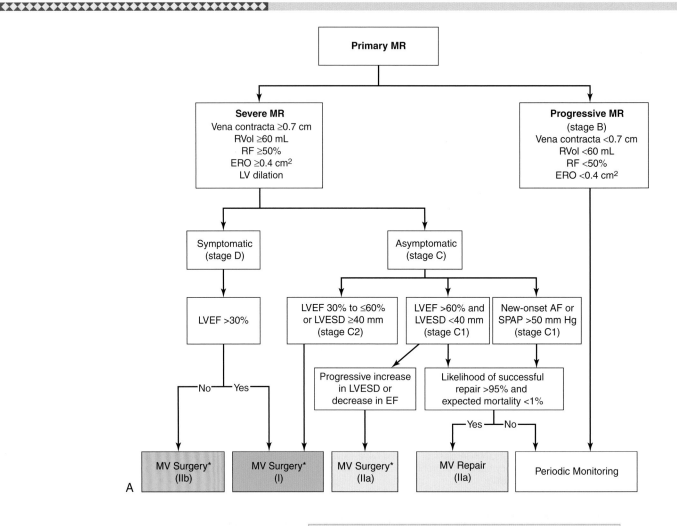

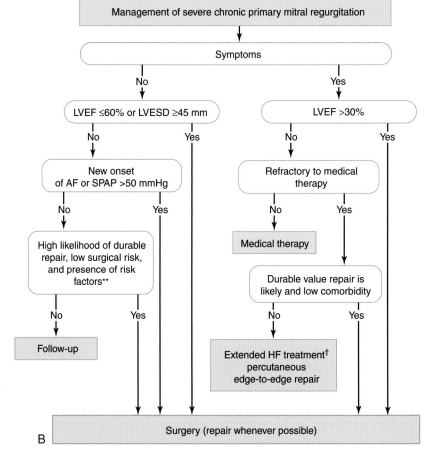

Fig. 17.11 Algorithm for the Management of Primary Mitral Regurgitation According to the 2017 American (AHA/ACC)[36] (A) and European (ESC)[35] Guidelines (B). (A) *Asterisk* indicates that MV repair is preferred over MV replacement when possible. (B) *Double asterisk,* When there is a high likelihood of durable valve repair at a low risk, valve repair should be considered (IIa C) in patients with LVESD ≥40 mm and one of the following is present: flail leaflet or LA volume ≥60 mL/m² BSA at sinus rhythm. *Dagger,* Extended HF management includes cardiac resynchronization therapy, ventricular assist devices, cardiac restraint devices, and heart transplantation. *AF,* Atrial fibrillation; *EF,* ejection fraction; *ERO,* effective regurgitant orifice; *HF,* heart failure; *LVEF,* left ventricular ejection fraction; *LVESD,* left ventricular end-systolic diameter; *MR,* mitral regurgitation; *MV,* mitral valve; *RF,* regurgitant fraction; *RVol,* regurgitant volume; *SPAP,* systolic pulmonary artery pressure.

asymptomatic MR. RV dysfunction at rest has been reported as a significant prognostic marker,[70] and similar findings were observed for RV function at peak exercise.[71] Change in MR degree has been evaluated, but evaluation is challenging, especially in patients with MVP, and requires further validation.[72]

Several studies have evaluated the role of biomarkers and brain natriuretic peptide (BNP) in the risk stratification of patients with degenerative MR. Activation of BNP reflects ventricular and atrial effects of the regurgitation and provides important prognostic information under conservative management.[73] One large, multicenter cohort of 1331 patients with degenerative MR further refined the prognostic value of BNP and showed that the BNP ratio (i.e., ratio of the BNP value to the upper limit of normal for age, sex, and assay) was a powerful, independent, and incremental predictor of long-term mortality rates.[74] The prognostic value of BNP has also been demonstrated by other groups.[75]

LA size is a major predictor of atrial fibrillation. Significant enlargement (≥ 60 mL/m^2) has been proposed as a strong indicator for surgery, especially if the probability of durable repair is high.[35]

Management of Asymptomatic Patients

Indications for asymptomatic patients are disputed because of the absence of large, randomized, controlled trials. Practice guidelines are based on outcome studies, and all have some degree of inherent bias. The rationale for early surgery in patients with MVP and severe MR who are in sinus rhythm and have a normal LVEF can be summarized as follows:

1. MR is not a benign condition and is associated with increased risks of death, stroke, and congestive heart failure.[52,54,76–79] The risk of sudden death, although low, is not negligible.
2. Several publications have shown that surgery is almost unavoidable in patients with severe MR, especially those with flail leaflets.[78] Therefore, the question seems to be more *when* the surgery should be performed than *if*.
3. Performance of surgery in patients with severe symptoms, LV dysfunction, atrial fibrillation, or systolic pulmonary hypertension does not restore the life expectancy and is associated with increased postoperative mortality and morbidity rates. Approaching the guideline-based triggers for surgery is not safe, and mitral surgery performed for class I or IIa indications is associated with poor outcomes (Fig. 17.12).[80] This is true for older and younger patients.[80,81] Therefore, surgery in this setting should be regarded as a rescue procedure, and although warranted, it cannot be considered as the preferred or optimal application for surgery.
4. In the setting of degenerative/MVP disease, valve repair (i.e., the procedure of choice for patients undergoing surgical intervention) can be performed for most patients (>95%) in experienced centers with a very low in-hospital mortality rate (<1%) and excellent long-term results.[82–84] MV repair provides better preservation of LV systolic function after surgery than replacement and avoids prosthetic valve–related complications (i.e., thromboembolism, need for anticoagulation, and structural deterioration).
5. Several studies, although not randomized, have compared early surgery with conservative management. The results in all cases favored early surgery with restoration of life expectancy similar to that expected for individuals of the same age and gender (Fig. 17.13).[45,80,85–87]
6. Early surgery prevents the risk that patients will be lost to follow-up or will delay seeing their physician until severe symptoms or LV dysfunction occurs.

However, to give a complete picture of the comparison with so-called watchful waiting,[88] several limitations of these studies should be underlined:

1. Survival without need for intervention was reported to be higher in several studies, up to 50% at 8 years, although patients in these

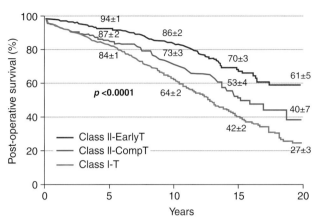

Fig. 17.12 Impact of Surgical Indications on Outcome. Outcome curves show a lower rate of postoperative survival for patients undergoing surgery for class I indications (class I-T: heart failure symptoms, EF < 60%, or end-systolic LV diameter > 40 mm) or class IIa indications (class II-compT: atrial fibrillation or systolic pulmonary pressure > 50 mmHg) compared with patients who underwent early surgery (class II-early T: high probability of valve repair in the absence of other class I or II indications). (From Enriquez-Sarano M, Suri RM, Clavel MA, et al. Is there an outcome penalty linked to guideline-based indications for valvular surgery? Early and long-term analysis of patients with organic mitral regurgitation. J Thorac Cardiovasc Surg 2015;150:50-58.)

studies seemed to have less severe disease at presentation, no quantification was provided, and patients with flail leaflet constituted a minority of the population.[88]

2. Although it is a requirement of the watchful waiting strategy, no systematic follow-up was performed, precluding the possibility of scheduling intervention after the appearance of only modest symptoms or parameters of LV size and function that have just reached the proposed threshold for surgery. The AHA/ACC guidelines clearly state that when longitudinal follow-up demonstrates a progressive decrease in LVEF toward 60% or a progressive increase in LV end-systolic diameter approaching 40 mm, it is reasonable to consider intervention.[89]
3. No specific triggers or precise guidelines for surgery were provided for patients conservatively managed (by design in these observational studies).
4. High rates of successful MV repair are achieved only in expert valve centers.[90] Although the risk of recurrent MR is low in centers of excellence,[83,91] this may not apply at a majority of centers worldwide or even in the United States.[92]

Increasing evidence favors early surgery, but the uncertainties presented here emphasize the need to identify subsets of asymptomatic patients with severe MR who may benefit from early surgery, possibly including those with flail leaflets, elevated BNP levels, or severely enlarged LAs. Early surgery should be considered only in patients at low surgical risk (i.e., no comorbidities) with favorable anatomy and no leaflet or mitral annular calcifications and when it can be performed in an expert valve center after obtaining thorough and accurate patient information.

Follow-Up of Conservatively Managed Patients

For asymptomatic patients with a normal LVEF and sinus rhythm who are conservatively managed, regular and close follow-up is recommended. These patients should be monitored every 6 months, including performance of repeat TTE, ideally in a heart valve center. There is no need for TEE in the follow-up of these patients. A closer follow-up is indicated in the absence of a reference test (i.e., new patient) or when

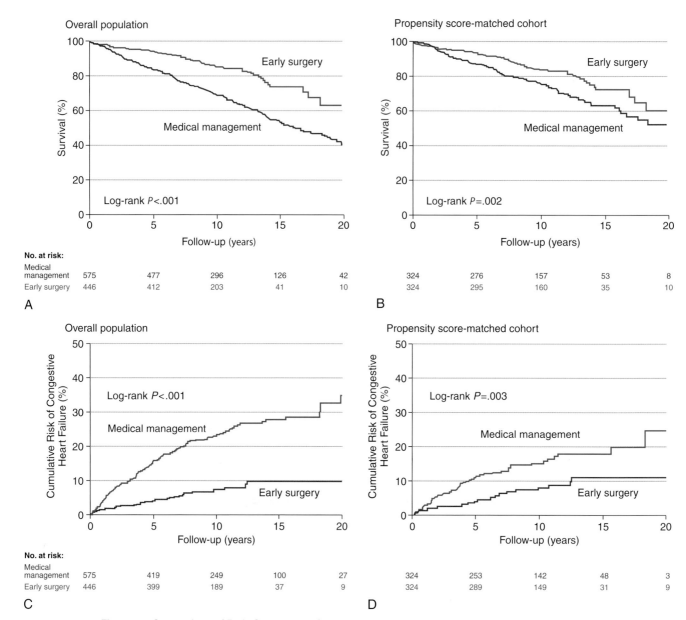

Fig. 17.13 **Comparison of Early Surgery and Conservative Management.** Incidences of survival (A and B) and of heart failure (C and D) after a diagnosis of mitral regurgitation due to flail leaflet in 1021 patients with no class I indication included in the Mitral Regurgitation International Database (MIDA) registry (i.e., six tertiary centers in the United States and Europe). Rates of mortality and congestive heart failure were lower for patients who underwent early surgery (within 3 months) compared with those who were conservatively managed, both for the overall population (A and C) and for the propensity score–matched cohort (B and D). (From Suri RM, Vanoverschelde JL, Grigioni F, et al. Association between early surgical intervention vs watchful waiting and outcomes for mitral regurgitation due to flail mitral valve leaflets. JAMA 2013;310:609-616.)

echocardiographic changes are observed or are close to the thresholds. When guideline indications for surgery are reached, it should be performed within 2 months. Yearly follow-up is recommended for patients with moderate MR.

SUMMARY

MVP is the leading cause of organic MR. It is a heterogeneous disease that can manifest with various phenotypes, from a single isolated scallop prolapse to diffuse Barlow disease. MVP is a common disorder affecting 2% to 3% of the general population. Its pathophysiology needs to be better understood so that therapy targeting the diseased

tissue to prevent MR occurrence or increase can be developed. MVP is a progressive disease but appears to be a benign condition, even if responsible for sudden death in rare cases. Most of the complications associated with MVP are related to MR severity and its effects on left-sided chambers and PAP; assessment of these factors mainly relies on echocardiography.

Precise MR quantification is critical because it is a main predictor of outcome. If left untreated and not timely and appropriately managed, MVP with severe MR confers excess morbidity, including congestive heart failure and stroke, and excess mortality. Surgery remains the only curative treatment for MVP with severe MR, although transcatheter therapy has emerged as an alternative in patients at prohibitive or high surgical risk. Patients with symptoms, LV dysfunction (i.e., EF ≤ 60% or end-systolic diameter > 40 mm), atrial fibrillation, or pulmonary hypertension (i.e., class I and IIa indications) should be promptly referred for surgery, but in this setting, surgery is associated with a poor outcome and therefore should be regarded as a rescue treatment.

In contrast, there is increasing evidence favoring early surgery, which allows restoration of a life expectancy similar to that expected for patients of the same age and gender. In expert centers, MV repair—the procedure of choice for patients undergoing surgical intervention—can be performed in most patients (>95%) with a very low in-hospital mortality rate (<1%) and excellent long-term results. For patients at low surgical risk with favorable anatomy, early surgery should be considered as the best option when performed in expert valve centers.

REFERENCES

1. Levine RA, Handschumacher MD, Sanfilippo AJ, et al. Three-dimensional echocardiographic reconstruction of the mitral valve, with implications for the diagnosis of mitral valve prolapse. Circulation 1989;80(3): 589-598.
2. Timek TA, Lai DT, Dagum P, et al. Ablation of mitral annular and leaflet muscle: effects on annular and leaflet dynamics. Am J Physiol Heart Circ Physiol 2003;285(4):H1668-H1674.
3. Clavel MA, Mantovani F, Malouf J, et al. Dynamic phenotypes of degenerative myxomatous mitral valve disease: quantitative 3-dimensional echocardiographic study. Circ Cardiovasc Imaging 2015;8(5).
4. Otsuji Y, Kumanohoso T, Yoshifuku S, et al. Isolated annular dilation does not usually cause important functional mitral regurgitation: comparison between patients with lone atrial fibrillation and those with idiopathic or ischemic cardiomyopathy. J Am Coll Cardiol 2002;39(10): 1651-1656.
5. Rabkin E, Aikawa M, Stone JR, et al. Activated interstitial myofibroblasts express catabolic enzymes and mediate matrix remodeling in myxomatous heart valves. Circulation 2001;104(21):2525-2532.
6. Levine RA, Hagege AA, Judge DP, et al. Mitral valve disease—morphology and mechanisms. Nat Rev Cardiol 2015;12(12):689-710.
7. Delling FN, Vasan RS. Epidemiology and pathophysiology of mitral valve prolapse: new insights into disease progression, genetics, and molecular basis. Circulation 2014;129(21):2158-2170.
8. Disse S, Abergel E, Berrebi A, et al. Mapping of a first locus for autosomal dominant myxomatous mitral-valve prolapse to chromosome 16p11.2-p12.1. Am J Hum Genet 1999;65(5):1242-1251.
9. Freed LA, Acierno JS, Jr., Dai D, et al. A locus for autosomal dominant mitral valve prolapse on chromosome 11p15.4. Am J Hum Genet 2003; 72(6):1551-1559.
10. Kyndt F, Gueffet JP, Probst V, et al. Mutations in the gene encoding filamin A as a cause for familial cardiac valvular dystrophy. Circulation 2007;115(1):40-49.
11. Kyndt F, Schott JJ, Trochu JN, et al. Mapping of X-linked myxomatous valvular dystrophy to chromosome Xq28. Am J Hum Genet 1998; 62(3):627-632.
12. Nesta F, Leyne M, Yosefy C, et al. New locus for autosomal dominant mitral valve prolapse on chromosome 13: clinical insights from genetic studies. Circulation 2005;112(13):2022-2030.
13. Oceandy D, Yusoff R, Baudoin FM, Neyses L, Ray SG. Promoter polymorphism of the matrix metalloproteinase 3 gene is associated with regurgitation and left ventricular remodelling in mitral valve prolapse patients. Eur J Heart Fail 2007;9(10):1010-1017.
14. Le Tourneau T, Merot J, Rimbert A, et al. Genetics of syndromic and non-syndromic mitral valve prolapse. Heart 2018;104(12):978-984.
15. Delling FN, Rong J, Larson MG, et al. Familial clustering of mitral valve prolapse in the community. Circulation 2015;131(3):263-268.
16. Freed LA, Levy D, Levine RA, et al. Prevalence and clinical outcome of mitral-valve prolapse. N Engl J Med 1999;341(1):1-7.
17. d'Arcy JL, Coffey S, Loudon MA, et al. Large-scale community echocardiographic screening reveals a major burden of undiagnosed valvular heart disease in older people: the OxVALVE Population Cohort Study. Eur Heart J 2016;37(47):3515-3522.
18. Delling FN, Gona P, Larson MG, et al. Mild expression of mitral valve prolapse in the Framingham offspring: expanding the phenotypic spectrum. J Am Soc Echocardiogr 2014;27(1):17-23.
19. Delling FN, Rong J, Larson MG, et al. Evolution of mitral valve prolapse: insights from the Framingham Heart Study. Circulation 2016;133(17): 1688-1695.
20. Avierinos JF, Detaint D, Messika-Zeitoun D, et al. Risk, determinants, and outcome implications of progression of mitral regurgitation after diagnosis of mitral valve prolapse in a single community. Am J Cardiol 2008; 101(5):662-667.
21. Enriquez-Sarano M, Basmadjian A, Rossi A, et al. Progression of mitral regurgitation: a prospective Doppler echocardiographic study. J Am Coll Cardiol 1999;34:1137-1144.
22. Avierinos JF, Gersh BJ, Melton LJ, 3rd, et al. Natural history of asymptomatic mitral valve prolapse in the community. Circulation 2002;106(11): 1355-1361.
23. Grigioni F, Clavel MA, Vanoverschelde JL, et al. The MIDA Mortality Risk Score: development and external validation of a prognostic model for early and late death in degenerative mitral regurgitation. Eur Heart J 2018;39(15):1281-1291.
24. Antoine C, Benfari G, Michelena HI, et al. Clinical outcome of degenerative mitral regurgitation. Circulation 2018;138(13):1317-1326.
25. Grigioni F, Enriquez-Sarano M, Ling LH, et al. Sudden death in mitral regurgitation due to flail leaflet. J Am Coll Cardiol 1999;34(7): 2078-2085.
26. Basso C, Perazzolo Marra M, Rizzo S, et al. Arrhythmic mitral valve prolapse and sudden cardiac death. Circulation 2015;132(7):556-566.
27. Sriram CS, Syed FF, Ferguson ME, et al. Malignant bileaflet mitral valve prolapse syndrome in patients with otherwise idiopathic out-of-hospital cardiac arrest. J Am Coll Cardiol 2013;62(3):222-230.
28. Perazzolo Marra M, Basso C, De Lazzari M, et al. Morphofunctional abnormalities of mitral annulus and arrhythmic mitral valve prolapse. Circ Cardiovasc Imaging 2016;9(8):e005030.
29. Ermakov S, Gulhar R, Lim L, et al. Left ventricular mechanical dispersion predicts arrhythmic risk in mitral valve prolapse. Heart 2019;105(14):1063-1069.
30. Hourdain J, Clavel MA, Deharo JC, et al. Common phenotype in patients with mitral valve prolapse who experienced sudden cardiac death. Circulation 2018;138(10):1067-1069.
31. Habib G, Lancellotti P, Antunes MJ, et al. 2015 ESC Guidelines for the management of infective endocarditis: the Task Force for the Management of Infective Endocarditis of the European Society of Cardiology (ESC). Endorsed by: European Association for Cardio-Thoracic Surgery (EACTS), the European Association of Nuclear Medicine (EANM). Eur Heart J 2015;36(44):3075-3128.
32. Levine RA, Stathogiannis E, Newell JB, Harrigan P, Weyman AE. Reconsideration of echocardiographic standards for mitral valve prolapse: lack of association between leaflet displacement isolated to the apical four chamber view and independent echocardiographic evidence of abnormality. J Am Coll Cardiol 1988;11(5):1010-1019.
33. MacMahon SW, Roberts JK, Kramer-Fox R, et al. Mitral valve prolapse and infective endocarditis. Am Heart J 1987;113(5):1291-1298.
34. Katan O, Michelena HI, Avierinos JF, et al. Incidence and predictors of infective endocarditis in mitral valve prolapse: a population-based study. Mayo Clin Proc 2016;91(3):336-342.
35. Baumgartner H, Falk V, Bax JJ, et al. 2017 ESC/EACTS Guidelines for the management of valvular heart disease: the Task Force for the Management of Valvular Heart Disease of the European Society of Cardiology (ESC) and the European Association for Cardio-Thoracic Surgery (EACTS). Eur Heart J 2017;38(36):2739-2791.
36. Nishimura RA, Otto CM, Bonow RO, et al. 2017 AHA/ACC focused update of the 2014 AHA/ACC guideline for the management of patients with valvular heart disease: a report of the American College of Cardiology/American Heart Association Task Force on Clinical Practice Guidelines. Circulation 2017; 135(25):e1159-e1195.

37. Alkadhi H, Wildermuth S, Bettex DA, et al. Mitral regurgitation: quantification with 16-detector row CT—initial experience. Radiology 2006; 238(2):454-463.

38. van Rosendael PJ, van Wijngaarden SE, Kamperidis V, et al. Integrated imaging of echocardiography and computed tomography to grade mitral regurgitation severity in patients undergoing transcatheter aortic valve implantation. Eur Heart J 2017;38(28):2221-2226.

39. Krieger EV, Lee J, Branch KR, Hamilton-Craig C. Quantitation of mitral regurgitation with cardiac magnetic resonance imaging: a systematic review. Heart 2016;102(23):1864-1870.

40. Zoghbi WA, Adams D, Bonow RO, et al. Recommendations for noninvasive evaluation of native valvular regurgitation: a report from the American Society of Echocardiography developed in collaboration with the Society for Cardiovascular Magnetic Resonance. J Am Soc Echocardiogr 2017;30(4):303-371.

41. Lancellotti P, Moura L, Pierard LA, et al. European Association of Echocardiography recommendations for the assessment of valvular regurgitation. Part 2: mitral and tricuspid regurgitation (native valve disease). Eur J Echocardiogr 2010;11(4):307-332.

42. Enriquez-Sarano M, Sinak L, Tajik A, et al. Changes in effective regurgitant orifice throughout systole in patients with mitral valve prolapse. A clinical study using the proximal isovelocity surface area method. Circulation 1995;92:2951-2958.

43. Topilsky Y, Michelena H, Bichara V, et al. Mitral valve prolapse with mid-late systolic mitral regurgitation: pitfalls of evaluation and clinical outcome compared with holosystolic regurgitation. Circulation 2012;125(13): 1643-1651.

44. Enriquez-Sarano M, Bailey K, Seward J, et al. Quantitative Doppler assessment of valvular regurgitation. Circulation 1993;87:841-848.

45. Enriquez-Sarano M, Avierinos JF, Messika-Zeitoun D, et al. Quantitative determinants of the outcome of asymptomatic mitral regurgitation. N Engl J Med 2005;352(9):875-883.

46. Nishimura RA, Otto CM, Bonow RO, et al. 2014 AHA/ACC Guideline for the management of patients with valvular heart disease: executive summary: a report of the American College of Cardiology/American Heart Association Task Force on Practice Guidelines. Circulation 2014; 129(23):2440-2492.

47. Little SH, Pirat B, Kumar R, et al. Three-dimensional color Doppler echocardiography for direct measurement of vena contracta area in mitral regurgitation: in vitro validation and clinical experience. JACC Cardiovasc Imaging 2008;1(6):695-704.

48. Tsang W, Weinert L, Sugeng L, et al. The value of three-dimensional echocardiography derived mitral valve parametric maps and the role of experience in the diagnosis of pathology. J Am Soc Echocardiogr 2011;24(8):860-867.

49. Tribouilloy C, Rusinaru D, Grigioni F, et al. Long-term mortality associated with left ventricular dysfunction in mitral regurgitation due to flail leaflets: a multicenter analysis. Circ Cardiovasc Imaging 2014; 7(2):363-370.

50. Tribouilloy C, Grigioni F, Avierinos JF, et al. Survival implication of left ventricular end-systolic diameter in mitral regurgitation due to flail leaflets a long-term follow-up multicenter study. J Am Coll Cardiol 2009;54(21):1961-1968.

51. Magne J, Mahjoub H, Pierard LA, et al. Prognostic importance of brain natriuretic peptide and left ventricular longitudinal function in asymptomatic degenerative mitral regurgitation. Heart 2012;98(7): 584-591.

52. Grigioni F, Avierinos JF, Ling LH, et al. Atrial fibrillation complicating the course of degenerative mitral regurgitation: determinants and long-term outcome. J Am Coll Cardiol 2002;40(1):84-92.

53. Kernis SJ, Nkomo VT, Messika-Zeitoun D, et al. Atrial fibrillation after surgical correction of mitral regurgitation in sinus rhythm: incidence, outcome, and determinants. Circulation 2004;110(16):2320-2325.

54. Ling L, Enriquez-Sarano M, Seward J, et al. Early surgery in patients with mitral regurgitation due to partial flail leaflet: a long-term outcome study. Circulation 1997;96:1819-1825.

55. Rusinaru D, Tribouilloy C, Grigioni F, et al. Left atrial size is a potent predictor of mortality in mitral regurgitation due to flail leaflets: results from a large international multicenter study. Circ Cardiovasc Imaging 2011; 4(5):473-481.

56. Messika-Zeitoun D, Bellamy M, Avierinos JF, et al. Left atrial remodelling in mitral regurgitation—methodologic approach, physiological determinants, and outcome implications: a prospective quantitative Doppler-echocardiographic and electron beam-computed tomographic study. Eur Heart J 2007;28(14):1773-1781.

57. Le Tourneau T, Messika-Zeitoun D, Russo A, et al. Impact of left atrial volume on clinical outcome in organic mitral regurgitation. J Am Coll Cardiol 2010;56(7):570-578.

58. Barbieri A, Bursi F, Grigioni F, et al. Prognostic and therapeutic implications of pulmonary hypertension complicating degenerative mitral regurgitation due to flail leaflet: a multicenter long-term international study. Eur Heart J 2011;32(6):751-759.

59. Feldman T, Foster E, Glower DD, et al. Percutaneous repair or surgery for mitral regurgitation. N Engl J Med 2011;364(15):1395-1406.

60. Sorajja P, Mack M, Vemulapalli S, et al. Initial experience with commercial transcatheter mitral valve repair in the United States. J Am Coll Cardiol 2016;67(10):1129-1140.

61. Messika-Zeitoun D, Johnson BD, Nkomo V, et al. Cardiopulmonary exercise testing determination of functional capacity in mitral regurgitation: physiologic and outcome implications. J Am Coll Cardiol 2006; 47(12):2521-2527.

62. Magne J, Lancellotti P, Pierard LA. Exercise pulmonary hypertension in asymptomatic degenerative mitral regurgitation. Circulation 2010;122(1):33-41.

63. Magne J, Donal E, Mahjoub H, et al. Impact of exercise pulmonary hypertension on postoperative outcome in primary mitral regurgitation. Heart 2015;101(5):391-396.

64. Ha JW, Choi D, Park S, et al. Determinants of exercise-induced pulmonary hypertension in patients with normal left ventricular ejection fraction. Heart 2009;95(6):490-494.

65. Mahjoub H, Levy F, Cassol M, et al. Effects of age on pulmonary artery systolic pressure at rest and during exercise in normal adults. Eur J Echocardiogr 2009;10(5):635-640.

66. Lancellotti P, Cosyns B, Zacharakis D, et al. Importance of left ventricular longitudinal function and functional reserve in patients with degenerative mitral regurgitation: assessment by two-dimensional speckle tracking. J Am Soc Echocardiogr 2008;21(12):1331-1336.

67. Leung D, Griffin B, Stewart W, et al. Left ventricular function after valve repair for chronic mitral regurgitation: predictive value of preoperative assessment of contractile reserve by exercise echocardiography. J Am Coll Cardiol 1996;28:1198-1205.

68. Donal E, Mascle S, Brunet A, et al. Prediction of left ventricular ejection fraction 6 months after surgical correction of organic mitral regurgitation: the value of exercise echocardiography and deformation imaging. Eur Heart J Cardiovasc Imaging 2012;13(11):922-930.

69. Magne J, Donal E, Mahjoub H, et al. Impact of exercise pulmonary hypertension on postoperative outcome in primary mitral regurgitation. Heart 2014;101(5):391-396.

70. Le Tourneau T, Deswarte G, Lamblin N, et al. Right ventricular systolic function in organic mitral regurgitation: impact of biventricular impairment. Circulation 2013;127(15):1597-1608.

71. Kusunose K, Popovic ZB, Motoki H, Marwick TH. Prognostic significance of exercise-induced right ventricular dysfunction in asymptomatic degenerative mitral regurgitation. Circ Cardiovasc Imaging 2013;6(2):167-176.

72. Magne J, Lancellotti P, Pierard LA. Exercise-induced changes in degenerative mitral regurgitation. J Am Coll Cardiol 2010;56(4):300-309.

73. Detaint D, Messika-Zeitoun D, Avierinos JF, et al. B-type natriuretic peptide in organic mitral regurgitation: determinants and impact on outcome. Circulation 2005;111(18):2391-2397.

74. Clavel MA, Tribouilloy C, Vanoverschelde JL, et al. Association of B-type natriuretic peptide with survival in patients with degenerative mitral regurgitation. J Am Coll Cardiol 2016;68(12):1297-1307.

75. Pizarro R, Bazzino OO, Oberti PF, et al. Prospective validation of the prognostic usefulness of brain natriuretic peptide in asymptomatic patients with chronic severe mitral regurgitation. J Am Coll Cardiol 2009;54(12):1099-1106.

76. Avierinos JF, Brown RD, Foley DA, et al. Cerebral ischemic events after diagnosis of mitral valve prolapse: a community-based study of incidence and predictive factors. Stroke 2003;34(6):1339-1344.

77. Grigioni F, Tribouilloy C, Avierinos JF, et al. Outcomes in mitral regurgitation due to flail leaflets a multicenter European study. JACC Cardiovasc Imaging 2008;1(2):133-141.

78. Ling H, Enriquez-Sarano M, Seward J, et al. Clinical outcome of mitral regurgitation due to flail leaflets. N Eng J Med 1996;335:1417-1423.

79. Tribouilloy C, Enriquez-Sarano M, Schaff H, et al. Impact of preoperative symptoms on survival after surgical correction of organic mitral regurgitation: rationale for optimizing surgical indications. Circulation 1999; 99:400-405.

80. Enriquez-Sarano M, Suri RM, Clavel MA, et al. Is there an outcome penalty linked to guideline-based indications for valvular surgery? Early and long-term analysis of patients with organic mitral regurgitation. J Thorac Cardiovasc Surg 2015;150(1):50-58.

81. Avierinos JF, Tribouilloy C, Grigioni F, et al. Impact of ageing on presentation and outcome of mitral regurgitation due to flail leaflet: a multicentre international study. Eur Heart J 2013;34(33):2600-2609.

82. Braunberger E, Deloche A, Berrebi A, et al. Very long-term results (more than 20 years) of valve repair with Carpentier's techniques in nonrheumatic mitral valve insufficiency. Circulation 2001;104(12 Suppl 1):I8-I11.

83. David TE, Armstrong S, McCrindle BW, Manlhiot C. Late outcomes of mitral valve repair for mitral regurgitation due to degenerative disease. Circulation 2013;127(14):1485-1492.

84. Lazam S, Vanoverschelde JL, Tribouilloy C, et al. Twenty-year outcome after mitral repair versus replacement for severe degenerative mitral regurgitation: analysis of a large, prospective, multicenter, international registry. Circulation 2016;135(5):410-422.

85. Kang DH, Kim JH, Rim JH, et al. Comparison of early surgery versus conventional treatment in asymptomatic severe mitral regurgitation. Circulation 2009;119(6):797-804.

86. Kang DH, Park SJ, Sun BJ, et al. Early surgery versus conventional treatment for asymptomatic severe mitral regurgitation: a propensity analysis. J Am Coll Cardiol 2014;63(22):2398-2407.

87. Suri RM, Vanoverschelde JL, Grigioni F, et al. Association between early surgical intervention vs watchful waiting and outcomes for mitral regurgitation due to flail mitral valve leaflets. JAMA 2013;310(6):609-616.

88. Rosenhek R, Rader F, Klaar U, et al. Outcome of watchful waiting in asymptomatic severe mitral regurgitation. Circulation 2006;113(18): 2238-2244.

89. Tribouilloy C, Rusinaru D, Szymanski C, et al. Predicting left ventricular dysfunction after valve repair for mitral regurgitation due to leaflet prolapse: additive value of left ventricular end-systolic dimension to ejection fraction. Eur J Echocardiogr 2011;12(9):702-710.

90. Bolling SF, Li S, O'Brien SM, et al. Predictors of mitral valve repair: clinical and surgeon factors. Ann Thorac Surg 2010;90(6):1904-1911; discussion 1912.

91. Suri RM, Clavel MA, Schaff HV, et al. Effect of recurrent mitral regurgitation following degenerative mitral valve repair: long-term analysis of competing outcomes. J Am Coll Cardiol 2016;67(5):488-498.

92. Chikwe J, Toyoda N, Anyanwu AC, et al. Relation of mitral valve surgery volume to repair rate, durability, and survival. J Am Coll Cardiol 2017; 69(19):2397-2406.

93. Adams DH, Rosenhek R, Falk V. Degenerative mitral valve regurgitation: best practice revolution. Eur Heart J 2010;31(16):1958-1966.

94. Messika-Zeitoun D, Topilsky Y, Enriquez-Sarano M. The role of echocardiography in the management of patients with myxomatous disease. Cardiol Clin 2013;31(2):217-229.

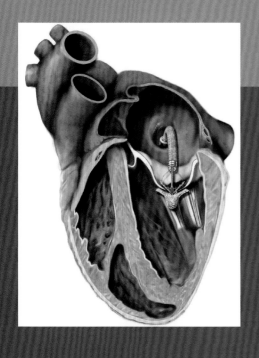

第18章
缺血性和扩张型心肌病的继发性（功能性）二尖瓣反流

本章重点介绍缺血性和非缺血性心肌病中慢性功能性二尖瓣反流的流行病学、发病机制、诊断、预后和治疗情况。

继发性（功能性）二尖瓣反流，是指瓣膜结构正常，由左心室功能障碍或二尖瓣瓣环扩张导致二尖瓣前后叶闭合不全而引起的反流，多由慢性缺血性或非缺血性心肌病引起。超声心动图是检测和评价继发性（功能性）二尖瓣反流最常用的方法，其可以确定继发性（功能性）二尖瓣反流的机制和严重程度，评价左心室的大小、形状和收缩功能。由于尚无单一的超声心动图参数可对继发性（功能性）二尖瓣反流的严重程度进行理想分级，因此建议采用多参数结合的综合方法进行评估。继发性（功能性）二尖瓣反流严重程度的加重与死亡率上升、左心室增大和左心室收缩功能降低有关，但继发性（功能性）二尖瓣反流是否是左心室功能障碍加重的标志或导致生存率下降的原因，目前仍不确定。针对继发性（功能性）二尖瓣反流的治疗主要包括对心力衰竭和左心室功能障碍进行最佳剂量的指南推荐药物治疗，必要时可在合适的患者中行心脏再同步化治疗或冠状动脉血运重建来进一步改善二尖瓣反流。二尖瓣外科手术治疗是否能降低死亡率，带来生存或生活质量方面的益处尚不清楚，经导管治疗的有效性也有待临床试验的进一步确认。

李秋忆

Secondary (Functional) Mitral Regurgitation in Ischemic and Dilated Cardiomyopathy

Paul A. Grayburn

CHAPTER OUTLINE

KEY POINTS

- Grading of mitral regurgitation (MR) severity by echocardiography should not be based on visual inspection of the color Doppler MR jet, but rather on integration of multiple qualitative and quantitative parameters.
- Secondary MR is dynamic, changing during systole in a biphasic pattern, and often varying dramatically with changes in loading conditions.
- Any degree of secondary MR is associated with an adverse prognosis; however, LV size and function are also worse with worsened degrees of secondary MR.
- Treatment of secondary MR begins with optimally tolerated doses of guideline-directed medical therapy for heart failure and/or left

ventricular dysfunction. Cardiac resynchronization therapy and coronary revascularization should be performed when indicated.
- Mitral valve surgery (replacement or repair) may be considered in selected patients with secondary MR but has not be shown to improve outcomes.
- In randomized clinical trials, transcatheter mitral valve repair with the MitraClip device has been shown to reduce heart failure hospitalization and mortality in patients with secondary MR and LV EF between 20% to 50%.

DEFINITION

Primary mitral regurgitation (MR) is caused by a lesion of the mitral valve leaflets, such as mitral valve prolapse, flail leaflet, endocarditis, rheumatic heart disease, radiation-induced heart disease, or various inflammatory conditions. Secondary MR, also known as functional MR (FMR), occurs when normal or nearly normal mitral leaflets are prevented from adequate coaptation by underlying left ventricular (LV) dysfunction or mitral annular dilation or both. Most cases of secondary MR are caused by chronic ischemic or nonischemic cardiomyopathy, but it occasionally results from pure annular dilation in chronic atrial fibrillation or restrictive cardiomyopathy. The term *ischemic mitral regurgitation* is often used to describe MR that occurs in chronic ischemic cardiomyopathy due to LV remodeling, although it can also refer to transient and reversible MR occurring during acute myocardial ischemia.

Acute MR due to papillary muscle rupture as a complication of acute myocardial infarction (MI) is not covered. This chapter focuses on the epidemiology, mechanism, prognostic implications, and treatment of chronic FMR in ischemic and nonischemic cardiomyopathies.

EPIDEMIOLOGY

MR is the most common form of valvular heart disease; the incidence is less than 1% before age 55 years but increases with each decade to more than 9% after age 75 years.[1] These estimates were based on an analysis of pooled data from three large epidemiologic studies and the Olmstead County database, in which moderate or severe MR was reported from qualitative echocardiographic grading. The study did not distinguish between moderate and severe MR, nor did it differentiate primary from secondary MR. A subsequent meta-analysis attempted to examine the prevalence of MR in the U.S. population using the

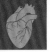

Carpentier classification of leaflet motion to determine mechanism. The study authors estimated that MR affected 2 to 2.5 million people in the United States in the year 2000. The most common underlying mechanism was restricted motion of the leaflets only during systole (i.e., Carpentier class IIIb), which is the classic condition for FMR.[2] The prevalence of FMR due to ischemic cardiomyopathy was estimated at 7500 to 9000 cases per 1 million people, and that of FMR due to nonischemic LV dysfunction was 16,250 cases per 1 million.

Although FMR is common, most cases are mild or moderate in severity. For example, in the Surgical Treatment of Ischemic Heart Failure (STICH) trial, an independent echocardiography core laboratory adjudicated the severity of FMR in ischemic cardiomyopathy as none in 27%, mild in 47%, moderate in 17%, and severe (grade 3+ or 4+) in 9% of 1852 patients with interpretable studies.[3] Moderate or severe MR seems to occur in roughly one fourth of patients with cardiomyopathy.

MECHANISM

The mitral apparatus consists of the leaflets, annulus, chordae tendineae, and papillary muscles with their supporting LV myocardium. Normal mitral valve closure is achieved by proper balance between closing forces that push the valve leaflets together during systole and tethering forces that prevent the valve from prolapsing into the left atrium (LA) (Fig. 18.1). The mechanisms underlying FMR were eloquently reviewed by Levine and Schwammenthal.[4] Closing forces are exerted on the mitral leaflets by systolic contraction of the LV myocardium and the mitral annulus. These forces are counterbalanced by the tethering forces exerted by the papillary muscles with their chordal attachments to the leaflets. In the normally shaped LV, the papillary muscles and chordae tendineae exert a vertical force on the leaflets, bringing them together during isovolumic contraction and preventing them from prolapsing into the LA during ejection. Spherical LV geometry due to remodeling causes the papillary muscles to migrate laterally and apically; as a result, they can no longer exert a vertical force during systole, leading to FMR.[5]

Because wall motion abnormalities may be regional rather than global, tethering forces are often asymmetric. For example, inferoposterior wall motion abnormalities commonly tether the posteromedial scallop (P3 segment) of the posterior leaflet and lead to asymmetric

dilation of the annulus on its medial aspect.[6] In addition to an imbalance between closing forces and tethering forces, annular dilation, flattening of the annulus, and loss of systolic annular contraction may contribute to FMR.[7] In some patients, LV dyssynchrony leads to discoordinated myocardial contraction that further distorts the balance between closing and tethering forces, resulting in a loss of normal mitral leaflet coaptation and competence.[8]

Despite the obvious fact that closing forces and tethering forces are abnormal in virtually all patients with chronic ischemic or nonischemic cardiomyopathy, many of these patients do not have FMR or have only mild FMR. The most obvious explanation is that the reduction in closing force and the increase in tethering force may be balanced so that MR remains absent or mild. Another reason is the potential for mitral leaflet tissue to expand over time, allowing more leaflet surface for coaptation.[9] In patients with chronic severe aortic regurgitation, who have very dilated LV chambers with leaflet tethering, the mitral leaflet surface is 30% larger than normal, and FMR is uncommon.[10] FMR may not simply be a disease of the LV but may also involve inadequate compensatory mitral leaflet enlargement due to lack of time for compensatory enlargement to occur (e.g., MR after MI) or to biologic abnormalities (e.g., advanced age, diabetes, genetic factors).[11]

Ischemic Mitral Regurgitation

During percutaneous coronary intervention (PCI), acute myocardial ischemia induced by balloon inflation causes prompt segmental myocardial dyskinesis, which reverses on balloon deflation.[12] Relief of ischemia by PCI has been shown to reduce or eliminate acute ischemic MR.[13] In the setting of acute MI, a significant wall motion abnormality may lead to FMR, particularly with inferoposterior MI.[14] Although this represents true ischemic MR, that term is most often used to refer to MR in the setting of chronic ischemic heart disease with LV dilation and dysfunction.

The mechanism of MR can vary, depending in part on the distribution of coronary artery disease (CAD). Right coronary disease typically leads to an inferoposterior wall motion abnormality, often with normal or only mildly reduced left ventricular ejection fraction (LVEF). On echocardiography, the posterior leaflet, particularly the posteromedial scallop, appears to be restricted, whereas the anterior leaflet appears to override the posterior leaflet without rising above the annulus plane (i.e., pseudoprolapse) (Fig. 18.2).[15] The mid-anterior leaflet may

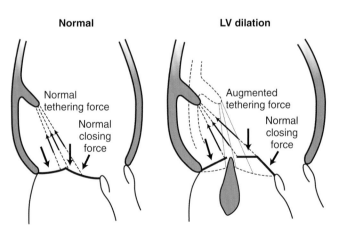

Fig. 18.1 Principles of Mitral Valve Tethering in Ischemic Mitral Regurgitation (MR). Basic principles of tethering mechanism for ischemic mitral regurgitation (MR) and balance of apposed closing and tethering forces acting on the leaflets. Augmented tethering force created by papillary muscle displacement apically *(dotted lines)* displaces the leaflets and causes MR. *LV,* Left ventricle.

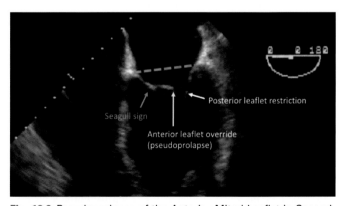

Fig. 18.2 Pseudoprolapse of the Anterior Mitral Leaflet in Secondary Mitral Regurgitation (MR) Due to Severely Restricted Posterior Leaflet Motion. TEE image in mid-systole shows pseudoprolapse of the anterior mitral leaflet in a patient with severe secondary MR. The posterior leaflet has severely restricted motion *(white arrow),* and the anterior leaflet overrides it *(yellow arrow).* The body of the anterior leaflet is tented by a strut chord (i.e., seagull sign) *(blue arrow).* This is not anterior leaflet prolapse because the anterior leaflet never moves above the annulus *(dashed blue line).*

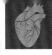

be tented by tension on strut chords, resulting in the so-called seagull sign (see Fig. 18.2). In anterior MI, FMR often results from spherical LV remodeling with reduced LVEF. The alterations in LV geometry change the papillary muscle position and the direction of tension exerted on mitral leaflets.[16]

Contrary to traditional teaching, isolated infarction of the papillary muscles does not cause FMR.[17] Rather, it is displacement of the papillary muscles by the underlying myocardium that increases tethering forces and results in ischemic FMR. This can occur with wall motion abnormalities in any myocardial territory or with global LV remodeling in ischemic heart disease.

Functional Mitral Regurgitation in the Absence of Coronary Artery Disease

MR is common in all forms of nonischemic cardiomyopathy, including dilated, hypertrophic, and restrictive cardiomyopathy. In dilated cardiomyopathy, the mitral annulus is dilated and the papillary muscles are outwardly and apically displaced as a result of the spherical LV remodeling.[18] The papillary muscle displacement causes an abnormal tethering of mitral leaflets so that the point of coaptation is inside the LV chamber, well beneath the MV plane.[19] In hypertrophic cardiomyopathy, FMR occurs in late systole as the mitral valve is displaced anteriorly.

In restrictive cardiomyopathy, the LV usually is not dilated and typically exhibits normal systolic function until late in the course of the disease. MR is usually caused by severe atrial enlargement with annular dilation rather than by tethering.

Atrial FMR is a subcategory of secondary MR that occurs in patients with chronic atrial fibrillation and a markedly dilated LA.[20] This form of FMR is caused by pure annular dilation with normal (i.e., Carpentier type I) leaflet motion. It occurs in a minority of patients with chronic atrial fibrillation.

DIAGNOSIS

MR may be suspected from the history and physical examination. Exertional dyspnea and fatigue are the predominant symptoms associated with MR. However, in most patients with secondary MR, it can be difficult to distinguish whether symptoms are the result of the underlying cardiomyopathy, FMR, or other common comorbidities such as chronic lung disease, obesity, or deconditioning.

In FMR, the typical holosystolic murmur of MR may be absent. In a small substudy of the Thrombolysis in Myocardial Infarction (TIMI) trial, a murmur was appreciated in only 50% of cases in which MR was clearly present on contrast-enhanced left ventriculography.[21] When the MR is directed posteriorly, as occurs with posterior leaflet tethering, the murmur may radiate to the back and may be missed on routine precordial examination. When LA pressures are severely elevated, the duration of MR is brief and the murmur may be missed or mistaken for an ejection murmur. Findings on chest radiographs are nonspecific and may include cardiomegaly with evidence of LV and LA enlargement and pulmonary vascular congestion.

Echocardiography

Transthoracic echocardiography (TTE) is the imaging modality most commonly used to detect and evaluate FMR. A comprehensive TTE study (Table 18.1) is required and should begin with accurate assessment of LV size and function, including LV volumes at end-diastole and end-systole, sphericity index, LVEF, and regional wall motion abnormalities. The most accurate and reproducible technique for measuring LV size and systolic function is three-dimensional (3D) TTE, which is recommended by American Society of Echocardiography (ASE) guidelines.[22]

Assessment	Measurements
TABLE 18.1 Comprehensive Echocardiographic Assessment of Secondary Mitral Regurgitation.	
LV size and function	• LV end-diastolic diameter and volume/volume index • LV end-systolic diameter and volume/volume index • LV ejection fraction • LV regional wall motion abnormalities, including dyssynchrony • LV sphericity index • LV global longitudinal strain
Mitral valve morphology	• Leaflets should be structurally normal (mild age-related focal thickening acceptable) • Restricted leaflet motion in systole (posterior leaflet, anterior leaflet, both) • Symmetric or asymmetric tethering (posteromedial scallop is most common) • Tenting height/area by 2D imaging and/or tenting volume by 3D imaging • Posterior leaflet tethering angle • Coaptation length • Mitral annulus diameter in anteroposterior (long-axis view) and intercommissural planes (intercommissural view on TEE) and/or mitral annulus area/perimeter by 3D imaging
Mitral regurgitation	• Presence or absence by color Doppler imaging • Number and direction of MR jets • Integrated assessment of MR severity (none/trace, mild, moderate, severe) • Vena contracta width (2D imaging) or vena contracta area (3D imaging) • EROA • Regurgitant volume • Regurgitant fraction • Continuous-wave Doppler profile of MR jet (faint, dense, triangular, duration of systole) • Pulmonary venous flow pattern • Mitral inflow pattern • Estimated RV systolic pressure (for tricuspid regurgitation) • LA volume/volume index • Secondary tricuspid regurgitation • Associated RV dilation and dysfunction
Dynamic assessment	• Reassess after blood pressure control, optimization of guideline-directed medical therapy for heart failure, revascularization, and/or cardiac resynchronization therapy • Evaluate MR severity, PA pressure response to exercise • Contractile reserve to identify hibernating or stunned myocardium

EROA, Effective regurgitant orifice area; *MR*, mitral regurgitation; *PA*, pulmonary artery.

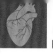

The mechanism of MR requires assessment of mitral leaflet morphology in multiple views and measurement of tenting area, coaptation depth, annular diameter, and posterior leaflet angle (Fig. 18.3). TTE is usually sufficient, but transesophageal echocardiography (TEE) may be required to identify the mechanism of MR or to define severity of MR in selected patients. Assessment of the severity of MR requires an integrated approach that combines multiple qualitative and quantitative methods because no single method is sufficiently precise or reproducible to serve as the sole determinant of MR severity. Echocardiographic findings with asymmetric versus symmetric tethering are presented in Table 18.2.

Grading Mitral Regurgitation Severity by Echocardiography

Severity of MR is most commonly assessed with the use of color-flow Doppler (CFD) imaging during TTE or TEE. CFD is misnamed: it is an image of the spatial distribution of velocities, not flow, within the image plane.

Jet size by CFD is profoundly affected by instrument settings and hemodynamic factors.[23,24] When those are held constant, the size of a jet is determined by its momentum flux, ρAV^2 (ρ is blood density, A is orifice area, and V^2 is velocity squared).[25] An MR jet with a 6 m/s driving velocity appears 44% larger by CFD than an MR jet with a 5 m/s driving velocity. High driving velocities occur when LV systolic pressure is abnormally high (i.e., hypertension, aortic stenosis, LV outflow tract obstruction), and this should be recognized by the interpreting physician when grading MR severity.

The tendency for CFD to overestimate MR severity was shown in a study comparing TTE with cardiac magnetic resonance (CMR) for quantitation.[26] This partially explains why healthy individuals with no heart murmur often have mild FMR on CFD.[27] However, MR can be significantly underestimated in the setting of a low driving velocity or when the MR jet is markedly eccentric. In the latter case, MR jets lose momentum as they slam into the LA wall.[28] Low-velocity jets (i.e., 4 m/s) are worrisome because they imply high LA pressure and low LV

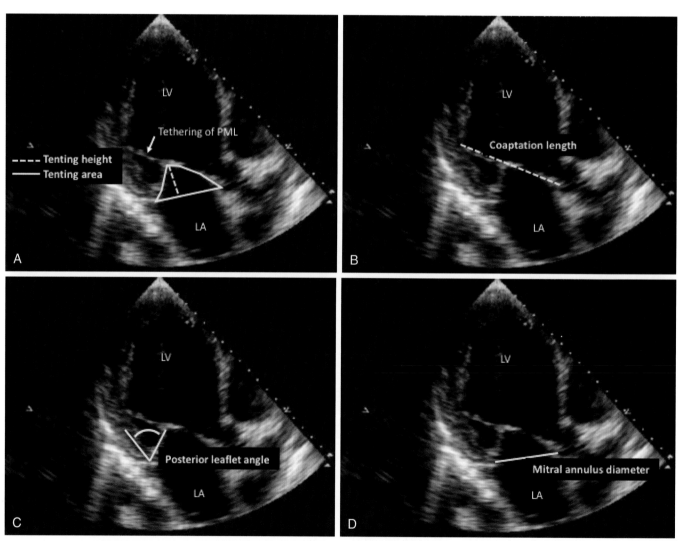

Fig. 18.3 Echocardiographic Measurements of Leaflet Tenting in Secondary Mitral Regurgitation (MR).
End-systolic frame from the apical long-axis view in a patient with ischemic cardiomyopathy and severe secondary MR. (A) Mitral leaflet coaptation is tented toward the LV apex. Tenting height *(dashed line)* and tenting area *(solid line)* are measured as shown. (B) Coaptation length is a measure of papillary muscle displacement *(dashed line)*. (C) Posterior leaflet angle is measured between the posterior leaflet itself and the underlying endocardial border. (D) The mitral annulus is best measured in the long-axis view (rather than the four-chamber view) because it is aligned with the minor (anteroposterior) axis of the mitral annulus. *PML,* Posterior mitral leaflet.

TABLE 18.2 Echocardiographic Findings in Secondary Mitral Regurgitation due to Asymmetric or Symmetric Tethering.

Feature	Asymmetric	Symmetric
Cause	Inferoposterior or lateral myocardial infarction (MI)	Large anterior or multiple MIs Nonischemic cardiomyopathy
Tethering	Posterior leaflet; often limited to or worse at posteromedial scallop (P3 segment)	Both leaflets; anterior leaflet may demonstrate seagull sign
Tenting	None or mildly increased	Markedly increased
Annulus	Dilation absent, mild, asymmetric	Dilated, flattened
Left ventricular remodeling	Limited to inferoposterior or lateral wall, often at base only	Global dilation with increased sphericity index
Mitral regurgitation jet direction	Posterior or posterolateral	Often central

pressure, consistent with severe MR with hemodynamic compromise (assuming proper alignment of the continuous-wave Doppler beam with the MR jet).

In addition to jet driving velocity and eccentricity, CFD jet size is affected by many other technical and hemodynamic factors.[29] The U.S. and European guidelines recommend that determinations of MR jet size by CFD not be used alone to assess MR severity.[23,24]

Quantitative Parameters

The use of quantitative measures, including effective regurgitant orifice area (EROA), regurgitant volume (RVol), and regurgitant fraction (RF), is strongly recommended by American Society of Echocardiography guidelines for assessing MR severity.[23] These parameters can be measured by several techniques, including the proximal isovelocity surface area (PISA) method, volumetric methods, and 3D imaging.[30]

It is crucial to recognize the technical limitations and imprecision of each method and the overlap of values obtained. Volumetric methods suffer from multiplication of the errors inherent in measurement of stroke volumes at different locations, but they can account for the whole of MR over the duration of systole. Single-frame measurements, such as PISA or vena contracta width or area, can markedly overestimate MR severity when the jet is limited to early or late systole.[31]

Assuming proper measurement, values of EROA equal to or greater than 0.4 cm², RVol equal to or greater than 60 mL, or RF equal to or greater than 50% are highly specific for severe MR; values of EROA equal to or less than 0.2 cm², RVol equal to or less than 30 mL, or RF less than 30% are highly specific for mild MR. Intermediate values can occur in severe FMR, but they lack specificity.

A common scenario in which lower values of EROA and RVol may represent severe MR includes markedly crescent-shaped orifice geometry in secondary MR: PISA yields a falsely low value for EROA due to its inherent assumption of a round orifice (Fig. 18.4).[32–41] Another example occurs in the setting of multiple MR jets: a measured EROA from a single jet does not reflect the totality of MR severity. Addition of EROA or vena contracta areas from multiple MR jets should be accurate, but this has not been well validated.

Integration of Multiple Parameters

A comprehensive approach is recommended so that multiple parameters are evaluated and integrated to form a final determination of MR severity.[23,24] No single echocardiographic parameter has the measurement precision or reproducibility to serve as the sole arbiter of MR severity, and all parameters have strengths and weaknesses. Nevertheless, it is recognized that most physicians interpreting an echocardiogram look at CFD to detect MR and form an initial impression of its severity. This type of assessment should be considered only as a starting point;

it requires further confirmation using a bayesian approach that integrates multiple factors to arrive at a final determination.

When multiple specific parameters for mild or severe MR are concordant, MR can be graded as mild or severe with high probability of being correct. This is often the case on TTE, especially with the common finding of mild MR and a structurally normal mitral valve. However, when different parameters are discordant among themselves or with the clinical findings, MR severity should be considered uncertain and further testing should be pursued. TEE may be sufficient to define leaflet pathology and quantitate MR severity. However, cine cardiac magnetic resonance (CMR) imaging should be strongly considered because it is more accurate and more reproducible for quantitating RVol and RF and for LV volumes and LVEF.[42–46]

Dynamic Nature of Mitral Regurgitation

It has long been recognized that MR severity varies significantly with loading conditions (Fig. 18.5).[47] Sedation and reduced blood pressure during TEE may result in a significant reduction in MR severity compared with TTE data. Patients with hypertensive urgency can have moderate or severe FMR at presentation that resolves completely with blood pressure control. Guideline-directed medical therapy (GDMT), revascularization, and cardiac resynchronization therapy (CRT) may improve MR severity in cardiomyopathy patients, particularly if the interventions result in reverse LV remodeling or improved regional wall motion.

In addition to changing over time, MR severity is dynamic within the cardiac cycle.[48,49] The classic example is late systolic MR due to prolapse. However, secondary MR may be limited to very early systole in the setting of bundle branch block or ventricular pacing. FMR also may exhibit a biphasic pattern (Fig. 18.6) in which MR severity diminishes during mid-systole, when closing forces are maximal, and is greater in early and late systole.[48] When MR is nonholosystolic, single-frame measurements such as vena contracta width or area or PISA tend to overestimate MR severity. In these cases, EROA or RVol should be measured with volumetric techniques that include all of systole. It is possible to correct EROA for duration of systole, but this method has not been validated.

CFD measures of MR severity can vary significantly during pronounced variations in the R-R interval (e.g., atrial fibrillation). Likewise, caution must be used to avoid measuring MR during premature ventricular contractions (PVCs) or after PVC beats.

Value of Exercise Testing

Stress testing is often used for patients with asymptomatic primary MR to elicit symptoms. In secondary MR, an exercise-induced increase in EROA of 0.13 cm² or more has been shown to predict worse

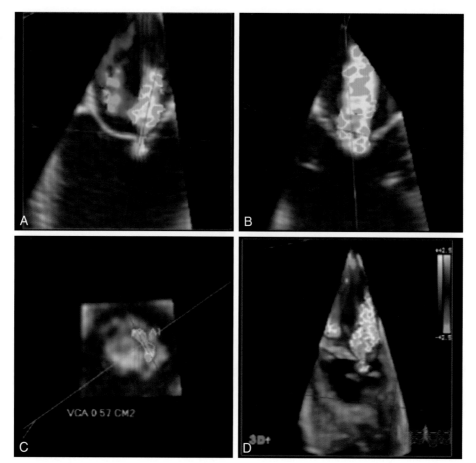

Fig. 18.4 Noncircular Orifice of Secondary Mitral Regurgitation (MR). A 3D reconstruction of color Doppler velocity images from a patient with secondary MR. (A) Long-axis orientation shows a narrow MR jet. The EROA by PISA measured 0.24 cm^2 (not shown). (B) Bicommissural orientation shows a wide MR jet. (C) Cross-sectional plane oriented through the vena contracta of the MR jet shows a markedly elliptical orifice with an EROA of 0.57 cm^2. The PISA formula assumes a round orifice and can underestimate MR severity if the orifice is markedly elliptical or crescent shaped. (D) The full 3D image from which the reconstructed data were made. *EROA*, Effective regurgitant orifice area; *PISA*, proximal isovelocity surface area.

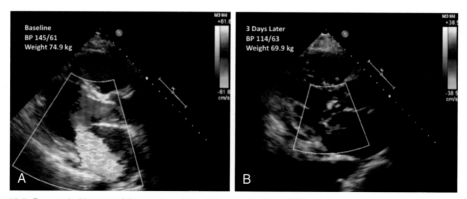

Fig. 18.5 Dynamic Nature of Secondary Mitral Regurgitation (MR). (A) Parasternal long-axis view shows a very large MR jet in a patient with acute decompensated heart failure with blood pressure of 145/61 mmHg, weight of 74.9 kg, and 4+ pedal edema. (B) After 3 days of inotropic therapy and diuresis, the patient weighed 69.9 kg, edema was gone, and the MR jet was very small. The effective regurgitant orifice area (EROA) had declined from 0.46 cm^2 at baseline to 0.08 cm^2 after 3 days of intensive heart failure therapy.

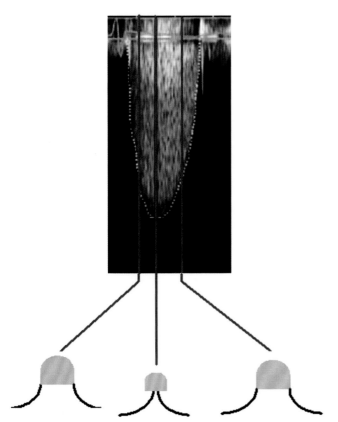

Fig. 18.6 Variation in Proximal Isovelocity Surface Area (PISA) During Systole in Functional Mitral Regurgitation. The variation in PISA *(yellow semi-circles)* is caused by the variation in the regurgitant orifice area (ROA) during systole. In early *(left)* and late *(right)* systole, closing forces are relatively low, and the ROA and PISA values are relatively large. In mid-systole at the point of peak regurgitant velocity *(center)*, the closing forces are maximal, forcing the leaflet tips closer together and reducing ROA and PISA. (From Ray S. The echocardiographic assessment of functional mitral regurgitation. Eur J Echocardiogr 2010;11:i11-i17.)

outcomes. This is another indication of the dynamic nature of FMR, which can be more severe during exercise than at rest.[50] Exercise stress echocardiography may be helpful to evaluate FMR in patients with LV systolic dysfunction who exhibit exertional dyspnea out of proportion to the severity of resting LV dysfunction or MR, in those who have acute pulmonary edema without obvious cause, and before surgical revascularization in patients with moderate MR.[51,52] It may also be helpful in selected patients with FMR for assessment of myocardial ischemia or viability before coronary revascularization.

PROGNOSIS

Observational studies have consistently shown that FMR is associated with an adverse prognosis. Hickey et al reported that for 11,748 patients undergoing cardiac catheterization after MI, increasing severity of MR on LV angiography was associated with worse outcomes, regardless of treatment.[53] In the Survival and Ventricular Enlargement (SAVE) trial,[54] patients with FMR detected by TTE after acute MI were more likely to experience cardiovascular mortality (29% vs. 12%) and severe heart failure (HF) (24% vs. 16%) than those without MR.

Grigioni et al studied patients in the post-MI period (>16 days) and showed an increasing risk of death with higher grades of MR.[55] Mentias et al reported the outcomes of MR for 4005 patients with ST-elevation acute MI (STEMI) treated with acute PCI. MR was graded by TTE using the current guideline-recommended integrated approach. The data confirmed that increasing grades of MR severity were associated with increasing mortality (Fig. 18.7).[56]

Similar findings are seen in MR caused by chronic LV dysfunction.[57–64] Results from the STICH trial are particularly compelling because it was a randomized trial comparing medical therapy with coronary artery bypass grafting (CABG) for HF due to ischemic cardiomyopathy and LVEF less than 35%; patients received current GDMT for HF; and events were adjudicated with prospectively defined end points. Mortality rates were worse with increasing degrees of MR (Fig. 18.8).[62]

Outcomes of HF patients with FMR are similar whether the cause of HF is ischemic or nonischemic cardiomyopathy. In the Beta-blocker Evaluation of Survival Trial (BEST trial), approximately 40% of

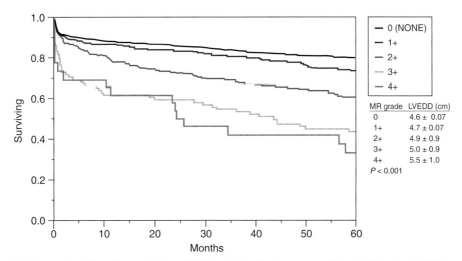

MR grade	LVEDD (cm)
0	4.6 ± 0.07
1+	4.7 ± 0.07
2+	4.9 ± 0.9
3+	5.0 ± 0.9
4+	5.5 ± 1.0

P < 0.001

Fig. 18.7 Survival by Mitral Regurgitation *(MR)* Grade for Contemporary Patients With Acute ST-Elevation Myocardial Infarction (STEMI) Treated With Percutaneous Coronary Intervention. Survival worsened with each increasing grade of MR (*P* = 0.001). Each increasing grade of MR also was associated with a larger LV end-diastolic diameter *(LVEDD)* on echocardiography, consistent with the hypothesis that secondary MR is predominantly a disease of the LV. (From Mentias A, Raza MQ, Barakat AF, et al. Outcomes of ischaemic mitral regurgitation in anterior versus inferior ST elevation myocardial infarction. Open Heart 2016;3:e000493.)

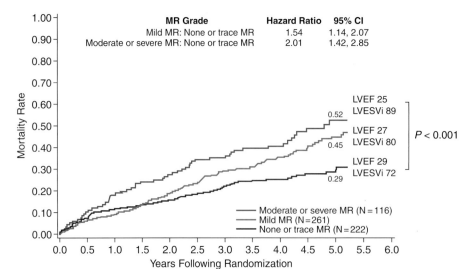

Fig. 18.8 Survival by Mitral Regurgitation *(MR)* Grade for Patients With Heart Failure and Ischemic Cardiomyopathy in the Surgical Treatment of Ischemic Heart Failure (STICH) Trial. Mortality rates increased with increasing severity of MR. Increasing MR grade was associated with larger LV size and lower LVEF, a finding that is consistent across multiple studies. *CI*, Confidence interval; *LVEF*, left ventricular ejection fraction; *LVSVi*, left ventricular stroke volume index. (From Deja MA, Grayburn PA, Sun B, et al. Influence of mitral regurgitation repair on survival in the surgical treatment for ischemic heart failure trial. Circulation 2012;125:2639-2648.)

patients had nonischemic cardiomyopathy. Three variables predicted the combined end point of death, hospitalization for HF, and transplantation: LV end-diastolic volume index equal to or greater than 120 mL/m², mitral deceleration time 150 ms or less, and MR vena contracta width equal to or greater than 0.4 cm.[60] Rossi et al studied 1256 patients with FMR due to ischemic and nonischemic cardiomyopathy, 27% of whom had no FMR, 49% mild to moderate MR, and 24% severe FMR.[62] FMR measured quantitatively was an independent predictor of poor survival, even when the EROA was 0.2 cm² (hazard ratio [HR] = 2.0), a finding typically considered to be the threshold for distinguishing mild from moderate MR.[62] There was a strong independent association between severe FMR and prognosis (HR = 2.0) after adjustment for LVEF and restrictive filling pattern.

Not all studies have shown that an EROA of 0.2 cm² predicts poor outcomes. Patel et al studied the use of EROA for predicting outcomes of FMR in an advanced HF clinic.[64] There was no difference in mortality rates for patients with EROAs larger or smaller than 0.2 cm². A potential explanation for this apparent discrepancy is that the values of EROA and RVol that define severe MR can vary, depending on LV volumes and LVEF.[65] Patients in studies that showed an EROA of 0.2 cm² to be associated with poor outcomes tended to have smaller LV volumes (resulting in a large RF), whereas the patients in the Patel study had very large LV volumes (i.e., producing a much larger EROA required to yield an RF > 50% and a markedly dilated LV that could be the main driver of outcomes) (Fig. 18.9).

Although it is clear from observational studies that any degree of FMR confers an adverse prognosis relative to absence of MR, LV size and systolic function were more abnormal with higher degrees of MR. It remains uncertain whether FMR is simply a marker of worse LV function and geometry.[66]

TREATMENT

Medical Therapy

Because FMR results from underlying LV dysfunction, GDMT for HF due to LV dysfunction is the first line of treatment. The goals are to optimize cardiac performance, reduce symptoms, and enhance survival

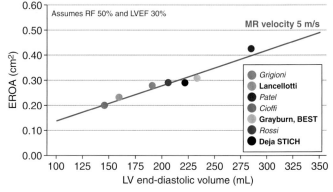

X–LVEDV values given in paper
Y–LVEDV not given in paper, calculated from LVEDD or LVEDVI (Cioffi)

Fig. 18.9 Effective Regurgitant Orifice Area *(EROA)* and Left Ventricular End-Diastolic Volume *(LVEDV)*. Plot shows the relationship of the EROA and LVEDV and assumes severe mitral regurgitation *(MR)* with a regurgitant fraction of 50% and a left ventricular ejection fraction *(LVEF)* of 30%. The relationship is linear: much higher EROAs are required to produce severe MR as LV volume increases. *Colored dots* represent studies of secondary MR. Studies showing that an EROA of 0.2 cm² represents severe MR fell on the left side of the relationship, where lower EROA values could represent 50% regurgitant volume. The Patel study, which did not find that a 0.2 cm² EROA predicted prognosis, lies on the upper right part of the EROA/LVEDV relationship, where severe MR would be expected at an EROA value of 0.4 cm². *BEST*, Beta-blocker Evaluation of Survival Trial; *STICH*, Surgical Treatment of Ischemic Heart Failure. (From Grayburn PA, Carabello B, Gillam LD, et al. Defining severe mitral regurgitation: emphasis on an integrated approach. J Am Coll Cardiol 2014;2014;64:2792-2801.)

by unloading the LV and maintaining euvolemia. GDMT includes carefully titrated therapy with diuretics, angiotensin-converting enzyme (ACE) inhibitors or angiotensin receptor antagonists, or the combination of an angiotensin receptor antagonist and a neprilysin inhibitor, β-blockers, and aldosterone inhibitors. The HF guidelines emphasize titration to dosages that have been effective in reducing mortality rates in randomized clinical trials.[67] The use of carvedilol has decreased severity of FMR and is associated with an increase in the forward aortic stroke volume.[68,69] In the setting of FMR, blood pressure control is particularly important. It is not uncommon to encounter patients with severe LV dysfunction who remain hypertensive. They are not on optimal GDMT and require increased doses or the addition of vasodilators.

Cardiac Resynchronization Therapy

CRT may improve LV systolic function and thereby reduce FMR severity in some cases.[70] CRT should be considered for symptomatic patients with FMR who meet the indications for device therapy as outlined in the American Hospital Association/American College of Cardiology (ACC/AHA) guidelines for valvular heart disease (i.e., class I, level of evidence A).[71] In a large trial of CRT-defibrillator in patients with FMR due to ischemic and noninschemic cardiomyopathy, 67% had improvements in MR grade, 28% had no change, and 5% had worsening of MR grade.[71] For patients with no MR at baseline, the development of MR at follow-up was uncommon (5%).

Although the finding of MR at baseline does not necessarily portend a worse response to CRT, those with severe MR after CRT have a worse prognosis.[72,73] Onishi et al reported three echocardiographic features independently associated with improved MR after CRT: anteroseptal to posterior wall radial strain dyssynchrony greater than 200 ms, lack of severe LV dilation (end-systolic dimension index < 29 mm/m^2), and lack of echocardiographic scar at papillary muscle insertion sites.[74]

The frequency of successful response to CRT in terms of reverse LV remodeling and MR reduction is two to three times greater in cases of nonischemic cardiomyopathy than ischemic cardiomyopathy. Inferior MI with scarring is a frequent cause of MR, and CRT has been less beneficial in patients with scarring.[75] Similar results were seen in the multicenter trial by Di Biase et al,[76] in which nonischemic patients had a significantly higher rate of CRT responses (i.e., LV reverse remodeling) than ischemic patients.

Coronary Revascularization

Patients with FMR due to acute or chronic ischemic heart disease should undergo appropriate revascularization as indicated for documented ischemia. In the setting of acute inferior or posterior MI, reperfusion with thrombolytic therapy reduced MR immediately and at 30 days.[77] Later data in the PCI era showed a similar reduction of MR by urgent PCI.[13] Although MR is more common in cases of inferoposterior MI, the prognosis for ischemic MR after anterior MI is worse, even in the PCI era.[78] In the Should We Emergently Revascularize Occluded Coronaries for Cardiogenic Shock (SHOCK) trial, moderate or severe MR was seen in 39% of patients.[79] The presence of moderate to severe MR increased the odds of death more than sixfold and was the only echocardiographic predictor of death other than LVEF. However, despite their much higher mortality rate, patients with moderate to severe MR still demonstrated a survival benefit with early revascularization.[79]

In chronic ischemic heart disease, there is support for revascularization by PCI and CABG, but randomized trials comparing GDMT, PCI, and CABG in patients with FMR are lacking. The STICH trial randomly assigned 1212 patients with HF due to ischemic cardiomyopathy to receive GDMT or GDMT plus CABG. There was a trend for improved all-cause mortality rates with CABG at 1 year of follow-up (HR = 0.86; 95% confidence interval [CI], 0.72–10.4; $P = 0.12$),[80] but at 10 years, the survival rate was statistically significantly better with CABG (HR = 0.84; 95% CI, 0.73–0.97; $P = 0.02$).[81] Post hoc analysis showed superiority of CABG compared with medical therapy in patients with mild MR (HR = 0.74; 95% CI, 0.60−0.92) but not in moderate or severe MR (HR = 0.94; 95% CI, 0.68–1.29).[81]

Kang et al reported a nonrandomized study of 185 patients with chronic ischemic FMR undergoing coronary revascularization by PCI ($n = 66$) or CABG ($n = 119$).[82] In a propensity-matched analysis, the number of cardiac events was lower with CABG than with PCI (HR = 0.499; 95% CI, 0.25–0.99; $P = 0.043$). However, the study was not randomized and was confounded by the fact that more than one half of the CABG patients also underwent mitral ring annuloplasty.

Castleberry et al reported the largest study of various treatment strategies for ischemic FMR in 4988 patients from the Duke database.[83] Compared with medical therapy only, patients treated with PCI, CABG alone, or CABG plus mitral valve surgery had improved long-term survival rates across the whole study group and when propensity matching was used to account for the nonrandomized study design. The addition of mitral valve repair to CABG did not improve survival compared with revascularization alone with CABG or PCI. Taken together, these studies provide strong support for revascularization in patients with ischemic MR.

Surgical Treatment of Functional Mitral Regurgitation

Surgical correction of FMR can be considered for patients who have significant symptomatic FMR despite optimal GDMT and revascularization (if indicated). However, there is no convincing evidence that surgical treatment of FMR improves mortality rates. The current recommendation is to repair moderate or severe FMR if the patient is already scheduled for CABG or AVR (i.e., class IIa, level of evidence C).[71] Mitral surgery can also be considered in two other situations: (1) in severely symptomatic patients (i.e., New York Health Association class III or IV) with chronic severe FMR (i.e., class IIb, level of evidence B) and (2) in patients with chronic moderate FMR who are undergoing other cardiac surgery (i.e., class IIb, level of evidence C).[71]

When considering mitral valve surgery for FMR, it is important to distinguish between ischemic and noninschemic causes. For moderate ischemic MR, CABG can lead to reversed LV remodeling and therefore improvement or elimination of FMR.[84] However, several studies have shown that CABG alone leaves 40% of patients with significant residual FMR.[85,86] A small, single-center, randomized clinical trial enrolling 102 patients reported no significant benefit for the addition of mitral valve annuloplasty to CABG.[87] This study was underpowered and did not exclude the possibility of a benefit.

In a substudy of the STICH trial, there was a strong trend for benefit with the addition of mitral valve repair to CABG compared with medical therapy alone.[63] Patients who received CABG plus mitral valve repair had a lower point estimate for death, but this difference was not statistically significant (HR = 0.62; 95% CI, 0.35–1.08). After adjustment for baseline prognostic variables, CABG with mitral surgery was superior to CABG alone (HR = 0.41; 95% CI, 0.22–0.77; $P = 0.006$). Although STICH was a randomized trial, the decision to treat the mitral valve during CABG was not randomized but was left to the discretion of the surgeon. Moreover, the aforementioned Castleberry study showed a statistically significant survival advantage with CABG alone compared with CABG plus mitral valve surgery.[83]

In the Randomized Ischemic Mitral Evaluation (RIME) trial, 73 patients with moderate FMR were randomized to CABG alone versus CABG plus mitral valve repair.[88] The trial was stopped early because of a benefit in the primary end point of peak oxygen consumption. LV remodeling, MR severity, and functional class were better with mitral valve repair, but the trial was not sufficiently powered to detect a mortality difference.

For nonischemic cardiomyopathy, a retrospective analysis failed to show a benefit of restrictive mitral valve annuloplasty over medical therapy.[89] However, in the ACORN CorCap Cardiac Support Device clinical trial, mitral valve repair, with or without an external cardiac

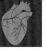
restraint device, was associated with progressive reduction in LV mass, increased LVEF, and increased sphericity index, all consistent with reverse remodeling.[90]

In a study of moderate MR, the Cardiothoracic Surgical Trials Network (CTSN) randomized 301 patients with moderate (2+) MR due to ischemic cardiomyopathy to CABG alone or to CABG plus an undersized complete mitral annuloplasty ring.[91] The primary end point was reduction in LV end-systolic volume index at 1 year; the trial was not powered to detect a difference in mortality rates. The primary end point was not met. Although MR reduction was more likely in the group receiving mitral annuloplasty, there was no difference at 1 year in the mortality rate, hospital readmission, functional class, or quality of life.

In a frequently cited observational study, an LV end-diastolic dimension of less than 65 mm was the best predictor of the extent of reverse remodeling and FMR reduction after restrictive mitral annuloplasty, suggesting that after severe LV dilation has occurred, it may be too late to successfully repair the mitral valve.[92]

Surgical Mitral Valve Repair Versus Replacement

The choice between repair and replacement is left to the surgeon's discretion. In primary MR, mitral valve repair is strongly preferred whenever possible.[71] The potential advantages of repair include lower perioperative mortality rates, avoidance of long-term anticoagulation and risk of structural valve deterioration, decreased endocarditis risk, and preservation of the native leaflet structure and function.

Many techniques for mitral valve repair in FMR have been reported. Ring annuloplasty is considered the cornerstone of repair. Partial-ring annuloplasty is thought to be inadequate because it fails to prevent progressive annular dilation.[93] Similarly, flexible rings permit annular distortion and have had a higher recurrence rate of MR compared with rigid rings.[94] Undersizing a complete rigid ring by 1 to 2 mm restores annular geometry, ensuring proper leaflet coaptation with minimal risk of stenosis.[92-95] However, mitral valve annuloplasty addresses only annular dilation; it does not directly correct mitral leaflet tethering, which is the primary mechanism of FMR. Recurrence of MR after mitral annuloplasty for ischemic FMR is 15% to 25% at 1 year and as high as 75% at 5 years.[96,97]

Additional procedures have been proposed to address leaflet tethering, but they have not been widely adopted by the surgical community. Papillary muscles may be approximated together or relocated to a more favorable position on the ventricular wall to help reduce leaflet tethering.[98] When the anterior leaflet is tethered by strut chords (i.e., seagull sign), the chords can be surgically ligated without detriment to LV systolic function.[99,100]

MVR is usually reserved for situations in which the valve cannot be reasonably repaired and those in which recurrent FMR seems likely based on anatomic considerations. MVR may be appropriate for complex valve disease with mixed primary and secondary MR. MVR is also usually faster than repair, with a shorter cardiopulmonary bypass time, and therefore may be more appropriate for selected high-risk surgical candidates for whom valve repair is considered difficult (i.e., those with severe mitral annular calcification). Biological prostheses are typically used for older patients, those with expected survival of less than 10 years, and patients who are unable to tolerate or maintain compliance with anticoagulation. The operative mortality rate for MVR in patients with FMR is approximately 3% to 4% in those selected to undergo surgery.[101-103]

It remains unclear whether surgical repair is superior to replacement in cases of FMR. The CTSN randomized 251 patients with moderate to severe ischemic MR and CAD to receive mitral valve repair or chord-sparing replacement.[104] The primary end point, LV reverse

remodeling assessed by change in LV end-systolic volume index at 12 months, was not significantly different between the groups (i.e., mean change from baseline of −6.6 and −6.8 mL/m² for annuloplasty vs. MVR, respectively). The 1-year mortality rate was 14.3% for the repair group and 17.6% for the replacement group, but the trial was not powered to detect a mortality rate difference. However, the repair group showed a significantly higher rate of recurrence of moderate or severe MR at 12 months (32.6% vs. 2.3%).

There were no significant differences between the groups in the rate of a composite of major adverse cardiac or cerebrovascular events, functional status, or quality of life at 12 months. The investigators concluded that although replacement provided a more durable correction of MR, there was no significant between-group difference in clinical outcomes. Long-term follow-up is ongoing. The high recurrence rate of significant MR despite the use of complete rigid rings in the hands of excellent surgeons may turn out to change the current practice of favoring annuloplasty over chord-sparing MVR. It may also dampen enthusiasm for percutaneous annuloplasty devices now in development. A post hoc analysis of the CTSN severe MR trial showed that recurrence of FMR after complete ring annuloplasty was more likely for patients who had severely restricted posterior leaflet motion due to posterobasal aneurysm.[105] These patients may benefit from chord-sparing MVR rather than restrictive annuloplasty because the latter may worsen posterior leaflet restriction (Fig. 18.10).

Transcatheter Mitral Valve Therapies

Various transcatheter approaches have been devised for the minimally invasive treatment of MR.[106] These devices attempt to mimic a specific surgical technique in a beating heart without cardiopulmonary bypass or aortic cross-clamping. The devices enable leaflet repair, chordal replacement, annular shape change, LV geometry change, and valve replacement. The most widely used of these is the MitraClip, a cloth-covered cobalt-chromium clip that pins the anterior and posterior leaflets together in a manner analogous to the Alfieri stitch. MitraClip has been used in more than 100,000 patients worldwide and is considered a class IIb indication for treatment of FMR in the AHA/ACC heart failure and valvular heart disease guidelines.[67,71]

Although MitraClip has improved MR severity and symptoms and caused reverse remodeling in primary MR and FMR,[107-112] it was initially approved in the United States only for use in patients with primary degenerative MR who are at prohibitive risk for surgical repair. A large European registry of ischemic and nonischemic FMR showed significantly improved MR severity and functional class for both groups, with no difference in survival or rehospitalization at 1 year.[113]

In a large, propensity-matched population of patients treated with MitraClip or medical therapy, there was a significant reduction in mortality rates at 30 days and at 1 year in a mixed population dominated by FMR.[114] Importantly, two large randomized clinical trials of MitraClip in FMR have recently been reported. In the MITRAFR study, the combined endpoint of all-cause mortality and unplanned heart failure hospitalization was not significantly reduced in patients randomized to MitraClip plus GDMT versus GDMT alone (54.6% vs. 51.3%, $p = 0.53$).[115] However, the entry criteria allowed either an EROA of at least 0.2 cm² or a regurgitant volume of at least 30 mL without the requirement for integration with multiple other parameters, as specified in all guidelines. More than half the patients in the trial had moderate MR by quantitative criteria, with EROA 0.2 to 0.3 cm², and only 16% had an EROA of 0.4 cm² or higher, which is highly specific for severe MR. LV end-diastolic volume index was quite large at 135 ± 35 mL/m². In addition, patients were randomized and then excluded for failure to meet entry criteria, which could lead to an unbalance of unmeasured variables in the MitraClip and control arms. Only 109 of 152 patients

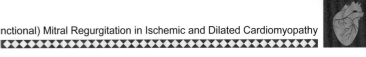

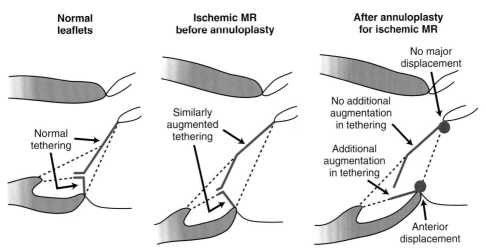

Fig. 18.10 Potential Mechanism of Persistent or Recurrent Mitral Regurgitation *(MR)* After Annuloplasty for Ischemic MR. LV remodeling with outward displacement of papillary muscles increases tethering angles similarly between the anterior leaflet or posterior mitral leaflet (PML) and the annular line *(middle image)*. Although surgical annuloplasty may not displace the anterior annulus fixed at the aortic root, this procedure hoists the posterior annulus anteriorly, which may specifically augment posterior leaflet tethering with recurrent MR *(right image)*. (Diagram by Yutaka Otsuji of University of Occupational and Environment Health, Japan. Reprinted from Beeri R, Otsuji Y, Schwammenthal E, et al. Ischemic mitral regurgitation. In Otto CM, Bonow RO, editors. Valvular heart disease: a companion to Braunwald's Heart Disease. 3rd ed. Philadelphia: Elsevier Science; 2009. p. 260-273.)

in the treatment arm underwent the MitraClip procedure, and the technical results were poor, with a high early complication rate (14.6%) and 17% of patients having residual 3+ or 4+ MR at 1 year. Despite these flaws, MITRAFR was an important study because it demonstrated that treatment of moderate FMR, which is associated with an adverse prognosis, does not improve mortality and HF hospitalization.

In the Cardiovascular Outcomes Assessment of the MitraClip Percutaneous Therapy for Heart Failure Patients With Functional Mitral Regurgitation (COAPT) trial, 614 patients with LVEF 20% to 50% and severe (3+ or 4+) MR were also randomized to MitraClip plus GDMT versus GDMT alone.[116] An expert review panel confirmed that patients were on optimally tolerated doses of GDMT prior to enrollment. The primary efficacy endpoint was cumulative heart failure hospitalizations over 24 months, which was reduced by 47% in the MitraClip arm (p <0.001) (Fig. 18.11). All-cause mortality, a prespecified secondary endpoint, was reduced by 38% in the MitraClip arm (p <0.001). MitraClip also resulted in significant improvement in MR severity, quality of life measures, and functional capacity. Reduction of MR severity to mild (1+) MR was 82%, which is the highest reported in any registry/trial to date. Moreover, only 5% had residual severe (3+ or 4+) MR at 2 years, suggesting high-quality technical skill with a durable response. COAPT is the first randomized clinical trial to demonstrate improved heart failure hospitalization and survival with treatment of FMR, and the magnitude of effect leaves no doubt that MitraClip was effective in the COAPT patient population. Compared with MITRAFR, COAPT randomized patients had smaller LV volume indexes (101 ± 34 mL/m² vs. 135 ± 35 mL/m²) and more severe FMR (EROA 0.41 ± 0.15 cm² vs. 0.31 ± 0.1 cm²). This suggests that careful identification of which FMR patients will benefit from MitraClip and which ones will not remains an important objective for future study. In the meantime, MitraClip was approved by the US Food and Drug Administration (FDA) for patients who continue to have severe, symptomatic FMR after optimization of GDMT and who meet the entry criteria for the COAPT trial. It is also likely that trials of newer devices will need to be compared with MitraClip rather than GDMT.

Several annuloplasty devices have been developed using a variety of approaches. Indirect annuloplasty through the coronary sinus has shown good preliminary results,[117] but this approach is limited because the coronary sinus overlies the left circumflex coronary artery in a substantial number of patients, is often farther than 1 cm from the mitral annulus, and does not allow complete ring repair. Direct annuloplasty can be performed through the LA with direct surgical approaches or transseptal approaches. The devices have anchoring systems to connect to the mitral annulus and can be tightened under TEE guidance to achieve maximal reduction of MR in a beating heart. Early results from the Cardioband Transfemoral Trial showed a 100% implant success rate in 31 patients and no perioperative deaths.[118] MR severity was reduced and functional class improved, but durability remains to be demonstrated.

A criticism of all percutaneous annuloplasty devices is that they are not complete rings. Given the 32% recurrence rate of significant MR in the CTSN trial with direct surgical implantation of complete rigid rings, percutaneous annuloplasty rings will be required to demonstrate durability. Chordal repair techniques are being developed, but they are more appropriate for primary degenerative MR than for FMR.

Several devices are being developed for transcatheter mitral valve replacement (TMVR) using transapical or transseptal approaches. Like transcatheter aortic valve replacement (TAVR), TMVR offers the potential to provide beating-heart valve replacement in high-risk patients and may be particularly suitable in those with FMR. In contrast to TAVR, TMVR will be harder to develop because of the noncircular shape of the mitral annulus, the potential for pushing the anterior mitral leaflet into the LV outflow tract, and difficulty anchoring the device to the anterior portion of the mitral annulus (i.e., aortomitral curtain).

Finally, there are several devices being developed for TMVR, either via transapical or transseptal approaches. Like TAVR, TMVR offers the potential to provide beating heart valve replacement to high-risk patients and may be particularly suitable for FMR. In contrast to TAVR, TMVR will be harder to develop because of the noncircular shape of

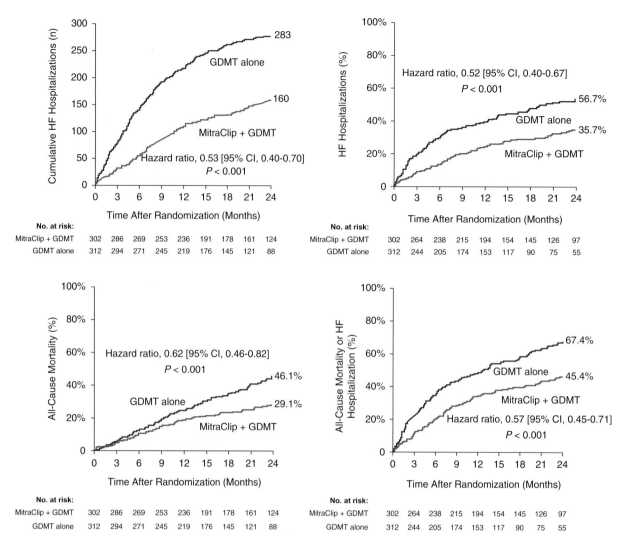

Fig. 18.11 Results From the COAPT Trial. (A) Primary endpoint of cumulative heart failure hospitalizations over 24 months. (B) Time to first heart failure hospitalization. (C) All-cause mortality. (D) Time to all-cause mortality or first heart failure hospitalization. *GDMT,* Guideline-directed medical therapy; *HF,* heart failure.(From Stone GW, Lindenfeld J, Abraham WT, et al for the COAPT Investigators. Transcatheter mitral-valve repair in patients with heart failure. N Engl J Med 2018;379:2307-2318.)

the mitral annulus, the potential for pushing the anterior mitral leaflet into the LV outflow tract, and the difficulty of anchoring the device to the anterior portion of the mitral annulus (the aorto-mitral curtain). An early feasibility trial with the Tendyne device, which is implanted transapically and has a D-shaped flexible skirt and a tether that anchors the device to the LV apex, has been recently reported in 30 subjects.[119] The device was successfully implanted in 28 patients with no acute mortality. One patient died at 13 days of pneumonia, and MR reduction was excellent, with only one patient having mild residual central MR at 30 days. Both LV end-diastolic volume and Kansas City Cardiomyopathy Questionnaire were significantly improved at 30 days. Longer term results are pending. Several other TMVR devices are currently in early feasibility trials. Given the safety profile of MitraClip, it is likely that these devices will evolve from transapical to transseptal delivery. As of this writing, all TMVR devices are experimental; FDA approval awaits completion of pivotal trials.

Spectrum of Functional Mitral Regurgitation

FMR occurs along a spectrum of severity of LV dysfunction (Fig. 18.12). At one end of the spectrum is a severely dilated, spherical LV with markedly depressed LV systolic function and FMR. Treatment of MR in these

patients may not improve symptoms, enhance quality of life, or reverse LV remodeling because the primary problem is severe LV dysfunction. Heart transplantation or a destination LV assist device may be a more effective treatment strategy than mitral valve surgery.

At the other end of the spectrum, a patient with an isolated inferobasal MI may develop severe FMR due to posterior leaflet tethering despite normal LV size, shape, and ejection fraction. In these patients, it may be clinically obvious that severe MR is the cause of HF, and surgery may be indicated.

In the middle of the spectrum, it can be very hard to distinguish whether the MR, the LV dysfunction, or both are contributing to HF symptoms. Current studies are confounded by inclusion of nonischemic and ischemic causes of FMR and a wide range of LV dysfunction. Future studies of therapy for FMR should define homogeneous patient populations so that any potential therapeutic benefit is not masked by including patients with irreversible LV myocardial dysfunction or end-stage HF.

CONCLUSIONS

FMR is a complex disorder in which MR occurs because of disordered LV geometry and contractile function or pure annular dilation due to

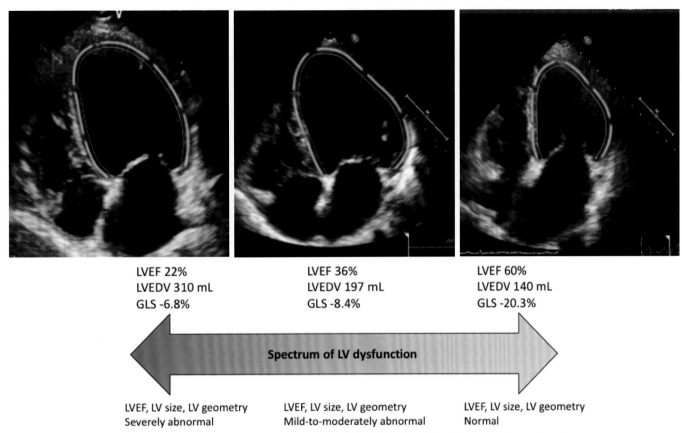

LVEF 22%   LVEF 36%   LVEF 60%
LVEDV 310 mL   LVEDV 197 mL   LVEDV 140 mL
GLS -6.8%   GLS -8.4%   GLS -20.3%

Spectrum of LV dysfunction

LVEF, LV size, LV geometry   LVEF, LV size, LV geometry   LVEF, LV size, LV geometry
Severely abnormal   Mild-to-moderately abnormal   Normal

Fig. 18.12 Spectrum of Secondary Mitral Regurgitation (MR). Secondary MR occurs along a broad spectrum of LV dysfunction from severely depressed LV systolic function, size, and spherical geometry *(left)* to mildly or moderately impaired LV systolic function, size, and geometry *(middle)* to normal LV systolic function, size, and geometry *(right)*. Patients who have a markedly dilated LV with an ejection fraction *(LVEF)* of 20% are unlikely to benefit from mitral valve intervention because they would likely still have severe heart failure from LV dysfunction, which could worsen after mitral valve surgery. In patients with normal LVEF, size, and geometry (i.e., small inferobasal myocardial infarction or atrial functional MR), it is often clear that heart failure results from the MR itself, and mitral valve surgery could resolve the heart failure. In the middle range, it remains unclear whether mitral valve surgery offers a survival benefit or improved quality of life. The inclusion of a heterogeneous population of patients across this spectrum confounds interpretation of most studies. *GLS*, Global longitudinal strain; *LVEDV*, left ventricular end-diastolic volume.

atrial enlargement. Treatment of FMR should first be targeted to the underlying LV dysfunction, using GDMT and CRT or coronary revascularization when indicated. Mitral valve surgery can be considered for patients who are already scheduled for CABG or other cardiac surgery and for those in whom symptoms persist and are attributable to FMR despite optimal GDMT. Advances in percutaneous devices for treatment of FMR are promising and will continue to evolve.

REFERENCES

1. Nkomo VT, Gardin JM, Skelton TN, et al. Burden of valvular heart diseases: a population-based study. Lancet 2006;368:1005-1011.
2. de Marchena E, Badiye A, Robalino G, et al. Respective prevalence of the different carpentier classes of mitral regurgitation: a stepping stone for future therapeutic research and development. J Card Surg 2011;26:385-392.
3. Oh J, Pellikka P, Panza JA, et al. Core lab analysis of baseline echocardiographic studies in the STICH trial and recommendation for use of echocardiography in future clinical trials. J Am Soc Echocardiogr 2012;25:327-336.
4. Levine RA, Schwammenthal E. Ischemic mitral regurgitation on the threshold of a solution: from paradoxes to unifying concepts. Circulation 2005;112:745-758.
5. Kono T, Sabbah HN, Stein PD, et al. Left ventricular shape as a determinant of functional mitral regurgitation in patients with severe heart failure secondary to either coronary artery disease or idiopathic dilated cardiomyopathy. Am J Cardiol 1991;68:355-359.
6. Kwan J, Shiota T, Agler DA, et al. Geometric differences of the mitral apparatus between ischemic and dilated cardiomyopathy with significant mitral regurgitation: real-time three-dimensional echocardiography study. Circulation 2003;107:1135-1140.
7. Golba K, Mokrzycki K, Drozdz J, et al. Mechanisms of functional mitral regurgitation in ischemic cardiomyopathy determined by transesophageal echocardiography (from the Surgical Treatment for Ischemic Heart Failure Trial). Am J Cardiol 2013;112:1812-1818.
8. Agricola E, Oppizzi M, Galderisi M, et al. Role of regional mechanical dyssynchrony as a determinant of functional mitral regurgitation in patients with left ventricular systolic dysfunction. Heart 2006;92:1390-1395.
9. Chaput M, Handschumacher MD, Tournoux F, et al. Mitral valve enlargement in chronic aortic regurgitation as a compensatory mechanism to prevent functional mitral regurgitation in the dilated left ventricle. Circulation 2008;118:845-852.
10. Beaudoin J, Handschumacher MD, Zeng X, et al. Mitral valve enlargement in chronic aortic regurgitation as a compensatory mechanism to prevent

functional mitral regurgitation in the dilated left ventricle. J Am Coll Cardiol 2013;61:1809-1816.

11. Grayburn PA. New concepts in functional mitral regurgitation: it is not just a disease of the left ventricle. J Am Coll Cardiol 2013;61:1817-1819.

12. Hauser AM, Ganghadharan V, Ramos RG, et al. Sequence of mechanical, electrocardiographic and clinical effects of repeated coronary artery occlusion in human beings: echocardiographic observations during coronary angioplasty. J Am Coll Cardiol 1985;5:193-197.

13. Nishino S, Watanabe N, Kimura T, et al. The course of ischemic mitral regurgitation in acute myocardial infarction after primary percutaneous coronary intervention: from emergency room to long-term follow-up. Circ Cardiovasc Imaging 2016;9(8):e004841.

14. Sharma SK, Seckler J, Israel DH, et al. Clinical, angiographic and anatomic findings in acute severe ischemic mitral regurgitation. Am J Cardiol 1992;70:277-280.

15. Hashim SW, Youssef SJ, Ayyash B, et al. Pseudoprolapse of the anterior leaflet in chronic ischemic mitral regurgitation: identification and repair. J Thorac Cardiovasc Surg 2012;143:S33-S37.

16. Yosefy C, Beeri R, Guerrero JL, et al. Mitral regurgitation after anteroapical myocardial infarction: new mechanistic insights. Circulation 2011;123:1529-1536.

17. Kaul S, Spotnitz WD, Glasheen WP, et al. Mechanism of ischemic mitral regurgitation: an experimental evaluation. Circulation 1991;84:2167-2180.

18. Kono T, Sabbah HN, Rosman H, et al. Left ventricular shape is the primary determinant of functional mitral regurgitation in heart failure. J Am Coll Cardiol 1992;20:1594-1598.

19. Yiu SF, Enriquez-Sarano M, Tribouilloy C, et al. Determinants of the degree of functional mitral regurgitation in patients with systolic left ventricular dysfunction: a quantitative clinical study. Circulation 2000;102:1400-1406.

20. Gertz ZM, Raina A, Saghy L, et al. Evidence of atrial functional mitral regurgitation due to atrial fibrillation: reversal with arrhythmia control. J Am Coll Cardiol 2011;58:1474-1481.

21. Lehmann KG, Francis CK, Dodge HT. Mitral regurgitation in early myocardial infarction: incidence, clinical detection, and prognostic implications. TIMI Study Group. Ann Intern Med 1992;117:10-17.

22. Lang RM, Badano LP, Mor-Avi V, et al. Recommendations for cardiac chamber quantification by echocardiography in adults: an update from the American Society of Echocardiography and the European Association of Cardiovascular Imaging. J Am Soc Echocardiogr 2015;28:1-39.e14.

23. Zoghbi WA, Adams D, Bonow RO, et al. ASE guidelines and standards recommendations for non-invasive evaluation of native valvular regurgitation from the American Society of Echocardiography in collaboration with the Society for Cardiovascular Magnetic Resonance. J Am Soc Echocardiogr 2017;30(4):303-371.

24. Lancellotti P, Moura L, Pierard L, et al. European Association of Echocardiography recommendations for the assessment of valvular regurgitation, part 2: mitral and tricuspid regurgitation (native disease). Eur J Echocardiogr 2010;11:307-332.

25. Thomas J, Liu C, Flachskampf F, et al. Quantification of jet flow by momentum analysis: an in vitro color Doppler flow study. Circulation 1990;81:247-259.

26. Uretsky S, Gillam L, Lang R, et al. Discordance between echocardiography and MRI in the assessment of mitral regurgitation severity: a prospective multicenter trial. J Am Coll Cardiol 2015;65:1078-1088.

27. Singh JP, Evans JC, Levy D, et al. Prevalence and clinical determinants of mitral, tricuspid, and aortic regurgitation (the Framingham Heart Study). Am J Cardiol 1999;83:897-902.

28. Chen CG, Thomas JD, Anconina J, et al., Impact of impinging wall jet on color Doppler quantification of mitral regurgitation. Circulation 1991;84:712-720.

29. Sahn D. Instrumentation and physical factors related to visualization of stenotic and regurgitant jets by Doppler color flow mapping. J Am Coll Cardiol 1988;12:1354-1365.

30. Grayburn PA, Weissman NJ, Zamorano JL. Quantitation of mitral regurgitation. Circulation 2012;126:2005-2017.

31. Topilsky Y, Michelena H, Bichara V, et al. Mitral valve prolapse with mid-late systolic mitral regurgitation: pitfalls of evaluation and clinical outcome compared with holosystolic regurgitation. Circulation 2012;125:1643-1651.

32. Altiok E, Hamada S, van Hall S, et al. Comparison of direct planimetry of mitral valve regurgitation orifice area by three-dimensional transesophageal echocardiography to effective regurgitant orifice area obtained by proximal flow convergence method and vena contracta area determined by color Doppler echocardiography. Am J Cardiol 2011;107:452-458.

33. Kahlert P, Plicht B, Schenk IM, et al. Direct assessment of size and shape of noncircular vena contracta area in functional versus organic mitral regurgitation using real-time three-dimensional echocardiography. J Am Soc Echocardiogr 2008;21:912-921.

34. Matsumura Y, Saracino G, Sugioka K, et al. Determination of regurgitant orifice area with the use of a new three-dimensional flow convergence geometric assumption in functional mitral regurgitation. J Am Soc Echocardiogr 2008;21:1251-1256.

35. Matsumura Y, Fukuda S, Tran H, et al. Geometry of the proximal isovelocity surface area in mitral regurgitation by 3-dimensional color Doppler echocardiography: difference between functional mitral regurgitation and prolapse regurgitation. Am Heart J 2008;155:231-238.

36. Iwakura K, Ito H, Kawano S, et al. Comparison of orifice area by transthoracic three-dimensional echocardiography versus proximal isovelocity surface area (PISA) method for assessment of mitral regurgitation. Am J Cardiol 2006;97:1630-1637.

37. Little SH, Pirat B, Kumar R, et al. Three-dimensional color Doppler echocardiography for direct measurement of vena contracta area in mitral regurgitation: in vitro validation and clinical experience. JACC Cardiovasc Imaging 2008;1:695-704.

38. Yosefy C, Hung J, Chua S, et al. Direct measurement of vena contracta area by real-time 3-dimensional echocardiography for assessing severity of mitral regurgitation. Am J Cardiol 2009;104:978-983.

39. Marsan NA, Westenberg JJ, Ypenburg C, et al. Quantification of functional mitral regurgitation by real-time 3D echocardiography: comparison with 3D velocity-encoded cardiac magnetic resonance. JACC Cardiovasc Imaging 2009;2:1245-1252.

40. Shanks M, Siebelink HMJ, Delgado V, et al. Quantitative assessment of mitral regurgitation: comparison between three-dimensional transesophageal echocardiography and magnetic resonance imaging. Circ Cardiovasc Imaging 2010;3:694-700.

41. Zeng X, Levine RA, Hua L, et al. Diagnostic value of vena contracta area in the quantification of mitral regurgitation severity by color Doppler 3D echocardiography. Circ Cardiovasc Imaging 2011;4:506-513.

42. Hundley WG, Li HF, Willard JE, et al., Magnetic resonance imaging assessment of the severity of mitral regurgitation. Comparison with invasive techniques. Circulation 1995;92:1151-1158.

43. Kon MW, Myerson SG, Moat NE, Pennell DJ. Quantification of regurgitant fraction in mitral regurgitation by cardiovascular magnetic resonance: comparison of techniques. J Heart Valve Dis 2004;13:600-607.

44. Fujita N, Chazouilleres AF, Hartiala JJ, et al. Quantification of mitral regurgitation by velocity-encoded cine nuclear magnetic resonance imaging. J Am Coll Cardiol 1994;23:951-958.

45. Maceira AM, Prasad SK, Khan M, Pennell DJ. Normalized left ventricular systolic and diastolic function by steady state free precession cardiovascular magnetic resonance. J Cardiovasc Magn Reson 2006;8:417-426.

46. Kizilbash AM, Hundley WG, Willett DL, et al. Comparison of quantitative Doppler with magnetic resonance imaging for assessment of the severity of mitral regurgitation. Am J Cardiol 1998;81:792-795.

47. Yoran C, Yellin EL, Becker RM, et al. Dynamic aspects of acute mitral regurgitation: effects of ventricular volume, pressure and contractility on the effective regurgitant orifice area. Circulation 1979;60:170-176.

48. Hung J, Otsuji Y, Handschumacher MD, et al. Mechanism of dynamic regurgitant orifice area variation in functional mitral regurgitation: physiologic insights from the proximal flow convergence technique. J Am Coll Cardiol 1999;33:538-545.

49. Buck T, Plicht B, Kahlert P, et al. Effect of dynamic flow rate and orifice area on mitral regurgitant stroke volume quantification using the proximal isovelocity surface area method. J Am Coll Cardiol 2008;52:767-778.

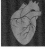

50. Lancellotti P, Troisfontaines P, Toussaint AC, Pierard LA. Prognostic importance of exercise-induced changes in mitral regurgitation in patients with chronic ischemic left ventricular dysfunction. Circulation 2003;108:1713-1717.

51. Pierard LA, Lancellotti P. The role of ischemic mitral regurgitation in the pathogenesis of acute pulmonary edema. N Engl J Med 2004;351:1627-1634.

52. Pierard LA, Lancellotti P. Stress testing in valve disease. Heart 2007;93:766-772.

53. Hickey MS, Smith LR, Muhlbaier LH, et al. Current prognosis of ischemic mitral regurgitation. Implications for future management. Circulation 1988;78(Suppl II):151-159.

54. Lamas GA, Mitchell GF, Flaker GC, et al. Clinical significance of mitral regurgitation after acute myocardial infarction. Survival and ventricular enlargement investigators. Circulation 1997;96:827-833.

55. Grigioni F, Enriquez-Sarano M, Zehr KJ, et al. Ischemic mitral regurgitation: long-term outcome and prognostic implications with quantitative Doppler assessment. Circulation 2001;103:1759-1764.

56. Mentias A, Raza MQ, Barakat AF, et al. Prognostic significance of ischemic mitral regurgitation on outcomes in acute ST-elevation myocardial infarction managed by primary percutaneous coronary intervention. Am J Cardiol 2017;119:20-26.

57. Koelling TM, Aaronson KD, Cody RJ, et al. Prognostic significance of mitral regurgitation and tricuspid regurgitation in patients with left ventricular systolic dysfunction. Am Heart J 2002;144:524-529.

58. Trichon BH, Felker GM, Shaw LK, et al. Relation of frequency and severity of mitral regurgitation to survival among patients with left ventricular systolic dysfunction and heart failure. Am J Cardiol 2003;91:538-543.

59. Bursi F, Enriquez-Sarano M, Nkomo VT, et al. Heart failure and death after myocardial infarction in the community. Emerging role of mitral regurgitation. Circulation 2005;111:295-301.

60. Grayburn PA, Appleton CP, DeMaria AN, et al. Echocardiographic predictors of morbidity and mortality in patients with advanced heart failure: The Beta-Blocker Evaluation of Survival Trial (BEST). J Am Coll Cardiol 2005;45:1064-1071.

61. Cioffi G, Tarantini L, De Feo S, et al. Functional mitral regurgitation predicts 1-year mortality in elderly patients with systolic chronic heart failure. Eur J Heart Fail 2005;7:1112-1117.

62. Rossi A, Dini FL, Faggiano P, Let al. Independent prognostic value of functional mitral regurgitation in patients with heart failure. A quantitative analysis of 1256 patients with ischaemic and non-ischaemic dilated cardiomyopathy. Heart 2011;97:1675-1680.

63. Deja MA, Grayburn PA, Sun B, et al. Influence of mitral regurgitation repair on survival in the surgical treatment for ischemic heart failure trial. Circulation 2012;125:2639-2648.

64. Patel JB, Borgeson DD, Barnes ME, et al. Mitral regurgitation in patients with advanced systolic heart failure. J Card Fail 2004;10:285-291.

65. Grayburn PA, Carabello B, Gillam LD, et al. Defining severe mitral regurgitation: emphasis on an integrated approach. J Am Coll Cardiol 2014;64:2792-2801.

66. Sannino A, Smith II RL, Schiattarrella GG, Trimarco B, Esposito G, Grayburn PA. Survival and cardiovascular outcomes of patients with secondary mitral regurgitation: a meta-analysis of 53 studies. JAMA Cardiol 2017;2:1130-1139.

67. Yancy CW, Jessup M, Bozkurt B, et al. 2013 ACCF/AHA guideline for the management of heart failure: a report of the American College of Cardiology Foundation/American Heart Association Task Force on Practice Guidelines. J Am Coll Cardiol 2013;62:e147-e239.

68. Comin-Colet J, Sanchez-Corral MA, Manito N, et al. Effect of carvedilol therapy on functional mitral regurgitation, ventricular remodeling, and contractility in patients with heart failure due to left ventricular systolic dysfunction. Transplant Proc 2002;34:177-178.

69. Lowes BD, Gill EA, Abraham WT, et al. Effect of carvedilol on left ventricular mass, chamber geometry and mitral regurgitation in chronic heart failure. Am J Cardiol 1999;83:1201-1205.

70. Sutton MG, Plappert T, Hilpisch KE, et al. Sustained reverse left ventricular structural remodeling with cardiac resynchronization at one year is a function of etiology: quantitative Doppler echocardiographic evidence from the Multicenter InSync Randomized Clinical Evaluation (MIRACLE). Circulation 2006;113:266-272.

71. Nishimura RA, Otto CM, Bonow RO, et al. 2014 AHA/ACC guideline for the management of patients with valvular heart disease: a report of the American College of CardiologyAmerican Heart Association Task Force on Practice Guidelines. J Am Coll Cardiol 2014;63:e57-e185.

72. Boriani G, Gasparini M, Landolina M, et al. Impact of mitral regurgitation on the outcome of patients treated with CRT-D: data from the Insync ICD Italian Registry. Pacing Clin Electrophysiol 2012;35:146-154.

73. Cabrera-Bueno F, Garcia-Pinilla JM, Pena-Hernandez J, et al. Repercussion of functional mitral regurgitation on reverse remodeling in cardiac resynchronization therapy. Europace 2007;9:757-761.

74. Onishi T, Onishi T, Marek JJ, et al. Mechanistic features associated with improvement in mitral regurgitation after cardiac resynchronization therapy and their relation to long-term patient outcome. Circ Heart Fail 2013;6:685-693.

75. Xu YZ, Cha YM, Feng D, et al. Impact of myocardial scarring on outcomes of cardiac resynchronization therapy: extent or location? J Nucl Med 2012;53:47-54.

76. Di Biase L, Auricchio A, Mohanty P, et al. Impact of cardiac resynchronization therapy on the severity of mitral regurgitation. Europace 2011;13:829-838.

77. Leor J, Feinberg MS, Vered Z, et al. Effect of thrombolytic therapy on the evolution of significant mitral regurgitation in patients with a first inferior myocardial infarction. J Am Coll Cardiol 1993;21:1661-1666.

78. Mentias A, Raza MQ, Barakat AF, et al. Outcomes of ischaemic mitral regurgitation in anterior versus inferior ST elevation myocardial infarction. Open Heart 2016;3:e000493.

79. Hochman JS, Sleeper LA, Webb JG, et al. Early revascularization in acute myocardial infarction complicated by cardiogenic shock. Shock investigators. Should we emergently revascularize occluded coronaries for cardiogenic shock. N Engl J Med 1999;341:625-634.

80. Velazquez EJ, Lee KL, Deja MA, et al. Coronary-artery bypass surgery in patients with left ventricular dysfunction. N Engl J Med 2011;364:1607-1616.

81. Velazquez EJ, Lee KL, Jones RH, et al. Coronary-artery bypass surgery in patients with ischemic cardiomyopathy. N Engl J Med 2016;374:1511-1520.

82. Kang DH, Sun BJ, Kim DH, et al. Percutaneous versus surgical revascularization in patients with ischemic mitral regurgitation. Circulation 2011;124(Suppl 11):S156-S162.

83. Castleberry AW, Williams JB, Daneshmand MA, et al. Surgical revascularization is associated with maximal survival in patients with ischemic mitral regurgitation: a 20-year experience. Circulation 2014;129:2547-2556.

84. Balu V, Hershowitz S, Zaki Masud A, et al. Mitral regurgitation in coronary artery disease. Chest 1982;81:550-555.

85. Harris KM, Sundt TM 3rd, Aeppli D, et al. Can late survival of patients with moderate ischemic mitral regurgitation be impacted by intervention on the valve? Ann Thorac Surg 2002;74:1468-1475.

86. Aklog L, Filsoufi F, Flores KQ, et al. Does coronary artery bypass grafting alone correct moderate ischemic mitral regurgitation? Circulation 2001;104:I68-I75.

87. Fattouch K, Guccione F, Sampognaro R, et al. Efficacy of adding mitral valve restrictive annuloplasty to coronary artery bypass grafting in patients with moderate ischemic mitral valve regurgitation: a randomized trial. J Thorac Cardiovasc Surg 2009;138:278-285.

88. Chan KM, Punjabi PP, Flather M, et al. Coronary artery bypass surgery with or without mitral valve annuloplasty in moderate functional ischemic mitral regurgitation: final results of the Randomized Ischemic Mitral Evaluation (RIME) trial. Circulation 2012;126:2502-2510.

89. Wu A, Aaronson K, Bolling S, et al. Impact of mitral valve annuloplasty on mortality risk in patients with mitral regurgitation and left ventricular systolic dysfunction. J Am Coll Cardiol 2005;45:381-387.

90. Acker MA, Bolling S, Shemin R, et al. Mitral valve surgery in heart failure: insights from the Acorn Clinical Trial. J Thorac Cardiovasc Surg 2006;132:568-577.

91. Smith PK, Puskas JD, Ascheim DD, et al. Surgical treatment of moderate mitral regurgitation. N Engl J Med 2014;371:2178-2188.

92. Braun J, van de Veire NR, Klautz RJ, et al. Restrictive mitral annuloplasty cures ischemic mitral regurgitation and heart failure. Ann Thorac Surg 2008;85:430-436.

93. Mihaljevic T, Lam B, Rajeswaran J, et al. Impact of mitral valve annuloplasty combined with revascularization in patients with functional ischemic mitral regurgitation. J Am Coll Cardiol 2007;49:2191-2201.

94. Ryan L, Jackson B, Hamamoto H, et al. The influence of annuloplasty ring geometry on mitral leaflet curvature. Ann Thorac Surg 2008;86:749-760.

95. Acker M. Should moderate or greater mitral regurgitation be repaired in all patients with LVEF <30%? Mitral valve repair in patients with advanced heart failure and severe functional mitral insufficiency reverses left ventricular remodeling and improves symptoms. Circ Heart Fail 2008;1:281-284.

96. Milano CA, Daneshmand MA, Rankin JS, et al. Survival prognosis and surgical management of ischemic mitral regurgitation. Ann Thorac Surg 2008;86:735-744.

97. Magne J, Senechal M, Dumesnil JG, Pibarot P. Ischemic mitral regurgitation: a complex, multifaceted disease. Cardiology 2009;112:244-259.

98. Kron I, Green G, Cope J. Surgical relocation of the posterior papillary muscle in chronic ischemic mitral regurgitation. Ann Thorac Surg 2002;74:600-601.

99. Borger MA, Murphy PM, Alam A, et al. Initial results of the chordal-cutting operation for ischemic mitral regurgitation. J Thorac Cardiovasc Surg 2007;133;1483-1492.

100. Lee AP, Acker M, Kubo SH, et al. Mechanisms of recurrent functional mitral regurgitation after mitral valve repair in nonischemic dilated cardiomyopathy: importance of distal anterior leaflet tethering. Circulation 2009;119:2606-2614.

101. Gillinov AM, Wierup PN, Blackstone EH, et al. Is repair preferable to replacement for ischemic mitral regurgitation? J Thorac Cardiovasc Surg 2001;122:1125-1241.

102. Filsoufi F, Salzberg S, Adams D. Current management of ischemic mitral regurgitation. Mt Sinai J Med 2005;72:105-115.

103. Adams D, Filsoufi F, Aklog L. Surgical treatment of the ischemic mitral valve. J Heart Valve Dis 2002;11:S21-S25.

104. Acker MA, Parides MK, Perrault LP, et al. Mitral-valve repair versus replacement for severe ischemic mitral regurgitation. N Engl J Med 2014;370:23-32.

105. Kron IL, Hung J, Overbey JR, et al. Predicting recurrent mitral regurgitation after mitral valve repair for severe ischemic mitral regurgitation. J Thorac Cardiovasc Surg 2015;149:752-761.

106. Feldman T, Young A. Percutaneous approaches to valve repair in mitral regurgitation. J Am Coll Cardiol 2014;63(20):2057-2068.

107. Feldman T, Foster E, Glower D, et al. Percutaneous repair or surgery for mitral regurgitation. N Engl J Med 2011;364:1395-1406.

108. Feldman T, Kar S, Elmariah S, et al. Randomized comparision of percutaneous repair and surgery for mitral regurgitation: 5-year results of EVEREST II. J Am Coll Cardiol 2015;66:2844-2854.

109. Foster E, Kwan D, Feldman T, et al. Percutaneous mitral valve repair in the initial EVEREST cohort: evidence of reverse left ventricular remodeling. Circ Cardiovasc Imaging 2013;6:522-530.

110. Grayburn PA, Sangli C, Massaro J, et al. The relationship between the magnitude of reduction in mitral regurgitation severity and left ventricular and left atrial reverse remodeling after MitraClip therapy. Circulation 2013;128:1667-1674.

111. Auricchio A, Schillinger W, Meyer S, et al. Correction of mitral regurgitation in nonresponders to cardiac resynchronization therapy by MitraClip improves symptoms and promotes reverse remodeling. J Am Coll Cardiol 2011;58:2183-2189.

112. Glower DD, Kar S, Trento A, et al. Percutaneous mitral valve repair for mitral regurgitation in high-risk patients: results of the EVEREST II Study. J Am Coll Cardiol 2014;64:172-181.

113. Pighi M, Estevez-Loureiro R, Maisano F, et al. Immediate and 12-month outcomes of ischemic versus nonischemic functional mitral regurgitation in patients treated with MitraClip (from the 2011 to 2012 Pilot Sentinel Registry of Percutaneous Edge-To-Edge Mitral Valve Repair of the European Society of Cardiology). Am J Cardiol 2017;119(4):630-637.

114. Velazquez EJ, Samad Z, Al-Khalidi H, et al. The Mitraclip and survival in patients with mitral regurgitation at high risk for surgery: a propensity-matched comparison. Am Heart J 2015;170:1050-1059.

115. Obadia JF, Messika-Zeitoun D, Leurent G, et al. Percutaneous repair or medical treatment for secondary mitral regurgitation. N Engl J Med 2018;379(24):2297-2306.

116. Stone GW, Lindenfeld J, Abraham WT, et al. Transcatheter mitral valve repair in patients with heart failure. N Engl J Med 2018;379(24):2307-2318.

117. Siminiak T, Wu JC, Haude M, et al. Treatment of functional mitral regurgitation by percutaneous annuloplasty: results of the TITAN Trial. Eur J Heart Fail 2012;14:931-938.

118. Nickenig G, Hammerstingl C, Schuler R, et al. Transcatheter mitral annuloplasty in chronic functional mitral regurgitation: 6 months results with the Cardioband™ percutaneous mitral repair system. JACC Cardiovasc Interv 2016;9:2039-2047.

119. Muller DWM, Pedersen WA, Jansz P, et al. Transcatheter mitral valve implantation with a self-expanding prosthesis for symptomatic native mitral regurgitation. J Am Coll Cardiol 2017;69:381-391.

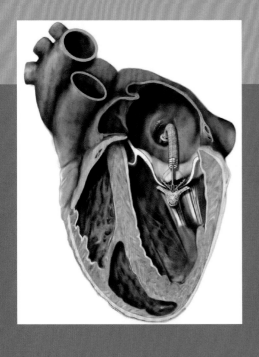

第19章
二尖瓣疾病的外科修复与置换

外科瓣膜修复或置换手术是二尖瓣疾病的主要治疗手段之一。本章首先介绍了二尖瓣的解剖结构及二尖瓣反流的病理生理学特征，而后详细讲述了二尖瓣外科手术入路，二尖瓣外科修复与置换的技术、适应证、研究进展及临床结局。

二尖瓣是复杂的三维解剖结构，其正常工作是瓣环、瓣叶、瓣叶交界、腱索、乳头肌与左心室协调作用的结果。任一解剖结构的异常都可能导致二尖瓣病变，引起二尖瓣反流或二尖瓣狭窄。目前来说，风湿性疾病仍是世界范围内二尖瓣反流的主要病因，然而，在西方发达国家，由退行性病变导致的二尖瓣疾病已占据主导。二尖瓣修复术是治疗退行性二尖瓣疾病的金标准。研究表明，在有经验的医学中心，退行性二尖瓣疾病修复术的围手术期风险和术后残余二尖瓣反流率极低。二尖瓣置换术在风湿性二尖瓣疾病中开展较多，对一部分缺血性二尖瓣反流患者来说，二尖瓣置换术也是一种可考虑的治疗方式。在人工心脏瓣膜的选择方面，对于中年患者来说，若无抗凝禁忌证，或有明确加速性瓣膜结构损害风险，采用机械瓣膜置换是合理的。然而，目前生物瓣膜的使用呈现显著增加趋势。推荐应用生物瓣膜置换的人群包括：无法接受高质量抗凝治疗的患者、最佳抗凝治疗下仍有机械瓣血栓形成需再次干预的患者、有生育需求的女性患者及不愿接受抗凝治疗的患者等。

吕俊兴

Surgical Mitral Valve Repair and Replacement

Javier G. Castillo, David H. Adams

CHAPTER OUTLINE

KEY POINTS

- The mitral valve is a complex, three-dimensional assembly of independent anatomic components, including the annulus, leaflets and commissures, chordae tendineae, papillary muscles, and left ventricle. Abnormalities (lesions with etiologic implications) in any of these components may cause alteration in closure (i.e., dysfunction) against left ventricular (LV) pressure and consequently mitral regurgitation (MR) or mitral stenosis (MS).

- Although rheumatic disease remains the most common cause of MR worldwide, it is no longer a frequent cause of mitral valve disease in developed countries. In Western countries, degenerative disease is the leading cause of mitral valve disease and MR. Ischemic MR (i.e., secondary MR) accounts for 10% to 20% of cases, but early percutaneous intervention in acute coronary syndromes will progressively limit this disease prevalence.

- Several variables have been identified that significantly affect the natural history of MR in the setting of mitral valve prolapse and can serve as surgical triggers. They include LV dysfunction with an ejection fraction of less than 60%, New York Heart Association functional class III or IV, regurgitant orifice area of 40 mm^2 or larger, LV end-systolic dimension greater than 40 mm, left atrial index of 60 mL/m^2 or less, left atrial dimension greater than 55 mm, pulmonary hypertension at rest or during exercise, and atrial fibrillation.

- Mitral valve repair is the gold standard treatment for patients with degenerative mitral valve disease. The literature demonstrates that it is possible to repair almost all prolapsing degenerative mitral

valves with a very low perioperative risk and absence of residual MR when the procedure is performed in reference centers. This is crucial because of the increasing number of asymptomatic patients referred for surgery. The latest practice guidelines introduced the referral to reference centers as an algorithm variable.

- Whereas mitral valve replacement (MVR) is rare in patients with degenerative disease, it is prevalent among patients with rheumatic disease and may be considered a viable option for selected patients with ischemic MR. In cases of ischemic MR, MVR may provide a good alternative because prosthetic valve function is not affected by the degree of LV dysfunction, although there is the early risk of prosthesis-related complications.

- If the decision to proceed with MVR is made, a chordal-sparing approach should be employed to preserve chordal-ventricular-annular continuity, which is important to maintain long-term LV shape and performance.

- Use of a mechanical prosthesis is reasonable in middle-aged patients if there are no contraindications to anticoagulation and if there is a clear risk of accelerated structural valve deterioration. However, there is a significant trend toward the use of bioprostheses. Bioprostheses should be recommended when good-quality anticoagulation is unlikely (due to compliance problems or contraindication), for reoperation for mechanical thrombosis despite excellent anticoagulant control, in women contemplating pregnancy, and in patients wishing to avoid anticoagulation.

The normal mitral valve is in the left atrioventricular groove and allows unidirectional flow of oxygenated blood from the left atrium into the left ventricle (LV) in a near-frictionless fashion during diastole.[1] The valve is a complex, three-dimensional assembly of independent anatomic components: the annulus, the leaflets and commissures, the chordae tendineae, the papillary muscles, and the LV. During systole, a coordinated interaction of these anatomic components seals the valve against LV pressure.[2] Even a normal, competent valve may permit a physiologically trivial amount of reversed flow into the left atrium; more than a trace of mitral regurgitation (MR) is considered pathologic.[3]

Although mild to moderate MR may be tolerated indefinitely, severe MR eventually leads to LV remodeling, heart failure, and death.[4] In this

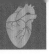

context, the natural history of MR depends intimately on its cause, the severity of LV volume overload, LV contractile performance,[5] and the appearance of overlapping clinical conditions due to reversal of flow, such as atrial fibrillation and pulmonary hypertension.[6]

Primary degenerative mitral valve disease is the most prevalent cause of isolated severe MR in the United States.[7] Distinct pathologic features of the disease include mitral valve billowing (i.e., intact valve coaptation) and prolapse (i.e., deficient valve coaptation) caused by myxomatous degeneration of the mitral leaflets, chordal elongation or rupture, or papillary muscle elongation or rupture.[8]

In the setting of severe MR, even in the absence of symptoms, mitral valve repair is the gold standard procedure for patients who require surgery for degenerative MR.[8–11] For this subset of patients, mitral valve repair has become feasible and safe, and repair techniques have demonstrated an excellent durability, especially when performed in high-volume institutions.[12–14]

The latest guidelines for managing valvular heart disease suggest targeted referral to reference centers with experienced surgeons to ensure a repair rate greater than 90% and a mortality rate of 1% or less.[15] Although these new standards have triggered a more liberal referral of asymptomatic patients, mitral valve repair is still underused in the United States. A data analysis from the Society of Thoracic Surgeons (STS) observed an average mitral valve repair rate of only 70%.[16]

Simple lesions such as posterior leaflet prolapse are associated with very high mitral valve repair rates in many centers,[17] but the overall repair rate for more complex scenarios, as defined by leaflet involvement (e.g., isolated anterior leaflet or bileaflet prolapse), lesion complexity (e.g., significant annular calcification, significant excess tissue), or patient comorbidities (e.g., older age, reoperations), remains uncertain and seems to be well below guideline recommendations.[18]

SURGICAL ANATOMY OF THE MITRAL VALVE

The normal mitral valve is a dynamic complex of independent anatomic structures. Abnormalities (i.e., lesions) in any of these components may lead to altered closure against LV pressure (i.e., dysfunction) and, consequently, MR. Structural abnormalities of the mitral valve are referred to as *primary mitral valve disease*, whereas valve dysfunction due to perturbations in LV geometry is called *ischemic MR* in ischemic cardiomyopathy and *functional MR* in dilated cardiomyopathy.

Mitral Annulus

The mitral annulus is a discontinuous, fibromuscular, D-shaped ring located in the left atrioventricular groove (between the LV and the left atrium) that serves as an anchor and hinge point for the mitral valve leaflets.[19] The mitral annulus can be subjectively divided into anterior and posterior segments according to the attachments of the anterior and posterior mitral leaflets. It can also be segmented by location into septal and lateral components. The anterior part of the mitral annulus is in continuity with the fibrous skeleton of the heart and is limited by the right and left fibrous trigones and the aortic mitral curtain (i.e., continuity at the level of the left and noncoronary aortic valve cusps).[20] The posterior part of the mitral annulus lacks a fibrous skeleton and is more prone to dilation and calcification.[21]

The resultant changes in annular dimensions lead to a more circular annulus compared with its normal kidney-bean shape, and this compromises the coaptation of the mitral leaflets. The normal mitral annulus also has a three-dimensional saddle shape with two lower points at the level of both trigones and one peak at the midpoint of the anterior leaflet. The peak point is always above the midpoint of the posterior leaflet, allowing bulging during systole to accommodate the aortic root and optimize stress distribution over both leaflets.

The overall circumference of the annulus may decrease by as much as 20% during systole (i.e., less eccentricity), promoting central leaflet coaptation.[22] Reduction in annular size begins with atrial contraction and reaches its maximum halfway through the systolic cycle.

Mitral Leaflets and Commissures

The mitral valve has two leaflets (anterior and posterior) with similar surface areas and thicknesses (≈1 mm) but significantly different shapes. The anterior leaflet is taller and has a shorter base than the posterior leaflet; it extends vertically and is anchored to one third of the annular circumference between the right and left fibrous trigones.[23] The posterior leaflet is broader based and has a shorter height than the anterior leaflet; it lies transverse to the mitral valve orifice, and together with the commissures, it is fixed to the remaining two thirds of the annulus. The posterior leaflet is closely related to the LV wall base, the point of greatest systolic stress.

The different orientations of the two leaflets ensures a competent closure line of the mitral valve during systole. The closure line is located in the posterior one third of the valve orifice, which naturally prevents systolic anterior motion.[24] Both leaflets have two zones from the base to the free border or margin: the *atrial or membranous zone,* which is smooth and translucent, and the *coaptation zone,* which is rough, nodular, and thicker due to the attachment and fusion of chordae tendineae.

As a surgical reference, the leaflets of the mitral valve can be distinguished by location of the clefts or indentations in the posterior leaflet. If both commissures are counted as individual segments, a total of eight segments can be identified. Unlike the anterior leaflet, the posterior leaflet has two clefts in its free margin that allow full opening during LV filling and demarcate three segments or scallops. The middle scallop of the posterior leaflet is designated *P2,* and the adjacent medial and lateral scallops are designated *P1* and *P3,* respectively. The corresponding areas of the anterior leaflet are designated by their opposition to the segments in the posterior leaflet as *A1, A2,* and *A3* (Fig. 19.1).

In addition to the anterior and posterior leaflet scallops or segments, the mitral valve has two triangular segments (i.e., commissures) that establish continuity between the two leaflets. These distinct areas of leaflet tissue are supported by chordal fans and are critical to achieving a good surface of coaptation at the junctions of the two leaflets. For their identification, the vertical axis of the papillary muscles and their corresponding chordae tendineae is used as a reference point, thereby obtaining an anterior commissure and a posterior commissure (Fig. 19.2).

Chordae Tendineae

The chordate tendineae are filament-like structures of fibrous connective tissue that join the LV surface and free border of the mitral leaflets to the papillary muscles and, by default, to the posterior wall of the LV. They create a suspension system that allows full opening of the leaflets during diastole and prevents excursion of the leaflets above the annular plane during systole.[25]

About 25 primary chordae begin in the papillary muscles and progressively subdivide to insert into the leaflets. Chordae tendineae are classified according to their insertion point between the free border and the base of the mitral leaflets. Primary or marginal chordae attach along the margin (every 3 to 5 mm) of the leaflets and are critical to prevent leaflet prolapse and to align the rough zones of the anterior and posterior leaflets during systole. Secondary or intermediate chordae, which are inserted in the ventricular side of the body of the leaflets, relieve excess tension during systole.[26] Tertiary or basal chordae are found only on the posterior leaflet; they connect its base and the posterior annulus to the papillary muscles, providing additional linkage to the ventricle (see Fig. 19.2).

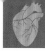

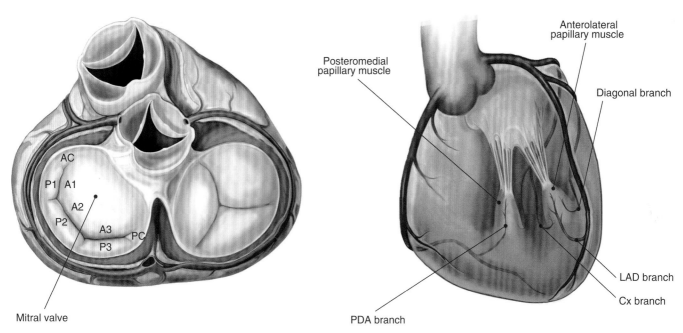

Fig. 19.1 Anatomic view of the cardiac valves in systole *(left)*. Anatomy and arterial supply of the papillary muscles of the left ventricle *(right)*. *A1*, *A2*, and *A3*, Anterior leaflet scallops; *AC*, anterior commissure; *Cx*, circumflex; *LAD*, left anterior descending artery; *P1*, *P2*, and *P3*, posterior leaflet scallops; *PC*, posterior commissure; *PDA*, posterior descending artery.

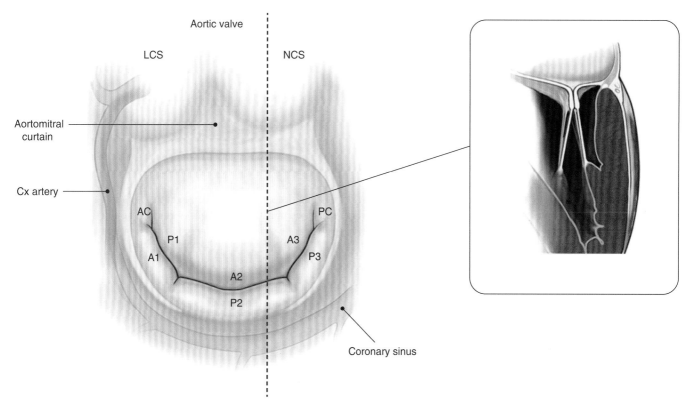

Fig. 19.2 Anatomic Structures Surrounding the Mitral Valve. Normal function of the mitral apparatus brings both leaflets together in systole and creates the coaptation zone. *A1*, *A2*, and *A3*, Anterior leaflet scallops; *AC*, anterior commissure; *Cx*, circumflex; *LCS*, left coronary sinus; *P1*, *P2*, and *P3*, posterior leaflet scallops; *NCS*, noncoronary sinus; *PC*, posterior commissure.

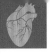

Papillary Muscles and the Left Ventricle

The mitral valve leaflets are attached by the chordae tendineae to the papillary muscles, which are considered an extension of the LV. The papillary muscles vary in number of heads and exact position in the ventricle, but two organized groups usually can be identified. Each papillary muscle is designated according to the relationship to the valve commissures, and each provides a fan chord to its corresponding commissure and to the anterior and posterior leaflets.

The anterior papillary muscle has a single body, is larger, and is perfused by the first obtuse marginal branch of the circumflex artery and the first diagonal branch of the left anterior descending artery (see Fig. 19.1). The posterior papillary muscle has two bodies, is smaller, and is supplied blood only by the posterior descending artery, a branch of the right coronary artery, in 90% of cases or by the circumflex artery in the other 10%. This arrangement explains the relative vulnerability of the posterior papillary muscle to ischemia and its subsequent involvement in localized remodeling in the setting of ischemic MR.[27]

The LV supports the entire mitral apparatus due to its continuation with the papillary muscles. LV dimensional changes in the setting of volume overload and remodeling, whether ischemic or not, can lead to leaflet tethering and MR.[28]

PATHOPHYSIOLOGIC TRIAD OF MITRAL VALVE REGURGITATION

MR is defined as the existence of blood flow in systole from the LV into the left atrium. Minimal structural lesions can cause MR by reducing mitral leaflet coaptation. Exhaustive interrogation of mitral lesions for identification, localization, and magnitude is essential to determining the chances of successful valve repair and proceeding with a tailored therapeutic plan for each patient.

Three decades ago, Carpentier described a systematic analytic approach to patients with MR known as the *pathophysiologic triad of MR*.[29] The triad emphasizes the importance of differentiating among the medical causes of MR, identifying the resulting lesions, and determining how the lesions affect leaflet motion (i.e., dysfunction). Besides promoting mutual understanding among surgeons and specialists in cardiac imaging, the triad also represents an organized and consistent way to elucidate the most appropriate techniques to achieve successful repair.

Dysfunction

Differentiation of valve dysfunctions (i.e., types I, II, and III) is based on the position of the leaflet margins with respect to the mitral annular plane. Type I dysfunction implies normal leaflet motion, and the most common cause of significant MR is perforation of one of the leaflets (e.g., endocarditis) or severe annular dilation with a central regurgitant jet (e.g., primary atrial fibrillation). Type II dysfunction denotes excess leaflet motion, which usually occurs due to chordal elongation or rupture or to myxomatous degeneration of the leaflets (i.e., regurgitant jet directed to the opposite side of the prolapsing leaflet).[30] Type III dysfunction designates restricted leaflet motion and typically results from retraction of the subvalvular apparatus (i.e., type IIIa, rheumatic valve disease, or other inflammatory scenarios that lead to scarring and calcification) or from papillary muscle displacement (i.e., leaflet tethering) due to LV remodeling or dilation (i.e., type IIIb, ischemic or dilated cardiomyopathy) (Fig. 19.3).

Etiology and Lesions

Worldwide, rheumatic disease remains the most common cause of MR,[31] but it has ceased to be the leading cause in developed countries.[32]

Ischemic disease, which is currently responsible for 20% of MR cases, may lose importance as a result of aggressive percutaneous treatment of coronary artery disease. Degenerative disease is the most frequent cause of MR in Western countries (Fig. 19.4).[33]

Degenerative mitral valve disease is characterized by a wide spectrum of lesions,[34] which vary from a simple chordal rupture leading to prolapse of an isolated segment (frequently P2) in an otherwise normal valve to multiple-segment prolapse of both leaflets in a valve with significant excess tissue.[35] The range of lesions gives rise to two opposing entities: fibroelastic deficiency and Barlow disease.[36]

Fibroelastic deficiency occurs in older patients (usually > 60 years of age) with a short history of severe holosystolic murmur. As the term implies, this disease is a condition associated with a deficit of the protein fibrillin that often leads to weakening, elongation, and ultimately rupture of chordae tendineae.[37] Chordal rupture of P2 is considered the most common lesion in patients with fibroelastic deficiency. The mitral leaflets are usually thin and translucent, although the prolapsing scallop may have a myxomatous aspect if the disease has existed for a long time. Distinguishing fibroelastic deficiency from other entities in the spectrum of degenerative mitral valve disease requires an exhaustive analysis of the segments immediately contiguous to the prolapsing one, which are usually normal in size, height, and tissue properties. The annular size in patients with this condition is often less than 32 mm.

At the opposite end of the spectrum of degenerative disease is Barlow disease.[38] Affected patients are usually younger than 60 years of age and have a long history of holosystolic murmur that has been monitored by the referring cardiologist for many years. Patients with Barlow disease have a more diffuse and complex redundancy of the leaflets. The most common lesions are excess leaflet tissue, leaflet thickening, and distention, with diffuse chordal elongation, thickening, or rupture.[39] In these patients, the annular size exceeds 36 mm, and it is not uncommon to find various degrees of annular calcification (often involving the anterior papillary muscle) and fibrosis of the subvalvular apparatus (Fig. 19.5).[40]

Rheumatic disease is the main cause of mitral disease in underdeveloped and developing countries. A systemic exudative inflammatory reaction involves the connective tissue of skin, joints, and heart.[32] Cardiac involvement has been described as a pancarditis with characteristic implications for the left-sided valves. Severe edema and cellular infiltration (i.e., severe leaflet thickening extending toward the commissures) is followed by the formation of rheumatic nodules along the free borders of the leaflets. All components of the subvalvular apparatus (i.e., papillary muscles and chordae tendineae) are also affected, leading to chordal thickening and retraction and to chordal and commissural fusion. The annulus then dilates in a very asymmetric fashion, predominantly along the P3 segment. The anterior leaflet is typically less affected than the posterior leaflet, which is often retracted. Because of the complexity of lesions, rheumatic mitral disease is not as amenable to valve repair as other lesions.[41]

Ischemic MR is a consequence of myocardial ischemia and remodeling. In this context, ischemic MR can manifest acutely after papillary muscle rupture (primary disease) or from LV remodeling and apical and inferior displacement of the papillary muscles.[42] In the setting of ischemic MR, the mitral leaflets are tethered, and their coaptation point is below the mitral annulus. When restricted leaflet movement occurs principally in systole, the pattern is asymmetric; this is mainly observed in patients with posterior infarction and posterior leaflet restriction (i.e., eccentric regurgitant jet).[43] In patients with dilated cardiomyopathy or anterior and posterior infarctions, both leaflets have a restrictive deficit, giving rise to a symmetric pattern (i.e., central jet).[44]

In planning the surgical approach to ischemic MR, it is critical to understand the mechanism (i.e., secondary classification) and dynamics

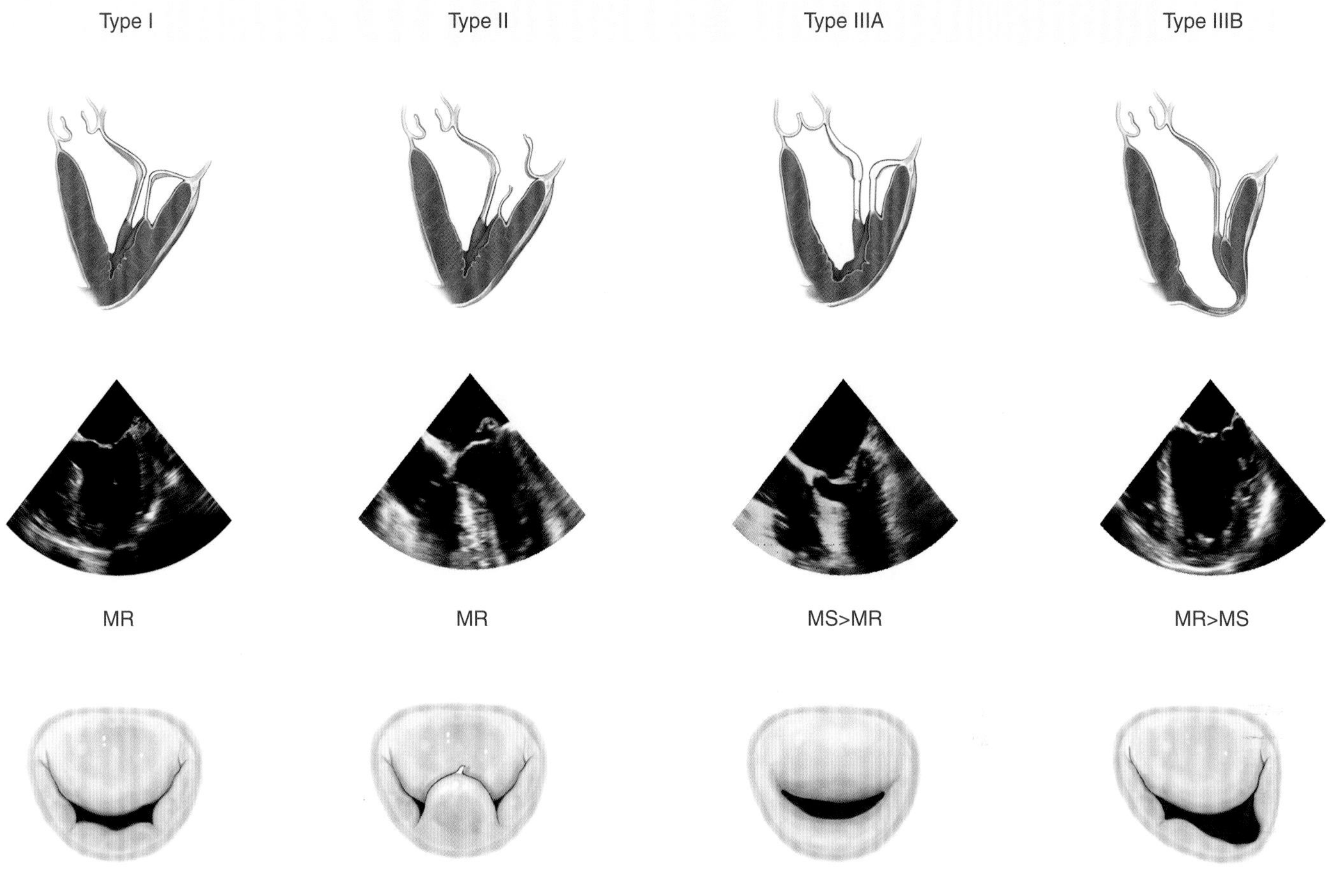

Type I	Type II	Type IIIA	Type IIIB
MR	MR	MS>MR	MR>MS
Normal Leaflet Motion (annular dilation)	Increased Leaflet Motion (leaflet prolapse)	Restricted Leaflet Motion (restricted opening)	Restricted Leaflet Motion (retsricted closure)
Annular dilation Annular deformation Leaflet perforation Leaflet cleft	Myxomatous degeneration Chordal elongation Chordal rupture Papillary muscle elongation Papillary muscle rupture	Leaflet thickening, retraction Chordal thickening, retraction Chordal fusion Calcification Commissural fusion Ventricular fibrosis	Leaflet tethering Displacement of PM Ventricular dilation Ventricular aneurysm Ventricular fibrosis
Ischemic cardiomyopathy Dilated cardiomyopathy Endocarditis Congenital	Degenerative disease Marfan syndrome Endocarditis Rheumatic disease Trauma Ischemic cardiomyopathy Ehlers-Danlos syndrome	Rheumatic disease Carcinoid disease Radiation Lupus eythematosus Ergotamine use Hypereosinophilic syndrome Mucoploysaccharidosis	Ischemic cardiomyopathy Dilated cardiomyopathy

Fig. 19.3 Pathophysiologic triad of mitral valve disease composed of (top to bottom in each column) the ventricular view, echocardiographic view, atrial view, leaflet dysfunction, valve lesions, and cause. *MR,* Mitral regurgitation; *MS,* mitral stenosis; *PM,* papillary muscle.

(i.e., possible progression) of the disease.[45] Analysis of the mechanism of MR answers several prognostic questions. How tethered and angulated are the leaflets? Is there a pseudoprolapse? Is the regurgitation jet eccentric or central? What are the ventricular dimensions? How reversible is the ischemic insult (Fig. 19.6)?[46]

MITRAL VALVE SURGERY

MR predisposes the LV to volume overload as compensation for the volume lost to regurgitation.[47] Although mild to moderate MR may be well tolerated for long periods, severe MR is fatal at a determined stage.[48] Severe MR can be divided into three clinical stages: acute,

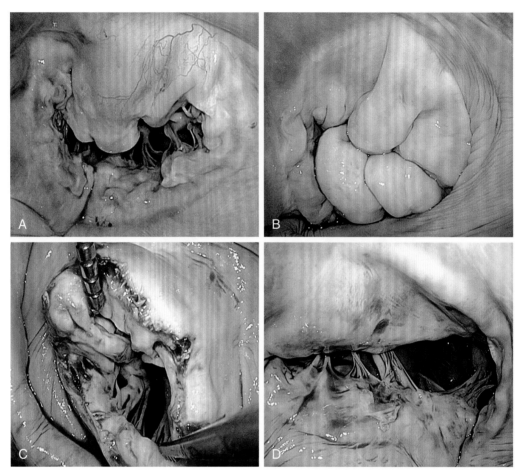

Fig. 19.4 Intraoperative views of the mitral valve in patients with annular dilation (A), degenerative disease (B), rheumatic disease (C), and ischemic disease (D).

chronic compensated, and chronic decompensated; each requires different management and has different surgical triggers (Fig. 19.7; see Chapter 17 and Fig. 17.11).[49]

Severe MR is a mechanical problem for which surgery (i.e., mitral valve repair or MVR) is the only definitive solution.[50] Although the lack of randomized trials comparing mitral valve repair with MVR has led to controversy,[51] particularly in the setting of secondary MR (Fig. 19.8), repair is favored over replacement for many reasons, especially in patients with degenerative mitral valve disease (see Chapter 18).[52] The reasons include a likely lower perioperative risk and improved event-free survival for most surgical patients, freedom from the various complications of prosthetic heart valves, and better postoperative LV function (Fig. 19.9).[53]

Surgical Approach

Several surgical approaches for access to the mitral valve have been described.[54] Although the earliest mitral valve procedures were performed through a right thoracotomy, the mitral valve has traditionally been exposed through a median sternotomy.[55] Median sternotomy remains the gold standard and is still the most popular approach.[56] Central cannulation and direct aortic clamping enable mitral surgery with generous exposure and excellent results.[57]

Some groups have significantly transformed the incision to a lower hemisternotomy, limiting the length of the incision to 7 to 9 cm. To reduce invasiveness and potential operative morbidity, cardiac surgeons adopted nonsternotomy approaches, also known as video-assisted approaches, including right thoracotomy and robotic surgery (Figs. 19.10

and 19.11).[58–60] Although the safety and efficacy of minimally invasive cardiac surgery have been established in several high-volume specialized centers, potential issues have been raised,[61] including a higher incidence of certain complications such as postoperative stroke.[62] One concern is the compromise of repair rates because minimally invasive cardiac surgery is most predictably effective when used in cases of simple pathology rather than in complex valve surgery.[63] There have been no clearly demonstrable clinical benefits of minimally invasive access other than cosmetic advantages.[64]

The most important goal for patients with MR and the physicians involved in their perioperative care is to achieve a good and durable repair of the mitral valve,[65] as emphasized in the latest guidelines from the European Society of Cardiology (ESC) and the European Association for Cardio-Thoracic Surgery (EACTS).[66] Achieving a competent and symmetric line of closure, a good surface of coaptation, and an effective preservation of leaflet mobility is key to providing the patient with a competent and durable repair.[67]

In ideal conditions, these axioms could be met in the setting of simple or complex lesions, regardless of the preferred surgical approach. However, in the real world, complex mitral valve repair remains challenging in patients undergoing median sternotomy in most centers and certainly is unpredictable when attempted with minimally invasive strategies. This issue is crucial when referring young asymptomatic patients, in whom durability of repair is critical and the occurrence of stroke is particularly devastating. As technology advances and training for surgical subspecialties develops, minimally invasive techniques may be applied to a wider spectrum of lesions. At this time, the

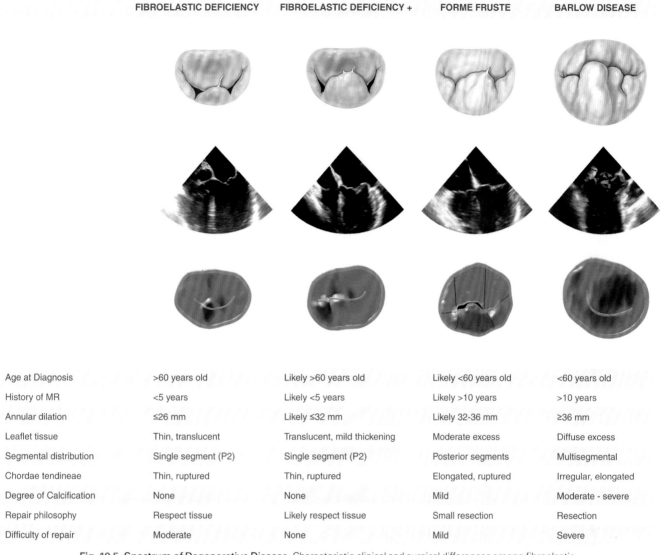

	FIBROELASTIC DEFICIENCY	FIBROELASTIC DEFICIENCY +	FORME FRUSTE	BARLOW DISEASE
Age at Diagnosis	>60 years old	Likely >60 years old	Likely <60 years old	<60 years old
History of MR	<5 years	Likely <5 years	Likely >10 years	>10 years
Annular dilation	≤26 mm	Likely ≤32 mm	Likely 32-36 mm	≥36 mm
Leaflet tissue	Thin, translucent	Translucent, mild thickening	Moderate excess	Diffuse excess
Segmental distribution	Single segment (P2)	Single segment (P2)	Posterior segments	Multisegmental
Chordae tendineae	Thin, ruptured	Thin, ruptured	Elongated, ruptured	Irregular, elongated
Degree of Calcification	None	None	Mild	Moderate - severe
Repair philosophy	Respect tissue	Likely respect tissue	Small resection	Resection
Difficulty of repair	Moderate	None	Mild	Severe

Fig. 19.5 Spectrum of Degenerative Disease. Characteristic clinical and surgical differences among fibroelastic deficiencies, Barlow disease, and forme fruste. *MR,* Mitral regurgitation.

use of these strategies to attempt mitral valve repair seems restricted to selected, high-volume, specialized centers.[64]

Mitral Valve Repair

Degenerative mitral valve disease encompasses a wide spectrum of lesions that requires a wide variety of surgical techniques for repair.[12] After a systematic valve analysis and identification of the lesions, mitral valve repair should be performed with a sequential approach as follows: (1) repair of the posterior leaflet; (2) ring annuloplasty preferably using a complete, semirigid remodeling ring; and (3) repair of any residual prolapse of the anterior leaflet or commissures after inspection of the line of closure during saline testing.[68]

If posterior leaflet prolapse results from fibroelastic disease, it is most commonly treated by a triangular or limited resection of the affected segment. The prolapsing segment is removed, and direct suturing of the leaflet remnants and edges restores leaflet continuity. Occasionally, annular plication techniques may be applied to relieve leaflet tension. In the setting of very limited or normal leaflet tissue, it may be preferable to avoid leaflet resection and proceed with a chordal transfer or surgical techniques using polytetrafluoroethylene (PTFE) (i.e., loop technique, loop-in-loop technique, or single neochordoplasty). If a more extensive leaflet resection is needed, it is usually performed where the prolapse is greatest or the leaflet is tallest. The width of this resection is typically 1 cm or less; additional excess tissue can be removed later. If the height is greater than 15 mm in any residual leaflet segment, a sliding leaflet plasty (including secondary chordal cutting) to reduce the residual leaflet height to 12 to 15 mm across the posterior leaflet can be performed.

Reattachment of the leaflet to the annulus reduces the leaflet height by several millimeters, depending on the depth of suture bites, and the leaflet height before suturing should ideally be about 15 mm in all segments. If the leaflet is taller than 2 cm, a horizontal wedge excision is made at the base of the appropriate segment to further reduce its height before reattachment. The margins of the reconstructed posterior leaflets are then examined to ensure that all segments are adequately supported. Any gaps in support or any areas supported by thinned-out chordae (even in the absence of prolapse) are reinforced by transposition of previously detached secondary chordae or artificial PTFE neochords.

After posterior leaflet repair, annular remodeling needs to be addressed because annular dilation is the most commonly associated lesion

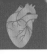

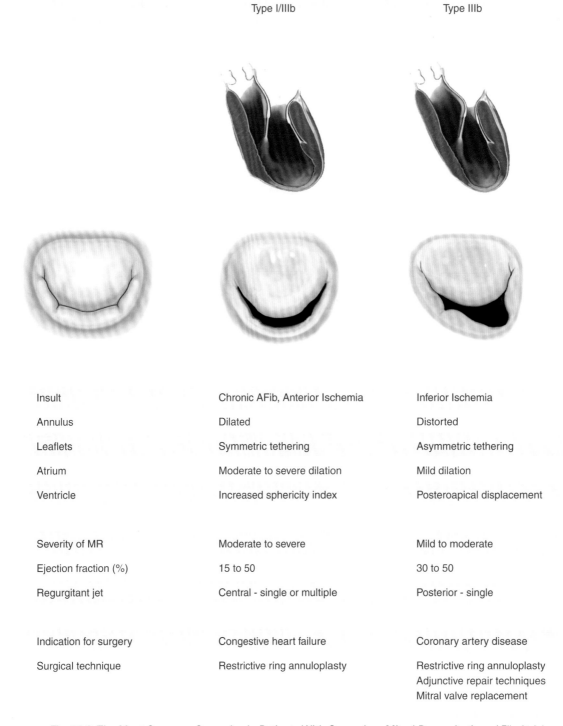

	Type I/IIIb	Type IIIb
Insult	Chronic AFib, Anterior Ischemia	Inferior Ischemia
Annulus	Dilated	Distorted
Leaflets	Symmetric tethering	Asymmetric tethering
Atrium	Moderate to severe dilation	Mild dilation
Ventricle	Increased sphericity index	Posteroapical displacement
Severity of MR	Moderate to severe	Mild to moderate
Ejection fraction (%)	15 to 50	30 to 50
Regurgitant jet	Central - single or multiple	Posterior - single
Indication for surgery	Congestive heart failure	Coronary artery disease
Surgical technique	Restrictive ring annuloplasty	Restrictive ring annuloplasty Adjunctive repair techniques Mitral valve replacement

Fig. 19.6 The Most Common Scenarios in Patients With Secondary Mitral Regurgitation. *AFib*, Atrial fibrillation; *MR*, mitral regurgitation.

in the setting of leaflet prolapse. Annuloplasty sutures are usually placed around the annulus before correction of leaflet height or prolapse. Annular sizing is performed by measuring the intercommissural distance and the surface area of the anterior leaflet. Sutures are passed through the annuloplasty ring, and the ring is tied down securely (Fig. 19.12).

Correction of anterior leaflet dysfunction is usually addressed after a remodeling ring is placed. The anatomic disposition of the anterior leaflet does not allow aggressive resection of the leaflet margins. The surgical strategy to fix opposing anterior leaflet prolapse includes minimal resection (i.e., limited to the rough area of the leaflet) or no resection. After saline testing with moderate pressurization of the LV, correction of the anterior leaflet prolapse using one or more of the following techniques may be performed: (1) chordal transfer of basal chords, secondary chords, or a small segment of posterior leaflet with attached chords (i.e., flip technique); (2) neochordoplasty with PTFE sutures; (3) PTFE loop or loop-in-loop technique to correct multiple

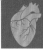

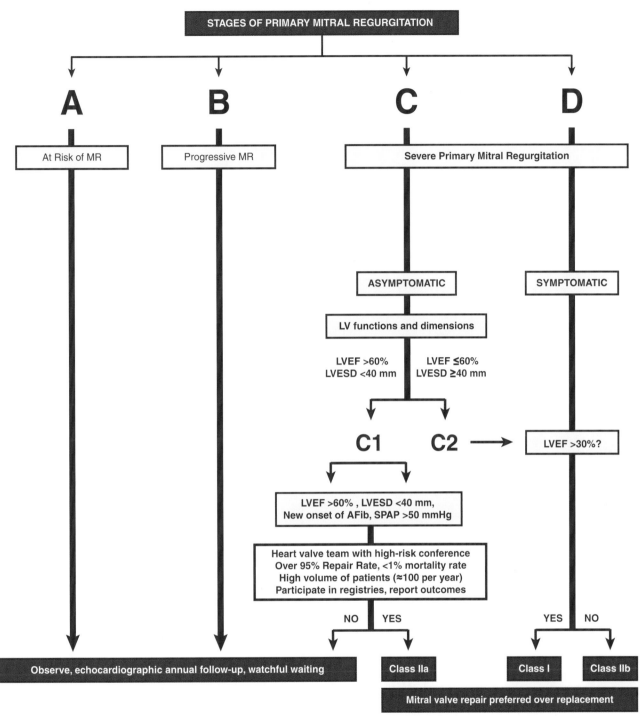

Fig. 19.7 Proposed Management Algorithm for Patients With Degenerative Mitral Valve Disease. *AFib,* Atrial fibrillation; *LVEF,* left ventricular ejection fraction; *LVESD,* left ventricular end-systolic dimension; *MR,* mitral regurgitation, *SPAP,* systolic pulmonary artery pressure. (Modified from Nishimura RA, Otto CM, Bonow RO, et al. 2014 AHA/ACC guideline for the management of patients with valvular heart disease: executive summary: a report of the American College of Cardiology/American Heart Association Task Force on Practice Guidelines. J Am Coll Cardiol. 2014;63:2438-2488.)

prolapsing segments; or (4) limited triangular resection of a prolapsing segment.

Commissural prolapse (often seen in patients with Barlow disease) may be corrected by placing one or two vertical mattress sutures (i.e., Carpentier's "magic" suture) to fix opposing segments of A1/P1 or A3/P3, advancing the commissures. As a useful alternative, PTFE neochords may be placed to support opposing segments at the commissures, with one arm of the suture passed through opposing anterior and posterior leaflet segments. An optimal mitral valve repair should meet the following criteria: (1) the valve is competent on saline

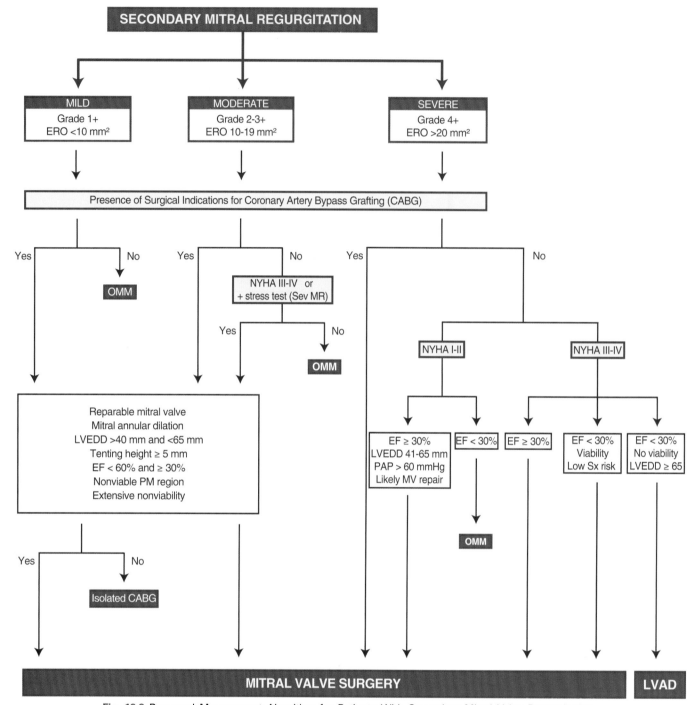

Fig. 19.8 Proposed Management Algorithm for Patients With Secondary Mitral Valve Regurgitation. *AFib*, Atrial fibrillation; *CABG*, coronary artery bypass grafting; *EF*, ejection fraction; *ERO*, effective regurgitant orifice; *LVAD*, left ventricular assist device; *LVEDD*, left ventricular end-diastolic diameter; *MR*, mitral regurgitation; *MV*, mitral valve; *NYHA*, New York Heart Association functional class; *OMM*, optimal medical management, including cardiac resynchronization therapy; *PAP*, pulmonary artery pressure; *PM*, papillary muscle; *Sev*, severe; *SPAP*, systolic pulmonary artery pressure; *Sx*, surgical. (Modified from Crestanello JA. Surgical approach to mitral regurgitation in chronic heart failure: when is it an option? Curr Heart Fail Rep 2012;9:40-50.)

testing; (2) there is a good surface of coaptation; (3) the line of closure where the anterior leaflet occupies 80% or more of the valve area is symmetric; (4) there is no residual billowing; and (5) there is no tendency to systolic anterior motion.

Evaluation of all these points may require two different intraoperative tests: the saline test and the ink test. The saline test is performed by filling the ventricle with saline. Examination of the valve confirms the absence of prolapse, billowing, and incompetence; a symmetric closure line; and an anterior leaflet that occupies most of the valve orifice. The ink test is performed by drawing a line on the valve closure line during maximum saline instillations.[69] The coaptation zone beyond the ink is examined and should be at least 6 mm long (which transforms to

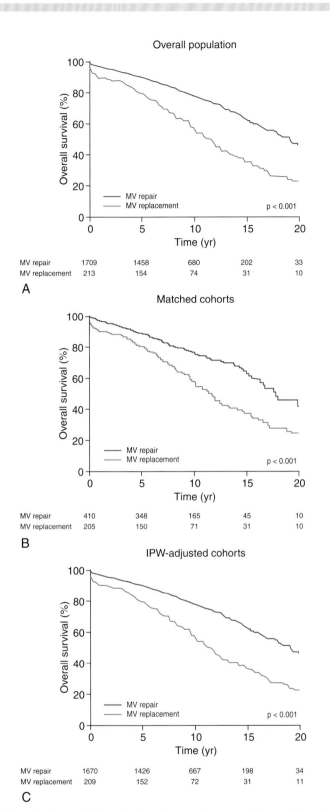

A

B

C

Fig. 19.9 Kaplan-Meier Survival Curves Compare 20-year Overall Postoperative Survival Among Patients Undergoing Mitral Valve (MV) Repair or MV Replacement. Survival curves for matched cohorts receiving MR repair or MR replacement (A) and for patients who were 75 years old or older at the time of treatment (B). Rates of thromboembolism (C) and freedom from valve-related complications after MR repair or replacement. (From Lazam S, Vanoverschelde JL, Tribouilloy C, et al. Twenty-year outcome after mitral repair versus replacement for severe degenerative mitral regurgitation: analysis of a large, prospective, multicenter international registry. Circulation 2017;135(5):410-422.)

approximately 10 mm on echocardiography because part of the ink is within the coaptation zone). There should be no more than 1 cm of anterior leaflet beyond the ink line; more than this amount would signify a risk of systolic anterior motion.

Practice guidelines separate recommendations for surgery according to the severity of MR and its symptoms rather than the cause.[70] Most patients with severe ischemic MR have symptoms of heart failure.[71] According to current guidelines, patients with severe, symptomatic MR have a class I indication for mitral valve surgery if the LV ejection fraction is greater than 30% and or the end-systolic LV dimension is 55 mm or smaller. The valvular apparatus is examined systematically to assess tissue pliability and identify leaflet restriction with P1 as a reference point.[72] The mitral annulus is also examined to assess the severity of annular dilation, which is very common.

If mitral valve repair is the procedure of choice, restrictive remodeling annuloplasty[73] should be used. Because leaflet restriction in ischemic MR results in less leaflet tissue available for coaptation, it is necessary to downsize a complete remodeling ring by one or two sizes or to use a true-sized Carpentier-McCarthy-Adams IMR Etlogix ring (Edwards Lifesciences Corp., Irvine, CA)[74] to ensure an adequate surface of coaptation after annuloplasty.[75] This ring combines the principles of undersizing with the specific asymmetric deformation (i.e., severe tethering along P3) observed in type IIIb ischemic MR.

In cases of severe leaflet tethering and moderate to severe LV dilation, restrictive annuloplasty and combined coronary artery bypass grafting (CABG) surgery may not provide durable results. Several adjunctive techniques and alternative procedures have been advocated, including division of secondary chords, posterior leaflet extension with a pericardial patch, repositioning of the papillary muscles, and MVR with chordal sparing.[76]

Rheumatic mitral valve disease is characterized mainly by mitral stenosis (MS) due to fibrotic restrictions of the subvalvular apparatus. Nonetheless, some patients present for treatment with MR resulting from various degrees of restriction, chordal thickening, and commissural fusion. If the valve is severely calcified and there is freezing of the chordal structures, mitral valve repair is extremely complex and often fruitless. If there is MS due to isolated commissural fusion or a more preserved subvalvular apparatus, as occurs in younger patients, mitral valve repair becomes feasible.[77]

Techniques for rheumatic repair include commissurotomy and commissural reconstruction, calcium debridement, chordal fenestration and cutting, and patch extension of both leaflets with glutaraldehyde-fixed pericardium, a technique that usually requires leaflet resuspension with PTFE neochords.

Mitral Valve Replacement

Although MVR should be uncommonly used for patients with degenerative mitral disease who are appropriately referred to experienced surgeons, it remains fairly prevalent among patients with complex lesions. This situation is reversed for patients with rheumatic disease, for whom MVR rates are as high as 50% in reference centers.

For patients with chronic ischemic MR, the best approach—MVR or mitral valve repair with annuloplasty—remains debatable. This is in part because prosthetic valve function is not affected by worsening LV function if there is further negative remodeling.[78] Studies have suggested better echocardiographic outcomes in those patients undergoing MVR, with no significant difference in mortality at 2.5 years.[79] Longer follow-up is needed to analyze the occurrence of classic complications of valve replacement, such as structural valve degeneration, nonstructural dysfunction, valve thrombosis, embolism, bleeding events, and endocarditis.

If the decision to proceed with MVR is made, a chord-sparing approach should be employed. The posterior leaflet with chords and often

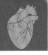
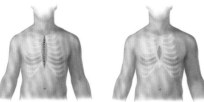
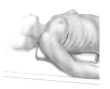
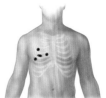

FEATURES	STERNOTOMY/MINISTERNOTOMY	VIDEO-ASSISTED APPROACHES
Arterial perfusion	Antegrade (aorta)	Retrograde (femoral artery)
Venous drainage	Central	Peripheral
Aortic clamping	Direct, site detected by direct palpation, epi-aortic US	Endoscopic clamp or balloon
Myocardial protection	Direct	Indirect by rapid injection
Visualization	Direct and wide for all memebrs of the team	Limited to the endoscopic device
Annuloplasty devices	As desired	Limited to adequacy
Annuloplasty sutures	Braided polyester	Braided polyester, running polypropylene, nitinol clips
Repair techniques	As desired	Predilection for nonresectional techniques
Ventilation	Two-lung ventilation	Single-lung ventilation

Fig. 19.10 Technical Variations and Limitations of Mitral Valve Surgery According to Surgical Approach. *US,* Ultrasound.

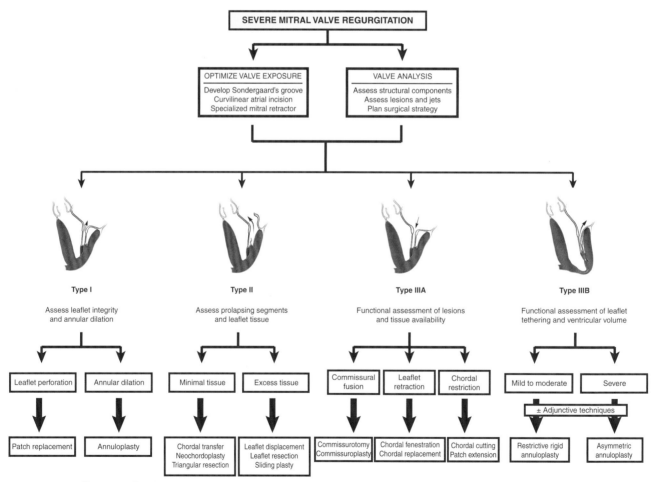

Fig. 19.11 Surgical approach to mitral valve disease includes optimization of valve exposure, valve analysis, and application of the most common technical resource according to the lesion encountered.

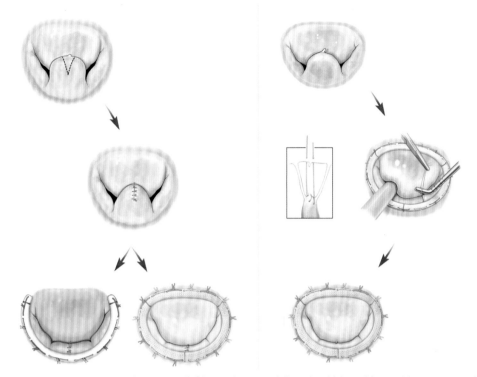

Fig. 19.12 After posterior leaflet repair *(left)*, annular remodeling should be addressed because annular dilation is the most commonly associated lesion in the setting of leaflet prolapse. Annuloplasty sutures are placed around the annulus before correction of leaflet height or prolapse correction. Sutures are passed through the annuloplasty ring *(right)*, and the ring is tied down securely.

all or portions of the anterior leaflet with chords are incorporated into the sutures used to secure the replacement valve prosthesis. This technique preserves chordal-ventricular-annular continuity, which is important to preserving long-term LV shape and performance.

Guidelines recommend that patient preference be considered in the decision to use a mechanical valve or a bioprosthetic valve in patients younger than 65 years of age.[15] In practice, more and more patients are selecting bioprostheses regardless of age because of their desire not to commit to a lifetime of warfarin therapy.

An important trend has favored the use of bioprostheses in the United States. Between 1999 and 2008, the implantation of mechanical valves in Medicare beneficiaries declined from 53% to 21%, and the implantation of bioprostheses increased from 22% to 34%.[80] This phenomenon occurred despite lack of data suggesting a significant difference in long-term survival associated with a specific type of prosthesis.

Two factors may play an important role in decision making when it comes to choosing the type of prosthesis. First, patients older than 65 years, who gain the most benefit from biologic prostheses, represent a growing proportion of patients undergoing valve surgery. Second, cardiologists and physicians in general have increased awareness of the lifetime risk of using anticoagulation. Moreover, variables that historically were considered strong reasons to implant a mechanical valve are no longer valid. They include atrial fibrillation, which has been ameliorated by the availability of more advanced intraoperative antiarrhythmic procedures, and dialysis-dependent renal failure, in which poor long-term survival with either choice may favor the use of bioprostheses.

Although the choice of prosthesis in elderly patients or young patients seems to be clear, there are no data suggesting any significant difference in survival benefit between mechanical and bioprosthetic valves in middle-aged patients. After a thorough discussion about the potential risks of reoperation compared with the lifelong risks of

thromboembolic and hemorrhagic complications, either choice seems reasonable for patients in this age range.[81] According to the latest guidelines on the management of valvular heart disease, mechanical prostheses are reasonable according to the desire of the informed patient if there are no contraindications to anticoagulation. Mechanical valves are preferred if there is risk of accelerated structural valve deterioration or the patient is already undergoing anticoagulation because of a mechanical prosthesis in another position. Bioprostheses should be recommended when good-quality anticoagulation is unlikely (i.e., compliance problems or contraindication) for reoperation for mechanical thrombosis despite excellent anticoagulant control, in women who are contemplating pregnancy, and in patients who wish to avoid anticoagulation.

OUTCOMES OF MITRAL VALVE REPAIR

Data show low mortality rates after mitral valve repair regardless of the cause.[60] In patients with degenerative mitral valve disease, the rate of long-term freedom from reoperation is very low,[82] although return of moderate to severe MR has been reported in later series to occur at a rate of 1% to 4% per year.[12,83–85] Failure to use an annuloplasty ring, use of chordal shortening techniques (which are now uncommon), anterior leaflet pathology, and unavailability of pliable leaflet tissue are associated with higher failure rate after mitral repair.[86,87] The following sections analyze the outcomes of mitral valve repair according to cause.

Degenerative Mitral Valve Disease

In many high-volume valve surgery centers, series of mitral valve procedures for degenerative disease have reported valve replacement rates of 5% to 15% in higher-risk groups such as elderly patients[88] and for more complex pathology, including anterior leaflet involvement.[89]

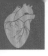
However, the latest reports have demonstrated that it is possible in high-volume reference centers to repair almost all prolapsing degenerative mitral valves with a low operative risk (mortality rate < 1%) and absence of residual MR (Fig. 19.13).[12–14,96]

As a growing number of asymptomatic patients with degenerative mitral valve disease are referred for surgery,[90] it seems mandatory that surgeons can reasonably ensure repair at minimal risk with good long-term results. This goal has proved feasible when repair is performed by specialized valve teams that include cardiologists, anesthesiologists, intensivists, and surgeons.[91]

Use of a systematic surgical strategy and a wide spectrum of surgical techniques to attempt repair in all valves should achieve very high repair rates in experienced hands. Subscribing to a particular technique[92,93] (e.g., use of PTFE) or philosophy (e.g., resect or monitor) may endanger repair rates because specific techniques and philosophies are not applicable to the full spectrum of lesions encountered. Repair of certain valves (e.g., calcified annulus, advanced Barlow disease, repeat repairs) may require long cross-clamp times, and the surgeon must be willing to take as long as necessary to achieve a successful repair.[94] Moreover, no patient should leave the operating room with more than trivial MR as shown by post-bypass transesophageal

echocardiography. If even mild MR remains, surgeons should resume bypass and perfect the repair because it usually requires chordal adjustments or closure of clefts, which take time.[95]

Postoperative mortality rates are affected by age, with an average risk of about 1% for patients younger than 65 years, 2% for those 65 to 80 years, and 4% to 5% for those older than 80 years of age.[96] Preoperative factors that significantly affect survival of patients with MR include LV dysfunction (ejection fraction < 60%), New York Heart Association functional class III or IV, regurgitant orifice area of 40 mm² or more, an LV end-systolic dimension greater than 40 mm, a left atrial index of 60 mL/m² or higher, a left atrial dimension greater than 55 mm, pulmonary hypertension at rest or with exercise, and atrial fibrillation.[97,98] After mitral valve repair, patients who had severe symptoms before surgery continue to have increased mortality rates despite symptom relief (especially those with an LV ejection fraction < 50%), whereas for those who had no or few preoperative symptoms, restoration of life expectancy can be achieved.[99,100]

Durability of mitral valve repair, defined as freedom from moderate or greater degree of MR, has been between 90% and 95% at 5 years in high-volume centers, with a recurrent MR rate of 1% to 1.5% per year (Fig. 19.13). If durability rates are stratified by leaflet involvement,

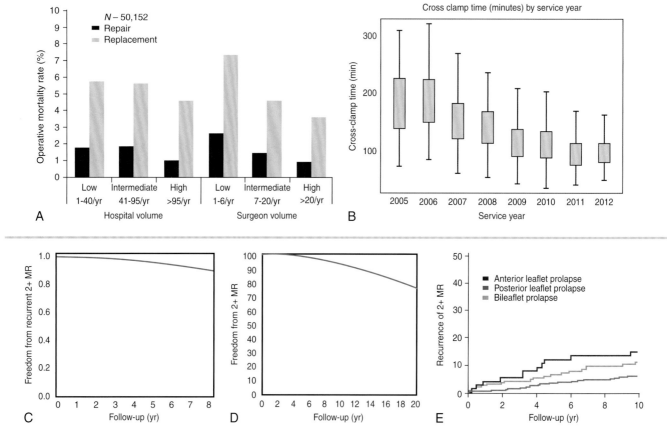

Fig. 19.13 (A) Impact of hospital and surgeon volume on operative outcomes. (B) Improvement in cross-clamp time, 2005 to 2012. (C–E) Long-term outcomes of mitral valve repair in reference centers. *MR*, Mitral regurgitation. (A, Modified from Kilic A, Shah AS, Conte JV, et al. Operative outcomes in mitral valve surgery: combined effect of surgeon and hospital volume in a population-based analysis. J Thorac Cardiovasc Surg 2013;146: 638-646; B, modified from Weiner MM, Hofer I, Lin HM, et al. Relationship among surgical volume, repair quality, and perioperative outcomes for repair of mitral insufficiency in a mitral valve reference center. J Thorac Cardiovasc Surg 2014;148[5]:2021-2026; C, modified from Castillo JG, Anyanwu AC, Fuster V, et al. A near 100% repair rate for mitral valve prolapse is achievable in a reference center: implications for future guidelines. J Thorac Cardiovasc Surg 2012;144:308-312; D, from David TE, Armstrong S, McCrindle BW, et al. Late outcomes of mitral valve repair for mitral regurgitation due to degenerative disease. Circulation 2013;127:1485-1492; E, from Suri RM, Clavel MA, Schaff HV, et al. Effect of recurrent mitral regurgitation following degenerative mitral valve repair: long-term analysis of competing outcomes. J Am Coll Cardiol 2016;67:488-498.)

patients with isolated anterior leaflet prolapse have lower durability rates, ranging between 75% and 85% at 5 years.[101] This fact has a potential etiologic explanation. Patients with isolated anterior leaflet prolapse usually have fibroelastic disease and have thin leaflets with limited tissue availability at presentation. After repair, the coaptation height is not as robust as it is in patients with a minimal degree of myxomatous degeneration, potentially affecting the durability of the repair.

Ischemic Mitral Regurgitation

The increasing life expectancy of the general population, together with the improved survival rates after myocardial infarction due to interventional advancements, is expected to contribute to even a higher prevalence of ischemic MR in the near future. Although mitral valve repair is considered more beneficial than valve replacement,[102] especially in patients with degenerative disease, the best approach for chronic ischemic MR remains debatable,[103] and therefore only a small number of patients are referred for surgery.[104] Postoperative improvement in functional class and LV dimensions have been demonstrated in patients who undergo restrictive annuloplasty,[105] but the lack of firm evidence of a survival benefit precludes surgical referral in many cardiology practices.[106]

Significant rates (15%–25%) of recurrent MR as early as 6 months after surgery prompted the search for alternative therapies, including MVR and percutaneous approaches.[107] Investigation was further stimulated by studies that reported a possible induction of MS after restrictive annuloplasty.[108]

The finding of immediate residual MR in the early postoperative period after restrictive annuloplasty is likely related to a progressive leaflet tethering in symmetric and asymmetric patterns. However, recurrence of MR is likely to be caused by negative LV remodeling and worsening sphericity. In this scenario, MVR may provide a good alternative because prosthetic valve function is not affected by changes in severity of LV dysfunction, although there is an increased risk of complications (see Mitral Valve Replacement).[109] In the setting of ischemic MR, even mild MR after surgery must be taken into consideration because mild MR is associated with reduced postoperative survival. In contrast, for other causes such as degenerative mitral valve disease, postoperative MR can be obviated by valve replacement instead of repair.[110]

Evidence demonstrates that CABG surgery alone does not correct ischemic MR.[111] One of the initial publications on ischemic MR found that 40% of patients with moderate MR who underwent CABG surgery alone were left with moderate or severe (3+ to 4+) residual

ischemic MR.[112] The results of the Randomized Ischemic Mitral Evaluation (RIME) trial, published in 2012, demonstrated a significantly better outcome when annuloplasty was added to CABG in patients with moderate MR and an ejection fraction greater than 30%.[113] A ring-remodeling annuloplasty with complete, rigid, or semirigid rings should be strongly recommended for patients with ischemic MR because the use of flexible rings or annuloplasty bands has been associated with recurrent moderate or greater MR rates of 29% and 30%, respectively, as early as 18 months after surgery. These failure rates in mitral valve repair, potentially related to the asymmetric tethering of the mitral valve toward P2 and P3, have been improved with the use of restrictive asymmetric rings; the rate of freedom from recurrent MR of 2+ severity or greater was 95% at 15 months and 89% at 25 months.[114]

Later publications demonstrated better midterm (2.5 years) echocardiographic outcomes with MVR in terms of freedom from mild to moderate MR, and similar results were reported when the variable analyzed was freedom from moderate to severe MR in other studies, supporting the use of MVR as a viable option.[115] The unadjusted survival rate is typically lower for patients undergoing MVR.[115] Two-year outcomes reported by the Cardiothoracic Surgery Trials Network (CTSN) randomized trial of mitral valve repair versus MVR in patients with severe ischemic MR revealed no significant difference in LV reverse remodeling or survival.[116] Moreover, MR recurred more frequently in the repair group, resulting in more heart failure–related adverse events and cardiovascular admissions. It is important in this regard to highlight the lack of uniformity among the repair techniques selected and applied by the different participating centers (Fig. 19.14).

Rheumatic Valve Disease

Although MVR has traditionally been considered the predominant procedure for patients with rheumatic valve disease, increased sophistication in reconstructive techniques has contributed to the expansion of mitral valve repair,[77,117,118] which has affected outcomes regardless the cause of disease.[119] The most recent series on rheumatic mitral valve repair reported an increase in the repair rate (within the same surgical group) of 42% to 69% over the past decade.[120] Previous series had reported repair rates of only about 25% in experienced hands.[121]

Close analysis of the literature reveals that series with lower repair rates included a significantly larger percentage of patients with MS (i.e., more complex lesions of uncertain durability if repaired) and of older patients (i.e., more likely to have subvalvular fibrosis and calcified lesions).[117] The estimated failure rate of mitral valve repair in

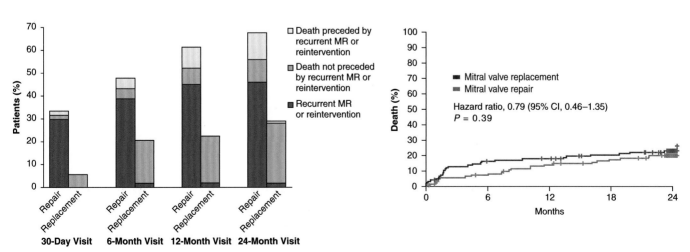

Fig. 19.14 Cumulative failure of mitral valve repair or replacement *(left)* and time-to-event curves for death. *MR,* Mitral regurgitation. (Modified from Goldstein D, Moskowitz AJ, Gelijns AC, et al. Two-year outcomes of surgical treatment of severe ischemic mitral regurgitation. N Engl J Med 2016;374:344-353.)

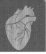

TABLE 19.1			Results of Mitral Valve Repair in Adult Patients With Rheumatic Mitral Valve Disease.									
			Age	TYPE OF DYSFUNCTION (%)						Mortality	Survival	Durability
Study	Year	N	(yr)	I	II	III	IIIa/IIIb	MS (%)	RR (%)	(%)[a]	(%)[b]	(%)[b]
Yau et al[121]	2000	573	54 ± 14	NA	NA	NA	NA	85	25	0.7	88 ± 1	72 ± 1 (R)
Choudhary et al[122]	2001	818	23 ± 11	6	5	88	1	None	NA[c]	4.0	93 ± 1	52 ± 3 (E)
Chauvaud et al[77]	2001	951	25 ± 18	7	33	36	24	None	NA	2.0	89 ± 2	82 ± 2 (R)
Kumar et al[118]	2006	898	22 ± 10	NA	NA	NA	NA	54	NA	3.6	92 ± 1	81 ± 5 (R)
Kim et al[117]	2010	540	49 ± 11	NA	NA	NA	NA	69	23	1.1	86 ± 5	97 ± 2 (R)
Yakub et al[120]	2013	627	32 ± 19	NA	NA	NA	NA	13	69	2.4	83 ± 4	72 ± 5 (E)

[a]Mortality rate for of mitral valve repair.
[b]Survival and durability are estimated up to 10 years.
[c]The absence of repair rate indicates a report on a selected patient population (i.e., mitral valve repairs were selected only).
E, Echocardiographic freedom from greater than moderate MR; *MR*, mitral regurgitation; *MS*, mitral stenosis (any degree of MS including combined MS and mitral regurgitation); *NA*, not applicable; *R*, freedom from reoperation; *RR*, repair rate;

patients with rheumatic mitral valve disease is 2% to 5% per year (compared with 1% to 2% per year for patients with degenerative mitral valve disease)[120,122] (Table 19.1).

OUTCOMES OF MITRAL VALVE REPLACEMENT

Disparities in reporting of morbidity and mortality rates after cardiac valve interventions led to the publication of consensus guidelines by the American Association for Thoracic Surgery and the STS to provide clear definitions of perioperative mortality, survival, structural and nonstructural valve dysfunction, valve thrombosis, embolism, hemorrhagic events, endocarditis, and freedom from reoperation.[123] The 2016 STS executive summary reported an unadjusted in-hospital mortality rate of 5% to 6% for patients undergoing isolated MVR. If concomitant CABG was performed, the in-hospital mortality rate increased up to 11%. Data from the National Inpatient Sample (*n* = 767,375) also showed an in-hospital mortality rate of 4.9% for patients undergoing isolated MVR.[124]

There are no data suggesting that the choice of a mechanical or bioprosthetic valve has a significant impact on operative mortality. However, there is a clear trend toward use of bioprostheses, particularly in high-volume centers.[125,126] For older patients and in patients with a life expectancy estimated to be less than 10 years, event-free survival is better with a bioprosthesis. These valves pose a very low lifetime risk of reoperation for structural degeneration, and they avoid most of the major thrombotic and hemorrhagic complications associated with mechanical prostheses and lifelong anticoagulation.[127]

Rates of mortality and long-term survival after valve replacement have been significantly linked to demographic variables such as age or to comorbidities such as coronary artery disease and LV dysfunction.[128] Randomized trials have failed to show any difference in long-term survival between bioprosthetic and mechanical valves.[129] The Edinburgh Heart Valve Trial reported 20-year survival rates of 28% and 31% (*P* = 0.57) for patients with mechanical and bioprosthetic valves, respectively[130] (Fig. 19.15).

Valve dysfunction is often divided into structural types (i.e., inevitable degeneration inherent to the valve, mostly seen in biologic prostheses) and nonstructural types (i.e., any abnormality not inherent to the valve, such as pannus formation, paravalvular leaks, or a technical error, but excluding endocarditis and thromboembolic complications).

Structural valve degeneration is considered the most common nonfatal complication in patients with bioprosthetic valves. Although there has been clear improvement in durability with each generation of valves, freedom from structural degeneration remains at 70% to 80% after 10 years and decreases rapidly thereafter, with ranges between 40% and 50% at 15 years.[128]

Even though renal failure may predispose to accelerated calcification of bioprosthetic valves, the lower life expectancy of patients in renal failure with either type of valve has probably biased observational studies, and no difference in outcome between mechanical and bioprosthetic valves in this subpopulation has been observed. Although structural degeneration is seldom seen in mechanical valves, nonstructural dysfunction is almost exclusively seen in mechanical valves. Rotating the valve (i.e., sewing the ring into a position in which the leaflet opening is not impinged) is thought to reduce the risk of this complication.

Valve thrombosis is thought to be more common with mechanical valves, especially in the mitral position (<0.2%/yr for mechanical valves versus < 0.1%/yr for biological valves). Large randomized trials have reported a probability of valve thrombosis of 1% to 2% up to 15 years after surgery, regardless of the type of valve.[129] Patients with mechanical valves are at a higher risk for embolic events. Major embolism occurs in approximately 9% of patients with prosthetic valves. If stratified by type of prosthesis, the incidence of systemic embolism at 15 years is 18% and 22% (*P* = 0.96) for mechanical valves and bioprostheses, respectively. Other long-term results have demonstrated the incidence of all embolism at 20 years to be 53% for mechanical valves versus and 32% for bioprostheses (*P* = 0.13).[130] It also seems reasonable that hemorrhagic events are more likely to occur in patients who receive mechanical valves and anticoagulation. However, as with thromboembolic complications, this likelihood strongly depends on adherence to anticoagulation and patient comorbidities.

Prosthetic valve endocarditis may occur years after surgery or early during the perioperative course (i.e., from field contamination, wound infection, or indwelling catheters and cannulas). In the latter case, the most frequent causative agents are *Staphylococcus aureus, Staphylococcus epidermidis*, and gram-negative bacteria. This complication is slightly more common in patients receiving mechanical valves, with an overall incidence of 1%.[130] Late endocarditis has an incidence of 0.2% to 0.4% per patient-year, and there is no difference in incidence between types of prostheses.

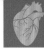

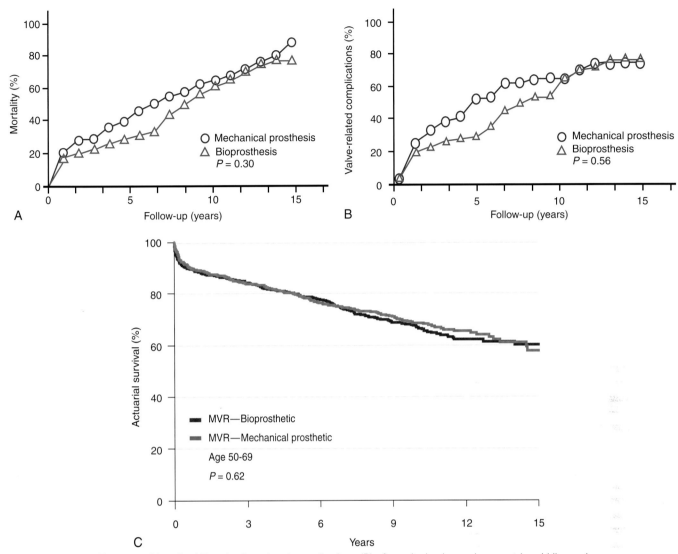

Fig. 19.15 Mortality (A) and valve-related complications (B) after mitral valve replacement in middle-aged patients. (C) Actuarial survival of patients undergoing mitral valve replacement *(MVR)*. (A, Modified from Hammermeister K, Sethi GK, Henderson WG, et al. Outcomes 15 years after valve replacement with a mechanical versus a bioprosthetic valve: final report of the Veterans Affairs randomized trial. J Am Coll Cardiol 2000;36:1152-1158. B, From Grunkemeier GL, Li HH, Naftel DC, et al. Long-term performance of heart valve prostheses. Curr Probl Cardiol 2000;25:73-154. C, Modified from Chikwe J, Chiang YP, Egorova NN, et al. Survival and outcomes following bioprosthetic vs mechanical mitral valve replacement in patients aged 50 to 69 years. JAMA 2015;313:1435-1442.)

REFERENCES

1. Quill JL, Hill AJ, Laske TG, et al. Mitral leaflet anatomy revisited. J Thorac Cardiovasc Surg 2009;137(5):1077-1081.
2. Pandis D, Sengupta PP, Castillo JG, et al. Assessment of longitudinal myocardial mechanics in patients with degenerative mitral valve regurgitation predicts postoperative worsening of left ventricular systolic function. J Am Soc Echocardiogr 2014;27(6):627-638.
3. Zoghbi WA, Adams D, Bonow RO, et al. Recommendations for noninvasive evaluation of native valvular regurgitation: a report from the American Society of Echocardiography developed in collaboration with the Society for Cardiovascular Magnetic Resonance. J Am Soc Echocardiogr 2017;30(4):303-371.
4. Basso C, Perazzolo Marra M, Rizzo S, et al. Arrhythmic mitral valve prolapse and sudden cardiac death. Circulation 2015;132(7):556-566.
5. O'Gara PT, Grayburn PA, Badhwar V, et al. 2017 ACC expert consensus decision pathway on the management of mitral regurgitation: a report of the American College of Cardiology Task Force on Expert Consensus Decision Pathways. J Am Coll Cardiol 2017;70(19):2421-2449.
6. Nishimura RA, Vahanian A, Eleid MF, Mack MJ. Mitral valve disease—current management and future challenges. Lancet 2016;387(10025):1324-1334.
7. Nkomo VT, Gardin JM, Skelton TN, et al. Burden of valvular heart diseases: a population-based study. Lancet 2006;368(9540):1005-1011.
8. Carpentier A. Cardiac valve surgery—the "French correction." J Thorac Cardiovasc Surg 1983;86(3):323-337.
9. Enriquez-Sarano M, Akins CW, Vahanian A. Mitral regurgitation. Lancet 2009;373(9672):1382-1394.
10. Enriquez-Sarano M, Suri RM, Clavel MA, et al. Is there an outcome penalty linked to guideline-based indications for valvular surgery? Early and

long-term analysis of patients with organic mitral regurgitation. J Thorac Cardiovasc Surg 2015;150(1):50-58.

11. Suri RM, Vanoverschelde JL, Grigioni F, et al. Association between early surgical intervention vs watchful waiting and outcomes for mitral regurgitation due to flail mitral valve leaflets. JAMA 2013;310(6):609-616.

12. Castillo JG, Anyanwu AC, Fuster V, Adams DH. A near 100% repair rate for mitral valve prolapse is achievable in a reference center: implications for future guidelines. J Thorac Cardiovasc Surg 2012;144(2):308-312.

13. David TE, Armstrong S, McCrindle BW, Manlhiot C. Late outcomes of mitral valve repair for mitral regurgitation due to degenerative disease. Circulation 2013;127(14):1485-1492.

14. Suri RM, Clavel MA, Schaff HV, et al. Effect of recurrent mitral regurgitation following degenerative mitral valve repair: long-term analysis of competing outcomes. J Am Coll Cardiol 2016;67(5):488-498.

15. Nishimura RA, Otto CM, Bonow RO, et al. 2014 AHA/ACC guideline for the management of patients with valvular heart disease: a report of the American College of Cardiology/American Heart Association Task Force on Practice Guidelines. J Am Coll Cardiol 2014;63(22):e57-e185.

16. Gammie JS, Sheng S, Griffith BP, et al. Trends in mitral valve surgery in the United States: results from the Society of Thoracic Surgeons Adult Cardiac Surgery Database. Ann Thorac Surg 2009;87(5):1431-1437; discussion 1437-1439.

17. Spoon JN, Nkomo VT, Suri RM, et al. Mechanisms of mitral valve dysfunction following mitral valve repair for degenerative disease. JACC Cardiovasc Imaging 2015;8(10):1223-1227.

18. Umakanthan R, Leacche M, Petracek MR, et al. Safety of minimally invasive mitral valve surgery without aortic cross-clamp. Ann Thorac Surg 2008;85(5):1544-1549; discussion 1549-1550.

19. De Bonis M, Lapenna E, Maisano F, et al. Long-term results (≤18 years) of the edge-to-edge mitral valve repair without annuloplasty in degenerative mitral regurgitation: implications for the percutaneous approach. Circulation 2014;130(11 suppl 1):S19-S24.

20. Abramowitz Y, Jilaihawi H, Chakravarty T, et al. Mitral annulus calcification. J Am Coll Cardiol 2015;66(17):1934-1941.

21. Levine RA. Dynamic mitral regurgitation—more than meets the eye. N Engl J Med 2004;351(16):1681-1684.

22. Levine RA, Handschumacher MD, Sanfilippo AJ, et al. Three-dimensional echocardiographic reconstruction of the mitral valve, with implications for the diagnosis of mitral valve prolapse. Circulation 1989;80(3):589-598.

23. Ranganathan N, Lam JH, Wigle ED, Silver MD. Morphology of the human mitral valve. II. The value leaflets. Circulation 1970;41(3):459-467.

24. Dent JM, Spotnitz WD, Nolan SP, et al. Mechanism of mitral leaflet excursion. Am J Physiol 1995;269(6 Pt 2):H2100-H2108.

25. Lam JH, Ranganathan N, Wigle ED, Silver MD. Morphology of the human mitral valve. I. Chordae tendineae: a new classification. Circulation 1970; 41(3):449-458.

26. Rodriguez F, Langer F, Harrington KB, et al. Importance of mitral valve second-order chordae for left ventricular geometry, wall thickening mechanics, and global systolic function. Circulation 2004;110 (11 suppl 1):II115-II122.

27. Kron IL, Green GR, Cope JT. Surgical relocation of the posterior papillary muscle in chronic ischemic mitral regurgitation. Ann Thorac Surg 2002; 74(2):600-601.

28. Kono T, Sabbah HN, Rosman H, et al. Left ventricular shape is the primary determinant of functional mitral regurgitation in heart failure. J Am Coll Cardiol 1992;20(7):1594-1598.

29. Carpentier A, Chauvaud S, Fabiani JN, et al. Reconstructive surgery of mitral valve incompetence: ten-year appraisal. J Thorac Cardiovasc Surg 1980;79(3):338-348.

30. Durst R, Sauls K, Peal DS, et al. Mutations in DCHS1 cause mitral valve prolapse. Nature 2015;525(7567):109-113.

31. Zuhlke L, Engel ME, Karthikeyan G, et al. Characteristics, complications, and gaps in evidence-based interventions in rheumatic heart disease: the Global Rheumatic Heart Disease Registry (the REMEDY study). Eur Heart J 2015;36(18):1115-1122a.

32. Essop MR, Nkomo VT. Rheumatic and nonrheumatic valvular heart disease: epidemiology, management, and prevention in Africa. Circulation 2005;112(23):3584-3591.

33. Iung B, Baron G, Butchart EG, et al. A prospective survey of patients with valvular heart disease in Europe: the Euro Heart Survey on Valvular Heart Disease. Eur Heart J 2003;24(13):1231-1243.

34. Fornes P, Heudes D, Fuzellier JF, et al. Correlation between clinical and histologic patterns of degenerative mitral valve insufficiency: a histomorphometric study of 130 excised segments. Cardiovasc Pathol 1999;8(2): 81-92.

35. Adams DH, Anyanwu AC. Seeking a higher standard for degenerative mitral valve repair: begin with etiology. J Thorac Cardiovasc Surg 2008;136(3): 551-556.

36. Anyanwu AC, Adams DH. Etiologic classification of degenerative mitral valve disease: Barlow's disease and fibroelastic deficiency. Semin Thorac Cardiovasc Surg 2007;19(2):90-96.

37. Carpentier A, Lacour-Gayet F, Camilleri J. Fibroelastic dysplasia of the mitral valve: an anatomical and clinical entity. Circulation 1982;3:307.

38. Barlow JB, Bosman CK. Aneurysmal protrusion of the posterior leaflet of the mitral valve. An auscultatory-electrocardiographic syndrome. Am Heart J 1966;71(2):166-178.

39. Barletta GA, Gagliardi R, Benvenuti L, Fantini F. Cerebral ischemic attacks as a complication of aortic and mitral valve prolapse. Stroke 1985;16(2): 219-223.

40. Adams DH, Anyanwu AC, Rahmanian PB, et al. Large annuloplasty rings facilitate mitral valve repair in Barlow's disease. Ann Thorac Surg 2006;82(6):2096-2100; discussion 2101.

41. Lee R, Li S, Rankin JS, et al. Fifteen-year outcome trends for valve surgery in North America. Ann Thorac Surg 2011;91(3):677-684; discussion 684.

42. Agricola E, Oppizzi M, Pisani M, et al. Ischemic mitral regurgitation: mechanisms and echocardiographic classification. Eur J Echocardiogr 2008;9(2):207-221.

43. Bax JJ, Braun J, Somer ST, et al. Restrictive annuloplasty and coronary revascularization in ischemic mitral regurgitation results in reverse left ventricular remodeling. Circulation 2004;110(11 suppl 1):II103-II108.

44. Levine RA, Hung J. Ischemic mitral regurgitation, the dynamic lesion: clues to the cure. J Am Coll Cardiol 2003;42(11):1929-1932.

45. Unger P, Magne J, Dedobbeleer C, Lancellotti P. Ischemic mitral regurgitation: not only a bystander. Curr Cardiol Rep 2012;14(2):180-189.

46. Mesana T. Ischemic mitral regurgitation: the challenge goes on. Curr Opin Cardiol 2012;27(2):108-110.

47. Lancellotti P, Tribouilloy C, Hagendorff A, et al. Recommendations for the echocardiographic assessment of native valvular regurgitation: an executive summary from the European Association of Cardiovascular Imaging. Eur Heart J Cardiovasc Imaging 2013;14(7):611-644.

48. Maslow A. Mitral valve repair: an echocardiographic review: part 2. J Cardiothorac Vasc Anesth 2015;29(2):439-471.

49. Coutinho GF, Garcia AL, Correia PM, et al. Negative impact of atrial fibrillation and pulmonary hypertension after mitral valve surgery in asymptomatic patients with severe mitral regurgitation: a 20-year follow-up. Eur J Cardiothorac Surg 2015;48(4):548-555; discussion 555-546.

50. Calleja A, Poulin F, Woo A, et al. Quantitative modeling of the mitral valve by three-dimensional transesophageal echocardiography in patients undergoing mitral valve repair: correlation with intraoperative surgical technique. J Am Soc Echocardiogr 2015;28(9):1083-1092.

51. Crestanello JA. Surgical approach to mitral regurgitation in chronic heart failure: when is it an option? Curr Heart Fail Rep 2012;9(1):40-50.

52. Suri RM, Schaff HV, Dearani JA, et al. Survival advantage and improved durability of mitral repair for leaflet prolapse subsets in the current era. Ann Thorac Surg 2006;82(3):819-826.

53. Lazam S, Vanoverschelde JL, Tribouilloy C, et al. Twenty-year outcome after mitral repair versus replacement for severe degenerative mitral regurgitation: analysis of a large, prospective, multicenter international registry. Circulation 2017;135(5):410-422.

54. Goldstone AB, Atluri P, Szeto WY, et al. Minimally invasive approach provides at least equivalent results for surgical correction of mitral regurgitation: a propensity-matched comparison. J Thorac Cardiovasc Surg 2013;145(3): 748-756.

55. Glauber M, Miceli A. State of the art for approaching the mitral valve: sternotomy, minimally invasive or total endoscopic robotic? Eur J Cardiothorac Surg 2015;48(5):639-641.

56. Gammie JS, Zhao Y, Peterson ED, et al. J. Maxwell Chamberlain Memorial Paper for adult cardiac surgery. Less-invasive mitral valve operations: trends and outcomes from the Society of Thoracic Surgeons Adult Cardiac Surgery Database. Ann Thorac Surg 2010;90(5):1401-1408.

57. Seder CW, Raymond DP, Wright CD, et al. The Society of Thoracic Surgeons General Thoracic Surgery Database 2017 update on outcomes and quality. Ann Thorac Surg 2017;103(5):1378-1383.

58. Casselman FP, Van Slycke S, Dom H, et al. Endoscopic mitral valve repair: feasible, reproducible, and durable. J Thorac Cardiovasc Surg 2003;125(2): 273-282.

59. Chitwood Jr WR, Rodriguez E, Chu MW, et al. Robotic mitral valve repairs in 300 patients: a single-center experience. J Thorac Cardiovasc Surg 2008;136(2):436-441.

60. Seeburger J, Borger MA, Falk V, et al. Minimal invasive mitral valve repair for mitral regurgitation: results of 1339 consecutive patients. Eur J Cardiothorac Surg 2008;34(4):760-765.

61. Holzhey DM, Seeburger J, Misfeld M, et al. Learning minimally invasive mitral valve surgery: a cumulative sum sequential probability analysis of 3895 operations from a single high-volume center. Circulation 2013;128(5):483-491.

62. Casselman FP, Van Slycke S, Wellens F, et al. Mitral valve surgery can now routinely be performed endoscopically. Circulation 2003;108(suppl 1): II48-II54.

63. Lazar HL. Robotic mitral valve repair for degenerative mitral valve regurgitation: is it for everyone? Circulation 2015;132(21):1941-1942.

64. Murphy DA, Moss E, Binongo J, et al. The expanding role of endoscopic robotics in mitral valve surgery: 1,257 consecutive procedures. Ann Thorac Surg 2015;100(5):1675-1682.

65. Castillo JG, Anyanwu AC, El-Eshmawi A, Adams DH. All anterior and bileaflet mitral valve prolapses are repairable in the modern era of reconstructive surgery. Eur J Cardiothorac Surg 2014;45(1):139-145; discussion 145.

66. Baumgartner H, Falk V, Bax JJ, et al. 2017 ESC/EACTS guidelines for the management of valvular heart disease. The Task Force for the Management of Valvular Heart Disease of the European Society of Cardiology (ESC) and the European Association for Cardio-Thoracic Surgery (EACTS). Eur Heart J 2017;38:2739-2791.

67. Castillo JG, Anyanwu AC, El-Eshmawi A, et al. Early rupture of an expanded polytetrafluoroethylene neochord after complex mitral valve repair: an electron microscopic analysis. J Thorac Cardiovasc Surg 2013;145(3):e29-e31.

68. Adams DH, Anyanwu AC, Rahmanian PB, Filsoufi F. Current concepts in mitral valve repair for degenerative disease. Heart Fail Rev 2006;11(3): 241-257.

69. Anyanwu AC, Adams DH. The intraoperative "ink test": a novel assessment tool in mitral valve repair. J Thorac Cardiovasc Surg 2007;133(6):1635-1636.

70. Bonow RO. Chronic mitral regurgitation and aortic regurgitation: have indications for surgery changed? J Am Coll Cardiol 2013;61(7):693-701.

71. Chan V, Ruel M, Elmistekawy E, Mesana TG. Determinants of left ventricular dysfunction after repair of chronic asymptomatic mitral regurgitation. Ann Thorac Surg 2015;99(1):38-42.

72. Uretsky S, Gillam L, Lang R, et al. Discordance between echocardiography and MRI in the assessment of mitral regurgitation severity: a prospective multicenter trial. J Am Coll Cardiol 2015;65(11):1078-1088.

73. Braun J, van de Veire NR, Klautz RJ, et al. Restrictive mitral annuloplasty cures ischemic mitral regurgitation and heart failure. Ann Thorac Surg 2008;85(2):430-436; discussion 436-437.

74. Filsoufi F, Castillo JG, Rahmanian PB, et al. [Remodeling annuloplasty using a prosthetic ring designed for correcting type-IIIb ischemic mitral regurgitation]. Rev Esp Cardiol 2007;60(11):1151-1158.

75. Daimon M, Fukuda S, Adams DH, et al. Mitral valve repair with Carpentier-McCarthy-Adams IMR ETlogix annuloplasty ring for ischemic mitral regurgitation: early echocardiographic results from a multi-center study. Circulation 2006;114(suppl 1):I588-I593.

76. Borger MA. Chronic ischemic mitral regurgitation: insights into Pandora's box. Circulation 2012;126(23):2674-2676.

77. Chauvaud S, Fuzellier JF, Berrebi A, et al. Long-term (29 years) results of reconstructive surgery in rheumatic mitral valve insufficiency. Circulation 2001;104(12 suppl 1):I12-I15.

78. Magne J, Mahjoub H, Dulgheru R, et al. Left ventricular contractile reserve in asymptomatic primary mitral regurgitation. Eur Heart J 2014; 35(24):1608-1616.

79. Chan V, Ruel M, Mesana TG. Mitral valve replacement is a viable alternative to mitral valve repair for ischemic mitral regurgitation: a case-matched study. Ann Thorac Surg 2011;92(4):1358-1365; discussion 1365-1356.

80. Dodson JA, Wang Y, Desai MM, et al. Outcomes for mitral valve surgery among Medicare fee-for-service beneficiaries, 1999 to 2008. Circ Cardiovasc Qual Outcomes 2012;5(3):298-307.

81. Rahimtoola SH. Choice of prosthetic heart valve in adults an update. J Am Coll Cardiol 2010;55(22):2413-2426.

82. Seeburger J, Borger MA, Doll N, et al. Comparison of outcomes of minimally invasive mitral valve surgery for posterior, anterior and bileaflet prolapse. Eur J Cardiothorac Surg 2009;36(3):532-538.

83. David TE. Outcomes of mitral valve repair for mitral regurgitation due to degenerative disease. Semin Thorac Cardiovasc Surg 2007;19(2):116-120.

84. Flameng W, Herijgers P, Bogaerts K. Recurrence of mitral valve regurgitation after mitral valve repair in degenerative valve disease. Circulation 2003;107(12):1609-1613.

85. Gillinov AM, Mihaljevic T, Blackstone EH, et al. Should patients with severe degenerative mitral regurgitation delay surgery until symptoms develop? Ann Thorac Surg 2010;90(2):481-488.

86. Javadikasgari H, Mihaljevic T, Suri RM, et al. Simple versus complex degenerative mitral valve disease. J Thorac Cardiovasc Surg 2018; 156(1):122-129.e16.

87. Ma W, Shi W, Zhang W, et al. Management of incomplete initial repair in the treatment of degenerative mitral insufficiency. Int Heart J 2018;59(3):510-517.

88. Badhwar V, Peterson ED, Jacobs JP, et al. Longitudinal outcome of isolated mitral repair in older patients: results from 14,604 procedures performed from 1991 to 2007. Ann Thorac Surg 2012;94(6):1870-1877; discussion 1877-1879.

89. Pfannmuller B, Seeburger J, Misfeld M, et al. Minimally invasive mitral valve repair for anterior leaflet prolapse. J Thorac Cardiovasc Surg 2013;146(1):109-113.

90. Tietge WJ, de Heer LM, van Hessen MW, et al. Early mitral valve repair versus watchful waiting in patients with severe asymptomatic organic mitral regurgitation; rationale and design of the Dutch AMR trial, a multicenter, randomised trial. Neth Heart J 2012;20(3):94-101.

91. El-Eshmawi A, Castillo JG, Tang GHL, Adams DH. Developing a mitral valve center of excellence. Curr Opin Cardiol 2018;33(2):155-161.

92. Lawrie GM, Earle EA, Earle NR. Nonresectional repair of the Barlow mitral valve: importance of dynamic annular evaluation. Ann Thorac Surg 2009;88(4):1191-1196.

93. Perier P, Hohenberger W, Lakew F, et al. Toward a new paradigm for the reconstruction of posterior leaflet prolapse: midterm results of the "respect rather than resect" approach. Ann Thorac Surg 2008;86(3): 718-725; discussion 718-725.

94. Chikwe J, Toyoda N, Anyanwu AC, et al. Relation of mitral valve surgery volume to repair rate, durability, and survival. J Am Coll Cardiol 2017; 69(19):2397-2406.

95. Bolling SF, Li S, O'Brien SM, et al. Predictors of mitral valve repair: clinical and surgeon factors. Ann Thorac Surg 2010;90(6):1904-1911; discussion 1912.

96. Kilic A, Shah AS, Conte JV, et al. Operative outcomes in mitral valve surgery: combined effect of surgeon and hospital volume in a population-based analysis. J Thorac Cardiovasc Surg 2013;146(3):638-646.

97. LaPar DJ, Speir AM, Crosby IK, et al. Postoperative atrial fibrillation significantly increases mortality, hospital readmission, and hospital costs. Ann Thorac Surg 2014;98(2):527-533; discussion 533.

98. Murashita T, Okada Y, Kanemitsu H, et al. Long-term outcomes after mitral valve repair for degenerative mitral regurgitation with persistent atrial fibrillation. Thorac Cardiovasc Surg 2015;63(3):243-249.

99. Enriquez-Sarano M, Avierinos JF, Messika-Zeitoun D, et al. Quantitative determinants of the outcome of asymptomatic mitral regurgitation. N Engl J Med 2005;352(9):875-883.

100. Enriquez-Sarano M, Nkomo V, Mohty D, et al. Mitral regurgitation: predictors of outcome and natural history. Adv Cardiol 2002;39:133-143.

101. David TE, Ivanov J, Armstrong S, et al. A comparison of outcomes of mitral valve repair for degenerative disease with posterior, anterior, and bileaflet prolapse. J Thorac Cardiovasc Surg 2005;130(5):1242-1249.

102. Reece TB, Tribble CG, Ellman PI, et al. Mitral repair is superior to replacement when associated with coronary artery disease. Ann Surg 2004;239(5):671-675; discussion 675-677.

103. Gillinov AM, Wierup PN, Blackstone EH, et al. Is repair preferable to replacement for ischemic mitral regurgitation? J Thorac Cardiovasc Surg 2001;122(6):1125-1141.

104. Kron IL, Hung J, Overbey JR, et al. Predicting recurrent mitral regurgitation after mitral valve repair for severe ischemic mitral regurgitation. J Thorac Cardiovasc Surg 2015;149(3):752-761.e1.

105. Deja MA, Grayburn PA, Sun B, et al. Influence of mitral regurgitation repair on survival in the surgical treatment for ischemic heart failure trial. Circulation 2012;125(21):2639-2648.

106. Vassileva CM, Boley T, Markwell S, Hazelrigg S. Meta-analysis of short-term and long-term survival following repair versus replacement for ischemic mitral regurgitation. Eur J Cardiothorac Surg 2011;39(3):295-303.

107. Penicka M, Linkova H, Lang O, et al. Predictors of improvement of unrepaired moderate ischemic mitral regurgitation in patients undergoing elective isolated coronary artery bypass graft surgery. Circulation 2009;120(15):1474-1481.

108. Magne J, Senechal M, Mathieu P, et al. Restrictive annuloplasty for ischemic mitral regurgitation may induce functional mitral stenosis. J Am Coll Cardiol 2008;51(17):1692-1701.

109. Glower DD. Surgical approaches to mitral regurgitation. J Am Coll Cardiol 2012;60(15):1315-1322.

110. Sandoval Y, Sorajja P, Harris KM. Contemporary management of ischemic mitral regurgitation: a review. Am J Med 2018.

111. Mihaljevic T, Lam BK, Rajeswaran J, et al. Impact of mitral valve annuloplasty combined with revascularization in patients with functional ischemic mitral regurgitation. J Am Coll Cardiol 2007;49(22):2191-2201.

112. Aklog L, Filsoufi F, Flores KQ, et al. Does coronary artery bypass grafting alone correct moderate ischemic mitral regurgitation? Circulation 2001;104(12 suppl 1):I68-I75.

113. Chan KM, Punjabi PP, Flather M, et al. Coronary artery bypass surgery with or without mitral valve annuloplasty in moderate functional ischemic mitral regurgitation: final results of the Randomized Ischemic Mitral Evaluation (RIME) trial. Circulation 2012;126(21):2502-2510.

114. de Varennes B, Chaturvedi R, Sidhu S, et al. Initial results of posterior leaflet extension for severe type IIIb ischemic mitral regurgitation. Circulation 2009;119(21):2837-2843.

115. Lorusso R, Gelsomino S, Vizzardi E, et al. Mitral valve repair or replacement for ischemic mitral regurgitation? The Italian Study on the Treatment of Ischemic Mitral Regurgitation (ISTIMIR). J Thorac Cardiovasc Surg 2013;145(1):128-139; discussion 137-138.

116. Goldstein D, Moskowitz AJ, Gelijns AC, et al. Two-year outcomes of surgical treatment of severe ischemic mitral regurgitation. N Engl J Med 2016;374(4):344-353.

117. Kim JB, Kim HJ, Moon DH, et al. Long-term outcomes after surgery for rheumatic mitral valve disease: valve repair versus mechanical valve replacement. Eur J Cardiothorac Surg 2010;37(5):1039-1046.

118. Kumar AS, Talwar S, Saxena A, et al. Results of mitral valve repair in rheumatic mitral regurgitation. Interact Cardiovasc Thorac Surg 2006;5(4):356-361.

119. Dillon J, Yakub MA, Kong PK, et al. Comparative long-term results of mitral valve repair in adults with chronic rheumatic disease and degenerative disease: is repair for "burnt-out" rheumatic disease still inferior to repair for degenerative disease in the current era? J Thorac Cardiovasc Surg 2015;149(3):771-777.

120. Yakub MA, Dillon J, Krishna Moorthy PS, et al. Is rheumatic aetiology a predictor of poor outcome in the current era of mitral valve repair? Contemporary long-term results of mitral valve repair in rheumatic heart disease. Eur J Cardiothorac Surg 2013;44(4):673-681.

121. Yau TM, El-Ghoneimi YA, Armstrong S, et al. Mitral valve repair and replacement for rheumatic disease. J Thorac Cardiovasc Surg 2000;119(1):53-60.

122. Choudhary SK, Talwar S, Dubey B, et al. Mitral valve repair in a predominantly rheumatic population. Long-term results. Tex Heart Inst J 2001;28(1):8-15.

123. Edmunds Jr LH, Clark RE, Cohn LH, et al. Guidelines for reporting morbidity and mortality after cardiac valvular operations. The American Association for Thoracic Surgery, Ad Hoc Liaison Committee for Standardizing Definitions of Prosthetic Heart Valve Morbidity. Ann Thorac Surg 1996;62(3):932-935.

124. Isaacs AJ, Shuhaiber J, Salemi A, et al. National trends in utilization and in-hospital outcomes of mechanical versus bioprosthetic aortic valve replacements. J Thorac Cardiovasc Surg 2015;149(5):1262-1269.e3.

125. Brown JM, O'Brien SM, Wu C, et al. Isolated aortic valve replacement in North America comprising 108,687 patients in 10 years: changes in risks, valve types, and outcomes in the Society of Thoracic Surgeons National Database. J Thorac Cardiovasc Surg 2009;137(1):82-90.

126. Dunning J, Gao H, Chambers J, et al. Aortic valve surgery: marked increases in volume and significant decreases in mechanical valve use—an analysis of 41,227 patients over 5 years from the Society for Cardiothoracic Surgery in Great Britain and Ireland National database. J Thorac Cardiovasc Surg 2011;142(4):776-782.e3.

127. van Geldorp MW, Eric Jamieson WR, Kappetein AP, et al. Patient outcome after aortic valve replacement with a mechanical or biological prosthesis: weighing lifetime anticoagulant-related event risk against reoperation risk. J Thorac Cardiovasc Surg 2009;137(4):881-886, 886e1-5.

128. Grunkemeier GL, Li HH, Naftel DC, et al. Long-term performance of heart valve prostheses. Curr Probl Cardiol 2000;25(2):73-154.

129. Hammermeister K, Sethi GK, Henderson WG, et al. Outcomes 15 years after valve replacement with a mechanical versus a bioprosthetic valve: final report of the Veterans Affairs randomized trial. J Am Coll Cardiol 2000;36(4):1152-1158.

130. Oxenham H, Bloomfield P, Wheatley DJ, et al. Twenty year comparison of a Bjork-Shiley mechanical heart valve with porcine bioprostheses. Heart 2003;89(7):715-721.

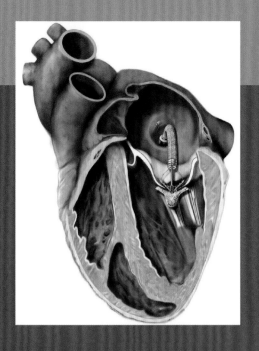

中文导读

第20章
经导管二尖瓣修复和置换

　　二尖瓣反流是一种异质性较强的疾病，其可由二尖瓣复合体任何部分结构或功能异常导致。二尖瓣复合体主要包括瓣叶、瓣环、腱索、乳头肌、左心房和左心室，其功能的复杂使得二尖瓣反流呈现不同的病理生理机制，导致经导管二尖瓣介入治疗器械种类繁多且发展相比于经导管主动脉置换较慢。然而，随着全球人口老龄化进程加速，心力衰竭的发病率越来越高，这些患者多数具有明显的二尖瓣反流，迫切的临床需求推动了更安全有效的经导管介入诊疗方案的持续创新。与外科医师拥有大量不同的手术器械不同，目前经导管介入治疗器械通常只重点解决二尖瓣复合体中的一种解剖结构异常，如瓣叶修复、瓣环成形或瓣膜置换等。本章将逐一介绍这些不同类型经导管二尖瓣介入治疗器械最新的研究进展，重点描述在美国和欧洲已经获批的器械，或已经进入临床试验阶段且发布的研究数据提示颇有应用前景的器械。在真实世界的临床实践中，构建多学科心脏团队是应用这些新技术处理复杂瓣膜病变的核心需求。随着医学科学家和工程专家共同协作创新，并在医学影像精准导航的助力下，经导管二尖瓣介入诊疗必然会成为二尖瓣反流患者的一个重要且安全可靠的选择。

卢志南

Transcatheter Mitral Valve Repair and Replacement

Howard C. Herrmann

CHAPTER OUTLINE

KEY POINTS

- The risks of surgery for severe mitral regurgitation (MR) in elderly patients and those with medical comorbidities, particularly with consideration of patient preference for quick recovery, have stimulated attempts to develop less invasive solutions.
- Unlike the extensive toolbox available to the mitral surgeon, transcatheter approaches are much more limited and often are able to address only a single major element of the dysfunctional valve that contributes to MR.
- Leaflet edge-to-edge repair is safe and effective treatment for primary MR; it has been approved for that purpose in patients

with high or prohibitive surgical risk, as well as for treatment of secondary MR and for guideline-directed medical therapy in patients not suitable for surgery.
- Investigations are underway to test the safety and efficacy of other nonsurgical devices, including mitral annuloplasty devices, left ventricular remodeling devices (to reduce severity of MR in patients with dilated left ventricles), and transcatheter mitral valve replacement.

Mitral regurgitation (MR) is a diverse disease that results from dysfunction of any of the portions of the complex mitral valve (MV) apparatus, including the leaflets, chordae, annulus, and left ventricle (LV). It is convenient to classify MR on the basis of two broad categories of dysfunction: primary diseases (i.e., organic or degenerative), which affect mainly the leaflets (e.g., fibromuscular dysplasia, MV prolapse, rheumatic disease), and secondary diseases (i.e., ischemic or functional), which spare the leaflets (e.g., diseases of the atrium and ventricle, including ischemic dysfunction and dilated cardiomyopathy) (see Chapters 17 and 18). Even in secondary functional or ischemic MR, there may be changes that affect the leaflets.[1] Some diseases such as ischemic MR may affect more than one portion of the valve apparatus. For example, leaflet tethering and annular dilation may coexist and contribute to MR.[2]

Whether symptomatic[3] or not,[4] patients with severe MR have decreased survival,[5] and surgery is often recommended. However, some studies have demonstrated that asymptomatic patients with severe MR and preserved LV function can be safely monitored with a watchful waiting approach until the development of symptoms, LV dysfunction, pulmonary hypertension, or atrial fibrillation, without a morbidity penalty at the time of surgery.[6] Current guidelines recommend surgery for symptomatic patients and for asymptomatic patients with abnormal LV function.[7] Surgery may also be considered for asymptomatic patients with normal LV function when there is a high likelihood of successful repair.

RATIONALE FOR TRANSCATHETER THERAPY

Surgery to repair or replace the MV in patients with severe MR appears to improve survival in observational studies.[8] The impetus for the development of transcatheter therapies for valvular heart disease arises from two major factors. First is the expectation that a transcatheter therapy can avoid the risks and discomfort associated with surgery, particularly the use of cardiopulmonary bypass and sternotomy or thoracotomy.[9] Second is the patient's desire to avoid the slower recovery associated with major surgery. However, these factors must be balanced with the efficacy of the transcatheter approach. A transcatheter approach that is less invasive, provides faster patient recovery, and has similar efficacy is always preferred to a surgical approach. However, a less efficacious approach, even if safer and associated with faster recovery, requires more complex shared decision making that takes into account the patient's age, frailty, comorbidities, and goals of care.

Surgery is associated with mortality rates of 1% to 5% and additional morbidity rates of 10% to 20%, with morbidity including stroke, reoperation, renal failure, and prolonged ventilation.[10] In one study of Medicare-age patients, more than 20% required rehospitalization during the first 30 days after surgery.[11] The risks of surgery are particularly high in patients who are elderly or have LV dysfunction.[10,12] In a study of more than 30,000 patients undergoing MV replacement, the mortality rate increased from 4.1% for those younger than 50 years of age to 17.0% for octogenarians (Fig. 20.1).

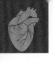

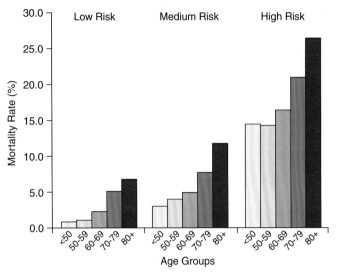

Fig. 20.1 Mortality Rate by Age for Low-, Medium-, and High-Risk Categories of Patients Undergoing Mitral Valve Replacement. (From Mehta RH, Eagle KA, Coombs LP, et al. Influence of age on outcomes in patients undergoing mitral valve replacement. Ann Thorac Surg 2002;74:1459-1467.)

Significant morbidity (i.e., stroke, prolonged ventilation, renal failure, reoperation, sternal infection) affected more than one third of the octogenarians. Predictors of risk in addition to age in this study included hemodynamic instability, severe symptoms, renal failure, and prior coronary artery bypass grafting surgery (CABG).[12]

For patients with LV dysfunction and secondary MR, whether ischemic or functional, survival with or without surgery is not as good as for patients with preserved LV function and a diagnosis of primary MR.[4] Whether the increased mortality rate is a consequence of the preexisting LV dysfunction or the MR contributes to the reduced

survival remains a controversial issue. In vitro studies have demonstrated progressive adverse LV remodeling in sheep even after successful MR repair.[13] Other studies have not shown benefit with annuloplasty repair of MR in dilated cardiomyopathy[14] or at the time of revascularization with CABG.[15] One study of MV repair during CABG reported a rate of recurrence for moderate or severe MR of close to 60% at 2 years.[16] In cases of ischemic and nonischemic functional MR, age and comorbidities are the most important predictors of survival.[17]

The major reason for surgery in most patients with ischemic MR is to provide symptomatic improvement, and in those with primary MR, the goal is to forestall the development of LV dysfunction. It also is essential to discuss the efficacy of surgery in terms of MR reduction. In relatively young patients (range, 55–60 years) with primary MR, long-term freedom from repeat surgery is well documented.[18,19] However, recurrent 3+ and 4+ MR may be observed in up to 30% of patients within 15 years.[18,19] Recurrent MR is even more common in patients with ischemic MR, providing a potential target for the development of transcatheter therapies.[20]

CLASSIFICATION OF PERCUTANEOUS REPAIR TECHNIQUES

In keeping with the complexity of the MV apparatus, it is useful to consider the percutaneous approaches according to the major structural abnormalities that they address.[21] Unlike the extensive toolbox available to the MV surgeon, transcatheter approaches are much more limited and often able to address only a single major element of the dysfunctional valve that contributes to MR.

The remainder of this chapter addresses these transcatheter approaches, with an emphasis on devices that have been approved in some part of the world, those that have entered first-in-human or phase 1 clinical investigation, and those with published data (i.e., clinical or preclinical). Some devices that have been evaluated in vivo without success or are no longer under development are discussed only as they relate to other current approaches. Table 20.1 lists the devices

TABLE 20.1 Devices for Transcatheter Mitral Valve Therapy.

Device	Manufacturer	Development Status	References
Leaflet or Chordal Procedure			
MitraClip	Abbott Vascular, Abbott Park, IL	CE Mark FDA approved	25–35
NeoChord DS1000 system	NeoChord, Inc., Eden Prairie, MN	CE Mark FDA pivotal trial underway	36
Harpoon TSD-5	Harpoon Medical Inc., Baltimore, MD	Phase 1 trial (outside U.S.)	37
Mitra-Spacer	Cardiosolutions, Inc., West Bridgewater, MA	Phase 1 trial (outside U.S.)	38
MitraFlex	TransCardiac Therapeutics, LLC, Atlanta, GA	Preclinical study	—
Indirect Annuloplasty			
Carillon XE2 mitral contour system	Cardiac Dimensions, Inc., Kirkland, WI	CE Mark FDA pivotal trial underway	41, 42
Cerclage annuloplasty	National Heart, Lung, and Blood Institute, Bethesda, MD	U.S. early feasibility trial	47
Direct or Left Ventricular Annuloplasty			
Mitralign percutaneous annuloplasty system	Mitralign, Inc., Tewksbury, MA	CE Mark	48, 49
AccuCinch system	Ancora Heart, Santa Clara, CA	Phase 1 trial (U.S.)	—
Cardioband	Edwards Lifesciences, Inc., Irvine, CA	CE Mark FDA pivotal trial underway	50
Millipede system	Boston Scientific Inc., Marlborough, MA	Phase 1 trial (outside U.S.)	—

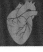

TABLE 20.1 Devices for Transcatheter Mitral Valve Therapy.—cont'd

Device	Manufacturer	Development Status	References
Hybrid Surgical Procedure			
Adjustable Annuloplasty Ring	Mitral Solutions, Fort Lauderdale, FL	Phase 1 trial	—
Dynaplasty ring	MiCardia Corporation, Irvine, CA	Phase 1 trial	—
Left Ventricular Remodeling			
Phoenix cardiac device (basal annuloplasty of the cardia externally [BACE])	Mardil Medical, Minneapolis, MN	Phase 1 trial	—
Tendyne repair	Abbott Vascular, Abbott Park, IL	Preclinical study	—
Transcatheter Mitral Valve Replacement			
Evoque	Edwards LifeSciences, Inc., Irvine, CA	Phase 1 trial	—
Tendyne	Abbott Vascular, Inc., Abbott Park, IL	FDA pivotal trial underway	74
Tiara	Neovasc, Inc., Richmond, British Columbia, Canada	Phase 1 trial	—
Intrepid	Medtronic, Inc., Minneapolis, MN	FDA pivotal trial underway	—
Caisson	Caisson Interventional, Inc., Maple Grove, MN	Phase 1 trial	—
Highlife	Highlife Medical, Inc., Irvine, CA	Phase 1 trial (outside U.S.)	

along with their manufacturers, state of development, and available published reports.

Leaflet and Chordal Technology

MitraClip

The major technology in this category, MitraClip (Abbott Vascular), was also the first transcatheter MV repair technology to receive CE Mark approval (Fig. 20.2). This system has its roots in the Alfieri stitch operation, in which the middle scallops of the posterior and anterior leaflets (P2 and A2, respectively) are sutured together to create a double-orifice MV. Although this operation is usually performed with adjunctive ring annuloplasty, it has proved effective and durable in a wide variety of pathologies and even in selected patients without annuloplasty.[22,23]

The concept of a percutaneous replicate of the Alfieri stitch was initially conceived by St. Goar and subsequently developed as Mitra-Clip by Evalve, Inc. (which was later acquired by Abbott Vascular).[24] A series of trials with this device confirmed its feasibility (Endovascular Valve Edge-to-Edge Repair Study [EVEREST] I), and its safety and efficacy were compared with those of surgical repair in a randomized trial (EVEREST II), providing a wealth of data on this technology (described later).[25,26]

The procedure is performed with standard catheterization techniques using a transseptal approach from the right femoral vein.[27] The clip delivery system is introduced through a 24-Fr sheath into the left atrium, where it can be guided using a series of turning knobs under transesophageal (two- and three-dimensional) echocardiographic guidance through the MV and into the LV. A properly aligned and oriented clip can be placed on the P2 and A2 segments of leaflets, grasping them from the ventricular side to create leaflet apposition. After leaflet insertion is confirmed by echocardiography, the clip can be released. If a suboptimal grasp occurs, the leaflet can be released, allowing repositioning before a second grasp attempt. Two or more clips can be placed as needed for optimal MR reduction (Fig. 20.3).[27]

In the 2:1 randomized EVEREST II trial, 184 patients were designated to receive MitraClip therapy and 95 to undergo surgical repair

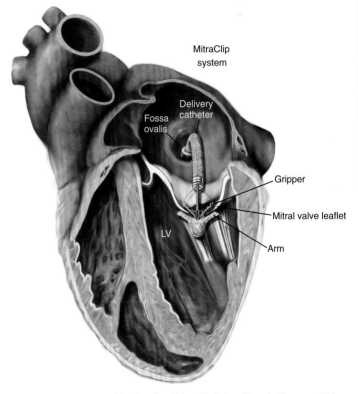

Fig. 20.2 The MitraClip Leaflet Edge-To-Edge Repair System. This device (Abbott Vascular) creates a bridge between the P2 and A2 segments of the mitral valve similar to that created in the Alfieri stitch operation. The clip delivery system is advanced across the atrial septum and through the mitral valve in the open position before the leaflets are grasped. (From Salcedo EE, et al. Transcatheter mitral valve repair. In: Otto CM, editor. The practice of clinical echocardiography. 5th ed. St Louis: Elsevier; 2016. p. 376.)

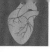

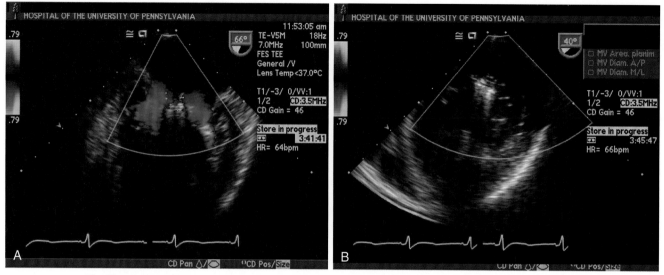

Fig. 20.3 Echocardiograms After Deployment of Two MitraClip Devices. (A) Mitral inflow view demonstrates flow around the MitraClips (Abbott Vascular) into the ventricle through both orifices. (B) Dual orifices in the transgastric view.

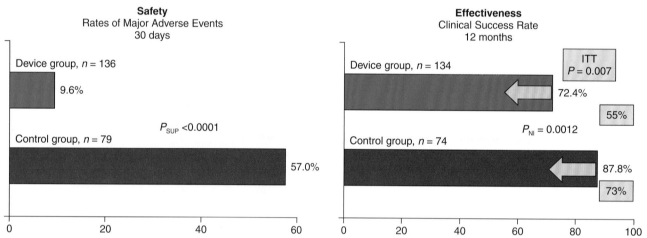

Fig. 20.4 Primary Safety and Efficacy End Points for EVEREST II. Rates of major adverse events at 30 days were reduced by MitraClip (Abbott Vascular) from 57.0% to 9.6% ($P < 0.0001$). The rates of clinical success at 12 months for patients with immediate procedural success were similar, although by intent-to-treat *(ITT)* analysis of all patients *(yellow arrows)*, effectiveness was better with surgery (73%) than with MitraClip (55%; $P = 0.007$). *EVEREST,* Endovascular Valve Edge-to-Edge Repair Study; *NI,* noninferiority; *SUP,* superiority. (Data from Feldman T, Foster E, Glower D, et al. Percutaneous repair or surgery for mitral regurgitation. N Engl J Med 2011;364:1395-1406.)

or replacement. These patients were almost a decade older (mean age, 67 years) than in usual surgical series and had more comorbidities. Major adverse events at 30 days were significantly less frequent with MitraClip therapy (9.6%, vs. 57% with surgery; $P < 0.0001$), although much of the difference could be attributed to the greater need for blood transfusions with surgery[28] (Fig. 20.4). Freedom from the combined outcome of death, MV surgery, and MR severity greater than 2+ at 12 months was higher with surgery (73%) than with MitraClip therapy (55%; $P = 0.0007$). For patients with acute MitraClip therapy success, the result appeared to be durable to 5 years, with 78% of surgeries occurring during the first 6 months and a very low rate of later MV surgery[29] (Fig. 20.5).

Subsequent analyses of this rich database have demonstrated persistent reductions in MR grade, improvement in New York Heart Association (NYHA) functional class, and reduction in LV dimensions[29] with MitraClip therapy. Other studies have demonstrated a lack of mitral stenosis, no effect of initial rhythm on results, and benefit in higher-risk subjects.[30–32]

In the EVEREST II high-risk study, 78 patients with an estimated surgical mortality rate of 12% or higher (mean, 14%) were treated with MitraClip, with an actual 30-day mortality rate of 8%. The survival rate at 12 months was 76% and significantly better than that of a concurrently screened comparison group, most (86%) of whom were treated medically. Patients treated with MitraClip had improved MR grade at 12 months (78% ≤ 2+), LV dimensions, NYHA functional class, and quality of life and they had a reduced need for hospitalization.[32] Similar benefit was demonstrated in another series of extreme-risk patients.[33] Based on the observed

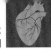

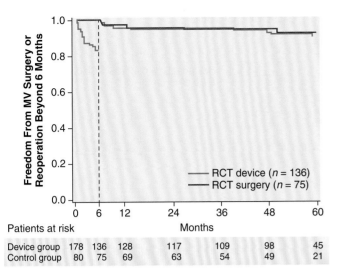

Fig. 20.5 Landmark Analysis of the Freedom From Mitral Valve (MV) Surgery or Reoperation Beyond 6 Months After MitraClip Implantation or Surgery for Patients in the Randomized EVEREST II Study. Patients with good results at 6 months after MitraClip (Abbott Vascular) appeared to have a durable outcome to 5 years. *EVEREST,* Endovascular Valve Edge-to-Edge Repair Study; *RCT,* randomized, controlled trial. (From Feldman T, Kar S, Elmariah S, et al. Randomized comparison of percutaneous repair and surgery for mitral regurgitation J Am Coll Cardiol 2015;66:2844-2854.)

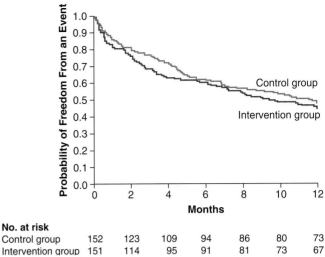

Fig. 20.6 Primary Outcome of Mitra-FR. The rates of freedom from death from any cause or unplanned hospitalization for heart failure are shown for the control and intervention groups. There was no significant difference in the event rate at 1 year. (Obadia JF, Messika-Zeitoun D, Leurent G, et al. Percutaneous repair or medical treatment for secondary mitral regurgitation. N Engl J Med 2018;379:2297-2306.)

benefit for high-risk patients with primary MR, MitraClip was granted approval by the U.S. Food and Drug Administration (FDA) for patients with primary MR, prohibitive surgical risk, and expected benefit from MR reduction.

Although the EVEREST II trial failed to demonstrate efficacy equivalent to that of surgery for a diverse group of patients with varied risk levels and causes, the EVEREST II High-Risk Registry and prohibitive-risk subset, combined with the experience outside the United States, points to a more appropriate role in high-risk patients and in those with secondary functional or ischemic MR. European investigators demonstrated the feasibility of MitraClip therapy in a group of 51 severely symptomatic patients with secondary ischemic or functional MR that had failed to respond to cardiac resynchronization therapy.[34] In addition to improved symptoms, a marked 50% to 70% reduction in hospitalization for heart failure during the year after MitraClip implantation compared with the previous year was observed in several studies, prompting a randomized trial (Clinical Outcomes Assessment of the MitraClip Percutaneous Therapy for High Surgical Risk Patients [COAPT]) to compare the device with medical therapy for patients with secondary MR.[35]

Published results of the COAPT trial and a similar European trial, Mitra-FR, have added significant new information on the use of MitraClip in patients with secondary MR. The Mitra-FR trial randomized 354 patients with severe secondary MR to MitraClip or medical therapy. The primary outcome of death from any cause or unplanned hospitalization for heart failure at 1 year did not differ between groups (Fig. 20.6).[36] The randomized COAPT trial also enrolled patients with severe secondary MR (*n* = 614) but demonstrated a striking reduction at 2 years in death from any cause (from 46% to 29%) and the annualized rate of all hospitalizations for heart failure (from 68% per patient-year to 36%) (Fig. 20.7).[37]

There are several possible explanations for the discrepant findings of these two trials, including enrollment of patients with less MR and more LV dysfunction in Mitra-FR, differences in the primary end point and timing of first versus all hospitalizations, greater adherence to optimized medical therapy in COAPT, and better acute and late MR reduction results in COAPT.[38,39]

Other Devices

Other devices in this category are the NeoChord, Harpoon, Mitra-Spacer, and MitraFlex (see Table 20.1). The NeoChord DS1000 system is a transapically inserted tool that can capture a flail leaflet segment and pierce it with a semidull needle to attach a standard polytetrafluoroethylene (PTFE) artificial chord, which is then anchored to the apical entry site with a pledgeted suture (Fig. 20.8). In the multicenter Transapical Artificial Chordae Tendineae (TACT) trial of 30 patients, acute procedural success was achieved in 87% of patients, with 59% achieving an MR grade of 2+ or less at 30 days, demonstrating safety and feasibility.[40]

A similar transapical chordal delivery device (Harpoon Medical TSD-5) reported high early success rates (100%) for 11 patients, with all but 1 having mild MR at 30 days.[41] A pivotal trial with NeoChord in the United States (ReChord) has been initiated (ClinicalTrials.gov: NCT02803957).

Mitra-Spacer (Cardiosolutions, Inc.) is an occluder device that is anchored in the LV apex by transseptal or transapical insertion with an anchor fixed outside the heart. The tethered balloon-like spacer floats in the mitral inflow pathway, providing a space occluder around which the mitral leaflets coalesce. This device has entered first-in-human evaluation outside the United States and has been deployed in four patients, with a reported reduction of one to two MR grades.[42] The MitraFlex device (TransCardiac Therapeutics) is designed as a transapically inserted thoracoscopic device to implant artificial chordae tendineae and is in preclinical development.

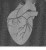

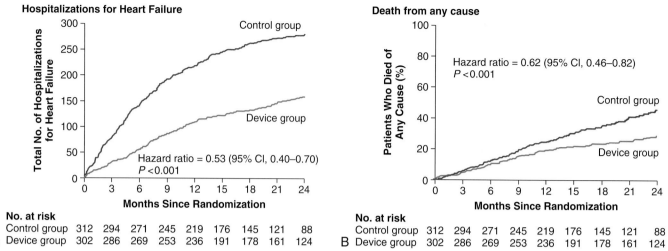

Fig. 20.7 Number of Hospitalizations for Heart Failure and Deaths From Any Cause for MitraClip and Medical Therapy. The primary outcomes for the COAPT trial of MitraClip *(device group)* and guideline-directed medical therapy *(control group)* are shown for the total number of hospitalizations *(top)* and all-cause mortality *(bottom).* There were significant reductions in both end points with MitraClip repair. (With permission from Stone GW, Lindenfeld JA, Abraham WT, et al. Transcatheter mitral-valve repair in patients with heart failure. N Engl J Med 2018;379:2307-2318.)

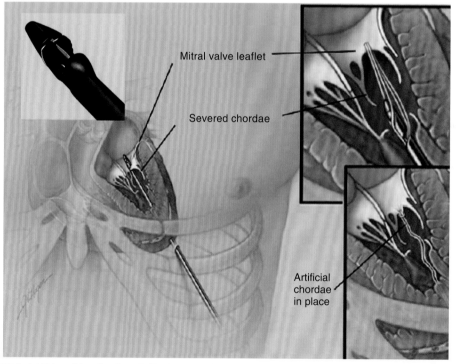

Fig. 20.8 Additional Leaflet Repair Technology. NeoChord DS 1000 insertion of a transapically anchored polytetrafluoroethylene chord (NeoChord, Inc., Eden Prairie, MN).

Indirect Annuloplasty

The venous anatomy of the heart is of particular interest for treatment of MR because of the ease of access (from the right internal jugular vein) and the location of the great cardiac vein in proximity to the posterior mitral annulus. Some of the first attempts to treat MR without surgery did so by mimicking surgical ring annuloplasty through placement of devices in the coronary sinus, so-called indirect or percutaneous coronary sinus annuloplasty. The goal of this approach is to

remodel the posterior annulus, cinching the great cardiac vein or pushing in on the posterior annulus from the vein to improve leaflet coaptation.

Two early attempts to do this highlighted some of the difficulties encountered with this approach. The Monarc annuloplasty system (Edward Lifesciences, Irvine, CA) consisted of two stent anchors with a shortening bridge between them that pulled the anchors together over several weeks with the intent to cinch the vein and shorten the circumference of the MV

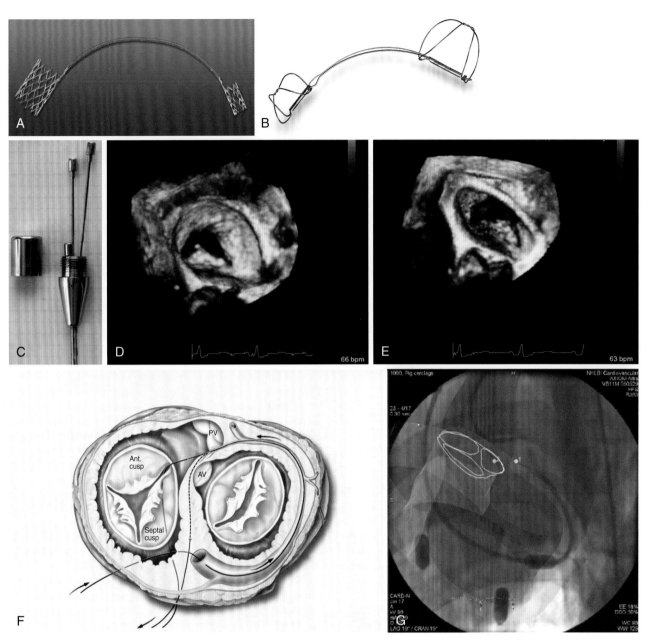

Fig. 20.9 Several Indirect Annuloplasty Devices. (A) Edwards Monarc annuloplasty system (Edwards Lifesciences LLC, Irvine, CA). (B) Carillon XE2 Mitral Contour System (Cardiac Dimension, Inc., Kirkland, WA) coronary sinus cinching device. (C) Viacor (Wilmington, MA) coronary sinus device. Three-dimensional transesophageal echocardiograms before (D) and after (E) use of the Viacor device in a patient in whom the device has pushed on the P2 segment to remodel the annulus and improve leaflet coaptation. The cerclage technique is shown in a schematic diagram (F) and in an angiogram with superimposed magnetic resonance images (G). *AV,* aortic valve; *PV,* pulmonary valve. (F and G From Kim JH, Kocaturk O, Ozturk C, et al. Mitral cerclage annuloplasty, a novel transcatheter treatment for secondary mitral valve regurgitation: initial results in swine. J Am Coll Cardiol 2009;54:638-651.)

in its posterior portion (Fig. 20.9A). The device was initially implanted in 59 of 72 patients, with a modest reduction in MR grade at 12 months: among 22 patients with matched echocardiograms at baseline and 12 months, 50% achieved at least 1 grade reduction in MR severity. More concerning was a high incidence of major adverse cardiovascular events, which included tamponade, early and late myocardial infarction, and nine deaths (at least one of which appeared to be device related).[43] The combination of modest efficacy and safety concerns caused the manufacturer to abandon subsequent development.

In another approach, the Viacor Percutaneous Transvenous Mitral Annuloplasty system (Viacor, Inc., Wilmington, MA) involved placement of a nitinol rod in the coronary sinus to push on the P2 segment of the annulus, thereby reducing the septal-lateral dimension and improving leaflet coaptation (see Fig. 20.9C–E). This device had the advantage of not requiring permanent implantation until after efficacy was determined in vivo, but it suffered from the same limitations as the Monarc: only mild efficacy, the potential risk for myocardial infarction, and the additional risk for rupture of the great cardiac vein.[44] This approach was also abandoned.

One coronary sinus approach has met with sufficient success and promise to obtain the CE Mark, and a U.S. investigational device exemption (IDE) trial is underway. The Carillon XE2 Mitral Contour

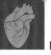

System (Cardiac Dimensions) uses novel anchors placed permanently in the coronary sinus that are pulled toward each other with a cinching device to reduce the mitral annular dimension by traction (see Fig. 20.9B). Early evaluation in the Carillon Mitral Annuloplasty Device European Union Study (AMADEUS) demonstrated feasibility, with implantation in 30 of 48 patients and modest improvement in quantitative measures of MR, with a small risk of coronary compromise (15%) and death (1 patient).[45]

A redesigned device was tested in the Transcatheter Implantation of Carillon Mitral Annuloplasty Device (TITAN) trial.[46] Among 65 enrolled subjects with secondary MR (62% ischemic), the device was implanted successfully in 36 patients with a mean age of 62 years, a mean ejection fraction of 29%, predominantly NYHA functional class III symptoms, and 2+ (30%), 3+ (55%), or 4+ (15%) grade MR. Quantitative measures of MR were better at 6 and 12 months than for 17 patients who were enrolled in the trial and did not receive implants. An FDA pivotal trial comparing the Carillon device with guideline-directed medical therapy in 400 patients has been initiated (ClinicalTrials.gov: NCT03142152).

Another device in this category is the Arto System, which places an anchor in the coronary sinus and the atrial septum to cinch the posterior annulus toward the septum. In a multicenter trial of 11 patients (MAVERIC trial), a 14% reduction in anteroposterior diameter was achieved with improvements in NYHA class and MR grade.[47]

In general, indirect annuloplasty devices do not reduce the septal-lateral annulus dimension to the same extent as surgical annuloplasty rings, but they may be able to provide modest MR reduction in selected patients. Whether this level of efficacy will result in sufficient symptomatic improvement and LV remodeling to justify the procedure requires further study. The limited efficacy is related to the location of the coronary sinus relative to the annulus (up to 10 mm more cranial), great individual anatomic variability, and the limited benefit of partial annular remodeling.[48,49] It is possible that some super-responders can be identified on the basis of anatomic considerations before the procedure.

The risks of this approach must also be considered. In addition to the risk for damage to the cardiac venous system, devices in this location can compress the left circumflex or diagonal coronary arteries, which traverse between the coronary sinus and the mitral annulus in most patients.[50]

A novel indirect approach to reduce the septal-lateral dimension that deserves further consideration is the cerclage annuloplasty technique (see Fig. 20.9F,G). This approach attempts to create a more complete circumferential annuloplasty by placing a suture from the coronary sinus through a septal perforator vein into the right atrium or right ventricle, where it is snared and tensioned with the proximal end from the right atrium to create a closed purse-string suture.[51] The procedure is guided by cardiac magnetic resonance imaging and uses a novel rigid protection device to avoid coronary compression. First-in-human preliminary results for five South Korean patients were presented, and a U.S. early feasibility trial has been initiated (ClinicalTrials.gov: NCT03929913).[51a]

Direct Annuloplasty and Hybrid Techniques

In part because of the limitations of the coronary sinus devices previously described, other attempts to more directly remodel the mitral annulus have been developed. They include transcatheter devices and hybrid devices that require surgical implantation with subsequent transcatheter adjustment.

The Mitralign Percutaneous Annuloplasty System (Mitralign, Inc.) was originally based on the surgical techniques of Paneth's posterior suture plicaton.[52] In this procedure, a transaortic catheter is advanced to the LV and used to deliver pledgeted anchors through the posterior annulus that can be pulled together to shorten (plicate) the annulus up

to 17 mm (with two implants). In 50 of 71 patients successfully treated in a phase 1 trial, the septal-lateral dimension was reduced by about 2 mm (<10%), MR grade at 6 months was reduced by a mean of 1.3 grades in 50% of patients, and modest symptomatic improvement was observed.[53] CE Mark was recently granted, and a phase 2 trial is underway.

The AccuCinch Ventricular Repair System (Ancora Heart, Santa Clara, CA) uses a similar catheter approach to place up to 12 anchors along the ventricular surface of the posterior mitral annulus. A cable running through the anchors is tensioned to create posterior plication. In a later development, the anchors have been placed in the ventricular myocardium just below the valve plane. This device has been characterized as more of a ventricular remodeling approach rather than one that is truly annular (i.e., percutaneous ventriculoplasty). It is being assessed in early feasibility trials to reduce MR and to improve LV function (Fig. 20.10).

Two devices that are under development represent a hybrid of surgical and transcatheter approaches. The Adjustable Annuloplasty Ring (Mitral Solutions) and the enCor Dynaplasty ring (MiCardia Corp.) are surgically implanted annuloplasty rings (see Table 20.1). The former can be adjusted (i.e., circumferentially reduced) with a mechanical catheter attachment. Similarly, the enCor ring is placed surgically and can be reshaped with radiofrequency energy supplied by removable leads passed externally from the left atrium through the incision for connection to an activation generator. The latter device has CE Mark approval and a U.S. IDE trial is underway. A subcutaneous version that may allow late activation and shape changing on an outpatient basis and a transcatheter version are under development. These devices may improve surgical annuloplasty outcomes by allowing for fine tuning of the ring size and shape under more physiologic conditions (e.g., not during cardiopulmonary bypass) or at a future time if further MR or ventricular enlargement develops.

In development are two devices that attempt to mimic surgical ring annuloplasty with a transcatheter approach. The Millipede nitinol ring (Boston Scientific Inc.) is envisioned as a self-expanding, catheter-delivered device. This device has begun first-in-human evaluation during open surgery, and transcatheter feasibility has been demonstrated.

The Cardioband (Edwards LifeSciences) is an adjustable, catheter-delivered, sutureless device that is inserted transseptally and directly anchored on the atrial side of the annulus with subsequent adjustment (see Fig. 20.10). In a phase 1 European study, 31 high-risk patients with severe secondary MR received treatment.[54] Mean septal-lateral dimension was markedly reduced, from 37 to 29 mm, with initial reduction in MR grade to trace or mild for 93% of patients and to moderate or less at 30 days for 88%.[54] This device received CE Mark approval, and a U.S. IDE trial is underway.

Left Ventricular Remodeling Techniques

The theoretical basis for devices to treat MR by affecting the shape of the LV arises from the pathophysiology of secondary ischemic or functional MR. Changes in the inferior and lateral LV due to infarction can lead to tethering or tenting of the posterior leaflet, allowing anterior leaflet override as the mechanism of MR.[1,2] Similarly, failure of leaflet coaptation due to global LV enlargement causing annular distention is the major mechanism for MR in dilated cardiomyopathy.[55] Ring annuloplasty can often ameliorate MR caused by LV distortion, and procedures that specifically address the underlying LV pathology may be beneficial.

The Coapsys annuloplasty system (Myocor Inc., Maple Grove, MN) was originally developed as an adjunct to surgical revascularization. This device has two extracardiac epicardial pads connected by a flexible, transventricular subvalvular chord that can be shortened intraoperatively. In the Randomized Evaluation of a Surgical Treatment for Off-Pump Repair

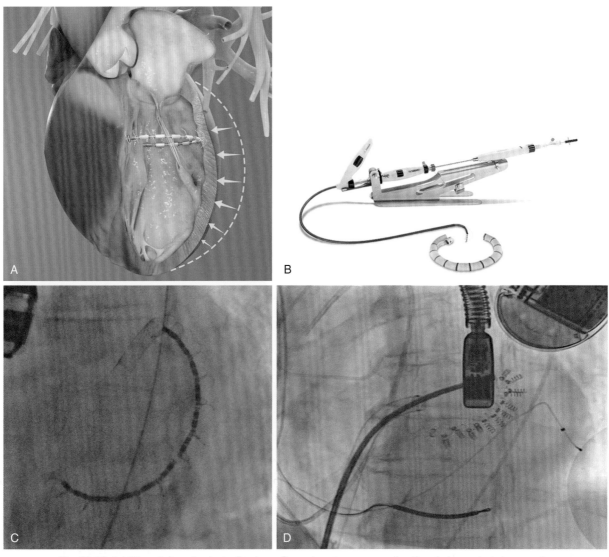

Fig. 20.10 Additional Annuloplasty Devices. Several systems more directly mimic surgical ring annuloplasty. (A) The AccuCinch ventricular implant (i.e., ventricular repair system) is primarily used for heart failure and cardiomyopathy. (B) The Cardioband (Edwards Lifesciences LLC, Irvine, CA) transcatheter annuloplasty system. (C and D) Fluoroscopic images of each device implanted in a patient.

of the Mitral Valve (RESTORE-MV) trial, 165 patients were randomly assigned to undergo CABG with or without Coapsys ventricular reshaping.[56] Patients treated with the device had greater reductions in LV end-diastolic dimension, lower MR grades, and better survival at 2 years. Despite the benefit and proof of concept demonstrated in this trial and the early success with a percutaneous prototype (iCoapsys), the company ran out of funding and ceased operations in 2008.

Other companies are developing approaches to LV remodeling (see Table 20.1). The Phoenix cardiac device (i.e., the basal annuloplasty of the cardia externally [BACE] device, Mardil Medical) is a surgically implanted external tension band that is placed around the heart externally at the time of CABG revascularization to treat ischemic MR. In a preliminary report of 11 patients treated in India, MR grade was reduced acutely from grade 3.3 to 0.6.[57]

The idea that a papillary muscle repair could assist in the durability of mitral annuloplasty for secondary MR is not new,[58] and it received additional validation in an Italian randomized surgical trial.[59] Preclinical work with a transcatheter approach to approximate the papillary muscles based on these concepts is in development (Tendyne Repair, Abbott Vascular).

TRANSCATHETER MITRAL VALVE REPLACEMENT

The rationale for transcatheter mitral valve replacement (TMVR) has as its basis in several lessons learned from surgical valve replacement.[60] Surgical valve replacement is the most effective method to reliably reduce MR. This is particularly evident in comparisons with transcatheter repairs, which do not appear to reduce MR to the same extent as surgical repairs. Despite its proven efficacy, the risks of surgery include significant morbidity and mortality related to the incision and the need for cardiopulmonary bypass.[10–12]

One of the most touted advantages of surgical repair compared with replacement is the improved survival related to better LV remodeling.[8] However, this and other observational comparisons may be confounded by differences in patient baseline characteristics and comorbid conditions. In one study using propensity scoring, 322 patients undergoing MV repair were matched with an equal number of patients undergoing valve replacement.[61] During a median follow-up of 3.4 years, a modest survival benefit was associated with repair, but the rate of freedom from reoperation was twofold higher with replacement. Importantly, only 15% of these patients had MR with an ischemic cause. In a comparison

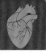

TABLE 20.2   Transcatheter Mitral Valve-in-Valve Implantation.

Study	N	Access Route (n)	Procedural Success (n/total)	Postprocedure MR Grade	Residual Mean Gradient (mmHg)	30-Day Mortality Rate (%)	Comments
Seiffert (2010)[67]	1	Transapical	1/1	0–1+	2	100	—
Webb (2010)[68]	7	Transseptal (1), transaortic (1), transapical (5)	6/7	0–1+	8	29	—
Cerillo (2011)[69]	3	Transapical	2/3	1+	5	33	—
Cheung (2011)[70]	11	Transaortic (1), transapical (10)	9/10	0–1+	7	10	Includes some patients from Maisano (2016)[54]
Van Garsse (2011)[71]	1	Transapical	1/1	0	3	0	—
de Weger (2011)[73]	1	Transapical	1/1	1+	4	0	Status after ring annuloplasty
Himbert (2011)[74]	1	Transseptal	1/1	1+	8	0	Status after ring annuloplasty
Gaia (2012)[72]	1	Transatrial	1/1	0	5	0	—
Himbert (2012)[75]	8	Transseptal	—	—	—	—	Status after ring annuloplasty (n = 6)
Yoon (2017)[76]	176	65% transseptal	89%	93% ≤ mild	6	6	Valve-in-valve
	72	28% transseptal	76%	81% ≤ mild	6	8	Valve-in-ring

MR, Mitral regurgitation.

of 397 patients with ischemic MR undergoing repair and 85 patients undergoing replacement, Gillinov et al[62] did not find a survival benefit for repair in patients with the most complex and severe conditions.

Randomized comparisons of repair and replacement are absent, and historical comparisons are limited by the use of older prostheses and the lack of chordal sparing techniques.[63,64] For this reason, a randomized trial comparing repair and replacement with complete subvalvular preservation in severe ischemic MR was sponsored by the National Heart, Lung, and Blood Institute. In this study, 251 patients with severe ischemic MR underwent surgical repair with annuloplasty or chord-sparing replacement.[65] At 12 months, there was no difference in the primary end point of LV end-systolic volume index, and recurrent MR was more frequent in the repair group (32.6% of those with moderate or severe MR vs. 2.3% after replacement), although the subset of patients with successful repair had the most favorable LV remodeling. Nonetheless, this finding provides a rationale to consider TMVR as an alternative to surgery.

Fueled by the success of transcatheter aortic valve replacement (TAVR), those interested in transcatheter treatment of MR hoped that TMVR might offer a more efficacious solution than transcatheter repair for the more divergent anatomic etiologies of MR.[66] These devices will likely first be used in elderly patients and others at high surgical risk, for whom the benefits of repair are unproven. Early experience using TAVR devices in previously implanted and now degenerating surgical bioprostheses and rings has confirmed the feasibility of this approach (Table 20.2). Balloon-expandable prostheses have been implanted in degenerating bioprostheses[67–72] and previous surgical annuloplasty rings,[73–75] predominantly with a transapical approach.

Transseptal delivery[68,74,75] and transatrial[68,70] delivery have also been demonstrated to be feasible[76] (Fig. 20.11). Initial reports of

success with TAVR devices in this setting prompted attempts to implant TAVR prostheses in a native calcified mitral annulus; despite anecdotal success, early mortality rate in a registry was as high as 30%, and complications included valve embolization, thrombosis, and LV outflow tract obstruction.[77]

More than 30 dedicated TMVR devices are under development with novel deployment approaches and insertion, folding, fixation, and sealing mechanisms.[78] At least five of these have entered early feasibility studies in the United States (Fig. 20.12). Initial results from the largest study, investigating the safety and efficacy of the Tendyne Mitral Valve System (Abbott Vascular), have been reported.[79] Muller et al treated 30 patients at eight sites who were at high risk for surgery with this transcatheter, transapical, self-expanding nitinol prosthesis supporting a trileaflet, porcine pericardial valve. Novel aspects of the Tendyne device include an outer D shape with an asymmetric sealing cuff and a braided polyethylene tether that helps to anchor the prosthesis to an apical epicardial pad.

All patients (mean age, 76 years; 83% male) had severe or moderately severe MR and a mean Society of Thoracic Surgery (STS) predicted risk of mortality at 30 days of 7.3%. The majority (77%) had secondary MR, and almost one half had LV ejection fractions of less than 30%. The device was successfully implanted in 28 patients (93%) and was retrieved without complications in the other 2 patients. Grade 0 MR was reported in all but one patient; there were no device embolizations, no strokes, and no LV outlet tract obstruction. At 30 days, there was 1 death due to pneumonia, and only 1 patient had mild MR. Overall freedom from major adverse events was 83%, and there was significant improvement in NYHA class, walk time, and quality of life.[79]

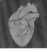

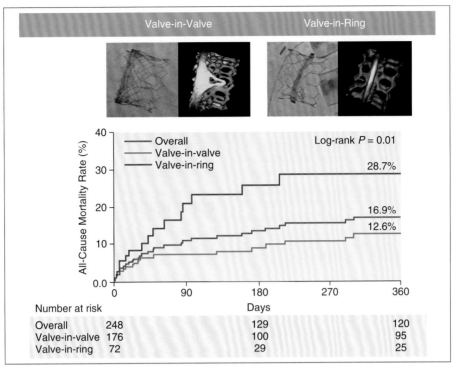

Fig. 20.11 Mortality Rates After Mitral Valve-in-Valve and Valve-in-Ring Procedures. *Top,* Procedural and postprocedural CT images of mitral valve-in-valve and valve-in-ring operations. *Bottom,* Cumulative mortality rates for the overall cohort (16.9%) and for valve-in-valve (12.6%) and valve-in-ring (28.75%) procedures. (From Yoon SH, Whisenant BK, Bleiziffer S, et al. Transcatheter mitral valve replacement for degenerated bioprosthetic valves and failed annuloplasty rings. J Am Coll Cardiol 2017;70:1121-1131.)

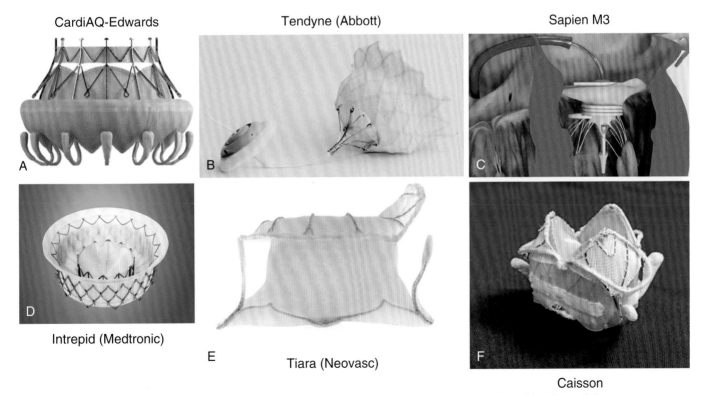

Fig. 20.12 Transcatheter Mitral Valve Replacement (TMVR). TMVR devices currently in trials. (A) CardiAQ-Edwards (Edwards LifeSciences). (B) Tendyne (Abbott Vascular). (C) Sapien M3 (Edwards LifeSciences). (D) Intrepid (with permission of Medtronic, Inc.). (E) Tiara (Tiara system, Neovasc, Inc.; all rights reserved.). (F) Caisson (with the permission of Livanova).

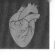

Bapat et al reported a high implant success rate (96%) with a 30-day mortality rate of 14% for 50 patients treated with the Intrepid (Medtronic, Inc.) transapical self-expanding prosthesis.[80] This TMVR device is the first to be investigated in a U.S. pivotal trial (APOLLO; clinicaltrials.gov NCT03242642).

Despite these early demonstrations of the feasibility of transcatheter mitral valve-in-valve implantation, it is likely that de novo placement of such devices in native valves will be more challenging.[81] The devices will need to be larger than most aortic devices, and fixation to the diseased mitral apparatus will be hampered by the greater valve complexity, the lack of calcium, the potential need for orientation, and the noncircular annular shape. Paravalvular leaks, already demonstrated to reduce survival after TAVR, are even less well tolerated in the MV, with its higher driving pressures and more common development of hemolysis.[82] There may be important effects of MV replacement on the normal LV twisting contraction pattern or on normal vortex inflow created by the anterior leaflet that could have adverse effects on LV function. All such devices will need to preserve the subvalvular apparatus and not create LV outflow tract obstruction.

Most current designs employ a stent-based bioprosthesis that is self-expanding and inserted transseptally (e.g., Evoque, Caisson) or transapically (e.g., Tendyne, Tiara, Intrepid) (see Fig. 20.12). It is anticipated that transseptal insertion will have advantages over transapical access if issues of delivery and placement can be solved. Some are two-stage deployments that involve separate steps for valve prosthesis insertion and anchoring fixation. Devices that do not rely on radial force for fixation in the annulus may be advantageous to reduce the risk of outflow tract obstruction.

Issues relating to study design and patient population will need to be solved before TMVR can become clinically relevant.[83] Phase 2 study investigators will wrestle with the fact that most patients with secondary MR do not have high short-term mortality rates and therefore are frequently medically managed. Overcoming procedural complications of TMVR will be essential to realize the symptomatic benefits compared with medical care. Cardiac and noncardiac comorbidities may hamper and confound comparative evaluations. For example, the treatment of concomitant tricuspid regurgitation, which occurs in most MR patients, will confound a surgical comparison group that also undergoes a tricuspid annuloplasty. It will be difficult to improve on the efficacy of current surgical repair results for primary MR if these patients are included in the study population.

The safety of transcatheter MV repair with MitraClip for suitable anatomic candidates with primary MR and high surgical risk will be hard to beat. The use of TMVR will require complex decision making on an individual patient level, incorporating patient age, frailty, comorbidities, goals of care (including patient preferences), specific valve anatomy, and each device's specific safety and efficacy profiles.

CONCLUSIONS

The complexity of the MV apparatus and the myriad types of MR have caused the field of transcatheter MV repair and TMVR to develop more slowly than treatments for aortic stenosis. The growing prevalence of heart failure in the aging U.S. population,[84] coupled with the fact that most of these patients have significant MR, will continue to drive efforts to develop safer and more efficacious treatments.

Transcatheter MV repair, particularly with the MitraClip, is very safe. TMVR results in more early complications but has the potential for more efficacious MR reduction acutely and in the long term. The multidisciplinary heart team, now established as a class I indication for the evaluation of complex patients with valvular heart disease, should play a central role in the use of these new technologies. The heart team and the patient should share decision making on how to balance in an individual patient the relative safety and efficacy of specific devices (Fig. 20.13). The opportunity for cardiologists and surgeons to learn from each other, practice together, and improve patient outcomes, aided by the ingenuity of physicians and engineers, gives confidence that transcatheter MV therapies will become an available option for many patients.

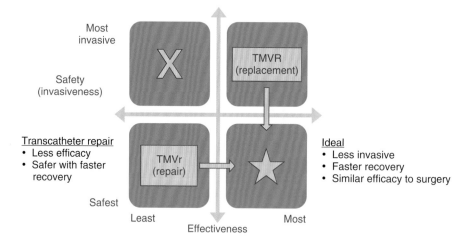

Complex decision making (on an individual basis) that takes into account
Patient age
Frailty
Comorbidities
Goals of care (incl patient preference)
Valve anatomy
Specific safety and efficacy of each device

Fig. 20.13 Balance in Clinical Decision Making. The relative safety of transcatheter mitral valve repair (TMVr) must be balanced against the greater efficacy of transcatheter mitral valve replacement (TMVR) in the context of specific patient and device characteristics.

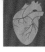

REFERENCES

1. Chaput M, Handschumacher MD, Tournoux F, et al. Mitral leaflet adaptation to ventricular remodeling: occurrence and adequacy in patients with functional mitral regurgitation. Circulation 2008;118:845-852.

2. Silbinger JJ. Mechanistic insights into ischemic mitral regurgitation: echocardiographic and surgical implications. J Am Soc Echocardiogr 2011;24:707-719.

3. Trichon BH, Felker GM, Shaw LK, et al. Relation of frequency and severity of mitral regurgitation to survival among patients with left ventricular systolic dysfunction and heart failure. Am J Cardiol 2003;91:538-543.

4. Enriquez-Sarano M, Avierinos JF, Messika-Zeitoun D, et al. Quantitative determinants of the outcome of asymptomatic mitral regurgitation. N Engl J Med 2005;352:875-883.

5. Bursi F, Enriquez-Sarano M, Nkomo VT, et al. Heart failure and death after myocardial infarction in the community: the emerging role of mitral regurgitation. Circulation 2005;111:295-301.

6. Rosenhek R, Rader F, Klaar U, et al. Outcome of watchful waiting in asymptomatic severe mitral regurgitation. Circulation 2006;113:2238-2244.

7. Bonow RO, Carabello BA, Chatterjee K, et al. 2008 focused update incorporated into the ACC/AHA 2006 guidelines for the management of patients with valvular heart disease: a report of the American College of Cardiology/ American Heart Association Task Force on Practice Guidelines (Writing Committee to revise the 1998 guidelines for the management of patients with valvular heart disease). Endorsed by the Society of Cardiovascular Anesthesiologists, Society for Cardiovascular Angiography and Interventions, and Society of Thoracic Surgeons. J Am Coll Cardiol 2008;52:e1-e142.

8. Enriquez-Sarano M, Schaff HV, Orszulak TA, et al. Valve repair improves the outcome of surgery for mitral regurgitation: a multivariate analysis. Circulation 1995;91:1022-1028.

9. Masson JB, Webb JG. Percutaneous treatment of mitral regurgitation. Circ Cardiovasc Interv 2009;2:140-146.

10. Gammie JS, O'Brien SM, Griffith BP, et al. Influence of hospital procedural volume on care process and mortality for patients undergoing elective surgery for mitral regurgitation. Circulation 2007;115:881-887.

11. Goodney PP, Stuke TA, Lucas FL, et al. Hospital volume, length of stay, and readmission rates in high-risk surgery. Ann Surg 2003;238:161-167.

12. Mehta RH, Eagle KA, Coombs LP, et al. Influence of age on outcomes in patients undergoing mitral valve replacement. Ann Thorac Surg 2002;74: 1459-1467.

13. Guy TS, Moainie SL, Gorman JH, et al. Prevention of ischemic mitral regurgitation does not influence the outcome of remodeling after posterolateral myocardial infarction. J Am Coll Cardiol 2004;43:377-383.

14. Wu AH, Aaronson KD, Bolling SF, et al. Impact of mitral valve annuloplasty on mortality risk in patients with mitral regurgitation and left ventricular systolic dysfunction. J Am Coll Cardiol 2005;45:381-387.

15. Mihaljevic T, Lam BK, Rajeswaran J, et al. Impact of mitral valve annuloplasty combined with revascularization in patients with functional ischemic mitral regurgitation. J Am Coll Cardiol 2007;49:2191-2201.

16. Goldstein D, Moskowitz AJ, Geligns AC, et al. Two-year outcomes of surgical treatment of severe ischemic mitral regurgitation. N Engl J Med 2016;374:344-353.

17. Glower DD, Tuttle RH, Shah LK, et al. Patient survival characteristics after routine mitral valve repair for ischemic mitral regurgitation. J Thorac Cardiovasc Surg 2005;129:860-868.

18. David TE. Outcomes of mitral valve repair for mitral regurgitation due to degenerative disease. Semin Thorac Cardiovasc Surg 2007;19:116-120.

19. Flameng W, Herijgers P, Bogaerts K. Recurrence of mitral valve regurgitation after mitral valve repair in degenerative valve disease. Circulation 2003; 107:1609-1613.

20. McGee EC, Gillino AM, Blackstone EH, et al. Recurrent mitral regurgitation after annuloplasty for functional ischemic mitral regurgitation. J Thorac Cardiovasc Surg 2004;128:916-924.

21. Chiam PT, Ruiz CE. Percutaneous transcatheter mitral valve repair: a classification of the technology. JACC Cardiovasc Interv 2011;4:1-13.

22. Alfieri O, Maisano F, DeBonis M, et al. The double-orifice technique in mitral valve repair: a simple solution for complex problems. J Thorac Cardiovasc Surg 2001;122:674-681.

23. Maisono F, Caldarola A, Blasio A, et al. Midterm results of edge-to-edge mitral valve repair without annuloplasty. J Thorac Cardiovasc Surg 2003;126:1987-1997.

24. St Goar FG, Fann JI, Komtebedde J, et al. Endovascular edge-to-edge mitral valve repair: short-term results in a porcine model. Circulation 2003;108:1990-1993.

25. Feldman T, Wasserman HS, Herrmann HC, et al. Percutaneous mitral valve repair using the edge-to-edge technique: six-month results of the EVEREST Phase 1 Clinical Trial. J Am Coll Cardiol 2005;46:2134-2140.

26. Herrmann HC, Feldman T. Percutaneous mitral valve edge-to-edge repair with the Evalve MitraClip System: rationale and phase 1 results. EuroIntervention 2006;1(Suppl A):A36-A39.

27. Silvestry FE, Rodriguez LL, Herrmann HC, et al. Echocardiographic guidance and assessment of percutaneous repair for mitral regurgitation with the Evalve MitraClip: lessons learned from EVEREST 1. J Am Soc Echocardiogr 2007;20:1131-1140.

28. Feldman T, Foster E, Glower D, et al. Percutaneous repair or surgery for mitral regurgitation. N Engl J Med 2011;364:1395-1406.

29. Feldman T, Kar S, Elmariah S, et al. Randomized comparison of percutaneous repair and surgery for mitral regurgitation. J Am Coll Cardiol 2015;66:2844-2854.

30. Herrmann HC, Kar S, Siegel R, et al. Effect of percutaneous mitral repair with the MitraClip device on mitral valve area and gradient. EuroIntervention 2009;4:437-442.

31. Herrmann HC, Gertz ZM, Silvestry FE, et al. Effects of atrial fibrillation on treatment of mitral regurgitation in the EVEREST II Randomized Trial. J Am Coll Cardiol 2012;59:A17-A20.

32. Whitlow PL, Feldman T, Pedersen WR, et al. Acute and 12-month results with catheter-based mitral valve leaflet repair. J Am Coll Cardiol 2012;59:130-139.

33. Rudolph V, Knap M, Frnazen O, et al. Echocardiographic and clinical outcomes of MitraClip therapy in patients not amenable to surgery. J Am Coll Cardiol 2011;58:2190-2195.

34. Auricchio A, Schillinger W, Meyer S, et al. Correction of mitral regurgitation in nonresponders to cardiac resynchronization therapy by MitraClip improves symptoms and promotes reverse remodeling. J Am Coll Cardiol 2011;58:2183-2189.

35. Asgar AW, Mack MJ, Stone GW. Secondary mitral regurgitation in heart failure. J Am Coll Cardiol 2015;65(12):1231-1248.

36. Obadia JF, Messika-Zeitoun D, Leurent G, et al. Percutaneous repair or medical treatment for secondary mitral regurgitation. N Engl J Med 2018;379:2297-2306.

37. Stone GW, Lindenfeld J, Abraham WT, et al. Transcatheter mitral-valve repair in patients with heart failure. N Engl J Med 2018;379:2307-2318.

38. Nishimura RA and Bonow RO. Percutaneous repair of secondary mitral regurgitation – a tale of two trials. N Engl J Med 2018;379:2374-2376.

39. Grayburn PA, Sannino A, Packer M. Proportionate and disproportionate functional mitral regurgitation. JACC Cardiovasc Imaging 2019;12: 353-362.

40. Seeburger J, Rinaldi M, Nielsen SL, et al. Off-pump transapical implantation of artificial neo-chordae to correct mitral regurgitation. J Am Coll Cardiol 2014;63:914-919.

41. Gammie JS, Wilson P, Bartus K, et al. Transapical beating-heart mitral valve repair with an expanded polytetraluoroethylene chordal implantation device. Circulation 2016;134:189-197.

42. Svensson L. Presentation at transcatheter therapeutics 23rd annual scientific symposium, November 7-11, 2011, San Francisco.

43. Harnek J, Webb JG, Kuck KH, et al. Transcatheter implantation of the MONARC coronary sinus device for mitral regurgitation. JACC Cardiovasc Interv 2011;4:115-122.

44. Sack S, Kahlert P, Bilodeau L, et al. Percutaneous transvenous mitral annuloplasty: initial human experience with a novel coronary sinus implant device. Circ Cardiovasc Interv 2009;2:277-284.

45. Schofer J, Siminiak T, Haude M, et al. Percutaneous mitral annuloplasty for functional mitral regurgitation: results of the Carillon Mitral Annuloplasty Device European Union Study. Circulation 2009;120:326-333.

46. Goldberg S. Presentation at transcatheter therapeutics 23rd annual scientific symposium, November 7-11, 2011, San Francisco.

47. Rogers JH, Thomas M, Morice MC, et al. Treatment of heart failure with associated functional mitral regurgitation using the ARTO system. JACC Cardiovasc Interv 2015;8:1095-1104.

48. Choure AJ, Barcia MJ, Hesse B, et al. In vivo analysis of the anatomical relationship of coronary sinus to mitral annulus and left circumflex coronary artery using cardiac multidetector computed tomography. J Am Coll Cardiol 2006;48:1938-1945.

49. Maselli D, Guarracino F, Chiaramonti F, et al. Percutaneous mitral annuloplasty: an anatomic study of human coronary sinus and its relation with mitral valve annulus and coronary arteries. Circulation 2006;114:377-380.

50. Spongo S, Bertrand OF, Philippon F, et al. Reversible circumflex coronary artery occlusion during percutaneous transvenous mitral annuloplasty with the Viacor system. J Am Coll Cardiol 2012;59:288.

51. Kim JH, Kocaturk O, Ozturk C, et al. Mitral cerclage annuloplasty, a novel transcatheter treatment for secondary mitral valve regurgitation: initial results in swine. J Am Coll Cardiol 2009;54:638-651.

51a. Park YH, Chon MK, Lederman RJ, et al. Mitral loop cerclage annuloplasty for secondary mitral regurgitation: first human results. JACC Cardiovasc Interv 2017;10(6):597-610.

52. Tibayan FA, Rodriguez F, Liang D, et al. Paneth suture annuloplasty abolishes acute ischemic mitral regurgitation but preserves annular and leaflet dynamics. Circulation 2003;108(Suppl II):II-128-II-133.

53. Nickenig G, Schueler R, Dager A, et al. Treatment of functional mitral valve regurgitation with a percutaneous annuloplasty system. J Am Coll Cardiol 2016;67:2927-2936.

54. Maisano F, Taramasso M, Nickenig G, et al. Cardioband, a transcatheter surgical-like direct mitral valve annuloplasty system: early results of the feasibility trial. Eur Heart J 2016;37:817-825.

55. Komeda M, Glasson JR, Bolger AF, et al. Geometric determinants of ischemic mitral regurgitation. Circulation 1997;96(Suppl 9):II-128-II-33.

56. Grossi EA, Patel N, Woo YJ, et al. Outcomes of the RESTOR-MV Trial (Randomized Evaluation of a Surgical Treatment for Off-Pump Repair of the Mitral Valve). J Am Coll Cardiol 2010;56:1984-1993.

57. Presentation at transcatheter therapeutics 23rd annual scientific symposium, November 7-11, 2011, San Francisco.

58. Langer F, Kunihara T, Hell K, et al. Ring and string: successful repair technique for ischemic mitral regurgitation with severe leaflet tethering. Circulation 2009;120:S85-S91.

59. Nappi F, Lusini M, Spdaccio C, et al. Papillary muscle approximation versus restrictive annuloplasty alone for severe ischemic mitral regurgitation. J am Coll Cardiol 2016;67:2334-2346.

60. Herrmann HC. Transcatheter mitral valve implantation. Cardiac Interventions Today, August/September 2009:82-85.

61. Moss RR, Humphries KH, Gao M, et al. Outcome of mitral valve repair or replacement: a comparison by propensity score analysis. Circulation 2003;108(Suppl II):II90-II97.

62. Gillinov AM, Wierup PN, Blackstone EH, et al. Is repair preferable to replacement for ischemic mitral regurgitation? J Thorac Cardiovasc Surg 2001;122:1125-1141.

63. Rozich JD, Carabello BA, Usher BW, et al. Mitral valve replacement with and without chordal preservation in patients with chronic mitral regurgitation: mechanisms for differences in postoperative ejection performance. Circulation 1992;86:1718-1726.

64. Yun KL, Sinteck CF, Miller DC, et al. Randomized trial comparing partial versus complete chordal-sparing mitral valve replacement: effects on left ventricular volume and function. J Thorac Cardiovasc Surg 2002;123:707-714.

65. Acker MA, Parides MK, Perrault LP, et al. Mitral-valve repair versus replacement for severe ischemic mitral regurgitation. N Engl J Med 2014;370:23-32.

66. Maisano F, Alfieri O, Banai S, et al. The future of transcatheter mitral valve interventions: competitive or complementary role of repair versus replacement? Eur Heart J 2015;38:1651-1659.

67. Seiffert M, Franzen O, Conradi L, et al. Series of transcatheter valve-in-valve implantations in high-risk patients with degenerated bioprostheses in aortic and mitral position. Catheter Cardiovasc Interv 2010;76:608-615.

68. Webb JG, Wood DA, Ye J, et al. Transcatheter valve-in-valve implantation for failed bioprosthetic heart valves. Circulation 2010;121:1848-1857.

69. Cerillo AG, Chiaramonti F, Murzi M, et al. Transcatheter valve in valve implantation for failed mitral and tricuspid bioprosthesis. Catheter Cardiovasc Interv 2011;78:987-995.

70. Cheung AW, Gurvitch R, Ye J, et al. Transcatheter transapical mitral valve-in-valve implantations for a failed bioprosthesis: a case series. J Thorac Cardiovasc Surg 2011;141:711-715.

71. Van Garsse LA, Gelsomino S, Van Ommen V, et al. Emergency transthoracic transapical mitral valve-in-valve implantation. J Interv Cardiol 2011;24:474-476.

72. Gaia DF, Palma JH, de Souza JAM, et al. Transapical mitral valve-in-valve implant: an alternative for high risk and multiple reoperative rheumatic patients. Int J Cardiol 2012;154:e6-e7.

73. de Weger A, Ewe SH, Delagado V, et al. First in man implantation of a transcatheter aortic valve in a mitral annuloplasty ring: novel treatment modality for failed mitral valve repair. Eur J Cardiothorac Surg 2011;39:1054-1056.

74. Himbert D, Brochet E, Radu C, et al. Transseptal implantation of a transcatheter heart valve in a mitral annuloplasty ring to treat mitral repair failure. Circ Cardiovasc Interv 2011;4:396-398.

75. Himbert D, Descoutures F, Brochet E, et al. Transvenous mitral valve replacement after failure of surgical ring annuloplasty. J Am Coll Cardiol 2012;60:1205-1206.

76. Yoon SH, Whisenant BK, Bleiziffer S, et al. Transcatheter mitral valve replacement for degenerated bioprosthetic valves and failed annuloplasty rings. J Am Coll Cardiol 2017;70:1121-1131.

77. Guerrero M, Urena M, Himbert D, et al. 1-Year outcomes of transcatheter mitral valve replacement in patients with severe mitral annular calcification. J Am Coll Cardiol 2018;71:1841-1853.

78. DeBacker O, Piazza N, Banai S, et al. Percutaneous transcatheter mitral valve replacement: an overview of devices in preclinical and early clinical evaluation. Circ Cardiovasc Interv 2014;7:400-409.

79. Muller D, Farivar RS, Jansz P, et al. Transcatheter mitral valve replacement for patients with symptomatic mitral regurgitation: global feasibility trial. J Am Coll Cardiol 2017;69:381-391.

80. Bapat V, Rajagopal V, Meduri C, et al. Early experience with new transcatheter mitral valve replacement. J Am Coll Cardiol 2017;71:12-21.

81. Herrmann HC, Chitwood WR. Transcatheter mitral valve replacement clears the first hurdle. J Am Coll Cardiol 2017;69:392-394.

82. Taramasso M, Maisano F, Denti P, et al. Surgical treatment of paravalvular leak: long-term results in a single center experience (up to 14 years). J Thorac Cardiovasc Surg 2015;149:1270-1275.

83. Anyanwu AC, Adams DH. Transcatheter mitral valve replacement. J Am Coll Cardiol 2014;64:1820-1824.

84. Roger VL, Go AS, Lloyd-Jones DM, et al. Heart disease and stroke statistics—2011 update. A report from the American Heart Association. Circulation 2011;123:e18-e209.

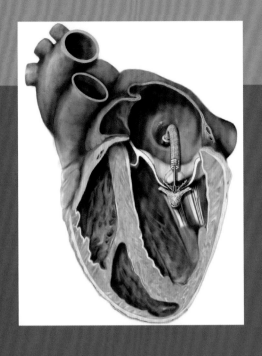

第21章
经导管二尖瓣手术的
影像指导

　　结构性心脏病介入治疗领域发展迅速，而二尖瓣介入治疗是其中最为前沿的行业热点。由于介入治疗"非直视"微创手术的特点，心脏影像评估技术在经导管二尖瓣治疗中起到了重要的指导作用。

　　近年来，基于二尖瓣介入治疗的多种影像评估技术得到快速发展，其中包括超声心动图、心脏MRI、心脏CT及图像融合技术等诸多方面，其中术中三维经食管超声心动图已成为经导管二尖瓣介入治疗影像评估指导的基本技术，可以准确指导术中器械的释放及效果评估。而以二尖瓣心脏超声为核心的心脏数字建模+术中造影影像实时融合成像新技术是目前最新的研发方向，其发展大大提高了心脏超声在二尖瓣介入治疗的应用价值。心脏MRI技术在量化经导管二尖瓣缘对缘修复术后患者二尖瓣反流严重程度方面弥补了超声心动图的缺陷，提高了量化的精确程度。而多层螺旋CT可高分辨率三维重建二尖瓣瓣环及相关形态，在经导管二尖瓣置换术的术前评估解剖毗邻，选择器械型号及预防流出道梗阻等并发症方面发挥重要作用。

　　本章条理清晰地向各位读者系统介绍了二尖瓣介入治疗影像评估及应用技术，相信会在这个崭新的领域为读者带来全面的知识与收获。

王墨扬

Imaging Guidance of Transcatheter Mitral Valve Procedures

Ernesto E. Salcedo, Robert A. Quaife, John D. Carroll

CHAPTER OUTLINE

KEY POINTS

- The field of structural heart disease interventions is expanding rapidly. Advances in cardiac imaging are playing a central role in patient selection, imaging guidance, and follow-up of patients undergoing transcatheter mitral valve procedures (TCMVPs).
- Three-dimensional transesophageal echocardiography has become the fundamental technique for imaging guidance of TCMVP.
- Advances in heart and mitral valve modeling and echocardiographic-fluoroscopic (echo/fluoro) fusion imaging have enhanced the

applicability of cardiac ultrasound in the cardiac catheterization laboratory and the hybrid operating room.
- There is significant interest in determining the role of cardiac magnetic resonance imaging in quantifying mitral regurgitation severity in patients after transcatheter mitral valve clip implantation, for which echocardiography may be imprecise.
- Multislice computed tomography provides high-resolution reconstructions of the mitral annulus and plays an important role in the nascent area of percutaneous mitral valve replacement.

BASIC PRINCIPLES

Mitral regurgitation (MR), the most common form of valvular heart disease, can result from disease of the mitral valve (MV) apparatus (i.e., primary MR) or from disease of the left ventricle (i.e., secondary MR). Mitral stenosis (MS), the least common form of valvular heart disease, can be related to rheumatic fever (i.e., rheumatic MS) or to calcific degenerative changes of the MV (i.e., calcific MS). Severe symptomatic MV disease has traditionally been treated surgically through MV repair or replacement.[1] In great part due to advances in cardiac imaging, transcatheter treatment of MV disease has become an alternative to surgery for patients with severe MV disease.

Types of Transcatheter Mitral Valve Intervention

Five major domains of transcatheter mitral valve procedures (TCMVPs) have emerged: (1) balloon-induced commissurotomy for rheumatic MS, (2) edge-to-edge repair with placement of one or more mechanical clips to enhance leaflet coaptation and induce annular modification for MR, (3) annular reduction by direct or indirect techniques for MR, (4) plugging of paraprosthetic leaks causing MR, and (5) insertion of bioprosthetic valves for MR and MS disease of the native MV or a degenerated bioprosthetic valve. Some therapies are well established with extensive insights into imaging guidance issues, and others are emerging technologies with experience limited to early feasibility

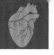

studies. The imaging guidance considerations for each of these five domains are discussed in the following sections.

Imaging guidance plays a central role in the successful and safe execution of all TCMVPs. New interventions have stimulated improvements in imaging guidance technologies and techniques, and advances in imaging guidance technologies and experience have enabled the development of new interventional therapies. This push-pull relationship between medical imaging and devices is a key aspect for the future of this field.

Goals of Imaging Guidance

Imaging guidance for the five domains of TCMVPs and for preprocedural planning has several common goals that provide an organizing principle for what can otherwise be diverse tasks that must be performed for different types of interventions. These include the following:

- Preprocedural, intraprocedural, and postprocedural assessment of the structure and function of the MV
- Planning and execution of the initial access to the left heart and MV, mainly with transseptal or transapical access
- Planning and execution of delivery system placement
- Planning and execution of therapeutic device deployment that involves sizing the device, targeting to a specific final location of the device, and aligning the device to key structures
- Prediction, detection, and actions in response to potential complications

These imaging-related goals of TCMVPs are addressed by an expanding array of imaging modalities with specialized applications that provide optimal visualization for performance of specific tasks, quantitation of key variables, and the ability to combine different modalities to enhance workflow efficiency, hand-eye coordination, and understanding of complex three-dimensional (3D) relationships.

Fluoroscopy, angiography, and hemodynamic assessment have been the main guiding tools in the catheterization laboratory, but as the field of structural heart disease interventions has developed, advanced cardiac imaging techniques, including echocardiography, cardiac magnetic resonance imaging (CMR), and computed tomography (CT) have complemented cine-angiography by providing soft tissue characterization not available with the radiographic techniques alone.[2,3] Noninvasive imaging guidance techniques provide superb visualization of the cardiac structures from perspectives previously seen only by the surgeon in the beating heart. Noninvasive imaging modalities, specifically echocardiography, have become the foundation for patient selection, imaging guidance, and evaluation of results in patients undergoing all structural heart disease interventions but especially MV interventions.

Education and Training for Procedural Imaging

Imaging guidance and preprocedural planning required new skill sets and a new focus in the careers of those who partner with catheter interventionalists. Several publications have reviewed transcatheter valve technology for the treatment of valvular heart disease[2,4-11] and have highlighted the central role played by cardiac imaging and imaging experts in achieving a successful intervention. The development of dedicated heart teams, composed of cardiac surgeons, interventionalists, anesthesiologists, and cardiac imagers, for the contemporary management of advanced valvular heart disease solidifies the importance of imaging in structural heart disease interventions.[12,13]

In response to these new therapeutic options for treating MV disease and the central role of imaging for planning and guiding interventions, professional societies have needed to expand training, other educational efforts, and facility requirements as experience and best practices have evolved. The 2014 American Heart Association (AHA)/American College of Cardiology (ACC) guidelines for the management of patients with valvular heart disease support the use of TCMVP for symptomatic patients with severe MS and for severely symptomatic patients with chronic severe primary MR who have a prohibitive surgical risk because of severe comorbidities.[14]

The European Association of Echocardiography (ESE), in partnership with the American Society of Echocardiography (ASE), published recommendations for the use of transcatheter interventions for valvular heart disease.[15,16] These updated the previous recommendations of the ASE on echocardiographic-guided interventions.[17] The expert consensus document of the Society for Cardiovascular Angiography and Interventions (SCAI), American Association for Thoracic Surgery (AATS), ACC, and Society for Thoracic Surgeons (STS) on the operator and institutional requirements for transcatheter valve repair and replacement[18] highlighted the importance of noninvasive imaging, requiring that institutions engaged in TCMVP have adequate noninvasive imaging facilities.

This chapter reviews the critical role played by cardiac imaging in TCMVP. It highlights TCMVP general imaging guidance issues, common and advanced imaging tools in use, and imaging guidance of specific TCMVPs and presents our view of the future of this field.

KEY STEPS FOR IMAGING GUIDANCE

Imaging guidance of TCMVPs requires detailed knowledge of MV anatomy and pathology, a clear understanding of the available interventional procedures used in MV interventions, and experience with the standard and advanced imaging techniques used to guide TCMVPs. Table 21.1 summarizes the fundamental imaging guidance principles related to TCMVPs. Thoughtful imaging guidance planning enhances the chance of a successful intervention.

Preprocedural planning requires precise characterization and assessment of MV morphology and function and of how the native or prosthetic MV will be affected by the intervention. Familiarity with catheters, devices, and interventional workflow is mandatory. Appropriate imaging guidance of TCMVP also requires detailed knowledge of the access pathways used to reach the interventional target. Choosing the appropriate imaging tools for preprocedural planning depends on the planned intervention and the advantages and disadvantages of each imaging modality for the specific TCMVP.

Intraprocedural guidance means determining the imaging modalities needed to perform each step of the intervention; defining key sequential steps in performing the MV intervention; developing a common language to facilitate communication between imager and interventionalist; familiarity with catheters, devices, and interventional workflow; recognizing specific imaging limitations; and considering available alternatives.

Anticipation of imaging guidance needs for the interventionalist is essential. Intraprocedural detection and understanding of complications is often first informed by imaging, and the imaging specialist must be familiar with potential complications such as thrombus on catheters, guidewires, and devices; pericardial effusion and tamponade; and embolization of equipment. At the completion of the intervention but before the patient leaves the procedure room, imaging is often combined with traditional catheter-based hemodynamics to assess the success of the intervention and identify when adjustments need to be made.

Postprocedural assessment is directed to the final assessment of the intervention, often after the patient has awakened and returned to a baseline hemodynamic state.

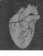

TABLE 21.1	Imaging Guidance Issues in Transcatheter Mitral Valve Procedures.	
Assessment of Mitral Anatomy and Function	Understanding of Catheters, Devices, and Access Pathways	Planning of Imaging Guidance
Preprocedural Planning		
1. What aspects of mitral valve anatomy and function need to be characterized for the intervention?	What type and size of device are needed?	What imaging modalities will be necessary?
• Characterization of mitral valve dysfunction severity • Defining degenerative versus functional mitral regurgitation	*Femoral vein access*, inferior vena cava, plane of interatrial septum, trajectory to align with mitral valve	Assess what imaging guidance challenges and limitations may exist for individual patients.
2. What are the goals of the intervention?	Choose the interatrial septum puncture site.	Determine which gantry locations will be needed to perform certain tasks.
3. What structure is the target of the intervention?	*Arterial access*, retrograde aortic pathway, trajectory to mitral valve targets	Is the procedure likely to carry a high radiation dose, and what steps can be taken to minimize this?
4. Where should the devices be placed?	*Transapical access*, left ventricular entry point, trajectory to mitral valve targets	Will contrast use be limited by renal dysfunction?
Intraprocedural Guidance		
1. Determine imaging modalities needed to perform each step of the intervention.	Define key sequential steps in performing the mitral valve intervention.	Clear and precise communication with interventionalist
2. Familiarity with catheters, devices, and interventional workflow is mandatory.	Guide intervention with a complication prevention frame of mind.	Anticipate imaging guidance needs for the interventionalist.
3. Knowledge of imaging appearance of catheters and devices is essential.	Recognize common and uncommon device-induced artifacts.	Suggest alternative imaging tool if the one being used proves inadequate.
Postprocedural Assessment		
1. Assess the success of the interventions.	Identify when adjustments or additional intervention should be made.	Detect and understand intraprocedural complications and how serious they are.

Standard Imaging Tools

Matching of the optimal imaging modality with advanced tools for optimal visualization is central to the planning, execution, and evaluation of TCMVPs.[19] Fig. 21.1 outlines the standard and advanced imaging tools used for the preprocedural, intraprocedural, and postprocedural stages of TCMVPs. The main applications and the advantages and disadvantages of each imaging modality are highlighted in Table 21.2.

X-Ray Imaging

Fluoroscopy and, to a lesser degree, angiography are the basic imaging guidance tools for the performance of TCMVPs. These imaging tools are part of the standard cardiac catheterization laboratory and are routinely used for most parts of the intervention: aiding in vascular access; guiding vascular and cardiac navigation of guidewires, catheters, and devices; and positioning and deploying devices on the structural targets (Fig. 21.2).

Because the x-ray field of view is large, encompassing the whole chest, it provides a comprehensive imaging perspective of the cardiovascular areas of interest. The main disadvantage of x-ray techniques for procedural guidance is the lack of detailed characterization of the soft tissues structures in the heart.

Fluoroscopy consists of projection of images of radiopaque structures that are flat or two-dimensional (2D) images with loss of depth. Only by changing the perspective can the clinician start to understand depth and 3D relationships. Another disadvantage of cine-fluoroscopy is radiation exposure and the use of potentially nephrotoxic and intravascular volume-expanding contrast agents.

Ventriculography can be used in the preprocedural and postprocedural evaluation of ventricular volumes and for evaluation of the severity of MR. Digital laboratories provide rapid, accurate measurements of left ventricular (LV) volume that have been validated with human heart casts and CMR. End-systolic and end-diastolic volumes predict outcomes in regurgitant valvular lesions and should be routinely obtained when left ventriculography is performed.[37] The radiation dose and contrast volume needed for repetitive ventriculograms reduce the usefulness of this imaging modality, especially for patients who have renal insufficiency or are already in a volume overload state.

Two- and Three-Dimensional Echocardiography

Echocardiography has become an indispensable tool for the imaging guidance of structural heart disease interventions. Transthoracic echocardiography (TTE) is usually sufficient to provide preprocedural characterization of MV morphology and function, and it aids immensely in patient selection for MV interventions. Because of the interference with fluoroscopy, the relatively limited acoustic windows, the inability to characterize details of the MV apparatus, the additional radiation exposure to the sonographer, and the use of nonsterile probes, the value of TTE for procedural imaging guidance is limited. TTE is the usual imaging modality for long-term follow-up after MV interventions.

Transesophageal echocardiography (TEE) has become the standard imaging guidance tool for TCMVP; both 2D and 3D techniques are employed (Fig. 21.3).[38] Color Doppler images of the mitral apparatus made with 2D TEE provide high resolution and high frame rates with

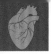

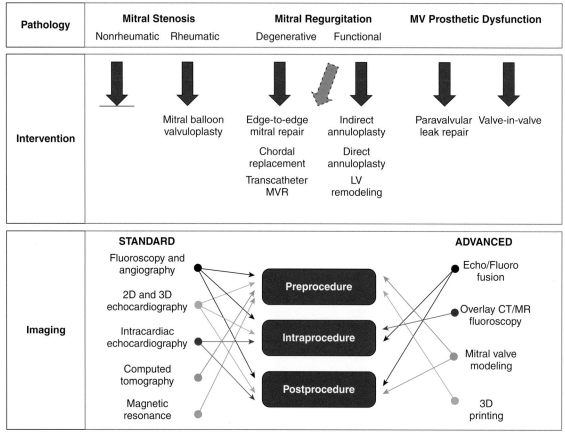

Fig. 21.1 Imaging Guidance of Transcatheter Mitral Valve Procedures. Imaging guidance of transcatheter mitral valve procedures is based on a clear understanding of the pathology of the mitral valve, the available interventions for each mitral disease process, and the standard and advanced imaging tools for the preprocedural, intraprocedural, and postprocedural phases of the transcatheter mitral valve intervention. *CT*, Computed tomography; *Echo/Fluoro*, echocardiographic-fluoroscopic; *MR*, magnetic resonance; *MV*, mitral valve; *MVR*, mitral valve regurgitation.

TABLE 21.2   Imaging Tools in Transcatheter Mitral Valve Procedures.

Modality	Main Application	Advantages	Disadvantages
Standard Imaging Tools			
X-ray imaging	Intraprocedural guidance	Standard equipment in catheter laboratory Best visualization of catheters and devices	Radiation exposure Need for contrast No soft tissue visualization
2D and 3D TEE[3,15,20]	Preprocedural planning Intraprocedural guidance Postprocedural assessment	Soft tissue visualization Provides real-time/multibeat anatomic and physiologic data	TEE is semi-invasive. Need for intubation Variability of image quality and imaging artifacts Operator dependence
Intracardiac echocardiography[21–24]	Intraprocedural guidance	No need for anesthesia and intubation	Added cost, small field of view, lacks 3D imaging
Magnetic resonance imaging[25,26]	Preprocedural planning Potential intraprocedural guidance Postprocedural assessment	No radiation Outstanding spatial resolution Gold standard for left ventricular volumes Noninvasive	Impractical for intraprocedural guidance Cardiac cycle dependence
CT[27–29]	Preprocedural planning	Comprehensive cardiac and vascular assessment Outstanding spatial resolution High reproducibility Calcium is well seen and characterized Noninvasive	Contrast required Radiation exposure Cardiac cycle dependence Poor temporal resolution

Continued

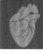

Modality	Main Application	Advantages	Disadvantages
Advanced Imaging Tools			
Echocardiographic-fluoroscopic fusion[30,31]	Intraprocedural guidance	Real-time overlay of catheters and devices (fluoroscopy) on cardiac anatomic structures (3D TEE)	Few studies have documented its value.
Overlay of 3D CT and fluoroscopy[32]	Intraprocedural guidance	Overlay of catheters and devices (fluoroscopy) on frozen cardiac anatomic structures (CT)	CT not in real time
Mitral valve 3D modeling[28,33–35]	Preprocedural planning Evaluation of results	Realistic model of mitral annulus	Few studies have documented its value.
Rapid prototyping[36]	Preprocedural planning	Actual physical model with which devices can be tried	Few studies have documented its value.

TABLE 21.2 Imaging Tools in Transcatheter Mitral Valve Procedures.—cont'd

CT, Computed tomography.

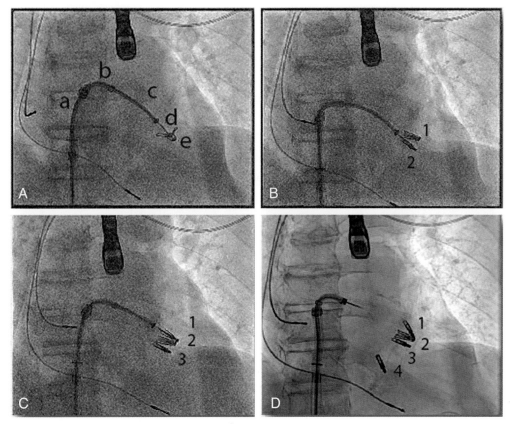

Fig. 21.2 MitraClip Fluoroscopy (Video 21.2 ▶). Fluoroscopic images from a patient undergoing a Mitra-Clip procedure that required four clips. In all images, the TEE probe, which is a required additional imaging guidance tool for the MitraClip procedure, is visible. The patient has a pacemaker with atrial and right ventricular leads. (A) The MitraClip system with its components: the guide catheter *(a)*, the sleeve *(b)*, the delivery catheter *(c)*, the tip of the delivery catheter *(d)*, and the clip *(e)*. (B–D) Progressive use of two, three, and four clips (numbered *1* through *4*, respectively). Notice the sharp tip of the delivery catheter (D), which needs to be followed carefully as it is withdrawn, with TEE and fluoroscopy, to avoid soft tissue damage.

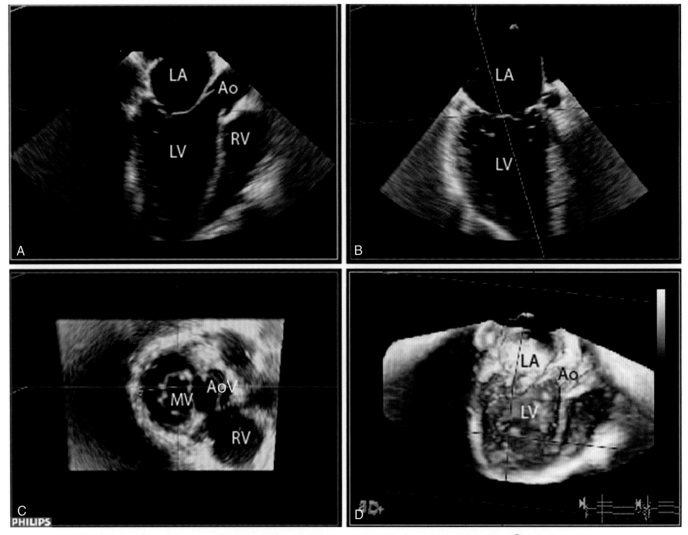

Fig. 21.3 3D Multiplane Reconstruction of Functional Mitral Regurgitation (Video 21.3 ▶). A 64-year-old man was referred for MitraClip treatment of severe functional mitral regurgitation. 3D TEE multiplane reconstruction revealed a normal mitral valve and severe LV dilation. (A) LV outflow tract view. (B) Bicommissural view. (C) Short-axis view shows the MV, AoV, and RV. (D) Global dilation of the LV and a structurally normal mitral valve. *Ao,* Aorta; *AoV,* aortic valve; *MV,* mitral valve.

well-standardized imaging views. 3D TEE provides unique anatomic detail of the MV and surrounding structures and greatly facilitates guidance of catheters and devices to the area of interest. Although 3D TEE color Doppler has been somewhat limited because of slow frame rates, this technology is rapidly improving and holds promise for enhanced imaging guidance for TCMVPs (Fig. 21.4).

The main strengths of echocardiographic methods for imaging guidance of TCMVP reside in their ability to provide real-time, continuous anatomic and physiologic data. The main limitation is the relatively small area of the heart that can be visualized at any given moment (compared with fluoroscopy, CT, or CMR). Quantification of MR severity after MV interventions, particularly after MitraClip deployment, is difficult, although quantification of the vena contracta area with 3D TEE shows some promise.[39,40]

The quality of the echocardiographic images is patient dependent, and patient cooperation is unpredictable. Although the clinician can usually obtain diagnostic information, some fine anatomic details may be difficult to characterize in some patients. Imaging artifacts and drop-out also may be produced by calcified structures, catheters,

prosthetic valves, and implanted devices. This highlights the importance of changing the position of the TEE probe (within the constraints of the esophagus and stomach), which may be needed for optimal visualization. Another shortcoming of echocardiography is that the image quality is operator dependent, and there is a significant learning curve.

Intracardiac Echocardiography

Intracardiac echocardiography (ICE) is increasingly used to guide percutaneous interventional procedures, principally to support electrophysiologic interventions and for closure of a patent foramen ovale and small atrial septal defects (ASDs). Imaging with ICE has evolved from cross-sectional imaging using a rotating transducer (similar to intravascular ultrasound) to sector-based imaging using a phased-array transducer. Phased-array ICE is the most common form of ICE used for TCMVPs because of its high-frequency range, large depth of field, steerability, and the possibility of acquiring Doppler and color-flow imaging.[21]

3D ICE is likely to play a significant role in the imaging guidance of TCMVPs.[41] Reports suggest that ICE may be used for primary guidance

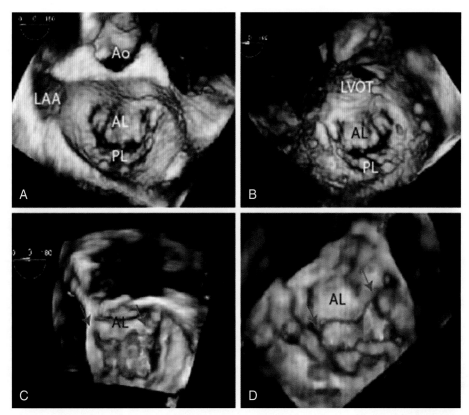

Fig. 21.4 Functional Mitral Regurgitation (MR). The mitral valve is depicted in 3D TEE images before MitraClip intervention as viewed from the left atrium (A; Video 21.4A ▶) and from the left ventricle (B; Video 21.4B ▶). Notice the absence of structural abnormalities in the leaflets and the lack of leaflet coaptation along the leaflet coaptation line. 3D TEE color images illustrate the presence of MR along the coaptation line *(red arrows)*, as seen from the left atrial perspective (C; Video 21.4C ▶) and from the left ventricle (D). *Ao,* Aorta; *AL,* anterior leaflet; *LAA,* left atrial appendage; *LVOT,* left ventricular outflow tract; *PL,* posterior leaflet.

or as a supplement to TEE for patients undergoing percutaneous MV repair and paravalvular leak (PVL) closure.[42]

The main advantages of ICE compared with TEE are that ICE eliminates the need for general anesthesia, provides very clear images (because it can be close to the target with no air to degrade image quality), and can result in shorter procedure times, potentially reducing hospital stay and radiation doses. The main disadvantage is the additional cost of the catheter, even with resterilization and reuse.[43] Operator skills must be developed, and the perspective of the image is limited by where the catheter can or cannot be located.

ICE can provide essential imaging guidance and procedural monitoring during percutaneous balloon mitral commisurotomy (BMC).[44] Although currently TEE is used more frequently for imaging guidance of BMC, ICE is a viable alternative. The use of ICE for imaging guidance of periprosthetic MR has been described, suggesting that ICE could become a second-line alternative to TEE.[45]

The MitraClip procedure is usually performed under TEE guidance. However, in some patients, TEE may not provide adequate imaging information, and the use of ICE from the left atrium (LA), both atria, or the LV for visualization and guidance of the MitraClip procedure has been described.[22,46,47] MV repair with the MitraClip system assisted by ICE has been demonstrated to be feasible in patients with prior surgical rings, achieving an excellent risk profile and satisfactory procedural success.[46] In patients with postsurgical anatomy, clear TEE imaging of the MV leaflets may be complicated by shadowing from the surgical annuloplasty ring, particularly

when assessing the adequacy of posterior leaflet insertion into the MitraClip arms. ICE guidance from the LV offers a feasible imaging guidance alternative.[48]

Cardiac Magnetic Resonance Imaging

Real-time CMR-guided catheterization offers a potentially effective, radiation-free alternative to comprehensive x-ray–guided right catheterization.[25] With improved tools and further optimization, CMR may become a realistic option for structural heart disease interventions.

CMR plays a limited role in the imaging guidance of TCMVPs; it is mainly confined to the preprocedural and postprocedural assessment of MR severity and the evaluation of ventricular and atrial remodeling.[49–51] One report highlighted the discordance existing between echocardiography and CMR in the assessment of MR severity.[52] The data suggested that CMR was more accurate than echocardiography in assessing the severity of MR and that CMR should be considered for patients in whom MR severity as assessed by echocardiography is determining the decision to undergo MV repair or replacement.

Another study compared the value of TEE versus CMR in evaluating residual MR severity after the MitraClip procedure.[26] CMR performed very well in the quantitation of MR after MitraClip insertion and had excellent reproducibility compared with echocardiographic methods. CMR is a potentially useful technique for the comprehensive evaluation of residual regurgitation in patients after MitraClip

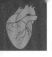

PreCTA

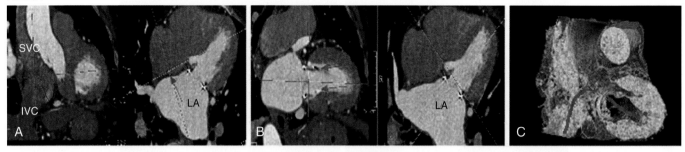

Procedural TEE

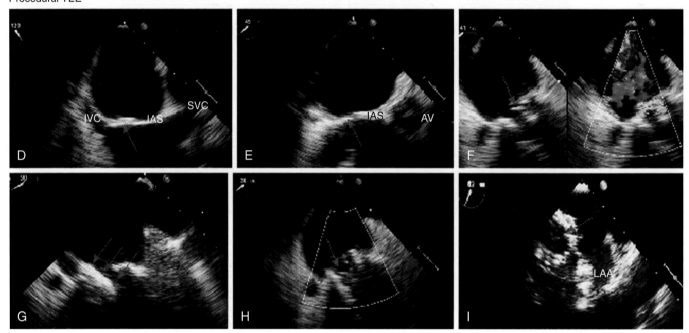

Fig. 21.5 Computed Tomographic Angiography (CTA) of Mitral Valve-in-Valve Procedures. CTA images *(dashed lines* and *red arrows)* are used for preprocedural planning. (A) Proposed position of the transseptal puncture in orthogonal views. The superior vena cava *(SVC)* and inferior vena cava *(IVC)* are shown with *arrows* defining the puncture position. The trajectories of the valve deployment catheters into the bioprosthetic struts are modeled from these images. (B) The relationship of the valve and the LV outflow tract is modeled for positioning the valve and determining the relative residual outflow tract size after the stent-mounted valve is deployed. (C) A 3D volumetric model of the pathway and trajectory *(red line)* of a catheter-mounted valve system is shown from the transseptal puncture to within the struts. Intraprocedural images were obtained with the use of a pediatric TEE probe to perform the valve-in-valve procedure. In orthogonal single views, bicaval (D) and short-axis (E) displays at the aortic valve *(AV)*, the *arrows* define the position of the transseptal puncture in relation to the prior atriotomy patch or suture. (F) With the use of a color-compare method, the prolapse of the bioprosthetic valve leaflet is shown *(arrows)*, along with the significant eccentrically directed regurgitant jet. (G) The stent-mounted valve is shown within the bioprosthetic valve struts *(arrows)*. The deployed stent and valve. (H and I) The deployed valve in valve *(red arrows)*. IAS, Interatrial septum; *LAA,* left atrial appendage.

intervention. Cross-sectional imaging, including CT and CMR, is increasingly being integrated into the evaluation of mitral and tricuspid valve disease.[53]

Campbell-Washburn et al. provided an overview of the imaging technology used in CMR-guided cardiac interventions. They outlined clinical targets, standard image acquisition and analysis tools, and the integration of these tools into the clinical workflow.[54]

Multislice Computed Tomography

Multislice computed tomography (MSCT) is a valuable technique in the preprocedural evaluation of patients being considered for TCMVP because it allows characterization of LV geometry and MV

anatomy and geometry.[27] It has been particularly helpful for patients undergoing mitral valve-in-valve procedures (Fig. 21.5). In patients with moderate to severe functional mitral regurgitation (FMR), asymmetric remodeling of the MV is observed, with tethering of the mitral leaflets at the central and posteromedial levels. MSCT provides anatomic and geometric analysis of the MV apparatus and may be of value to guide surgical treatment of FMR.

Shanks et al.[28] demonstrated the accuracy and clinical feasibility of the assessment of MV geometry with 3D TEE; they were comparable to those of the MSCT measurements. 3D TEE and MSCT provide accurate and complementary information in the evaluation of patients with MV disease.

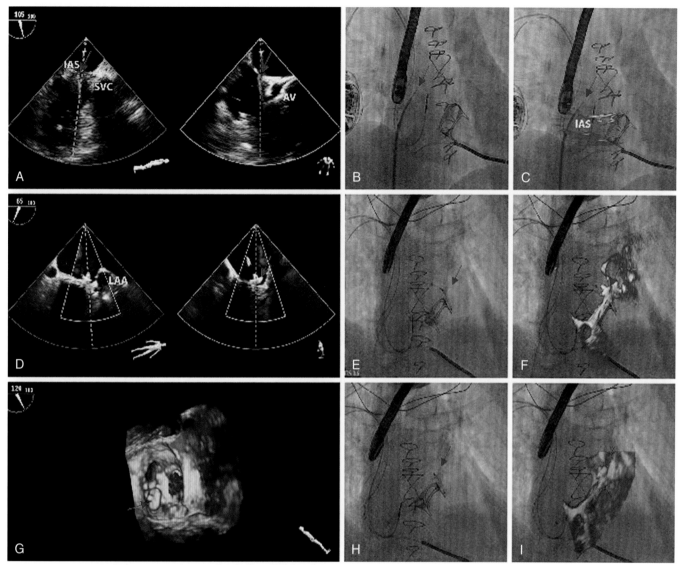

Fig. 21.6 EchoNavigator System Applied to Closure of a Paravalvular Leak. Procedural images for closure of a mitral valve paravalvular leak are shown. (A) Transseptal puncture positioning *(arrows)* is shown in a biplane display of orthogonal views of the interatrial septum *(IAS)*. (B) The needle is visible *(arrow)*, but it is hard to know where in space it is positioned without tissue verification. (C) Using an echocardiographic and fluoroscopic IAS overlay, the septum and needle are viewed together *(arrow)* with confidence of position. (D) The bioprosthetic valve ring is shown with biplane imaging and color-flow Doppler. Notice the vascular plug within the paravalvular leak *(arrow)*, with minimal residual leak after closure. (E) Fluoroscopic image shows the plug adjacent to the sewing ring of the valve. (F) Overlay-fused image shows the device location *(arrow)* and the lack of residual leak after the device has been appropriately positioned. (G) A 3D image from the atrium shows the vascular plug device at a 7-o'clock position in the paravalvular leak *(arrow)*. (H) The metal from the mitral valve sewing ring is seen with the adjacent plug *(arrow)*. (I) The fused tissue with metal valve structure is shown *(arrow)* in the overlay images. *AV,* Aortic valve; *LAA,* left atrial appendage; *SVC,* superior vena cava.

Mak et al. compared 3D TEE and MSCT in patients with severe MR being considered for transcatheter mitral valve implantation (TMVI).[29] The results supported use of 3D TEE as a complementary tool to CT assessment of the D-shaped mitral annulus to determine mitral annulus size.

Advanced Imaging Tools
Echocardiographic-Fluoroscopic Fusion Imaging
X-ray fluoroscopy provides high-contrast and high-definition images of catheters and devices, whereas 3D TEE is better for visualizing soft tissue cardiac anatomy. EchoNavigator (Philips Healthcare, Andover, MA) is a system in which the two modalities are combined, with a 3D TEE volume registered to and overlaid on an x-ray projection image in real time[30,31,55–59] (Figs. 21.6 and 21.7).

Because both fluoroscopic and echocardiographic images are obtained in real time, the fused image is ideal for performing many of the tasks required for various mitral interventions. The operator can focus on the composite image with all important objects being visualized rather than glancing back and forth between two separate image displays. Eye-hand coordination is facilitated because fluoroscopic

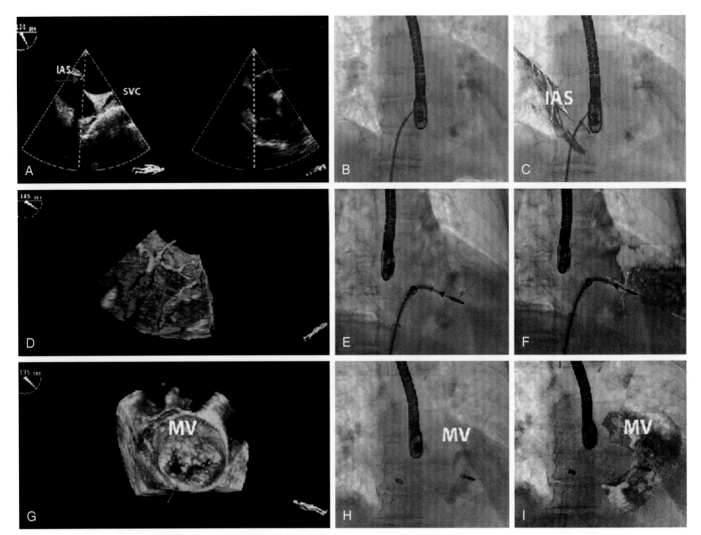

Fig. 21.7 EchoNavigator System Used in MitraClip Repair. (A–C) The transseptal puncture process for a mitral valve *(MV)* clipping procedure was used to treat valvular regurgitation. Biplane echocardiographic images (A) depict a transseptal puncture *(arrows)* with the needle across the interatrial septum *(IAS)*. The fluoroscopic image (B) and the EchoNavigator fused echocardiographic-fluoroscopic image (C) show the interatrial septum and needle superimposed for tissue structure image concordance. This provides the interventional cardiologist a view of the tissue landmarks in conjunction with device positioning within a 3D space. (D) A 3D image shows the clip with grasp of the anterior and posterior leaflets *(arrow)*. Only the closed clip *(arrow)* can be appreciated in the fluoroscopic image (E), whereas both the tissue grasp and the closed clip *(arrow)* are shown in the EchoNavigator overlay image of the two methods (F). (G) Successful mitral clip placement is shown *(arrow)* in a focused 3D echocardiographic image viewed from the left atrial perspective with the dual-orifice MV. (H) The clip is located in the center of the ring of mitral annular calcification. (I) In the overlay of mitral valve tissue, the calcification ring and the clip have identical positions *(arrow)*. *SVC,* Superior vena cava.

perspective is what most interventionalists use for navigation tasks. Kim et al. reported the use of echocardiographic-fluoroscopic (echo-fluoro) fusion imaging to guide transcatheter aortic valve replacement.[60] Guidance of transseptal puncture with real-time fusion imaging during the MitraClip procedure and left atrial appendage closure proved to be safe and efficient in terms of reduction of time until transseptal puncture.[61]

Faletra et al.[62] described their experience with echo-fluoro fusion imaging in patients undergoing MitraClip, Cardioband, and PVL closure interventions and highlighted the potential of this technique to become the main imaging modality in catheter-based structural heart disease interventions.

Overlay of Computed Tomography and Fluoroscopy

Because of its 2D nature, fluoroscopic imaging alone often does not provide adequate anatomic detail for guiding structural heart disease interventions. The modern C-arm is capable of acquiring CT-like 3D images by rotational image acquisition with 3D reconstruction algorithms and overlaying them on the fluoroscopic image. This new technology provides a substantial degree of anatomic guidance for catheter and device manipulation.[63]

Overlay of 3D CT data onto real-time procedural fluoroscopic images in the cardiac catheterization laboratory is feasible to aid procedural guidance. Registration between the two images needs to be completed, but even with this action, the real-time fluoroscopic image

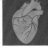

VOLUME   SLICES   MODEL

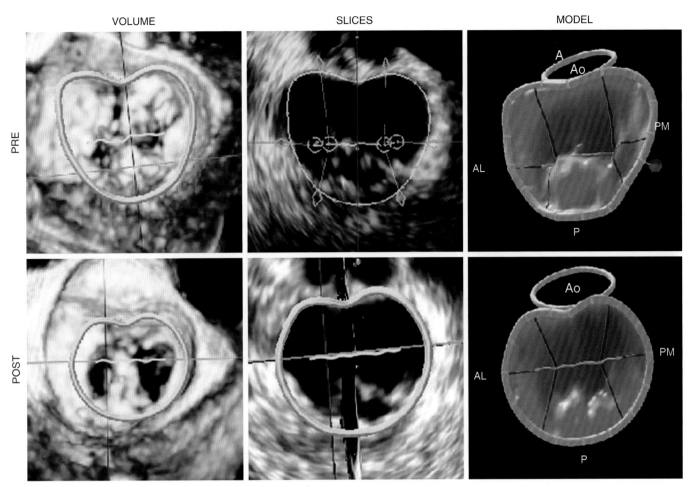

Fig. 21.8 Mitral Valve 3D Model (Video 21.8 ▶). Mitral valve modeling obtained before and after MitraClip repair. The volume format *(left column)* demonstrates the 3D appearance of the mitral valve as seen from the left atrium with the mitral annulus outlined in *yellow*. The slices format *(center column)* illustrates the 2D appearance with the annulus demarcated in *yellow*. The *yellow wavy line* in the center of the images represents the line of coaptation of the mitral valve. The *small green circles* represent the commissures and the position of the papillary muscles. The model format *(right column)* is a computer-generated model of the mitral apparatus as seen from the left atrium perspective. The anteroposterior diameter of the mitral valve decreased from 42 to 37 mm, the mediolateral diameter increased from 46 to 48 mm, and the annular circumference decreased from 162 to 147 mm after Mitra-Clip application. The MitraClip had a therapeutic effect due to two mechanisms: enhancement of leaflet coaptation and modification of the mitral annulus. *A,* Anterior; *AL,* anterior leaflet; *Ao,* aorta; *P,* posterior; *PM,* postero-medial.

is only intermittently registered to the static CT-derived image. This overlay is considered most helpful for patients undergoing PVL closure and pulmonary vein stenting.[32]

CT fusion overlay represents another iterative advancement in the application of advanced imaging technology aimed at achieving the goal of enhanced procedural safety and efficacy.[64] Schulz et al. reported the transapical implantation of a transcatheter aortic valve prosthesis into a mitral annuloplasty ring guided by real-time 3D cardiac CT-fluoroscopic fusion imaging.[65]

Mitral Valve 3D Modeling

Full-volume 3D TEE datasets can be digitally stored and transferred to a workstation with Philips Q-Laboratory MV quantification software (Philips Healthcare) for off-line analysis (Fig. 21.8). Complete 3D delineation of the annulus is obtained, and the software calculates the annular parameters in 3D space, including annular area, circumference, intercommissural diameter, anteroposterior diameter, and height.[66]

Using 3D TEE MV modeling, Al Amri et al. demonstrated that percutaneous MitraClip therapy affects MV geometry in patients with

FMR by increasing coaptation length and area due to a larger contribution of the anterior mitral leaflet to coaptation after the procedure.[33] Patzelt et al. demonstrated mechanical approximation of both MV annulus edges with improved MV annular coaptation by percutaneous mitral valve replacement (PMVR) using the MitraClip system, correlating with the degree of residual MR in patients with MR.[67]

Rapid Prototyping

Rapid prototyping, a process by which 3D digital surface models are converted into physical models, represents the next evolution in advanced image display and may serve as a means to improve TC-MVP guidance.[68–70] Ultimately, the technology may be used to enhance the level of care provided to the growing number of patients with structural heart defects.[36] With the unique capabilities afforded by modern imaging modalities such as MSCT, CMR, and 3D echocardiography, rapid prototyping has begun an expansion into medical applications in which it may directly affect patient care. The use of rapid prototyping in a patient with prosthetic mitral PVL has been described.[71]

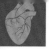

A physical model of a patient's heart can help the proceduralist understand 3D relationships, plan the intervention, and practice deployment of devices. The major barriers to the use of rapid prototyping have been the need to segment the image and produce the file format for printing and the cost of printing, which is often several thousand dollars.

GENERAL APPROACH

Assessment of Mitral Valve Morphology and Function

When considering a patient for TCMVP, the surgeon needs to first determine that the MV morphology and degree of dysfunction are suitable for the intervention. A detailed echocardiographic examination of the MV anatomy and pathology provides the framework to characterize the severity and type of MV dysfunction and its hemodynamic consequences.[72-75] The imager must have a comprehensive understanding of the anatomy of interest and the intended transcatheter device to be used.

In patients with rheumatic MS, the echocardiographic markers that support the use of BMC include (1) decreased mitral orifice size (usually < 1.5 cm^2), (2) commissural fusion, (3) absence of excessive leaflet thickening and calcification, (4) nonobstructive chordae tendineae, (5) absence of LA thrombus, and (6) absence of significant MR. Echocardiography permits the recognition of nonrheumatic MS, including degenerative MS (i.e., annular calcification), radiation-induced valvular MS, congenital MS, and pharmacologically induced MS.[75] These conditions can be characterized by echocardiography and usually are not amenable to transcatheter interventions.

Patients with MR being considered for TCMVP usually have significant MR[76] and have one of two categories of disease: *degenerative* (i.e., organic or primary) MR, which arises as a result of pathology affecting one or more components of the MV apparatus (see Fig. 21.8), or *functional* (i.e., secondary) MR. FMR is a consequence of annular dilation and geometric distortion of the subvalvular apparatus caused by LV dilation or dysfunction and dyssynchrony, usually associated with LV remodeling due to ischemic or nonischemic cardiomyopathy (see Figs. 21.3 and 21.4). Mixed situations involving a degenerative leaflet abnormality and a functional abnormality can also occur.

Interatrial Septum Puncture

Transseptal heart catheterization was initially used for hemodynamic assessment of the left side of the heart.[77] With the advent of echocardiography, this was no longer needed, and transseptal catheterization was rarely used for a decade, except for BMC and some ablation procedures. The advent of atrial fibrillation ablations and structural heart disease interventions has rekindled interest in transseptal puncture, and simultaneously there has been a switch from fluoroscopy and angiography as the exclusive guidance tools to TEE[78,79] and ICE[80] as complementary transseptal imaging guidance tools.

The use of echocardiography to assist transseptal puncture has improved determination of the precise location in the septum where the puncture will take place. Precision in site selection facilitates the navigation of catheters in the LA and the delivery of devices to the intended anatomic site[81]; for example, for the MitraClip procedure, a puncture site in the posterosuperior aspect of the fossa ovalis is preferred (Fig. 21.9). TEE and ICE guidance of septal puncture also provides visual clues to the soft tissue cardiac anatomy, improving the efficiency and safety of the procedure. This is particularly relevant in patients with enlarged atria or an enlarged ascending aorta because direct visualization of the interatrial septum is crucial for a safe transseptal puncture.

Catheters and Devices

The default imaging guidance technique for wires, catheters, and devices for transcatheter structural heart disease interventions is fluoroscopy. These catheters and devices have been designed to have optimal radiographic visualization. It is also possible to visualize them with echocardiography, CT, and CMR, but their rendition is not ideal, artifacts are common, and experience is required to optimally follow these devices during an interventional procedure.

IMAGING GUIDANCE OF SPECIFIC TRANSCATHETER MITRAL VALVE INTERVENTIONS

An overview of available transcatheter MV interventions is presented in Table 21.3. The following discussion focuses on the more pertinent interventions (because of frequency, relevance, and commercially available technology), including BMC, MitraClip edge-to-edge repair, paravalvular mitral prosthesis leak repair, and percutaneous replacement of a mitral prosthesis. For information on less frequent interventions that have not yet reached common clinical use, there are review articles summarizing these investigative interventions[4,5,9,82,83] and the references listed in Table 21.3.

Balloon Mitral Commissurotomy

Transthoracic and transesophageal 2D and 3D echocardiography play a central role in patient selection, procedural imaging guidance, and evaluation of results in patients with rheumatic MS who may benefit from the balloon-induced commissurotomy. Other imaging modalities, such as computed tomographic angiography (CTA) and CMR, play a minor role in the evaluation and management of patients with MS and are rarely necessary or used in these patients.

TTE is usually sufficient to characterize MS cause, severity, and suitability for BMC. TEE and fluoroscopy are the usual imaging modalities for imaging guidance during BMC and for the intraprocedural evaluation of results and detection of acute complications. TTE is used for long-term follow-up after BMC, including detection of restenosis and need for repeat BMC or surgery.

Mitral Valve Edge-to-Edge Repair
Preprocedural Imaging Planning

The MitraClip procedure has been approved for transcatheter treatment of moderate/severe or severe primary MR in symptomatic patients at high surgical risk.[108] This indication is being expanded for the treatment of symptomatic FMR.[109]

For preprocedural evaluation, TTE is usually sufficient to detect MV dysfunction; to characterize MV morphology, permitting differentiation of degenerative versus functional and mixed MR; and to define MR as moderate/severe (3+) or severe (4+), which are the grades required for MitraClip repair. TTE permits assessment of ventricular size, global and segmental function, LA volume, and the presence and severity of associated pulmonary hypertension.

Both 2D and 3D TEE provide additional structural information and aid in final selection of appropriate candidates for MitraClip repair. TEE is integral to the success of the procedure. Its role extends from assessment of suitability to intraprocedural guidance, confirmation of success, and exclusion of complications.[110]

Criteria suggesting patient suitability for MitraClip repair include a nonrheumatic cause, absence of calcification in the grasping areas, absence of severe mitral annulus calcification, absence of a cleft, absence of intracardiac mass thrombus or vegetation, a central MR jet, and an MV orifice area of at least 4 cm^2. In degenerative MR with a flail leaflet, the flail gap should be less than 10 mm and the flail width less than 15 mm. The posterior leaflet length should be 10 mm or more. In patients who have FMR with leaflet tethering, coaptation

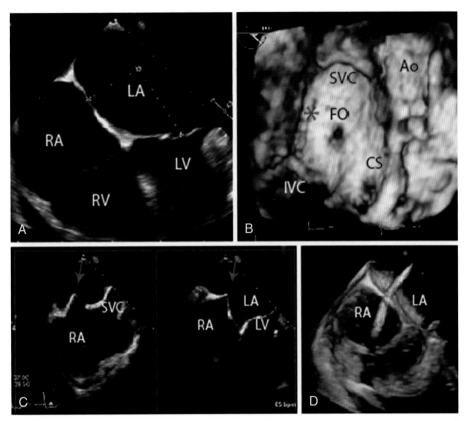

Fig. 21.9 Septal Puncture Performed for a MitraClip Procedure. (A) The vertical distance (4 cm in this case) from the mitral coaptation line to the interatrial septum *(dotted line)* is shown. (B) A 3D zoom view shows the interatrial septum from the right atrial side (Video 21.9B ▶). The tip of the catheter *(red asterisk)* is placed in the posterosuperior aspect of the fossa ovalis *(FO)*; a puncture in this area facilitates navigation of the MitraClip to the mitral valve orifice. (C) X-plane bicaval and four-chamber views of the interatrial septum illustrate tenting *(red arrows)* of the interatrial septum in the area to be punctured (Video 21.9C ▶). (D) The guide catheter is depicted with the dilator advancing from the RA to the LA (Video 21.9D ▶). *Ao,* Aorta; *CS,* coronary sinus; *IVC,* inferior vena cava; *SVC,* superior vena cava.

TABLE 21.3 Imaging Guidance of Specific Transcatheter Native Mitral Valve Interventions.		
Intervention	**Comments/Current Status**	**Imaging Comments**
Mitral Stenosis MV balloon valvuloplasty[84]	Common clinical use Has replaced surgery in most patients	Suitable anatomy and absence of significant MR characterized by echocardiography
Mitral Regurgitation ***Edge-to-Edge Mitral Repair*** MitraClip (Abbott Vascular, Abbott Park, IL)[85]	Degenerative MR: cleared for use in patients with significant symptomatic MR FMR: COAPT trial ongoing enrollment	Central role of echocardiography for patient selection, TEE procedural guidance, and evaluation of results
Transcatheter Indirect Annuloplasty (Through Coronary Sinus) Monarc (Edwards Lifesciences, Irvine CA)[86]	The Monarc device in the coronary sinus is feasible and may reduce MR, but coronary artery compression may occur in patients in whom the great cardiac vein passes over a coronary artery. Discontinued	CT to determine relation between coronary sinus and Cx TEE/fluoroscopy for determining MR severity and mechanism, procedural guidance, and evaluation of results
Viacor (Viacor, Inc., Wilmington, MA)[87]	Discontinued	TTE for preprocedural and postprocedural MR evaluation Fluoroscopy and TEE for intraprocedural guidance
Carillon Mitral Contour System (Cardiac Dimensions Inc., Kirkland, WA)[88]	TITAN trial CE mark approval	CT to determine relation between coronary sinus and Cx TEE/fluoroscopy for intraprocedural guidance

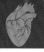

TABLE 21.3   Imaging Guidance of Specific Transcatheter Native Mitral Valve Interventions.—cont'd

Intervention	Comments/Current Status	Imaging Comments
Transcatheter Direct Annuloplasty		
Cardioband (Valtech Cardio Ltd., Or Yehuda, Israel)[89,90]	Ongoing clinical trial	Fluoroscopy and 3D TEE guidance required
GDS AccuCinch Annuloplasty System (Graduated Delivery Systems, Santa Clara, CA)[91]	Another direct annuloplasty device using the retrograde transventricular approach. A series of anchors are implanted in the subannular space beneath the MV in the base of the LV	Reduction of MR quantified as regurgitant volume and effective regurgitant area by echocardiography
Adjustable Annuloplasty Ring (Mitral Solutions, Fort Lauderdale, FL)[92]	This new deformable nickel–titanium (nitinol)–based annuloplasty ring is heated for 45 s, which induces a change of geometry to a preformed shape, reducing the anterior-posterior diameter.	TTE evaluations conducted at the follow-up time points. TEE evaluations are conducted during the surgical procedure and during the ring adjustment.
Dynamic Annuloplasty Ring System (MiCardia, Irvine, CA)[93]	Nitinol-based dynamic complete ring that allows modification of the septal-lateral diameter	TEE guidance in the loaded beating heart after MV repair
ReCor (QuantumCor, Inc., Lake Forest, CA)[94]	Therapeutic ultrasound energy application to the mitral annulus is feasible percutaneously. A reduction in annular dimensions occurs immediately and appears to be durable without peri-annular damage. Animal model	Relative to baseline, MV annular diameter reduction (measured by TTE) was 8.4% immediately after application
Transcatheter Chordal Replacement		
NeoChord (Neochord, Inc., Minnetonka, MN)[95]	The NeoChord DS1000 consists of a handheld instrument designed to load and deploy sutures through the LV apex.	The NeoChord DS1000 is directed toward the left atrium with 2D TEE guidance, avoiding native subvalvular apparatus coupling
Transcatheter LV Remodeling		
iCoapsys (Myocor, Inc., Maple Grove, MN)[96]	Analysis of RESTOR-MV trial indicates patients with FMR requiring revascularization treated with ventricular reshaping rather than standard surgery had improved survival and a significant decrease in major adverse outcomes.	MR was evaluated in a core laboratory by one of two observers. MR was graded as 1 (mild), 2 (moderate), 3 (moderate to severe), or 4 (severe).
Parachute (CardioKinetix, Palo Alto, CA)[97]	A novel catheter-based LV partitioning device is available for the treatment of patients with severe systolic dysfunction after anteroapical myocardial infarction with regional wall motion abnormalities.	CT demonstrated a significant reduction in volume of the dynamic LV compartment (that which was not excluded by the device) after implantation, accompanied by a significant reduction in dyskinetic motion and a trend toward an improved ejection fraction.

CT, Computed tomography; *Cx*, circumflex artery; *FMR*, functional mitral regurgitation; *MR*, mitral regurgitation; *MV*, mitral valve; *RESTOR-MV*, Randomized Evaluation of a Surgical Treatment for Off-Pump Repair of the Mitral Valve.

depth should be less than 11 mm, and coaptation length should be at least 2 mm.[11,111]

In patients undergoing MitraClip therapy, a transmitral pressure gradient of 4 mmHg or greater, an effective regurgitant area of 70.8 mm^2 or greater, or an MV orifice area of 3.0 cm^2 or less indicates an increased risk of procedural failure.[112] The 3D TEE–derived MV orifice area predicts postprocedural MS after one-clip implantation; however, the preprocedural mediolateral diameter of the LV inflow orifice is more useful to predict the result after two-clip implantation.[113]

The use of percutaneous edge-to-edge mitral repair for patients with worse baseline echocardiographic features appears to have similar rates of safety and efficacy when compared with the standard echocardiographic inclusion criteria previously described.[114] These results suggest that as experience is gained with the edge-to-edge repair, there will be opportunities to expand its use. The technology is undergoing improvements, including the MitraClip XTR system (Abbott Vascular, Santa Clara, CA),[115] and other device manufacturers are developing their own systems for edge-to-edge repair.

Among predictors of mortality after edge-to-edge PMVR, severe tricuspid regurgitation (TR) at baseline is the most important. Patients with no improvement of TR at 30 days after PMVR have a significantly higher mortality rate at follow-up.[116] This fact is prompting increasing interest in the potential combined use of the MitraClip procedure for MR and TR[117,118] and in the use of the MitraClip system for transcatheter treatment of severe TR.[119]

Intraprocedural Guidance

Imaging guidance of the MitraClip procedure is done with fluoroscopy and 2D and 3D TEE (Figs. 21.10, 21.11, and 21.12). It is good practice to obtain an intraprocedural baseline TEE to reassess MV morphology, MR severity under general anesthesia, LV size and function, MV gradients, presence or absence of pulmonary flow reversal, absence of left atrial appendage thrombus, TR severity, and pulmonary artery systolic pressure.

After conventional peripheral access through the right femoral vein and under direct fluoroscopic guidance, a guidewire is advanced into the superior vena cava. This is followed by advancement of the

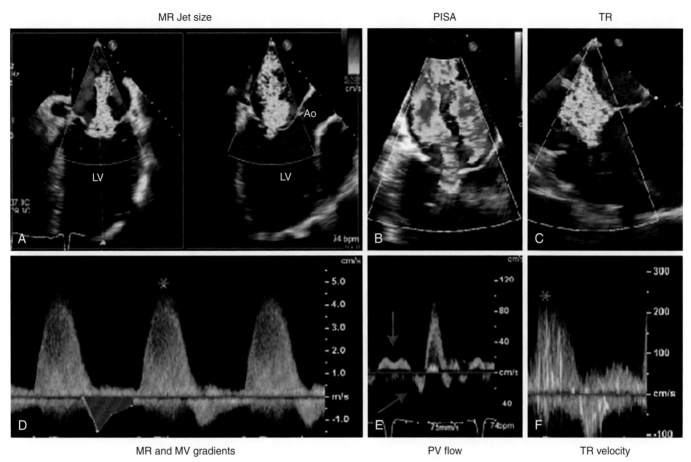

Fig. 21.10 Assessment of Mitral Regurgitation (MR) Severity and Hemodynamics Before Percutaneous Mitral Valve Repair. (A) Severe MR is assessed by the color-flow area filling the left atrium (Video 21.10A ▶). MR is demonstrated in the bicommissural and LV outflow tract views. (B) A large-diameter (8-mm) proximal isovelocity surface area (PISA) is demonstrated, consistent with severe MR. (C) Associated severe tricuspid regurgitation *(TR)*. The TR velocity is only 2.5 m/s (see F), but the severe TR, because of right ventricular/right atrial pressure equalization, makes TR velocity estimates unreliable for pulmonary artery pressure determination. (D) MR jet velocity of about 5 m/s *(red asterisk)*. The mean mitral valve (MV) gradient (2 mmHg) and the maximal mitral gradient (5 mmHg) are estimated from the mitral inflow velocity time integral *(red)*; in this case, neither gradient is of concern for MitraClip implantation. (E) A left upper pulmonary vein *(PV)* pulsed-Doppler recording illustrates systolic blunting *(top arrow)* and mild systolic flow reversal *(bottom arrow)*, consistent with severe MR. (F) TR velocity graph; *asterisk* indicates peak TR velocity. *Ao*, Aorta.

catheter or needle that, under fluoroscopic and TEE guidance, is slowly withdrawn until it drops under the limbic edge. With TEE guidance, the location of the septal puncture is selected using three 2D TEE planes: the bicaval view at 90 to 120 degrees for superior-inferior orientation, a short-axis view at the base of 40 to 60 degrees, and a four-chamber view at 0 degrees to determine the correct height above the mitral annulus.

The optimal septal puncture height above the MV is different in degenerative MR and FMR. In patients with degenerative MR, the puncture site should be 4 to 5 cm above the annulus to provide adequate space to maneuver the catheter and device. In patients with FMR, because of the additional distance that tenting provides, the puncture site needs to be somewhat lower, approximately 3.5 cm from the annulus or 4 to 4.5 cm from the leaflet coaptation point. Care is taken to visualize the tip of the needle in the apex of the tenting septum produced by the pressure exerted by the catheter or needle on the interatrial septum. In patients in whom the MR is more lateral, the distance from the puncture site and the target mitral coaptation plane

is increased, the septal puncture should be on the lower range of the optimal puncture point. The opposite (i.e., septal puncture on the upper range of the optimal puncture point) needs to be considered if there is medial MR.

After the catheter or needle is confirmed to be in the right location and pointing posteriorly away from the aorta, the needle is advanced or radiofrequency energy is used to cross the septum. When the needle crosses the interatrial septum, a small "give" motion is felt; the tip of the needle is visualized in the LA by TEE, and microbubbles are frequently seen in the LA. An LA pressure curve becomes evident on the hemodynamic registration.

TEE is particularly helpful in the setting of atrial septal abnormalities such as a resistant septum, a very large left or right atrium, a bulging septum, an atrial septal aneurysm, or a dilated aorta. In these situations, TEE adds confidence for the operator in puncturing the septum in a safe and appropriate location.

After the septal puncture has been accomplished, the catheter is advanced across the septum, the needle is withdrawn, and, under

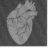

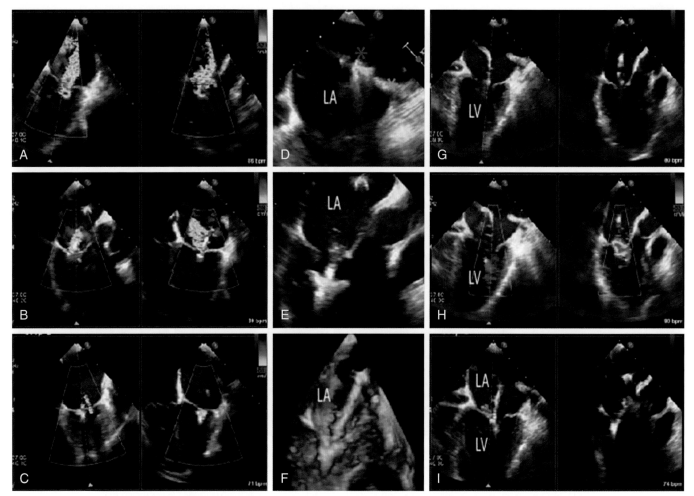

Fig. 21.11 MitraClip Procedure With TEE Guidance. This MitraClip procedure for severe functional mitral regurgitation (MR) required two clips. (A–C) X-plane views with color (bicommissural and left ventricular [LV] outflow tract views) illustrate MR severity at different times during the procedure. (A) Baseline image shows severe central MR (Video 21.11A ▶). (B) Persistent moderate MR after application of one clip (Video 21.11B ▶). (C) Trace MR after application of the second clip (Video 21.11C ▶). (D) The clip (red asterisk) is being navigated in the LA, bypassing the Coumadin ridge (green asterisk) (Video 21.11D ▶). (E) The clip with open arms (i.e., arrowhead appearance) is in the LV, just inferior to the mitral valve (MV) (Video 21.11E ▶). (F) A 3D rendition of the MitraClip grasping the mitral leaflets (Video 21.11F ▶). (G) The MitraClip approximates the central part of the MV orifice. (H) Color Doppler imaging is used to direct the clip to the area of the MV where the MR originates. (I) The MitraClip is grasping the leaflets.

fluoroscopic and TEE guidance, a guidewire is advanced into the left superior pulmonary vein to serve as an anchor for advancement of the large delivery catheter. Subsequently, the clip delivery system is advanced out of the guiding catheter and, with TEE and fluoroscopic guidance, the entire system is navigated using the knobs to change the curvature of the system to align it to the MV while avoiding contact with the atrial walls and the Coumadin ridge (see Fig. 21.11D).

Under fluoroscopy and 2D and 3D TEE guidance, the clip delivery system is navigated toward the MV orifice with a trajectory appropriate for the location of the regurgitant jet. Using biplane TEE, the left ventricular outflow tract (LVOT) and bicommissural views are simultaneously presented and used for further precise alignment of the clip into the MV region of interest. The LVOT perspective allows anteroposterior corrections of the clip path, and the bicommissural view allows correction of the mediolateral path.

Before the clip is advanced into the LV, an additional step to orient the clip perpendicular to the line of coaptation of the MV is needed. This can be best accomplished when guided by an *en-face* view of the

MV from the LA perspective. Clockwise or counter-clockwise rotation of the open clip is performed until the clip arms are perpendicular to the MV coaptation line and in the area of maximal MR. Next, the clip is advanced with the arms open into the LV and is then closed to a 120-degree angle for subsequent grasping. In the LVOT view, the clip has an arrowhead appearance, confirming that the arms are perpendicular to the MV coaptation line.

After the MitraClip is in the LV and after confirmation that it is not entrapped by chordae tendineae, it is pulled back toward the MV in an attempt to grasp the mitral leaflets. After the leaflets are apposed to the open clip arms, they are grasped by lowering the nitinol grippers, and the clip is closed, but not to its tightest extent. Attention is then turned to assessment of the adequacy of leaflet capture using both 2D and 3D echocardiography. Key findings of a successful capture of both leaflets include reduced movement of leaflets in the grasped region, visualization of each leaflet inserting into the clip, and documentation of a tissue bridge using a 3D *en-face* view from the LA perspective.

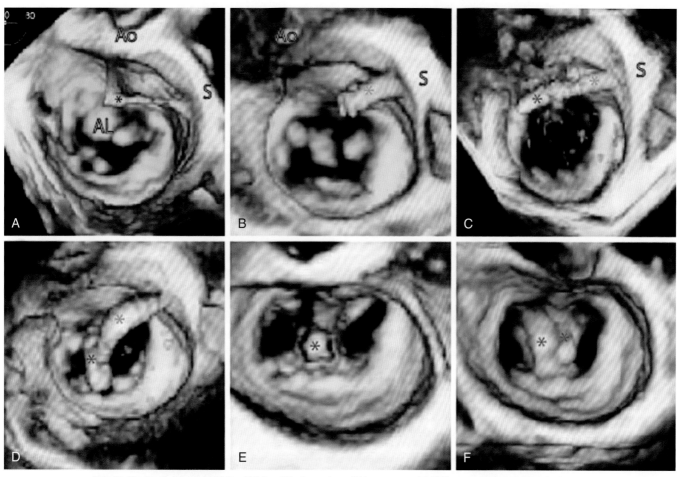

Fig. 21.12 3D Guidance of Mitral Valve Clip Insertion. All images are 3D TEE zoom views of the mitral valve as seen from the left atrium (LA). The aorta *(Ao)* is anterior; the interatrial septum *(S)* is medial. (A) The guidewire *(asterisk)* is seen in the LA. (B) The delivery catheter *(asterisk)* has been advanced into the LA (Video 21.12B ▶). (C) The MitraClip *(red asterisk)* has been advanced through the delivery catheter *(green asterisk)* into the LA. (D) The MitraClip *(red asterisk)* has been directed toward the mitral valve orifice, guided by the delivery catheter *(green asterisk)*. (E) The MitraClip *(asterisk)* has grasped the anterior and posterior mitral leaflets, producing a double-orifice mitral valve, and is ready to be realized. (F) Because the patient had significant residual MR after placement of the first clip, an additional clip was deployed; *asterisks* indicate the two clips.

After adequate grasp of both leaflets is confirmed, the presence and severity of residual MR is documented from multiple views, and the clip is completely tightened, which typically results in further reduction of the MR. At this point, the MV has a double orifice, and the transmitral gradient in each of the orifices is documented. Most patients have a mild degree of stenosis; ideally, the gradient through each orifice should be less than 5 to 8 mmHg.

The clip is released if the following criteria are met: there is minimal residual MR; no other significant MR jets are produced at a different location; and there is no significant MS. Under fluoroscopy and TEE guidance, the clip delivery system is removed, with care taken to avoid contact of the metal spear at the end of the system with the LA wall, and then LA pressure is measured using the guiding catheter. The guiding catheter is then pulled back into the right atrium, and the iatrogenic ASD is assessed. The guiding catheter is removed, and hemostasis is achieved with various approaches, including percutaneous suture closure.

If there is residual 2+ or greater MR medial or lateral to the first clip, the surgeon must consider either moving the clip to a more favorable position or placing one or more additional clips. Occasionally, there is another jet quite distant from the first clip that needs to

be treated. The placement of additional clips follows procedural steps similar to those for implantation of the first clip; however, the advancement of the clip into the LV is done with the clip arms closed to avoid dislodging the first clip, and the arrowhead appearance of the clip is not seen.

When there is more than one clip in the echocardiographic field of view, it is challenging to differentiate between them. It is helpful to search for the clip that is still connected to the delivery catheter to recognize which is the clip of interest. It is increasingly common to place two clips but quite unusual to place three or more clips. Before releasing an additional clip, it is important to assess the resultant mean mitral gradient and determine the MV area by using planimetry for the size of both orifices. The mitral gradient needs to be assessed in the context of the heart rate because a mean gradient of 7 mmHg with a heart rate of 60 beats/min may be significantly higher when the patient is awake and physically active.

Reports have documented the feasibility of implanting the Amplatzer Vascular Plug II (AVP-II, St. Jude Medical, St. Paul, MN) between two MitraClips (i.e., intraclip) and of treating commissural periclip MR when only one MitraClip is placed[120,121] (Figs. 21.13 and 21.14).

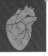

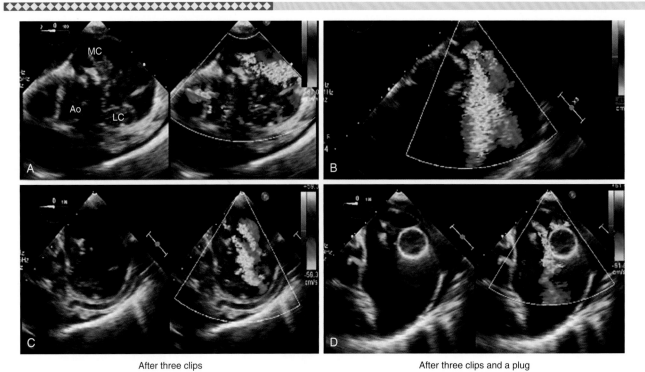

After three clips   After three clips and a plug

Fig. 21.13 Three Clips and a Vascular Plug. An 87-year-old patient had severe degenerative mitral regurgitation (MR). Transgastric TEE views were obtained during a MitraClip procedure. (A) Before clip placement, imaging demonstrates severe MR originating near the middle commissure *(MC)* (Video 21.13A ▶). (B) Within a few minutes after deployment of the first clip, worsening of MR was observed (Video 21.13B ▶). (C) After deployment of three clips, persistent moderate/severe MR was still present (Video 21.13C ▶). (D) A 20-mm Amplatzer vascular plug *(circle)* was placed between the medial clips, reducing the MR to a mild level (Video 21.13D ▶). *Ao,* Aorta; *LC,* lateral commissure.

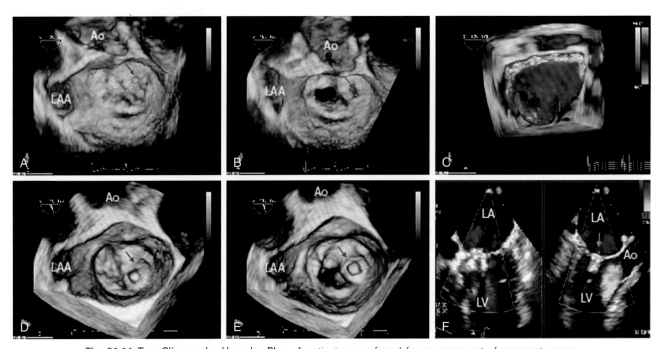

Fig. 21.14 Two Clips and a Vascular Plug. A patient was referred for management of recurrent severe mitral regurgitation (MR) after placement of two MitraClips. (A) A systolic frame of the mitral valve as seen from the left atrium. A MitraClip *(asterisk)* and residual flail chordae in the medial commissure *(arrow)* are seen (Video 21.14A ▶). (B) A diastolic frame demonstrates a double-orifice mitral valve with a miniscule medial orifice *(arrow)* between the two MitraClips *(asterisks)* and a larger lateral orifice lateral to the medial clip. (C) An eccentric MR jet *(arrows)* is seen originating between the clips and traversing the entire left atrial width, ending in the left atrial appendage *(LAA)* (Video 21.14C ▶). The medial mitral orifice was thought to be too small to take an additional clip, and a 10-mm Amplatzer Vascular Plug II was placed between the MitraClips, obliterating the residual MR. (D) The deployed vascular plug *(arrow)* during systole (Video 21.14D ▶). (E) The vascular plug *(arrow)* during diastole. (F) A color X-plane view illustrates the absence of MR after deployment of the vascular plug *(red arrow)* (Video 21.14F ▶). The *green arrow* points to the medial MitraClip. *Ao,* Aorta.

Postprocedural Assessment

After the delivery catheter is removed, documentation of the residual ASD in the area of septal puncture is documented.[122] Usually, this is small with unidirectional left-to-right shunting, and it can be left alone because it is likely to spontaneously close in a few months. However, in some patients, a large residual ASD exists, and if it persists 1 year after the procedure, there is an increased chance of right-sided heart enlargement, worsening TR, and a higher rate of rehospitalization for heart failure.[122] Placement of a percutaneous ASD occluder should be considered if there is acute right ventricular dysfunction[123] or if the ASD shunt is large, especially with torn septal tissue or significant right-to-left shunting that could result in systemic hypoxemia (Fig. 21.15).

Before the TEE probe is removed, a systematic search for potential complications is performed. Assessment of the MV area by 3D TEE can predict hemodynamic response and postprocedural prognosis after Mitra-Clip therapy.[124] The surgeon needs to search for a pericardial effusion and possible tamponade, which usually results from the transseptal puncture (i.e., due to puncture of the aorta or back wall of the atrium) (Fig. 21.16). Throughout the procedure, it is important to be on the lookout for thrombus, particularly near the area of the septal puncture (Fig. 21.17).

It is important to obtain a TTE study before the patient is discharged. This provides a final assessment in the waking state of the degree of residual MR, the transmitral gradient, changes in LV function, the nature of shunting through the iatrogenic ASD, and estimated pulmonary artery systolic pressure.

Paravalvular Mitral Prosthesis Leak Repair

A significant mitral PVL, without infection, can develop soon after surgery or many years after mitral valve replacement; 96.2% of patients are free of major PVLs at 10 years and 86.9% at 20 years.[125] Because reoperation for PVL in some patients carries substantial mortality and morbidity risks, catheter-based procedures have emerged.[98,126,127] In the most recent AHA/ACC guidelines on valvular heart disease, percutaneous repair of paravalvular prosthetic regurgitation is recommended for patients with severe symptoms or hemolysis who are at high surgical risk and who have suitable anatomic features (i.e., class IIa recommendation).[1]

Percutaneous PVL repair requires special interventional skills and unique equipment. Imaging guidance is required before and during the procedure to characterize the location, number, and size of the leaks; to determine the approach to be employed to cross the defect (transseptal, retrograde transaortic, or direct transapical); and to aid with the complexities of intraprocedural guidance.[128–131]

Preprocedural Imaging Planning

The main goals of preprocedural characterization of mitral PVL are (1) to determine the presence, size, and severity of a PVL; (2) to define

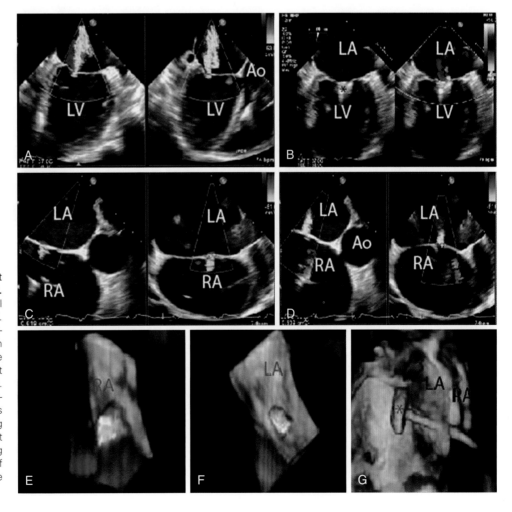

Fig. 21.15 Large Atrial Septal Defect (ASD) After MitraClip Placement. (A) A patient had severe mixed mitral regurgitation (MR) (Video 21.15A). (B) He underwent a successful Mitra-Clip procedure (Video 21.15B), with resulting trace residual MR. After the procedure, an ASD with a significant bidirectional shunt was detected. (C) The left-to-right shunt. (D) The right-to-left shunt. (E) The left-to-right shunt is demonstrated with color 3D imaging (Video 21.15E). (F) The right-to-left shunt is depicted with color 3D imaging (Video 21.15F). (G) Deployment of an 8-mm Amplatzer ASD closure device (asterisk) (Video 21.15G).

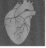
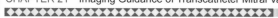

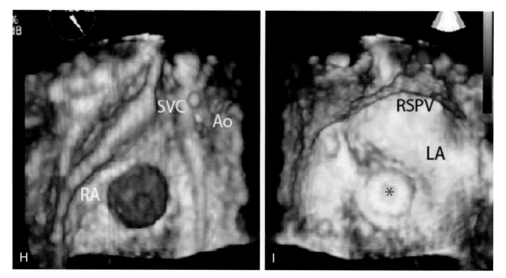

Fig. 21.15, cont'd (H) The deployed device (*asterisk*) is seen from the right atrium (Video 21.15H ▶). (I) The deployed device is seen from the left atrium. *Ao*, Aorta; *RSPV*, right superior pulmonary vein; *SVC*, superior vena cava.

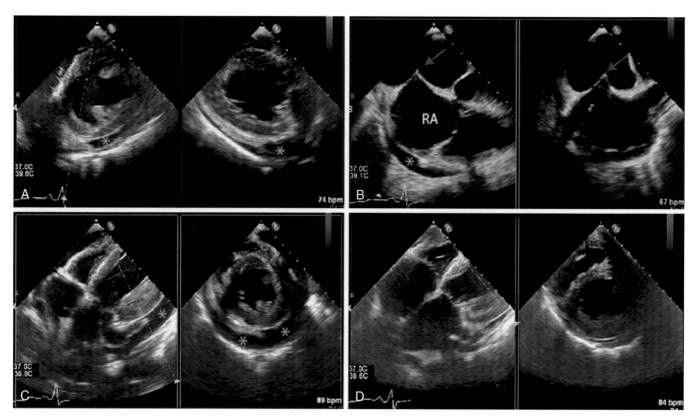

Fig. 21.16 Pericardial Effusion After a Mitraclip Procedure. A patient with severe functional mitral regurgitation (MR) underwent a MitraClip procedure and developed a large pericardial effusion of unclear cause. Cardiac tamponade was resolved after drainage of 270 mL of a bloody pericardial effusion. The MitraClip procedure was successfully completed with amelioration of the MR from severe to mild. (A) A small pericardial effusion (*asterisk*) was present at the beginning of the case, highlighting the need to document and follow the size of any pericardial effusion from the start of an intervention (Video 21.16A ▶). (B) Septal tenting (*arrow*) occurred in the middle of the fossa and away from the aorta and posterior left atrial wall (Video 21.16B ▶). The *asterisk* denotes the pericardial effusion. (C) Development of a large circumferential effusion (*asterisks*) (Video 21.16C ▶). (D) A residual trivial pericardial effusion (*asterisk*) was detected after drainage of 270 mL of pericardial fluid (Video 21.16D ▶).

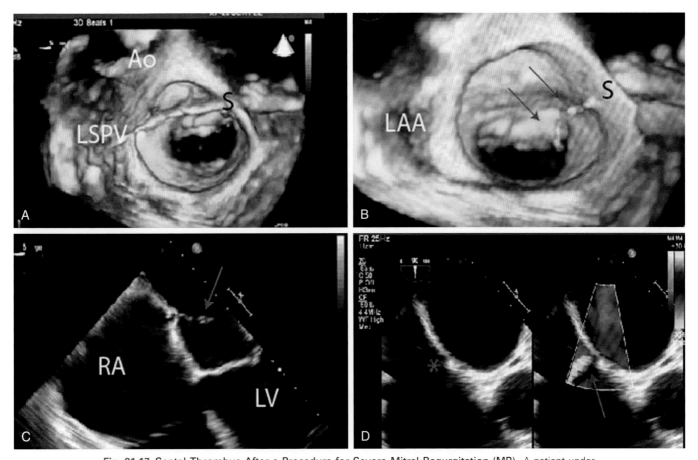

Fig. 21.17 Septal Thrombus After a Procedure for Severe Mitral Regurgitation (MR). A patient underwent a MitraClip procedure for severe MR. A mobile mass in the LA and attached to the interatrial septum was observed in the area of a septal puncture soon after cannulation of the left superior pulmonary vein *(LSPV)* through the septal puncture site. The differential diagnosis included a thrombus on the area of the septal puncture and septal tissue from a catheter-induced septal tear. The mass appeared stable, and the decision was made to proceed with the MitraClip procedure, which was completed successfully, reducing the MR from 3+ to 1+. (A) The guide catheter in the LSPV and the area of the septum *(S)* that was punctured are shown. (B) 3D TEE view of the mass *(arrows)* from the LA (Video 21.17B ▶). (C) 2D TEE four-chamber view depicts the mass *(arrow)* in the LA, originating from the area of the septal puncture. The plan was to use an atrial septal defect (ASD) occluder device at the end of the procedure to close the ASD and immobilize the LA mass. (D) However, this was aborted because the mass was no longer present and there was only mild unidirectional left-to-right shunting at the end of the procedure. The *asterisk* demarcates the area of ASD, and the *arrow* points to the left-to-right shunt. The patient did not have any clinical evidence of systemic embolization. *Ao,* Aorta; *LAA,* left atrial appendage.

the presence or absence of associated central prosthetic insufficiency or stenosis; and (3) to assess the potential location of transseptal puncture to optimize catheter trajectories to the PVL. This is usually done with TEE guidance, which can determine the exact location of the defect using helpful anatomic landmarks for reference.

TEE assessment uses the surgical view and a triangulation method[127] (i.e., anterior aorta, lateral left atrial appendage, and medial interatrial septum) or an orientation based on the face of a clock with the aorta in the 12-o'clock position.[128,130] CTA is also used for this purpose and may yield complementary information on the size, shape, borders, and number of defects (see Fig. 21.5). Most PVLs are irregular rather than circular and serpentine rather than cylindrical; tissue calcification may be present on one side of the sewing ring. Defects that are larger than one-fourth of the annular circumference or that are associated with rocking of the prosthetic valve are unlikely to be amenable to percutaneous repair.

After the precise location of the PVL is determined, the next step is deciding which approach is best to percutaneously fix this defect. The most common approach is transseptal puncture and antegrade cannulation of the defects from the LA. Direct transapical puncture or a retrograde approach with cannulation from the LV also can be used.[126]

Intraprocedural Guidance

There are no PVL-specific devices. A variety of off-label devices are used, including atrial septal occluders, the Amplatzer Vascular Plug II, patent ductal occluders, and ventricular septal occluders.[98] Familiarity with these devices and their imaging appearance facilitates imaging guidance.

Clear and precise anatomic landmark characterization and 3D spatial orientation are essential for procedure performance, as is communication between imager and interventionalist. Access to the left side of the heart is obtained under fluoroscopy and color 2D and 3D TEE guidance. The guidewire and catheters are advanced to the PVL area under fluoroscopy and TEE guidance. Subsequently, the catheter used for crossing the PVL is exchanged for a delivery catheter, and a plugging device is inserted.

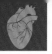

Imaging is essential during deployment of the device to position it correctly across the leaking orifice and to verify that there is no interference with prosthetic valve function when treating a PVL around a mechanical valve. After the selected closure device is verified to have a satisfactory position and to be stable, the MR reduction is deemed adequate, and lack of interference with the prosthetic valve is confirmed, the device is released. Depending on the presence and size of a residual PVL as determined by color TEE, an additional occluder device may be considered. Before the procedure is ended, indications of potential complications are sought, including pericardial effusion or tamponade, change in LV systolic function and pulmonary pressure, and characterization of iatrogenic ASD in cases of septal puncture.

Postprocedural Assessment

TTE is frequently used to assess the result of a procedure before patient discharge. Depending on the location of the PVL, residual MR and the deployed plug or plugs may or may not be well assessed with TTE, and TEE should be considered if necessary.

Transcatheter Mitral Valve Implantation and Valve-in-Valve Percutaneous Therapy

The use of bioprosthetic valves for MV disease is increasingly popular. However, these valves are known to degenerate over time.

Historically, reoperation was the only recourse for a failing bioprosthetic valve. Today, percutaneous options exist with the use of TMVI. This less-invasive option requires preprocedural, intraprocedural, and postprocedural evaluation during valve insertion.[132] TMVI is being developed for treatment of MR in patients who are not eligible for surgery because their surgical risk is considered prohibitive.[133–135] No transcatheter MVs have yet received approval by the U.S. Food and Drug Administration. The transcatheter aortic prosthesis Edwards Sapien (Edwards Lifesciences, Irvine, CA) is used in an off-label fashion for degenerated surgically implanted mitral bioprosthetic valves, failed surgical repairs with annular rings, and severe native MR and MS due to mitral annular calcification.[106,132,136–138]

Several dedicated TMVR technologies are undergoing early feasibility studies. Table 21.4 summarizes the trials investigating the potential clinical applications of TMVI for MR. Most of these devices require an apical puncture and use fluoroscopy and TEE for procedural guidance. The role of CT and 3D TEE MV modeling to assist with TMVI has been reported.[29] Preprocedural CTA has an essential role in patient selection and planning of the intervention. The assessment of potential LVOT obstruction is a major need with all forms of TMVR. Intraprocedural fluoroscopy and TEE are needed to optimally align the new valve with the old valve and to monitor its correct placement. Assessments of residual MR, LVOT gradients, and MV gradients are essential after valve implantation.

TABLE 21.4 Imaging Guidance of Specific Prosthetic Mitral Valve Interventions.

Intervention	Current Status	Imaging Comments
Paravalvular Leak Repair No specific device available: off-label devices, Amplatzer Vascular Plug II, patent ductal occluder, and ventricular septal occluder[98]	Has replaced surgery for most patients Essential for characterization of size, location, and number of PVL defects Determination of approach needed to close the leak	TEE guidance essential in transseptal and apical approaches TTE of limited value: color Doppler images obscured by annular calcium and sewing rings CT and TEE preferred imaging tools
Transcatheter Mitral Valve Replacement *For Mitral Regurgitation* Fortis (Edwards Lifesciences, Irvine, CA)[99] CardiAQ-Edwards (Edwards Lifesciences, Irvine, CA)[100] Tiara Mitral Valve System (Neovasc Inc., Vancouver, Canada)[101] Tendyne (Tendyne Holdings LLC, a subsidiary of Abbott Laboratories, Chicago, IL)[102] Medtronic Intrepid TMR device (Medtronic, Minneapolis, MN)[103]	Attractive alternative option for functional and degenerative MR Apical and transseptal approaches have been described. Fixation systems and avoidance of PVLs are main challenges.	3D TEE is complementary to CT assessment of the D-shaped mitral annulus to determine transcatheter MV implantation size. Fluoroscopy and TEE guidance is required; TEE is used to obtain delivery system coaxiality with annulus.
For Mitral Stenosis and Mitral Annular Calcification Sapien Valve (Edwards Lifesciences, Irvine, CA)[104] Direct Flow valves (Direct Flow Medical, Santa Clara, CA)[105]	TMVR with balloon-expandable valves in patients with MS or severe MAC is feasible but may be associated with significant adverse events. This strategy may be an alternative for selected high-risk patients with limited treatment options.	CT and TTE are used for MV and annular characterization. Fluoroscopy and TEE are used for intraprocedural guidance.
Transcatheter Valve-in-Valve Repair Sapien Valve (Edwards Lifesciences, Irvine, CA)[106] Lotus (Boston Scientific Corp., Marlborough, MA)[107]	Malfunctioning MVR Malfunctioning MV ring Percutaneous transvenous MV implantation in high-surgical-risk patients with degenerated bioprosthesis or failed annuloplasty ring is an attractive alternative to open heart surgery.	TTE is used to characterize preprocedural mitral prosthetic dysfunction. Fluoroscopy and 2D/3D TEE are used for intraprocedural guidance.

CT, Computed tomography; *MAC,* mitral annular calcification; *MR,* mitral regurgitation; *MS,* mitral stenosis; *MV,* mitral valve; *MVR,* mitral valve replacement; *PVL,* paravalvular leak; *TMVR,* transcatheter mitral valve replacement.

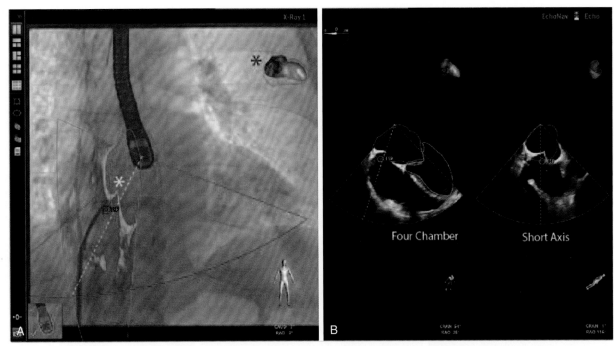

Fig. 21.18 Heart Model Fluoroscopic Overlay in Septal Puncture (Video 21.18 ○). In a patient undergoing MitraClip repair, whole heart modeling with fluoroscopic overlay was used during the interatrial septal puncture. (A) A thumbnail rendering of the heart model is marked by the *blue asterisk*. The catheter is marked by a *red square*. Septal tenting is indicated by the *yellow asterisk*. (B) Heart model thumbnail depictions with correct anatomic orientation are seen in the upper part of the figure. The four-chamber view with outlines of the left atrium and left ventricle are seen on the *left*, and an orthogonal short-axis view (bicaval) is shown on the *right*. Tenting of the septum is visible on both images. Having access to the heart model images simultaneously with the echo/fluoro fusion images facilitates guidance of the intervention.

CONCLUSIONS AND FUTURE DIRECTIONS

The field of structural heart disease interventions is expanding rapidly because advances in cardiac imaging are playing a central role in patient selection, imaging guidance, and follow-up of patients undergoing TCMVP. Because of the real-time rendition of detailed structural and functional information provided by 3D TEE, this tool has become the principal technique for imaging guidance of TCMVP.

Work in transducer design, hardware, and software will continue to improve the echocardiographic image quality for guidance of structural heart disease interventions. Advances in heart and MV modeling and echo-fluoro fusion imaging are expanding the applicability of cardiac ultrasound in the cardiac catheterization laboratory and in the hybrid operating room. Examples include whole-heart modeling with fluoroscopic overlay, MV modeling with fluoroscopic overlay, and enhanced tissue rendering with selective illumination (Figs. 21.18 through 21.20).

For patients in whom TEE is not feasible or the images are substandard, it is likely that ICE will continue to be a viable alternative, especially after 3D ICE becomes the norm.

CMR is the gold standard for LV remodeling evaluation, and there is increasing confidence in its capacity to characterize MR severity. There is significant interest in determining the role of CMR in MR severity quantification in patients after MitraClip implantation, when echocardiography may be imprecise.

MSCT provides high-resolution reconstructions of the mitral annulus and is playing an increasing role in the morphologic characterization of the mitral apparatus. This application will continue to expand, especially in the nascent area of PMVR. MSCT will continue to be the basis for rapid prototyping, and as 3D printing becomes less

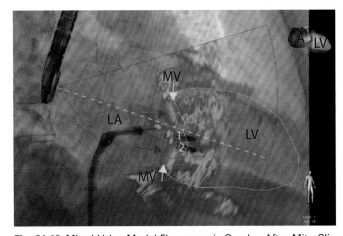

Fig. 21.19 Mitral Valve Model Fluoroscopic Overlay After MitraClip placement (Video 21.19 ○). Image obtained immediately after placement of two MitraClips depicts a heart model overlaid on the fluoroscopic view with the outline of the LA in purple and the outline of the LV and mitral valve (MV) in *pink* (*yellow arrows*). Filling of the LV through a double-orifice MV (*red arrows*) is shown by color Doppler; the two clips (*1 and 2*) are seen in the center.

expensive and more available, MSCT will play a central role in this imaging modality.

The marriage of TCMVP and advanced cardiac imaging has been very successful, and one can predict with confidence that this union will be a lasting one.

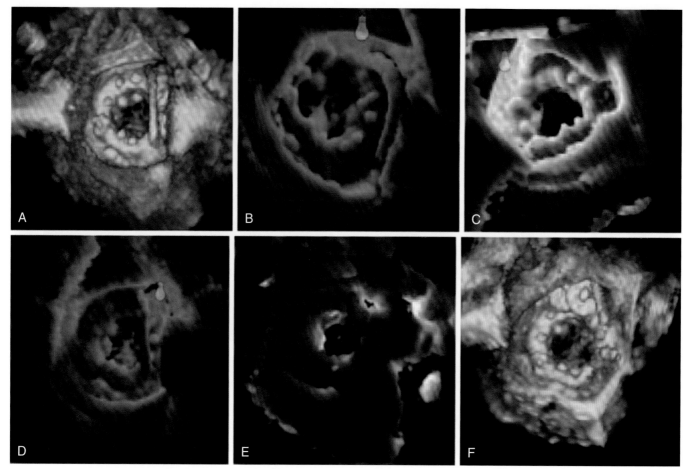

Fig. 21.20 Realistic Rendering of a Periprosthetic Mitral Leak Repair (Video 21.20 ⏵). Serial 3D TEE images of a patient undergoing paravalvular mitral leak (PVL) repair. All images are *en-face* views of a bioprosthesis as seen from the left atrial perspective. (A and F) Usual color rendition is used; all other illustrations represent enhanced anatomic rendition with various angles of illumination. (B) The light source, marked by the *light bulb*, comes from a 12-o'clock position. (C) The light source is at the 11-o'clock position. (D) The light source is at 1-o'clock. (E) The light source is coming from the left ventricle, highlighting the PVL at 1 o'clock.

REFERENCES

1. Nishimura RA, Otto CM, Bonow RO, et al. 2014 AHA/ACC guideline for the management of patients with valvular heart disease: a report of the American College of Cardiology/American Heart Association Task Force on Practice Guidelines. J Thorac Cardiovasc Surg 2014;148(1):e1-e132.
2. Salcedo E, Carroll J. Echocardiography in patient assessment and procedural guidance in structural heart disease interventions. In: Carroll J, Webb J, eds. *Structural Heart Disease Interventions*. Philadelphia, PA: Lippincott Williams & Wilkins; 2012:79-96.
3. Quaife RA, Salcedo EE, Carroll JD. Procedural guidance using advance imaging techniques for percutaneous edge-to-edge mitral valve repair. Curr Cardiol Rep 2014;16(2):452.
4. Figulla HR, Webb JG, Lauten A, Feldman T. The transcatheter valve technology pipeline for treatment of adult valvular heart disease. Eur Heart J 2016;37(28):2226-2239.
5. Sarraf M, Feldman T. Percutaneous intervention for mitral regurgitation. Heart Fail Clin 2015;11(2):243-259.
6. De Bonis M, Taramasso M, Lapenna E, et al. MitraClip therapy and surgical edge-to-edge repair in patients with severe left ventricular dysfunction and secondary mitral regurgitation: mid-term results of a single-centre experience†. Eur J Cardiothorac Surg 2016;49(1):255-262.
7. Pope NH, Ailawadi G. Transcatheter mitral valve repair. Oper Tech Thorac Cardiovasc Surg 2014;19(2):219-237.
8. Munkholm-Larsen S, Wan B, Tian DH, et al. A systematic review on the safety and efficacy of percutaneous edge-to-edge mitral valve repair with the Mitra-Clip system for high surgical risk candidates. Heart 2014;100(6):473-478.
9. Feldman T, Young A. Percutaneous approaches to valve repair for mitral regurgitation. J Am Coll Cardiol 2014;63(20):2057-2068.
10. Doshi JV, Agrawal S, Garg J, et al. Percutaneous mitral heart valve repair—MitraClip. Cardiol Rev 2014;22(6):289-296.
11. Beigel R, Wunderlich NC, Kar S, Siegel RJ. The evolution of percutaneous mitral valve repair therapy: lessons learned and implications for patient selection. J Am Coll Cardiol 2014;64(24):2688-2700.
12. Treede H, Schirmer J, Rudolph V, et al. A heart team's perspective on interventional mitral valve repair: percutaneous clip implantation as an important adjunct to a surgical mitral valve program for treatment of high-risk patients. J Thorac Cardiovasc Surg 2012;143(1):78-84.
13. Holmes Jr DR, Rich JB, Zoghbi WA, Mack MJ. The heart team of cardiovascular care. J Am Coll Cardiol 2013;61(9):903-907.
14. Nishimura RA, Otto CM, Bonow RO, et al. 2014 AHA/ACC Guideline for the Management of Patients With Valvular Heart Disease: executive summary: a report of the American College of Cardiology/American Heart Association Task Force on Practice Guidelines. Circulation 2014;129(23):2440-2492.
15. Zamorano JL, Badano LP, Bruce C, et al. EAE/ASE recommendations for the use of echocardiography in new transcatheter interventions for valvular heart disease. Eur J Echocardiogr 2011;12(8):557-584.

16. Zamorano J, Gonçalves A, Lancellotti P, et al. The use of imaging in new transcatheter interventions: an EACVI review paper. Eur Heart J Cardiovasc Imaging 2016;17(8):835-835af.

17. Silvestry FE, Kerber RE, Brook MM, et al. Echocardiography-guided interventions. J Am Soc Echocardiogr 2009;22(3):213-231; quiz 316-317.

18. Tommaso CL, Fullerton DA, Feldman T, et al. SCAI/AATS/ACC/STS operator and institutional requirements for transcatheter valve repair and replacement. Part II. mitral valve. J Am Coll Cardiol 2014;64(14):1515-1526.

19. Wunderlich NC, Beigel R, Ho SY, et al. Imaging for mitral interventions: methods and efficacy. JACC Cardiovasc Imaging 2018;11(6):872-901.

20. Foster E, Wasserman HS, Gray W, et al. Quantitative assessment of severity of mitral regurgitation by serial echocardiography in a multicenter clinical trial of percutaneous mitral valve repair. Am J Cardiol 2007;100(10):1577-1583.

21. Kim SS, Hijazi ZM, Lang RM, Knight BP. The use of intracardiac echocardiography and other intracardiac imaging tools to guide noncoronary cardiac interventions. J Am Coll Cardiol 2009;53(23):2117-2128.

22. Patzelt J, Seizer P, Zhang YY, et al. Percutaneous mitral valve edge-to-edge repair with simultaneous biatrial intracardiac echocardiography: first-in-human experience. Circulation 2016;133(15):1517-1519.

23. de Sousa L. Intracardiac echocardiography in structural heart disease: current prospects. Rev Port Cardiol 2012;31(6):413-414.

24. Bartel T, Bonaros N, Müller L, et al. Intracardiac echocardiography: a new guiding tool for transcatheter aortic valve replacement. J Am Soc Echocardiogr 2011;24(9):966-975.

25. Ratnayaka K, Faranesh AZ, Hansen MS, et al. Real-time MRI-guided right heart catheterization in adults using passive catheters. Eur Heart J 2013;34(5):380-389.

26. Hamilton-Craig C, Strugnell W, Gaikwad N, et al. Quantitation of mitral regurgitation after percutaneous MitraClip repair: comparison of Doppler echocardiography and cardiac magnetic resonance imaging. Ann Cardiothorac Surg 2015;4(4):341-351.

27. Delgado V, Tops LF, Schuijf JD, et al. Assessment of mitral valve anatomy and geometry with multislice computed tomography. JACC Cardiovasc Imaging 2009;2(5):556-565.

28. Shanks M, Delgado V, Ng AC, et al. Mitral valve morphology assessment: three-dimensional transesophageal echocardiography versus computed tomography. Ann Thorac Surg 2010;90(6):1922-1929.

29. Mak GJ, Blanke P, Ong K, et al. Three-dimensional echocardiography compared with computed tomography to determine mitral annulus size before transcatheter mitral valve implantation. Circ Cardiovasc Imaging 2016;9(6):e004176.

30. Housden RJ, Arujuna A, Ma Y, et al. Evaluation of a real-time hybrid three-dimensional echo and X-ray imaging system for guidance of cardiac catheterisation procedures. Med Image Comput Comput Assist Interv 2012;15(Pt 2):25-32.

31. Carroll JD, Salcedo EE. Fusion of 3D echocardiography with fluoroscopy for interventional guidance. In: Lang RM, ed. *Dynamic Echocardiography*. Philadelphia, PA: Saunders Elsevier; 2015.

32. Krishnaswamy A, Tuzcu EM, Kapadia SR. Integration of MDCT and fluoroscopy using C-arm computed tomography to guide structural cardiac interventions in the cardiac catheterization laboratory. Catheter Cardiovasc Interv 2015;85(1):139-147.

33. Al Amri I, Debonnaire P, van der Kley F, et al. Acute effect of MitraClip implantation on mitral valve geometry in patients with functional mitral regurgitation: insights from three-dimensional transoesophageal echocardiography. EuroIntervention 2016;11(13):1554-1561.

34. Schmidt FP, von Bardeleben RS, Nikolai P, et al. Immediate effect of the MitraClip procedure on mitral ring geometry in primary and secondary mitral regurgitation. Eur Heart J Cardiovasc Imaging 2013;14(9):851-857.

35. Schueler R, Momcilovic D, Weber M, et al. Acute changes of mitral valve geometry during interventional edge-to-edge repair with the MitraClip system are associated with midterm outcomes in patients with functional valve disease: preliminary results from a prospective single-center study. Circ Cardiovasc Interv 2014;7(3):390-399.

36. Kim MS, Hansgen AR, Carroll JD. Use of rapid prototyping in the care of patients with structural heart disease. Trends Cardiovasc Med 2008;18(6):210-216.

37. Gigliotti OS, Babb JD, Dieter RS, et al. Optimal use of left ventriculography at the time of cardiac catheterization: a consensus statement from the Society for Cardiovascular Angiography and Interventions. Catheter Cardiovasc Interv 2015;85(2):181-191.

38. Faletra FF, Berrebi A, Pedrazzini G, et al. 3D transesophageal echocardiography: A new imaging tool for assessment of mitral regurgitation and for guiding percutaneous edge-to-edge mitral valve repair. Prog Cardiovasc Dis 2017;60(3):305-321.

39. Dietl A, Prieschenk C, Eckert F, et al. 3D vena contracta area after MitraClip© procedure: precise quantification of residual mitral regurgitation and identification of prognostic information. Cardiovasc Ultrasound 2018;16(1):1.

40. Goebel B, Heck R, Hamadanchi A, et al. Vena contracta area for severity grading in functional and degenerative mitral regurgitation: a transoesophageal 3D colour Doppler analysis in 500 patients. Eur Heart J Cardiovasc Imaging 2018;19(6):639-646.

41. Wildes D, Lee W, Haider B, et al. 4-D ICE: A 2-D Array Transducer with Integrated ASIC in a 10-Fr Catheter for Real-Time 3-D Intracardiac Echocardiography. IEEE Trans Ultrason Ferroelectr Freq Control 2016;63(12):2159-2173.

42. Basman C, Parmar YJ, Kronzon I. Intracardiac echocardiography for structural heart and electrophysiological interventions. Curr Cardiol Rep 2017;19(10):102.

43. Asrress KN, Mitchell AR. Intracardiac echocardiography. Heart 2009;95(4):327-331.

44. Green NE, Hansgen AR, Carroll JD. Initial clinical experience with intracardiac echocardiography in guiding balloon mitral valvuloplasty: technique, safety, utility, and limitations. Catheter Cardiovasc Interv 2004;63(3):385-394.

45. Defteros S, Giannopoulos G, Raisakis K, et al. Intracardiac echocardiography imaging of periprosthetic valvular regurgitation. Eur J Echocardiogr 2010;11(5):E20.

46. Saji M, Rossi AM, Ailawadi G, et al. Adjunctive intracardiac echocardiography imaging from the left ventricle to guide percutaneous mitral valve repair with the MitraClip in patients with failed prior surgical rings. Catheter Cardiovasc Interv 2016;87(2):E75-E82.

47. Henning A, Mueller II, Mueller K, et al. Percutaneous edge-to-edge mitral valve repair escorted by left atrial intracardiac echocardiography (ICE). Circulation 2014;130(20):e173-e174.

48. Lim DS, Kunjummen BJ, Smalling R. Mitral valve repair with the MitraClip device after prior surgical mitral annuloplasty. Catheter Cardiovasc Interv 2010;76(3):455-459.

49. Delgado V, Hundley WG. Added value of cardiovascular magnetic resonance in primary mitral regurgitation. Circulation 2018;137(13):1361-1363.

50. Penicka M, Vecera J, Mirica DC, et al. Prognostic implications of magnetic resonance-derived quantification in asymptomatic patients with organic mitral regurgitation: comparison with doppler echocardiography-derived integrative approach. Circulation 2018;137(13):1349-1360.

51. Sturla F, Onorati F, Puppini G, et al. Dynamic and quantitative evaluation of degenerative mitral valve disease: a dedicated framework based on cardiac magnetic resonance imaging. J Thorac Dis 2017;9(Suppl 4):S225-S238.

52. Uretsky S, Gillam L, Lang R, et al. Discordance between echocardiography and MRI in the assessment of mitral regurgitation severity: a prospective multicenter trial. J Am Coll Cardiol 2015;65(11):1078-1088.

53. Naoum C, Blanke P, Cavalcante JL, Leipsic J. Cardiac computed tomography and magnetic resonance imaging in the evaluation of mitral and tricuspid valve disease: implications for transcatheter interventions. Circ Cardiovasc Imaging 2017;10(3):e005331.

54. Campbell-Washburn AE, Tavallaei MA, Pop M, et al. Real-time MRI guidance of cardiac interventions. J Magn Reson Imaging 2017;46(4):935-950.

55. Balzer J, Zeus T, Blehm A, et al. Intraprocedural online fusion of echocardiography and fluoroscopy during transapical mitral valve-in-valve implantation. Can J Cardiol 2015;31(3):364.e9-364.e11.

56. Jone PN, Ross MM, Bracken JA, et al. Feasibility and safety of using a fused echocardiography/fluoroscopy imaging system in patients with congenital heart disease. J Am Soc Echocardiogr 2016;29(6):513-521.

57. Balzer J, Zeus T, Veulemans V, Kelm M. Hybrid imaging in the catheter laboratory: real-time fusion of echocardiography and fluoroscopy during

percutaneous structural heart disease interventions. Interv Cardiol 2016;11(1):59-64.

58. Gafoor S, Schulz P, Heuer L, et al. Use of EchoNavigator, a novel echocardiography-fluoroscopy overlay system, for transseptal puncture and left atrial appendage occlusion. J Interv Cardiol 2015;28(2):215-217.

59. Sundermann SH, Biaggi P, Grünenfelder J, et al. Safety and feasibility of novel technology fusing echocardiography and fluoroscopy images during MitraClip interventions. EuroIntervention 2014;9(10):1210-1216.

60. Kim MS, Bracken J, Nijhof N, et al. Integrated 3D Echo-X-Ray navigation to predict optimal angiographic deployment projections for TAVR. JACC Cardiovasc Imaging 2014;7(8):847-848.

61. Afzal S, Veulemans V, Balzer J, et al. Safety and efficacy of transseptal puncture guided by real-time fusion of echocardiography and fluoroscopy. Neth Heart J 2017;25(2):131-136.

62. Faletra FF, et al. Echocardiographic-fluoroscopic fusion imaging for transcatheter mitral valve repair guidance. Eur Heart J Cardiovasc Imaging 2018;19(7):715-726.

63. Krishnaswamy A, Tuzcu EM, Kapadia SR. Three-dimensional computed tomography in the cardiac catheterization laboratory. Catheter Cardiovasc Interv 2011;77(6):860-865.

64. Eng MH, Kim MS. Fluoroscopy and CT fusion overlay—greater than the sum of their parts. Catheter Cardiovasc Interv 2015;85(1):148-149.

65. Schulz E, Tamm A, Kasper-König W, et al. Transapical implantation of a transcatheter aortic valve prosthesis into a mitral annuloplasty ring guided by real-time three-dimensional cardiac computed tomography-fluoroscopy fusion imaging. Eur Heart J 2018;39(4):327-328.

66. Grewal J, Suri R, Mankad S, et al. Mitral annular dynamics in myxomatous valve disease: new insights with real-time 3-dimensional echocardiography. Circulation 2010;121(12):1423-1431.

67. Patzelt J, Zhang Y, Magunia H, et al. Improved mitral valve coaptation and reduced mitral valve annular size after percutaneous mitral valve repair (PMVR) using the MitraClip system. Eur Heart J Cardiovasc Imaging 2018;19(7):785-791.

68. El Sabbagh A, Eleid MF, Matsumoto JM, et al. Three-dimensional prototyping for procedural simulation of transcatheter mitral valve replacement in patients with mitral annular calcification. Catheter Cardiovasc Interv 2018;92(7):E537-E549.

69. Sardari Nia P, Heuts S, Daemen J, et al. Preoperative planning with three-dimensional reconstruction of patient's anatomy, rapid prototyping and simulation for endoscopic mitral valve repair. Interact Cardiovasc Thorac Surg 2017;24(2):163-168.

70. Vaquerizo B, Theriault-Lauzier P, Piazza N. Percutaneous transcatheter mitral valve replacement: patient-specific three-dimensional computer-based heart model and prototyping. Rev Esp Cardiol (Engl Ed) 2015;68(12):1165-1173.

71. Kim MS, Hansgen AR, Wink O, et al. Rapid prototyping: a new tool in understanding and treating structural heart disease. Circulation 2008;117(18):2388-2394.

72. Zamorano JL, González-Gomez A, Lancellotti P. Mitral valve anatomy: implications for transcatheter mitral valve interventions. EuroIntervention 2014;10(Suppl U):U106-U111.

73. Salcedo EE, Quaife RA, Seres T, Carroll JD. A framework for systematic characterization of the mitral valve by real-time three-dimensional transesophageal echocardiography. J Am Soc Echocardiogr 2009;22(10):1087-1099.

74. Ho SY. Anatomy of the mitral valve. Heart 2002;88(Suppl 4):iv5-iv10.

75. Krapf L, Dreyfus J, Cueff C, et al. Anatomical features of rheumatic and non-rheumatic mitral stenosis: potential additional value of three-dimensional echocardiography. Arch Cardiovasc Dis 2013;106(2):111-115.

76. Grayburn PA, Weissman NJ, Zamorano JL. Quantitation of mitral regurgitation. Circulation 2012;126(16):2005-2017.

77. Ross Jr J. Transseptal left heart catheterization a 50-year odyssey. J Am Coll Cardiol 2008;51(22):2107-2115.

78. Mahmoud HM, Al-Ghamdi MA, Ghabashi AE, Anwar AM. A proposed maneuver to guide transseptal puncture using real-time three-dimensional transesophageal echocardiography: pilot study. Cardiol Res Pract 2015;2015:174051.

79. Ardashev AV, Mangutov DA, Rybachenko MS, et al. Comparison of transthoracic, transesophageal, and intracardiac echocardiography

80. Cafri C, de la Guardia B, Barasch E, et al. Transseptal puncture guided by intracardiac echocardiography during percutaneous transvenous mitral commissurotomy in patients with distorted anatomy of the fossa ovalis. Catheter Cardiovasc Interv 2000;50(4):463-467.

81. Alkhouli M, Rihal CS, Holmes Jr DR. Transseptal techniques for emerging structural heart interventions. JACC Cardiovasc Interv 2016;9(24):2465-2480.

82. Young A, Feldman T. Percutaneous mitral valve repair. Curr Cardiol Rep 2014;16(1):443.

83. von Bardeleben RS, Colli A, Schulz E, et al. First in human transcatheter COMBO mitral valve repair with direct ring annuloplasty and neochord leaflet implantation to treat degenerative mitral regurgitation: feasibility of the simultaneous toolbox concept guided by 3D echo and computed tomography fusion imaging. Eur Heart J 2018;39(15):1314-1315.

84. Palacios IF, Sanchez PL, Harrell LC, et al. Which patients benefit from percutaneous mitral balloon valvuloplasty? Prevalvuloplasty and postvalvuloplasty variables that predict long-term outcome. Circulation 2002;105(12):1465-1471.

85. Feldman T, Foster E, Glower DD, et al. Percutaneous repair or surgery for mitral regurgitation. N Engl J Med 2011;364(15):1395-1406.

86. Harnek J, Webb JG, Kuck KH, et al. Transcatheter implantation of the MONARC coronary sinus device for mitral regurgitation: 1-year results from the EVOLUTION phase I study (Clinical Evaluation of the Edwards Lifesciences Percutaneous Mitral Annuloplasty System for the Treatment of Mitral Regurgitation). JACC Cardiovasc Interv 2011;4(1):115-122.

87. Sack S, Kahlert P, Bilodeau L, et al. Percutaneous transvenous mitral annuloplasty: initial human experience with a novel coronary sinus implant device. Circ Cardiovasc Interv 2009;2(4):277-284.

88. Siminiak T, Wu JC, Haude M, et al. Treatment of functional mitral regurgitation by percutaneous annuloplasty: results of the TITAN Trial. Eur J Heart Fail 2012;14(8):931-938.

89. Maisano F, Taramasso M, Nickenig G, et al. Cardioband, a transcatheter surgical-like direct mitral valve annuloplasty system: early results of the feasibility trial. Eur Heart J 2016;37(10):817-825.

90. Ferrero Guadagnoli A, De Carlo C, Maisano F, et al. Cardioband system as a treatment for functional mitral regurgitation. Expert Rev Med Devices 2018;15(6):415-421.

91. Gooley RP, Meredith IT. The Accucinch transcatheter direct mitral valve annuloplasty system. EuroIntervention 2015;11(Suppl W):W60-W61.

92. Andreas M, Doll N, Livesey S, et al. Safety and feasibility of a novel adjustable mitral annuloplasty ring: a multicentre European experience. Eur J Cardiothorac Surg 2016;49(1):249-254.

93. Langer F, Borger MA, Czesla M, et al. Dynamic annuloplasty for mitral regurgitation. J Thorac Cardiovasc Surg 2013;145(2):425-429.

94. Jilaihawi H, Virmani R, Nakagawa H, et al. Mitral annular reduction with subablative therapeutic ultrasound: pre-clinical evaluation of the ReCor device. EuroIntervention 2010;6(1):54-62.

95. Colli A, Zucchetta F, Torregrossa G, et al. Transapical off-pump mitral valve repair with Neochord Implantation (TOP-MINI): step-by-step guide. Ann Cardiothorac Surg 2015;4(3):295-297.

96. Grossi EA, Patel N, Woo YJ, et al. Outcomes of the RESTOR-MV Trial (Randomized Evaluation of a Surgical Treatment for Off-Pump Repair of the Mitral Valve). J Am Coll Cardiol 2010;56(24):1984-1993.

97. Ielasi A, Tespili M, Repossini A, et al. Percutaneous implantation of a left ventricular restoration device [Parachute(TM)] for the treatment of ischemic heart failure. G Ital Cardiol (Rome) 2015;16(1):52-57.

98. Sorajja P, Cabalka AK, Hagler DJ, Rihal CS. The learning curve in percutaneous repair of paravalvular prosthetic regurgitation: an analysis of 200 cases. JACC Cardiovasc Interv 2014;7(5):521-529.

99. Abdul-Jawad Altisent O, Dumont E, Dagenais F, et al. Initial experience of Transcatheter Mitral Valve Replacement with a novel transcatheter mitral valve: procedural and 6-month follow-up results. J Am Coll Cardiol 2015;66(9):1011-1019.

100. Barbanti M, Tamburino C. Transcatheter mitral valve implantation: CardiAQ. EuroIntervention 2016;12(Y):Y73-Y74.

101. Verheye S, Cheung A, Leon M, Banai S. The Tiara transcatheter mitral valve implantation system. EuroIntervention 2015;11(Suppl W): W71-W72.

102. Perpetua EM, Reisman M. The Tendyne transcatheter mitral valve implantation system. EuroIntervention 2015;11(Suppl W):W78-W79.

103. Meredith I, Bapat V, Morriss J, et al. Intrepid transcatheter mitral valve replacement system: technical and product description. EuroIntervention 2016;12(Y):Y78-Y80.

104. El Sabbagh A, Foley T, Rihal C, et al. TCT-644 transcatheter balloon expandable SAPIEN valve implantation using transatrial approach in patients with mitral stenosis and severe mitral annular calcification. J Am Coll Cardiol 2016;68(Suppl 18):B262.

105. Sinning C, Conradi L, Deuschl FG, et al. Combined rendezvous approach with the Direct Flow Medical® aortic valve prosthesis to treat aortic and mitral stenosis. Int J Cardiol 2016;214:284-285.

106. Eleid MF, Cabalka AK, Williams MR, et al. Percutaneous transvenous transseptal transcatheter valve implantation in failed bioprosthetic mitral valves, ring annuloplasty, and severe mitral annular calcification. JACC Cardiovasc Interv 2016;9(11):1161-1174.

107. Feldman T, Reardon MJ. Mitral valve-in-valve with the Lotus mechanically expanding platform. Catheter Cardiovasc Interv 2015;86(7):1287-1288.

108. Feldman T, Kar S, Rinaldi M, et al. Percutaneous mitral repair with the MitraClip system: safety and midterm durability in the initial EVEREST (Endovascular Valve Edge-to-Edge REpair Study) cohort. J Am Coll Cardiol 2009;54(8):686-694.

109. Mendirichaga R, Singh V, Blumer V, et al. Transcatheter mitral valve repair with mitraclip for symptomatic functional mitral valve regurgitation. Am J Cardiol 2017;120(4):708-715.

110. Nyman CB, Mackensen GB, Jelacic S, et al. Transcatheter mitral valve repair using the edge-to-edge clip. J Am Soc Echocardiogr 2018;31(4):434-453.

111. Mauri L, Garg P, Massaro JM, et al. The EVEREST II Trial: design and rationale for a randomized study of the evalve mitraclip system compared with mitral valve surgery for mitral regurgitation. Am Heart J 2010;160(1):23-29.

112. Lubos E, Schlüter M, Vettorazzi E, et al. MitraClip therapy in surgical high-risk patients: identification of echocardiographic variables affecting acute procedural outcome. JACC Cardiovasc Interv 2014; 7(4):394-402.

113. Itabashi Y, Utsunomiya H, Kubo S, et al. Different indicators for postprocedural mitral stenosis caused by single- or multiple-clip implantation after percutaneous mitral valve repair. J Cardiol 2018;71(4):336-345.

114. Attizzani GF, Ohno Y, Capodanno D, et al. Extended use of percutaneous edge-to-edge mitral valve repair beyond EVEREST (Endovascular Valve Edge-to-Edge Repair) criteria: 30-day and 12-month clinical and echocardiographic outcomes from the GRASP (Getting Reduction of Mitral Insufficiency by Percutaneous Clip Implantation) registry. JACC Cardiovasc Interv 2015;8(1 Pt A):74-82.

115. Jorbenadze R, Schreieck J, Barthel C, et al. Percutaneous edge-to-edge mitral valve repair using the new MitraClip XTR System. JACC Cardiovasc Interv 2018;11(12):e93-e95.

116. Yzeiraj E, Bijuklic K, Tiburtius C, et al. Tricuspid regurgitation is a predictor of mortality after percutaneous mitral valve edge-to-edge repair. EuroIntervention 2017;12(15):e1817-e1824.

117. Besler C, Blazek S, Rommel KP, et al. Combined mitral and tricuspid versus isolated mitral valve transcatheter edge-to-edge repair in patients with symptomatic valve regurgitation at high surgical risk. JACC Cardiovasc Interv 2018;11(12):1142-1151.

118. Panaich SS, Eleid MF. Current status of MitraClip for patients with mitral and tricuspid regurgitation. Trends Cardiovasc Med 2018; 28(3):200-209.

119. Nickenig G, Kowalski M, Hausleiter J, et al. Transcatheter treatment of severe tricuspid regurgitation with the edge-to-edge MitraClip technique. Circulation 2017;135(19):1802-1814.

120. Alkhouli M, El Sabbagh A, Villarraga HR, et al. Novel treatment of residual Peri-MitraClip Regurgitation with an Amplatzer Vascular Plug II. JACC Cardiovasc Interv 2016;9(17):e171-e175.

121. Taramasso M, Zuber M, Gruner C, et al. First-in-man report of residual "intra-clip" regurgitation between two MitraClips treated by AMPLATZER Vascular Plug II. EuroIntervention 2016;11(13):1537-1540.

122. Toyama K, Rader F, Kar S, et al. Iatrogenic atrial septal defect after percutaneous mitral valve repair with the MitraClip System. Am J Cardiol 2018;121(4):475-479.

123. Yeh L, Mashari A, Montealegre-Gallegos M, et al. Immediate closure of iatrogenic ASD After MitraClip Procedure Prompted by Acute Right Ventricular Dysfunction. J Cardiothorac Vasc Anesth 2017;31(4):1304-1307.

124. Utsunomiya H, Itabashi Y, Kobayashi S, et al. Effect of percutaneous edge-to-edge repair on mitral valve area and its association with pulmonary hypertension and outcomes. Am J Cardiol 2017;120(4):662-669.

125. Hwang HY, Choi JW, Kim HK, et al. Paravalvular leak after mitral valve replacement: 20-year follow-up. Ann Thorac Surg 2015;100(4):1347-1352.

126. Sorajja P, Bae R, Lesser JA, Pedersen WA. Percutaneous repair of paravalvular prosthetic regurgitation: patient selection, techniques and outcomes. Heart 2015;101(9):665-673.

127. Rihal CS, Sorajja P, Booker JD, et al. Principles of percutaneous paravalvular leak closure. JACC Cardiovasc Interv 2012;5(2):121-130.

128. Quader N, Davidson CJ, Rigolin VH. Percutaneous closure of perivalvular mitral regurgitation: how should the interventionalists and the echocardiographers communicate? J Am Soc Echocardiogr 2015; 28(5):497-508.

129. Spoon DB, Malouf JF, Spoon JN, et al. Mitral paravalvular leak: description and assessment of a novel anatomical method of localization. JACC Cardiovasc Imaging 2013;6(11):1212-1214.

130. Mahjoub H, Noble S, Ibrahim R, et al. Description and assessment of a common reference method for fluoroscopic and transesophageal echocardiographic localization and guidance of mitral periprosthetic transcatheter leak reduction. JACC Cardiovasc Interv 2011;4(1):107-114.

131. Horton KD, Whisenant B, Horton S. Percutaneous closure of a mitral perivalvular leak using three dimensional real time and color flow imaging. J Am Soc Echocardiogr 2010;23(8):903.e5-7.

132. Mankad SV, Aldea GS, Ho NM, et al. Transcatheter mitral valve implantation in degenerated bioprosthetic valves. J Am Soc Echocardiogr 2018; 31(8):845-859.

133. Moat N, Duncan A, Lindsay A, et al. Transcatheter mitral valve replacement for the treatment of mitral regurgitation: in-hospital outcomes of an apically tethered device. J Am Coll Cardiol 2015;65(21):2352-2353.

134. Cheung A, Webb J, Verheye S, et al. Short-term results of transapical transcatheter mitral valve implantation for mitral regurgitation. J Am Coll Cardiol 2014;64(17):1814-1819.

135. Bapat V, Buellesfeld L, Peterson MD, et al. Transcatheter mitral valve implantation (TMVI) using the Edwards FORTIS device. EuroIntervention 2014;10(Suppl U):U120-U128.

136. El Sabbagh A, Eleid MF, Foley TA, et al. Direct transatrial implantation of balloon-expandable valve for mitral stenosis with severe annular calcifications: early experience and lessons learned. Eur J Cardiothorac Surg 2018;53(1):162-169.

137. Hachinohe D, Latib A, Montorfano M, Colombo A. Transcatheter mitral valve implantation in rigid mitral annuloplasty rings: Potential differences between complete and incomplete rings. Catheter Cardiovasc Interv 2019;93(1):E71-E74.

138. Gualis J, Estévez-Loureiro R, Alonso D, et al. Transapical Transcatheter Mitral Valve-In-Valve Implantation Using an Edwards SAPIEN 3 Valve. Heart Lung Circ 2018;27(3):e23-e24.

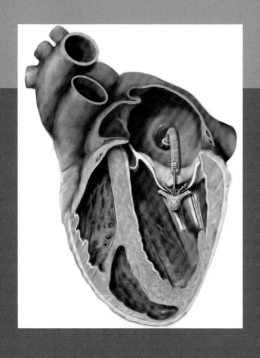

第22章
二尖瓣手术的术中超声心动图技术

　　不论是常规二尖瓣成形、瓣膜置换或是二尖瓣介入成形，术中经食管超声心动图检查作为手术医师的"第三只眼睛"发挥了不可替代的作用，术中实时经食管超声心动图检查，尤其是实时三维经食管超声心动图检查能够更直观地观察瓣叶形态，更精准评估病变区域，使得超声医师与手术医师能够更顺畅的沟通。

　　术前评估二尖瓣病变应注意麻醉及机械通气对循环状态的影响，二者会干扰经食管超声心动图的评估，因此不管是术前评估二尖瓣反流程度或是术后对二尖瓣手术效果的评估均应注意调整患者的血管张力、循环容量以达到最接近生理状态。

　　评估二尖瓣反流病因、病变部位及严重程度有利于做出二尖瓣成形或置换的决策，尤其是对二尖瓣反流病变的处理。二尖瓣反流程度的评估涉及多个定量指标，如缩流颈宽度、有效反流口面积、反流容积等，精准的评估有赖于结合形态学病变及多个定量指标。

　　二尖瓣病变术后即刻的超声评估主要为二尖瓣成形及置换效果的评估，二尖瓣成形术后少量反流是可接受的，术后存在明显反流时，经食管超声心动图，尤其是三维经食管超声心动图应协助评估原因及定位反流部位。二尖瓣成形术后少见的SAM现象与术前二尖瓣及其周边结构特点相关，术后要密切观察。二尖瓣置换术后需要密切评估瓣叶启闭状态及精准区别瓣环内及瓣周反流，三维经食管超声心动图可定位瓣周反流位置。另外，毗邻结构（如主动脉瓣）需除外医源性损伤。

　　本章主要介绍了评估二尖瓣的常规切面、二尖瓣病变分型、术前及术后需要评估的重点内容。相信该章节能够让读者对经食管超声心动图在二尖瓣手术围手术期的应用有一个全面且直观的了解。

王建德

Intraoperative Echocardiography for Mitral Valve Surgery

Donald C. Oxorn

KEY POINTS

- Mitral regurgitation (MR) and mitral stenosis (MS) may result from abnormalities of the mitral valvular complex—leaflets, annulus, chordae, and papillary muscles—and the left atrium and ventricle.
- Intraoperative echocardiography is a vital diagnostic technique for mitral valve (MV) surgery and is recommended for all valve repair procedures. Three-dimensional (3D) echocardiography, with or without color Doppler, may aid the clinician in localizing valvular pathology before and after cardiopulmonary bypass.
- The alterations in loading conditions resulting from general anesthesia and positive-pressure ventilation have dramatic effects on indices of MR and MS severity. The high-flow state after the use of cardiopulmonary bypass may falsely raise pressure gradients across prosthetic mitral valves.
- Each prosthetic valve type (i.e., mechanical or biological) has unique echocardiographic patterns on transesophageal echocardiography (TEE) after bypass.

- Epicardial echocardiography may be employed by the surgeon to evaluate the MV in its dynamic state if questions still exist about the mechanism of MV dysfunction after sternotomy.
- Residual MR after MV repair portends a poor prognosis. The location of MR (i.e., central or eccentric) and its mechanism (undercorrection of annulus, failure of neochords, residual leaflet abnormalities, repair breakdown, ring dehiscence, or systolic anterior motion [SAM]) are just as important as the degree of regurgitation.
- Common prosthetic valve abnormalities are impairment of leaflet opening and closing (due to thrombus, pannus, calcification, or entrapment by subvalvular tissue) and paravalvular regurgitation. Native mitral tissue left after valve replacement has the potential to create SAM. Small paravalvular leaks after valve replacement usually resolve after heparin reversal.

NOMENCLATURE

One key to successful communication between the echocardiographer and the surgeon is to make sure they speak the same procedural language.[1] A structure may be named differently depending on the anatomic terms of reference used. For example, the lateral and medial commissures are sometimes referred to as the anterior and posterior commissures, respectively. Whereas the echocardiographer readily identifies the annulus as the hinge point at the base of the leaflets, the surgical identification is the level of the visible transition between the

left atrial (LA) myocardium and the denser white leaflet (Fig. 22.1). When communication is optimal and the echocardiographic assessment is consistent, superior outcomes may result.[2]

The anterior leaflet is intimately associated with the aortic-mitral curtain and is sometimes referred to as the aortic leaflet. At the outside margins of the aortic-mitral curtain lie the fibrous trigones, which are important surgical landmarks. The posterior leaflet may be referred to as the mural leaflet, due to its proximity to the left ventricular (LV) wall. The classification endorsed by the American Society of Echocardiography and Society of Cardiovascular Anesthesiologists is shown in

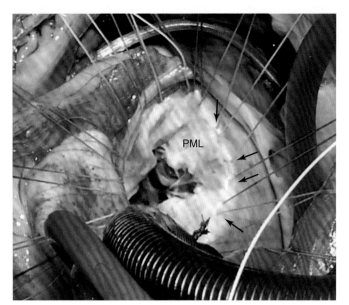

Fig. 22.1 Surgical Exposure of the Mitral Valve. The surgeon has placed sutures in the posterior annulus, which is identified as the transition between the pink atrial myocardium and the white leaflet *(arrows)*. *PML,* Posterior mitral leaflet.

Fig. 22.2. From left to right (or lateral to medial), the posterior leaflet is divided into scallops P1, P2, and P3, and the corresponding segments of the nonscalloped anterior leaflet into segments A1, A2, and A3. Deviant clefts are found in up to 30% of posterior leaflet specimens.[3]

THE INTRAOPERATIVE MILIEU

The intraoperative setting can be daunting, even to experienced practitioners who do not spend the bulk of their clinical time in the operating room. Numerous factors constrain optimal image acquisition, including bright lights and noise. Time may be limited because several different physicians and nurses have responsibilities in surgical preparation and the surgical procedure. If feasible, the echocardiographer

should request that room lighting be dimmed or, at a minimum, that any overhead surgical lighting be directed away from the echocardiographic system screen.

Most general anesthetic medications diminish vascular tone and decrease contractility. Patients are often taking preoperative vasodilator medications such as angiotensin-converting enzyme (ACE) inhibitors and angiotensin receptor blockers (ARBs). The echocardiographer must take the effects of decreased afterload into account when quantifying the degree of mitral regurgitation (MR). Positive-pressure ventilation and cardiopulmonary bypass have numerous hemodynamic effects with the potential to alter echocardiographic findings.

After the surgical procedure commences, electrocautery is used, which causes interference with the quality of two-dimensional (2D) echocardiography, spectral Doppler echocardiography, and especially color-flow Doppler imaging data. Electrocautery also creates stitching artifacts during multiple-beat acquisitions on three-dimensional (3D) transesophageal echocardiography (TEE). The distortion of the electrocardiogram may prevent appropriate triggering of cine loop recording from the QRS complex; instead, the echocardiography instrument should be set to store data for a set length of time (e.g., 2 s), rather than a set number of beats. The use of electrocautery may preclude the use of 3D multibeat acquisition modes.

PRE-BYPASS ASSESSMENT

Preoperative Preparation

The variety and acuity of diagnoses of patients coming to the operating room for treatment of valve disease has increased considerably as surgical options and the timing of surgery have changed over the past few decades.[4,5] Patients may require repeat surgery because of complications from a previous valve replacement (i.e., operative or interventional) or repair.

Remaining uncertainties after preoperative evaluation should be defined, with a plan for their resolution. Along with clinical data and results from other imaging modalities, the preoperative transthoracic echocardiography (TTE) data should be reviewed; if possible, the actual images should be examined to assess data quality. If, as often

Fig. 22.2 Anatomic View of the Cardiac Valves From the Perspective of the Base of the Heart With the Left and Right Atria Cut Away and the Great Vessels Transected. Notice the close anatomic relationships of all four cardiac valves. In particular, the aortic valve is adjacent to the mitral valve along the midsegment of the anterior mitral valve leaflet. The pulmonic valve is slightly superior to the aortic valve, and the aortic and pulmonic valve planes are almost perpendicular to each other. The three scallops of the posterior mitral leaflet are the lateral *(P1),* central *(P2),* and medial *(P3)* scallops; the corresponding segments for the anterior leaflet are the *A1, A2,* and *A3* segments. *Asterisk with arrows* indicates the aortic-mitral curtain. *L,* Left; *LAD,* left anterior descending artery; *R,* right.

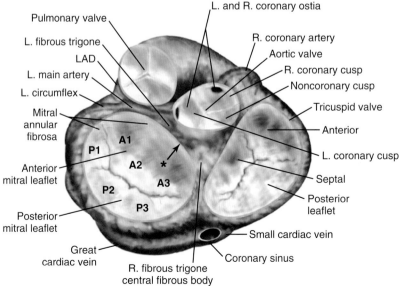

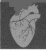

TABLE 22.1 Perioperative Implications of Lesions Associated With Mitral Valve Disease.

Secondary Condition	Preoperative Significance	Postoperative Significance
Pulmonary hypertension	May indicate LV failure, LV outflow tract obstruction, aortic valve disease, severe mitral regurgitation	Aortic valve surgery may be needed. Pharmacologic therapy may be needed.
Right heart failure	Often due to elevated left-sided filling pressures	Aggressive pharmacologic support may be needed.
Tricuspid regurgitation	Often due to elevated left-sided filling pressures; consideration for reparative procedure at time of mitral surgery	Must be differentiated from primary tricuspid valve disease
Mitral leaflet systolic anterior motion	Consideration for reparative procedure (i.e., myomectomy)	Aggressive pharmacologic manipulation may be needed; may necessitate valve replacement
Rheumatic valvular disease	Aortic stenosis, aortic regurgitation, tricuspid stenosis/regurgitation may necessitate intervention. Aortic regurgitation may confound mitral valve area calculation by the pressure half-time method.	Reassessment of native valves or of repaired/replaced valves after mitral valve surgery is required.

occurs, previously undiagnosed pathology is discovered on TEE, this information should be promptly shared with the surgeon.

Systematic Examination

A comprehensive baseline intraoperative TEE examination is recommended to confirm or refute the mechanism and severity of the MV abnormality, assess valve reparability, and provide comparison images for the postoperative evaluation. The baseline TEE examination includes 2D, spectral, and color-flow Doppler studies with quantitation of mitral stenosis (MS) and MR using standard approaches (see Chapters 15 and 16). 3D imaging, if available, enhances the understanding of abnormal mitral function.

Secondary effects on other structures, specifically the left-sided chambers and the tricuspid valve, may help determine the chronicity of the process. Some lesions are often associated primarily and secondarily with MV disease (Table 22.1), and they may require correction at the time of mitral surgery. Of paramount importance is recognition of the profound impact that alterations of loading conditions and ventricular function can have on the severity of MR.

Two-Dimensional Imaging

2D imaging allows assessment of the general condition of the leaflets, including the degree of thickness, mobility, calcification, and subvalvular disease. The LA is assessed for thrombus and ruptured chordae. The finding of LA or LV dilation may speak to the chronicity of the mitral abnormality, and it is assessed using published guidelines.[6] Spontaneous echocardiographic contrast or "smoke" indicates relative stasis of blood in the LA; it is often seen in patients with significant MS and may portend a high likelihood of LA appendage thrombus. Detection of masses should alert the echocardiographer to the possibility of endocarditis, with the potential for extension, leaflet perforation, involvement of other valves, and pseudoaneurysm formation (see Chapter 25).

A systematic examination of the MV is performed next. Assessment plans have been described by Shanewise et al,[7] Foster et al,[8] Bhatia et al,[9] and Hahn et al[10] (Figs. 22.3 and 22.4; Table 22.2). Hahn's report combines a description of standard 2D and 3D views with a general summary of indications, contraindications, and training requirements for TEE. Using these guides, the intraoperative echocardiographer can

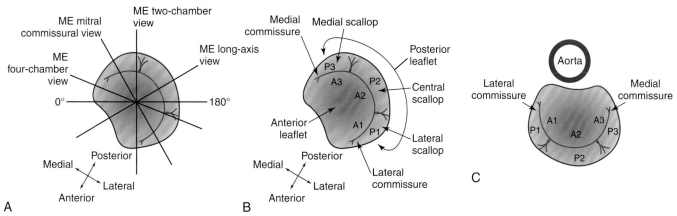

Fig. 22.3 TEE Views of the Mitral Valve. (A) Short-axis view of the mitral valve illustrates how it is transected by mid-esophageal *(ME)* views. Rotation through multiplane angles from 0 to 180 degrees moves the imaging plane axially through the entire mitral valve. (B) Anatomy of the mitral valve. (C) The surgeon's view of the mitral valve. *A1,* Lateral third of anterior leaflet; *A2,* central third of anterior leaflet; *A3,* medial third of anterior leaflet; *P1,* lateral scallop of posterior leaflet; *P2,* central scallop of posterior leaflet; *P3,* medial scallop of posterior leaflet. (From Shanewise JS, Cheung AT, Aronson S, et al. ASE/SCA guidelines for performing a comprehensive intraoperative multiplane transesophageal echocardiography examination: recommendations of the American Society of Echocardiography Council for Intraoperative Echocardiography and the Society of Cardiovascular Anesthesiologists Task Force for Certification in Perioperative Transesophageal Echocardiography. J Am Soc Echocardiogr 1999;12:884-900.)

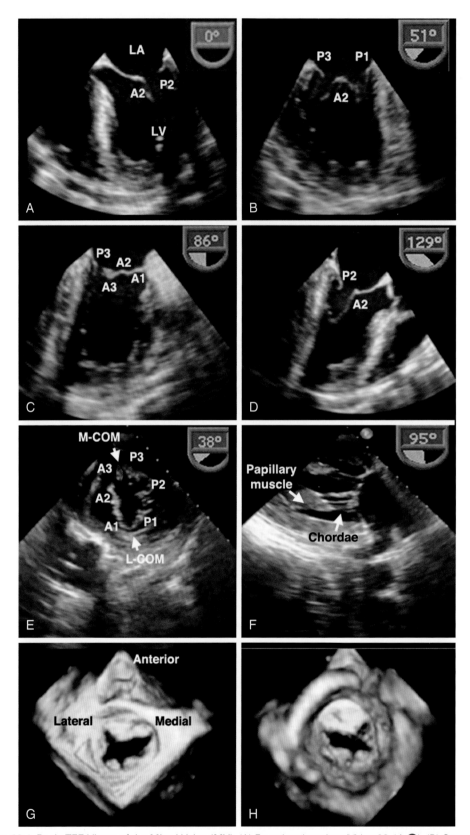

Fig. 22.4 Basic TEE Views of the Mitral Valve (MV). (A) Four-chamber view (Video 22.4A ▶). (B) Commissural view (Video 22.4B ▶). (C) Mid-esophageal two-chamber view (Video 22.4C ▶). (D) Mid-esophageal long-axis view (Video 22.4D ▶). (E) Transgastric short-axis view (Video 22.4E ▶). (F) Transgastric two-chamber view (Video 22.4F ▶). (G) 3D *en face* view from the LA (Video 22.4G ▶). (H) 3D view from the LV (Video 22.4H ▶). *A1, A2, A3,* Anterior leaflet sections; *L-COM,* anterolateral commissure; *M-COM,* posteromedial commissure; *P1, P2, P3,* posterior leaflet sections.

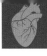

TABLE 22.2 Systematic Mitral Examination.

Name of View	Description of View	2D TEE Appearance
ME four-chamber view (≈0–10 degrees)	AML is on left side, adjacent to aortic valve. PML is on right side. Area of PML and AML that are visible are mostly P2 and A2. Probe flexion and slight withdrawal will bring A1 and P1 into view; retroflexion and slight advancement will bring A3 and P3 into view	See Fig. 22.4A and Video 22.4A
ME commissural view (≈50–70 degrees)	Two apparent coaptation points From left to right, visible mitral segments are P3, A2, and P1.	See Fig. 22.4B and Video 22.4B
ME two-chamber view (≈80–100 degrees)	Small P3 on left side and large AML on right side Segment that coapts with P3 is A3. Rest of visible AML varies.	See Fig. 22.4C and Video 22.4C
ME long-axis view (≈120–140 degrees)	PML on left side and AML on right side If plane of scan is centered, P2 and A2 are visible. May scan from side to side.	See Fig. 22.4D and Video 22.4D
TG short-axis view (≈0–20 degrees)	AML on left side and PML on right side Posterior commissure at top and anterior commissure at bottom	See Fig. 22.4E and Video 22.4E
TG two-chamber view (≈90–110 degrees)	Inferior wall at top Anterior wall at bottom Slight movement from side to side reveals papillary muscles and chordae.	See Fig. 22.4F and Video 22.4F
3D LA view	This view looks down at the valve from the LA and is closest to the surgeon's actual view of the valve. By convention	See Fig. 22.4G and Video 22.4G
3D LV view	This view looks up at the valve from the LV apex. The AML is at top, and the PML is at bottom.	See Fig. 22.4H and Video 22.4H

A1, A2, A3, Anterior leaflet sections; *AML,* anterior mitral leaflet; *ME,* mid-esophageal; *P1, P2, P3,* posterior leaflet sections; *PML,* posterior mitral leaflet; *TG,* transgastric.

recognize where the pathologic aspects of the valve lie. Basic views of the MV leaflets are obtained from a mid-esophageal position (see Fig. 22.4). As each view is obtained, slight movements of the probe—withdrawal and advancement, rotation left and right, and flexion and extension—are used to completely examine each leaflet segment. At this stage of the examination, color-flow Doppler imaging may be used, but this is more to help clarify the mechanism of MR (Figs. 22.5 and 22.6).

The subvalvular apparatus is best seen with transgastric views, which allow visualization of chordal thickening, redundancy, or frank rupture along with the orientation of the papillary muscles. On the basis of these images, the Carpentier classification can be used to define the mechanism and cause of MR, which may be helpful in planning the surgical approach[11] (Fig. 22.7 and Table 22.3).

Measurement of annular diameter guides the surgeon in the selection of a prosthesis or annuloplasty ring. The saddle shape of the annulus is demonstrated with 3D reconstructions (see Fig. 22.4). The low points of the saddle are at the commissures, seen in the commissural view, and the high points are in the anteroposterior axis, seen in the mid-esophageal long-axis view.

On the basis of comparison with cardiac computed tomography, the best approach for annular measurement is the commissure-to-commissure peak systolic diameter in the TEE commissural view the and anteroposterior diameter in the long-axis view.[12] This may also be accomplished with 3D imaging with or without the use of mitral

reconstruction software. The annulus is also assessed for the degree of calcification, which may predict paravalvular leaks,[13] perioperative stroke,[14] and whether extensive annular debridement is performed; it is also assessed for left ventricular rupture at the atrioventricular groove[15] and for left atrial dissection.[16]

Examination of global and segmental LV function is also needed in the evaluation of the mechanism of MR. Secondary MR is caused by global or regional LV systolic dysfunction or by altered LV geometry. However, chronic primary MR also leads to LV dilation with the potential for progressive LV dysfunction (see Chapter 5), which may complicate the perioperative management of MV surgery.

Epicardial Echocardiography

If TEE images are suboptimal, the surgeon can employ the technique of epicardial echocardiography before and after cardiopulmonary bypass.[17] A transthoracic probe is placed inside a sterile sheath, which is then placed directly on the heart. Most standard transthoracic views can be obtained, with excellent resolution. The use of 3D epicardial echocardiography has been shown to be both feasible, an productive of high-quality images.[18]

Three-Dimensional Echocardiography

Numerous reports have described techniques for intraoperative 3D acquisition and assessment.[19–22] Potential benefits include a mechanistic explanation of a given patient's MR, better assessment of the pathologic

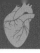

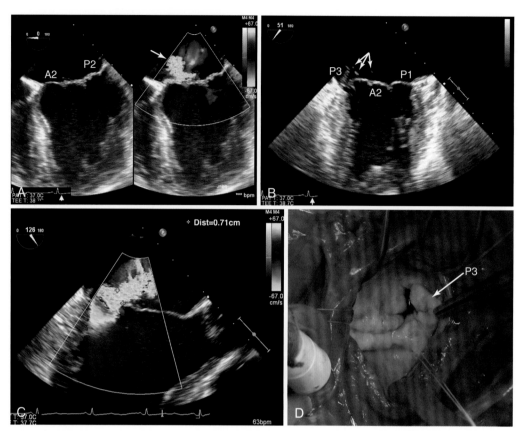

Fig. 22.5 Anteriorly Directed Mitral Regurgitant Jet. The 46-year-old patient had increasing shortness of breath over several years and an acute increase in dyspnea over the last week. (A) A four-chamber view *(left)* demonstrates normal coaptation, but a color-flow Doppler image *(right)* shows an anteriorly directed jet of mitral regurgitation (MR) *(arrow)*, indicative of posterior leaflet prolapse or anterior leaflet restriction. (B) The commissural view shows a flail *P3* scallop with numerous ruptured chordae *(arrows)*. (C) A vena contracta of 0.71 cm, indicative of severe MR. (D) Surgical exposure revealed involvement of the P3 scallop *(arrow)*. *A2,* Second anterior leaflet section; *P1, P2, P3,* Posterior leaflet sections.

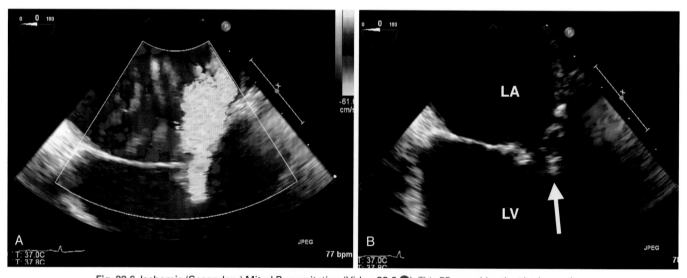

Fig. 22.6 Ischemic (Secondary) Mitral Regurgitation (Video 22.6 ▶). This 55-year-old patient had a previous history of inferior wall myocardial infarction. (A) The posteriorly directed jet of mitral regurgitation indicates anterior leaflet prolapse or posterior leaflet restriction. (B) Systolic restriction of the posterior leaflet *(arrow)*.

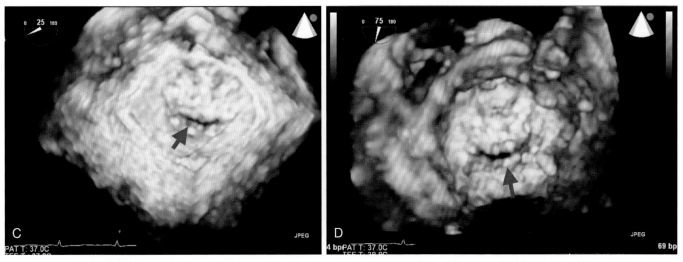

Fig. 22.6, cont'd The systolic coaptation defects *(red arrows)* are seen in the LA perspective (C) and in the LV perspective (D).

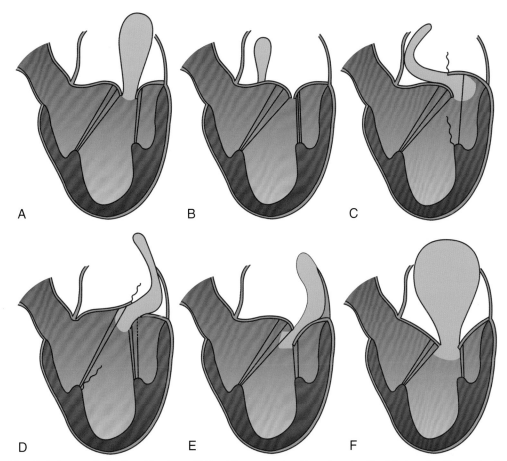

Fig. 22.7 Carpentier's Classification of Mitral Regurgitation Based on Leaflet Motion. Leaflet motion is classified as normal (type I), excessive (type II), or restricted (type III). (A and B) In type I, the leaflet motion is normal and the jet tends to be central. The cause of mitral regurgitation is usually annular dilatation (A) or leaflet perforation (B). (C and D) In type II, there is excessive leaflet motion and the jet is directed away from the diseased leaflet. (E and F) In type III lesions, the leaflet motion is restricted. Type III lesions are further subdivided into IIIA (i.e., restricted leaflet motion in diastole and systole) and IIIB (i.e., restricted leaflet motion in systole). The jet can be directed toward the affected leaflet (E), or it can be central if both leaflets are equally affected (F). (Modified from Perrino AC, Reeves ST. The practice of perioperative transesophageal echocardiography. Philadelphia: Lippincott William & Wilkins; 2003.)

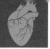

TABLE 22.3 Common Causes of Mitral Regurgitation Seen in the Operating Room.

Type of Mitral Regurgitation	Common Causes
Structural MR	Mitral valve prolapse Rheumatic disease Congenital valve disease Mitral valve endocarditis
Secondary MR	Ischemic heart disease Nonischemic dilated cardiomyopathy
MR associated with obstruction of left ventricular outflow tract	HCM Underfilled or hyperdynamic left ventricle (rare without HCM) After mitral valve repair (usually in the setting of underfilling/hyperdynamic states)

HCM, Hypertrophic cardiomyopathy; *MR,* mitral regurgitation.

components of the valve that need to be addressed surgically, evaluation of MV repair and replacement, and localization of postprocedural leaks.[23]

Although 3D TEE is commonly used in a complementary fashion to 2D TEE, few studies have attempted to define the incremental value added by 3D TEE. Although few would dispute that intraoperative 3D TEE for MV surgery is an established technique, no amount of perioperative imaging can make up for inadequate surgical exposure.[24]

Grewal et al[25] compared 2D TEE and 3D TEE in the setting of MV surgery and found that the two methods were equally reliable in diagnosing the cause; however, 3D TEE had greater sensitivity and specificity for disease involving the P1 segment of the posterior leaflet or the A3 segment of the anterior leaflet and for bileaflet disease. Similarly, Ben Zekry et al[26] reported that the 2D and 3D methods of TEE were highly accurate in diagnosing mitral disease but that 3D TEE could localize the lesion more predictably. Both studies acknowledged the limitations inherent in such comparisons. Surgical observation is considered to be the gold standard even though it is performed with the heart in a flaccid state.

In an elegant study, Maffessanti et al[27] evaluated a large group of patients with Carpentier type II disease and found improved localization of leaflet abnormalities with 3D TEE and a greater ability to define annular shape before and after surgical repair. Other studies have reported higher accuracy with 3D TEE in the evaluation of mitral pathology,[28–32] especially when there was involvement of the commissures[33] (Fig. 22.8).

3D TEE has enhanced our understanding of mitral leaflet and annular mechanics and the ability to define complex lesions before and after bypass (see Chapter 2). The valve can be imaged from the LA and LV sides. MV quantification software may improve the ability to fully define MV lesions and may help the surgeon better plan the procedure[2]: what to resect, the shape of annular ring to choose, and the predicted effect of remodeling procedures such as papillary muscle repositioning.[34] The limitations on the use of 3D TEE in the operating room are related to the negative effect of electrocautery on multibeat acquisition and the lower resolution compared with 2D TEE. The two techniques remain complementary.

Mitral Regurgitant Severity
Loading Conditions
The most important confounding variables in the intraoperative assessment of MR are the loading conditions, which are affected to a great

degree by (1) the depressive effects of general anesthesia on myocardial contractility[35] and vascular tone and (2) the effects of positive-pressure ventilation on systemic venous return in open heart and closed chest procedures.[36] For these reasons, the degree of intraoperative MR is often significantly less than what is than seen on preoperative transthoracic studies. This finding sometimes creates uncertainty about the proper surgical course of action.

Several strategies have been proposed to replicate findings in the preoperative state after TEE. In a prospective study of patients with at least moderate MR due to a variety of causes, TEE was performed at three stages: with conscious sedation before induction of anesthesia, after induction, and after use of phenylephrine to bring the blood pressure back to pre-induction levels.[37] Blood pressure dropped significantly after induction and was raised above baseline with phenylephrine. Compared with pre-induction findings, there were decreases in measurements of vena contracta, regurgitant orifice area (ROA), and regurgitant volume, although the decreases were not statistically significant. Phenylephrine resulted in the return of regurgitant parameters to baseline, with a significant increase in MR severity compared with values after induction, regardless of the underlying cause. This was likely a result of the combination of increased blood pressure, changes in preload, and possible myocardial ischemia.

In another study of patients with ischemic MR, phenylephrine and fluids were used to restore preinduction hemodynamics. The parameters of MR severity dropped after anesthesia induction, although not significantly. With loading, blood pressure, ROA, and regurgitant volume superseded baseline measurements.[38] However, these effects have not been seen uniformly in all patients. In a diverse group of patients with MR, values for MR severity remained less than at baseline in 20% of patients despite the use of vasoactive agents to bring blood pressure back to baseline.[39]

These studies in combination with clinical experience emphasize that intraoperative Doppler estimation of MR is complex. Measures of MR severity are affected by the degree of blood pressure drop, the use of pacemakers in the post-bypass period, changes in preload and afterload, LV contractility, LV dyssynchrony, mitral closing force, the cause of the mitral disease, other concurrent valve lesions, and the possible induction of myocardial ischemia. The use of pharmacologic manipulation to reestablish baseline conditions is to some extent artificial, and the significance of increased MR severity with overdriving of loading parameters is uncertain. Parenthetically, the use of phenylephrine may reduce the amount of MR in patients with dynamic obstruction of the left ventricular outflow tract (LVOT).

It is axiomatic that a high-quality preoperative echocardiogram performed without general anesthesia should be readily available for review in the operating room. Decisions based on the patient's clinical course and symptoms, degree of LV dilation and systolic dysfunction, and quantitation of MR on the preoperative study should rarely be overruled simply on the basis of differences in the quantitative parameters of MR severity on intraoperative TEE.

Color Doppler Imaging
The MR jet as defined by color Doppler imaging is complex. The size of the jet as it fans out into the LA is of limited quantitative value because of numerous technical and physiologic factors.[40] The direction of the jet gives useful information about the mechanism of the MR (see Fig. 22.8), and the presence of multiple jets may indicate leaflet perforation (Fig. 22.9). However, eccentric jets appear smaller than central jets because they flatten out against the wall of the receiving chamber. Physiologic factors such as the driving pressure across the valve or changes in LA compliance related to chronicity of regurgitation also affect the size of the jet. Instrument settings (e.g., color gain, pulse repetition frequency) affect jet size independently of ROA.

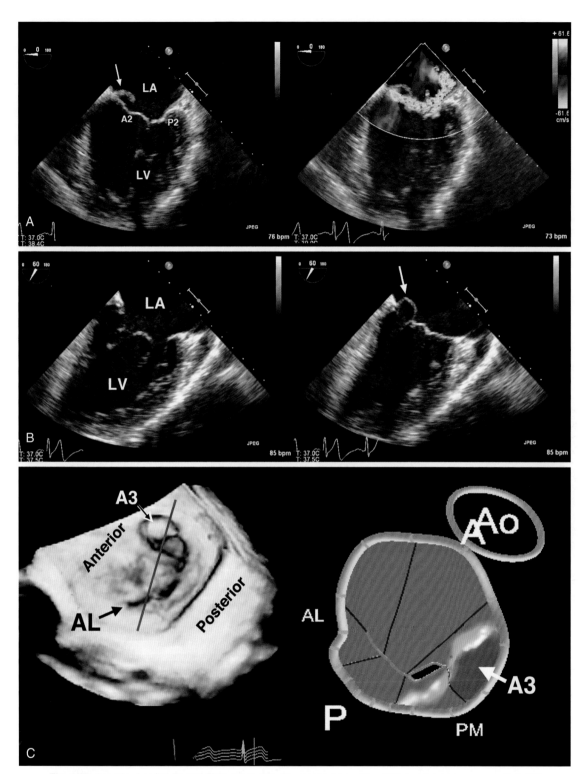

Fig. 22.8 Anterior Leaflet Partial Flail. (A) In this 42-year-old man with a history of dyspnea on exertion, 2D imaging *(left)* in a posteriorly angulated four-chamber view at 0 degrees rotation during systole demonstrates normally functioning *A2* and *P2* segments; there is, however, what is presumably a flail segment of one of the mitral leaflets *(arrow)* (Video 22.8A ▶). Color-flow imaging *(right)* shows a posteriorly directed mitral regurgitant jet, which is most consistent with anterior leaflet disease. (B) In a commisural view at 60 degrees, the valve opens normally in diastole *(left)* and during systole *(right)* (Video 22.8B ▶). There is prolapse *(arrow)* of what would appear to be the P3 scallop, but this is contradicted by the posterior direction of the MR jet as seen in A. (C) 3D quantification shows how this paradox can arise (Video 22.8C ▶). From the LA perspective *(left)*, the *red line* approximates the TEE commissural plane; however, the A3 segment can be seen to prolapse, intersect the commissural plane, and obscure the P3 segment. Quantification *(right)* shows that the *A3* segment is primarily affected. *A*, Anterior; *AL*, anterolateral, *Ao*, aortic valve; *P*, posterior; *PM*, posteromedial.

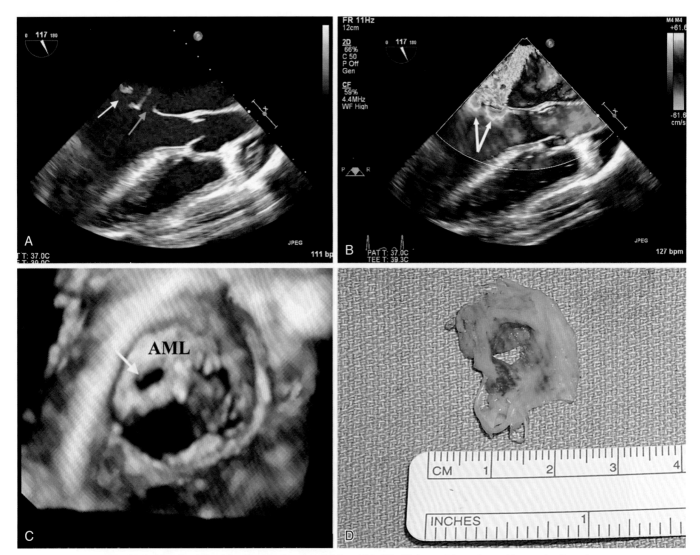

Fig. 22.9 Anterior Mitral Leaflet Perforation (Video 22.9 ▶). (A) In a mid-esophageal long-axis view, the *white arrow* indicates the normal point of coaptation, whereas the *green arrow* indicates another regurgitant orifice. (B) Color Doppler in the same view. Two jets of mitral regurgitation *(double arrow)* can be seen—a normal central jet and another jet that appears to come through a leaflet perforation. (C) 3D transesophageal echocardiography confirms a perforation *(arrow)* in the anterior mitral leaflet *(AML).* (D) The excised mitral leaflet.

Vena Contracta

The vena contracta (see Fig. 6.15) is the narrowest central flow region of a jet that occurs at or just downstream from the orifice of a regurgitant valve.[41] The vena contracta measurement is easily obtained in the operating room and can be used to assess regurgitation severity. The vena contracta is measured as the narrow neck between the proximal flow convergence area and expansion of the jet in the receiving chamber, at or distal to the valve orifice. Vena contracta measurements correlate with invasive measures of MR, regardless of the cause of regurgitation, and they compare favorably with more complex measures such as regurgitant volume and ROA.[42,43]

Current guidelines recommend that vena contracta widths between 3 and 7 mm need to be confirmed by more quantitative methods when feasible.[44,45] They include other Doppler imaging–based techniques, such as proximal isovelocity surface area (PISA), and volumetric methods based on calculations of stroke volume through the mitral and aortic annuli.[44] However, these methods can be challenging with intraoperative TEE.

There has been interest in 3D methods of MR quantification.[46] The measurement of 3D vena contracta area is appealing because it theoretically overcomes some of the noncircular geometric differences in patients with secondary MR. Cutoff values for severe MR range from 0.4 to 0.6 cm². However, the inherent limitations of intraoperative 3D imaging previously described apply here: need for multiple beats, stitching artifacts, need for precise orientation of the intersecting planes, and variation depending on the phase of systole chosen.[46] Although many studies have shown good agreement with other methods of MR quantitation,[47] vena contracta area measurement has not yet found its way into published guidelines.[44,45]

Spectral Doppler Imaging

Continuous-wave Doppler echocardiography is used to examine the temporal characteristics of the MR jet and jet density. Dense, early-peaking, and triangular jets are more indicative of significant MR (Fig. 22.10).

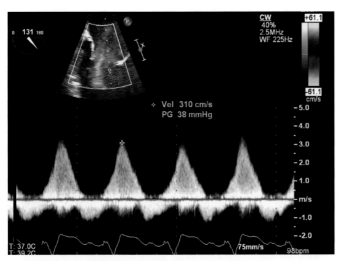

Fig. 22.10 Continuous-Wave Doppler Echocardiography of Mitral Regurgitation. The velocity profile is very dense and triangular, indicating significant mitral regurgitation.

Pulsed-wave Doppler echocardiography interrogation of the pulmonary veins is easy to perform. The finding of systolic reversal has high specificity but low sensitivity for severe MR; systolic blunting may indicate moderate MR, but it often coexists with other causes of elevated LA pressure.

Mitral inflow velocities are measured with either pulsed-wave or continuous-wave Doppler echocardiography to assess for MS. Advantages and limitations of various quantitative techniques are described elsewhere (see Chapters 15 and 16).

Reparability

Numerous techniques of MV repair exist and are in constant evolution (see Chapter 19). The reparability of a given valve depends on the lesion (Tables 22.4 and 22.5) and, more importantly, the skill of the surgeon. The echocardiographer must present the information needed to make the appropriate surgical decision. This involves a complete 2D MV examination (described earlier), and if proper equipment and a skilled operator are available, a comprehensive 3D examination. The Carpentier classification[11] is widely used to describe the subgroups of MR and has relevance regarding the choice of surgical procedure.

Carpentier type I: normal leaflet motion. In the case of leaflet perforation, MR with normal leaflet motion (see Figs. 22.7 and 22.9) often is repaired with a patch, unless the degree of leaflet destruction precludes this approach. The indications for MV surgery with or without coronary artery bypass grafting (CABG) in patients with dilated cardiomyopathy are discussed elsewhere (see Chapter 18). If desired, repair may be accomplished with ring annuloplasty or valve replacement.

Carpentier type II: excessive leaflet motion. Excessive leaflet motion, as in MV prolapse, is often repairable, most frequently with resection of redundant posterior leaflet segments and placement of an annuloplasty ring (Fig. 22.11; see Fig. 22.7). Altering the leaflet lengths and annular diameter may change the distance between the coaptation point and the interventricular septum and therefore has the potential to produce postoperative systolic anterior motion (SAM) of the MV. The pathophysiology of SAM after valve replacement is related to anatomic factors, which set the stage for the anterior leaflet to obstruct the (LVOT),[48] and post-bypass physiologic abnormalities (discussed later). The anatomic factors include excess posterior leaflet movement causing anterior displacement of the coaptation plane and a long anterior leaflet with or without an undersized annuloplasty ring.

Maslow et al[49] and Varghese et al[50] stressed the importance of the pre-bypass examination and emphasized the significance of a small LV, an enlarged basal septum, a small anterior-to-posterior leaflet ratio, a narrow aortomitral angle, and a small coaptation point–to-septal distance—all factors that portend outflow obstruction. Surgical modifications that can be used to decrease the likelihood of SAM include posterior leaflet reduction with a sliding annuloplasty,[51] triangular resection of the posterior leaflet prolapse,[52] anterior leaflet shortening, and LVOT myomectomy[53]

TABLE 22.4 Probability of Successful Mitral Valve Repair for Primary Mitral Regurgitation Based on Echocardiographic Findings.

Type	Dysfunction (Carpentier Class)	Calcification	Mitral Annulus Dilation	Probability of Repair
Degenerative	II: Localized prolapse (leaflet P2 and/or A2)	No/localized	Mild/moderate	Feasible
Ischemic or secondary	I or IIIb	No	Moderate	Feasible
Barlow disease	II: Extensive prolapse (≥3 scallops, posterior commissure)	Localized (annulus)	Moderate	Difficult
Rheumatic	IIIa but pliable anterior leaflet	Localized	Moderate	Difficult
Severe Barlow disease	II: Extensive prolapse (>3 scallops, anterior commissure)	Extensive (annulus + leaflets)	Severe	Unlikely
Endocarditis	II: Prolapse but destructive lesions	No	No/mild	Unlikely
Rheumatic	IIIa but stiff anterior leaflet	Extensive (annulus + leaflets)	Moderate/severe	Unlikely
Ischemic or secondary	IIIb but severe valvular deformation	No	No or severe	Unlikely

From Lancellotti, P, Tribouilloy C, Hagendorff A, et al. Recommendations for the echocardiographic assessment of native valvular regurgitation: an executive summary from the European Association of Cardiovascular Imaging. Eur Heart J Cardiovasc Imaging 2013;14(7):611-644.

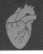

TABLE 22.5 Transthoracic Echocardiographic Characteristics Unfavorable for Mitral Valve Repair in Secondary Mitral Regurgitation.

Coaptation distance > 1 cm

Tenting area > 2.5 cm^2

Posterolateral angle > 45 degrees (high posterior leaflet tethering)

Distal anterior mitral leaflet angle > 25 degrees

LV end-diastolic diameter > 65 mm

LV end-systolic diameter > 51 mm

End-systolic interpapillary muscle distance > 20 mm

Systolic sphericity index > 0.7

From Lancellotti P, Tribouilloy C, Hagendorff A, et al. Recommendations for the echocardiographic assessment of native valvular regurgitation: an executive summary from the European Association of Cardiovascular Imaging. Eur Heart J Cardiovasc Imaging 2013;14(7):611-644.

(see Chapter 19). Patients with Barlow disease and bileaflet prolapse at presentation are often not candidates for repair.

Correction of anterior leaflet prolapse is more complex because of its association with the rigid aortic-mitral curtain (see Fig. 22.2). Options include placement of synthetic chordae or chordal transfer[54] and edge-to-edge plication of the anterior and posterior leaflets.

If excessive leaflet motion is the result of endocarditis, valve replacement is usually indicated. Rarely, papillary muscle rupture complicates myocardial infarction, usually involving the inferoposterior wall. The flail segment may or may not be visualized in the LA. Surgical treatment is usually valve replacement.

Carpentier type IIIB: restricted systolic leaflet motion. Symmetric or asymmetric leaflet tethering often occurs in the setting of ischemic heart disease (Table 22.6; see Fig. 22.7). The greater the degree of leaflet restriction, the less likely it is that a surgical repair will be successful. Because the abnormality is not in the valve leaflets but in the LV and subvalvular apparatus, novel restorative approaches are being slowly introduced into the therapeutic realm.[34] The techniques of surgical treatment of ischemic MR vary greatly and are summarized in the American Association for Thoracic Surgery consensus guidelines for treatment of ischemic MR.[55]

Carpentier type IIIA: restricted systolic and diastolic leaflet motion. Adults with rheumatic MV disease usually undergo valve replacement, especially if there is coexistent MS (see Fig. 22.7).[56] They typically are individuals who have extensive distortion of the valve apparatus, often with extensive chordal involvement, and for whom balloon valvuloplasty has been rejected. However, when valve thickening and chordal fusion are not as prominent but valvuloplasty is judged as inappropriate because of excessive regurgitation, ring annuloplasty may be feasible.

The probability of successful MV repair in primary and secondary MR based on echocardiographic findings is presented in Tables 22.4 and 22.5. The MR that accompanies hypertrophic obstructive cardiomyopathy does not fit neatly into any of the previously defined categories. Surgical treatment involves septal myectomy and concomitant procedures on the MV[57] and subvalvular apparatus.[58]

Prosthetic Valves

Problems with prosthetic valves such as perivalvular regurgitation due to valve dehiscence or stuck leaflets may be detected before chest closure, and these problems should be rectified before the patient leaves the operating room (see later discussion).

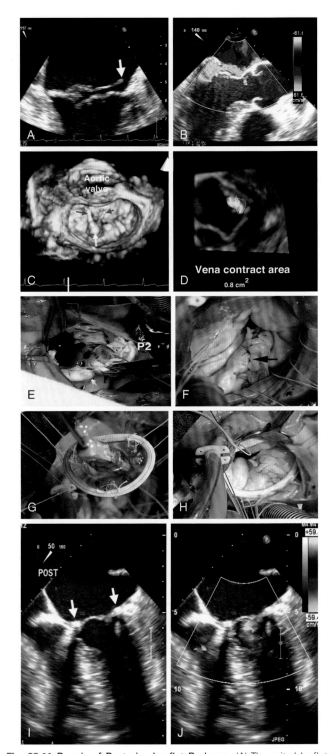

Fig. 22.11 Repair of Posterior Leaflet Prolapse. (A) The mitral leaflets are only mildly thickened with prolapse of P2 with a torn chord *(arrow)* seen in the mid-esophageal long-axis view (Video 22.11A ►). (B) Color-flow Doppler imaging shows an anteriorly directed jet of mitral regurgitation (Video 22.11B ►). All three components of the jet are seen. The vena contracta width measures 0.7 cm. (C) Real-time 3D echocardiography of the mitral valve from the surgeon's view shows the P2 prolapse *(white arrow)* with torn chordae *(red arrows)* (Video 22.11C ►). (D) A 3D vena contracta area is measured at 0.8 cm^2. (E) At surgery, the affected P2 segment is grasped by the surgeon. (F) After excision of the P2 segment, P1 and P3 are sutured together *(arrow)*. The annuloplasty ring has been sized to the anterior leaflet (G) and sutured in place (H). (I) The *arrows* indicate the position of the annuloplasty ring after bypass. (J) No residual regurgitation is seen (Video 22.11 I and J ►).

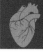

TABLE 22.6   Examination of the Mitral Valve After Cardiopulmonary Bypass.

Structure or Subject of Interest	Examination	Views	Focus
Mitral Valve Repair			
LV	Regional and global function, volume status	Mid-esophageal two- and four-chamber, mid-esophageal long-axis, transgastric long- and short-axis views	Adequate contractility important for valve closure; hypovolemia or hypercontractility predispose to SAM. Examine LV restraint, papillary repositioning if performed
Right ventricle	Regional and global function	Mid-esophageal four-chamber, transgastric long- and short-axis views	New dysfunction may indicate right coronary artery air, significant residual MR
MV competence	Define residual jets for severity, direction. Assess coaptation length, residual prolapse, flail, tethering	Views as outlined in Fig. 22.4 and Table 22.2. Color-flow Doppler with appropriate technical settings. PW Doppler of pulmonary veins	Trace central jets usually acceptable. Eccentric jets may indicate breakdown of valve repair
MV gradients	Excessive gradients may indicate undersized annuloplasty ring	PW and CW Doppler of mitral inflow	Gradients may be present due to high flow state after cardiopulmonary bypass
Annulus	Assess for seating, MR outside the annuloplasty ring	Views outlined in Fig. 22.4 and Table 22.2	Regurgitation outside the ring always abnormal, may indicate separation from native annulus, poor valve seating
LVOT	LVOT obstruction	Mid-esophageal four-chamber and long-axis, deep transgastric, transgastric long-axis views with color-flow and CW Doppler views	Abnormal flow acceleration may indicate LVOT obstruction. Look for SAM
Surrounding structures	Aortic valve, circumflex artery, AV nodal artery[a]	Check aortic valve competence, circumflex territory, heart block views	
Prosthetic Valve Replacement			
Mechanical valve	Evaluate proper bileaflet motion. Color-flow Doppler, PW and CW Doppler gradients	Scan valve from mid-esophageal position. Leaflet best viewed at about 0–20 degrees if valve placement is anatomic, 50–70 degrees if anti-anatomic; 3D TEE may help identify adequacy of leaflet motion.	Small washing jets acceptable. Paravalvular MR, if small, often disappears after heparin reversal
	LVOT obstruction	Mid-esophageal four-chamber and long-axis, deep transgastric, transgastric long-axis with color and CW Doppler views	Preserved anterior leaflet may result in SAM
Tissue valve	Evaluate leaflet motion, color Doppler, Doppler-derived gradients	Midesophageal 4-chamber and long-axis	Small central MR often present
	LVOT obstruction	Mid-esophageal four-chamber and long-axis, deep transgastric, transgastric long-axis with color and CW Doppler views	Preserved anterior leaflet may result in SAM (see Fig. 22.17). Prosthetic struts may protrude into LVOT, infrequently a cause of LVOT obstruction

[a]Berdajs D, Schurr UP, Wagner A, et al. Incidence and pathophysiology of atrioventricular block following mitral valve replacement and ring annuloplasty. Eur J Cardio-Thorac Surg 2008;34:55-61.

AV, Atrioventricular; *Doppler,* Doppler echocardiography/imaging; *MR,* mitral regurgitation; *MV,* mitral valve; *OT,* outflow tract; *PW,* pulsed-wave; *SAM,* systolic anterior motion of the mitral valve.

Patients with prosthetic MVs may return later for replacement of the valves. The pattern of presentation depends on the type of prosthesis. Tissue valves become fibrotic and calcified over time. Leaflet degeneration may lead to regurgitation, whereas calcification often results in stenosis. Abnormalities of leaflet motion in mechanical valves may be caused by pannus or thrombus formation and may lead to various degrees of stenosis and regurgitation, often acute; the differentiation

between pannus and thrombus is often challenging and may require additional preoperative imaging modalities such as 64-section cardiac computed tomography.[59]

Endocarditis is a concern for mechanical and tissue prosthetic valves and may lead to emboli, leaflet dysfunction, and paravalvular infectious complications resulting in valve dehiscence and fistula formation. On echocardiographic imaging, the issue of distal shadowing

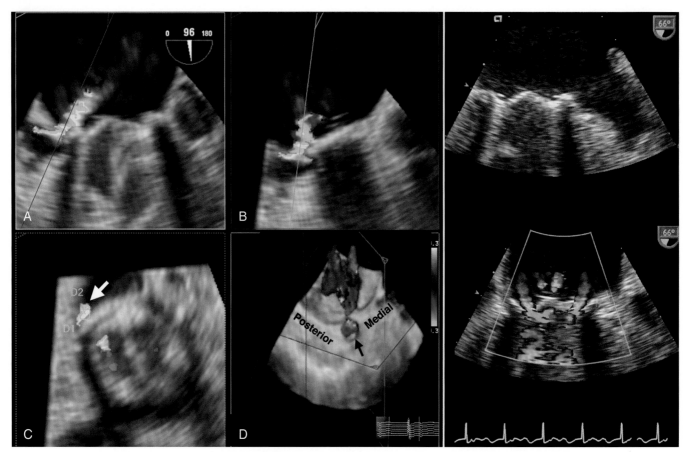

Fig. 22.12 Paravalvular Prosthetic Mitral Valve Regurgitation. This 62-year-old man with a bileaflet mechanical mitral prosthesis underwent TEE as part of a workup of hemolysis. (A and B) Orthogonal images of a jet of paravalvular regurgitation show vena contracta diameters of 0.65 and 0.4 cm and a vena contracta area of 0.4 cm² (Videos 22.12A ▶ and B ▶). (C) The jet within the ring is a cleaning jet. (D) 3D imaging accurately localizes the jet (arrow) as being located posteromedial to the valve ring. The patient underwent surgical revision of the valve. On the right, the two images show a normal bileaflet prosthesis with four cleaning jets identified within the sewing ring.

is more of a concern for mechanical valves. With TTE, the LA and the MR jet may be obscured, whereas with TEE, the LV and LVOT are not well visualized. The two techniques are complementary, and typically both are needed in patient evaluation.

A complete intraoperative evaluation requires careful scanning of the prosthetic MV from stomach and esophagus and from different angles of interrogation. The appearance of the valve leaflets and whether tissue leaflet motion is excessive or restricted are documented. Spectral Doppler imaging is used to obtain the mean pressure gradient and pressure half-time, and 2D and 3D color-flow Doppler echocardiography allows quantification of the severity of MR and the relationship of the jet to the sewing ring (Fig. 22.12). 3D TEE may be helpful in the evaluation and percutaneous closure of mitral paravalvular leaks[60] (see Chapter 21).

Tricuspid Regurgitation

Tricuspid regurgitation (TR) commonly results from the right ventricular and tricuspid annular dilation that often accompanies MV disease. The pathophysiology of secondary TR is complex. In some instances, lesser degrees of TR in relatively healthy patients can regress after mitral surgery alone. However, with TR of moderate or greater severity, consideration should be given to annular reduction, especially in the setting of dilated cardiomyopathy.[61] This approach

is justified by the consequently reduced rate of TR progression, reverse remodeling of the dysfunctional right ventricle, and better outcomes.[62,63]

Severe tethering, increased age, and severe TR preoperatively indicate a high likelihood of residual TR after annuloplasty (Fig. 22.13). The risk of underestimating TR in the anesthetized patient, which is theoretically an issue because of a change in right ventricular loading conditions, must be considered in clinical decision making. In patients whose tricuspid valve disease is caused by disease of the leaflets, there is a higher likelihood of a need for valve replacement.

POST-BYPASS EVALUATION

Native Valve Assessment

MV repair in properly selected patients has excellent long-term durability. However, residual regurgitation after MV repair relates to the complexity of the procedure and portends a poor long-term outcome in terms of rate of reoperation, recurrence of MR, LV dysfunction, and death.[64,65]

Anyanwu and Adams[66] broadly categorized the causes of MV repair failure as resulting from technical inadequacies (e.g., inappropriate annular ring selection) or progression of underlying disease with

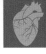

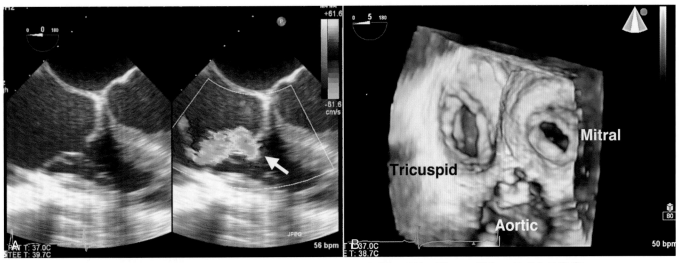

Fig. 22.13 Tricuspid Regurgitation Accompanying Rheumatic Mitral Valve Disease (Videos 22.13A, B ▶ ▶). (A and B) Severe TR was noticed on TEE in a 31-year-old man with rheumatic heart disease who was scheduled for mitral valve replacement. In real time, leaflet mobility was diminished *(arrow)*. (B) 3D TEE shows that the tricuspid leaflets are thickened and fused. Both atrioventricular valves were replaced. *TR,* Tricuspid regurgitation.

global or localized LV remodeling. The echocardiographer must recognize both conditions, which require immediate attention in the operating room, and situations in which late failure is predictable.

After MV repair and before removal of the cross-clamps, the surgeon distends the ventricle with saline to address gross inadequacies of the repair. The postprocedural evaluation begins in earnest after separation from cardiopulmonary bypass is complete. At that point, the echocardiographer should have a complete understanding of what the surgeon did and what problems can be anticipated. Because this is a time of rapid hemodynamic change, the final opinion on the result should await restoration of baseline conditions. The components of the examination after cardiopulmonary bypass are outlined in Table 22.6.

Left and right ventricular function should be carefully assessed, especially if coronary bypass with or without a ventricular remodeling procedure has been performed. Right ventricular dysfunction may be the result of persistent severe MR, intracoronary air emboli, or inadequate ventricular protection during the period of aortic cross-clamping. Any ancillary procedures, such as tricuspid annuloplasty, must be carefully evaluated.

The detection of residual MR is the most important component of the postoperative examination. As with the pre-bypass evaluation, multiple views of the MV, including off-axis views, 3D TEE if available, must be examined to determine the presence or absence of residual MR. Severity is assessed with use of the same criteria as for native valves on the baseline study. Normal loading conditions must be established before the final determination.

Residual MR may be caused by several factors. Failure of synthetic chordae or chordal transfer may result in persistence of MR. If the annulus has not been downsized appropriately, inadequate coaptation length and residual central MR may occur. If the MR is eccentric, the valve must be reexamined to determine whether there are persistent coaptation abnormalities. If the residual jet occurs outside the zone of coaptation, the suture used to close the leaflet defect after excision may have broken down. If the MR jet lies outside the annuloplasty ring, the ring may have become detached from the native annulus. The direction of the postoperative jet is often different from that seen preoperatively.

If the postoperative regurgitation is graded as greater than mild or if it results from a significant technical breakdown, the patient should be returned to cardiopulmonary bypass and the valve re-repaired or an MV replacement performed.[67] Only in exceptional circumstances, such as patient instability, should a second session of bypass be denied.

Mitral Valve Systolic Anterior Motion

SAM after MV repair is often first suspected from color-flow Doppler aliasing in the LVOT with residual MR, evident on four-chamber and long-axis views (Fig. 22.14). The late-peaking high-velocity (dagger) appearance on continuous-wave Doppler echocardiography can often be demonstrated in the transgastric long-axis and deep transgastric views and may allow calculation of the gradient across the outflow tract, although the gradient may be underestimated because of a nonparallel angle between the Doppler beam and the high-velocity jet. SAM is less of a problem in ischemic MR because the outflow tract is usually large.

Decreased preload and afterload along with increased heart rate and contractility can predispose to SAM and should be addressed through manipulations of vascular tone, volume, and inotropy. If MR cannot be ameliorated, cardiopulmonary bypass should be reinitiated and the valve repaired again or replaced. Patients who have intraoperative SAM that resolves with medical management in the operating room have low rates of recurrent SAM when evaluated at follow-up, with and without stress testing.[68,69]

In rare instances, certain congenital abnormalities may predispose to post-bypass LVOT obstruction. The anteriorly displaced aortic valve and gooseneck deformity of the LVOT seen in atrioventricular septal defect is an example.[70] Placement of a mitral annuloplasty ring may be sufficient to cause a fixed obstruction after bypass that may necessitate removal of the ring (Fig. 22.15).

Assessment must be made in a timely fashion to rectify problems before systemic heparin anticoagulation is reversed and the bypass cannulas are removed.

Prosthetic Valve Assessment

After replacement, the prosthetic valve should be imaged by 2D, 3D (if available), spectral, and color-flow Doppler echocardiography. This

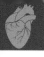

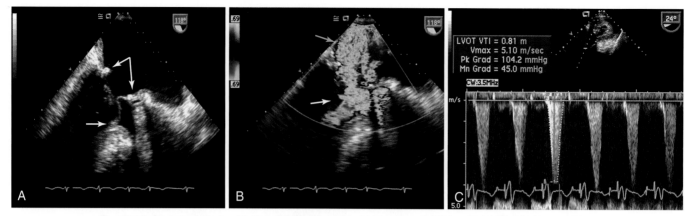

Fig. 22.14 Systolic Anterior Motion (SAM) After Mitral Valve Repair (Video 22.14 ▶). (A) After excision of the P2 segment and ring annuloplasty *(double arrow),* SAM developed *(single arrow)* due to hypovolemia. (B) Color-flow Doppler imaging shows mitral regurgitation (MR) *(purple arrow)* and left ventricular outflow tract (LVOT) obstruction manifested as color Doppler aliasing *(white arrow).* (C) Deep transgastric imaging allowed parallel alignment of the continuous-wave Doppler echocardiography beam with the outflow tract, showing an ice pick–shaped jet, evidence of dynamic obstruction. The MR and outflow obstruction resolved with measures to increase blood volume and a decrease in inotropic support. In real-time, SAM *(left)* can be seen and compared with its resolution *(right)* after hemodynamic optimization.

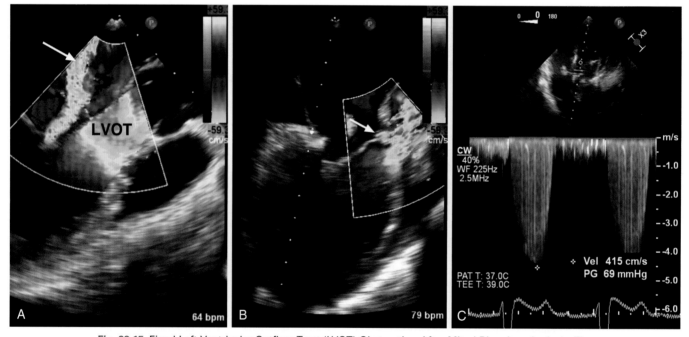

Fig. 22.15 Fixed Left Ventricular Outflow Tract (LVOT) Obstruction After Mitral Ring Annuloplasty. The patient with an atrioventricular septal defect presented for mitral valve repair. A gooseneck deformity of the LVOT was identified. (A) A mid-esophageal, long-axis view during systole shows a central jet of mitral regurgitation *(arrow)* and flow in the left ventricular outflow tract (Video 22.15A ▶). (B) Postoperatively, a mid-esophageal long-axis view shows anterior displacement of the ring annuloplasty *(arrow),* producing narrowing and turbulence in the LVOT (Video 22.15B ▶). (C) A deep transgastric view shows a pattern of fixed LVOT obstruction with a peak gradient of 69 mmHg. The patient was returned to bypass, and the ring was removed with subsequent resolution of the LVOT obstruction.

process is more straightforward for tissue prostheses, which are trileaflet valves. For mechanical valves, scanning from 0 to 180 degrees in the mid-esophageal position enables the optimal angle for leaflet assessment to be determined. Both leaflets should move in an unrestricted fashion (Fig. 22.16).

Pressure gradients across a newly placed prosthetic valve are often higher than expected. Assessment of pressure gradients after cardiopulmonary bypass may be confounded by several factors: increased post-bypass cardiac output and anemia, pressure recovery, complex flow patterns of prosthetic valves, and use of the simplified Bernoulli equation (pressure gradient $= 4v^2$), which does not take into account high velocities proximal to the MV.[71] Any increased gradient takes on significance if there is obvious valvular dysfunction. The posts of a tissue prosthesis have the potential to obstruct the LVOT, especially if it is small and the valve has a high profile. Later in follow-up, the finding of high gradients as defined in the literature[71,72] should prompt

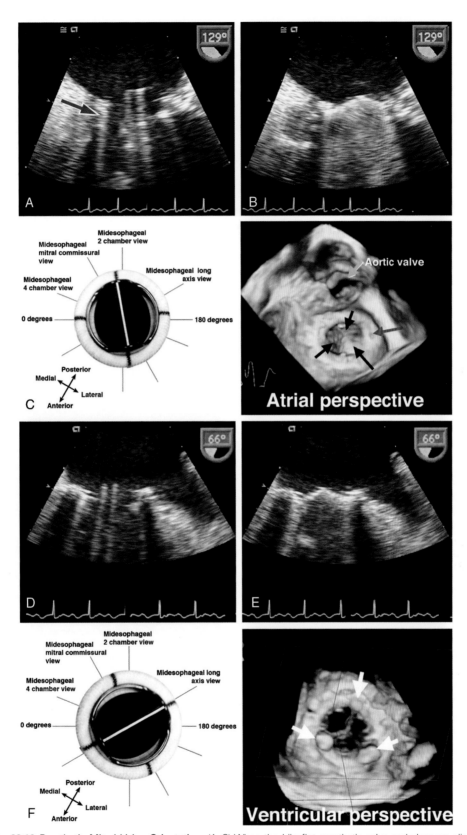

Fig. 22.16 Prosthetic Mitral Valve Orientation. (A–C) When the bileaflet prosthetic valve occluders are aligned parallel to the position of the native valve leaflets (i.e., anatomic position), mid-esophageal images in a long-axis plane show both leaflets opening normally in diastole (A) and closing in systole (B) (Video 22.16A, B. C ▶▶▶). The *arrow* (A) indicates a reverberation or comet tail artifact originating from the sewing ring. (D–F) When the prosthetic occluders are aligned perpendicular to the normal leaflet alignment (i.e., anti-anatomic position), the transesophageal echocardiography image plane must be rotated to about 65 degrees to show normal occluder motion in diastole (D) and systole (E) (Video 22.16D ▶). In the two panels on the right, a normal bioprosthetic valve is seen. The three leaflets are indicated by *black arrows,* the sewing ring by a *red arrow,* and the three struts by *white arrows.*

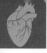

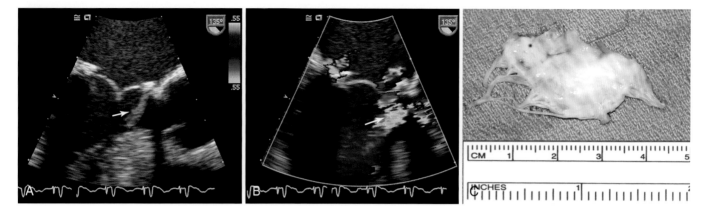

Fig. 22.17 Subaortic Obstruction (Video 22.17 ▶). (A) After prosthetic tissue mitral valve replacement and subvalvular preservation, native anterior leaflet tissue can be seen obstructing the left ventricular outflow tract (LVOT) *(arrow)*. (B) With color-flow Doppler, aliasing in the LVOT is seen, indicating flow acceleration. (C) Cardiopulmonary bypass was reinstituted, and after the native anterior leaflet was excised, the left ventricular outflow gradient resolved. The excised leaflet is shown.

examination for pathologic valve obstruction or patient prosthesis mismatch (see Chapter 26).

Color-flow Doppler evidence of MR is seen with most prosthetic valves. With a tissue prosthesis, there is often a small jet of central MR, and a bileaflet mechanical prosthesis has small intravalvular cleaning jets (see Fig. 22.12). Echocardiographic interrogation at multiple angles helps determine whether the jets are physiologic or pathologic.

Abnormally large intravalvular jets may result if valve closure is impeded by retained mitral tissue.[73] Return to cardiopulmonary bypass is usually needed so that rotation of the valve within the sewing ring or excision of the redundant tissue may be performed. Paravalvular jets are always abnormal (see Fig. 22.12) and result from inadequate seating in the native annulus, especially in the setting of mitral annular calcification. Small paravalvular leaks often disappear after heparin reversal, but larger leaks should be addressed in the operating room before decannulation. 3D TEE may help pinpoint their location.

If the patient cannot tolerate another bypass or attempted closure of the leak is technically too challenging, consideration may be given to transcatheter closure at a later date. SAM can compound mitral valve replacement if native anterior leaflet preservation is undertaken, and this can occur after bioprosthetic and mechanical valve replacements (Fig. 22.17).

Assessment of Proximate Structures

Several vulnerable anatomic structures lie near the mitral annulus. Sutures placed in the MV sewing ring may entrap the left and/or noncoronary leaflets of the aortic valve. The circumflex artery is also vulnerable as it passes posterior to the MV annulus (Fig. 22.18).[74,75] Appropriate 2D TEE and Doppler echocardiography examinations should be performed to rule out injury to these structures.

GUIDELINES AND OUTCOMES

The American Heart Association (AHA)/American College of Cardiology (ACC)/American Society of Echocardiography (ASE) guidelines[5] recommend the use of intraoperative TEE (class Ib recommendation) for all surgical valve repair and complex valve replacement procedures.

Several important questions arise. What is the additive value of TEE before bypass in clarifying MV pathology? What is the impact of post-bypass TEE on the rates of immediate and late reoperation, and does it result in improved outcomes?

If pre-bypass findings contradict preoperative TTE findings, should the surgical plan be changed? The answer is yes, but only if it can be

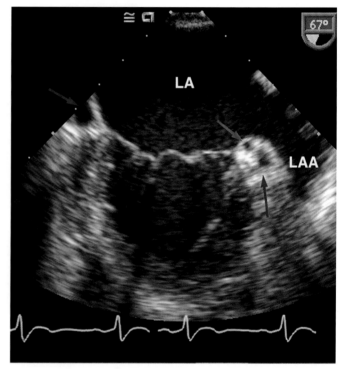

Fig. 22.18 Para-annular Anatomy. In this commissural view, the circumflex artery can be seen adjacent to the mitral annulus *(red arrow)*. The *blue arrow* indicates the coronary sinus. *LAA,* Left atrial appendage.

demonstrated that the new finding was not the result of changes in loading conditions but something that could reasonably have been missed on preoperative TTE, such as leaflet perforation. Comparison of the intraoperative TEE with the preoperative TTE should shed light on any differences.

If post-bypass imaging identifies abnormalities, should the finding prompt a second bypass session to allow correction? A gross technical failure of repair or an obvious abnormality of a prosthetic valve (e.g., stuck leaflet, large paravalvular leak, persistent SAM after medical optimization) should be addressed in the operating room, but more subtle degrees of MR in the adequately loaded patient present a greater challenge. Evidence seems to support an aggressive strategy to correct anything more serious than trivial MR because this is an independent predictor of recurrent MR and poor subsequent outcome.[65] In the intraoperative setting, the ability of a patient to tolerate a second pump run must be an important consideration.

CONCLUSIONS

Decision making in MV surgery is a complex task that must incorporate the clinical history, examination findings, and precise imaging with knowledge of current surgical techniques and outcomes. Recognizing what constitutes an acceptable result or a surgical failure is the most important aspect of intraoperative echocardiography. Ongoing developments of 3D technology and a better understanding of the pathophysiology of MV disease make this an exciting area of clinical practice and research.

REFERENCES

1. Anderson RH, Loukas M. The importance of attitudinally appropriate description of cardiac anatomy. Clin Anat 2009;22(1):47-51.
2. Drake DH, Zimmerman KG, Hepner AM, Nichols CD. Echo-guided mitral repair. Circ Cardiovasc Imaging 2014;7(1):132-141.
3. Quill JL, Hill AJ, Laske TG, et al. Mitral leaflet anatomy revisited. J Thorac Cardiovasc Surg 2009;137(5):1077-1081.
4. De Bonis M, Al-Attar N, Antunes M, et al. Surgical and interventional management of mitral valve regurgitation: a position statement from the European Society of Cardiology Working Groups on Cardiovascular Surgery and Valvular Heart Disease. Eur Heart J 2016;37(2):133-139.
5. Nishimura RA, Otto CM, Bonow RO, et al. 2014 AHA/ACC guideline for the management of patients with valvular heart disease: a report of the American College of Cardiology/American Heart Association Task Force on Practice Guidelines. J Thorac Cardiovasc Surg 2014;148(1):e1-e132.
6. Lang RM, Badano LP, Mor-Avi V, et al. Recommendations for cardiac chamber quantification by echocardiography in adults: an update from the American Society of Echocardiography and the European Association of Cardiovascular Imaging. J Am Soc Echocardiogr 2015;28(1):1-39.e14.
7. Shanewise JS, Cheung AT, Aronson S, et al. ASE/SCA guidelines for performing a comprehensive intraoperative multiplane transesophageal echocardiography examination: recommendations of the American Society of Echocardiography Council for Intraoperative Echocardiography and the Society of Cardiovascular Anesthesiologists Task Force for Certification in Perioperative Transesophageal Echocardiography. Anesth Analg 1999;89(4):870-884.
8. Foster GP, Isselbacher EM, Rose GA, et al. Accurate localization of mitral regurgitant defects using multiplane transesophageal echocardiography. Ann Thorac Surg 1998;65(4):1025-1031.
9. Bhatia M, Kumar P, Martinelli SM. Surgical echocardiography of the mitral valve: focus on 3D. Semin Cardiothorac Vasc Anesth 2019;23(1):26-36.
10. Hahn RT, Abraham T, Adams MS, et al. Guidelines for performing a comprehensive transesophageal echocardiographic examination: recommendations from the American Society of Echocardiography and the Society of Cardiovascular Anesthesiologists. J Am Soc Echocardiogr 2013;26(9):921-964.
11. Carpentier A. Cardiac valve surgery—the "French correction". J Thorac Cardiovasc Surg 1983;86(3):323-337.
12. Foster GP, Dunn AK, Abraham S, et al. Accurate measurement of mitral annular dimensions by echocardiography: importance of correctly aligned imaging planes and anatomic landmarks. J Am Soc Echocardiogr 2009;22(5):458-463.
13. Wasowicz M, Meineri M, Djaiani G, et al. Early complications and immediate postoperative outcomes of paravalvular leaks after valve replacement surgery. J Cardiothorac Vasc Anesth 2011;25(4):610-614.
14. Eleid MF, Foley TA, Said SM, et al. Severe mitral annular calcification: multimodality imaging for therapeutic strategies and interventions. JACC Cardiovasc Imaging 2016;9(11):1318-1337.
15. Sersar SI, Jamjoom AA. Left ventricular rupture post mitral valve replacement. Clin Med Cardiol 2009;3:101-113.
16. Moise OL, Loghin C, Tran SF, et al. Left atrium dissection: a rare cardiac surgery complication. J Cardiothorac Vasc Anesth 2017;31(3):1119-1122.
17. Reeves ST, Glas KE, Eltzschig H, et al. Guidelines for performing a comprehensive epicardial echocardiography examination: recommendations of the American Society of Echocardiography and the Society of Cardiovascular Anesthesiologists. Anesth Analg 2007;105(1):22-28.
18. Salandin V, De Castro S, Cavarretta E, et al. Epicardial real-time 3-dimensional echocardiography with the use of a pediatric transthoracic probe: a technical approach. J Cardiothorac Vasc Anesth 2010;24(1):43-50.
19. Tsang W, Freed BH, Lang RM. The role of 3-dimensional echocardiography in the diagnosis and management of mitral valve disease: myxomatous valve disease. Cardiol Clin 2013;31(2):203-215.
20. Tsang W, Lang RM. Three-dimensional echocardiography is essential for intraoperative assessment of mitral regurgitation. Circulation 2013;128(6):643-652; discussion 652.
21. Sidebotham DA, Allen SJ, Gerber IL, Fayers T. Intraoperative transesophageal echocardiography for surgical repair of mitral regurgitation. J Am Soc Echocardiogr 2014;27(4):345-366.
22. Mahmood F, Warraich HJ, Shahul S, et al. En face view of the mitral valve: definition and acquisition. Anesth Analg 2012;115(4):779-784.
23. Kronzon I, Sugeng L, Perk G, et al. Real-time 3-dimensional transesophageal echocardiography in the evaluation of post-operative mitral annuloplasty ring and prosthetic valve dehiscence. J Am Coll Cardiol 2009;53(17):1543-1547.
24. McCarthy PM. Three-dimensional echocardiography is not essential for intraoperative assessment of mitral regurgitation. Circulation 2013;128(6):653-658; discussion 658.
25. Grewal J, Mankad S, Freeman WK, et al. Real-time three-dimensional transesophageal echocardiography in the intraoperative assessment of mitral valve disease. J Am Soc Echocardiogr 2009;22(1):34-41.
26. Ben Zekry S, Nagueh SF, Little SH, et al. Comparative accuracy of two- and three-dimensional transthoracic and transesophageal echocardiography in identifying mitral valve pathology in patients undergoing mitral valve repair: initial observations. J Am Soc Echocardiogr 2011;24(10):1079-1085.
27. Maffessanti F, Marsan NA, Tamborini G, et al. Quantitative analysis of mitral valve apparatus in mitral valve prolapse before and after annuloplasty: a three-dimensional intraoperative transesophageal study. J Am Soc Echocardiogr 2011;24(4):405-413.
28. La Canna G, Arendar I, Maisano F, et al. Real-time three-dimensional transesophageal echocardiography for assessment of mitral valve functional anatomy in patients with prolapse-related regurgitation. Am J Cardiol 2011;107(9):1365-1374.
29. Mahmood F, Hess PE, Matyal R, et al. Echocardiographic anatomy of the mitral valve: a critical appraisal of 2-dimensional imaging protocols with a 3-dimensional perspective. J Cardiothorac Vasc Anesth 2012;26(5):777-784.
30. Hien MD, Rauch H, Lichtenberg A, et al. Real-time three-dimensional transesophageal echocardiography: improvements in intraoperative mitral valve imaging. Anesth Analg 2013;116(2):287-295.
31. Izumo M, Shiota M, Kar S, et al. Comparison of real-time three-dimensional transesophageal echocardiography to two-dimensional transesophageal echocardiography for quantification of mitral valve prolapse in patients with severe mitral regurgitation. Am J Cardiol 2013;111(4):588-594.
32. Huang HL, Xie XJ, Fei HW, et al. Real-time three-dimensional transesophageal echocardiography to predict artificial chordae length for mitral valve repair. J Cardiothorac Surg 2013;8:137.
33. Pepi M, Tamborini G, Maltagliati A, et al. Head-to-head comparison of two- and three-dimensional transthoracic and transesophageal echocardiography in the localization of mitral valve prolapse. J Am Coll Cardiol 2006;48(12):2524-2530.
34. Fattouch K, Murana G, Castrovinci S, et al. Mitral valve annuloplasty and papillary muscle relocation oriented by 3-dimensional transesophageal echocardiography for severe functional mitral regurgitation. J Thorac Cardiovasc Surg 2012;143(4):S38-S42.
35. Chin JH, Lee EH, Choi DK, Choi IC. The effect of depth of anesthesia on the severity of mitral regurgitation as measured by transesophageal echocardiography. J Cardiothorac Vasc Anesth 2012;26(6):994-998.

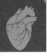
36. Kubitz JC, Annecke T, Kemming GI, et al. The influence of positive end-expiratory pressure on stroke volume variation and central blood volume during open and closed chest conditions. Eur J Cardiothorac Surg 2006;30(1):90-95.

37. Gisbert A, Souliere V, Denault AY, et al. Dynamic quantitative echocardiographic evaluation of mitral regurgitation in the operating department. J Am Soc Echocardiogr 2006;19(2):140-146.

38. Shiran A, Merdler A, Ismir E, et al. Intraoperative transesophageal echocardiography using a quantitative dynamic loading test for the evaluation of ischemic mitral regurgitation. J Am Soc Echocardiogr 2007;20(6):690-697.

39. Mihalatos DG, Gopal AS, Kates R, et al. Intraoperative assessment of mitral regurgitation: role of phenylephrine challenge. J Am Soc Echocardiogr 2006;19(9):1158-1164.

40. Zoghbi W. Recommendations for evaluation of the severity of native valvular regurgitation with two-dimensional and Doppler echocardiography. J Am Soc Echocardiogr 2003;16(7):777-802.

41. Tribouilloy C, Shen WF, Quere JP, et al. Assessment of severity of mitral regurgitation by measuring regurgitant jet width at its origin with transesophageal Doppler color flow imaging. Circulation 1992;85(4):1248-1253.

42. Lesniak-Sobelga A, Kostkiewicz M, Olszowska M, et al. Chronic mitral regurgitation—significance of the echocardiographic determinants in predicting severity. Acta Cardiol 2009;64(2):187-193.

43. Lesniak-Sobelga A, Olszowska M, Pienazek P, et al. Vena contracta width as a simple method of assessing mitral valve regurgitation. Comparison with Doppler quantitative methods. J Heart Valve Dis 2004;13(4):608-614.

44. Lancellotti P, Tribouilloy C, Hagendorff A, et al. Recommendations for the echocardiographic assessment of native valvular regurgitation: an executive summary from the European Association of Cardiovascular Imaging. Eur Heart J Cardiovasc Imaging 2013;14(7):611-644.

45. Zoghbi WA, Adams D, Bonow RO, et al. Recommendations fornoninvasive evaluation of native valvular regurgitation. J Am Soc Echocardiogr 2017;30(4):303-371.

46. Thavendiranathan P, Phelan D, Thomas JD, et al. Quantitative assessment of mitral regurgitation: validation of new methods. J Am Coll Cardiol 2012;60(16):1470-1483.

47. Buck T, Plicht B. Real-time three-dimensional echocardiographic assessment of severity of mitral regurgitation using proximal isovelocity surface area and vena contracta area method. Lessons we learned and clinical implications. Curr Cardiovasc Imaging Rep 2015;8(10):38.

48. Kahn RA, Mittnacht AJC, Anyanwu AC. Systolic anterior motion as a result of relative "undersizing" of a mitral valve annulus in a patient with Barlow's disease. Anesth Analg 2009;108(4):1102-1104.

49. Maslow AD, Regan MM, Haering JM, et al. Echocardiographic predictors of left ventricular outflow tract obstruction and systolic anterior motion of the mitral valve after mitral valve reconstruction for myxomatous valve disease. J Am Coll Cardiol 1999;34(7):2096-2104.

50. Varghese R, Itagaki S, Anyanwu AC, et al. Predicting systolic anterior motion after mitral valve reconstruction: using intraoperative transoesophageal echocardiography to identify those at greatest risk. Eur J Cardiothorac Surg 2014;45(1):132-137; discussion 137-138.

51. Adams DH, Anyanwu AC, Rahmanian PB, Filsoufi F. Current concepts in mitral valve repair for degenerative disease. Heart Fail Rev 2006;11(3):241-257.

52. George KM, Mihaljevic T, Gillinov AM. Triangular resection for posterior mitral prolapse: rationale for a simpler repair. J Heart Valve Dis 2009;18(1):119-121.

53. Said SM, Schaff HV, Suri RM, et al. Bulging subaortic septum: an important risk factor for systolic anterior motion after mitral valve repair. Ann Thorac Surg 2011;91(5):1427-1432.

54. Bourguignon T, Mazine A, Laurin C, et al. Repair of anterior mitral leaflet prolapse: comparison of mid-term outcomes with chordal transposition and chordal replacement techniques. J Heart Valve Dis 2016;25(2):187-194.

55. American Association for Thoracic Surgery Ischemic Mitral Regurgitation Consensus Guidelines Writing Committee, Kron IL, Acker MA, et al. 2015 the American Association for Thoracic Surgery Consensus Guidelines: ischemic mitral valve regurgitation. J Thorac Cardiovasc Surg 2016; 151(4):940-956.

56. Zakkar M, Amirak E, Chan KM, Punjabi PP. Rheumatic mitral valve disease: current surgical status. Prog Cardiovasc Dis 2009;51(6):478-481.

57. Hong JH, Schaff HV, Nishimura RA, et al. Mitral regurgitation in patients with hypertrophic obstructive cardiomyopathy: implications for concomitant valve procedures. J Am Coll Cardiol 2016;68(14):1497-1504.

58. Nampiaparampil RG, Swistel DG, Schlame M, et al. Intraoperative two- and three-dimensional transesophageal echocardiography in combined myectomy-mitral operations for hypertrophic cardiomyopathy. J Am Soc Echocardiogr 2018;31(3):275-288.

59. Gunduz S, Ozkan M, Kalcik M, et al. Sixty-four-section cardiac computed tomography in mechanical prosthetic heart valve dysfunction: thrombus or pannus. Circ Cardiovasc Imaging 2015;8(12).

60. Rana BS, Calvert PA, Punjabi PP, Hildick-Smith D. Role of percutaneous mitral valve repair in the contemporary management of mitral regurgitation. Heart 2015;101(19):1531-1539.

61. Gatti G, Dell'Angela L, Morosin M, et al. Tricuspid annuloplasty for tricuspid regurgitation secondary to left-sided heart valve disease: immediate outcomes and risk factors for late failure. Can J Cardiol 2016;32(6): 760-766.

62. Pozzoli A, Elisabetta L, Vicentini L, et al. Surgical indication for functional tricuspid regurgitation at initial operation: judging from long term outcomes. Gen Thorac Cardiovasc Surg 2016;64(9):509-516.

63. Di Mauro M, Bezante GP, Di Baldassarre A, et al. Functional tricuspid regurgitation: an underestimated issue. Int J Cardiol 168(2):707-715.

64. Bonow RO, Adams DH. The time has come to define centers of excellence in mitral valve repair. J Am Coll Cardiol 2016;67(5):499.

65. Suri RM, Clavel MA, Schaff HV, et al. Effect of recurrent mitral regurgitation following degenerative mitral valve repair. J Am Coll Cardiol 2016;67(5):488.

66. Anyanwu AC, Adams DH. Why do mitral valve repairs fail? J Am Soc Echocardiogr 2009;22(11):1265-1268.

67. Adams DH, Anyanwu A. Pitfalls and limitations in measuring and interpreting the outcomes of mitral valve repair. J Thorac Cardiovasc Surg 2006;131(3):523-529.

68. Kuperstein R, Spiegelstein D, Rotem G, et al. Late clinical outcome of transient intraoperative systolic anterior motion post mitral valve repair. J Thorac Cardiovasc Surg 2015;149(2):471-476.

69. Ad N. Transient systolic anterior motion after mitral valve repair: does it affect long-term outcomes? J Thorac Cardiovasc Surg 2015;149(2):477-478.

70. De Mey N, Couture P, Denault AY, et al. Subaortic stenosis after atrioventricular septal defect repair. Anesth Analg 2011;113(2):236-238.

71. Zoghbi WA, Chambers JB, Dumesnil JG, et al. Recommendations for evaluation of prosthetic valves with echocardiography and doppler ultrasound: a report from the American Society of Echocardiography's Guidelines and Standards Committee and the Task Force on Prosthetic Valves, developed in conjunction with the American College of Cardiology Cardiovascular Imaging Committee, Cardiac Imaging Committee of the American Heart Association, the European Association of Echocardiography, a registered branch of the European Society of Cardiology, the Japanese Society of Echocardiography and the Canadian Society of Echocardiography, endorsed by the American College of Cardiology Foundation, American Heart Association, European Association of Echocardiography, a registered branch of the European Society of Cardiology, the Japanese Society of Echocardiography, and Canadian Society of Echocardiography. J Am Soc Echocardiogr 2009;22(9):975-1014; quiz 1082-1014.

72. Pibarot P, Dumesnil JG. Doppler echocardiographic evaluation of prosthetic valve function. Heart 2012;98(1):69-78.

73. Oxorn D, Verrier ED. Echocardiographic diagnosis of incomplete St. Jude's bileaflet valvular closure after mitral valve replacement with subvalvular preservation. Eur J Cardiothorac Surg 2003;24(2):298.

74. Ender J, Singh R, Nakahira J, et al. Echo didactic: visualization of the circumflex artery in the perioperative setting with transesophageal echocardiography. Anesth Analg 2012;115(1):22-26.

75. Ender J, Selbach M, Borger MA, et al. Echocardiographic identification of iatrogenic injury of the circumflex artery during minimally invasive mitral valve repair. Ann Thorac Surg 2010;89(6):1866-1872.

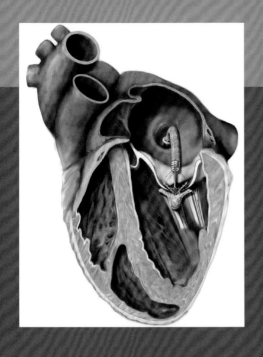

中文导读

第23章
三尖瓣疾病

　　三尖瓣被称为"被遗忘的心瓣膜"。尽管三尖瓣反流，尤其是继发性三尖瓣反流发病率极高，但传统观点认为纠正基础病因，其可自行改善。然而，多项研究证实，无论原发性或继发性三尖瓣反流，中度及以上三尖瓣反流均会引起右心室容量负荷增加，进而导致右心室功能损伤。部分左心瓣膜疾病合并三尖瓣反流患者，单纯左心瓣膜手术并未改善三尖瓣反流程度，甚至有加重趋势。欧洲与美国指南强调了临床表现、右心室形态及功能、三尖瓣瓣环扩张及是否同期行左心瓣膜手术等因素在三尖瓣反流干预决策中的重要性。然而，三尖瓣反流患者早期常无明显症状，晚期出现右心衰竭时，外科手术的围手术期死亡风险又极高，因此，三尖瓣反流的最佳干预时机目前仍不明确。在术式选择方面，一般认为，当存在三尖瓣瓣环扩张而无明显瓣叶结构异常时，优先选择三尖瓣修复术；对于存在瓣叶结构异常，不适合外科修复的患者，应进行瓣膜置换，并首选生物瓣。近年来，经导管三尖瓣反流介入治疗蓬勃发展，为外科手术高风险人群提供了新的治疗方式。由于三尖瓣瓣环结构独特，理想的干预治疗应恢复三尖瓣瓣环正常的动态三维椭圆形状，同时还要避免损伤邻近传导系统及冠状动脉。三尖瓣介入治疗技术和相关器械的研发目前仍处于探索阶段。三尖瓣狭窄极为罕见，其治疗策略缺乏数据支持。

　　本章首先向读者介绍了三尖瓣疾病的病理生理学特征和三尖瓣的解剖结构，而后详细讲述了三尖瓣反流的病因、诊断、疾病自然史与治疗策略。本章亦对三尖瓣狭窄的疾病特点进行了讨论。

王玮玮　吕俊兴

Diseases of the Tricuspid Valve

Grace Lin

CHAPTER OUTLINE

KEY POINTS

- Tricuspid regurgitation (TR) is most frequently functional, not related to primary tricuspid leaflet pathology but secondary to another disease process that produces right ventricular dilation, distortion of the subvalvular apparatus, tricuspid annular dilation, or a combination of these.
- Severe TR due to a flail leaflet is associated with adverse outcomes favoring early surgical repair.
- TR negatively impacts clinical outcome and survival, regardless of left ventricular ejection fraction or severity of pulmonary hypertension.

- Tricuspid valve repair is the preferred treatment for TR in the absence of severely dysplastic or damaged leaflets.
- When tricuspid valve replacement is required, bioprosthetic valves are usually preferred over mechanical valves, although long-term mortality rates are similar for both.
- Transcatheter tricuspid valve interventions are an emerging therapy for patients with functional TR.
- Tricuspid stenosis occurs infrequently and is rarely seen in isolation.

PATHOPHYSIOLOGY OF TRICUSPID VALVE DISEASE

Primary Versus Secondary Tricuspid Valve Disease

Differentiation of primary valve abnormalities from valve dysfunction that is secondary to pulmonary hypertension or primary right-sided heart disease is an important first step in the evaluation and management of tricuspid valve disease. Primary tricuspid disease may be caused by rheumatic or carcinoid heart disease, tricuspid valve prolapse, endocarditis, trauma, or congenital heart disease. Tricuspid regurgitation (TR) is most frequently secondary or functional, occurring as a consequence of tricuspid annular dilation and right ventricular (RV) remodeling due to right-sided chronic pressure or volume overload.

Response of the Right Heart to Pressure and Volume Overload

Changes in RV structure and function occur in response to pressure and volume overload and the extent of RV remodeling. Chronic volume overload results from TR and causes RV enlargement, primarily in the radial rather than the longitudinal direction,[1,2] which can lead to further tricuspid annular dilation and worsening TR. RV systolic function occurs earlier in the disease course than is typical for left-sided volume overload conditions.[3,4] However, as with left-sided valve disease, RV volume and systolic function are expected to improve after intervention for primary valvular disease unless an irreversible decline in contractility has occurred.

RV volume overload is also associated with abnormal or paradoxical ventricular septal motion; the septum moves toward the center of the RV in systole and moves rapidly posteriorly in diastole—a pattern opposite of normal.[5–7] In these patients, the reversed curvature of the septum is most marked in end-diastole. In contrast, in patients with pressure overload, the maximum reversed curvature is more evident and occurs early in diastole.[8]

The response of the RV to chronic pressure overload (e.g., from pulmonary hypertension or pulmonary stenosis) differs from that of the left ventricle (LV). Although the initial response is an increase in wall thickness, ventricular dilation may occur, depending on the acuteness and severity of the pressure overload. If there is a gradual increase in RV pressure, RV size and systolic function may remain normal with a compensatory increase in RV wall thickness.[9] After intervention to relieve pressure overload, an improvement in RV systolic function may occur as a result of the decreased RV afterload. RV dimensions and systolic function improve in most patients after lung transplantation, supporting the concept that systolic function improves with decreased afterload.[10,11]

With an acute increase in RV pressure, such as with acute pulmonary embolism, decreased RV systolic function and clinical right heart failure may be seen, with mean pulmonary pressures of only 20 to 40 mmHg.[12] Acute or subacute RV pressure overload often results in RV dilation with secondary annular dilation and TR. This superimposes a volume overload state, engendering a vicious cycle of RV dilation and worsening TR.

Principles of Diagnosis
Tricuspid Valve Stenosis and Regurgitation
After a thorough history and physical examination, echocardiography remains the cornerstone of diagnosis of tricuspid valve disease. The same principles as for evaluation for other valves are followed to confirm the presence and severity of valvular stenosis and regurgitation. Correct diagnosis of the mechanism of tricuspid stenosis (TS) or TR and assessment of the extent of RV modeling are critical to determine the most appropriate treatment strategy. Specific echocardiographic assessment of TR and TS is described later.

Stages of Tricuspid Valve Disease
The American Heart Association (AHA)/American College of Cardiology (ACC) guidelines and the European Society of Cardiology (ESC) valvular heart disease guidelines recommend staging of valve lesions to define progression and severity of valvular heart disease. Stage A represents patients at risk for valve dysfunction; stage B represents those with progressive valve disease; and stages C (asymptomatic) and D (symptomatic) represent those with severe valve dysfunction (Tables 23.1 and 23.2).[13–16]

TABLE 23.1   Stages of Tricuspid Regurgitation.

Structural Abnormality	Valve Hemodynamics	Hemodynamic Consequences	Symptoms
Stage A: At Risk			
Primary	None or trivial	Normal right-sided chambers and filling pressures	None due to TR
Mild structural abnormality (e.g., rheumatic or prolapse)			
Functional (secondary)			
None or mild annular dilation			
Stage B: Progressive			
Primary	*Mild*	*Mild*	None due to TR
Progressive structural abnormality (e.g., moderate-severe prolapse)	Jet area < 5 cm²	Normal right sided chambers	
	Parabolic CW contour	*Moderate*	
Functional (secondary)	*Moderate*	Normal RV size	
Mild annular dilation, moderate leaflet tethering	Jet area < 5–10 cm²	Normal–mild RA enlargement	
	VC < 0.7 cm	Normal–mild IVC dilation, normal RA pressure	
	Dense CW jet, varied contour		
	Blunted systolic hepatic vein flow		
Stage C: Asymptomatic Severe TR			
Primary	Jet area > 10 cm²	Dilated RV/RA/IVC	None due to TR
Flail or severely damaged leaflets	VC > 0.7 cm	↑RA pressure	
Functional (secondary)	Dense CW jet, early-peaking dagger-shaped contour	V-wave on examination	
Severe annular dilation		Diastolic septal flattening	
	Systolic hepatic vein flow reversal		
Stage D: Symptomatic Severe TR			
Primary	Jet area > 10 cm²	Dilated RV/RA/IVC	*Right heart failure*
Flail or severely damaged leaflets	VC > 0.7 cm	↑RA pressure	Fatigue
Functional (secondary)	Dense CW jet, early peaking dagger shaped contour	V-wave on examination	Ascites
Severe annular dilation (>40 mm or >21 mm/m²), severely tethered leaflets	Systolic hepatic vein flow reversal	Diastolic septal flattening	Abdominal discomfort
		Decreased RV systolic function	Dyspnea
			Anorexia
			Edema

CW, Continuous wave Doppler; *IVC,* inferior vena cava; *TR,* tricuspid regurgitation; *VC,* vena contracta.
From Nishimura RA, Otto CM, Bonow RO et al. 2014 AHA/ACC guideline for the management of patients with valvular heart disease: a report of the American College of Cardiology/American Heart Association Task Force on Practice Guidelines. J Thorac Cardiovasc Surg 2014;148:e1-e132.

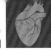

Stage	Structural Abnormality	TS Severity	Consequences	Symptoms
C and D: severe TS	Thickened, distorted, or calcified leaflets	PHT ≥ 190 ms Valve area ≤ 1.0 cm^2 Gradient > 5–10 mmHg at HR of 70 beats/min[a]	Dilated RA/IVC	Asymptomatic or right heart failure, affected by associated valve disease severity: Fatigue Hepatic congestion Abdominal discomfort Dyspnea Edema

TABLE 23.2 Stages of Tricuspid Stenosis.

[a]Tricuspid valve gradients vary and are affected by cardiac output, heart rate, and respiratory phases.
HR, Heart rate; *IVC*, inferior vena cava; *PHT*, pressure half-time; *TS*, tricuspid stenosis.
From Nishimura RA, Otto CM, Bonow RO et al. 2014 AHA/ACC guideline for the management of patients with valvular heart disease: a report of the American College of Cardiology/American Heart Association Task Force on Practice Guidelines. J Thorac Cardiovasc Surg 2014;148:e1-e132.

Trivial or mild TR, which may be incidentally identified by transthoracic echocardiography (TTE) obtained for other purposes, is a common physiologic finding in patients with structurally normal tricuspid valves. In contrast, patients with structural tricuspid valve abnormalities are at risk for progressive valve disease and even those with trivial TR should be staged and monitored for symptoms and severity of valve disease, including extent of RV remodeling. Whereas there are guideline recommendations for all stages of TR, only stage C and D criteria are described for TS (see Table 23.2).

Assessment of Right Ventricular Size and Function
Advanced RV dysfunction resulting in worsening heart failure is associated with increased mortality rates after tricuspid valve surgery.[17] Although echocardiography can provide morphologic assessment of RV dimensions and function, accurate measurements are difficult because of the complex three-dimensional (3D) anatomy of the RV.[18,19] 3D echocardiographic imaging improves estimation of RV volumes over two-dimensional (2D) imaging, but cardiac magnetic resonance (CMR) imaging is more accurate and reproducible.[20–22] However, assessment of RV function by CMR is less accurate than assessment of the LV.[23]

Tricuspid annular plane systolic excursion using M-mode echocardiography is a simple and reproducible measurement of RV longitudinal function that correlates well with other echocardiographic measures of RV function, including RV ejection fraction, but it may be less accurate in special populations such as those with congenital heart disease.[18–20,24]

Other measures of RV function, including the right-sided index of myocardial performance (Tei index)[25] and measurements of peak systolic velocity and displacement of the tricuspid annulus using tissue Doppler imaging,[26–28] are feasible and have prognostic value for patients with pulmonary hypertension and other pathologies.[18,19] RV longitudinal strain, as measured by echocardiography, can be used to evaluate global and regional RV contractility; reduced longitudinal strain predicts disease progression in pulmonary arterial hypertension.[18,19,29]

The extent of RV hypertrophy can be assessed qualitatively based on the thickness of the RV free wall.[18,19] Timing of ventricular septal motion also provides insight into RV function (discussed earlier) but is often better appreciated by M-mode rather than 2D echocardiography. In cases of RV enlargement, careful assessment of the atrial septum and pulmonary veins is critical to exclude a left-to-right shunt. Transesophageal echocardiography (TEE) should be performed if uncertainty remains after TTE imaging.

Pulmonary Artery Pressures
Estimation of pulmonary pressures is an essential component of the examination of patients with right-sided valve disease. RV pressures can be estimated noninvasively from the velocity of the tricuspid regurgitant jet (V_{TR}) and the appearance of the inferior vena cava. Most patients have some degree of TR that permits estimation of the right ventricular-to-atrial pressure gradient (ΔP_{RV-RA}), as described in the simplified Bernoulli equation:

$$\Delta P_{RV-RA} - 4(V_{TR})^2$$

where ΔP = change in pressure; RA = right atrium; RV = right ventricle; TR = tricuspid regurgitation; and V = velocity.

This Doppler-derived pressure gradient is added to an estimate of right atrial pressure based on the size and respiratory variation of the inferior vena cava caliber. However, in severe, wide-open TR, in which the right ventricular-to-atrial pressure gradient may be reduced by equilibration of pressures between the chambers, RV systolic pressure may be underestimated by echocardiography.

TRICUSPID VALVE ANATOMY

Normal Anatomy and Variants
The normal tricuspid valve is characterized by three sail-like leaflets: anterior, posterior, and septal (Fig. 23.1). The anterior leaflet is the largest and most anatomically constant of the three; the posterior and septal leaflets are smaller and vary more in size and position. The number of tricuspid valve papillary muscles varies. The larger anterior papillary muscle is most consistently present and supplies chordae to the anterior and posterior leaflets. A septal papillary muscle is absent in up to 20% of normal subjects,[30,31] and the septal leaflet may insert directly into the RV free wall, typically more apically (≤10 mm) than the septal portion of the anterior mitral valve leaflet.[30,32,33] It is the least mobile of the three leaflets and has the most support from the fibrous trigone.[33]

Changes in Anatomy with Disease States
The normal tricuspid annulus is elliptical and nonplanar or saddle-shaped. It is longer in the septal-to-lateral dimension (from the aortic valve to the lateral free wall) than in the anterior-to-posterior dimension, with high points at the anteroseptal aspect (adjacent to the aortic valve and RV outflow tract) and the posterolateral aspect (adjacent to the free wall) and low points at the posteroseptal and anterolateral aspects[34,35] (Figs. 23.2 and 23.3). The septal part of the tricuspid annulus includes the fibrous trigone, and as the RV dilates, the tricuspid annulus enlarges primarily outward along the free wall of the RV laterally, adjacent to the anterior and posterior leaflets.[33,35,36] It becomes more circular and flattens, affecting coaptation of the anterior and posterior leaflets.[33,35,36]

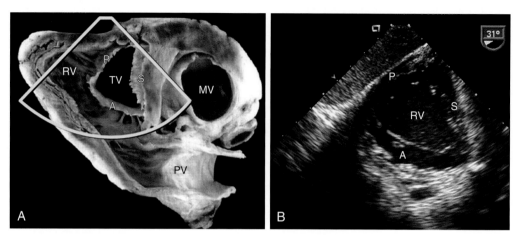

Fig. 23.1 Normal Tricuspid Valve Anatomy. (A) Pathology image demonstrates the right ventricle *(RV)* with tricuspid valve *(TV)* in the short axis. The pathologic section is oriented to replicate the transesophageal transgastric view obtained at a transducer angle of 31 degrees. Notice the septal *(S)*, anterior *(A)*, and posterior *(P)* leaflets. (B) Transesophageal transgastric echocardiographic image using the same imaging plane demonstrates the RV in short axis with TV leaflets S, A, and P. *MV,* Mitral valve. (A, Image courtesy of Dr. William D. Edwards, Department of Laboratory Medicine and Pathology, Mayo Clinic College of Medicine.)

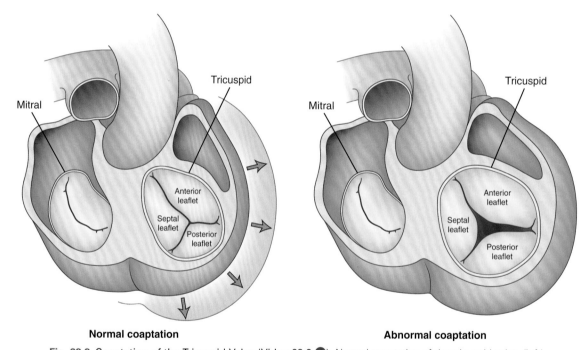

Fig. 23.2 Coaptation of the Tricuspid Valve (Video 23.2 ⏵). Normal coaptation of the tricuspid valve *(left)* and abnormal coaptation in functional tricuspid regurgitation *(right).* As the right ventricle dilates laterally *(arrows)* along the free wall adjacent to the anterior and posterior leaflets, central coaptation is affected.

Recommendations for surgical intervention for severe functional TR are based on the severity of tricuspid annular dilation (see Table 23.1). The AHA/ACC and ESC valvular heart disease guidelines define severe tricuspid annular dilation (stage C or D) as a tricuspid annulus of at least 40 mm or greater than 21 mm/m². [13–16] However, tricuspid annular size varies among normal individuals throughout the cardiac cycle and with different echocardiographic views. [37]

Consistent measurement of the tricuspid annulus is critical for making decisions about surgical and transcatheter interventions. The tricuspid annulus is typically measured from its mid-septal to mid-anterior points in the apical four-chamber view in early diastole, when the annulus size is largest. [37,38] Whereas 2D TTE is the most widely used technique to assess tricuspid annular size, cardiac computed tomography (CT) and CMR can also demonstrate proximity to surrounding structures for planning of surgical and transcatheter procedures and may provide precise annular measurements when 2D echocardiographic images are technically difficult or not feasible [30,39,40] (Fig. 23.4).

Imaging of Tricuspid Valve Leaflets

The three tricuspid valve leaflets can rarely be seen simultaneously by standard 2D TTE; this usually requires angling through different views: parasternal long-axis of the RV inflow, short-axis at the aortic valve level, apical four-chamber, and subcostal windows. [41] Typically, only two leaflets can be imaged in one view, and the anterior leaflet is the one most consistently visualized by echocardiography. [42]

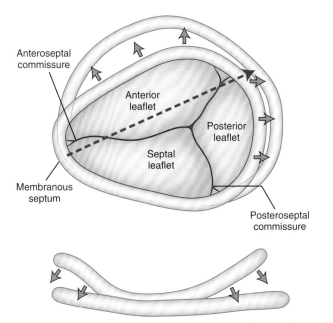

Fig. 23.3 Tricuspid Annular Dilation With Functional Tricuspid Regurgitation (Video 23.3 ▶). The annulus dilates *(arrows)* along the septal-to-lateral axis *(dashed line)*. As it dilates, the normal saddle shape with high and low points is lost; the annulus becomes circular and flattens *(bottom)*.

In the apical four-chamber view, the anterior leaflet is adjacent to the RV free wall, and the septal leaflet is opposite and adjacent to the septum. In the parasternal RV inflow view, the anterior leaflet is visualized in the near field, but the opposite leaflet may be the septal or the posterior leaflet.[42] Accurate identification of the three leaflets can be difficult unless a short-axis image of the tricuspid valve can be obtained from a modified subcostal view or from a transgastric view by TEE.[38,41] Real-time 3D echocardiography may be required to correctly and consistently identify all three tricuspid valve leaflets,[41,43] and cardiac CT or CMR may be useful, particularly in patients with congenital heart disease such as Ebstein anomaly.[42,44]

TRICUSPID REGURGITATION

Etiology

TR that is moderate or greater in severity is most frequently functional in nature. Functional TR by definition is not caused by primary tricuspid leaflet pathology but results from another disease process that causes RV dilation, atrial and tricuspid annular dilation, distortion of the subvalvular apparatus, and incomplete leaflet coaptation.[38] Moderate or greater TR, regardless of cause, usually leads to worsening TR due to the adverse hemodynamic consequences of RV volume overload; this results in a slow and inexorable clinical and hemodynamic deterioration. Causes of clinically significant TR are outlined in Box 23.1.

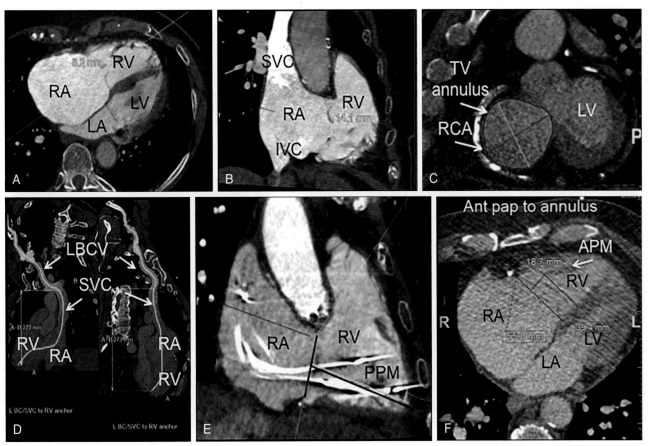

Fig. 23.4 Computed Tomography for Procedural Planning for Transcatheter Tricuspid Valve Repair. (A–C) Multiple imaging planes are obtained for measurement of tricuspid annular dimensions and area. (D) The distance from vascular structures to the RV wall anchoring point can be measured *(green line and arrows)*. (E) Additional structures, including device leads, can be identified and localized to prevent damage during procedural interventions. (F) The anterior papillary muscle *(arrow)* is identified to permit measurement of the distance to the tricuspid annulus. *APM,* Anterior papillary muscle; *IVC,* inferior vena cava; *LBCV,* left brachiocephalic vein; *PPM,* posterior papillary muscle; *RCA,* right coronary artery; *SVC,* superior vena cava; *TV,* tricuspid valve.

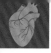

BOX 23.1 Causes of Tricuspid Valve Regurgitation

Congenital Causes
Ebstein anomaly
Tricuspid valve dysplasia
Tricuspid valve hypoplasia
Tricuspid valve cleft
Double-orifice tricuspid valve
Unguarded tricuspid valve orifice

Right Ventricular Disease
Right ventricular dysplasia
Endomyocardial fibrosis

Acquired Causes
Annular dilation
Left-sided valvular heart disease
Ischemic heart disease with papillary muscle disruption or rupture
Endocarditis, infectious or marantic
Trauma
Tricuspid valve prolapse or flail
Carcinoid heart disease
Rheumatic heart disease
Iatrogenic (e.g., irradiation, drugs, biopsy, pacemaker, implantable cardioverter-defibrillator)

Right Ventricular Dilation
Pulmonary hypertension
    Primary pulmonary hypertension
    Secondary to left-sided heart disease (e.g., valvular heart disease, cardiomyopathy)
Right ventricular volume overload
Atrial septal defect
Anomalous pulmonary venous drainage

Functional TR occurs in patients with pulmonary venous hypertension caused by significant left-sided heart disease, pulmonary arterial hypertension, or pulmonary hypertension due to pulmonary disease causing cor pulmonale.[30,33,38] As a general rule, when systolic pulmonary artery pressures increase beyond 55 mmHg, TR can occur despite anatomically normal tricuspid leaflets, whereas more-than-mild TR occurring in the setting of lower systolic pulmonary pressures (<55 mmHg) likely reflects a structural abnormality of the valve leaflets or the subvalvular apparatus.[45] Tricuspid annular dilation also results from chronic atrial fibrillation; RV dilation due to myocardial infarction or cardiomyopathy; or a chronic left-to-right shunt in the setting of an atrial septal defect (ASD) or anomalous pulmonary venous drainage—all leading to leaflet tethering or malcoaptation and functional TR.[30,38,44,46]

Primary tricuspid valve pathology leading to TR may result from blunt trauma, iatrogenic injury, or specific diseases. When caused by permanent pacemaker or internal cardiac defibrillator leads, the mechanism of valve injury varies and is related to lead entrapment in the tricuspid apparatus, direct leaflet perforation, fibrotic adhesion of the lead to the leaflet, or avulsion or laceration of the tricuspid valve leaflets on lead removal.[47] Because leaflet injury may be underappreciated, a high clinical index of suspicion is warranted, particularly when these patients later present with worsening right-sided heart failure. Echocardiography, including 3D imaging, may be useful in localizing the leads relative to the tricuspid valve leaflets (Fig. 23.5). The device leads can be visualized on CT imaging,[48] but their position relative to the tricuspid valve leaflets can be difficult to determine because of artifact from the leads.

Tricuspid valve repair or replacement may be required in symptomatic patients.[47] The role of pacemaker or defibrillator extraction to improve TR in patients without infection is less clear because the leaflets may be damaged by a chronic indwelling device lead.[49]

Direct tricuspid valve leaflet or chordal trauma is a known risk with transvenous endomyocardial biopsy, particularly in cardiac transplantation patients who undergo repeated biopsies for rejection surveillance[50] (Fig. 23.6). Echocardiographic guidance using real-time

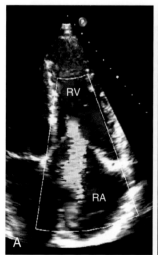
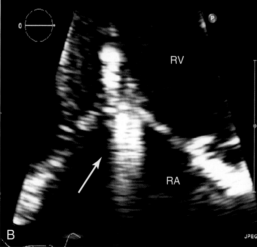
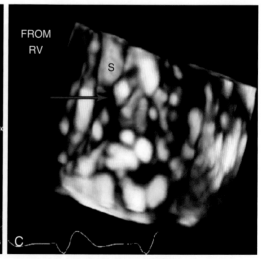

Fig. 23.5 Device Lead–Associated Tricuspid Regurgitation (TR). (A) Color-flow Doppler echocardiographic image demonstrates TR related to multiple device leads. (B) Zoomed view of tricuspid valve in apical four-chamber view with multiple leads *(arrow)* crossing the valve (Video 23.5B ▶). (C) 3D echocardiographic image of the tricuspid valve (Video 23.5C ▶). Full volume was obtained, and the image was cropped to obtain a short-axis view of the tricuspid valve, shown here from the right ventricular aspect of the valve. The device leads *(arrow)* impinge on the motion of the septal leaflet. *S*, Septal leaflet.

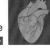

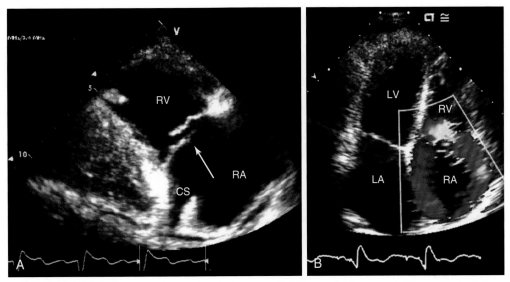

Fig. 23.6 Flail Tricuspid Valve Leaflet After Endomyocardial Biopsy. (A) Parasternal right ventricular inflow view (Video 23.6A ▶). The posterior leaflet is flail *(arrow)*. (B) Apical four-chamber view with color-flow Doppler. An eccentric, laterally directed jet of tricuspid regurgitation is shown (Video 23.6B ▶). *CS,* Coronary sinus.

3D imaging during the biopsy may prevent damage to the tricuspid valve or subvalvular apparatus.[51]

The tricuspid leaflets and supporting structures may also be damaged by blunt chest trauma, most often after a motor vehicle accident resulting in papillary muscle, valve, or chordal rupture. Affected patients may remain asymptomatic for years after the trauma, and the murmur of TR is often not initially recognized.[52] Conduction abnormalities, including right and left bundle branch block and left anterior hemiblock, occur in more than 90% of patients with traumatic TR. Severe TR due to a flail leaflet is associated with adverse outcomes favoring early surgical repair (discussed later).[50]

Right-sided infective endocarditis causing TR is rare and is usually a consequence of intravenous drug abuse, indwelling dialysis or chemotherapy venous catheters, or infected pacemakers or implantable cardioverter-defibrillators[53–58] (Fig. 23.7). The tricuspid valve is affected in 90% of right-sided infective endocarditis cases. *Staphylococcus aureus* accounts for 80% of infections, although coagulase-negative staphylococcus is more common in pacemaker- or defibrillator-associated endocarditis.[53,54,57,58] Antimicrobial therapy is directed at the causative microorganism.

Indications and timing of surgical intervention are less well defined than for left-sided infective endocarditis but should be considered if (1) tricuspid valve vegetations are larger than 20 mm with recurrent septic pulmonary emboli with or without right heart failure; (2) bacteremia persists longer than 7 days despite appropriate antimicrobial therapy or the causative organism is difficult to eradicate (i.e., fungi); or (3) right heart failure due to TR is refractory to diuretics (class IIa, level C)[57,58] (Fig. 23.8).

In-hospital mortality rates after surgical intervention are improving and may be equal to or lower than that for patients treated conservatively.

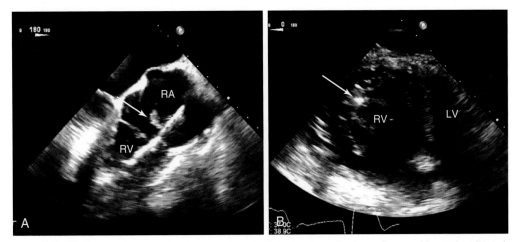

Fig. 23.7 Device Lead–Associated Endocarditis. (A) Transesophageal echocardiogram. Vegetation *(arrow)* is attached to the right atrial *(RA)* portion of the right ventricular *(RV)* defibrillator lead and the posterior leaflet of the tricuspid valve. (B) Transgastric short-axis image demonstrates the tricuspid valve; the defibrillator lead and vegetation *(arrow)* were visualized moving together with the posterior leaflet (Video 23.7B ▶). After device extraction, the vegetation was still attached to the posterior leaflet. *LV,* Left ventricle.

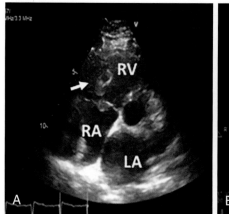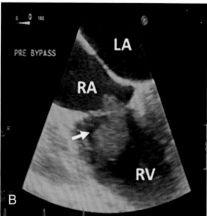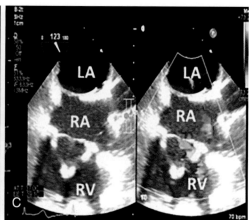

Fig. 23.8 Native Tricuspid Valve Endocarditis due to *Staphylococcus aureus* **Infection with Intravenous Drug Use.** (A) Transthoracic echocardiogram, short-axis view at aortic valve level. A large, multilobulated, heterogenous vegetation *(arrow)* is attached to the tricuspid valve anterior leaflet (Video 23.8A ►). (B) Intraoperative transesophageal echocardiogram. Large vegetation *(arrow)* is attached to the anterior leaflet (Video 23,8B ►). (C) During intraoperative inspection, the vegetation was found to involve most of the anterior leaflet and part of the posterior leaflet; the anterior leaflet was excised, and the valve was replaced (Video 23.8C ►).

Early surgery should be considered in cases of concomitant left-sided valve infection, ASDs, or indwelling catheters or cardiac devices.[59] In cases of infection related to an implantable cardiac device or indwelling catheter, early device extraction reduces mortality rates. The pacemaker or defibrillator usually can be explanted safely, even in cases with large vegetations.[54,60]

Infrequently, marantic (non-infective) endocarditis that occurs in the setting of malignancy, systemic lupus erythematosus, rheumatoid arthritis, or antiphospholipid antibody syndrome can involve the tricuspid valve.[61] The tricuspid valve may also be affected in 7% to 8% of patients with rheumatic valve disease.[62]

Serotonin-active drugs can induce fibroproliferative changes to valve tissue mediated by the serotonin 2B (5-HT$_{2B}$) receptor; although they are more common on the left-sided valves, these changes also can occur on the tricuspid valve.[63] Pathologic and echocardiographic features are similar to those seen in carcinoid heart disease (i.e., thickened tethered leaflets without significant calcification or commissural fusion), which can lead to TR.[64] This association was first described for the ergot alkaloids, ergotamine and methysergide, which were used for migraine therapy.[65] The anorectic drugs fenfluramine and dexfenfluramine, the dopamine agonists pergolide and cabergoline, the recreational drug methylenedioxymethamphetamine (MDMA, Ecstasy), and benfluorex, a weight-loss drug prescribed for diabetic patients, were subsequently found to induce valve thickening by a similar mechanism.[64,66–69]

Carcinoid heart disease is a rare but distinctive form of valve disease that affects primarily the right-sided cardiac valves; it occurs in 40% to 50% of patients with carcinoid syndrome.[70] Tumors arise from argentaffin cells. The primary tumor usually is located in the small bowel and metastasizes to the liver, producing serotonin, which leads to development and progression of valve disease.[71] Rarely, carcinoid valve disease occurs without hepatic metastases; an ovarian carcinoid tumor should be sought in this setting.[72] The tricuspid valve is typically thickened, with retracted leaflets and limited mobility, resulting in regurgitation and, rarely, stenosis (Fig. 23.9). Pulmonic valve changes are similar. Left-sided valvular involvement occurs in approximately 10% of carcinoid patients, usually related to right-to-left shunting of serotonin-rich blood through a patent foramen ovale or to primary lung metastases.[73]

A level of N-terminal pro-brain natriuretic peptide (NT-pro-BNP) greater than 260 pg/mL has emerged as a useful screening tool for carcinoid valve disease. Additional screening with echocardiography is recommended for those with elevated levels of NT-pro-BNP and/or 5-hydroxyindoleacetic acid (5-HIAA) and those with clinical symptoms suggesting valve disease or heart failure.[70]

Although aortic and mitral valve abnormalities are most common after mediastinal irradiation, the tricuspid valve can also be affected (Fig. 23.10). The leaflets become thickened and calcified, resulting in restricted motion leading to stenosis and regurgitation. The tricuspid annulus may also dilate in the setting of radiation-induced mitral valve disease, necessitating tricuspid valve repair.[74] These changes can manifest years after radiation treatment. One series of patients with Hodgkin lymphoma reported an 8% cumulative risk of radiation-related valvular heart disease 30 years after diagnosis; the risk increased with radiation doses greater than 30 Gy.[75] Although valve repair is feasible, replacement may be preferable because of the limited durability of repairs to irradiated valve leaflets.[74]

Endomyocardial fibrosis, which is prevalent in tropical Africa, causes fibrosis of the papillary muscle tip and thickening and shortening of the leaflets and chordae, leading to regurgitation. This process may affect mitral and tricuspid valves.

Congenital causes of TR are rare and include tricuspid valve prolapse (isolated or, more commonly, in conjunction with mitral valve prolapse) and tricuspid dysplasia (e.g., in Ebstein anomaly)[76,77] (Fig. 23.11). In Ebstein anomaly, there is apical displacement of the septal and posterior tricuspid valve leaflets into the RV, along with various degrees of tethering of the anterior leaflet and variation in the severity of TR. A patent foramen ovale or ASD occurs in more than 50% of patients; accessory conduction pathways, pulmonic stenosis, and ventricular septal defect may also be present.[78] TR can also occur in the setting of congenital heart conditions that affect the RV or tricuspid annulus, such the Uhl anomaly, pulmonary atresia, or tetralogy of Fallot.[79]

Diagnosis

The course and presentation of TR vary; moderate to severe TR is often well tolerated, and patients can remain asymptomatic for years.

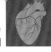

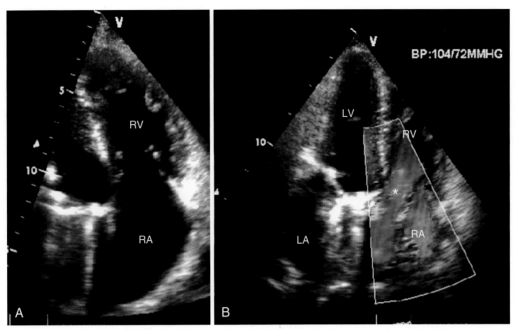

Fig. 23.9 Carcinoid Tricuspid Valve Disease. (A) Apical four-chamber view demonstrates thickened septal and anterior tricuspid valve leaflets with right ventricular *(RV)* enlargement and dysfunction in a patient with carcinoid heart disease (Video 23.9A ▶). This patient had previously undergone mitral valve replacement. (B) Color-flow Doppler image demonstrates severe tricuspid regurgitation in the same patient (Video 23.9B ▶). Notice laminar color-flow *(asterisk)* filling an enlarged right atrium *(RA)*.

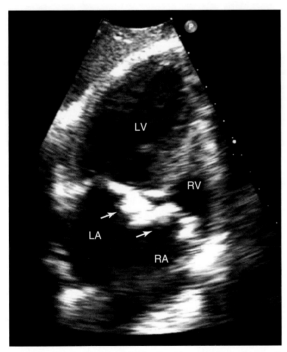

Fig. 23.10 Radiation-Induced Valvular Heart Disease in a Patient Treated for Lymphoma. Extensive thickening and calcification of the mitral and tricuspid annulus *(arrows)* and leaflets.

Symptoms depend on the acuity and chronicity of valve dysfunction and resultant dilation of the right chambers. Symptoms are usually related to hemodynamic changes that occur due to elevated right atrial pressure as a consequence of TR. Chronic, severe TR can lead to right heart failure and, eventually, to low cardiac output. Fatigue,

decreased exercise tolerance, peripheral edema, hepatic congestion with associated anorexia and abdominal fullness, ascites, and even anasarca may develop.

Physical examination findings are characterized by jugular venous distention with a systolic v wave.[80–82] Hepatomegaly occurs in 90% of patients, but palpable systolic pulsation of the liver is less common. Classically, the holosystolic murmur of TR is heard along the left sternal border with radiation to the hepatic region and increases in intensity with inspiration due to increased systemic venous return.[81] However, the murmur is often inaudible, and it can be auscultated in less than 20% of patients with documented TR.[80–82] Atrial fibrillation further confounds interpretation of the characteristic respiratory variation in murmur intensity.[80–83]

TR can be graded qualitatively, using color-flow Doppler imaging based on the extent of the systolic color-flow disturbance in the right atrium, and semiquantitatively, based on the density of the continuous-wave Doppler signal (Fig. 23.12A). Severe TR is characterized by a dense and dagger-shaped appearance on continuous-wave Doppler imaging that is caused by rapid equalization of pressures between the right atrium and RV (see Fig. 23.12B). Ancillary echocardiographic findings in patients with severe TR include inferior vena cava dilation greater than 2 cm and systolic flow reversals in the hepatic veins[15,16,42] (see Fig. 23.12C).

The effective regurgitant orifice (ERO) area can be estimated by measuring the vena contracta using color-flow Doppler imaging. A vena contracta of greater than 0.7 cm indicates severe TR.[15,16,42] Quantitative Doppler assessment is also feasible with use of the proximal isovelocity surface area (PISA) method, although this method requires angle correction.[42] A PISA radius of 0.9 cm (at a Nyquist limit of 30–40 cm/s), an ERO of 0.4 cm^2 or greater, and a regurgitant volume (RVol) of 45 mL or greater indicate severe TR.[42] Other qualitative echocardiographic criteria for severe TR are shown in Table 23.1.

As with auscultation, respiratory changes affect Doppler quantification of TR. Both ERO and RVol increase with inspiration, independent

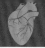

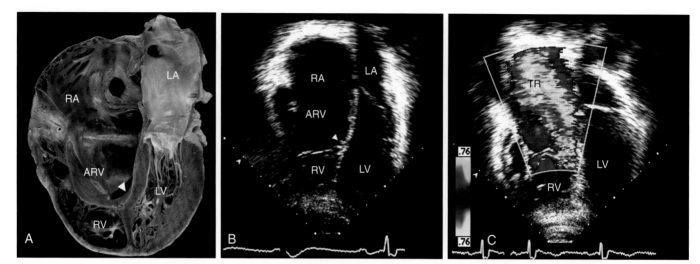

Fig. 23.11 Ebstein Anomaly. Characteristic apical displacement of the septal leaflet of the tricuspid valve *(arrowhead)* and varied tethering of the anterior leaflet. The segment of right ventricular *(RV)* myocardium between the leaflet insertion and the anatomic annulus is atrialized *(ARV)*, as demonstrated in this pathology specimen in the apical four-chamber, apex-down imaging format (A) and in a 2D echocardiographic image in the same format (B). Because of associated valve disease, severe tricuspid regurgitation *(TR)* had developed, as demonstrated by color-flow imaging (C), resulting in severely enlarged right heart chambers. (A, Image courtesy of Dr. William D. Edwards, Department of Laboratory Medicine and Pathology, Mayo Clinic College of Medicine.)

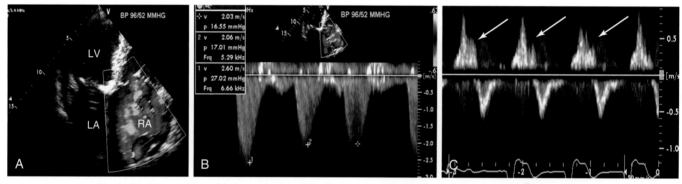

Fig. 23.12 Severe Tricuspid Regurgitation (TR). (A) Apical four-chamber view (Video 23.12A ▶). With color-flow Doppler imaging, the tricuspid regurgitant jet fills at least 30% of the right atrium *(RA)*, more than 10 cm². (B) Continuous-wave Doppler signal across the tricuspid valve demonstrates a dagger-shaped signal consistent with rapid equalization of RV and RA pressures. (C) Hepatic vein pulse-wave Doppler signal with accompanying electrocardiographic tracing demonstrates systolic flow reversals *(arrows)*, reflecting retrograde flow in the hepatic veins that can be appreciated clinically as a pulsatile liver and a v wave on jugular venous examination. Hepatic vein systolic reversals may not be specific for severe TR in the setting of atrial fibrillation.

of the severity or pathophysiology of TR or the degree of pulmonary hypertension.[84]

Natural History

The natural history of severe TR is often one of a prolonged latent period with eventual progressive RV volume overload and later right atrial volume overload. Atrial arrhythmias are common due to right atrial enlargement and may be difficult to treat in the setting of persistent TR. Initially, symptoms of right heart failure and volume overload can be palliated with diuretics, but as hepatic congestion and anorexia develop, patients may become nutritionally depleted.

The negative clinical impact of TR has been demonstrated in series of patients with cardiovascular disease. The mortality rate is increased by TR, regardless of ejection fraction or severity of pulmonary

hypertension, and it increases with greater severity of TR.[85] Survival of patients with an ERO of 0.4 cm² or greater is significantly worse than for those with less severe TR (38% vs. 70% at 10 years).[86] Severe TR after intervention for mitral valve disease with percutaneous mitral balloon valvuloplasty or mitral valve replacement is also associated with worse survival and decreased exercise capacity.[87,88]

Pacemaker-related TR is not benign. In a cohort of more than 58,000 patients, the survival rate was worse for those with significant TR with or without a pacemaker than for those without TR.[89]

Excess mortality and morbidity rates associated with TR due to flail tricuspid valve leaflets were demonstrated for a cohort of 60 patients at the Mayo Clinic. One half of the patients underwent operative intervention (27 tricuspid valve repair, 6 tricuspid valve replacement).[50] Unoperated patients experienced a higher than expected mortality rate (4.5%/yr,

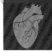

TABLE 23.3 2017 European Society of Cardiology Guidelines for Intervention in Tricuspid Valve Disease.

Indication	Class and Level of Evidence[a,b]
Severe primary or secondary TR in patients undergoing left-sided valve surgery	I, C
Severe symptomatic isolated primary TR without severe right ventricular dysfunction	I, C
Severe symptomatic TS; percutaneous balloon valvuloplasty can be considered in isolated TS	I, C
Severe symptomatic TS in a patient undergoing left-sided valve surgery; percutaneous balloon valvuloplasty can be considered if percutaneous mitral commissurotomy can also be performed	I, C
Moderate primary TR in a patient undergoing left-sided valve surgery	IIa, C
Asymptomatic severe isolated primary TR and progressive right ventricular enlargement or dysfunction	IIa, C
Mild or moderate secondary TR with dilated tricuspid annulus ($\geq$40 mm or >21 mm/m^2) in a patient undergoing left-sided valve surgery	IIa
Severe symptomatic TR in patients with previous left-sided surgery who have progressive right ventricular dysfunction in the absence of severe left or right ventricular dysfunction and without severe pulmonary hypertension	IIa, C
Mild or moderate secondary TR without annular dilation when there is evidence of recent right heart failure	IIb, C

[a]*Classification of recommendations:* I, Evidence and/or general agreement that a given treatment or procedure is beneficial, useful, and effective; II, Conflicting evidence and/or a divergence of opinion about the usefulness/efficacy of a given treatment or procedure; IIa, Weight of evidence/opinion is in favor of usefulness/efficacy; IIb, Usefulness/efficacy is less well established by evidence/opinion.
[b]*Levels of evidence:* A, Data derived from multiple randomized clinical trials or meta-analyses; B, Data derived from a single randomized trial or large nonrandomized studies; C, Consensus opinion of the experts and/or small studies, retrospective studies, registries.
TR, Tricuspid regurgitation; *TS,* tricuspid stenosis.

BOX 23.2 2014 AHA/ACC Recommendations for Tricuspid Valve Surgery

Class I[a]
1. Severe TR at the time of left-sided valve surgery (level of evidence C)[b]
2. Severe TS at the time of left-sided valve surgery (level of evidence C)
3. Isolated severe TS (level of evidence C)

Class IIa
1. Tricuspid valve repair may be considered for mild or moderate functional TR at the time of left-sided valve surgery with tricuspid annular dilation or evidence of right heart failure (level of evidence B)
2. Tricuspid valve surgery is reasonable for severe symptomatic primary TR unresponsive to medical therapy (level of evidence C)
3. Percutaneous balloon commissurotomy may be considered in severe symptomatic isolated TS without TR (level of evidence C)

Class IIb
1. Tricuspid valve repair may be appropriate for mild or moderate functional TR and pulmonary hypertension at the time of left-sided valve surgery (level of evidence C)
2. Tricuspid valve surgery can be considered for asymptomatic severe primary TR and progressive moderate or greater right ventricular enlargement or systolic dysfunction (level of evidence C)
3. Isolated tricuspid valve surgery can be considered in patients with previous left-sided valve surgery and severe symptomatic TR in the absence of severe pulmonary hypertension or right heart dysfunction or failure (level of evidence C)

[a]*Classification of recommendations:* I, The procedure or treatment is recommended and should be performed or administered; IIa, It is reasonable to perform or administer the treatment; IIb, The procedure or treatment can be considered; III, There is no benefit from the treatment or procedure, or the treatment may be harmful.
[b]*Levels of evidence:* A, Data were derived from multiple randomized clinical trials or meta-analysis; B, Data were derived from a single randomized trial or nonrandomized studies; C, Only consensus opinion of experts, case studies, or standard of care.
ACC, American College of Cardiology; *AHA,* American Hospital Association; *TR,* tricuspid regurgitation; *TS,* tricuspid stenosis.

$P < 0.01$) compared with a U.S. matched population. In this series, operative risk was low, and symptomatic improvement was observed in 88% of operated patients. Right-sided chamber enlargement, even in asymptomatic patients, was associated with a marked increase in morbidity.[50] Risk of atrial arrhythmia may persist even after successful repair.

Medical and Surgical Treatment

Overview

The patient's clinical status and the cause of the tricuspid valve regurgitation determine the appropriate therapeutic strategy (Table 23.3 and Box 23.2).[13,15] Correctable causes of TR should be identified and addressed. Medical management of symptomatic TR centers on treatment of right heart failure and primarily involves the use of diuretics combined with fluid and sodium restriction to manage volume status.

For patients with LV dysfunction, additional medical therapy may be required for management of left heart failure. As heart failure advances, however, symptoms of low cardiac output such as fatigue and hypotension may predominate, limiting use of these medications.

Indications for Surgery

Although medical therapy is indicated to treat symptoms of right heart failure related to severe TR or to reduce pulmonary hypertension that contributes to functional TR, tricuspid valve surgery is the only demonstrated effective treatment for symptomatic severe tricuspid valve regurgitation.[13,15] The AHA/ACC and ESC indications for tricuspid valve repair and replacement are summarized in Table 23.3 and Box 23.2.[13,15] Both guidelines emphasize the presence of symptoms of right-sided heart failure, right heart dilation and dysfunction, or tricuspid annular dilation (>40 mm or $\geq$ 21 mm/m^2 by echocardiography or > 70 mm during intraoperative inspection) and the need for concomitant cardiac surgery for left-sided valve disease as important considerations when determining whether to proceed with surgery for TR.

Tricuspid Regurgitation With Left-Sided Valve Disease

Surgery is recommended for severe TR at the time of mitral or aortic valve surgery, regardless of the cause of the TR.[13,15] This reflects observations that TR and RV dysfunction do not always improve after correction of left-sided valve disease, despite improvement in RV afterload (pulmonary hypertension).

Because even mild or moderate TR may progress after left-sided valve surgery,[90] tricuspid valve surgery can also be considered (class IIa recommendation; see Table 23.3 and Box 23.2) for these patients with right heart failure or tricuspid annular dilation. However, the long-term survival benefit of this approach is less clear.[13,15,91] A 2017 meta-analysis suggested that concomitant tricuspid valve repair in this population is associated with a lower risk of cardiovascular death (odds ratio = 0.38; 95% confidence interval: 0.32–1.05; $P = 0.07$) and lesser degrees of TR at long-term follow-up. However, the meta-analysis comprised primarily observational or retrospective data, and the study authors acknowledged that prospective and randomized trials may be needed to more definitively support this approach.[92]

Some investigators have argued for a more selective approach in this patient population. In a single-center experience of 699 patients undergoing mitral valve repair for degenerative mitral valve prolapse with associated less-than-severe TR, TR improved after surgery and remained clinically insignificant after 5 years of follow-up.[93] However, the likelihood of developing or worsening functional TR is affected by the cause of the mitral valve disease, and because the causes are not homogenous, these results cannot be generalized.[93]

Another reason to consider concomitant tricuspid valve surgery for less severe regurgitation is that reoperation for late secondary TR occurring after left-sided surgery has been associated with high rates of mortality and morbidity, especially for those with advanced age and multiple previous cardiac operations.[94] Acute mortality rates (6%–8% at 30 days) are acceptable if the valve surgery is performed before the onset of significant right heart dysfunction; however, long-term mortality rates remain uncertain and are worse if patients have significant preoperative pulmonary hypertension.[30,95]

The early mortality rate may be improved with minimally invasive approaches using a right thoracotomy. This avoids the risks of repeat median sternotomy and extensive dissection of adhesions around the RV that could predispose to postoperative RV dilation.[96]

Isolated Tricuspid Valve Surgery

Although the number of tricuspid valve surgeries performed annually is increasing, most are still performed at the time of mitral valve surgery.[97,98] Isolated tricuspid valve surgery accounts for only 20% of tricuspid valve operations, and the in-hospital mortality rate is high, reported as 8% to 10% in most contemporary series and up to 20% in some single-center studies.[97–100] Because of limited outcome data, guideline recommendations for isolated surgery for tricuspid valve regurgitation are less robust and are based on experiences with small cohorts of patients with flail tricuspid leaflets or carcinoid heart disease, in whom the outcomes after surgery were superior to those after medical therapy.[50,70,73] Surgery is considered reasonable if symptoms do not improve with medical therapy and if it can be performed before the onset of significant right heart dysfunction.[13,15]

Timing of surgery for isolated TR in asymptomatic patients remains controversial, in part because of limited and heterogenous data on postoperative outcomes. Current guideline recommendations favor proceeding only when some degree of RV dysfunction exists. This caution may reflect the concerns that although severe isolated TR imparts higher mortality rates regardless of RV function, the reported long-term postoperative mortality rates from tricuspid surgery remain high, up to 50% at 10 years.[17,86,101–103] This likely reflects the latent course of TR, with operation often occurring late in patients with advanced RV dysfunction and heart failure.

Older age, emergent status, associated atrial fibrillation, and pulmonary hypertension are preoperative predictors of poor outcome,[102] but advanced heart failure symptoms (New York Heart Association

[NYHA] class III–IV) are a critical determinant of poor postoperative outcome.[17,104] These findings add to the argument for earlier intervention in cases of severe isolated TR, even in those who are asymptomatic, before the onset of severe RV dysfunction and heart failure.

Tricuspid Valve Repair Versus Replacement

Accurate imaging of the tricuspid valve anatomy before surgery is paramount because the decision to proceed with repair or replacement often rests on the severity of leaflet damage or annular dilation. Intraoperative TEE may allow refinement of annuloplasty techniques to optimize outcome,[105–107] but this can be difficult due to limited Doppler angles of interrogation and periprocedural hemodynamic alterations that may reduce the severity of TR. A comprehensive assessment of the severity of TR is best undertaken by careful preoperative TTE.

In the setting of tricuspid annular dilation in the absence of significant abnormalities of the tricuspid valve leaflets, tricuspid valve repair usually is the preferred approach, particularly in those who are also undergoing left-sided valve surgery, to minimize bypass time.[13,15] A review of the Nationwide Inpatient Sample database suggested that more than 70% of tricuspid valve surgeries were repairs, and most were performed during left-sided valve surgery.[97] In contrast, tricuspid valve replacements were performed more frequently than repairs during isolated tricuspid valve surgery (59.2% vs. 40.8%).[98]

The evidence regarding survival benefit and durability of tricuspid repair versus replacement is conflicting, which may reflect in part different causes of TR.[108–110] Singh et al. compared tricuspid valve replacement with repair in primary tricuspid valve disease and demonstrated that repair was associated with better perioperative and medium-term event-free survival than replacement; despite the increased severity of recurrent TR, there was no difference in reoperation rates or in NYHA functional class during follow-up.[111] In contrast, a propensity analysis of 315 patients, including a significant number with functional or secondary TR, observed high 10-year mortality rates with both replacement and repair; although the mortality rate was higher with tricuspid valve replacement (49% vs. 66% survival at 10 years; $P = 0.66$), the difference was not significant. Zack et al. reported higher in-hospital mortality rates with tricuspid valve replacement compared with repair for those undergoing isolated tricuspid valve surgery.[98]

Options for tricuspid valve repair include ringed or flexible band annuloplasty, pursestring (DeVega) annuloplasty, edge-to-edge (Alfieri-type) repairs, and posterior annular (Kay) bicuspidization.[112,113] Robotic-assisted and other minimally invasive approaches by right thoracotomy have been employed and as a potential alternative may offer improved rates of early mortality.[96,114] Compared with a pursestring annuloplasty, ringed annuloplasty is associated with improved long-term event-free survival and freedom from recurrent TR.[115] The degree of tricuspid valve tethering and the severity of early postoperative LV dysfunction and recurrent TR are important determinants of residual and persistent TR after tricuspid valve repair.[116,117] Although preoperative and postoperative pulmonary hypertension reportedly were not predictive of recurrent TR, postoperative increase in pulmonary artery pressures was a risk factor.[117]

Tricuspid valve replacement is indicated for patients who have abnormal tricuspid valve leaflets not amenable to repair, including those with carcinoid heart disease or rheumatic heart disease, some patients with Ebstein anomaly, and those with recurrent TR after prior repair. Most commonly, tricuspid valve replacement is undertaken with a bioprosthesis because this obviates the need for long-term anticoagulation and because the durability of right-sided bioprostheses is superior to that of left-sided prostheses, likely related to lower transvalvular pressure gradients.[118] Pericardial bioprostheses are avoided in the tricuspid position because of leaflet stiffness and the associated risk of obstruction.

Mechanical tricuspid valve prostheses can be considered in patients with an established indication for long-term anticoagulation, such as concomitant mechanical left-sided prostheses or atrial fibrillation. Although there is a risk of thrombosis or bleeding due to long-term anticoagulation with mechanical valves, several large series have reported no difference in long-term mortality rates with bioprosthetic valves compared with mechanical tricuspid valves, although early mortality rates may still be high.[101,119–121]

Percutaneous options to address TR include transcatheter valve replacement and coaptation devices to reduce the severity of TR.[122,123] Valve replacement can be performed by placement of a percutaneous

bioprosthetic valve into a dysfunctional tricuspid bioprosthesis (valve-in-valve), which has yielded promising results with reduction in TR and clinical improvement[124–126] (Fig. 23.13), or by placement of stented valves in the inferior and superior venae cavae to address regurgitant flow into the caval veins.[127] Coaptation devices include those that permit edge-to-edge (Alfieri-type) repair (MitraClip system, Abbott Vascular, Santa Clara, CA); annuloplasty systems that approximate a Kay biscupidization (Trialign, Mitralign Inc., Tewksbury, MA); an annuloplasty band (Cardioband, Edwards LifeSciences, Irvine, CA); and a spacer device to reduce the regurgitant orifice area (FORMA system, Edwards LifeSciences) (Fig. 23.14).[128–131] Results from the Transcatheter

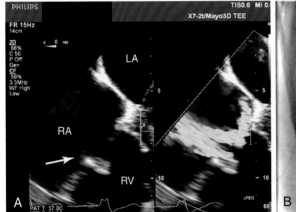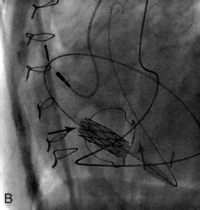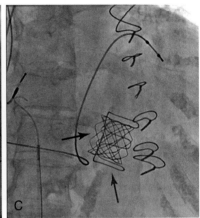

Fig. 23.13 Dysfunctional Tricuspid Valve Prosthesis Treated With a Melody Stented Valve (i.e., valve-in-valve procedure). (A) Transesophageal echocardiography *(left)* demonstrates a transverse view of the right atrium *(RA)*, the left atrium *(LA)*, the right ventricle *(RV)*, and a tricuspid valve bioprosthesis *(arrow)*. Severe prosthetic tricuspid regurgitation is indicated by color-flow Doppler imaging *(right)*. (B) Fluoroscopy image, left lateral view. A catheter carrying the Melody valve *(black arrow)* is placed through the tricuspid valve bioprosthesis *(red arrow)*. Notice the dual-chamber pacemaker with a coronary sinus lead as the primary ventricular pacing lead; no right ventricular lead was placed through the tricuspid valve bioprosthesis. (C) Right anterior oblique view after completed placement of the Melody valve *(black arrow)* with the stent fully deployed through the tricuspid valve bioprosthetic valve *(red arrow)*.

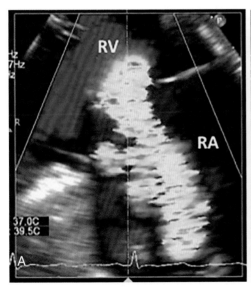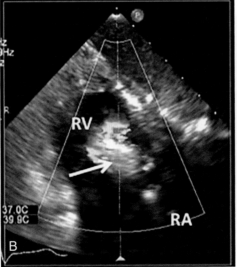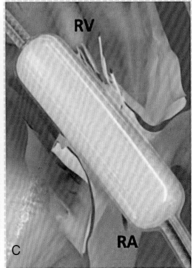

Fig. 23.14 Transcatheter Tricuspid Valve Repair of Severe Functional Tricuspid Regurgitation. Transthoracic echocardiographic guidance for placement of a spacer device (Forma system, Edwards Life Sciences, Irvine, CA) before (A; Video 23.14A ▶) and after (B; Video 23.14B ▶) intervention. The spacer device is shown crossing the tricuspid valve *(arrow)* and improving coaptation with reduction in tricuspid regurgitation by color-flow imaging. (C) Placement of the spacer device across the tricuspid valve. (C, Image courtesy of Dr. Mackram Eleid, Depart of Cardiovascular Diseases, Mayo Clinic College of Medicine.)

Tricuspid Valve Therapies (TriValve) Registry and early feasibility studies suggest that transcatheter interventions for severe TR in high-risk patients is feasible, but long-term outcomes and clinical efficacy need to be determined.[129]

Specific Considerations Based on Etiology

Flail Tricuspid Valve Leaflets

Early surgery should be considered for patients with severe TR resulting from flail leaflets because the long-term prognosis is poor and the likelihood of repair is high.[50]

Ebstein Anomaly

Although tricuspid valve replacement may be required, repair options are possible for patients with Ebstein anomaly.[76] Appropriate patient selection is critical, and these procedures should be performed at tertiary care centers by surgeons specializing in congenital cardiac conditions. Although different approaches have been described, contemporary repair techniques emphasize mobilization and joining of all available leaflet tissue to form a cone (i.e., cone repair), which is then anchored to the true tricuspid annulus, followed by plication of the atrialized portion of the RV. Echocardiographic markers of difficult repair include severe RV or tricuspid annular dilation, absence of septal leaflets, and older age.[132,133] When replacement is considered, bioprosthetic valves are preferred.[132]

Carcinoid Heart Disease

Carcinoid heart disease is best treated surgically with valve replacement, and operative intervention has a beneficial impact on patient survival and functional class.[71,134,135] Indications for operative intervention in patients with controlled carcinoid disease include progressive fatigue, dyspnea or right heart failure, and progressive right heart enlargement or dysfunction. Asymptomatic patients with severe carcinoid heart disease may be candidates for valve replacement in anticipation of partial hepatic resection or liver transplantation.[70] Optimization of carcinoid therapy after tricuspid valve surgery may be required to prevent damage to a bioprosthetic valve from vasoactive peptides.[70]

Secondary Tricuspid Regurgitation due to Pulmonary Thromboembolic Disease or Pulmonary Arterial Hypertension

In patients with pulmonary hypertension due to pulmonary thromboembolic disease, pulmonary thromboendarterectomy alone has been shown to reduce pulmonary hypertension and reduce TR without the need for concomitant tricuspid annuloplasty even if the tricuspid valve annulus is dilated.[136] TR due to severe primary pulmonary hypertension is usually treated with pulmonary vasodilator and diuretic therapy alone because of the risks associated with cardiac surgical intervention and the poor overall prognosis.

Pacemaker- or Defibrillator-Induced Tricuspid Regurgitation

Patients with severe TR due to pacemaker or implantable cardioverter-defibrillator lead impingement or perforation demonstrate symptomatic improvement after tricuspid valve repair or replacement.[47] Repair involves suture repair of a defect in the leaflet and positioning of the RV lead by suture fixation in the recess of the posteroseptal or anteroposterior commissure. However, some experts have advocated for explantation of the endovascular RV lead and placement of an epicardial or coronary sinus lead to prevent recurrence of TR.[108,137]

When tricuspid valve replacement is required because of more extensively damaged leaflets, the RV lead is placed outside the sewing ring. When pacing is required in the setting of an existing tricuspid mechanical prosthetic valve, a ventricular lead cannot be placed across the valve, and an epicardial lead or endovascular coronary sinus pacing lead is required (Fig. 23.15A,B). In selected patients, device leads can be placed across a tricuspid bioprosthetic valve without causing significant valve dysfunction (see Fig. 23.15C).[138]

Tricuspid Regurgitation in Patients Undergoing Left Ventricular Assist Device Implantation

LV assist devices are increasingly used to treat advanced heart failure, but postoperative RV dysfunction is a frequent early complication that results in increased mortality rates.[139] Because severe TR has been associated with increased risk of postoperative RV failure,[140] concomitant tricuspid valve repair may be performed at the time of LV assist device implantation. However, tricuspid valve surgery prolongs

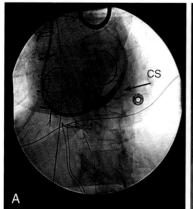
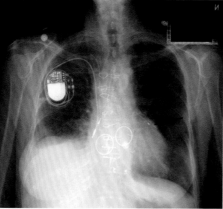
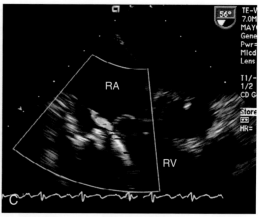

Fig. 23.15 Pacemaker Lead Placement Options in Patients with Tricuspid Valve Prostheses. (A) Venogram of the coronary sinus *(CS) (black arrow)* in a patient with radiation-induced valvular heart disease and mitral and tricuspid mechanical prostheses. Notice the abandoned epicardial pacing leads *(red arrow)*. (B) CS lead *(arrow)* placed for ventricular pacing in the same patient. (C) Transesophageal echocardiographic transverse view of the right atrium *(RA)* and right ventricle *(RV)* demonstrates trivial tricuspid regurgitation (TR) by color-flow Doppler after a pacemaker lead was placed through the tricuspid valve bioprosthesis (Video 23.15C ⏵). Two years later, only trivial TR remained.

cardiopulmonary bypass time, and the benefit of tricuspid valve repair on outcomes after LV assist device implantation is unclear. The optimal approach to TR in this setting remains debatable.[141]

Atrial Septal Defect

The management of functional TR in adult patients with an ASD or other shunt lesion causing tricuspid annular dilation is controversial. Because reduction in TR after ASD closure alone is unpredictable, those with more-than-moderate TR are often considered for tricuspid valve repair in addition to operative ASD closure to decrease the degree of right heart enlargement, although robust data to support this approach are lacking.

Data suggest a durable improvement in TR and right heart dimensions after percutaneous closure of a secundum ASD with a median follow-up period of 30 months.[142] Whether these findings are applicable to the wider population of patients who undergo surgical repairs of shunt lesions or to those who have very severe TR and severe RV enlargement remains to be seen.[143]

TRICUSPID STENOSIS

Etiology

In developed countries, TS is an exceptionally rare clinical condition. Although rheumatic heart disease accounts for about 90% of all cases of TS, concurrent TS occurs in only 3% to 8% of patients with rheumatic mitral valve disease.[62,144,145]

Other, more unusual causes of TS include carcinoid heart disease,[146] congenital anomalies, infective or marantic endocarditis, trauma or fibrosis from pacemaker implantation or endomyocardial biopsy, hypereosinophilia, and Whipple disease.[147] Bioprosthetic tricuspid valves can degenerate and become stenotic or thrombosed.[148] A right atrial myxoma or other tumors can manifest with signs and symptoms mimicking obstruction at the tricuspid valve level (Fig. 23.16A,B; Box 23.3).

Diagnosis

Because patients with rheumatic TS invariably have coexisting mitral valve disease, it is difficult to separate symptoms specific to tricuspid valve obstruction from those of mitral valve stenosis or regurgitation, which include fatigue, dyspnea, ascites, hepatic congestion, and peripheral edema or anasarca.[145,149,150] On physical examination, jugular

BOX 23.3 Causes of Tricuspid Stenosis

Rheumatic heart disease
Congenital tricuspid stenosis
Right atrial tumors
Carcinoid heart disease
Endomyocardial fibrosis
Valvular vegetations
Extracardiac tumors

venous pressure is elevated with a prominent a wave and characteristically an opening snap, followed by a diastolic rumbling murmur at the right sternal border that varies with respiration.[151] As with TR, the murmur is often inaudible.

Atrial fibrillation occurs in 50% of cases, but right atrial enlargement may be evident on electrocardiography in patients who are in sinus rhythm.[145,149–151] An enlarged right atrium is often seen on chest radiography of patients with normal pulmonary artery size and clear lung fields. The transvalvular pressure gradient and valve area of the stenotic tricuspid valve can be measured by hemodynamic catheterization, but Doppler evaluation by echocardiography has replaced the need for routine catheterization.[152–154]

Echocardiography enables a definitive diagnosis of the cause and severity of TS. Rheumatic involvement parallels the changes seen with rheumatic mitral valve disease, including commissural fusion and diastolic doming with thickened and shortened chordae (Fig. 23.17). Even on echocardiography, findings can be subtle, and tricuspid valve involvement may be overlooked unless specific attention is directed toward the tricuspid valve in patients with rheumatic mitral valve disease. Unlike mitral stenosis, short-axis 2D imaging of the valve orifice in TS is rarely feasible; 3D imaging may be useful to better define the valve anatomy and orifice size.[155]

Evaluation of the degree of TS includes calculation of the mean pressure gradient and valve area. TS is considered hemodynamically significant when the mean gradient is 5 mmHg or greater, valve area is 1.0 cm² or less, and the pressure half-time is 190 ms or longer.[155] When the mean gradient is assessed, measurements should be averaged throughout the respiratory cycle. If atrial fibrillation is detected, a minimum of five cardiac cycles should be recorded and measurements averaged. The valve area can be calculated by the pressure

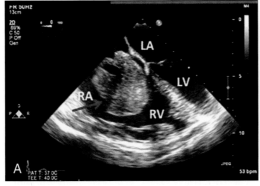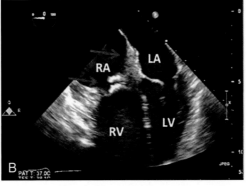

Fig. 23.16 Masses Contributing to Tricuspid Inflow Obstruction. Transesophageal intraoperative echocardiographic images of a large myxoma (A) and a calcified amorphous tumor (B) causing tricuspid inflow obstruction. (A) The large right atrial myxoma *(arrow)* has a heterogenous appearance and prolapses into the right ventricle during systole, obstructing flow (Video 23.16A ▶). (B) Surgical inspection demonstrated extensive calcification involving the tricuspid annulus and extending to the leaflets *(arrows)*, restricting leaflet mobility (Video 23.16B ▶).

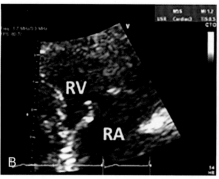
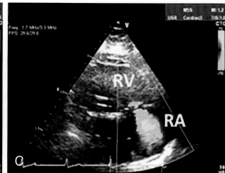

Fig. 23.17 Transthoracic Echocardiography During Serial Follow-Up of Rheumatic Tricuspid Stenosis.
(A) At early follow-up, there is subtle thickening, more prominent at the leaflet tips, with doming and a typical hockey-stick deformity (Video 23.17A ▶). (B) Eight years later, the hockey-stick deformity is more prominent (Video 23.17B ▶). (C) There is progression in tricuspid stenosis and tricuspid regurgitation (Video 23.17C ▶).

half-time method, as in mitral stenosis, using a constant of 190; alternatively, in the absence of significant TR, the continuity equation may be used.[155] TS is usually assessed by TTE, but invasive hemodynamic catheterization can also be considered in cases of symptomatic disease if the clinical presentation and echocardiographic parameters are not consistent.[15]

Natural History

Few data are available on the natural history of isolated TS because it typically accompanies rheumatic mitral valve disease. In a retrospective study of 13 patients with severe rheumatic TS, 12 underwent surgery for mitral and/or aortic valve involvement, and 6 of those had concurrent tricuspid valve surgery.[156] As in mitral stenosis, tricuspid valve obstruction is the result of a chronic, slowly progressive disease process correlating with a gradual increase in stenosis severity and gradual symptom onset. The 2014 AHA/ACC guidelines staged severity of TS but primarily addressed symptomatic (stage D) versus asymptomatic (stage C) disease for severe TS based on echocardiographic criteria (see Table 23.2).[15] In contrast to TR, there were no criteria to describe progressive or early (at-risk) TS.

Medical and Surgical Treatment

Medical therapy for hemodynamically significant TS consists of diuresis to improve systemic venous congestion and heart rate control to promote effective diastolic filling; otherwise, treatment may be given for the primary cause or systemic disease (e.g., infectious endocarditis). However, these methods are only temporizing, and tricuspid valve surgery is the definitive treatment for severe symptomatic disease those with for isolated severe TS and those undergoing left-sided valve surgery[13,15] (see Table 23.3 and Box 23.2).

Tricuspid valve repair can be attempted, but if the leaflets are extensively damaged or there is significant subvalvular involvement, tricuspid valve replacement is usually required.[157,158] Considerations for bioprosthetic versus mechanical prosthetic valves are similar to those applied to TR; in general, bioprosthetic valves are preferred because of the increased thrombotic risk and need for anticoagulation with mechanical valves.[157]

Tricuspid percutaneous balloon valvotomy can be considered for patients with isolated TS of various causes who do not have significant TR or leaflet calcification and are not candidates for surgery due to high operative risk.[13,15] However, severe TR is a common consequence of this procedure, and results are poor when severe TR develops.[159,160]

Percutaneous valve replacement (i.e., valve-in-valve) may be an option in selected patients with previous valve replacement and bioprosthetic valve stenosis; short- and medium-term outcomes are good, but there are limited data on long-term outcomes.[125,126,161] Among 156 patients in the Valve-in-Valve International Database Registry who underwent valve-in-valve intervention for bioprosthetic tricuspid valve dysfunction (29% for bioprosthetic valve stenosis and 47% for mixed regurgitation and stenosis), 10 required tricuspid valve re-intervention, and 3 others had recurrent valve dysfunction during a median follow-up period of 13.3 months.[126] Surviving patients had an improvement in symptoms and in valve gradient and regurgitation, but survival was significantly worse among those with advanced heart failure symptoms and those who were acutely ill at the time of intervention.[126]

SUMMARY

Tricuspid valve diseases have been historically underappreciated, but improved diagnostic testing and increasing awareness have led to substantial advances in diagnosis and treatment. Development and application of CMR imaging has facilitated more accurate characterization of RV size and function and the impact of tricuspid valvular heart disease. Newer techniques for percutaneous valve intervention allow for tricuspid valve repair and replacement with improved outcomes in increasingly complex cases. Appropriate application of these new technologies and vigilance in recognizing the consequences of tricuspid valvular heart disease will continue to improve patient outcomes.

REFERENCES

1. Bommer W, Weinert L, Neumann A, et al. Determination of right atrial and right ventricular size by two dimensional echocardiography. Circulation 1979;60:91-100.
2. Watanabe T, Katsume H, Matsukubo H, et al. Estimation of right ventricular volume with two dimensional echocardiography. Am J Cardiol 1982;49:1946-1953.
3. Dell'Italia L. The right ventricle: anatomy, physiology, and clinical importance. Curr Probl Cardiol 1991;16:653-720.
4. Lee F. Hemodynamics of the right ventricle in normal and disease states. Cardiol Clin 1992;10:59-67.
5. Dell'Italia L, Walsh R. Right ventricular diastolic pressure-volume relations and regional dimensions during acute alterations in loading conditions. Circulation 1988;77:1276-1282.
6. Feneley M, Gavaghan T. Paradoxical and pseudoparadoxical interventricular septal motion in patients with right ventricular volume overload. Circulation 1986;74:230-238.

7. Pearlman A, Clark C, Henry W, et al. Determinants of ventricular septal motion. Influence of relative right and left ventricular size. Circulation 1976;54:83-91.

8. Louie E, Rich S, Levitsky S, Brundage B. Doppler echocardiographic demonstration of the differential effects of right ventricular pressure and volume overload on left ventricular geometry and filling. J Am Coll Cardiol 1992;19:84-90.

9. Spann J, Buccino R, Sonnenblick E, Braunwald E. Contractile state of cardiac muscle obtained from cats with experimentally produced ventricular hypertrophy and heart failure. Circ Res 1967;21:341-354.

10. Kramer M, Valantine H, Marshall S, et al. Recovery of the right ventricle after single-lung transplantation in pulmonary hypertension. Am J Cardiol 1994;73:494-500.

11. Scuderi L, Bailey S, Calhoon J, et al. Echocardiographic assessment of right and left ventricular function after single-lung transplantation. Am Heart J 1994;127:636-642.

12. Jardin F, Dubourg O, Gueret P, et al. Quantitative two-dimensional echocardiography in massive pulmonary embolism: emphasis on ventricular interdependence and leftward septal displacement. J Am Coll Cardiol 1987;10:1201-1206.

13. Baumgartner H, Falk V, Bax JJ, et al. 2017 ESC/EACTS guidelines for the management of valvular heart disease. Eur Heart J 2017;38:2739-2791.

14. Nishimura RA, Otto CM, Bonow RO, et al. 2017 AHA/ACC focused update of the 2014 AHA/ACC guideline for the management of patients with valvular heart disease. J Am Coll Cardiol 2017;70:252-289.

15. Nishimura RA, Otto CM, Bonow RO, et al. 2014 AHA/ACC guideline for the management of patients with valvular heart disease: a report of the American College of Cardiology/American Heart Association Task Force on Practice Guidelines. J Thorac Cardiovasc Surg 2014;148:e1-e132.

16. Vahanian A, Alfieri O, Andreotti F, et al. Guidelines on the management of valvular heart disease (version 2012): the Joint Task Force on the Management of Valvular Heart Disease of the European Society of Cardiology (ESC) and the European Association for Cardio-Thoracic Surgery (EACTS). Eur J Cardiothorac Surg 2012;42:S1-S44.

17. Topilsky Y, Khanna AD, Oh JK, et al. Preoperative factors associated with adverse outcome after tricuspid valve replacement/clinical perspective. Circulation 2011;123:1929-1939.

18. Lang RM, Badano LP, Mor-Avi V, et al. Recommendations for cardiac chamber quantification by echocardiography in adults: an update from the American Society of Echocardiography and the European Association of Cardiovascular Imaging. Eur Heart J Cardiovasc Imaging 2015;16: 233-270.

19. Rudski LG, Lai WW, Afilalo J, et al. Guidelines for the echocardiographic assessment of the right heart in adults: a report from the American Society of Echocardiography: endorsed by the European Association of Echocardiography, a registered branch of the European Society of Cardiology, and the Canadian Society of Echocardiography. J Am Soc Echocardiogr 2010;23:685-713.

20. Kjaergaard J, Petersen CL, Kjaer A, et al. Evaluation of right ventricular volume and function by 2D and 3D echocardiography compared to MRI. Eur J Echocardiogr 2006;7:430-438.

21. Mooij CF, de Wit CJ, Graham DA, et al. Reproducibility of MRI measurements of right ventricular size and function in patients with normal and dilated ventricles. J Magn Reson Imaging 2008;28:67-73.

22. van der Zwaan HB, Geleijnse ML, McGhie JS, et al. Right ventricular quantification in clinical practice: two-dimensional vs. three-dimensional echocardiography compared with cardiac magnetic resonance imaging. Eur J Echocardiogr 2011;12:656-664.

23. Caudron J, Fares J, Lefebvre V, et al. Cardiac MRI assessment of right ventricular function in acquired heart disease: factors of variability. Acad Radiol 2012;19:991-1002.

24. Bonnemains L, Mandry D, Marie PY, et al. Assessment of right ventricle volumes and function by cardiac MRI: quantification of the regional and global interobserver variability. Magn Reson Med 2012;67:1740-1746.

25. Tei C, Dujardin KS, Hodge DO, et al. Doppler echocardiographic index for assessment of global right ventricular function. J Am Soc Echocardiogr 1996;9:838-847.

26. LaCorte JC, Cabreriza SE, Rabkin DG, et al. Correlation of the Tei index with invasive measurements of ventricular function in a porcine model. J Am Soc Echocardiogr 2003;16:442-447.

27. Meluzin J, Spinarova L, Bakala J, et al. Pulsed Doppler tissue imaging of the velocity of tricuspid annular systolic motion; a new, rapid, and non-invasive method of evaluating right ventricular systolic function. Eur Heart J 2001;22:340-348.

28. Miller D, Farah MG, Liner A, et al. The relation between quantitative right ventricular ejection fraction and indices of tricuspid annular motion and myocardial performance. J Am Soc Echocardiogr 2004;17:443-447.

29. Sachdev A, Villarraga HR, Frantz RP, et al. Right ventricular strain for prediction of survival in patients with pulmonary arterial hypertension. Chest 2011;139:1299-1309.

30. Rodes-Cabau J, Taramasso M, O'Gara PT. Diagnosis and treatment of tricuspid valve disease: current and future perspectives. Lancet 2016; 388:2431-2442.

31. Xanthos T, Dalivigkas I, Ekmektzoglou KA. Anatomic variations of the cardiac valves and papillary muscles of the right heart. Ital J Anat Embryol 2011;116:111-126.

32. Tretter JT, Sarwark AE, Anderson RH, Spicer DE. Assessment of the anatomical variation to be found in the normal tricuspid valve. Clin Anat 2016;29:399-407.

33. Huttin O, Voilliot D, Mandry D, et al. All you need to know about the tricuspid valve: tricuspid valve imaging and tricuspid regurgitation analysis. Arch Cardiovasc Dis 2016;109:67-80.

34. Fukuda S, Saracino G, Matsumura Y, et al. Three-dimensional geometry of the tricuspid annulus in healthy subjects and in patients with functional tricuspid regurgitation: a real-time, 3-dimensional echocardiographic study. Circulation 2006;114:I492-I498.

35. Ton-Nu TT, Levine RA, Handschumacher MD, et al. Geometric determinants of functional tricuspid regurgitation: insights from 3-dimensional echocardiography. Circulation 2006;114:143-149.

36. Fukuda S, Gillinov AM, Song JM, et al. Echocardiographic insights into atrial and ventricular mechanisms of functional tricuspid regurgitation. Am Heart J 2006;152:1208-1214.

37. Miglioranza MH, Mihaila S, Muraru D, et al. Dynamic changes in tricuspid annular diameter measurement in relation to the echocardiographic view and timing during the cardiac cycle. J Am Soc Echocardiogr 2015;28: 226-235.

38. Dreyfus GD, Martin RP, Chan KM, et al. Functional tricuspid regurgitation: a need to revise our understanding. J Am Coll Cardiol 2015;65:2331-2336.

39. Saremi F, Hassani C, Millan-Nunez V, Sanchez-Quintana D. Imaging evaluation of tricuspid valve: analysis of morphology and function with CT and MRI. AJR Am J Roentgenol 2015;204:W531-W542.

40. Takaoka H, Funabashi N, Kataoka A, et al. Utilities of 320-slice computed-tomography for evaluation of tricuspid valve annular diameter before tricuspid-valve-plasty compared with the direct-measurement of tricuspid valve annular diameter during open heart-surgery. Int J Cardiol 2013;168:2889-2893.

41. Lancellotti P, Magne J. Tricuspid valve regurgitation in patients with heart failure: does it matter? Eur Heart J 2013;34:799-801.

42. Zoghbi WA, Adams D, Bonow RO, et al. Recommendations for noninvasive evaluation of native valvular regurgitation: a report from the American Society of Echocardiography developed in collaboration with the Society for Cardiovascular Magnetic Resonance. J Am Soc Echocardiogr 2017; 30:303-371.

43. Anwar AM, Geleijnse ML, Soliman OI, et al. Assessment of normal tricuspid valve anatomy in adults by real-time three-dimensional echocardiography. Int J Cardiovasc Imaging 2007;23:717-724.

44. Antunes MJ, Rodriguez-Palomares J, Prendergast B, et al. Management of tricuspid valve regurgitation: position statement of the European Society of Cardiology Working Groups of Cardiovascular Surgery and Valvular Heart Disease. Eur J Cardiothorac Surg 2017;52:1022-1030.

45. Waller BF, Moriarty AT, Eble JN, et al. Etiology of pure tricuspid regurgitation based on anular circumference and leaflet area: analysis of 45 necropsy patients with clinical and morphologic evidence of pure tricuspid regurgitation. J Am Coll Cardiol 1986;7:1063-1074.

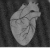

46. Najib MQ, Vinales KL, Vittala SS, et al. Predictors for the development of severe tricuspid regurgitation with anatomically normal valve in patients with atrial fibrillation. Echocardiography 2012;29:140-146.

47. Lin G, Nishimura RA, Connolly HM, et al. Severe symptomatic tricuspid valve regurgitation due to permanent pacemaker or implantable cardioverter-defibrillator leads. J Am Coll Cardiol 2005;45:1672-1675.

48. Piekarz J, Lelakowski J, Rydlewska A, Majewski J. Heart perforation in patients with permanent cardiac pacing - pilot personal observations. Arch Med Sci 2012;8:70-74.

49. Nazmul MN, Cha YM, Lin G, et al. Percutaneous pacemaker or implantable cardioverter-defibrillator lead removal in an attempt to improve symptomatic tricuspid regurgitation. Europace 2013;15:409-413.

50. Messika-Zeitoun D, Thomson H, Bellamy M, et al. Medical and surgical outcome of tricuspid regurgitation caused by flail leaflets. J Thorac Cardiovasc Surg 2004;128:296-302.

51. Sloan KP, Bruce CJ, Oh JK, Rihal C. Complications of echocardiography-guided endmyocardial biopsy. J Am Soc Echocardiogr 2009;22:324.

52. Marvin R, Schrank J, Nolan S. Traumatic tricuspid insufficiency. Am J Cardiol 1973;32:723-726.

53. Sohail MR, Uslan DZ, Khan AH, et al. Management and outcome of permanent pacemaker and implantable cardioverter-defibrillator infections. J Am Coll Cardiol 2007;49:1851-1859.

54. Sohail MR, Uslan DZ, Khan AH, et al. Infective endocarditis complicating permanent pacemaker and implantable cardioverter-defibrillator infection. Mayo Clin Proc 2008;83:46-53.

55. Greenspon AJ, Prutkin JM, Sohail MR, et al. Timing of the most recent device procedure influences the clinical outcome of lead-associated endocarditis: results of the MEDIC (Multicenter Electrophysiologic Device Infection Cohort). J Am Coll Cardiol 2012;59:681-687.

56. FitzGerald SF, O'Gorman J, Morris-Downes MM, et al. A 12-year review of *Staphylococcus aureus* bloodstream infections in haemodialysis patients: more work to be done. J Hosp Infect 2011;79:218-221.

57. Habib G, Lancellotti P, Antunes MJ, et al. 2015 ESC guidelines for the management of infective endocarditis: the Task Force for the Management of Infective Endocarditis of the European Society of Cardiology (ESC). Endorsed by: European Association for Cardio-Thoracic Surgery (EACTS), the European Association of Nuclear Medicine (EANM). Eur Heart J 2015;36:3075-3128.

58. Hussain ST, Witten J, Shrestha NK, et al. Tricuspid valve endocarditis. Ann Cardiothorac Surg 2017;6:255-261.

59. Dawood MY, Cheema FH, Ghoreishi M, et al. Contemporary outcomes of operations for tricuspid valve infective endocarditis. Ann Thorac Surg 2015;99:539-546.

60. Le KY, Sohail MR, Friedman PA, et al. Impact of timing of device removal on mortality in patients with cardiovascular implantable electronic device infections. Heart Rhythm 2011;8:1678-1685.

61. Biller J, Challa VR, Toole JF, Howard VJ. Nonbacterial thrombotic endocarditis. A neurologic perspective of clinicopathologic correlations of 99 patients. Arch Neurol 1982;39:95-98.

62. Sultan FA, Moustafa SE, Tajik J, et al. Rheumatic tricuspid valve disease: an evidence-based systematic overview. J Heart Valve Dis 2010;19: 374-382.

63. Rothman RB, Baumann MH, Savage JE, et al. Evidence for possible involvement of 5-HT(2B) receptors in the cardiac valvulopathy associated with fenfluramine and other serotonergic medications. Circulation 2000;102:2836-2841.

64. Andrejak M, Tribouilloy C. Drug-induced valvular heart disease: an update. Arch Cardiovasc Dis 2013;106:333-339.

65. Redfield MM, Nicholson WJ, Edwards WD, Tajik AJ. Valve disease associated with ergot alkaloid use: echocardiographic and pathologic correlations. Ann Intern Med 1992;117:50-52.

66. Connolly HM, Crary JL, McGoon MD, et al. Valvular heart disease associated with fenfluramine-phentermine. N Engl J Med 1997;337: 581-588.

67. Pritchett AM, Morrison JF, Edwards WD, et al. Valvular heart disease in patients taking pergolide. Mayo Clin Proc 2002;77:1280-1286.

68. Schade R, Andersohn F, Suissa S, et al. Dopamine agonists and the risk of cardiac-valve regurgitation. N Engl J Med 2007;356:29-38.

69. Zanettini R, Antonini A, Gatto G, et al. Valvular heart disease and the use of dopamine agonists for Parkinson's disease. N Engl J Med 2007;356:39-46.

70. Davar J, Connolly HM, Caplin ME, et al. Diagnosing and managing carcinoid heart disease in patients with neuroendocrine tumors: an expert statement. J Am Coll Cardiol 2017;69:1288-1304.

71. Moller JE, Pellikka PA, Bernheim AM, et al. Prognosis of carcinoid heart disease: analysis of 200 cases over two decades. Circulation 2005;112: 3320-3327.

72. Chaowalit N, Connolly HM, Schaff HV, et al. Carcinoid heart disease associated with primary ovarian carcinoid tumor. Am J Cardiol 2004;93:1314-1315.

73. Connolly HM, Schaff HV, Mullany CJ, et al. Surgical management of left-sided carcinoid heart disease. Circulation 2001;104:I36-I40.

74. Crestanello JA, McGregor CG, Danielson GK, et al. Mitral and tricuspid valve repair in patients with previous mediastinal radiation therapy. Ann Thorac Surg 2004;78:826-831; discussion 826-831.

75. Cutter DJ, Schaapveld M, Darby SC, et al. Risk of valvular heart disease after treatment for Hodgkin lymphoma. J Natl Cancer Inst 2015;107.

76. Attenhofer Jost CH, Connolly HM, Dearani JA, et al. Ebstein's anomaly. Circulation 2007;115:277-285.

77. Weinreich D, Burke J, Bharati S, Lev M. Isolated prolapse of the tricuspid valve. J Am Coll Cardiol 1985;6:475-481.

78. Celermajer D, Bull C, Till J, et al. Ebstein's anomaly: presentation and outcome from fetus to adult. J Am Coll Cardiol 1994;23:170-176.

79. Said SM, Burkhart HM, Dearani JA. Surgical management of congenital (non-Ebstein) tricuspid valve regurgitation. Semin Thorac Cardiovasc Surg Pediatr Card Surg Annu 2012;15:46-60.

80. Muller O, Shillingford J. Tricuspid incompetence. Br Heart J 1954;16:195.

81. Salazar E, Levine H. Rheumatic tricuspid regurgitation. Am J Med 1962;33:111.

82. Sepulveda G, Lukas D. The diagnosis of tricuspid insufficiency—clinical features in 60 cases with associated mitral valve disease. Circulation 1955;11:552.

83. Hansing C, Rowe G. Tricuspid insufficiency. A study of hemodynamics and pathogenesis. Circulation 1972;45:793-799.

84. Topilsky Y, Tribouilloy C, Michelena HI, et al. Pathophysiology of tricuspid regurgitation/clinical perspective. Circulation 2010;122:1505-1513.

85. Nath J, Foster E, Heidenreich PA. Impact of tricuspid regurgitation on long-term survival. J Am Coll Cardiol 2004;43:405-409.

86. Topilsky Y, Nkomo VT, Vatury O, et al. Clinical outcome of isolated tricuspid regurgitation. JACC Cardiovasc Imaging 2014;7:1185-1194.

87. Sagie A, Schwammenthal E, Newell J, et al. Significant tricuspid regurgitation is a marker for adverse outcome in patients undergoing percutaneous balloon mitral valvuloplasty. J Am Coll Cardiol 1994;24:696-702.

88. Groves P, Lewis N, Ikram S, et al. Reduced exercise capacity in patients with tricuspid regurgitation after successful mitral valve replacement for rheumatic mitral valve disease. Br Heart J 1991;66:295-301.

89. Delling FN, Hassan ZK, Piatkowski G, et al. Tricuspid regurgitation and mortality in patients with transvenous permanent pacemaker leads. Am J Cardiol 2016;117:988-992.

90. Kim JB, Yoo DG, Kim GS, et al. Mild-to-moderate functional tricuspid regurgitation in patients undergoing valve replacement for rheumatic mitral disease: the influence of tricuspid valve repair on clinical and echocardiographic outcomes. Heart 2012;98:24-30.

91. Ro SK, Kim JB, Jung SH, et al. Mild-to-moderate functional tricuspid regurgitation in patients undergoing mitral valve surgery. J Thorac Cardiovasc Surg 2013;146:1092-1097.

92. Pagnesi M, Montalto C, Mangieri A, et al. Tricuspid annuloplasty versus a conservative approach in patients with functional tricuspid regurgitation undergoing left-sided heart valve surgery: a study-level meta-analysis. Int J Cardiol 2017;240:138-144.

93. Yilmaz O, Suri RM, Dearani JA, et al. Functional tricuspid regurgitation at the time of mitral valve repair for degenerative leaflet prolapse: the case for a selective approach. J Thorac Cardiovasc Surg 2011;142:608-613.

94. Staab ME, Nishimura RA, Dearani JA. Isolated tricuspid valve surgery for severe tricuspid regurgitation following prior left heart valve surgery: analysis of outcome in 34 patients. J Heart Valve Dis 1999;8:567-574.

95. Buzzatti N, Iaci G, Taramasso M, et al. Long-term outcomes of tricuspid valve replacement after previous left-side heart surgery. Eur J Cardiothorac Surg 2014;46:713-719; discussion 719.

96. Pfannmuller B, Misfeld M, Borger MA, et al. Isolated reoperative minimally invasive tricuspid valve operations. Ann Thorac Surg 2012;94:2005-2010.

97. Vassileva CM, Shabosky J, Boley T, et al. Tricuspid valve surgery: the past 10 years from the Nationwide Inpatient Sample (NIS) database. J Thorac Cardiovasc Surg 2012;143:1043-1049.

98. Zack CJ, Fender EA, Chandrashekar P, et al. National trends and outcomes in isolated tricuspid valve surgery. J Am Coll Cardiol 2017;70:2953-2960.

99. Ejiofor JI, Neely RC, Yammine M, et al. Surgical outcomes of isolated tricuspid valve procedures: repair versus replacement. Ann Cardiothorac Surg 2017;6:214-222.

100. Bevan PJ, Haydock DA, Kang N. Long-term survival after isolated tricuspid valve replacement. Heart Lung Circ 2014;23:697-702.

101. Garatti A, Nano G, Bruschi G, et al. Twenty-five year outcomes of tricuspid valve replacement comparing mechanical and biologic prostheses. Ann Thorac Surg 2012;93:1146-1153.

102. Filsoufi F, Anyanwu AC, Salzberg SP, et al. Long-term outcomes of tricuspid valve replacement in the current era. Ann Thorac Surg 2005;80:845-850.

103. Chang BC, Lim SH, Yi G, et al. Long-term clinical results of tricuspid valve replacement. Ann Thorac Surg 2006;81:1317-1324.

104. Raikhelkar J, Lin HM, Neckman D, et al. Isolated tricuspid valve surgery: predictors of adverse outcome and survival. Heart Lung Circ 2013;22:211-220.

105. De Simone R, Lange R, Tanzeem A, et al. Adjustable tricuspid valve annuloplasty assisted by intraoperative transesophageal color Doppler echocardiography. Am J Cardiol 1993;71:926-931.

106. Pellegrini A, Colombo T, Donatelli F, et al. Evaluation and treatment of secondary tricuspid insufficiency. Eur J Cardiothorac Surg 1992;6:288-296.

107. Yada I, Tani K, Shimono T, et al. Preoperative evaluation and surgical treatment for tricuspid regurgitation associated with acquired valvular heart disease. The Kay-Boyd method vs the Carpentier-Edwards ring method. J Cardiovasc Surg (Torino) 1990;31:771-777.

108. McCarthy PM, Bhudia SK, Rajeswaran J, et al. Tricuspid valve repair: durability and risk factors for failure. J Thorac Cardiovasc Surg 2004;127:674-685.

109. Moraca RJ, Moon MR, Lawton JS, et al. Outcomes of tricuspid valve repair and replacement: a propensity analysis. Ann Thorac Surg 2009;87:83-88; discussion 88-89.

110. Jang JY, Heo R, Lee S, et al. Comparison of results of tricuspid valve repair versus replacement for severe functional tricuspid regurgitation. Am J Cardiol 2017;119:905-910.

111. Singh SK, Tang GH, Maganti MD, et al. Midterm outcomes of tricuspid valve repair versus replacement for organic tricuspid disease. Ann Thorac Surg 2006;82:1735-1741; discussion 1741.

112. Thapa R, Dawn B, Nath J. Tricuspid regurgitation: pathophysiology and management. Curr Cardiol Rep 2012;14:190-199.

113. Rogers JH, Bolling SF. The tricuspid valve. Circulation 2009;119:2718-2725.

114. Panos A, Myers P, Kalangos A. Thorascopic and robotic tricuspid valve annuloplasty with a biodegradeable ring: an initial experience. J Heart Valve Dis 2010;19:201-205.

115. Tang TG, David TE, Singh SK, et al. Tricuspid valve repair with an annuloplasty ring results in improved long-term outcomes. Circulation 2006;114:I577-I581.

116. Fukuda S, Song JM, Gillinov AM, et al. Tricuspid valve tethering predicts residual tricuspid regurgitation after tricuspid annuloplasty. Circulation 2005;111:975-979.

117. Fukuda S, Gillinov AM, McCarthy PM, et al. Determinants of recurrent or residual functional tricuspid regurgitation after tricuspid annuloplasty. Circulation 2006;114:I582-I587.

118. Ohata T, Kigawa I, Tohda E, Wanibuchi Y. Comparison of durability of bioprostheses in tricuspid and mitral positions. Ann Thorac Surg 2001;71:S240-S243.

119. Rizzoli G, Vendramin I, Nesseris G, et al. Biological or mechanical prostheses in tricuspid position? A meta-analysis of intra-institutional results. Ann Thorac Surg 2004;77:1607-1614.

120. Said SM, Burkhart HM, Schaff HV, et al. When should a mechanical tricuspid valve replacement be considered? J Thorac Cardiovasc Surg 2014;148:603-608.

121. Liu P, Qiao WH, Sun FQ, et al. Should a mechanical or biological prosthesis be used for a tricuspid valve replacement? A meta-analysis. J Card Surg 2016;31:294-302.

122. Rodes-Cabau J, Hahn RT, Latib A, et al. Transcatheter therapies for treating tricuspid regurgitation. J Am Coll Cardiol 2016;67:1829-1845.

123. Bouleti C, Juliard JM, Himbert D, et al. Tricuspid valve and percutaneous approach: no longer the forgotten valve! Arch Cardiovasc Dis 2016;109:55-66.

124. Boudjemline Y, Agnoletti G, Bonnet D, et al. Steps toward the percutaneous replacement of atrioventricular valves: an experimental study. J Am Coll Cardiol 2005;46:360-365.

125. Roberts PA, Boudjemline Y, Cheatham JP, et al. Percutaneous tricuspid valve replacement in congenital and acquired heart disease. J Am Coll Cardiol 2011;58:117-122.

126. McElhinney DB, Cabalka AK, Aboulhosn JA, et al. Transcatheter tricuspid valve-in-valve implantation for the treatment of dysfunctional surgical bioprosthetic valves: an international, multicenter registry study. Circulation 2016;133:1582-1593.

127. Lauten A, Doenst T, Hamadanchi A, et al. Percutaneous bicaval valve implantation for transcatheter treatment of tricuspid regurgitation: clinical observations and 12-month follow-up. Circ Cardiovasc Interv 2014;7:268-272.

128. Hahn RT, Meduri CU, Davidson CJ, et al. Early feasibility study of a transcatheter tricuspid valve annuloplasty: SCOUT trial 30-day results. J Am Coll Cardiol 2017;69:1795-1806.

129. Taramasso M, Hahn RT, Alessandrini H, et al. The International Multicenter TriValve Registry: which patients are undergoing transcatheter tricuspid repair? JACC Cardiovasc Interv 2017;10:1982-1990.

130. Ohno Y, Attizzani GF, Capodanno D, et al. Association of tricuspid regurgitation with clinical and echocardiographic outcomes after percutaneous mitral valve repair with the MitraClip System: 30-day and 12-month follow-up from the GRASP Registry. Eur Heart J Cardiovasc Imaging 2014;15:1246-1255.

131. Perlman G, Praz F, Puri R, et al. tricuspid valve repair with a new transcatheter coaptation system for the treatment of severe tricuspid regurgitation: 1-year clinical and echocardiographic results. JACC Cardiovasc Interv 2017;10:1994-2003.

132. Brown ML, Dearani JA, Danielson GK, et al. The outcomes of operations for 539 patients with Ebstein anomaly. J Thorac Cardiovasc Surg 2008;135:1120-1136.e7.

133. Holst KA, Dearani JA, Said S, et al. Improving results of surgery for Ebstein anomaly: where are we after 235 cone repairs? Ann Thorac Surg 2018;105:160-168.

134. Bhattacharyya S, Raja SG, Toumpanakis C, et al. Outcomes, risks and complications of cardiac surgery for carcinoid heart disease. Eur J Cardiothorac Surg 2011;40:168-172.

135. Mokhles P, van Herwerden LA, de Jong PL, et al. Carcinoid heart disease: outcomes after surgical valve replacement. Eur J Cardiothorac Surg 2011.

136. Sadeghi HM, Kimura BJ, Raisinghani A, et al. Does lowering pulmonary arterial pressure eliminate severe functional tricuspid regurgitation? Insights from pulmonary thromboendarterectomy. J Am Coll Cardiol 2004;44:126-132.

137. Pfannmueller B, Hirnle G, Seeburger J, et al. Tricuspid valve repair in the presence of a permanent ventricular pacemaker lead. Eur J Cardiothorac Surg 2011;39:657-661.

138. Eleid MF, Blauwet LA, Cha YM, et al. Bioprosthetic tricuspid valve regurgitation associated with pacemaker or defibrillator lead implantation. J Am Coll Cardiol 2012;59:813-818.

139. Kormos RL, Teuteberg JJ, Pagani FD, et al. Right ventricular failure in patients with the HeartMate II continuous-flow left ventricular assist device: incidence, risk factors, and effect on outcomes. J Thorac Cardiovasc Surg 2010;139:1316-1324.

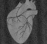
140. Piacentino V, 3rd, Williams ML, Depp T, et al. Impact of tricuspid valve regurgitation in patients treated with implantable left ventricular assist devices. Ann Thorac Surg 2011;91:1342-1346; discussion 1346-1347.

141. Dunlay SM, Deo SV, Park SJ. Impact of tricuspid valve surgery at the time of left ventricular assist device insertion on postoperative outcomes. ASAIO J 2015;61:15-20.

142. Takaya Y, Akagi T, Kijima Y, et al. Functional tricuspid regurgitation after transcatheter closure of atrial septal defect in adult patients: long-term follow-up. JACC Cardiovasc Interv 2017;10:2211-2218.

143. Webb GD, Opotowsky AR. Strategies for managing functional tricuspid regurgitation in adults with a secundum atrial septal defect. JACC Cardiovasc Interv 2017;10:2219-2221.

144. Bousvaros G, Stubington D. Some auscultatory and phonocardiographic features of tricuspid stenosis. Circulation 1964;29:26.

145. Kitchin A, Turner R. Diagnosis and treatment of tricuspid stenosis. Br Heart J 1964;16:354.

146. Pellikka PA, Tajik AJ, Khandheria BK, et al. Carcinoid heart disease. Clinical and echocardiographic spectrum in 74 patients. Circulation 1993;87:1188-1196.

147. Waller B, Howard J, Fess S. Pathology of tricuspid valve stenosis and pure tricuspid regurgitation—part III. Clin Cardiol 1995;18:225-230.

148. Egbe AC, Pislaru SV, Pellikka PA, et al. Bioprosthetic valve thrombosis versus structural failure: clinical and echocardiographic predictors. J Am Coll Cardiol 2015;66:2285-2294.

149. Gibson R, Wood P. The diagnosis of tricuspid stenosis. Br Heart J 1955;17:552.

150. Killip T, Lukas D. Tricuspid stenosis—clinical features in twelve cases. Am J Med 1958;24:836.

151. el-Sherif N. Rheumatic tricuspid stenosis. A haemodynamic correlation. Br Heart J 1971;33:16-31.

152. Guyer D, Gillam L, Foale R, et al. Comparison of the echocardiographic and hemodynamic diagnosis of rheumatic tricuspid stenosis. J Am Coll Cardiol 1984;3:1135-1144.

153. Perez J, JLudbrook P, Ahumada G. Usefulness of Doppler echocardiography in detecting tricuspid valve stenosis. Am J Cardiol 1985;55:601-603.

154. Shimada R, Takeshita A, Nakamura M, et al. Diagnosis of tricuspid stenosis by M-mode and two-dimensional echocardiography. Am J Cardiol 1984;53:164-168.

155. Baumgartner H, Hung J, Bermejo J, et al. Echocardiographic assessment of valve stenosis: EAE/ASE recommendations for clinical practice. J Am Soc Echocardiogr 2009;22:1-23.

156. Roguin A, Rinkevich D, Milo S, et al. Long-term follow-up of patients with severe rheumatic tricuspid stenosis. Am Heart J 1998;136:103-108.

157. Cevasco M, Shekar PS. Surgical management of tricuspid stenosis. Ann Cardiothorac Surg 2017;6:275-282.

158. Gur AK, Odabasi D, Kunt AG, Kunt AS. Isolated tricuspid valve repair for Libman-Sacks endocarditis. Echocardiography 2014;31:E166-E168.

159. Onate A, Alcibar J, Inguanzo R, et al. Balloon dilation of tricuspid and pulmonary valves in carcinoid heart disease. Tex Heart Inst J 1993;20:115-119.

160. Orbe LC, Sobrino N, Arcas R, et al. Initial outcome of percutaneous balloon valvuloplasty in rheumatic tricuspid valve stenosis. Am J Cardiol 1993;71:353-354.

161. Taggart NW, Cabalka AK, Eicken A, et al. Outcomes of transcatheter tricuspid valve-in-valve implantation in patients with Ebstein anomaly. Am J Cardiol 2018;121:262-268.

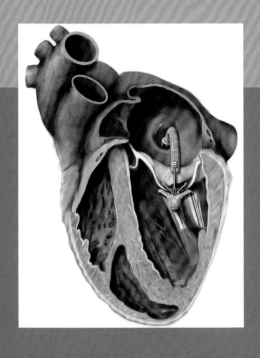

中文导读

第24章
成年人的肺动脉瓣疾病

　　先天性心脏病是一种严重的心脏或大血管在宫内发育期因某种不良因素影响而出现结构发育缺陷的先天畸形。全球发病率为4‰~30‰，亚洲发病率最高，约9.3‰，中国发病率为5‰~16‰。部分类型的先天性心脏病表现或合并表现出右心室流出道梗阻（如法洛四联症，肺动脉闭锁，右心室双出口，重度肺动脉狭窄等），右心室流出道梗阻发病率约为0.78‰。法洛四联症是最常见的发绀型心脏缺陷，发病率为每1000例活产婴儿中出现0.33例，其占所有形式先天性心脏病的6.7%。法洛四联症修复后的晚期生存率极佳，术后40年可达到86%，然而发病率极高，近一半的患者需要再次干预。肺动脉瓣置换是最常见的手术方式。

　　本章对肺动脉瓣病变的病理生理、常见病变位置、临床表现和治疗方法（包括手术修复和肺动脉瓣置换的临床背景、适应证、预后及目前所使用的器械）进行了详细介绍。

吴永健

Pulmonic Valve Disease in Adults

Yuli Y. Kim

KEY POINTS

- Congenital valvular pulmonic stenosis (PS) that is mild in severity is well tolerated and has a benign natural history.
- Balloon angioplasty is the first-line treatment for severe valvular PS, especially for doming pulmonic valves.
- Double-chambered right ventricle is an uncommon form of right ventricular outflow tract obstruction in which the right ventricle is divided into a proximal high-pressure and a distal low-pressure chamber. Surgical repair is effective and has low morbidity and mortality rates.
- Supravalvular PS can involve the main and/or branch pulmonary arteries and may be associated with genetic syndromes. Repair of main pulmonary artery stenosis is often surgical, but percutaneous stenting may be an option for some, whereas catheter-based treatments are considered first-line treatment for peripheral pulmonary artery stenosis.
- Repaired tetralogy of Fallot and valvular PS after surgical valvotomy are commonly associated with pulmonic regurgitation (PR),

which can be tolerated for years or decades before symptoms manifest.
- Cardiac magnetic resonance imaging (CMR) is the technique of choice for imaging tetralogy of Fallot, especially for quantification of PR and right ventricular size and function.
- Indications for pulmonic valve replacement (PVR) are continuing to evolve and are based on symptoms, right ventricular size, and systolic function with a heavy reliance on CMR assessment.
- PVR can improve symptoms but does not consistently improve right ventricular systolic function, and there are no data demonstrating a mortality benefit.
- Transcatheter PVR has emerged as an alternative therapy for some patients, and rapidly evolving technologies hold promise for expanding eligibility to others. No head-to-head studies have directly compared surgical versus transcatheter approaches, but short- to medium-term outcomes regarding right ventricular remodeling and symptomatic improvement are similar.

OVERVIEW OF PULMONIC VALVE DISEASE

Etiology

Pulmonic valve disease in the adult is most commonly a congenital defect, but it also can manifest as part of an acquired condition such as rheumatic heart disease, carcinoid, or infective endocarditis, or it can result from trauma. Pulmonic regurgitation (PR) in an anatomically normal pulmonic valve can be caused by pulmonary hypertension or dilated pulmonary artery (PA) in Marfan syndrome.[1] This chapter focuses on congenital diseases of the pulmonic valve, including tetralogy of Fallot (TOF).

Pathophysiology

The physiologic consequence of pressure overload to the right ventricle (RV) caused by pulmonic valve stenosis (PS) or by subvalvular pulmonic or supravalvular pulmonary stenosis is increased contractility and dilation that leads to increased wall stress and compensatory RV hypertrophy. Increased muscle mass enables the hypertrophied RV to maintain RV output. Severe hypertrophy leads to diminished compliance of the RV, resulting in increased RV end-diastolic pressure and right atrial pressure.[2] Right-to-left shunting may occur if there is an interatrial communication. Over time, progressive RV hypertrophy and stiffness can give rise to RV diastolic dysfunction, which manifests as dyspnea or effort intolerance.

Volume overload to the RV from PR results in RV dilation, and there is a linear relationship between the degree of PR and RV end-diastolic volume.[3] Increased RV end-diastolic volume allows for a compensatory increase in stroke volume to maintain cardiac output. Long-standing RV volume overload can result in RV diastolic dysfunction with elevation in RV end-diastolic pressure.[4]

Although the conditions are physiologically distinct, lessons learned from the effects of chronic aortic regurgitation on the left ventricle (LV) suggest that chronic severe PR may follow a similar course. After an asymptomatic compensatory phase in which semilunar valve regurgitation is well tolerated for many years, there is a maladaptive phase consisting of progressive ventricular remodeling and eventually ventricular dysfunction that can be accompanied by symptoms.[5] Dilation of the RV and the tricuspid annulus forms the substrate for functional tricuspid regurgitation, which compounds the volume overload.

PULMONIC, SUBPULMONIC, AND SUPRAVALVULAR PULMONARY STENOSIS

Pulmonic Valve Stenosis

Background

PS is usually an isolated lesion; it occurs in approximately 8% to 10% of congenital heart disease cases and is the most common form of right-sided obstruction.[6] The pulmonic valve is often dome shaped in systole with a narrow central opening and leaflet fusion; it can be calcified in older adults.

Pulmonic valve dysplasia is a less common form of PS; leaflets are thickened and poorly mobile, and there is no commissural fusion. It can be associated with a hypoplastic annulus and supravalvular PA narrowing. Dysplastic pulmonic valves are more often found in the setting of other cardiac and noncardiac anomalies. Unicuspid and bicuspid pulmonic valves rarely occur in isolation; they are usually found in complex congenital heart disease conditions such as TOF (Fig. 24.1). PS is associated with genetic syndromes, including Noonan, Alagille, and Williams syndromes, and with congenital rubella[6] (Table 24.1).

Valvular PS can be accompanied by aneurysmal dilation of the PA, with the poststenotic jet favoring the left PA. However, the degree of PA dilation is not necessarily related to the severity of PS. Most patients do not require operative repair unless there is PR resulting in RV dilation or symptoms attributable to compression of adjacent structures. The risk of dissection or rupture in the absence of pulmonary hypertension, left-to-right shunting, or connective tissue disorder is low, and conservative management is appropriate.[7]

Clinical Presentation and Assessment

Most patients with PS are asymptomatic and come to attention when a murmur is auscultated. Symptoms rarely occur in childhood but become more common with age and severity of disease. Symptoms of moderate to severe PS include exercise intolerance and dyspnea resulting from inadequate augmentation of cardiac output with exertion and can progress to frank right-sided heart failure if not addressed. Exertional chest discomfort can arise from relative RV ischemia or coexistent coronary atherosclerosis. Rarely, patients can experience syncope or even sudden death due to ischemia from decreased myocardial perfusion of a hypertrophied RV and resultant arrhythmia. Desaturation can result from right-to-left shunting across an atrial-level communication, such as an atrial septal defect or patent foramen ovale.

Physical examination findings in the adult with valvular PS depends on the severity of the stenosis and any associated lesions. In mild PS, the jugular venous waveforms are normal, and the precordium is quiet. A systolic crescendo-decrescendo murmur is heard in the pulmonic position; it increases with inspiration and usually ends in midsystole but can extend further with increasing severity of obstruction.[8] There may be a pulmonic ejection click that decreases with inspiration. The second heart sound (S_2) is usually split.

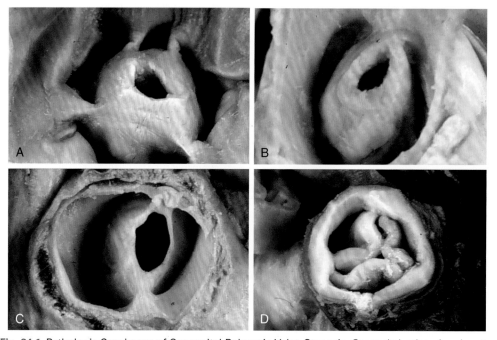

Fig. 24.1 Pathologic Specimens of Congenital Pulmonic Valve Stenosis. Congenital pulmonic valve stenosis is most often doming with a narrow central opening, rudimentary raphes, and no apparent commissure (A). Unicuspid (B) and bicuspid (C) valves can be seen in complex congenital heart disease. (D) Dysplastic valves are thickened with immobile leaflets.

TABLE 24.1 Genetic Syndromes Associated With Pulmonic Valve and Supravalvular Pulmonary Stenosis.

Genetic Syndrome	Genetic Defect	Cardiac Features	Noncardiac Features
Noonan	*PTPN11, SOS1, RAF1, RIT1* → aberrant RAS-MAPK signaling, autosomal dominant trait	Dysplastic pulmonic valve, supravalvular pulmonary stenosis, hypertrophic cardiomyopathy	Short stature, hypertelorism, micrognathia, high arched palate, low-set ears, webbed neck
Leopard (Noonan syndrome with multiple lentigines)	*PTPN11, RAF1, BRAF, MAP2K1*, autosomal dominant trait	Hypertrophic cardiomyopathy, valvular pulmonic or supravalvular pulmonary stenosis	Lentigines, ocular hypertelorism, ptosis, pectus deformity, genital abnormalities, growth retardation, deafness
Williams	7q11.23 deletion, autosomal dominant trait but most cases sporadic	Supravalvular aortic or pulmonic stenosis	Elfin facies, short stature, cognitive and developmental delay, endocrine disorders, genitourinary abnormalities
DiGeorge	22q11.2 deletion, autosomal dominant trait but most cases sporadic	Conotruncal anomalies such as tetralogy of Fallot	Hypertelorism, low-set and posteriorly rotated ears, palatal abnormalities, micrognathia, developmental delay, hypoplastic thymus, hypocalcemia, immunologic and neuropsychiatric disorders
Alagille	*JAG1, NOTCH2*, autosomal dominant trait	Peripheral pulmonary stenosis, tetralogy of Fallot	Dysmorphic facies with triangular face, wide nasal bridge, deep-set eyes, intrahepatic cholestasis, butterfly vertebrae
Keutel	*MGP* mutations, autosomal recessive trait	Peripheral pulmonary stenosis	Abnormal cartilage calcifications, brachytelephalangia, intellectual disability, hearing loss
Congenital rubella	—	Peripheral pulmonary stenosis, patent ductus arteriosus	Congenital cataract/glaucoma, deafness, pigmentary retinopathy

Modified from Cuypers JA, Witsenburg M, van der Linde D, et al. Pulmonary stenosis: update on diagnosis and therapeutic options. Heart 2013; 99:339-347.

In severe PS, the jugular venous pressure can be elevated with a prominent a wave. There may be an RV lift and a loud, harsh ejection murmur with associated thrill that radiates to the back. The degree of S_2 splitting is proportional to the degree of stenosis; it may be widely split and fixed. However, the pulmonic (P_2) component of the S_2 may be reduced or absent in severe stenosis, which can make splitting difficult to appreciate. A right-sided fourth heart sound (S_4) gallop may be auscultated.

The electrocardiogram (ECG) of PS is often normal in cases of mild disease, but with increasing severity the axis rotates rightward and features of RV hypertrophy and right atrial enlargement emerge. The chest radiograph typically demonstrates an enlarged main PA. The cardiac silhouette and vascularity are often normal in mild to moderate PS, but with severe PS cardiomegaly, right atrial enlargement, and decreased pulmonary vascular markings are seen (Fig. 24.2).

Echocardiography is considered the mainstay of imaging valvular PS (Fig. 24.3). The definition of severe valvular PS according to the 2018 American Hospital Association (AHA)/American College of Cardiology (ACC) guidelines for the management of adults with congenital heart disease[9] is a maximum velocity (V_{max}) greater than 4 m/s or a peak instantaneous gradient greater than 64 mmHg, whereas mild PS is defined as a V_{max} lower than 3 m/s or a peak instantaneous gradient lower than 36 mmHg (Table 24.2).

Physiologic conditions that alter flow across the pulmonic valve affect the accuracy of gradient calculation by the modified Bernoulli equation. For example, if there is severe RV systolic dysfunction, the RV cannot generate sufficient pressure to overcome significant PS, yielding a peak instantaneous gradient that underestimates the true severity of the stenosis. Similarly, left-to-right flow across a septal defect or concomitant PR increases flow across the pulmonic valve, thereby increasing the transpulmonary gradient and overestimating the severity of

pulmonic valve stenosis. Long-segment stenosis and serial obstructions (i.e., associated subvalvular PS and/or supravalvular PA stenosis) are other conditions in which Doppler-derived gradients are less reliable.

Peak instantaneous gradients measured by echocardiography overestimate peak-to-peak gradients in the catheterization laboratory and may be exaggerated by the effects of sedation. RV systolic pressure estimates based on tricuspid regurgitation peak velocity, qualitative assessment of septal position, and degree of RV hypertrophy can provide additional information on PS severity. Correlation between the Doppler gradient derived by echocardiography and clinical findings is recommended.

If there is a question, the gold standard in assessing the severity of valvular PS is cardiac catheterization, during which hemodynamic data, including pressure gradient across the pulmonic valve, RV systolic pressure compared with systemic pressure, and right-sided filling pressure, are obtained. In patients with normal cardiac output, mild stenosis is defined as a gradient lower than 35 to 40 mmHg or an RV pressure less than one half of the systemic pressure. Moderate stenosis is a gradient between 40 and 60 mmHg with RV pressure between one half and three fourths of the systemic pressure. Severe PS is defined as a gradient greater than 60 mmHg or an RV pressure equal to or greater than three fourths of the systemic pressure.[6]

Angiography can demonstrate the morphologic characteristics of the pulmonic valve, including leaflet thickening, mobility and excursion, and leaflet tethering, as well as associated lesions, including annular hypoplasia, infundibular obstruction, and distal main or branch PA stenosis.

There are mixed data on the accuracy of peak instantaneous gradients derived by echocardiography compared with gradients obtained by invasive cardiac catheterization for PS. Some studies have demonstrated excellent correlation with peak-to-peak gradients,[10,11] whereas others have shown that peak instantaneous gradients overestimate peak-to-peak

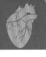

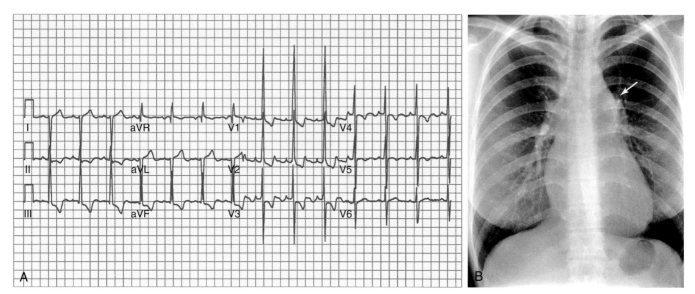

Fig. 24.2 Electrocardiogram and Chest Radiograph of a Patient With Severe Valvular Pulmonic Stenosis. (A) The electrocardiogram demonstrates right axis deviation and right ventricular hypertrophy with a strain pattern. (B) The chest radiograph shows right atrial and right ventricular enlargement, dilation of the main pulmonary artery *(arrow)*, and diminished vascular markings.

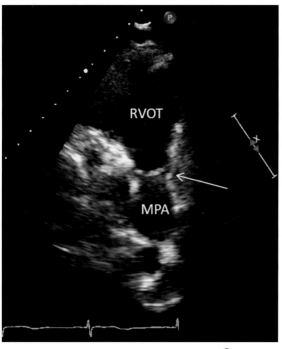

Fig. 24.3 Valvular Pulmonic Stenosis (Video 24. 3 ⏵). The transthoracic echocardiogram, a parasternal short-axis view focused over the main pulmonary artery *(MPA)*, shows a thickened pulmonic valve that domes in systole *(arrow). RVOT,* Right ventricular outflow tract.

TABLE 24.2 Severity of Pulmonic Valve Stenosis.

Assessment Measure	Mild	Moderate	Severe
Peak Doppler velocity (m/s)	<3	3–4	>4
Peak Doppler gradient (mmHg)	<36	36–64	>64
Mean Doppler gradient (mmHg)	—	—	>40
RV systolic pressure/LV systolic pressure	<50%	50%–74%	≥75%

Modified from Cuypers JA, Witsenburg M, van der Linde D, et al. Pulmonary stenosis: update on diagnosis and therapeutic options. Heart 2013;99:339-347.

population, regardless of a medical or surgical management strategy, with most patients being asymptomatic. Those with a gradient between 25 and 49 mmHg had a 20% chance of needing an intervention, and most of those with gradients equal to or greater than 50 mmHg had progressive stenosis and required intervention.[16]

Indications for intervention in valvular PS are summarized in Table 24.3. Successful percutaneous balloon valvuloplasty was initially reported in 1982, and it is the treatment of choice for classic domed valvular PS[17] (Fig. 24.4). The mechanism for relief of stenosis is commissural splitting, and the outcomes are usually excellent.[18,19] Moreover, although the outcomes are not as optimal as with classic domed PS, balloon valvuloplasty may provide some degree of relief for dysplastic pulmonic valves and is a reasonable first-line option.[20]

A large, multicenter registry of 533 patients followed for a median of 33 months (range, 1 month to 8.7 years) after balloon valvuloplasty showed that 23% had suboptimal results, defined as a residual gradient of 36 mmHg or greater or repeat balloon valvuloplasty or surgical valvotomy. Predictors of suboptimal outcome included earlier study year of intervention, higher residual postprocedural gradient, and unfavorable valvular anatomy.[21] Long-term outcomes were reported for 139 patients who underwent balloon valvuloplasty with a median

gradients but are comparable to catheter-derived maximal instantaneous gradients.[12,13] Mean Doppler gradients have the best correlation with peak-to-peak gradients in isolated[14] and complex[15] valvular PS.

Management and Outcomes

Progression of mild PS is unusual after early childhood. The Second Natural History Study of Congenital Heart Defects demonstrated comparable survival rates for patients with mild PS and the general

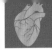

TABLE 24.3 Recommendations for Intervention in RVOT Obstruction, Pulmonic Valve Stenosis, and Supravalvular Pulmonary Stenosis.

Lesion	ACC/AHA		ESC	
	Class/LOE	Recommendation	Class/LOE	Recommendation
RVOT obstruction (any level)			I/C	Repair for severe RVOT obstruction ($\Delta P_{max} > 64$ mmHg) if RV function normal and valve substitute not needed, regardless of symptoms
			IIa/C	Repair for RV outflow obstruction with $\Delta P_{max} < 64$ mmHg in symptomatic patients, decreased RV function, important arrhythmias or right-to-left shunting across an ASD or VSD
DCRV	I/C-LD	Surgical repair for symptomatic patients with DCRV and at least moderate obstruction	I/C	Surgical repair for DCRV ($\Delta P_{max} > 64$ mmHg) if RV function normal and valve substitute not needed, regardless of symptoms
	IIb/C-LD	Surgical repair may be considered for asymptomatic patients with DCRV and severe obstruction	IIa/C	Consider surgical repair for patients with DCRV ($\Delta P_{max} < 64$ mmHg)
Valvular PS	I/B-NR	Balloon valvuloplasty for symptomatic patients (heart failure, cyanosis from right-to-left shunting across atrial communication, and/or exercise intolerance) with moderate or severe valvular PS	I/C	Balloon valvuloplasty for severe valvular PS ($\Delta P_{max} > 64$ mmHg) if RV function normal and valve substitute not needed, regardless of symptoms
	I/B-NR	Surgical repair for symptomatic patients with moderate or severe valvular PS who are not eligible for or failed balloon valvuloplasty	I/C	Surgical repair for asymptomatic patients with severe valvular PS with RVSP > 80 mmHg in whom balloon valvuloplasty is ineffective and surgical valve replacement is only option
	IIa/C-EO	Intervention is reasonable for asymptomatic valvular PS	IIa/C	Repair for patients with $\Delta P_{max} < 64$ mmHg with symptomatic valvular PS, important arrhythmias, or right-to-left shunting across an ASD or VSD
Peripheral branch PS	IIa/B-NR	Balloon angioplasty or stenting can be useful in peripheral PA stenosis	IIa/C	Repair for peripheral PA stenosis with diameter narrowing > 50% and RVSP > 50 mmHg and/or lung perfusion abnormalities, regardless of symptoms

ACC, American College of Cardiology; *AHA*, American Heart Association; *ASD*, atrial septal defect; *DCRV*, double-chambered right ventricle; *EO*, expert opinion; *ESC*, European Society of Cardiology; *LD*, limited data; *LOE*, level of evidence; *NR*, nonrandomized; *PA*, pulmonary artery; *PS*, pulmonic stenosis; *RVOT*, right ventricular outflow tract; *RVSP*, right ventricular systolic pressure; *VSD*, ventricular septal defect; ΔP_{max}, maximum instantaneous Doppler gradient.
Data from Stout KK, Daniels CJ, Aboulhosn JA, et al. 2018 AHA/ACC guideline for the management of adults with congenital heart disease: a report of the American College of Cardiology/American Heart Association Task Force on Clinical Practice Guidelines. J Am Coll Cardiol 2019;73:1494-1563; Bergersen L, Foerster F, Marshall AC, Meadows J, editors. Pulmonary angioplasty. In: Congenital heart disease: the catheterization manual. New York: Springer; 2009.

follow-up of 6 years (range, 0–21 years); reintervention was required in only 9.4% of patients, mostly for restenosis.[22] Mild PR is common, but moderate or greater PR can occur after balloon valvuloplasty and was observed in up to 60% of patients after a median follow-up of 15.1 years (range, 10.1–26.3 years).[22,23]

Surgical relief of PS involves commissurotomy or valvotomy by an incision through the pulmonary trunk using an open or closed technique. Valvectomy is reserved for situations in which simple valvotomy is inadequate (i.e., dysplastic pulmonic valves). A transannular patch using autologous pericardium may be required to enlarge the annulus and supravalvular area. Outcomes of surgical valvotomy have demonstrated excellent survival rates of 90% to 96% up to 40 years after surgery but with a significant incidence of PR necessitating repeat surgical intervention (e.g., pulmonic valve replacement [PVR]) later in life.[24–28]

Worsening of infundibular obstruction after relief of valvular PS by surgical valvotomy or balloon valvuloplasty is well documented, but this improves over time with regression of RV hypertrophy.[29,30] PR is not uncommon, especially after surgical intervention for valvular PS, and indications for PVR in cases of severe PR after surgical valvotomy are not well established. PVR may be appropriate in the setting of progressive RV dilation and dysfunction.[9,31] Management of residual PR is discussed later (see Tetralogy of Fallot).[32]

Subpulmonic Stenosis

Background

The anatomic RV is tripartite, comprising an inflow, a trabecular apex or sinus portion, and an outflow, also known as the infundibulum. Subpulmonic stenosis is an uncommon form of right-sided congeni-

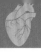

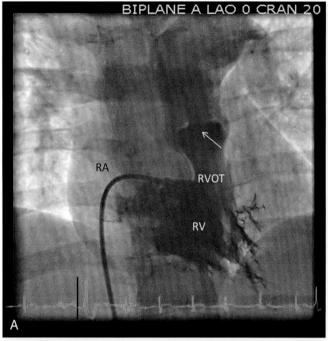

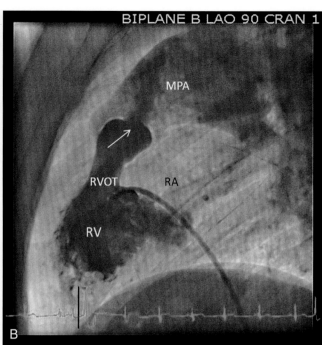

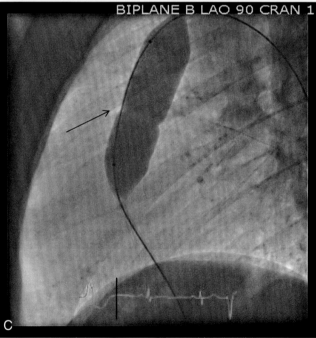

Fig. 24.4 Valvular Pulmonic Stenosis. Anteroposterior (A) and lateral (B) projections of a right ventriculogram demonstrate doming pulmonic valve leaflets *(arrows)*. Notice the dilated main pulmonary artery *(MPA)*. (C) Balloon valvuloplasty of pulmonic stenosis. Lateral projection of balloon inflation across the pulmonic valve. There is a mild waist at the level of pulmonic valve obstruction *(arrow)*. *RVOT,* Right ventricular outflow tract.

tal heart disease; it is caused by an infundibular right ventricular outflow tract (RVOT) stenosis due to a discrete fibromuscular ridge or ring or by hypertrophied muscle bundles resulting in a double-chambered RV. Infundibular stenosis can be located anywhere within the RVOT, from the ostium of the infundibulum to just below the pulmonary valve, whereas obstruction in double-chambered RV occurs at the os infundibulum, effectively dividing the RV into a proximal high-pressure sinus chamber and a distal low-pressure infundibular chamber (Fig. 24.5).

Infundibular stenosis can result from muscular thickening and hypertrophy of the infundibular wall due to PS, but it is also commonly associated with TOF, transposition of the great arteries, and

ventricular septal defects (VSDs). The cause of a double-chambered RV is not known. Muscle bundles may result from local hypertrophy of muscular tissue or from alterations in maturation of the primitive bulbus cordis during fetal development of the RV.[6,33]

Double-chambered RV is an uncommon lesion, accounting for 0.5% to 2% of all congenital heart disease.[34] It is associated with a VSD in 60% to 90% of cases, most commonly the membranous type with a communication usually between the LV and the proximal high-pressure chamber. It is associated with valvular PS in approximately 40% of cases and with atrial septal defect in approximately 17%. Double-chambered RV can also occur with complex congenital heart disease such as double-outlet RV or TOF.[34,35]

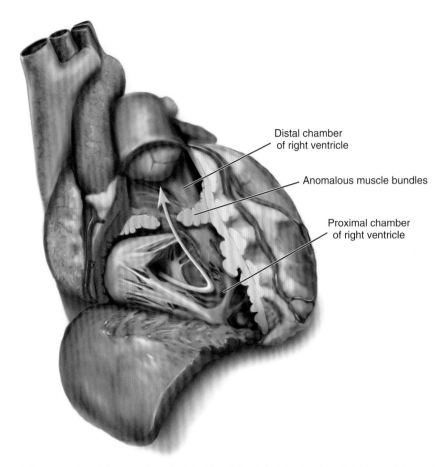

Fig. 24.5 Diagram of Double-Chambered Right Ventricle. A double-chambered right ventricle results from anomalous muscle bundles that divide the right ventricle into proximal and distal chambers. (From Otto C, editor. Practice of clinical echocardiography. 5th ed. Philadelphia: Elsevier; 2016.)

Clinical Presentation and Assessment

Either form of subpulmonic stenosis can have a presentation similar to that of PR, depending on the degree of obstruction and the associated VSD or other anomalies. The RV obstruction in double-chambered RV is progressive due to muscle bundle hypertrophy over time, but the rate of obstruction varies.[36,37] It is hypothesized that adults who have a double-chambered RV in isolation later in life may have had an associated VSD that spontaneously closed. In the setting of a VSD located proximal to the obstruction, elevated RV pressures can diminish the degree of left-to-right shunting, resulting in severe cases in right-to-left shunting and cyanosis.

The physical examination of patients with subpulmonic stenosis is notable for a systolic murmur located lower along the left sternal border than in patients with PS. There is no pulmonic ejection click, and the P_2 component of the S_2 is normal. With severe hypertrophy, there may be an RV heave. The ejection murmur across the obstruction is associated with a thrill in approximately 25% of patients with double-chambered RV.[34] The murmur of an associated VSD may be auscultated.

As in PS, the ECG in subpulmonic stenosis shows RV hypertrophy in most patients, but incomplete right bundle branch and right axis deviation have been observed. The chest radiograph is also similar to that seen in PS unless there is an associated significant VSD. Transthoracic echocardiography is usually diagnostic, especially in the young patient but can be challenging in older adults, and transesophageal echocardiography can be helpful[35] (Fig. 24.6).

Elevated RV systolic pressures measured by tricuspid regurgitation jet velocity and severe RV hypertrophy in the setting of a normal pulmonary valve may be mistakenly diagnosed as pulmonary hypertension if this form of RVOT obstruction is not recognized. It is important to define the location of a VSD in relation to the obstructive muscle bundles. If it is communicating with the proximal high-pressure RV sinus, the transseptal velocity across the VSD will be relatively low in cases of significant RVOT obstruction, even if the VSD is small and restricts flow.

Cardiac magnetic resonance (CMR) imaging is increasingly used to provide excellent visualization of anatomy.[38,39] Cardiac catheterization occasionally may be needed for diagnostic reasons and is valuable in determining the pressures proximal and distal to the obstruction. The diagnosis can be missed if the catheter is advanced across the RV sinus into the outflow tract without careful attention to the waveform.

Management and Outcomes

Treatment of discrete infundibular obstruction caused by a membranous ridge or obstructive muscle bundles is surgical. Because of the progressive nature of the disease, delaying surgical repair for double-chambered RV is not recommended unless the degree of obstruction is mild. Surgery is most commonly undertaken by a transatrial approach but may require a right ventriculotomy; outcomes are excellent with minimal residua.[40,41] Indications for surgical repair are summarized in Table 24.3.

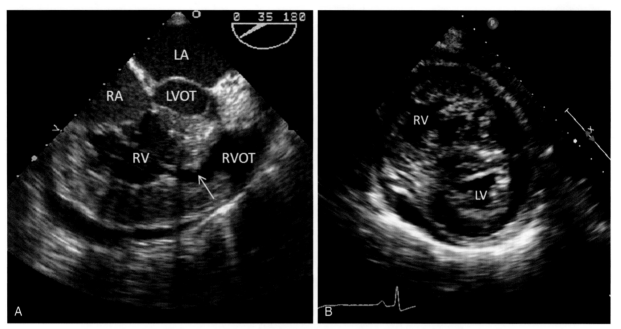

Fig. 24.6 Double-Chambered Right Ventricle. (A) Transesophageal echocardiogram on mid-esophageal short-axis view demonstrates obstruction in the right ventricle *(RV)* at the os infundibulum *(arrow)* (Video 24.6A ▶). (B) Transthoracic echocardiogram with a parasternal short-axis view at the mid-ventricle shows RV dilation and severe RV hypertrophy with a flattened, D-shaped septum in systole (Video 24.6B ▶). *LVOT,* Left ventricular outflow tract; *RVOT,* right ventricular outflow tract.

Supravalvular and Peripheral Pulmonary Artery Stenosis

Background

Supravalvular stenosis of the PA trunk occurs in 1% to 2% of patients with congenital heart disease, and peripheral branch PA stenosis occurs in 2% to 5%.[42,43] Although isolated peripheral pulmonary stenosis can occur, in 60% of cases it is seen with other congenital cardiac malformations such as valvular PS, atrial septal defect, VSD, and patent ductus arteriosus.[42]

Developmental and genetic factors play a role in the pathogenesis of main and branch PA stenosis, and these lesions are associated with Noonan, Williams, Alagille, and Keutel syndromes and with complex congenital heart disease such as TOF.[6] Teratogenesis has also been implicated, as in congenital rubella syndrome (see Table 24.1).

Supravalvular pulmonary stenosis may be seen postoperatively at the site of a prior PA band or after arterial switch operation for dextro (D)-transposition of the great arteries. Morphology and severity can range from a focal single stenosis to multiple stenoses of the main PA out to the peripheral branches; diffuse hypoplasia or near-atresia can occur.

Clinical Presentation and Assessment

Patients with mild to moderate bilateral or unilateral branch PA stenosis are usually asymptomatic. In cases of severe obstruction, exertional intolerance or even right heart failure may exist, similar to the situation in pulmonic or subpulmonic valve stenosis, as a result of increased RV afterload.

The auscultatory findings are notable for lack of an ejection click. The S₂ is usually split and can have a prominent P₂ component. In cases of severe stenosis, RV ejection is prolonged, and the pulmonic valve closure is delayed. The systolic ejection murmur is appreciated at the left upper sternal border and transmits to the back and peripheral lung fields. A continuous murmur may be heard, representing a significant diastolic gradient of severe obstruction.

The ECG of supravalvular or peripheral pulmonary stenosis is usually normal, but RV hypertrophy can be demonstrated in cases of severe obstruction. Similarly, chest radiographs are usually normal, and unless there is a coexistent left-to-right shunt in the setting of severe obstruction, abnormalities of pulmonary vascularity may not be apparent.[6]

The echocardiographic evaluation of supravalvular and peripheral pulmonary stenosis can be challenging in the adult with suboptimal windows. The right PA can be seen along its length in the high left parasternal short-axis or suprasternal short-axis view (Fig. 24.7), but the left PA is often difficult to visualize. Branch pulmonary arteries are readily assessed by CMR, which is comparable in diagnostic capability to x-ray angiography by catheterization.[44] For these reasons, alternative modes of imaging such as CMR or computed tomography are recommended.[9]

Invasive hemodynamic catheterization with x-ray angiography may be required for diagnostic purposes. In the case of unilateral branch PA stenosis, the contralateral PA can accommodate increased flow with no significant increase in pressure.[20] In the affected PA, systolic pressure differences across the stenosis can underestimate the severity of obstruction due to decreased blood flow, whereas diastolic pressure differences reflect the degree of obstruction.[6] Complete assessment of branch PA stenosis may require measurement of relative blood flow as assessed by nuclear perfusion scanning or CMR velocity cine imaging for branch flow splits.

Management and Outcomes

Repair of supravalvular stenosis of the main pulmonary trunk is usually surgical, especially with lesions that involve the bifurcation of the branch pulmonary arteries. However, stent angioplasty may be appropriate, provided the stent does not compromise valve function or impinge on the branch pulmonary arteries.[20]

Most cases of mild to moderate, unilateral or bilateral branch PA stenosis in adults do not require treatment. Indications for intervention

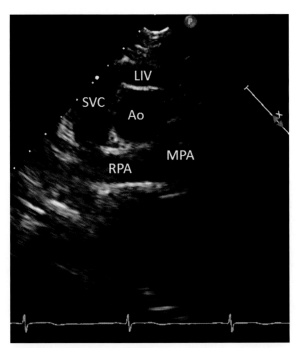

Fig. 24.7 Right Pulmonary Artery. Suprasternal short-axis view by transthoracic echocardiography demonstrates the right pulmonary artery *(RPA)* along its length. *Ao,* Aorta; *MPA,* main pulmonary artery; *LIV,* left innominate vein; *SVC,* superior vena cava.

for peripheral pulmonary stenosis include gradients greater than 20 mmHg across the stenosis, decreased lung perfusion (<35% of flow to one lung), RV hypertension at least one half of systemic pressure or greater than 50 mmHg, greater than 50% diameter narrowing, or symptoms[20,45,46] (see Table 24.3).

Catheter-based techniques are considered the treatment of choice for peripheral PA stenosis, with surgery reserved for lesions that are not amenable to percutaneous therapy and situations in which coexistent defects require repair.[41] Balloon angioplasty, introduced clinically in 1983,[47] can improve the angiographic appearance and gradient across the lesion, but results are often not durable.[48] Cutting balloons have been efficacious in the treatment of branch PA stenosis resistant to conventional high-pressure balloon techniques.[49] PA stenting is indicated when anatomically appropriate, especially if balloon dilation is unsuccessful.

In a large multicenter registry examining procedural outcomes of 1183 PA stenting procedures in children and adults, success (i.e., a 20% reduction in RV pressure or a 50% increase in PA diameter) was achieved in 76% of patients with a biventricular circulation. Complications occurred in 14%, major adverse events in 9%, and there was a procedural mortality rate of 0.2%.[50] Longer-term outcomes of branch PA stenting have been published mostly in the pediatric literature. Short-term results are good, but reintervention is common, particularly in those with Williams or Alagille syndrome or TOF.[51–54] For this reason, longitudinal surveillance and follow-up are essential.

TETRALOGY OF FALLOT

Congenital abnormalities of the infundibulum, pulmonic valve, and branch pulmonary arteries are characteristic of TOF. There is wide variation in the anatomy and resultant physiology. PR in repaired TOF is commonly encountered in the adult, and its evaluation and management are discussed here.

Background

TOF is the most common cyanotic heart defect, with an incidence of 0.33 cases per 1000 live births; it accounts for 6.7% of all forms of congenital heart disease.[55,56] It is a conotruncal anomaly comprising (1) VSD, (2) aorta overriding the VSD, (3) RVOT obstruction, and (4) RV hypertrophy (Fig. 24.8A).

Although the cause of TOF is not well understood, there is a genetic component with known associated chromosomal anomalies, single-gene defects, and syndromes such as DiGeorge or velocardiofacial syndrome (i.e., 22q11 deletion), Down syndrome, Alagille syndrome, and VATER or VACTERL association, a condition defined by at least three of the following congenital malformations: *v*ertebral defects, *a*nal atresia, *c*ardiac anomaly, *t*racheo-*e*sophageal fistula, *r*enal and *l*imb anomalies).[57]

The malalignment VSD in TOF results from deviation of the infundibular septum anteriorly and superiorly out of the plane with the rest of the ventricular septum (see Fig. 24.8B). This causes infundibular obstruction, which can be exacerbated by anomalous muscle bundles crossing the RVOT (see Fig. 24.8C). The anatomy and morphology of the pulmonic valve can vary greatly. The pulmonic valve is often hypoplastic and may be bicuspid or unicuspid with various degrees of PS.

The most extreme form is TOF with pulmonary atresia, which may be accompanied by discontinuous branch pulmonary arteries and major aortopulmonary collateral arteries that supply portions of the lung. TOF with absent pulmonic valve is a rare condition in which the valve leaflets are absent or rudimentary, resulting in aneurysmal dilation of the main and branch pulmonary arteries. Supravalvular and branch PA stenosis is common in TOF, especially left PA stenosis as a result of a ductal sling at its insertion site.[58]

Surgical Repair and Residuae

Most adults with TOF have undergone surgical repair. In the era when neonatal cardiopulmonary bypass was not readily available, a staged approach was used in which an aortopulmonary shunt procedure to augment pulmonary blood flow was performed before the complete repair. Primary complete repair became the standard of care in the 1980s, but a modified Blalock-Taussig shunt procedure may still be performed in infants with pulmonary atresia, in symptomatic neonates, and in centers where neonatal primary repair is not conducted. Although the procedure is no longer routinely performed, initial forms of palliative shunts are still encountered in the surgical history of older TOF patients (Table 24.4 and Fig. 24.9).

Complete repair consists of VSD closure, relief of RVOT obstruction, and take-down of the shunt, if previously palliated. RVOT obstruction and PS are addressed in a variety of ways, including muscle bundle resection, patch augmentation of the RVOT, transannular patch, pulmonic valvotomy/valvectomy, or a conduit between the RV and the PA in cases of pulmonary atresia or an anomalous coronary artery crossing the RVOT.

Residual structural and functional abnormalities are the norm after repair of TOF. Historically, patients underwent repair by right ventriculotomy with a generous transannular patch that effectively relieved the RVOT obstruction but resulted in severe PR. Although it was once thought to be benign, the natural history of chronic severe PR is progressive RV dilation and dysfunction, which has been associated with exercise intolerance, heart failure, arrhythmias, and sudden death in the third and fourth decades of life.[59–62] Branch PA stenosis can cause dyspnea on exertion and exacerbation of PR.[63]

A minority of patients has residual PS as the dominant lesion and may have undergone valve-sparing techniques to minimize PR.[64] Another subgroup of patients who have undergone repair in childhood with an RV-to-PA conduit (instead of a native RVOT) requires revision

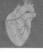

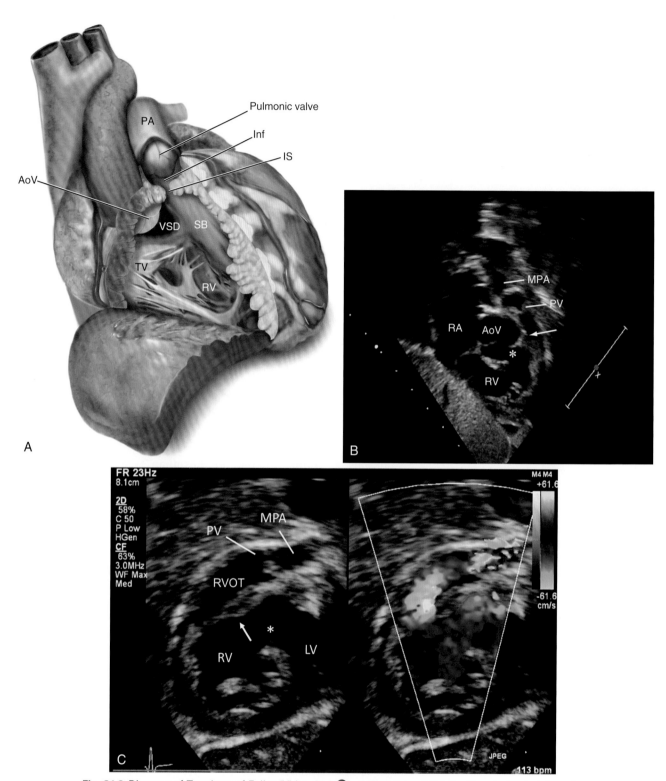

Fig. 24.8 Diagram of Tetralogy of Fallot (Video 24.8 ▶). (A) Tetralogy of Fallot with anterior deviation of the infundibular septum *(Inf)*, infundibular stenosis *(IS)*, malalignment ventricular septal defect *(VSD)*, overriding aortic valve *(AoV)*, and right ventricular *(RV)* hypertrophy. (B) Unrepaired tetralogy of Fallot. Transthoracic echocardiographic image, subcostal right anterior oblique view, demonstrates anteriorly malaligned Inf *(arrow)* with resulting VSD *(asterisk)*, overriding aorta *(AoV)*, and hypoplastic pulmonic valve *(PV)*. (C) Subcostal short-axis view with color compare shows the anteriorly malaligned infundibular septum, *(arrow)* resulting in systolic color-flow turbulence in the right ventricular outflow tract *(RVOT)* and VSD *(asterisk)*. Notice the thickened dysplastic leaflets with color Doppler aliasing across the PV. *MPA,* Main pulmonary artery; *PA,* pulmonary artery; *SB,* septal band; *TV,* tricuspid valve. (From Otto C, editor. Practice of clinical echocardiography. 5th ed. Philadelphia: Elsevier; 2016.)

TABLE 24.4   Palliative Shunt Procedures in Tetralogy of Fallot.

Shunt	Description	Notes
Classic Blalock-Taussig shunt	End-to-side anastomosis of subclavian artery to ipsilateral pulmonary artery	Lack of brachial and radial pulses on ipsilateral side Rarely can have excessive pulmonary blood flow and pulmonary hypertension Usually performed on the side opposite of arch sidedness First palliative heart surgery for cyanotic heart disease
Modified Blalock-Taussig shunt	Gore-Tex interposition tube graft of subclavian artery to ipsilateral pulmonary artery	0.5–4 mm in the neonate Better control of pulmonary blood flow than classic shunt May have weak upper extremity pulse on ipsilateral side
Waterston shunt	Side-to-side anastomosis between ascending aorta and right pulmonary artery	May have excessive pulmonary blood flow and pulmonary hypertension Pulmonary artery distortion or acquired atresia
Potts shunt	Side-to-side anastomosis between descending aorta and left pulmonary artery	Similar issues as above
Central shunt	Gore-Tex interposition tube graft between ascending aorta and pulmonary artery	Uncontrolled pulmonary blood flow and pulmonary hypertension

Modified from Babu-Narayan SV, Gatzoulis M. Tetralogy of Fallot. In: Gatzoulis M, Webb G, Daubeney PE, editors. Diagnosis and management of adult congenital heart disease. 2nd ed. Philadelphia: Elsevier Saunders; 2011:316-327.

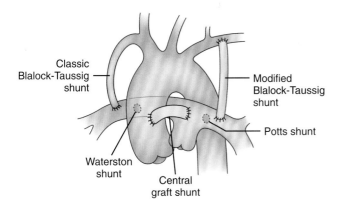

Fig. 24.9. Palliative Aortopulmonary Shunts. Anatomic descriptions of the aortopulmonary shunts used for tetralogy of Fallot are given in Table 24.4.

or upsizing in accord with somatic growth. These conduits degenerate over time, leading to stenosis, regurgitation, or a combination thereof.

Clinical Presentation and Assessment

Pulmonic insufficiency can be tolerated for many years without symptoms.[65] Depending on age and residual lesions, adults with TOF can have dyspnea on exertion, exercise intolerance, or even frank heart failure at presentation. The physical examination may be notable for elevated jugular venous pressures and large v waves if tricuspid regurgitation exists. Thoracotomy scars with absent or diminished ipsilateral brachial or radial pulses may indicate a prior Blalock-Taussig shunt. The precordium can be active with an RV lift. The S_2 can be single or widely split due to conduction delays related to RV dilation and right bundle branch block.

Often, a systolic ejection murmur is heard in the pulmonic area, representing acceleration of flow across the RVOT that can be accompanied by a diastolic decrescendo murmur of PR, creating a to-and-fro cadence. If there is free PR, the diastolic murmur may be short or practically inaudible due to rapid equilibration of diastolic pressures. A holosystolic murmur of tricuspid regurgitation or a right-sided S^3 gallop may be auscultated. Residual patch margin VSDs are often small and restrictive; they may lead to a high-frequency, holosystolic murmur at the left sternal border, if heard at all.

The characteristic ECG of the adult with repaired TOF demonstrates a right bundle branch block. A QRS duration greater than 180 ms is associated with malignant ventricular arrhythmias and sudden cardiac death in TOF.[66] Chest radiography may show central PA enlargement, cardiomegaly, and obliteration of the retrocardiac space on lateral view, consistent with RV enlargement (Fig. 24.10).

Echocardiography is the primary form of imaging in the routine assessment of TOF, although CMR is considered to be the reference standard in the assessment of PR and RV size and function.[67] Cardiac catheterization is rarely used as a first-line diagnostic modality but is necessary in situations in which the data obtained by other methods are inconclusive or contradictory. Guidelines for imaging in TOF have been published and emphasize an integrated multimodality approach for the complete assessment of TOF.[68]

Residual right-sided obstruction should be sought with a goal of defining the levels and extent of obstruction, akin to the evaluation of infundibular or valvular PS discussed earlier. Aneurysm of the RVOT can be seen by echocardiography as a large, echo-free space anterior or lateral to the outflow tract and main PA with associated thinning and dyskinesia.

The pulmonic valve annulus or conduit diameter should be measured for surgical or interventional planning in the native outflow tract or RV-to-PA conduit. Normal pulmonic annulus size ranges from 17 to 26 mm.[69] Conduits are notoriously difficult to profile in the adult by echocardiography because of their retrosternal, sometimes varied, location. Multiple views are required to adequately profile the conduit, and Doppler echocardiography is necessary for conduit localization and gradient measurements. Branch PA assessment should be part of the routine evaluation, and left branch PA stenosis is a known postoperative sequela of TOF repair.[70]

The severity of PR in TOF is determined by orifice size, RV compliance, and RV afterload.[63] Echocardiographic assessment of PR severity is qualitative, and it is the best method for distinguishing between mild and severe PR. Diastolic flow reversal in the branch pulmonary arteries[71,72] and a regurgitant jet width greater than 70% of the annulus diameter[71,73] are associated with severe PR (Fig. 24.11A).

One grading scheme defines mild PR as a jet width less than or equal to one third of the annulus diameter, moderate PR as one third to two thirds of the diameter, and severe PR as equal to or greater than two thirds of the annulus diameter.[74] A pressure half-time of less than 100 ms correlates with hemodynamically significant PR,[75] but noncompliant

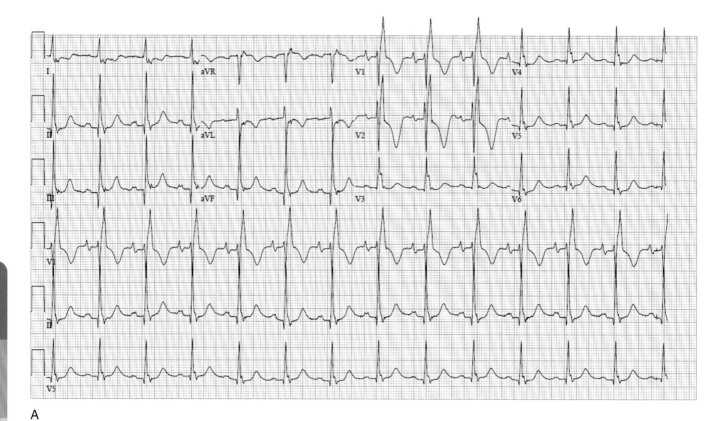

A

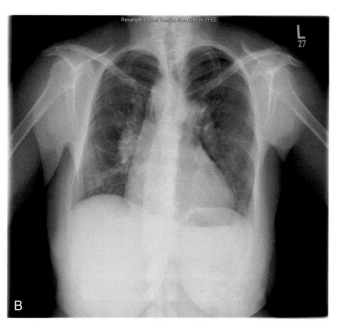

B

Fig. 24.10 Electrocardiogram and Chest Radiograph of a Patient With Repaired Tetralogy of Fallot. (A) Electrocardiogram classically demonstrates right bundle branch block. (B) Chest radiograph shows cardiomegaly, a dilated main pulmonary artery, and a right aortic arch, which is found in 25% of patients with tetralogy of Fallot. (From Roche SL, Greenway SC, Redington AN. Tetralogy of Fallot with pulmonary stenosis, pulmonary atresia, and absent pulmonary valve. In: Allen HD, Shaddy RE, Penny DJ, et al, editors: Moss and Adams' heart disease in infants, children, and adolescents: including the fetus and young adult. Vol 2, 9th ed. Philadelphia: Lippincott Williams & Wilkins; 2016:1029-1052.)

RV chambers with diastolic dysfunction can lead to overestimation of the degree of regurgitation by this measure because of rapid equilibration of end-diastolic pressures (see Fig. 24.10B). Other echocardiographic indices have been explored; they have various degrees of sensitivity and specificity or have not been validated.[76–79]

The assessment of PR severity by CMR is quantitative, and the regurgitant fraction can be calculated by dividing retrograde flow volume by antegrade flow volume as measured by phase-contrast cine across the main PA (Fig. 24.12). This technique yields a value comparable to that calculated by measuring the stroke volume difference between the

RV and LV unless there is concomitant tricuspid regurgitation, aortic regurgitation, or residual shunt. There is no standard grading scheme for severity of PR by CMR, but mild PR can be defined as a regurgitant fraction of less than 20%, moderate as 20% to 40%, and severe as greater than 40%.[78] Regurgitant volume (as opposed to regurgitant fraction) may be better for distinguishing moderate from severe RV dilation as measured by CMR, but it is not widely used clinically.[80]

Restrictive RV physiology is characterized by poor diastolic compliance in the setting of RV hypertrophy due to chronic pressure overload or decreased ventricular compliance. Late surgical repair has been

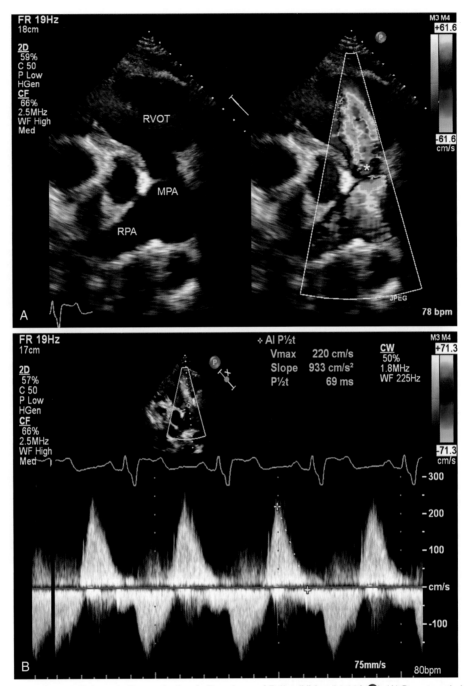

Fig. 24.11 Severe Pulmonic Regurgitation in Tetralogy of Fallot (Video 24.11A ⊙). (A) Parasternal short-axis view at the base with color Doppler demonstrates severe pulmonic regurgitation with color-flow reversal in the right pulmonary artery *(RPA)* by transthoracic echocardiography. Notice that the width of the regurgitant jet occupies the entire pulmonic annulus *(asterisk)* and aneurysmal right ventricular outflow tract *(ROVT)*. (B) Spectral Doppler pattern of severe pulmonic regurgitation. Continuous-wave Doppler across the pulmonary annulus demonstrates early diastolic pressure equalization with a pressure half-time of 69 ms *(dashed line)*. *MPA*, Main pulmonary artery;

identified as a risk factor.[81] Restrictive physiology can limit the degree of PR because of increased mid-diastolic to late-diastolic pressure that equilibrates with PA pressure; end-diastolic forward flow may be observed after atrial contraction. The restrictive RV acts as a passive conduit between the right atrium and PA during systole. There are mixed data on the relationship between restrictive RV physiology and RV size and outcomes such as exercise tolerance, likely due to differences in patient age and era of repair.[82-84]

Chronic PR is associated with RV enlargement and results in progressive RV dilation and dysfunction. Assessment of the RV by echocardiography is challenging because of its complex and highly varied geometry compared with the LV and its retrosternal location. For these reasons, CMR is considered the gold standard for imaging the RV in TOF[68,69] (Fig. 24.13). ECG-gated cine, steady-state free-precession imaging of the RV in short-axis slices can be contoured at end-systole and end-diastole to provide RV volumes, ejection fraction, and myocardial mass.[68]

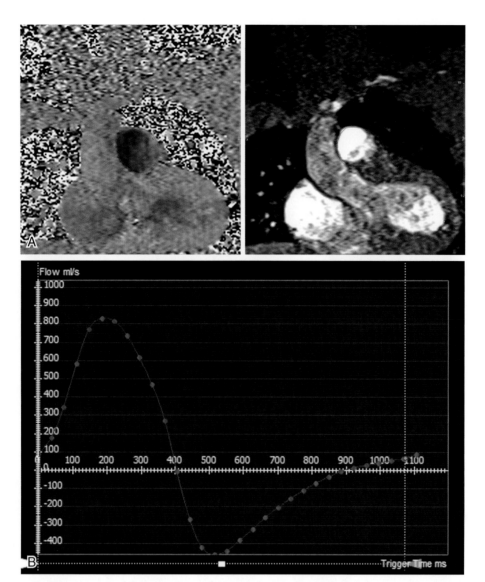

Fig. 24.12 Quantification of Pulmonic Regurgitation by Cardiac Magnetic Resonance Imaging. (A) Electrocardiographically gated cine phase-contrast *(left)* and magnitude *(right)* imaging of a region of interest across the proximal main pulmonary artery flow signal. (B) Flow rate (y-axis) plotted against time (x-axis) demonstrates antegrade flow volume (i.e., area above baseline) and retrograde flow volume (i.e., area below baseline). The pulmonic regurgitant fraction is calculated by dividing retrograde flow volume by antegrade flow volume.

Pulmonic Regurgitation and Timing of Pulmonic Valve Replacement

Late survival after TOF repair is excellent, reaching 86% up to 40 years after surgery.[60,85,86] However, morbidity is substantial, with almost one half of patients requiring reintervention. PVR is the most common procedure.[86] Although there is no debate concerning PVR in symptomatic patients, there is continued discussion regarding optimal timing of surgery in those who are asymptomatic.

Thierren et al. introduced the notion of "operating too late" for recovery or maintenance of RV contractility in patients whose RV function has already begun to deteriorate in the face of chronic PR.[87] In addition to the contribution to right heart failure, RV dysfunction can influence LV function and has independent prognostic value for long-term outcomes. The INDICATOR cohort, a large, multicenter registry of patients with TOF, compiled CMR data on 873 patients.

RV dysfunction was associated with death or sustained ventricular tachycardia in addition to LV dysfunction, atrial tachycardia, and RV hypertrophy.[88]

There are mixed data, however, about whether PVR itself improves RV ejection fraction. A meta-analysis found no significant improvement in RV ejection fraction.[89] Geva et al. found that a preoperative RV ejection fraction lower than 45% was associated with persistent RV dysfunction postoperatively, suggesting that PVR should occur before RV dysfunction develops.[90]

Attention has turned to using PVR before irreversible structural changes in RV size occur. The advent of CMR for quantification of RV size and function has enabled and perpetuated the concept of a threshold value for RV size, beyond which PVR is less likely to result in reverse RV remodeling. Initial studies suggested an indexed RV end-diastolic volume of 170 mL/m^2 or an end-systolic volume of 85 mL/m^2

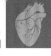

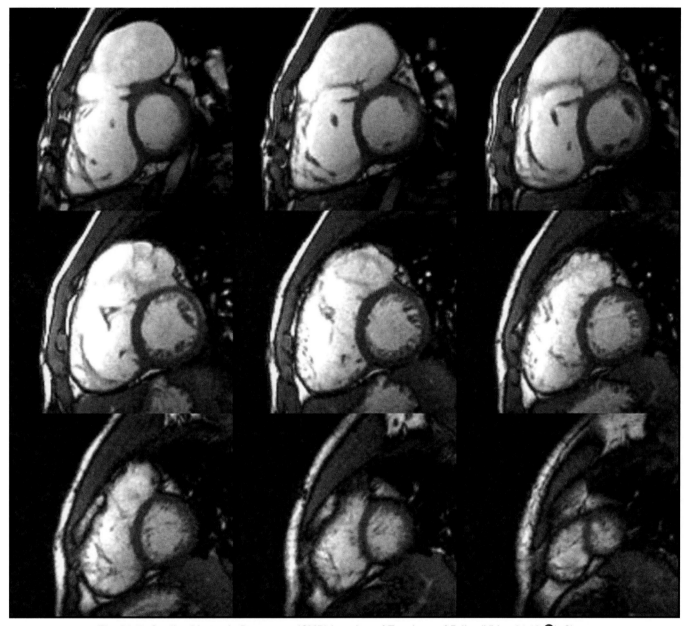

Fig. 24.13 Cardiac Magnetic Resonance (CMR) Imaging of Tetralogy of Fallot (Video 24.13 ▶). Short-axis stack of cine steady-state, free precession CMR images in repaired tetralogy of Fallot. Right ventricular volume and ejection fraction are calculated by tracing the endocardial border at end-diastole and end-systole for each slice. Notice the severely dilated right ventricle and thin-walled anterior infundibulum *(top row)*, consistent with a prior patch.

as threshold values, but the concept has evolved with a push toward smaller RV dimensions.[91–94] As with chronic aortic regurgitation, more emphasis has been placed on end-systolic volume.[95,96] Table 24.5[97,98] is a summary of the evidence on size threshold for PVR with a goal of attaining normal RV size.

In addition to parameters of RV size (including an RV-to-LV end-diastolic size ratio ≥ 2), RV dysfunction (RV ejection fraction < 47%), LV dysfunction (ejection fraction <55%), and other clinical parameters such as RVOT aneurysm, QRS duration greater than 160 ms, progressive exercise intolerance, sustained tachyarrhythmia, and other residual hemodynamic lesions can all be considered in the timing of PVR.[9,99]

Some patients have predominant PS, and indications for intervention are similar to those for isolated valvular PS. PVR is recommended for at least moderate RVOT obstruction or RV pressure greater than two thirds of the systemic pressure.[9] Catheter-based valvuloplasty may be an alternative to surgery in patients with appropriate anatomy.

There are few data to guide clinicians on the management of mixed pulmonic valve disease. Conventional recommendations are geared toward intervention based on the dominant lesion. However, branch PA stenosis increases afterload to the RV and is associated with worsening PR.[100] For this reason, addressing branch PA stenosis first, with reassessment of PR afterward, is recommended.[9]

TABLE 24.5 Evolution of Preoperative Right Ventricular Size Thresholds for Pulmonary Valve Replacement in Tetralogy of Fallot to Attain Normal Right Ventricular Size.

Study	Year	N	RV End-Diastolic Size (mL/m²)	RV End-Systolic Size (mL/m²)
Therrien et al.[91]	2005	17	170	85
Buechel et al.[97]	2005	20	150	—
Oosterof et al.[93]	2007	71	160	82
Frigiola et al.[98]	2008	71	150	—
Geva et al.[90]	2010	64	—	90
Lee et al.[95]	2012	170	163	80
Bokma et al.[96]	2016	157	—	80
Heng et al.[94]	2017	57	158	82

Exercise testing has long been used as an objective way to monitor functional capacity in patients with TOF before PVR, and it can support a referral for intervention. Babu-Narayan et al. reviewed 220 patients at a single center who underwent PVR and found that peak oxygen consumption (Vo₂), the relationship between minute ventilation and carbon dioxide production (VE/Vco₂ slope), and heart rate reserve on preoperative cardiopulmonary exercise stress testing predicted early death after PVR if the measured values were poor.[101] The data show that referral for PVR when patients still have reasonable functional capacity is associated with improved postoperative outcomes and support routine use of cardiopulmonary exercise testing to determine optimal surgical timing. Current guidelines for PVR are summarized in Table 24.6.

Pulmonic Valve Replacement Surgery and Outcomes

PVR surgery in repaired TOF requires an assessment of the RVOT and the main and branch pulmonary arteries. The standard approach is a transverse pulmonary arteriotomy, but a vertical incision is made if the RVOT is obstructed or requires revision due to calcified patch material. The incision can be extended to the branch pulmonary arteries, allowing augmentation, especially of the left PA.[102]

Bioprosthetic heterografts (usually porcine or bovine pericardial valves) are most commonly used but are marked by limited durability. In a single-center cohort of 227 children and adults with TOF who underwent stented bioprosthetic PVR, the rate of freedom from reintervention and structural valve deterioration was 74% at 5 years, with a median time to intervention of 6.4 years (range, 2–10.1 years). Age at PVR was an independent predictor of prosthetic valve deterioration.[103] A follow-up study from the same institution describing outcomes of 611 patients undergoing PVR between 1996 and 2014 (68.6% of whom were TOF patients) found that the Sorin Mitroflow valve (LivaNova, London) had a faster time to reintervention compared with the Carpentier-Edwards Magna/Magna Ease or Perimount valve (Edwards Lifesciences, Irvine, CA).[104]

Homograft RV-to-PA conduits made from cryopreserved aortic and pulmonary tissue are also at risk for degeneration and are not typically chosen, especially for use in younger patients, in whom smaller conduit size is a risk factor for homograft conduit failure.[105,106] Mechanical prostheses have been implanted in the pulmonic position with good short- and medium-term durability,[107,108] but they are at risk for thrombosis and pannus, especially in the setting of inadequate anticoagulation, pregnancy, or RV dysfunction.[109,110]

PVR eliminates PR and improves RV dimensions but does not consistently improve RV ejection fraction (Fig. 24.14). Clinically, patients feel better despite lack of improvement in objective measures of exercise capacity. Table 24.7[111–113] summarizes the clinical and hemodynamic response to PVR.

It is not known whether PVR timing based on the goal of normalizing RV size postoperatively translates into a hard clinical end point.[114] No study has demonstrated that PVR alone is associated with a reduction in rates of death or ventricular tachycardia postoperatively,[115,116] although patients who undergo cryoablation at the time of PVR have a decrease in atrial and ventricular arrhythmias postoperatively.[117,118] Patients seem to remain at risk for sudden cardiac death and ventricular arrhythmias despite PVR.[115,116]

Patients with primarily residual PS represent the minority of adult patients undergoing PVR, and their outcomes may be different. In contrast to TOF patients with PR, those with PS have improvement in the RV ejection fraction due to improvement in afterload and significant improvements in exercise capacity and RV ejection fraction on exercise stress testing.[119,120]

In the long term, TOF patients who undergo PVR generally do well, although often there are residual lesions that require intervention. Prosthetic pulmonic valve durability is limited, with the average lifespan estimated to be 10 to 15 years.[89,99] Although the RV initially improves in size, there is evidence of progressive prosthetic pulmonic valve dysfunction and RV deterioration with return to preoperative RV size over the ensuing 10 years.[121] Given this fact and the variations in RV remodeling after restoration of RVOT and pulmonic valve competence, it is difficult to know what criteria clinicians should use to refer patients for repeat PVR in the absence of symptoms.

TRANSCATHETER PULMONIC VALVE REPLACEMENT

Background

Since its initial introduction in 2000,[122] transcatheter PVR has gained widespread acceptance as a nonsurgical alternative for patients with congenital heart disease who have prior PVR or RV-to-PA conduits that have become dysfunctional (Fig. 24.15). Current valve options are limited, but innovations are rapidly evolving and expanding patient eligibility. Table 24.6 summarizes the recommendations for intervention in patients with dysfunctional RV-to-PA conduits.

The Medtronic Melody transcatheter pulmonary valve (Medtronic Inc., Minneapolis, MN) is a balloon-expandable device that has been commercially available in the United States since 2010. It received premarket approval in 2015 by the U.S. Food and Drug Administration (FDA). Use of the device was initially marked by struggles with stent fracture, but altering the approach with systematic prestenting of the conduit has reduced this complication significantly.[123,124] A limitation of this valve is its relatively small size; it is marketed for conduits equal to or greater than 16 mm, with two possible diameters expandable to 20 or 22 mm. Successful implantation at 24 mm has also been reported.[125]

The Edwards Sapien system (Edwards Lifesciences), used extensively in the aortic position, was first reported in the pulmonic position in 2006.[126] It is appropriate for larger conduits with expandable valve diameters of 23 and 26 mm and has been reported in a phase 1 multicenter trial.[127]

Plessis et al. published outcomes of 71 patients with the Edwards Sapien valve in the pulmonic position, most of which were Sapien XT valves (available up to 29 mm), with good technical success.[128] The newest iteration is the Sapien 3, which has an outer skirt designed to minimize paravalvular leak that can theoretically provide additional

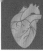

TABLE 24.6 **Recommendations for Intervention in Repaired Pulmonic Stenosis, Tetralogy of Fallot, and Right Ventricle-to-Pulmonary Artery Conduits.**

Lesion	ACC/AHA		ESC	
	Class/LOE	Recommendation	Class/LOE	Recommendation
Repaired PS	I/C-EO	PVR for symptomatic patients with at least moderate PR as a result of treated PS with dilated RV or RV dysfunction		
	IIb/C-EO	PVR may be reasonable for asymptomatic patients with at least moderate PR as a result of treated PS with dilated RV or RV dysfunction		
Repaired TOF	I/B-NR	PVR (surgical or transcatheter) for symptomatic patients with repaired TOF and at least moderate PR	I/C	PVR for symptomatic patients with repaired TOF and severe PR and/or PS (RVSP > 60 mmHg)
	IIa/B-NR	PVR (surgical or transcatheter) is reasonable for asymptomatic patients with repaired TOF for preservation of RV size and function who have at least moderate PR with at least two of the following: • RV or LV dysfunction • Severe RV dilation (RVEDV ≥ 160 ml/m², RVESV ≥ 80 ml/m²) • RVEDV/LVEDV ≥ 2 • RV systolic pressure ≥ ⅔ systemic due to RV outflow tract obstruction • Progressive reduction in objective exercise intolerance	IIa/C	PVR for asymptomatic patients with repaired TOF and severe PR and/or PS with any of the following: • decline in exercise function testing • progressive RV dilation • progressive RV dysfunction • progressive TR (at least moderate) • RVOT obstruction with RVSP > 80 mmHg • sustained atrial or ventricular arrhythmias
	IIb/C-EO	Surgical PVR may be reasonable for repaired TOF with at least moderate PR and other lesions requiring surgical intervention		
	IIb/C-EO	PVR and arrhythmia management may be considered for repaired TOF and at least moderate PR and ventricular tachyarrhythmia		
RV-PA conduits	IIa/B-NR	Surgical or transcatheter intervention is reasonable for at least moderate conduit stenosis or conduit regurgitation and reduced functional capacity or arrhythmia	I/C	Surgical or transcatheter intervention for symptomatic patients with RV-PA conduits and RVSP > 60 mmHg and/or moderate/severe conduit regurgitation
	IIb/B-NR	Surgical or transcatheter intervention may be reasonable for asymptomatic patients with severe conduit stenosis or conduit regurgitation with reduced RV systolic function or RV dilation	IIa/C	Surgical or transcatheter intervention for asymptomatic patients with RV-PA conduits and severe conduit stenosis and/or conduit regurgitation with any of the following: • decline in exercise function testing • progressive RV dilation • progressive RV dysfunction • progressive TR (at least moderate) • RVOT obstruction with RVSP > 80 mmHg • sustained atrial or ventricular arrhythmias

ACC, American College of Cardiology; *AHA*, American Heart Association; *ASD*, atrial septal defect; *DCRV*, double-chambered right ventricle; *EO*, expert opinion; *ESC*, European Society of Cardiology; *LD*, limited data; *LOE*, level of evidence; *LVEDV*, left ventricular end-diastolic volume; *NR*, nonrandomized; *PA*, pulmonary artery; *PR*, pulmonic regurgitation; *PS*, pulmonic stenosis; *PVR*, pulmonic valve replacement; *RVEDV*, right ventricular end-diastolic volume; *RVESV*, right ventricular end-systolic volume; *RVOT*, right ventricular outflow tract; *RVSP*, right ventricular systolic pressure; *TOF*, tetralogy of Fallot; *TR*, tricuspid regurgitation

Data from Stout KK, Daniels CJ, Aboulhosn JA, et al. 2018 AHA/ACC guideline for the management of adults with congenital heart disease: a report of the American College of Cardiology/American Heart Association Task Force on Clinical Practice Guidelines. J Am Coll Cardiol 2019;73:1494-1563; Baumgartner H, Bonhoeffer P, De Groot NM, et al. ESC guidelines for the management of grown-up congenital heart disease (new version 2010). Eur Heart J 2010;31:2915-2957.

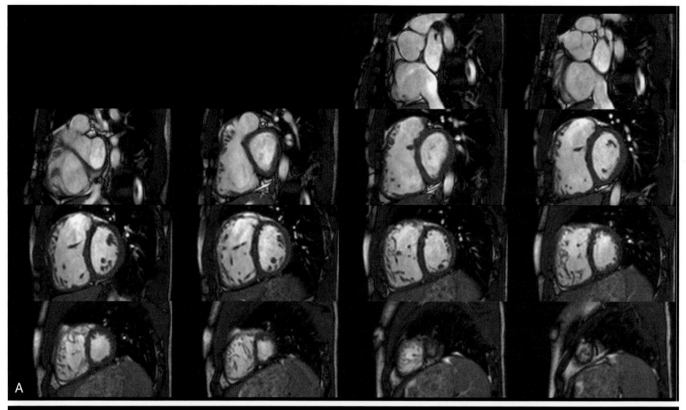

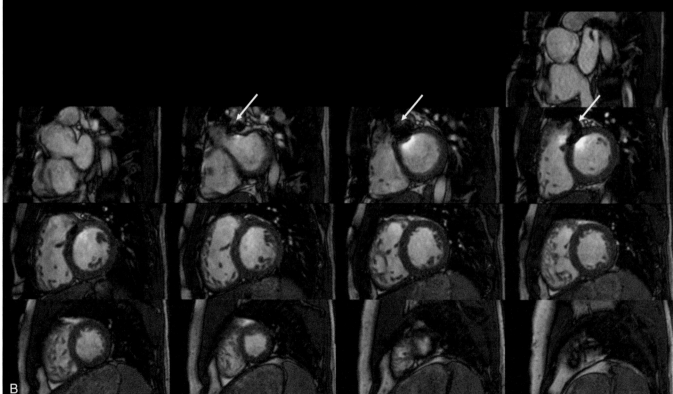

Fig. 24.14 Reverse Right Ventricular Remodeling After Pulmonic Valve Replacement. Short-axis stack of cine steady-state, free precession cardiac magnetic resonance images in repaired tetralogy of Fallot before (A; Video 24.14A ▶) and after (B; Video 24.14B ▶) pulmonic valve replacement. Diastolic septal flattening consistent with right ventricular overload is seen preoperatively. Notice the decrease in right ventricular size postoperatively. Signal artifact from the bioprosthetic pulmonic valve is seen *(arrows)*.

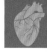

TABLE 24.7 Clinical Response to Pulmonary Valve Replacement.

Clinical Parameter	References for Studies Supporting Improvement After PVR[a]	References for Studies Supporting No Change After PVR[a]
NYHA class	90, 93, 98, 111, 112	
RV systolic function	95, 98	90, 93, 94, 111, 113
LV systolic function	94, 95, 98	90, 93, 111
Tricuspid regurgitation	9, 111	93
Peak Vo_2		90, 98, 111, 119
QRS duration	93, 95, 112	90, 111, 115

[a]Includes studies with 50 or more patients published in 2005 or later.
NYHA, New York Heart Association; PVR, pulmonary valve replacement; Vo_2, oxygen consumption.

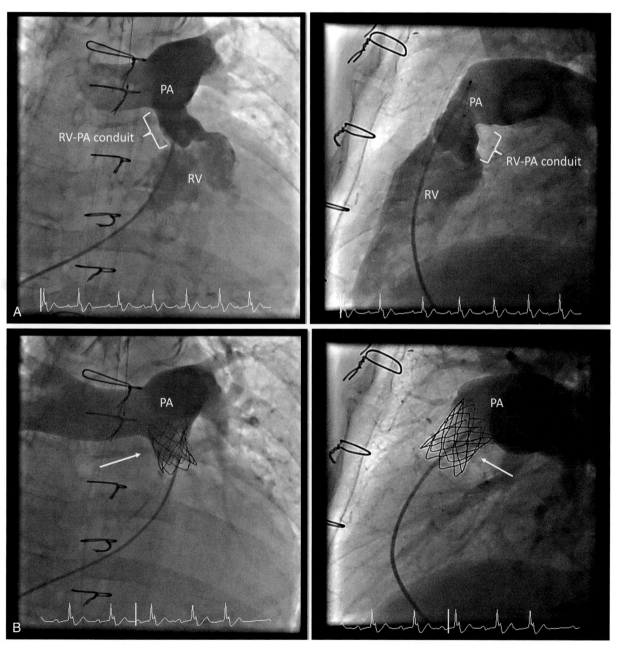

Fig. 24.15 Implantation of Melody Valve (Medtronic Inc., Minneapolis, MN) Into a Dysfunctional Right Ventricle *(RV)*–to–Pulmonary Artery *(PA)* Conduit. (A) Anteroposterior and lateral views of catheter across the right ventricle RV-PA conduit. (B) Anteroposterior and lateral views after placement of a Melody valve *(arrow)*. Notice the lack of conduit regurgitation on these diastolic still-frame images.

stability in the RVOT. FDA approved in June 2015 for the aortic position, it was first implanted in the pulmonic position in 2016.[129]

Although initially approved only for use in prior surgically placed circumferential RV-to-PA conduits, the Melody and the Edwards Sapien valve systems are being used off-label with increasing regularity in native outflow tracts with good short- to medium-term results.[130–132] Novel hybrid procedures have been described that combine transcatheter and minimally invasive surgical approaches[133,134]; however, the applicability and widespread use of such techniques have yet to be determined.

Two self-expanding valves are being tested; the target population is the majority of patients with repaired TOF who do not have a conduit or prosthetic valve. The first successful deployment of a self-expanding pulmonic valve was reported in 2010.[135] The Harmony Transcatheter Pulmonary Valve (Medtronic Inc.) was effective in an ovine model of PR.[136] Results from an early feasibility study were encouraging,[137] and an investigational device exemption (IDE) trial is planned for enrollment.

The Venus-P valve (Venus Medtech, Shanghai, China) is a novel pericardial tissue valve on a self-expanding nitinol frame with flared ends that conform to a dilated RVOT.[138] Initial experience with this native RVOT device showed short-term procedural success, but a frame fracture rate of 27% was observed on follow-up.[139–141]

The Alterra Adaptive Prestent (Edwards Lifesciences) is a native RVOT stent deployed as a landing zone for a 29-mm Sapien 3 valve to address native outflow tract dysfunction. The first human implant was reported in 2018,[142] and a clinical feasibility trial is ongoing.

Transcatheter techniques and technology are evolving rapidly, with at least 15 active trials in various stages examining transcatheter PVR (https://clinicaltrials.gov/). Table 24.8 summarizes the specifications of transcatheter pulmonic valves that are available or being investigated.

Outcomes

Supportive data on the short- and medium-term outcomes of the Melody valve and Edwards Sapien systems show good procedural success, low risk, improved CMR-defined ventricular parameters, reduction of tricuspid regurgitation, and improved exercise capacity.[123,143–146] Procedural complications are rare but have included coronary artery compression, valve embolization, conduit rupture, and PA obstruction. Stent fracture is the most common complication at follow-up; it occurred in 12.4% of cases in a pooled study of 12 observational trials but was minimized when presenting was used.[144,147] In the Melody transcatheter PVR postapproval study describing real-world outcomes, there was excellent short-term function, with freedom from transcatheter PVR dysfunction of 96.9% at 1 year.[148]

Patients undergoing transcatheter PVR anticipate a shorter recovery, lower risk, and outcomes similar to those obtained with surgical PVR. No head-to-head studies have directly compared transcatheter with surgically implanted pulmonic valves, but the reductions in PR and RV size appear to be comparable.[143,149]

TABLE 24.8 Transcatheter Pulmonic Valve Replacement Options.

Device	Manufacturer	Type	Approved Use	Off-Label Use	Expandable Diameter (mm)	Delivery System (Fr)
Melody Transcatheter Pulmonary Valve	Medtronic	Bovine jugular venous valve sutured in covered Cheatham platinum stent	RVOT conduits > 16 mm	Native RVOT, smaller conduits	20, 22	22
Edwards Sapien	Edwards	Bovine pericardial tissue valve mounted on stainless steel stent	RVOT conduits > 21 mm	Native RVOT	23, 26	22–24
Sapien XT	Edwards	Bovine pericardial tissue valve mounted on cobalt chromium alloy stent	RVOT conduits, native aortic valve, aortic valve-in-valve, mitral valve-in-valve	Native RVOT	23, 26, 29	18–19
Sapien 3	Edwards	Bovine pericardial tissue valve mounted on cobalt chromium alloy stent with polyethylene terephthalate outer skirt	Native aortic valve, RVOT conduit (investigational)	Native RVOT	20, 23, 26, 29	14–16
Harmony	Medtronic	Porcine pericardial valve mounted on self-expanding nitinol stent with hourglass contour	Native RVOT (investigational)		23.5	25
Venus-P valve	Venus Medtech	Porcine pericardium valve in covered self-expanding stent with flared ends	Native RVOT (investigational)		20–32	14–22
Alterra Adaptive Prestent	Edwards	Polyethylene fabric–covered self-expanding nitinol stent with flared ends as docking adaptor for 29-mm Sapien 3 valve	Native RVOT (investigational)		27	16

RVOT, Right ventricular outflow tract.

One issue of concern is the relatively high incidence of endocarditis after placement of Melody valves. In a single-center study of 147 patients who underwent Melody valve implantation between 2007 and 2012, 14 patients (9.5%) developed bloodstream infections after the procedure, 4 (2.7%) of whom had Melody valve endocarditis.[150] The same year, a multicenter study of 311 patients reported 16 cases (5.1%) of infective endocarditis.[151]

Multiple studies have suggested a rate of endocarditis greater than what is expected in surgical PVR; it is estimated to be as high as 10% to 15% in the medium term, compared with 1% to 2% for surgically implanted valves.[150–153] Risk factors include RVOT obstruction, incomplete stent apposition, and abrupt cessation of aspirin therapy.[153] Dental evaluation before transcatheter PVR (akin to dental clearance for surgical valves) is imperative, as are strict attention to good dental hygiene and antibiotic prophylaxis before routine cleaning.

Impact on Management of Pulmonic Valve Disease

Historically, timing for surgical referral involved balancing the goal of avoiding RV deterioration (i.e., going too late) and the need for repeat surgical interventions (i.e., going too soon). The latter is of particular relevance to a young congenital heart disease population who would otherwise look forward to decades of good health. In my institution, it is standard practice to surgically implant bioprosthetic pulmonic valves at least 27 mm in size, with the expectation that the next valve will be placed with the use of a transcatheter technique, thereby eliminating the risks and morbidity of repeat open heart surgery. Currently, the indication for transcatheter PVR is the same as that for surgical PVR.

This paradigm has been challenged by data suggesting that earlier percutaneous pulmonic valve implantation in younger patients—especially those with mixed pulmonic valve disease—resulted in incremental improvement in RV size and function and in parameters of exercise stress testing.[154] Given the safety profile, low morbidity rate, and good short- and medium-term rates of freedom from reintervention with the Melody valve,[123] waiting until patients reach surgical thresholds for PVR may not be appropriate, and some experts recommend a more aggressive strategy.[155]

The long-term data on transcatheter pulmonic valve durability are not known. Depending on the anatomy and rate of prosthetic valve dysfunction, the implication of multiple valve-in-valve procedures in a patient's lifetime may translate into need for surgical conduit revision later in life. However, there may be significant benefits to going early, with increased chances of RV preservation and avoidance of the untoward outcomes of heart failure, arrhythmia, and death.

REFERENCES

1. Waller BF, Howard J, Fess S. Pathology of pulmonic valve stenosis and pure regurgitation. Clin Cardiol 1995;18(1):45-50.
2. Borgdorff MA, Dickinson MG, Berger RM, Bartelds B. Right ventricular failure due to chronic pressure load: what have we learned in animal models since the NIH working group statement? Heart Fail Rev 2015;20(4):475-491.
3. Redington AN, Oldershaw PJ, Shinebourne EA, Rigby ML. A new technique for the assessment of pulmonary regurgitation and its application to the assessment of right ventricular function before and after repair of tetralogy of Fallot. Br Heart J 1988;60(1):57-65.
4. Reddy S, Zhao M, Hu DQ, et al. Physiologic and molecular characterization of a murine model of right ventricular volume overload. Am J Physiol Heart Circ Physiol 2013;304(10):H1314-H1327.
5. Nishimura RA, Otto CM, Bonow RO, et al. 2014 AHA/ACC guideline for the management of patients with valvular heart disease: executive summary: a report of the American College of Cardiology/American Heart Association Task Force on Practice Guidelines. J Am Coll Cardiol 2014;63(22):2438-2488.
6. Prieto LR, Latson LA. Pulmonary stenosis. In: Allen HD, Shaddy RE, Penny DJ, et al., editors. Moss and Adams' Heart disease in infants, children, and adolescents: including the fetus and young adult. Vol 2, 9th ed. Philadelphia: Lippincott Williams & Wilkins; 2016:983-1007.
7. Veldtman GR, Dearani JA, Warnes CA. Low pressure giant pulmonary artery aneurysms in the adult: natural history and management strategies. Heart 2003;89(9):1067-1070.
8. Dimond EG, Benchimol A. Phonocardiography in pulmonary stenosis: special correlation between hemodynamics and phonocardiographic findings. Ann Intern Med 1960;52:145-162.
9. Stout KK, Daniels CJ, Aboulhosn JA, et al. 2018 AHA/ACC guideline for the management of adults with congenital heart disease: a report of the American College of Cardiology/American Heart Association Task Force on Clinical Practice Guidelines. J Am Coll Cardiol 2019;73:e81-e192.
10. Lima CO, Sahn DJ, Valdes-Cruz LM, et al. Noninvasive prediction of transvalvular pressure gradient in patients with pulmonary stenosis by quantitative two-dimensional echocardiographic Doppler studies. Circulation 1983;67:866-871.
11. Frantz EG, Silverman NH. Doppler ultrasound evaluation of valvar pulmonary stenosis from multiple transducer positions in children requiring pulmonary valvuloplasty. Am J Cardiol 1988;61(10):844-849.
12. Aldousany AW, DiSessa TG, Dubois R, et al. Doppler estimation of pressure gradient in pulmonary stenosis: maximal instantaneous vs peak-to-peak, vs mean catheter gradient. Pediatr Cardiol 1989;10(3):145-149.
13. Currie PJ, Hagler DJ, Seward JB, et al. Instantaneous pressure gradient: a simultaneous Doppler and dual catheter correlative study. J Am Coll Cardiol 1986;7(4):800-806.
14. Silvilairat S, Cabalka AK, Cetta F, et al. Echocardiographic assessment of isolated pulmonary valve stenosis: which outpatient Doppler gradient has the most clinical validity? J Am Soc Echocardiogr 2005;18(11):1137-1142.
15. Silvilairat S, Cabalka AK, Cetta F, et al. Outpatient echocardiographic assessment of complex pulmonary outflow stenosis: Doppler mean gradient is superior to the maximum instantaneous gradient. J Am Soc Echocardiogr 2005;18(11):1143-1148.
16. Hayes CJ, Gersony WM, Driscoll DJ, et al. Second natural history study of congenital heart defects. Results of treatment of patients with pulmonary valvar stenosis. Circulation 1993;87(Suppl 2):I28-I37.
17. Kan JS, White Jr RI, Mitchell SE, Gardner TJ. Percutaneous balloon valvuloplasty: a new method for treating congenital pulmonary-valve stenosis. N Engl J Med 1982;307(9):540-542.
18. Chen CR, Cheng TO, Huang T, et al. Percutaneous balloon valvuloplasty for pulmonic stenosis in adolescents and adults. N Engl J Med 1996;335(1):21-25.
19. Ananthakrishna A, Balasubramonium VR, Thazhath HK, et al. Balloon pulmonary valvuloplasty in adults: immediate and long-term outcomes. J Heart Valve Dis 2014;23(4):511-515.
20. Feltes TF, Bacha E, Beekman RH III, et al. Indications for cardiac catheterization and intervention in pediatric cardiac disease: a scientific statement from the American Heart Association. Circulation 2011;123(22):2607-2652.
21. McCrindle BW. Independent predictors of long-term results after balloon pulmonary valvuloplasty. Valvuloplasty and Angioplasty of Congenital Anomalies (VACA) Registry Investigators. Circulation 1994;89(4):1751-1759.
22. Devanagondi R, Peck D, Sagi J, et al. Long-term outcomes of balloon valvuloplasty for isolated pulmonary valve stenosis. Pediatr Cardiol 2017;38:242-254.
23. Voet A, Rega F, de Bruaene AV, et al. Long-term outcome after treatment of isolated pulmonary valve stenosis. Int J Cardiol 2012;156(1):11-15.
24. Earing MG, Connolly HM, Dearani JA, et al. Long-term follow-up of patients after surgical treatment for isolated pulmonary valve stenosis. Mayo Clin Proc 2005;80(7):871-876.
25. O'Connor BK, Beekman RH, Lindauer A, Rocchini A. Intermediate-term outcome after pulmonary balloon valvuloplasty: comparison with a matched surgical control group. J Am Coll Cardiol 1992;20(1):169-173.
26. Roos-Hesselink JW, Meijboom FJ, Spitaels SE, et al. Long-term outcome after surgery for pulmonary stenosis (a longitudinal study of 22-33 years). Eur Heart J 2006;27(4):482-488.

27. Peterson C, Schilthuis JJ, Dodge-Khatami A, et al. Comparative long-term results of surgery versus balloon valvuloplasty for pulmonary valve stenosis in infants and children. Ann Thorac Surg 2003;76(4):1078-1082; discussion 1082-1083.

28. Cuypers JA, Menting ME, Opić P, et al. The unnatural history of pulmonary stenosis up to 40 years after surgical repair. Heart 2017;103:273-279.

29. Engle MA, Holswade GR, Goldberg HP, et al. Regression after open valvotomy of infundibular stenosis accompanying severe valvular pulmonic stenosis. Circulation 1958;17(5):862-873.

30. Ben-Shachar G, Cohen MH, Sivakoff MC, et al. Development of infundibular obstruction after percutaneous pulmonary balloon valvuloplasty. J Am Coll Cardiol 1985;5(3):754-756.

31. Bokma JP, Winter MM, Oosterhof T, et al. Pulmonary valve replacement after repair of pulmonary stenosis compared with tetralogy of Fallot. J Am Coll Cardiol 2016;67(9):1123-1124.

32. Babu-Narayan SV, Gatzoulis M. Tetralogy of Fallot. In: Gatzoulis M, Webb G, Daubeney PE, eds. Diagnosis and Management of Adult Congenital Heart Disease. 2nd ed. Philadelphia: Elsevier Saunders; 2011:316-327.

33. Loukas M, Housman B, Blaak C, et al. Double-chambered right ventricle: a review. Cardiovasc Pathol 2013;22(6):417-423.

34. Singh MN, McElhinney DB. Double-chambered right ventricle. In: Gatzoulis MA, Webb G, Daubeney PEF, eds. Diagnosis and Management of Adult Congenital Heart Disease. 2nd ed. Philadelphia: Elsevier Saunders; 2011:308-313.

35. Hoffman P, Wojcik AW, Rozanski J, et al. The role of echocardiography in diagnosing double chambered right ventricle in adults. Heart 2004;90(7):789-793.

36. Pongiglione G, Freedom RM, Cook D, Rowe RD. Mechanism of acquired right ventricular outflow tract obstruction in patients with ventricular septal defect: an angiocardiographic study. Am J Cardiol 1982;50(4):776-780.

37. Oliver JM, Garrido A, Gonzalez A, et al. Rapid progression of midventricular obstruction in adults with double-chambered right ventricle. J Thorac Cardiovasc Surg 2003;126(3):711-717.

38. Bashore TM. Adult congenital heart disease: right ventricular outflow tract lesions. Circulation 2007;115(14):1933-1947.

39. Kilner PJ, Geva T, Kaemmerer H, et al. Recommendations for cardiovascular magnetic resonance in adults with congenital heart disease from the respective working groups of the European Society of Cardiology. Eur Heart J 2010;31(7):794-805.

40. Kahr PC, Alonso-Gonzalez R, Kempny A, et al. Long-term natural history and postoperative outcome of double-chambered right ventricle—experience from two tertiary adult congenital heart centres and review of the literature. Int J Cardiol 2014;174(3):662-668.

41. Said SM, Burkhart HM, Dearani JA, et al. Outcomes of surgical repair of double-chambered right ventricle. Ann Thorac Surg 2012;93(1):197-200.

42. Bacha EA, Kreutzer J. Comprehensive management of branch pulmonary artery stenosis. J Interv Cardiol 2001;14(3):367-375.

43. Cuypers JA, Witsenburg M, van der Linde D, Roos-Hesselink JW. Pulmonary stenosis: update on diagnosis and therapeutic options. Heart 2013;99(5):339-347.

44. Geva T, Greil GF, Marshall AC, et al. Gadolinium-enhanced 3-dimensional magnetic resonance angiography of pulmonary blood supply in patients with complex pulmonary stenosis or atresia: comparison with x-ray angiography. Circulation 2002;106(4):473-478.

45. Bergersen L, Foerster S, Marshall AC, Meadows J, eds. Pulmonary angioplasty. In: Congenital Heart Disease: The Catheterization Manual. New York, NY: Springer US; 2009.

46. Baumgartner H, Bonhoeffer P, De Groot NM, et al. ESC guidelines for the management of grown-up congenital heart disease (new version 2010). Eur Heart J 2010;31(23):2915-2957.

47. Lock JE, Castaneda-Zuniga WR, Fuhrman BP, Bass JL. Balloon dilation angioplasty of hypoplastic and stenotic pulmonary arteries. Circulation 1983;67(5):962-967.

48. Rothman A, Perry SB, Keane JF, Lock JE. Early results and follow-up of balloon angioplasty for branch pulmonary artery stenoses. J Am Coll Cardiol 1990;15(5):1109-1117.

49. Bergersen L, Gauvreau K, Justino H, et al. Randomized trial of cutting balloon compared with high-pressure angioplasty for the treatment of resistant pulmonary artery stenosis. Circulation 2011;124(22):2388-2396.

50. Lewis MJ, Kennedy KF, Ginns J, et al. Procedural success and adverse events in pulmonary artery stenting: insights from the NCDR. J Am Coll Cardiol 2016;67(11):1327-1335.

51. Gonzalez I, Kenny D, Slyder S, Hijazi ZM. Medium and long-term outcomes after bilateral pulmonary artery stenting in children and adults with congenital heart disease. Pediatr Cardiol 2013;34(1):179-184.

52. Ing FF, Khan A, Kobayashi D, et al. Pulmonary artery stents in the recent era: immediate and intermediate follow-up. Catheter Cardiovasc Interv 2014;84(7):1123-1130.

53. Hallbergson A, Lock JE, Marshall AC. Frequency and risk of in-stent stenosis following pulmonary artery stenting. Am J Cardiol 2014;113(3):541-545.

54. McMahon CJ, El-Said HG, Grifka RG, et al. Redilation of endovascular stents in congenital heart disease: factors implicated in the development of restenosis and neointimal proliferation. J Am Coll Cardiol 2001;38(2):521-526.

55. Hoffman JI, Kaplan S. The incidence of congenital heart disease. J Am Coll Cardiol 2002;39(12):1890-1900.

56. Nies M, Brenner JI. Tetralogy of Fallot: epidemiology meets real-world management: lessons from the Baltimore-Washington Infant Study. Cardiol Young 2013;23(6):867-870.

57. Roche SL, Greenway SC, Redington AN. Tetralogy of Fallot with pulmonary stenosis, pulmonary atresia, and absent pulmonary valve. In: Allen HD, Shaddy RE, Penny DJ, et al., editors. Moss and Adams' Heart disease in infants, children, and adolescents: including the fetus and young adult. Vol 2. 9th ed. Philadelphia: Lippincott Williams & Wilkins; 2016:1029-1052.

58. Harikrishnan S, Tharakan J, Titus T, et al. Central pulmonary artery anatomy in right ventricular outflow tract obstructions. Int J Cardiol 2000;73(3):225-230.

59. Gatzoulis MA, Balaji S, Webber SA, et al. Risk factors for arrhythmia and sudden cardiac death late after repair of tetralogy of Fallot: a multicentre study. Lancet 2000;356(9234):975-981.

60. Nollert G, Fischlein T, Bouterwek S, et al. Long-term survival in patients with repair of tetralogy of Fallot: 36-year follow-up of 490 survivors of the first year after surgical repair. J Am Coll Cardiol 1997;30(5):1374-1383.

61. d'Udekem Y, Ovaert C, Grandjean F, et al. Tetralogy of Fallot: transannular and right ventricular patching equally affect late functional status. Circulation 2000;102(19 Suppl 3):III116-III122.

62. Khairy P, Aboulhosn J, Gurvitz MZ, et al. Arrhythmia burden in adults with surgically repaired tetralogy of Fallot: a multi-institutional study. Circulation 2010;122(9):868-875.

63. Redington AN. Determinants and assessment of pulmonary regurgitation in tetralogy of Fallot: practice and pitfalls. Cardiol Clin 2006;24(4):631-639, vii.

64. Sen DG, Najjar M, Yimaz B, et al. Aiming to preserve pulmonary valve function in tetralogy of Fallot repair: comparing a new approach to traditional management. Pediatr Cardiol 2016;37(5):818-825.

65. Shimazaki Y, Blackstone EH, Kirklin JW. The natural history of isolated congenital pulmonary valve incompetence: surgical implications. Thorac Cardiovasc Surg 1984;32(4):257-259.

66. Gatzoulis MA, Till JA, Somerville J, Redington AN. Mechanoelectrical interaction in tetralogy of Fallot. QRS prolongation relates to right ventricular size and predicts malignant ventricular arrhythmias and sudden death. Circulation 1995;92(2):231-237.

67. Kilner PJ, Geva T, Kaemmerer H, et al. Recommendations for cardiovascular magnetic resonance in adults with congenital heart disease from the respective working groups of the European Society of Cardiology. Eur Heart J 2010;31(7):794-805.

68. Valente AM, Cook S, Festa P, et al. Multimodality imaging guidelines for patients with repaired tetralogy of Fallot: a report from the American Society of Echocardiography: developed in collaboration with the Society for Cardiovascular Magnetic Resonance and the Society for Pediatric Radiology. J Am Soc Echocardiogr 2014;27(2):111-141.

69. Rudski LG, Lai WW, Afilalo J, et al. Guidelines for the echocardiographic assessment of the right heart in adults: a report from the American Society of Echocardiography endorsed by the European Association of Echocardiography, a registered branch of the European Society of Cardiology,

and the Canadian Society of Echocardiography. J Am Soc Echocardiogr 2010;23(7):685-713; quiz 786-788.

70. McElhinney DB, Parry AJ, Reddy VM, et al. Left pulmonary artery kinking caused by outflow tract dilatation after transannular patch repair of tetralogy of Fallot. Ann Thorac Surg 1998;65(4):1120-1126.

71. Puchalski MD, Askovich B, Sower CT, et al. Pulmonary regurgitation: determining severity by echocardiography and magnetic resonance imaging. Congenit Heart Dis 2008;3(3):168-175.

72. Renella P, Aboulhosn J, Lohan DG, et al. Two-dimensional and Doppler echocardiography reliably predict severe pulmonary regurgitation as quantified by cardiac magnetic resonance. J Am Soc Echocardiogr 2010; 23(8):880-886.

73. Williams RV, Minich LL, Shaddy RE, et al. Comparison of Doppler echocardiography with angiography for determining the severity of pulmonary regurgitation. Am J Cardiol 2002;89(12):1438-1441.

74. Srivastava S, Parness IA. Tetralogy of Fallot. In: Lai WW, Mertens L, Cohen MS, et al., eds. Echocardiography in Pediatric and Congenital Heart Disease From Fetus to Adult. Hoboken: Wiley-Blackwell; 2009: 362-384.

75. Silversides CK, Veldtman GR, Crossin J, et al. Pressure half-time predicts hemodynamically significant pulmonary regurgitation in adult patients with repaired tetralogy of Fallot. J Am Soc Echocardiogr 2003;16(10): 1057-1062.

76. Li W, Davlouros PA, Kilner PJ, et al. Doppler-echocardiographic assessment of pulmonary regurgitation in adults with repaired tetralogy of Fallot: comparison with cardiovascular magnetic resonance imaging. Am Heart J 2004;147(1):165-172.

77. Pothineni KR, Wells BJ, Hsiung MC, et al. Live/real time three-dimensional transthoracic echocardiographic assessment of pulmonary regurgitation. Echocardiography 2008;25(8):911-917.

78. Mercer-Rosa L, Yang W, Kutty S, et al. Quantifying pulmonary regurgitation and right ventricular function in surgically repaired tetralogy of Fallot: a comparative analysis of echocardiography and magnetic resonance imaging. Circ Cardiovasc Imaging 2012;5(5):637-643.

79. Festa P, Ait-Ali L, Minichilli F, et al. A new simple method to estimate pulmonary regurgitation by echocardiography in operated Fallot: comparison with magnetic resonance imaging and performance test evaluation. J Am Soc Echocardiogr 2010;23(5):496-503.

80. Wald RM, Redington AN, Pereira A, et al. Refining the assessment of pulmonary regurgitation in adults after tetralogy of Fallot repair: should we be measuring regurgitant fraction or regurgitant volume? Eur Heart J 2009;30(3):356-361.

81. Munkhammar P, Cullen S, Jogi P, et al. Early age at repair prevents restrictive right ventricular (RV) physiology after surgery for tetralogy of Fallot (TOF): diastolic RV function after TOF repair in infancy. J Am Coll Cardiol 1998;32(4):1083-1087.

82. Gatzoulis MA, Clark AL, Cullen S, et al. Right ventricular diastolic function 15 to 35 years after repair of tetralogy of Fallot. Restrictive physiology predicts superior exercise performance. Circulation 1995;91(6):1775-1781.

83. Samyn MM, Kwon EN, Gorentz JS, et al. Restrictive versus nonrestrictive physiology following repair of tetralogy of Fallot: is there a difference? J Am Soc Echocardiogr 2013;26(7):746-755.

84. Lee W, Yoo SJ, Roche SL, et al. Determinants and functional impact of restrictive physiology after repair of tetralogy of Fallot: new insights from magnetic resonance imaging. Int J Cardiol 2013;167(4):1347-1353.

85. Murphy JG, Gersh BJ, Mair DD, et al. Long-term outcome in patients undergoing surgical repair of tetralogy of Fallot. N Engl J Med 1993;329(9): 593-599.

86. Cuypers JA, Menting ME, Konings EE, et al. Unnatural history of tetralogy of Fallot: prospective follow-up of 40 years after surgical correction. Circulation 2014;130(22):1944-1953.

87. Therrien J, Siu SC, McLaughlin PR, et al. Pulmonary valve replacement in adults late after repair of tetralogy of Fallot: are we operating too late? J Am Coll Cardiol 2000;36(5):1670-1675.

88. Valente AM, Gauvreau K, Assenza GE, et al. Contemporary predictors of death and sustained ventricular tachycardia in patients with repaired tetralogy of Fallot enrolled in the INDICATOR cohort. Heart 2014;100(3): 247-253.

89. Ferraz Cavalcanti PE, Sá MP, Santos CA, et al. Pulmonary valve replacement after operative repair of tetralogy of Fallot: meta-analysis and meta-regression of 3,118 patients from 48 studies. J Am Coll Cardiol 2013;62(23):2227-2243.

90. Geva T, Gauvreau K, Powell AJ, et al. Randomized trial of pulmonary valve replacement with and without right ventricular remodeling surgery. Circulation 2010;122(Suppl 11):S201-S208.

91. Therrien J, Provost Y, Merchant N, et al. Optimal timing for pulmonary valve replacement in adults after tetralogy of Fallot repair. Am J Cardiol 2005;95(6):779-782.

92. Geva T. Indications and timing of pulmonary valve replacement after tetralogy of Fallot repair. Semin Thorac Cardiovasc Surg Pediatr Card Surg Annu 2006:11-22.

93. Oosterhof T, van Straten A, Vliegen HW, et al. Preoperative thresholds for pulmonary valve replacement in patients with corrected tetralogy of Fallot using cardiovascular magnetic resonance. Circulation 2007; 116(5):545-551.

94. Heng EL, Gatzoulis MA, Uebing A, et al. Immediate and midterm cardiac remodeling after surgical pulmonary valve replacement in adults with repaired tetralogy of Fallot: a prospective cardiovascular magnetic resonance and clinical study. Circulation 2017;136(18):1703-1713.

95. Lee C, Kim YM, Lee CH, et al. Outcomes of pulmonary valve replacement in 170 patients with chronic pulmonary regurgitation after relief of right ventricular outflow tract obstruction: implications for optimal timing of pulmonary valve replacement. J Am Coll Cardiol 2012;60(11): 1005-1014.

96. Bokma JP, Winter MM, Oosterhof T, et al. Preoperative thresholds for mid-to-late haemodynamic and clinical outcomes after pulmonary valve replacement in tetralogy of Fallot. Eur Heart J 2016;37(10):829-835.

97. Buechel ER, Dave HH, Kellenberger CJ, et al. Remodelling of the right ventricle after early pulmonary valve replacement in children with repaired tetralogy of Fallot: assessment by cardiovascular magnetic resonance. Eur Heart J 2005;26(24):2721-2727.

98. Frigiola A, Tsang V, Bull C, et al. Biventricular response after pulmonary valve replacement for right ventricular outflow tract dysfunction: is age a predictor of outcome? Circulation 2008;118(Suppl 14):S182-S190.

99. Geva T. Indications for pulmonary valve replacement in repaired tetralogy of Fallot: the quest continues. Circulation 2013;128(17):1855-1857.

100. Chaturvedi RR, Kilner PJ, White PA, et al. Increased airway pressure and simulated branch pulmonary artery stenosis increase pulmonary regurgitation after repair of tetralogy of Fallot. Real-time analysis with a conductance catheter technique. Circulation 1997;95(3):643-649.

101. Babu-Narayan SV, Diller GP, Gheta RR, et al. Clinical outcomes of surgical pulmonary valve replacement after repair of tetralogy of Fallot and potential prognostic value of preoperative cardiopulmonary exercise testing. Circulation 2014;129(1):18-27.

102. Fuller S. Tetralogy of Fallot and pulmonary valve replacement: timing and techniques in the asymptomatic patient. Semin Thorac Cardiovasc Surg Pediatr Card Surg Annu 2014;17(1):30-37.

103. Chen PC, Sager MS, Zurakowski D, et al. Younger age and valve oversizing are predictors of structural valve deterioration after pulmonary valve replacement in patients with tetralogy of Fallot. J Thorac Cardiovasc Surg 2012;143(2):352-360.

104. Nomoto R, Sleeper LA, Borisuk MJ, et al. Outcome and performance of bioprosthetic pulmonary valve replacement in patients with congenital heart disease. J Thorac Cardiovasc Surg 2016;152(5):1333-1342.e3.

105. Boethig D, Goerler H, Westhoff-Bleck M, et al. Evaluation of 188 consecutive homografts implanted in pulmonary position after 20 years. Eur J Cardiothorac Surg 2007;32(1):133-142.

106. Zubairi R, Malik S, Jaquiss RD, et al. Risk factors for prosthesis failure in pulmonary valve replacement. Ann Thorac Surg 2011;91(2):561-565.

107. Dehaki MG, Ghavidel AA, Omrani G, Javadikasgari H. Long-term outcome of mechanical pulmonary valve replacement in 121 patients with congenital heart disease. Thorac Cardiovasc Surg 2015;63(5): 367-372.

108. Stulak JM, Dearani JA, Burkhart HM, et al. The increasing use of mechanical pulmonary valve replacement over a 40-year period. Ann Thorac Surg 2010;90(6):2009-2014; discussion 2014-2015.

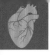
109. Freling HG, van Slooten YJ, van Melle JP, et al. Pulmonary valve replacement: twenty-six years of experience with mechanical valvar prostheses. Ann Thorac Surg 2015;99(3):905-910.

110. Dos L, Munoz-Guijosa C, Mendez AB, et al. Long term outcome of mechanical valve prosthesis in the pulmonary position. Int J Cardiol 2011;150(2):173-176.

111. Gengsakul A, Harris L, Bradley TJ, et al. The impact of pulmonary valve replacement after tetralogy of Fallot repair: a matched comparison. Eur J Cardiothorac Surg 2007;32(3):462-468.

112. Scherptong RW, Hazekamp MG, Mulder BJ, et al. Follow-up after pulmonary valve replacement in adults with tetralogy of Fallot: association between QRS duration and outcome. J Am Coll Cardiol 2010;56(18):1486-1492.

113. Graham Jr TP, Bernard Y, Arbogast P, et al. Outcome of pulmonary valve replacements in adults after tetralogy repair: a multi-institutional study. Congenit Heart Dis 2008;3(3):162-167.

114. Greutmann M. Tetralogy of Fallot, pulmonary valve replacement, and right ventricular volumes: are we chasing the right target? Eur Heart J 2016;37(10):836-839.

115. Harrild DM, Berul CI, Cecchin F, et al. Pulmonary valve replacement in tetralogy of Fallot: impact on survival and ventricular tachycardia. Circulation 2009;119(3):445-451.

116. Bokma JP, Geva T, Sleeper LA, et al. A propensity score-adjusted analysis of clinical outcomes after pulmonary valve replacement in tetralogy of Fallot. Heart 2018;104(9):738-744.

117. Therrien J, Siu SC, Harris L, et al. Impact of pulmonary valve replacement on arrhythmia propensity late after repair of tetralogy of Fallot. Circulation 2001;103(20):2489-2494.

118. Sabate Rotes A, Connolly HM, Warnes CA, et al. Ventricular arrhythmia risk stratification in patients with tetralogy of Fallot at the time of pulmonary valve replacement. Circ Arrhythm Electrophysiol 2015;8(1):110-116.

119. Lurz P, Nordmeyer J, Giardini A, et al. Early versus late functional outcome after successful percutaneous pulmonary valve implantation: are the acute effects of altered right ventricular loading all we can expect? J Am Coll Cardiol 2011;57(6):724-731.

120. Lurz P, Muthurangu V, Schuler PK, et al. Impact of reduction in right ventricular pressure and/or volume overload by percutaneous pulmonary valve implantation on biventricular response to exercise: an exercise stress real-time CMR study. Eur Heart J 2012;33(19):2434-2441.

121. Hallbergson A, Gauvreau K, Powell AJ, Geva T. Right ventricular remodeling after pulmonary valve replacement: early gains, late losses. Ann Thorac Surg 2015;99(2):660-666.

122. Bonhoeffer P, Boudjemline Y, Saliba Z, et al. Percutaneous replacement of pulmonary valve in a right-ventricle to pulmonary-artery prosthetic conduit with valve dysfunction. Lancet 2000;356(9239):1403-1405.

123. Cheatham JP, Hellenbrand WE, Zahn EM, et al. Clinical and hemodynamic outcomes up to 7 years after transcatheter pulmonary valve replacement in the US Melody valve investigational device exemption trial. Circulation 2015;131(22):1960-1970.

124. Cardoso R, Ansari M, Garcia D, et al. Prestenting for prevention of Melody valve stent fractures: a systematic review and meta-analysis. Catheter Cardiovasc Interv 2016;87(3):534-539.

125. Cheatham SL, Holzer RJ, Chisolm JL, Cheatham JP. The Medtronic Melody(R) transcatheter pulmonary valve implanted at 24-mm diameter—it works. Catheter Cardiovasc Interv 2013;82(5):816-823.

126. Garay F, Webb J, Hijazi ZM. Percutaneous replacement of pulmonary valve using the Edwards-Cribier percutaneous heart valve: first report in a human patient. Catheter Cardiovasc Interv 2006;67(5):659-662.

127. Kenny D, Hijazi ZM, Kar S, et al. Percutaneous implantation of the Edwards Sapien transcatheter heart valve for conduit failure in the pulmonary position: early phase 1 results from an international multicenter clinical trial. J Am Coll Cardiol 2011;58(21):2248-2256.

128. Plessis J, Hascoët S, Baruteau A, et al. Edwards SAPIEN transcatheter pulmonary valve implantation: results from a French registry. JACC Cardiovasc Interv 2018;11:1909-1916.

129. Rockefeller T, Shahanavaz S, Zajarias A, Balzer D. Transcatheter implantation of SAPIEN 3 valve in native right ventricular outflow tract for severe pulmonary regurgitation following tetralogy of Fallot repair. Catheter Cardiovasc Interv 2016;88(1):E28-E33.

130. Levi DS, Sinha S, Salem MM, Aboulhosn JA. Transcatheter native pulmonary valve and tricuspid valve replacement with the Sapien XT: Initial experience and development of a new delivery platform. Catheter Cardiovasc Interv 2016;88(3):434-443.

131. Cools B, Brown SC, Heying R, et al. Percutaneous pulmonary valve implantation for free pulmonary regurgitation following conduit-free surgery of the right ventricular outflow tract. Int J Cardiol 2015;186:129-135.

132. Meadows JJ, Moore PM, Berman DP, et al. Use and performance of the Melody Transcatheter Pulmonary Valve in native and postsurgical, nonconduit right ventricular outflow tracts. Circ Cardiovasc Interv 2014;7(3):374-380.

133. Phillips AB, Nevin P, Shah A, et al. Development of a novel hybrid strategy for transcatheter pulmonary valve placement in patients following transannular patch repair of tetralogy of Fallot. Catheter Cardiovasc Interv 2016;87(3):403-410.

134. Sosnowski C, Matella T, Fogg L, et al. Hybrid pulmonary artery plication followed by transcatheter pulmonary valve replacement: comparison with surgical PVR. Catheter Cardiovasc Interv 2016;88(5):804-810.

135. Schievano S, Taylor AM, Capelli C, et al. First-in-man implantation of a novel percutaneous valve: a new approach to medical device development. EuroIntervention 2010;5(6):745-750.

136. Schoonbeek RC, Takebayashi S, Aoki C, et al. Implantation of the Medtronic Harmony transcatheter pulmonary valve improves right ventricular size and function in an ovine model of postoperative chronic pulmonary insufficiency. Circ Cardiovasc Interv 2016;9(10).

137. Bergersen L, Benson LN, Gillespie MJ, et al. Harmony feasibility trial: acute and short-term outcomes with a self-expanding transcatheter pulmonary valve. JACC Cardiovasc Interv 2017;10(17):1763-1773.

138. Cao QL, Kenny D, Zhou D, et al. Early clinical experience with a novel self-expanding percutaneous stent-valve in the native right ventricular outflow tract. Catheter Cardiovasc Interv 2014;84(7):1131-1137.

139. Promphan W, Prachasilchai P, Siripornpitak S, et al. Percutaneous pulmonary valve implantation with the Venus P-valve: clinical experience and early results. Cardiol Young 2016;26(4):698-710.

140. Garay F, Pan X, Zhang YJ, et al. Early experience with the Venus P-valve for percutaneous pulmonary valve implantation in native outflow tract. Neth Heart J 2017;25(2):76-81.

141. Morgan G, Prachasilchai P, Promphan W, et al. Medium-term results of percutaneous pulmonary valve implantation using the Venus P-valve: international experience. EuroIntervention 2019;14(13):1363-1370.

142. Zahn EM, Chang JC, Armer D, Garg R. First human implant of the Alterra Adaptive Prestent(TM): a new self-expanding device designed to remodel the right ventricular outflow tract. Catheter Cardiovasc Interv 2018;91(6):1125-1129.

143. McElhinney DB, Hellenbrand WE, Zahn EM, et al. Short- and medium-term outcomes after transcatheter pulmonary valve placement in the expanded multicenter US Melody valve trial. Circulation 2010;122(5):507-516.

144. Virk SA, Liou K, Chandrakumar D, et al. Percutaneous pulmonary valve implantation: a systematic review of clinical outcomes. Int J Cardiol 2015;201:487-489.

145. Jones TK, Rome JJ, Armstrong AK, et al. Transcatheter pulmonary valve replacement reduces tricuspid regurgitation in patients with right ventricular volume/pressure overload. J Am Coll Cardiol 2016;68(14):1525-1535.

146. Hasan BS, Lunze FI, Chen MH, et al. Effects of transcatheter pulmonary valve replacement on the hemodynamic and ventricular response to exercise in patients with obstructed right ventricle-to-pulmonary artery conduits. JACC Cardiovasc Interv 2014;7(5):530-542.

147. McElhinney DB, Cheatham JP, Jones TK, et al. Stent fracture, valve dysfunction, and right ventricular outflow tract reintervention after transcatheter pulmonary valve implantation: patient-related and procedural risk factors in the US Melody Valve Trial. Circ Cardiovasc Interv 2011;4(6):602-614.

148. Armstrong AK, Balzer DT, Cabalka AK, et al. One-year follow-up of the Melody transcatheter pulmonary valve multicenter post-approval study. JACC Cardiovasc Interv 2014;7(11):1254-1262.

149. Fraisse A, Aldebert P, Malekzadeh-Milani S, et al. Melody (R) transcatheter pulmonary valve implantation: results from a French registry. Arch Cardiovasc Dis 2014;107(11):607-614.

150. Buber J, Bergersen L, Lock JE, et al. Bloodstream infections occurring in patients with percutaneously implanted bioprosthetic pulmonary valve: a single-center experience. Circ Cardiovasc Interv 2013;6(3):301-310.

151. McElhinney DB, Benson LN, Eicken A, et al. Infective endocarditis after transcatheter pulmonary valve replacement using the Melody valve: combined results of 3 prospective North American and European studies. Circ Cardiovasc Interv 2013;6(3):292-300.

152. Van Dijck I, Budts W, Cools B, et al. Infective endocarditis of a transcatheter pulmonary valve in comparison with surgical implants. Heart 2015; 101(10):788-793.

153. Patel M, Malekzadeh-Milani S, Ladouceur M, et al. Percutaneous pulmonary valve endocarditis: incidence, prevention and management. Arch Cardiovasc Dis 2014;107(11):615-624.

154. Borik S, Crean A, Horlick E, et al. Percutaneous pulmonary valve implantation: 5 years of follow-up: does age influence outcomes? Circ Cardiovasc Interv 2015;8(2):e001745.

155. Tretter JT, Friedberg MK, Wald RM, McElhinney DB. Defining and refining indications for transcatheter pulmonary valve replacement in patients with repaired tetralogy of Fallot: contributions from anatomical and functional imaging. Int J Cardiol 2016;221:916-925.

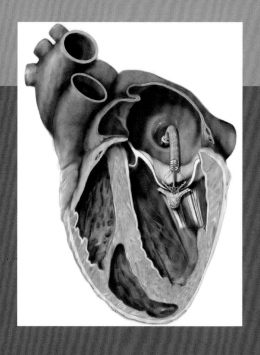

第25章
感染性心内膜炎

  感染性心内膜炎的概念目前已由心内膜的感染扩大至发生于心脏瓣膜、心内膜表面、人工瓣膜和起搏器等心脏植入式电子设备的急性或亚急性感染。尽管诊疗手段不断提升，感染性心内膜炎的院内死亡率仍高达20%。老年人群的感染性心内膜炎发病率不断上升，继发于医源性和心脏植入式电子设备的感染性心内膜炎亦不断增加。发生于左侧原生心脏瓣膜部位的感染性心内膜炎最为常见，而退行性病变是继发感染性心内膜炎最常见的瓣膜损害。金黄色葡萄球菌和链球菌是最常见的致病菌。由于缺乏临床证据支持，目前指南对在口腔科、外科和其他医学诊疗过程中使用抗生素预防感染性心内膜炎的推荐更为严格。采用Duke标准诊断感染性心内膜炎被证实具有良好的临床应用价值，而改良Duke标准对医源性感染性心内膜炎诊断更加准确。感染性心内膜炎的常见临床表现包括发热、心脏杂音、血管损害与黏膜损害等。血培养对感染性心内膜炎的诊断治疗具有重要价值，血清学检查、生物标志物和聚合酶链反应是对血培养的有效补充。经胸或经食管超声心动图是诊断感染性心内膜炎的一线影像学手段。正电子发射计算机体层显像仪对诊断人工瓣膜和心脏植入式电子设备相关的感染性心内膜炎具有较高价值。感染性心内膜炎的常见并发症包括因瓣膜反流导致的心力衰竭和脑卒中等栓塞事件。对感染性心内膜炎的治疗需要包括心脏科医师、传染病医师和心血管外科医师在内的多学科诊疗团队的决策。对患者进行最佳的抗生素应用、外科手术等治疗手段可降低患者的院内死亡率。感染性心内膜炎患者的10年死亡率仍>50%，因此感染性心内膜炎患者出院后应坚持定期随访。

孟　真

Infective Endocarditis

Andrew Wang, Thomas Michael Bashore

CHAPTER OUTLINE

KEY POINTS

- Infective endocarditis (IE) is a subacute or acute infection of a heart valve, endocardial surface, prosthetic valve or material, or cardiac implantable electronic device (CIED).

- Despite improvements in IE diagnosis and treatment, in-hospital mortality has not decreased and persists at almost 20%. Changes in the epidemiology, including older patients, more health care–associated infections, and more infections of CIEDs, reflect worsening host factors that may contribute to the persistently high mortality rate.

- *Staphylococcus aureus* and streptococcal species are the most common causative microorganisms, and clinical characteristics of IE patients are associated with these organisms.

- Recommendations for antibiotic prophylaxis for dental, surgical, or other medical procedures have been significantly restricted by the American Heart Association (AHA) and the European Society of Cardiology (ESC) due to lack of evidence that prophylaxis reduces the incidence of IE.

- Major criteria for the diagnosis of IE by modified Duke criteria are (1) multiple blood cultures positive for an organism that typically causes IE and (2) evidence of endocardial involvement, most commonly by echocardiography. Echocardiographic evidence of IE includes new valvular regurgitation, vegetations, intracardiac abscess, new prosthetic paravalvular regurgitation, prosthetic valve dehiscence, and fistula formation. Transthoracic echocardiography (TTE) has lower sensitivity than transesophageal echocardiography (TEE) for these findings; TEE is therefore an appropriate first-line diagnostic test when there is intermediate or high suspicion of IE.

- In patients with possible prosthetic or CIED endocarditis after echocardiography, ^{18}F-flurodeoxyglucose positron emission tomography/computed tomography (PET/CT) has high sensitivity for diagnosing IE and for reclassifying possible IE cases as definite or rejected.

- Multidisciplinary care of patients with IE that includes consultation with cardiologists, infectious disease specialists, and cardiac surgeons is recommended to optimize antibiotic and surgical treatment of IE and reduce in-hospital mortality rates.

- Heart failure due to severe valvular regurgitation is a complication in about one third of IE cases and is the most common indication for surgical treatment, particularly in left-sided IE. In patients with a CIED, complete device extraction is indicated in the setting of IE or occult bacteremia even without definitive evidence of device infection.

- Embolic events in IE are another common complication and are associated with large vegetations (>10 mm), *S. aureus*, and mitral valve involvement. A high percentage of embolic events in patients with IE occurs at the time of presentation or within the first week thereafter. To reduce the risk of embolic events, prompt surgical intervention for vegetations larger than 10 mm is indicated.

- About one half of patients with IE undergo cardiac surgery during the index hospitalization. Most patients with IE will develop an indication for surgery, but one in four patients with an indication will not undergo surgery due to operative risk or poor prognosis. Valve surgery may be considered in IE patients with stroke or subclinical cerebral emboli and residual vegetation without delay if intracranial hemorrhage has been excluded by imaging studies and neurologic damage is not severe.

Infective endocarditis (IE) was traditionally defined as an infection of the endocardium of the heart, specifically the valves and chordae within the cardiac chambers. This definition has been broadened to include infection on any structure within the heart including normal endothelial surfaces (e.g., myocardium, valvular structures), prosthetic heart valves (e.g., mechanical, bioprosthetic, homograft, autograft), and implanted devices (e.g., pacemakers, implantable defibrillators, ventricular assist devices).

Despite major improvements in the diagnosis and medical and surgical therapy for this disease, the high in-hospital mortality rate persists at almost 20%. This rate reflects many influences in this complex disease, including epidemiologic and microbiologic changes and challenges in diagnosis and treatment.

EPIDEMIOLOGY

The reported incidence of IE strongly depends on the study or host population. In a Swedish urban setting, Hogevik et al. found an incidence of 5.9 episodes per 100,000 person-years from 1984 to 1988.[1] During a similar period in a Philadelphia metropolitan study, the total incidence was calculated as 9.29 episodes per 100,000 person-years.[2] When patients with injection drug use (IDU) were excluded, this incidence fell to 5.02 episodes per 100,000 person-years. In urban and rural settings in France, the incidence was estimated to be 2.43 episodes per 100,000 person-years in 1991,[3] increasing to 3.1 episodes per 100,000 person-years in 1999, with a peak incidence of 14.5 episodes per 100,000 person-years among the elderly.[4]

The growing incidence among older individuals, who typically have more comorbid conditions, has been confirmed in the Medicare population in the United States, with 20.4 episodes per 100,000 person-years in 1998 (a 13.7% increase from 1986).[5] More than one half of all cases of IE in the United States and Europe are patients older than 60 years of age, and the median age of patients has increased steadily during the past 40 years.[6] Gender is also associated with the incidence of IE, with male-to-female ratios ranging from 3.2:1 to 9:1.[6,7]

Among all heart valve diseases, IE is a relatively uncommon disease process. In the Euro Heart Survey of various valvular diseases in a general population, IE was the major diagnosis in less than 1% of patients who were found to have aortic or mitral stenosis; in only 7.5% of those with aortic regurgitation; and in 3.5% of those who had mitral regurgitation.[8] Table 25.1 summarizes cardiac conditions and the associated incidences of IE per 100,000 patient-years.

Endocarditis involving left-sided native heart valves is the most common presentation, accounting for about 70% of all IE cases. Most patients do have identifiable underlying structural heart disease at the time of diagnosis of IE.[9,10] Earlier reports (before 1967) showed that rheumatic heart disease was the most common cardiac abnormality, being present in 39% of patients with IE,[11] and it typically affected young or middle-aged adults.

In the current era, degenerative valve conditions are the predominant predisposing cardiac lesions, and the prevalence of these conditions as a risk for IE increases with age.[12] Degenerative mitral valve disease (i.e., mitral valve prolapse) is the leading predisposing valve lesion, and the risk is particularly high among patients older than 50 years of age. Patients with degenerative aortic valve disease are also at risk, and this predisposing valve lesion may help account for the advancing age of patients diagnosed with IE over time.

Estimates of specific valvular lesion involvement are summarized in Table 25.2. Between 50% and 70% of children younger than 2 years of age who develop IE have no apparent underlying heart disease, whereas older children usually have a congenital heart condition.[13] Endocarditis in IDU patients also may occur when there is no apparent underlying valvular pathologic lesions.[14]

TABLE 25.1 Estimated Incidence of Endocarditis.

Group	Estimated Incidence (%) per 100,000 Patient-Years
General population	5–7
Underlying cardiac condition	
Mitral valve prolapse with no murmur	4.6
Mitral valve prolapse with mitral regurgitation	52
Ventricular septal defect	145 (risk is halved if the lesion is closed)
Aortic stenosis	271
Rheumatic heart disease	380–440
Prosthetic heart valve	308–383
Cardiac surgery for native infective endocarditis	630
Prior native endocarditis	740
Surgery for prosthetic infective endocarditis	2160

From Pallasch TJ. Antibiotic prophylaxis: problems in paradise. Dent Clin North Am 2003;47:665-679.

TABLE 25.2 Estimated Predisposing Valvular Lesions in Patients With Endocarditis.

Lesion	Endocarditis Cases (%)
Native valve disease, left-sided	70
Mitral regurgitation	21–33
Aortic regurgitation	17–30
Aortic stenosis	10–18
Congenital heart disease	4–18
Cyanotic heart disease	8
Tetralogy of Fallot	2
Ventricular septal defect	1.5
Patent ductus arteriosus	1.5
Eisenmenger syndrome	1.2
Atrial septal defect, coarctation of aorta	<1
Right-sided (including device infection)	5–10
Prosthetic valve	20

Prosthetic valve endocarditis (PVE) accounted for up to 20% of the IE patients reported in a series from the International Collaboration on Endocarditis–Prospective Cohort Study.[15] More than one half of PVE cases occur within the first year after implantation; it is estimated that 1.4% to 3.1% of all prosthetic valve patients will develop IE by 1 year and 3% to 5.7% by 5 years.[16]

PVE can develop early or late after prosthetic valve implantation. The early period is defined as IE occurring within the first 60 days after implantation, and most of the implicated organisms are considered nosocomial, especially *Staphylococcus aureus*. The late period involves organisms similar to those causing IE in native valves. Some investigators have proposed differentiating early (2 months), intermediate (2–12 months), and late (>12 months) PVE because of a more gradual change in causative organisms over time.[16] The microbiology in intermediate-term PVE suggests both nosocomial and community acquisition, and coagulase-negative staphylococci predominate.

Although there has always been a suggestion that mechanical valves are more susceptible to PVE, during the first 5 years, there seem to be similar rates of IE in mechanical and biologic prosthetic valves; most series do not suggest a difference in the risk by model, position, or type (i.e., mechanical or bioprosthetic) of valve.[17] Some patient factors have been associated with PVE, including renal dysfunction, young age, prior IE, and perioperative wound infections.[18] Health care–associated PVE is identified in 37% of all cases, and most infections (71%) occur within the first year after valve implantation.[19]

Among patients treated with transcatheter aortic valve replacement (TAVR) for aortic stenosis, the incidence of IE is approximately 1% per year, and IE manifests often in the first 6 months after TAVR.[20] Clinical factors associated with TAVR IE include younger age, male gender, diabetes mellitus, and more than moderate aortic valve regurgitation.[20] The most common organisms were enterococci and *S. aureus*. Because of advanced age and other comorbid conditions in this patient population, less than 20% of patients with TAVR endocarditis undergo cardiac surgery. These factors likely contribute to the very high in-hospital mortality rate of 36%.[20]

The increased use of cardiac implantable electronic devices (CIEDs), particularly in older patients with more comorbidities and greater health care exposure, has been associated with an increase in CIED infection.[21–23] Device infections have been associated with host factors or conditions such as older age (>65 years), heart failure, respiratory failure, diabetes mellitus, and renal dysfunction.[21] CIED IE, defined as an infection involving the electrode leads with or without involvement of a cardiac valve or endocardial surface, may not be associated with evidence of device pocket infection if the origin of infection is hematogenous seeding during transient bacteremia.

A report from the Multicenter Electrophysiologic Device Infection Cohort (MEDIC) registry covering 2009 to 2011 found that early device infections (<6 months after implantation) were typically related to pocket infections, whereas later IE resulted from other bacteremias.[24] A study from the Medicare database found that the device implantation rate rose 42% during the 1990s, whereas the rate of IE rose 124%.[25] Although permanent pacemakers and implantable cardioverter-defibrillators are available without the need for a transvenous lead, the impact of these systems on the CIED infection rate is unknown. Most cases of CIED IE are caused by *S. aureus* or coagulase-negative staphylococcal organisms.[23,26]

Health care–associated IE is defined by the following criteria: (1) onset of symptoms more than 48 hours after hospitalization with no evidence of IE at the time of hospital admission or within 6 months after hospital discharge (i.e., nosocomial IE) or (2) diagnostic or therapeutic manipulations in the ambulatory setting within 6 months before symptom onset (i.e., nosohusial IE), including long-term central venous catheter use; autologous or prosthetic arteriovenous fistula for hemodialysis; invasive intravascular techniques (i.e., cardiac catheterization, pacemaker insertion, or other intravascular devices); urologic, gynecologic, or digestive procedures; and acupuncture.[27] Health care–associated IE accounts for up to 30% of IE in cohort studies and is predominantly caused by *S. aureus* infection.[27] Among patients with *S. aureus* IE, health care–associated infection is detected in 39%.[28] Adverse host factors, including older age and more comorbid medical conditions requiring medical intervention, are obvious contributors to health care–associated IE.

The rate of IE among drug users continues to increase.[29] Older studies estimated that the overall incidence of IE among individuals with IDU to be 1.5 to 20 cases per 1000 persons per year.[30,31] It has been estimated that up to 76% of cases of IE among patients with IDU

occur on the right side, compared with only 9% of cases among nonusers.[30,31] The tricuspid valve is involved in 40% to 69% of cases, the aortic and mitral valves in 20% to 30%, and multiple valves in 5% to 10%.[32]

Nonbacterial thrombotic endocarditis (NBTE) is a rare condition characterized by valvular vegetations that do not contain bacteria. It is associated with other diseases, particularly malignancy, autoimmune conditions, and hypercoagulable conditions (e.g., anti-phospholipid antibody syndrome). NBTE is associated with a high rate of recurrent embolic events and may be considered in such cases when an infectious cause has been excluded or is considered very unlikely. Treatment of the primary condition is recommended; unlike cases of IE, anticoagulant treatment of NBTE may be beneficial to reduce embolic events. Surgery may be considered in NBTE with large vegetations, severe valvular dysfunction, or recurrent embolic events despite anticoagulant therapy.

Noncardiac predisposing clinical conditions and the organisms frequently associated with them are summarized in Table 25.3.

PATHOGENESIS

The normal heart valve is a three-layer histologic structure consisting of endothelium, spongiosa, and ventricularis. Its endothelium is in continuity with endothelium over the arterial, atrial, and ventricular walls. The endothelial lining is resistant to bacterial or fungal infection except for a few highly virulent organisms. Events that result in IE entail a complex interaction between the host and the invading microorganisms involving the vascular endothelium, host immune system, hemostatic mechanisms, cardiac anatomic characteristics, surface properties, enzyme and toxin production by the microorganisms, and peripheral events that have caused the bacteremia.[16]

Endothelial damage is the inciting event, followed by a platelet-fibrin deposition that provides the milieu for bacterial colonization. The role of endothelial damage as the inciting event is supported by the fact that the most likely areas of vegetation formation are similar to those where blood flow injury is most likely to occur: on the ventricular side of edges of the semilunar valves and the atrial side of atrioventricular valves.[33] Jet lesions from insufficient valves may also damage endothelium, and vegetations may form on such sites of injury, including the mitral chordae in aortic regurgitation, atrial wall (i.e., McCallum patch) in mitral regurgitation, and septal leaflet of the tricuspid valve in a ventricular septal defect. Fig. 25.1 shows the classic locations of endocardial and valvular lesions and the process of vegetation formation.

Interaction of damaged endothelium or microorganisms with intact endothelium results in exposure of the thrombogenic subendothelial valve collagen. As platelet and fibrin deposition occurs at the site, an NBTE lesion develops. The vegetation is an amorphous platelet and fibrin mass; for it to evolve into an infective vegetation, microorganisms must adhere. If transient bacteremia occurs and the organisms can adhere to the NBTE lesion, an infective vegetation may be formed.

A critical component in the formation of the infected vegetation is adherence of organisms to the endothelium or to the NBTE lesion. Adherence is facilitated by adhesive surface matrix molecules on the microorganism. Bacteria that commonly cause IE possess mechanisms that allow them to adhere to the endothelial surfaces of the heart. For example, *S. aureus* possesses unique surface proteins that enable it to adhere particularly well to host tissue. Ligand proteins, such as protein A on the N-terminus of the bacterial cell, function as adhesins.[34] Adhesins that bind to extracellular matrix molecules are called microbial surface components recognizing adhesive matrix molecules (MSCRAMMs).

TABLE 25.3   Epidemiologic Factors Associated With Development of Infective Endocarditis and Commonly Associated Organisms.

Epidemiologic Feature	Common Microorganisms
Injection drug use	*Staphylococcus aureus*, coagulase-negative staphylococci, β-hemolytic streptococci, fungi, aerobic gram-negative bacilli (including *Pseudomonas*), polymicrobial
Indwelling medical device	*S. aureus*, coagulase-negative staphylococci, β-hemolytic streptococci, fungi, aerobic gram-negative bacilli, *Corynebacterium* spp.
Poor dental health	Viridans group streptococci, HACEK group coccobacilli, nutritionally deficient streptococci, *Abiotrophia defectiva*, *Granulicatella* spp., *Gemella* spp.
Diabetes mellitus	*S. aureus*, β-hemolytic streptococci, *Streptococcus pneumoniae*
HIV/AIDS	*Salmonella* spp., *S. pneumoniae*, *S. aureus*
Chronic skin infections, burns	*S. aureus*, β-hemolytic streptococci, aerobic gram-negative bacilli, fungi
Genitourinary infection or manipulation, including pregnancy, abortion, delivery	*Enterococcus* spp., group B streptococci, *Listeria monocytogenes*, aerobic gram-negative bacilli, *Neisseria gonorrhoeae*
Alcoholic cirrhosis	*Bartonella* spp., *Aeromonas* spp., *Listeria* spp., *S. pneumoniae*, β-hemolytic streptococci
Gastrointestinal lesions	*Streptococcus bovis*, *Enterococcus* spp., *Clostridium septicum*
Solid organ transplant	*S. aureus*, *Aspergillus fumigatus*, *Candida* spp., *Enterococcus* spp.
Homelessness, body lice	*Bartonella* spp.
Pneumonia, meningitis	*S. pneumoniae*
Contact with containerized milk or infected farm animals	*Brucella* spp., *Pasteurella* spp., *Coxiella burnetii*, *Erysipelothrix* spp.
Dog or cat exposure	*Bartonella* spp., *Pasteurella* spp., *C. septicum*

HACEK, Haemophilus, Aggregatibacter, Cardiobacterium hominis, Eikenella corrodens, and *Kingella* spp.
Modified from Baddour LM, Wilson WR, Bayer AS, et al. Infective endocarditis: diagnosis, antimicrobial therapy, and management of complications. Circulation 2005;111:e394-e434.

When *S. aureus* is phagocytized by endothelial cells, the organism is protected against host defenses and antibiotics in the intracellular environment.[35] *S. aureus* produces a procoagulant enzyme that promotes conversion of fibrinogen to fibrin. Formation of a fibrin coat protects the organism within the vegetation and enhances its ability to propagate and invade surrounding tissue while avoiding host defenses.[32]

All of these interacting processes eventually lead to proliferation of the infecting organism in the vegetation. The cycle of adherence, organism growth, and platelet-fibrin deposition is repeated again and again as the vegetation grows and develops. Neutrophils and bacteria reside in untreated infected vegetations, and elastin and collagen become disrupted, quickly leading to valvular destruction. Extremely high concentrations of bacteria (e.g., 10^9–10^{11} bacteria per gram of tissue) may accumulate within the endocarditis vegetation. This process can become fulminant, extending into surrounding tissue and at times forming large friable vegetations that embolize. As the process continues, abscess formation may occur.

After treatment, capillaries and fibroblasts may appear in the lesion, whereas untreated lesions tend to be avascular. Necrosis, with various stages of healing, may occur along with vasculitic components in the healed lesion. Even after successful antimicrobial therapy, many sterile vegetation masses persist indefinitely.[36]

PREVENTION

Recognition of transient bacteremia as a critical factor in the cause of IE has driven IE prophylaxis recommendations. Viridans group streptococci are part of normal oral flora, and enterococci are part of the normal gastrointestinal and genitourinary tract flora. These organisms are common causes of IE, and they are generally susceptible to oral antibiotics recommended for prophylaxis.

Several principles have guided the prophylaxis recommendations by the American Heart Association (AHA)[37]:
1. Because IE is a life-threatening, morbid condition, prevention, if possible, is preferable to treatment.
2. Underlying cardiac conditions or pathology (e.g., rheumatic heart disease) predispose to IE development.
3. Transient bacteremia with organisms known to cause IE occurs commonly and predictably during dental and medical procedures involving the oral, gastrointestinal, and genitourinary tracts.
4. Antibacterial prophylaxis, which effectively reduces experimental IE occurrence in animal models, may also reduce IE in humans undergoing dental, gastrointestinal, or genitourinary procedures.

The recommendations for IE prophylaxis have evolved over half of a century, albeit based largely on expert consensus rather than stronger, randomized data. The overall trend has been a reduction in IE prophylaxis recommendations. In 1997, there was a major revision of IE prophylaxis recommendations by the AHA that significantly restricted its use.[38] The rationale cited for these reduced recommendations included the following points:
1. IE is more likely to result from random, frequent bacteremias during daily activities (e.g., chewing food, brushing teeth) than from bacteremia caused by a dental, gastrointestinal tract, or genitourinary tract procedure.
2. Antimicrobial prophylaxis therefore can prevent only a very small number of IE cases in individuals undergoing these procedures.
3. The risk of antibiotic-associated adverse events exceeds the small benefit, if any, from prophylactic antibiotic use.
4. Maintenance of good oral health and hygiene may reduce the incidence of bacteremia during daily activities to a greater extent than prophylactic antibiotics for a dental procedure.

Despite reduced recommendations for IE prophylaxis use, the AHA committee recognized that the occurrence of IE in certain

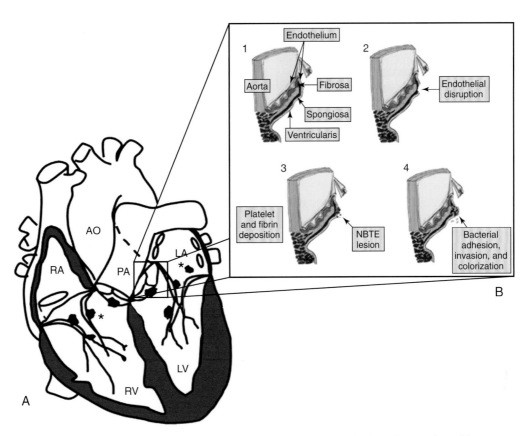

Fig. 25.1 Pathogenesis of Infective Endocarditis. (A) Sites of high-velocity jets where endocarditis vegetations occur. Notice that they are on the lower-pressure, atrial side of atrioventricular valves and on the ventricular side of semilunar valves. Jet lesions from semilunar valves can result in lesions on chordae. *Asterisk* marks areas of jet lesions (i.e., McCallum patches) on endocardium from lesions such as a ventricular septal defect (on tricuspid septal leaflet) or on the left atrium from a mitral regurgitation jet. (B) Progression of the endocarditis lesion on the aortic valve is shown. *Step 1,* The normal aortic valve leaflet. A thickened portion below the commissural line is the area where the leaflets coapt and where trauma is most likely to occur. Endothelium covers the valve and is an extension of aortic and ventricular endothelium. The fibrosa provides major support for the leaflet. The ventricularis underlies the free edge, and the spongiosa lies between the other two layers in the central portion. *Step 2,* The initial insult with endothelial injury and exposure of valve collagen. *Step 3,* Platelet and fibrin deposition with formation of the nonbacterial thrombotic endocardial lesion *(NBTE). Step 4,* Adhesion of microorganisms and then invasion into the NBTE lesion and colonization. Inflammatory cells become evident, elastin and collagen disruption occurs, and valve destruction begins. *AO,* Aorta; *PA,* pulmonary artery. (Modified from Bashore TM, Cabell C, Fowler V Jr. Update on infective endocarditis. Curr Probl Cardiol 2006;31:274-352.)

predisposing heart conditions could be associated with higher mortality and morbidity rates than native valve IE in a relatively healthy host. IE prophylaxis continues to be recommended for patients with these heart conditions before dental procedures involving manipulation of gingival tissue or the periapical region of teeth or perforation of the oral mucosa.[37] For dental procedures, the recommended regimens include amoxicillin as 2 g orally or intravenously; clindamycin as 600 mg orally or intravenously; or azithromycin as 500 mg orally or intravenously 1 hour before the procedure.

The U.K. National Institute for Health and Clinical Excellence (NICE) working group in 2008 took the final step in this evolving process and suggested restricting all prophylaxis before any procedure.[39] The NICE guidelines acknowledged that certain conditions predisposing to IE, including acquired valvular heart disease, valve replacement, structural congenital disease (i.e., surgically corrected or palliated structural conditions, fully repaired ventricular septal defect or patent ductus arteriosus, and closure devices), previous IE, and hypertrophic cardiomyopathy, may increase the risk of IE if bacteremia occurs. However, based on their review of all available data, the NICE

guidelines recommended eliminating antibiotic prophylaxis for all dental and nondental procedures.[39] They also stated that there is no preventive advantage to chlorhexidine mouthwash.

The various recommendations from these guideline committees are compared in Table 25.4.[40] The high-risk predisposing conditions for IE were confirmed in a study from Danish nationwide registries in which patients with prior IE or a prosthetic valve had a significantly increased associated risk of IE compared with matched controls.[41–43]

Based on these more restricted recommendations for IE prophylaxis, several population-based studies have evaluated the incidence of IE. An analysis of the Rochester Epidemiology Project data found that the incidence of IE due to viridans group streptococci was not increased after this change.[42,43] Other studies confirmed that no change in IE incidence was temporally related to the changes in AHA guidelines.[44,45] In contrast, in the United Kingdom, the significant decline in antibiotic prescriptions for prophylaxis was associated with a significant increase in cases of IE.[46] However, data were not available regarding the causative organisms of IE, particularly the rate of oral streptococcal infection.[46]

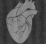

TABLE 25.4 Clinical Conditions That Pose Greatest Risk for Infective Endocarditis: Comparison of Recommendations for Endocarditis Prophylaxis Therapy After Dental Procedures.[a]

American Heart Association	British Cardiac Society
Prosthetic heart valve or prosthetic material used for valve repair	Prosthetic heart valve
Prior endocarditis	Prior endocarditis
Cyanotic heart disease	Cyanotic heart disease
Congenital heart disease	Transposition of the great vessels
• Unrepaired cyanotic heart disease (including palliative shunts and conduits)	Tetralogy of Fallot
• For 6 months after complete repair with prosthetic material or percutaneous device	Surgical systemic-to-pulmonary conduit
	Left ventricle–to–right atrium fistula
• Repaired with residual defect (jet lesion) at site or adjacent to prosthetic material	Mitral valve prolapse with regurgitation or thickened valve leaflet
Cardiac transplant valvulopathy with regurgitation	—

[a]The 2009 National Institute for Health and Care Excellence (NICE) guidelines recommend no antibiotic coverage in any situation.
Data from Wilson W, Taubert KA, Gewitz M, et al. Prevention of infective endocarditis: guidelines from the American Heart Association: a guideline from the American Heart Association Rheumatic Fever, Endocarditis, and Kawasaki Disease Committee, Council on Cardiovascular Disease in the Young, and the Council on Clinical Cardiology, Council on Cardiovascular Surgery and Anesthesia, and the Quality of Care and Outcomes Research Interdisciplinary Working Group. Circulation 2007;116(15): 1736-1754; and Richey R, Wray D, Stokes T; Guideline Development Group. Prophylaxis against infective endocarditis: summary of NICE guidance. BMJ 2008;336(7647):770-771.

DIAGNOSIS

Clinical Manifestations

The presentation of IE varies widely. The prevalence of the clinical features observed in patients with IE is summarized in Table 25.5. Many of these symptoms and signs were described by Osler in the Gulstonian lectures[47,48] but are less common now because of changes in epidemiology and improved diagnostic testing.

Fever is the most common symptom, occurring in 64% to 93% of patients with native valve IE, 85% of those with PVE, and 75% to 88% of IDU patients with IE. It is less common in elderly patients and in those with congestive heart failure, renal failure, severe debility, or previous antibiotic therapy.[49] A murmur is apparent in 80% to 85% of patients.[16] However, in acute valve regurgitation, the quality and intensity of the murmur may be less apparent than in cases of chronic valve regurgitation. This is particularly challenging in cases of acute aortic insufficiency, in which the diastolic murmur is brief due to tachycardia and marked elevation of left ventricular diastolic pressure.

A variety of peripheral cutaneous manifestations highlight the classic endocarditis examination (Fig. 25.2). However, these findings are present in only a small minority of IE cases in the current era,[50] and they lack sensitivity and specificity for the diagnosis of IE. Janeway lesions are painless, erythematous, nonraised skin lesions that often appear in crops on the hands or feet. They represent embolic events similar to splinters.

TABLE 25.5 Clinical Manifestations of Infective Endocarditis.

Symptom or Physical Finding	Incidence (%)
Fever	58–90
Weight loss	25–35
Headache	15–40
Musculoskeletal pain	15–40
Altered mentation	10–20
Murmur	80–85
Peripheral stigmata	
Petechiae	10–40
Janeway lesions	6–10
Osler nodes	7–23
Splinter hemorrhages	5–15
Clubbing	10–15
Neurologic manifestations	30–40
Roth spots	4–10
Splenomegaly or infarct	15–50

Biopsies reveal that they are microabscesses without arteritis, and organisms can often be cultured from them. In contrast, Osler nodes are painful, palpable lesions that manifest as nodules on the pads of the toes or fingertips and may persist for days. The cause of Osler nodes is unclear, but the fact that they may be seen in other settings such as systemic lupus erythematosus (and there is histologic evidence for perivasculitis on biopsy) has led many to consider them to be immunologic phenomena. Rarely, organisms have been cultured from Osler nodes, suggesting that emboli may at least be the inciting mechanism.[51]

Roth spots are retinal hemorrhages with a white center. They most likely represent septic emboli, but like Osler nodes, they have been described in other clinical settings, especially as a manifestation of systemic lupus erythematosus, anemia, diabetes, multiple myeloma, or human immunodeficiency virus (HIV) infection.[52]

Emboli can be observed in many other areas, including mouth or conjunctival petechiae, nail bed splinters, and skin, eye, or visceral organs. Splinter hemorrhages tend to occur in the proximal one half of the nail bed, whereas splinters caused by trauma occur in the distal portion.

Neurologic symptoms are common and are seen in as many as 30% to 50% of patients with IE. Symptoms appear to be more common in IDU patients and in those with staphylococcal IE.[53] Embolic stroke is the most common and most serious manifestation. Intracranial hemorrhage may occur from a ruptured arterial vessel, a ruptured mycotic aneurysm, or bleeding into a thrombotic stroke distribution.[54] Neurologic symptoms may be related to cerebritis or meningitis or to toxic or immune-mediated injury. Brain abscess is rare, but microabscesses from virulent organisms, such as S. aureus, occur with some frequency.[55] Meningitis may be a major feature in IE caused by Streptococcus pneumoniae.

Diagnostic Criteria

Although the association between infective lesions on the endocardium and the clinical manifestations of IE were well recognized historically, the clinical manifestations of the disease remained nonspecific and challenged accurate clinical diagnosis of the disease antemortem.[56] In 1977, Pelletier and Petersdorf proposed case definitions for IE that relied mainly on clinical characteristics and focused on the presence of continuous bacteremia.[57] Although these criteria provided a first step in standardization of the diagnosis of IE and were highly specific, they lacked sensitivity. In 1981, Von Reyn et al.

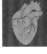

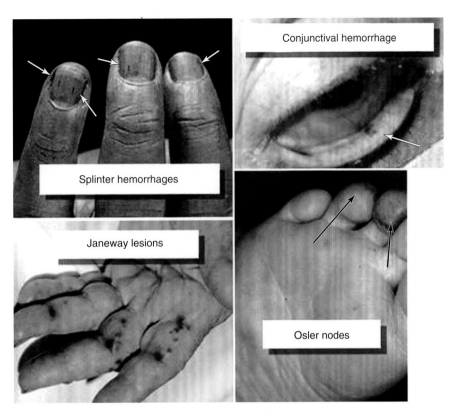

Fig. 25.2 Peripheral Manifestations of Infective Endocarditis. Cutaneous manifestations include splinter hemorrhages *(arrows)* in the nail beds, conjunctival hemorrhages *(arrow)*, Janeway lesions, and Osler nodes *(arrows)*.

expanded on these clinical criteria and offered levels of diagnostic certainty (i.e., rejected, possible, probable, and definite) for suspected IE.[58] These modifications improved sensitivity and specificity but did not incorporate evidence of endocardial involvement.

In 1994, the Duke criteria, proposed by Durack et al.,[40] incorporated visualization of endocardial involvement by echocardiography with microbiologic and clinical criteria for the first time. *Definite endocarditis* is diagnosed if there is pathologic evidence (i.e., surgical pathologic or vegetation histology or culture) or if there is clinical evidence as demonstrated by two major criteria, one major criterion plus three minor criteria, or five minor criteria. *Possible endocarditis* is defined as one major criterion plus one minor criterion or as three minor criteria. *Rejected endocarditis* is identified if there is a firm alternative diagnosis, sustained resolution of the evidence for IE after 4 or fewer days of antibiotic therapy, or no pathologic evidence for IE at surgery or autopsy after 4 or fewer days of therapy.

The major criteria focus on identifying an organism and providing evidence that there is valvular, cardiac, or device infection from that organism. Positive blood cultures play an important role. One major diagnostic criterion is met if two separate blood cultures show a typical organism, such as *S. aureus*, viridans *Streptococcus* species, *Streptococcus bovis*, HACEK group coccobacilli (*Haemophilus, Aggregatibacter, Cardiobacterium hominis, Eikenella corrodens,* and *Kingella* spp.), or enterococci in the absence of a primary focus or if blood culture results are persistently positive (i.e., two or more positive cultures from specimens collected > 12 hours apart or three positive cultures among three or four specimens drawn within a 1-hour period). The other major criterion is evidence of localized cardiac infection, such as cardiac or device vegetation or valve destruction as demonstrated by echocardiographic evidence of a vegetation, abscess, or dehiscence of a prosthetic valve; the clinical presence of a new (not changing) regurgitant valve lesion on examination also meets the criterion.

The minor criteria focus on the epiphenomena that often exist in IE but represent less specific clinical findings. They include a predisposition to IE (from a known heart condition or IDU), fever, vascular phenomena (major arterial emboli, septic pulmonary infarction, mycotic aneurysm, intracranial hemorrhage, conjunctival hemorrhage, or Janeway lesions), immunologic phenomena (glomerulonephritis, Osler nodes, Roth spots, rheumatoid factor), and other microbiologic evidence (i.e., positive blood culture results that do not meet the major criterion or serologic evidence for an active infection with an organism consistent with IE).

Several comparative studies of the Von Reyn and Duke criteria in various cohorts have established the superior sensitivity of the Duke criteria compared with earlier case definitions.[59–66] The negative predictive value of these criteria was greater than 92%, with a high sensitivity (100%) and high specificity (88%).[67,68] Later modifications of the Duke criteria (Table 25.6) have improved these operating characteristics.[69] The modified Duke criteria include *S. aureus* bacteremia as a major criterion regardless of acquisition in the community or in a health care setting, recognizing the rise in health care–associated infection in the epidemiology of IE.[69]

In addition to positive blood cultures, specific serologic criteria in the modified Duke criteria include culture-negative cases. These serologic criteria improve the sensitivity in cases in which a pathogenic organism is slow growing in routine blood cultures (e.g., *Brucella* species) or requires special blood culture media (e.g., *Bartonella* species, *Tropheryma whipplei*) or is not culturable (e.g., *Coxiella burnetii*).[71] In cases of culture-negative endocarditis, serologic testing for *C. burnetii* (Q fever) and *Bartonella* species identifies a causative organism in about one half of cases.[72]

Because possible IE was diagnosed in a high percentage of patients based on the original Duke criteria, the modified criteria were changed

TABLE 25.6 The Modified Duke Criteria.[a]

I. Major criteria

  A. Microbiologic

- Typical microorganisms isolated or identified from a pathologic specimen *or* found in positive blood cultures (all 3 or 3 of 4 drawn over 1 hour or 2 positive cultures separated by >12 hours), *or* a single positive blood culture for *Coxiella burnetii* (*or* phase I immunoglobulin G [IgG] antibody titer to *C. burnetii* >1:800).

  B. Evidence of endocardial involvement

- Positive echocardiogram results (oscillating intracardiac mass on valve or supporting structures, in the path of regurgitant jets, or on an implanted cardiac device in the absence of other anatomic cause, *or* para-annular abscess, *or* new dehiscence of a prosthetic valve) *or* new valvular regurgitation

II. Minor criteria

  A. Predisposition to infective endocarditis

- Previous infective endocarditis
- Injection drug use
- Prosthetic heart valve
- Mitral valve prolapse
- Cyanotic congenital heart disease
- Other cardiac lesions creating turbulent flow within the intracardiac chambers

  B. Fever > 38° C (100.4° F)

  C. Vascular phenomena (e.g., embolic event, mycotic aneurysm, Janeway lesion)

  D. Immunologic phenomena (e.g., glomerulonephritis, Osler nodes, Roth spots, positive rheumatoid factor)

  E. Microbiologic findings not meeting major criteria *or* serologic evidence for an active infection with a typical organism

[a]Definite infective endocarditis = 2 major criteria or 1 major criterion plus 3 minor criteria or 5 minor criteria. Possible infective endocarditis = 1 major criterion plus 1 minor criterion or 3 minor criteria.

From Li JS, Sexton DJ, Mick N et al. Proposed modifications to the Duke criteria for the diagnosis of infective endocarditis. Clin Infect Dis 2000;30:633-638.

to require a minimum of one major plus one minor criterion or three minor criteria. As a result, a proportion of possible IE cases were reclassified as rejected IE but without future evidence of IE in these patients.[69] These criteria, originally developed for use in epidemiologic and clinical research studies for case definitions, have proved useful in these settings and also for clinical care.

Blood Cultures

As a major diagnostic criterion, the identification of bacteremia is essential for the diagnosis and appropriate treatment of IE. At least three sets of blood cultures obtained from different venipuncture sites should be obtained, recording the time between first and last cultures drawn.[71] These cultures should be obtained before the initiation of empiric antibiotic therapy because prior antibiotic therapy is a known factor related to culture-negative IE. The ESC has outlined recommendations for microbiologic evaluation of suspected IE (Fig. 25.3).

Biomarkers and Polymerase Chain Reaction

A C-reactive protein (CRP) level that is elevated at baseline and normalizes with therapy is associated with good outcomes,[73] whereas a CRP level that remains persistently elevated despite therapy signals an increased incidence of cardiovascular events.[74] Procalcitonin, a marker of systemic bacterial infection, is also elevated in IE and may be an early marker of the disease.[75] Troponin T has been identified in 93% of patients with IE, and its maximal level has been correlated with a poor outcome.[76] An elevated brain natriuretic peptide (BNP) value has been associated with poor outcomes, both alone and in association with the troponin level.[77]

It has been proposed that certain biomarkers, specifically the erythrocyte sedimentation rate and CRP, should be added to the Duke criteria to improve the sensitivity. The major limitation is the nonspecific nature of these levels, particularly in patients with other medical conditions.

As discussed earlier, serologic testing is indicated. It can provide accepted diagnostic criteria for certain organisms known to cause IE, particularly in culture-negative endocarditis.

The bacterial 16S ribosomal RNA gene has both highly conserved and variable regions, and polymerase chain reaction (PCR) can detect bacteria at the genus level and provide identification.[78] Although PCR of blood samples has increased the diagnosis of causative organisms in culture-negative IE cases, most of the organisms detected were zoonotic species also detectable by serologic testing.[72] PCR has improved the sensitivity and specificity of diagnosis in excised heart valves.[78,79] However, even with the use of endocardial samples from surgery, the sensitivity (67%) is suboptimal.[80]

Transthoracic and Transesophageal Echocardiography
Indications

Transthoracic echocardiography (TTE) and transesophageal echocardiography (TEE) play significant roles in the diagnosis and management of patients with suspected IE. TTE is widely available and can rapidly provide important diagnostic information. Under ideal conditions, TTE can reliably identify structures as small as 5 mm in diameter, although TEE can depict structures as small as 1 mm. Specific subsets of patients for whom TEE should be performed, even as the primary imaging modality (without preceding TTE) for diagnosis of IE, include (1) those with prosthetic heart valves and suspected IE, (2) those with persistent staphylococcal bacteremia without known source or nosocomial staphylococcal bacteremia, and (3) those with suspected CIED infection. In these clinical situations, pretest probability is not low and visualization of suspected endocardial or device vegetation and complications may not be optimal.

For patients with suspected culture-negative IE (approximately 10% of all cases of definite IE), TEE has higher sensitivity than TTE for visualizing diagnostic findings of endocardial involvement.[81] TTE has a sensitivity of 50% to 90% for the diagnosis of native valve IE and a specificity of 90%. The sensitivity of TTE for prosthetic valve IE is significantly lower. TEE has a reported sensitivity of 90% to 100% and a specificity of 90% in native valve IE, with a slightly lower sensitivity in prosthetic valve IE.

The clinical utility of any diagnostic tool such as echocardiography is optimal in the appropriate clinical context or pretest probability of disease (2%–3%). Although there are few empiric data to quantify the pretest probability of disease, there is general consensus that certain characteristics increase the likelihood of disease (Table 25.7).

Studies suggest that imaging technologies such as echocardiography can be overused in certain clinical scenarios, such as in the evaluation of suspected IE. Kurupuu et al. showed that 53% of echocardiograms could be avoided without loss of diagnostic accuracy with the use of a simple algorithm in patients with a low pretest probability of disease. Similarly, Greaves et al. showed that the absence of five simple clinical criteria is associated with a zero probability that TTE will

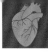

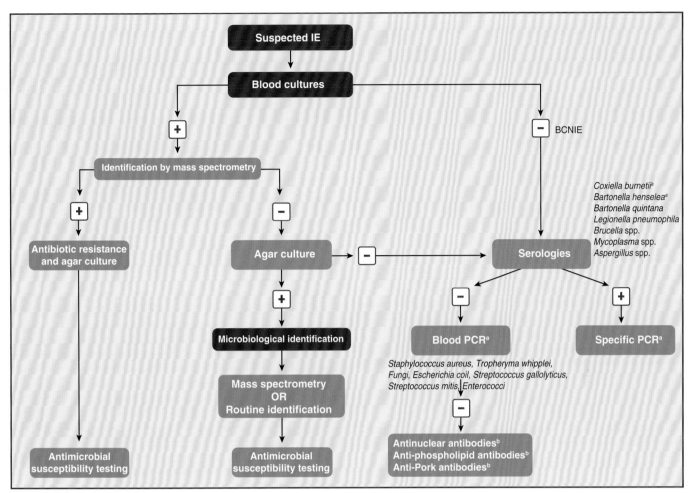

Fig. 25.3 Recommendations for the Microbiologic Evaluation of Suspected Endocarditis *(IE)*. The European Society of Cardiology outlined recommendations for microbiologic evaluation of suspected IE. *BCNIE*, Blood culture–negative infective endocarditis; *PCR*, polymerase chain reaction. *a*, PCR tests are performed in a qualified microbiological laboratory. *b*, Antinuclear, anti-phospholipid, and anti-pig antibodies are measured in an immunologic laboratory. (From Habib G, Lancellotti P, Antunes MJ, et al. 2015 ESC guidelines for the management of infective endocarditis: the Task Force for the Management of Infective Endocarditis of the European Society of Cardiology (ESC). Endorsed by European Association for Cardio-Thoracic Surgery (EACTS), the European Association of Nuclear Medicine (EANM). Eur Heart J 2015;36:3075-1128.)

demonstrate evidence of IE: (1) vasculitic/embolic phenomena, (2) central venous access, (3) recent history of IDU, (4) prosthetic heart valve, and (5) positive blood cultures.[82] Collectively, these studies showed that for patients with a very low pretest probability of disease, echocardiography may be avoided without loss of diagnostic accuracy.

Fig. 25.4 outlines the guidelines for appropriate use of TTE and TEE in the diagnosis and follow-up of patients with IE.[83] This algorithm reflects studies showing that an initial strategy of TEE imaging is the most cost-effective approach in many clinical situations. A diagnostic strategy that focused on TEE as the initial imaging modality in suspected IE was found to be more cost-effective than a staged procedure with TTE.[84] In this study, TEE was optimal for patients who had a prior probability of IE that is observed commonly in clinical practice (i.e., 4%–60%), with a modestly reduced cost compared with the use of TTE as initial study.[85]

In a similar study of catheter-associated bacteremia, three management strategies were compared: (1) empiric treatment with 4 weeks of antibiotics (i.e., long course); (2) empiric treatment with 2 weeks of antibiotic therapy (i.e., short course); and (3) TEE-guided therapy. In the TEE strategy, positive results dictated long-course therapy and

negative results dictated short-course therapy. The effectiveness of an empiric long-course strategy and that of a TEE-guided strategy were both superior to empiric short-course therapy. When costs were accounted for, the TEE-guided strategy was superior to the empiric long-course strategy, for which an estimated cost of more than $1,500,000 per quality-adjusted life-year saved was calculated.

If the initial TEE is not diagnostic but there continues to be high clinical suspicion for IE, a repeat TEE is recommended in 3 to 5 days or sooner if clinical findings change. A repeat TEE may be clinically indicated during treatment of IE if there is concern about a new intracardiac complication.[71] After completion of antibiotic treatment, repeat TTE may be helpful to establish new baseline levels of valve and cardiac function for subsequent comparisons.[71]

Echocardiographic Findings

Echocardiographic features of IE include vegetation, abscess, aneurysm, fistula, leaflet perforation, and valvular dehiscence (Table 25.8). Vegetations occur at regions of endocardial denudation and often result from preexisting valvular disease (Fig. 25.5). Disruption of the endocardial surface results in platelet adhesion and fibrin deposition,

TABLE 25.7 Pretest Probability Estimates for Infective Endocarditis According to Patient Characteristics.

Clinical Feature	Estimate of Pretest Probability
Viridans group streptococcal bacteremia	14% (95% CI: 6%–22%)
Unexplained bacteremia	5%–40%
Bacteremia and recent injection drug use	31% (95% CI: 19%–44%)
Admission with fever and recent injection drug use	13% (95% CI: 7%–19%)
Persistently positive blood cultures and predisposing heart disease	>50%
Persistently positive blood cultures and a new regurgitant murmur	>90%
Collective absence of vasculitic/embolic phenomena, central venous access, recent history of injection drug use, a prosthetic valve, and positive blood cultures	0%
Firm alternative diagnosis or resolution of endocarditis syndrome within 4 days	<2%
Gram-negative bacteremia with a clear noncardiac source of infection	<2%

CI, Confidence interval.
Data from Heidenreich PA, Masoudi FA, Maini B, et al. Echocardiography in patients with suspected endocarditis: a cost-effectiveness analysis. Am J Med 1999;107:198-208; Greaves K, Mou D, Patel A, Celermajer DS. Clinical criteria and the appropriate use of transthoracic echocardiography for the exclusion of infective endocarditis. Heart 2003;89:273-275.

to which microorganisms adhere during transient bacteremia to form an infected vegetation.

Vegetations are visualized in almost 90% of patients with definite IE.[50] On echocardiography, vegetations appear as irregularly shaped, discrete, oscillating, echogenic masses that adhere to valves, chordae, or other endocardial surfaces in the path of turbulent jets passing through regurgitant valves or septal defects. They are typically located on the low-pressure side of high-velocity jets, and in cases of regurgitation, they are located on the atrial aspect of the mitral and tricuspid valves and the ventricular aspect of the aortic and pulmonic valves. They often display the same echogenicity as midmyocardial structures and may be heterogenous with echodense or echolucent areas. Vegetations may also be found on noncardiac structures such as intracardiac devices. In the setting of a vegetation, perforation of a valve leaflet may be visualized as a defect in the body of the leaflet with evidence of flow through the defect. A valve perforation is often associated with severe valvular regurgitation.

Machine settings such as frame rate, sector arc size, gray scale, and focal zones must be optimized, and a careful examination, including nonstandard views, should be conducted to exclude the presence of vegetations. Increased gain settings and improper focal zones can make vegetations appear larger than their actual size. Color flow imaging may change pulse repetition frequency and impair visualization of the vegetation. The size of the vegetations should be measured within the resolution characteristics of the transducer so that machine settings can be duplicated for future comparative studies, if clinically indicated. Large vegetations are defined as those with a maximum diameter greater than 10 mm.

Vegetations need to be differentiated from other masses with similar appearance on echocardiography, such as Libman-Sacks (noninfective)

endocarditis, degenerative changes (e.g., ruptured chord of mitral valve), Lambl excrescences, thrombus, or tumors. Because there are no echocardiographic features that can reliably differentiate infective from noninfective endocardial lesions, the key to a proper diagnosis lies in integrating imaging data and clinical information. Visualization of distinct vegetations may be impaired by severe, underlying valvular degeneration and particularly by prominent calcification of valve leaflets.

Tissue destruction in IE may result in other structural complications that can be identified on echocardiography. Paravalvular abscesses complicated 30% to 40% of cases of IE in earlier reports,[86] but in a larger subsequent study, they were found in 14% of patients with definite IE.[50] An abscess is a result of invasive infection that typically spreads along contiguous tissue planes, particularly in the case of aortic valve infection. Development of a new atrioventricular conduction abnormality, a worsening clinical picture, persistent bacteremia or fever in the setting of aortic valve IE, injection drug use, infection with an invasive pathogen (staphylococcal), and prosthetic valves should prompt a search for an aortic root abscess.[87]

TEE is the diagnostic test of choice when an abscess is suspected clinically. An abscess is diagnosed by TEE as the visualization of a thickened area or mass with a heterogeneous echogenic or echolucent appearance within the myocardium or annular region.[86] On color Doppler imaging, flow within the area supports the diagnosis. Abscesses complicating native valve IE most commonly involve the aortic valve annulus at the junction of the aortic root and the anterior mitral valve leaflet. They may extend into the adjacent interventricular septum, the right ventricular outflow tract, the interatrial septum, and the anterior mitral valve leaflet. Location of the abscess, particularly in the posterior annulus of the mitral valve when calcification exists, may limit its visualization by echocardiography.[88]

In the International Collaboration on Endocarditis (ICE) cohort, 22% of cases of definite aortic valve IE were complicated by a periannular abscess.[87] These patients were more likely to have prosthetic valves and coagulase-negative staphylococcal infection. Surgical experience suggests an even higher prevalence of abscess formation not visualized by TEE.[88] New paravalvular regurgitation around a prosthetic valve may also suggest an abscess or infected sewing ring of the prosthesis.

An example of an annular abscess is shown in Fig. 25.6. When valvular infection is visualized, thorough echocardiographic examination is required to rule out extension into the annulus because the presence of abscess has considerable implications regarding the need for and extent of surgical treatment. Loss of structural integrity of the valve, valvular regurgitation and vegetations, and thickening of adjacent tissues help differentiate a native aortic valve abscess from fluid in the transverse pericardial sinus. These associated findings are also helpful in detecting an abscess in patients with prosthetic valves in the aortic position. Postsurgical changes, including an echolucent space between a prosthetic valve sewing ring and the aortic root with or without paravalvular regurgitation, may pose a diagnostic dilemma in a patient with a prosthetic valve and fever. Comparison with intraoperative TEE images, if available, can be very helpful in determining the chronicity of the abnormality.

In rare cases, exposure of abscesses to high intravascular pressures and progressive burrowing infection may lead to pseudoaneurysm formation (color-flow imaging demonstrates flow in echolucent space that is contiguous with the bloodstream). Because of further tissue invasion, the paravalvular cavities or pseudoaneurysms can form fistulous connections (aortoatrial or aortoventricular) and can result in leaflet perforation or even myocardial perforation.

Fistula formation complicated 1.6% of cases of native valve IE and 3.5% of cases of PVE in a cohort of 4681 cases of definite IE.[89] These lesions occurred with similar frequency in the three sinuses of Valsalva.

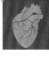

IE SUSPECTED

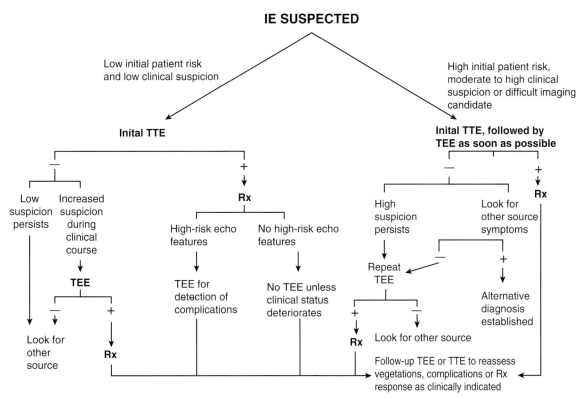

Fig. 25.4 Algorithm for the Effective Use of Transthoracic Echocardiography *(TTE)* and Transesophageal Echocardiography *(TEE)* Echocardiography. The algorithm reflects studies showing that an initial strategy of TEE imaging is the most cost-effective approach in many clinical situations. *echo,* Echocardiographic; *IE,* infective endocarditis; *Rx,* prescription. (From Baddour LM, Wilson WR, Bayer AS, et al. Infective endocarditis in adults: diagnosis, antimicrobial therapy, and management of complications: a scientific statement for healthcare professionals from the American Heart Association. Circulation 2015;132:1435-1486. ©2015 American Heart Association, Inc.)

Fistulas from the right or noncoronary sinus usually track or exit into the right ventricle, whereas fistulas from the left sinus exit to the left atrium.[90] TEE is the modality of choice to investigate these structural complications. Color-flow Doppler imaging demonstrates flow turbulence, abnormal flow in echolucent spaces, and shunting of blood flow in cases of fistulous connection between cardiac chambers. Aortocavitary communications, especially to right heart structures, create intracardiac shunts, which may result in further clinical deterioration and hemodynamic instability (Fig. 25.7).

Progressive tissue destruction due to infection can result in mitral chordal rupture in native valve IE and valve dehiscence in prosthetic valve IE. Valvular dehiscence is an uncommon, serious complication and portends a poor outcome for the patient. On echocardiography, valvular dehiscence is defined as a rocking motion of the valve with excursion of 15 degrees or more in at least one direction. An example of prosthetic valve dehiscence demonstrated by echocardiography is shown in Fig. 25.8. This structural deterioration is often accompanied by severe paravalvular regurgitation.

In addition to these complications of IE, new valvular regurgitation may represent endocardial infection and is a major diagnostic Duke criterion for IE. It is important to determine the mechanism of regurgitation and quantify its severity; severe regurgitation is poorly tolerated clinically due to acute onset without time for ventricular compensation and is an indication for surgical intervention.

In patients with prosthetic valves, a complete examination requires use of a combination of TTE and TEE approaches. The imaging of prosthetic valve infection can be challenging because the pathology

often involves the paravalvular tissue, and the usual complications such as periprosthetic leaks, dehiscence, ring abscesses, and fistula formation can be masked by acoustic shadowing and reverberation artifacts caused by the prosthetic material. TTE allows visualization of the ventricular aspect of the valve but is limited for the purpose of examining the atrial aspect because of beam attenuation and shadowing. Doppler echocardiography may be used to interrogate prosthetic valves for regurgitation using the velocity-time integral. TEE allows for much better assessment of valvular regurgitation and evaluation for vegetations on the atrial side of valve prostheses.

In patients with a CIED, there is substantial artifact generation, and TEE is superior to TTE if CIED infection is suspected.[91–93] Visualization of the lead in the proximal superior vena cava from TEE views may identify vegetations attached to CIED leads that are difficult to visualize by other modalities. During the examination, it is important to visualize the entire course of the prosthetic device throughout the vasculature and cardiac structures. Careful evaluation of the cardiac valves is also important because of the high rate of concomitant valve infection, particularly the tricuspid valve. Fig. 25.9 shows vegetations attached to pacemaker leads. In suspected CIED infection, visualization of a mass adherent to a cardiac lead by echocardiography may indicate a thrombus or an infected vegetation. Because it is impossible to distinguish between these two entities by echocardiography alone and recognizing that 5% of adherent masses were deemed thrombus in one retrospective survey,[94] careful clinical judgment must be employed for the diagnosis of CIED infection.

TABLE 25.8   Pathologic Features of Infective Endocarditis: Echocardiographic Appearance and Clinical Significance.

Echocardiographic Finding	Pathology	Echocardiographic Appearance and Measurements	Pitfalls	Clinical Significance
Vegetation	Collection of microorganisms embedded in platelets, fibrin, and other inflammatory cellular material adherent to an endothelial surface within the heart	Irregularly shaped, discrete echogenic mass / Adherent to but distinct from the cardiac surface / Oscillation of mass is supportive, not mandatory / Measure maximum size	False-negative result: / Small size; sessile, not oscillating; degenerated valve; inappropriate gain setting / False-positive result: / Postoperative changes; valve calcification; Libman-Sacks endocarditis; Lambl excrescence; thrombus; tumor	Size and location associated with embolic risk / Large size may suggest lower likelihood of cure with antibiotics alone
Abscess	A cavity with purulent exudates formed by liquefactive necrosis	Thickened area or mass within the myocardium or annular region / Appearance is nonhomogenous, with echogenic and echolucent characteristics	False-negative: / Absence of flow; early in abscess formation; gain settings; posterior mitral valve annulus when calcification is present / False-positive result: / Postoperative change after valve replacement, including paravalvular regurgitation; gain settings	May be associated with new conduction abnormality / Indication for surgery
Fistula	Abnormal connection between two distinct cardiac blood spaces through a nonanatomic channel	Left-to-right shunt visible on color Doppler imaging / Recorded loops should contain sweeps of the region of interest / Continuous-wave Doppler imaging to show high-velocity jet across defect	False-negative result: / Small defect; masking by valvular regurgitation or flow turbulence / False-positive result: / Valvular regurgitation or other turbulent flow; no confirmation by high Doppler jet velocity across defect	Heart failure due to left-to-right shunting / Indication for surgery
Leaflet perforation	Defect in body of a valve leaflet with evidence of flow through defect	Color Doppler imaging to document regurgitant flow through perforation / Multiple views to differentiate perforation from leaflet regurgitation / 3DE may help locate precise location preoperatively / Quantify regurgitation	False-negative result: / High gain setting; small defect; regurgitant jet masks flow through perforation / False-positive result: / Echo drop-out; commissure or cleft	Increases severity of regurgitation and possibility of heart failure
Prosthetic valve dehiscence	Rocking motion of prosthetic valve with excursion >15° in at least one direction	Regurgitant jets visible by color Doppler imaging / Quantify regurgitation	False-negative result: / No paravalvular regurgitation visualized / False-positive result: / Normal annulus motion during cardiac cycle	Paravalvular regurgitation may result in heart failure, hemolysis / Urgent indication for surgery
CIED infection	Mobile mass seen on intracardiac device (lead) in setting of fever, bacteremia, and/or embolic events	Vegetation seen adherent to device lead / Careful search for vegetations throughout intracardiac course of device / Evaluate for concomitant valve infection	False-negative result: / Vegetation on extracardiac region of device / False-positive result: / Thrombus	Generally treated with device extraction plus antibiotic therapy

3DE, Three-dimensional echocardiography; *CIED*, cardiac implantable electronic device.
From Otto C. The practice of clinical echocardiography. 5th ed. St Louis: Elsevier; 2016.

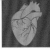

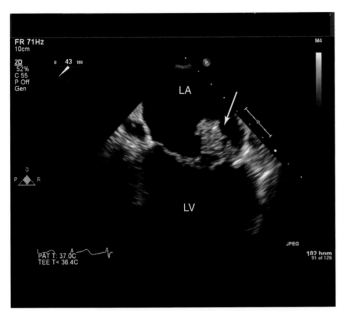

Fig. 25.5 Typical Endocarditis Vegetative Lesion on a Native Mitral Valve, as Seen on a Transesophageal Echocardiogram. The echocardiographic density of the vegetation *(arrow)* is similar to that of the myocardium. (From Bashore TM, Cabell C, Fowler V Jr. Update on infective endocarditis. Curr Probl Cardiol 2006;31:274-352.)

Other Imaging Modalities

Other imaging modalities may provide evidence in specific situations of suspected or confirmed IE. Cardiac computed tomography (CT) has excellent spatial resolution for the diagnosis and delineation of paravalvular complications such as abscess or aneurysm, with potentially

less imaging artifact in prosthetic valve IE,[95,96] but it requires radiation exposure and iodinated contrast administration. Cardiac CT has a class II recommendation for the diagnosis of paravalvular complications in endocarditis.

The combination of CT imaging and metabolic imaging by [18]-fluorodeoxyglucose positron emission tomography ([18]FDG-PET) or leukocyte scintigraphy allows detection of cardiac structural abnormalities and inflammatory activity. In the setting of suspected prosthetic valve or CIED infection, radiolabeled leukocyte scintigraphy or [18]FDG-PET/CT scanning improved the sensitivity of the modified Duke criteria by reclassifying a high percentage of possible IE cases as definite IE.[97] In a cohort of patients with suspected prosthetic or CIED endocarditis, [18]FDG-PET/CT demonstrated an overall sensitivity of 87% and a specificity of 90% and increased the sensitivity of the modified Duke criteria from 51% to 90%.[98] The ESC included these complementary imaging modalities along with echocardiography in their diagnostic criteria for IE. Fig. 25.10 provides an example of a PET/CT image in prosthetic valve IE.

MANAGEMENT

The AHA and ESC guidelines strongly recommend that IE cases be managed by a multidisciplinary team that includes cardiologists, infectious disease specialists, and cardiac surgeons. Multidisciplinary care of IE has been associated with appropriate antibiotic and surgical therapy and higher in-hospital survival rates.[99,100]

Medical Therapy
Antibiotic Therapy

A broad spectrum of microorganisms has been implicated in IE, but staphylococci and streptococci account for most cases. The International Collaboration on Endocarditis–Prospective Cohort Study identified the microbiologic agent in 1779 patients from 39 medical centers

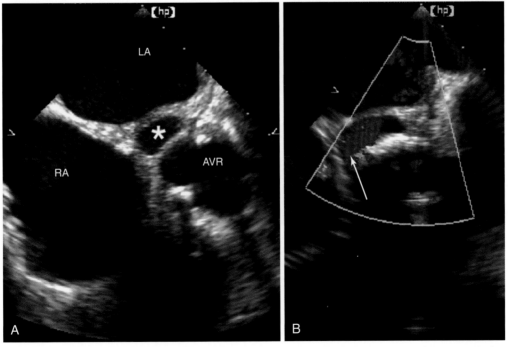

Fig. 25.6 Annular Abscess Formation in Endocarditis. (A) *Asterisk* denotes the area of the paravalvular abscess between the aortic valve replacement *(AVR)* and the left atrium *(LA)*. (B), The color-flow Doppler echocardiogram shows the flow in and out of the abscess *(arrow)*. *RA,* Right atrium. (From Bashore TM, Cabell C, Fowler V Jr. Update on infective endocarditis. Curr Probl Cardiol 2006;31:274-352.)

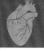

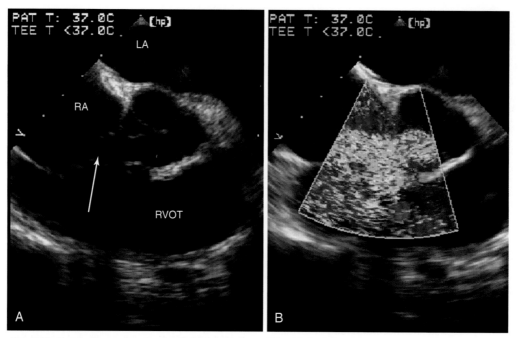

Fig. 25.7 Fistula Formation During Infective Endocarditis. (A) An infected sinus of Valsalva aneurysm *(arrow)* ruptured into the right ventricular outflow tract *(RVOT)* and right atrium *(RA)*. (B) Color-flow Doppler imaging shows a pattern of high-velocity flow from the high-pressure aorta into the lower-pressure RA and RV. *LA*, Left atrium. (From Bashore TM, Cabell C, Fowler V Jr. Update on infective endocarditis. Curr Probl Cardiol 2006;31:274-352.)

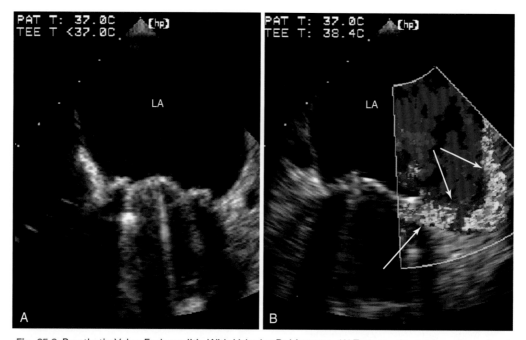

Fig. 25.8 Prosthetic Valve Endocarditis With Valvular Dehiscence. (A) Transesophageal two-dimensional echocardiogram of a St. Jude mitral valve. (B) Color-flow Doppler echocardiogram shows severe paravalvular mitral regurgitation *(arrows)* into the left atrium *(LA)* due to dehiscence of the mitral valve replacement. (From Bashore TM, Cabell C, Fowler V Jr. Update on infective endocarditis. Curr Probl Cardiol 2006;31:274-352.)

in 16 countries with definite IE and found that staphylococci were the etiologic agents in 42% and streptococci in 40%.[50] Table 25.3 outlines the prevalence of the various microorganisms involved in different clinical scenarios.

Based on the suspected pathogen and the severity of the presentation, empiric antibiotic therapy may be initiated while blood culture and other diagnostic testing results are pending. The recommended empiric antibiotic treatment is summarized in Table 25.9. In general, empiric antibiotic therapy should be guided by the type of IE (native or prosthetic valve) and risk factors for resistant or less common organisms. If the patient with suspected IE is clinically stable, antibiotic therapy may be withheld pending the results of blood cultures, which

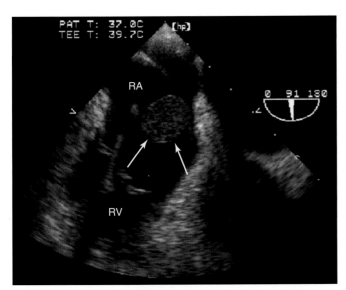

Fig. 25.9 Endocarditis on a Pacemaker or Defibrillator Lead. Ball-like, *Staphylococcus aureus* vegetation *(arrows)* on a pacemaker lead (vertical echoes seen in the right atrium *[RA]*). Horizontal echoes between the RA and right ventricle *(RV)* represent the tricuspid valve. (From Bashore TM, Cabell C, Fowler V Jr. Update on infective endocarditis. Curr Probl Cardiol 2006;31:274-352.)

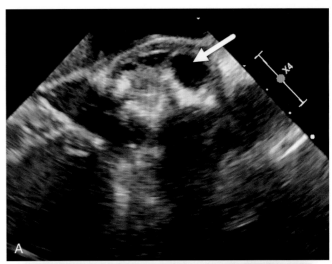

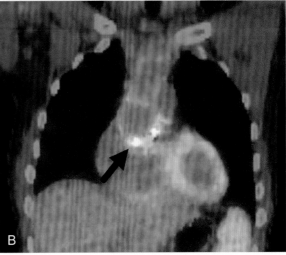

Fig. 25.10 Aortic Annular Abscess. (A) TEE short-axis view of a bio-prosthetic aortic valve replacement with paravalvular echolucent areas *(arrow)*. (B) A [18]-Fluorodeoxyglucose positron emission tomography/computed tomographic (PET/CT) image shows increased uptake surrounding prosthetic aortic valve *(arrow)*, consistent with paravalvular abscess.

may identify the organism and its antibiotic susceptibilities within a few days. If empiric antibiotic therapy is initiated but the diagnosis of IE remains uncertain, antibiotic therapy may be discontinued and repeat blood cultures performed if the patient remains stable.[101]

Prolonged, parenteral, bactericidal antibiotic therapy is considered to be needed to cure infection in IE. This dogma is based on the unique features of an infected vegetation, including focal infection with high bacterial density, slow rate of bacterial growth in biofilms, and low microorganism metabolic activity.[102] The inoculum effect is described as reduced antibiotic activity against highly dense bacterial populations. In the setting of dense bacterial populations, the organisms may be tolerant of the bactericidal effect of antibiotics. High inocula may also have antibiotic-resistant subpopulations that can arise in the setting of antibiotic treatment.[71] Antibiotic therapy should therefore focus on bactericidal agents with prolonged therapy to ensure complete eradication of bacteria within vegetations. Duration of parenteral therapy is 4 weeks for native valve, left-sided IE and 6 weeks for prosthetic valve IE.

Antibiotic regimens specific to the infecting bacteria have been recommended by the AHA and ESC guidelines.[71,103] Consultation with an infectious disease specialist should be obtained in cases of IE to define an optimal treatment regimen. Some broader principles include the following:

1. Aminoglycosides are no longer recommended for staphylococcal native valve endocarditis because of questionable benefit and the potential for renal toxicity. However, aminoglycosides continue to be recommended for IE caused by viridans group streptococci or enterococci and for staphylococcal prosthetic valve IE.

2. Rifampin is not recommended for the treatment of staphylococcal native valve IE but remains part of the treatment regimen for staphylococcal PVE.

3. Daptomycin, approved for the treatment of *S. aureus* bacteremia and right-sided IE, is recommended as an alternative to vancomycin in patients with native valve, methicillin-sensitive or methicillin-resistant *S. aureus* endocarditis.

Shorter courses of parenteral antibiotic treatment have been safe and effective in a few specific clinical situations. In patients with highly penicillin-susceptible viridans group streptococcal IE, a 2-week regimen that includes gentamicin may be considered for patients with uncomplicated IE, rapid response to treatment, and no underlying renal disease.[71] In patients with native valve IE who undergo valve replacement surgery, if the valve culture is negative, an additional 2 weeks of intravenous antibiotic therapy may be considered (in addition to the antibiotic treatment duration before valve replacement).[71]

In a Danish multicenter randomized clinical trial with strict inclusion and monitoring criteria, patients with left-sided IE and stable clinical status were randomized to oral or continued intravenous antibiotic treatment after at least 10 days of initial parenteral antibiotic therapy (median time to randomization was 17 days in both groups). For the primary composite end point of all-cause mortality, unplanned cardiac surgery, embolic events, or relapse of bacteremia, changing to an oral antibiotic regimen was noninferior to continuing intravenous treatment.[104]

TABLE 25.9 Empiric Antibiotic Therapy for Infectious Endocarditis.

Antimicrobial	Dose/Route	Comment
1. NVE: Indolent Presentation		
Amoxicillin[a] *and*	2 g q4h IV	If patient is stable, ideally await blood cultures. Better activity against enterococci and many HACEK microorganisms compared with benzylpenicillin Use regimen 2 if genuine penicillin allergy
(optional) gentamicin[a]	1 mg/kg ABW	The role of gentamicin is controversial before culture results are available.
2. NVE: Severe Sepsis (No Risk Factors for Enterobacteriaceae, *Pseudomonas*)		
Vancomycin[a] *and*	Dosed according to local guidelines	In severe sepsis, staphylococci (including methicillin-resistant staphylococci) need to be covered. If allergic to vancomycin, replace with daptomycin 6 mg/kg q24h IV.
gentamicin[a]	1 mg/kg IBW q12h IV	If there are concerns about nephrotoxicity or acute kidney injury, use ciprofloxacin in place of gentamicin.[a]
3. NVE: Severe Sepsis and Risk Factors for Multiresistant Enterobacteriaceae, *Pseudomonas*		
Vancomycin[a] *and*	Dosed according to local guidelines, IV	Provides cover against staphylococci (including methicillin-resistant staphylococci), streptococci, enterococci, HACEK, Enterobacteriaceae and *P. aeruginosa*.
Meropenem[a]	2 g q8h IV	
4. PVE: Pending Blood Cultures or With Negative Blood Cultures		
Vancomycin[a] *and*	1 g q12h IV	
gentamicin[a] *and*	1 mg/kg q12h IV	
rifampicin[a]	300–600 mg q12h PO/IV	Use lower dose of rifampicin in severe renal impairment.

[a]Doses require adjustment according to renal function.
ABW, Actual body weight; *HACEK*, *Haemophilus, Aggregatibacter, Cardiobacterium hominis, Eikenella corrodens*, and *Kingella* spp.; *IBW*, ideal body weight; *IV*, intravenous; *NVE*, native valve endocarditis; *PVE*, prosthetic valve endocarditis; *PO*, orally; *q4h*, every 4 h; *q8h*, every 8 h; *q12h*, every 12 h.
From Gould FK, Denning DW, Elliott TS, et al. Guidelines for the diagnosis and antibiotic treatment of endocarditis in adults: a report of the Working Party of the British Society for Antimicrobial Chemotherapy. J Antimicrob Chemother 2012;67:269-289.

Anticoagulant and Antiplatelet Therapies

For patients on chronic anticoagulation, there is appropriate concern that continued anticoagulation may promote conversion of brain embolic events to hemorrhagic strokes. For patients with mechanical heart valve replacements, this concern is balanced by the concern for thromboembolism due to prosthetic valve thrombosis. Some experts have recommended discontinuation of all forms of anticoagulation in patients with IE, regardless of type of valve prosthesis. AHA recommendations include discontinuation of anticoagulation for at least 2 weeks in patients with mechanical valve IE who have experienced a central nervous system embolic event.[71]

Continuation of long-term aspirin therapy at the time of development of IE may be considered if no bleeding complications have occurred. However, initiation of aspirin specifically for reducing IE-related complications is not recommended because a randomized trial of aspirin (325 mg/day) showed no benefits on vegetation resolution or embolic events but a trend toward more bleeding events.[105]

Complications

IE may be associated with a number of serious complications, which are outlined in Table 25.10.

Valve Regurgitation and Heart Failure

The most common complication and indication for surgical treatment in IE is heart failure. Heart failure in IE is usually the result of acute, left-sided valvular regurgitation rather than ventricular dysfunction. In acute valvular regurgitation, the lack of adaptive left ventricular

TABLE 25.10 Estimated Incidence of Complications From Infective Endocarditis in the Modern Era.

Complication	Incidence (%)
Death	12–45 (24% average)
Congestive heart failure (aortic regurgitation > mitral regurgitation > tricuspid regurgitation)	50–60
Embolization (mitral > aortic valve)	20–25
Stroke	15
Other major emboli	
Limb	2–3
Mesenteric	2
Splenic	2–3
Glomerulonephritis	15–25
Annular abscess	10–15
Mycotic aneurysm	10–15
Conduction system involvement	5–10
Central nervous system abscess	3–4
Other less common complications (pericarditis, myocarditis, myocardial infarction, intracardiac fistula, metastatic abscess)	1–2

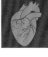

hypertrophy to accommodate the increase in left ventricular volume without marked increase in diastolic filling pressures leads to heart failure, including pulmonary edema and reduced cardiac output. In severe cases, hemodynamic deterioration and cardiogenic shock may ensue. The ability of the heart to compensate for the acute valvular regurgitation depends on several factors: the severity of the regurgitation, which valve is involved, the rapidity of valvular dysfunction, and the size and function of the chamber receiving the regurgitant volume.

Heart failure is a complication in about one third of IE cases.[106] Although heart failure was reported in the 1970s to be more common in aortic valve IE than when other valves were involved,[107] a more recent registry showed that new aortic and new mitral regurgitation occurred with similar frequencies.[106] In this large, multinational study of IE, other variables associated with heart failure included older age, health care–associated infection, and paravalvular complications. Among patients who developed heart failure in IE, two thirds had severe symptoms (New York Heart Association class III–IV).[106]

Heart failure in IE is an urgent indication for surgery because of the lack of ventricular adaptation and potential for worsening regurgitation. Severe heart failure in IE is independently associated with higher in-hospital and 1-year mortality rates, but surgery during the index hospitalization is associated with lower mortality rates at both time points.[106] In a large, observational, multinational registry of IE, the mortality rate was 29% at 1 year for patients who underwent surgery during their index hospitalization for heart failure in IE; in contrast, the rate was 58% for patients who did not undergo surgery.

In general, surgery for heart failure symptoms should not be delayed for stabilization. If there is a delay before surgical intervention, short-acting, intravenous vasodilatory agents may be considered, but their use and effect may be limited by hypotension. In patients with acute, severe mitral valve regurgitation, intraaortic balloon pump counterpulsation may offer hemodynamic support.

Embolic Events

The second most common complication of endocarditis is embolization. Stroke is the most frequently observed major clinical consequence of embolization. Cerebral infarction due to emboli or mycotic aneurysm is the presenting sign of IE for up to 14% of patients.[108,109] Magnetic resonance imaging (MRI) is useful in detecting stroke and for distinguishing an ischemic infarct from a hemorrhagic stroke (Fig. 25.11).

The rate of embolic events declines rapidly after the initiation of effective antibiotics, dropping from 13 events per 1000 patient-days in the first week to fewer than 1.2 events per 1000 patient-days after 2 weeks of therapy.[110,111] Pulmonary emboli, usually septic in nature, occur in 66% to 75% of IDU patients who have tricuspid valve endocarditis.[14] Emboli may involve virtually any systemic organ, including the liver, spleen, kidney, and abdominal mesenteric vessels. Renal emboli can cause hematuria and flank pain. Splenic infarction may lead to abscess development and cause prolonged fevers, left upper quadrant abdominal pain, or left shoulder pain from diaphragmatic irritation. Coronary emboli can result in myocardial infarction. Distal emboli can produce peripheral metastatic abscesses, especially of the spine or other bony structures. Muscular and joint pains are not uncommon in IE, but severe osteoarticular pain may indicate a septic embolus to bone.[112]

Vegetation size greater than 10 mm and increased mobility of the vegetation have been shown in several series to predict embolic events.[113,114] In a meta-analysis, in addition to vegetation size, other major predictors of embolic events included intravenous drug use, *S. aureus* infection, and mitral valve vegetation.[115] Embolic events in IE have been found to be a strong, independent predictor of in-hospital death.[116] In one multicenter prospective study of 384 patients with definite IE, vegetation length greater than 15 mm was independently

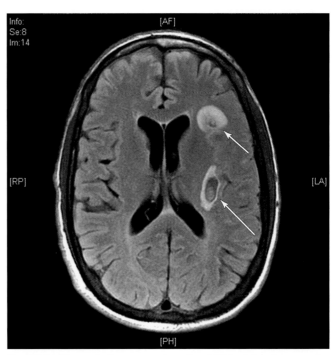

Fig. 25.11 Magnetic Resonance Imaging (MRI) of Cerebrovascular Hemorrhage in Endocarditis. Brain MRI shows an intracranial hemorrhage *(arrows)* from a ruptured mycotic aneurysm.

associated with death by 1 year.[117] In an observational study of 132 patients with left-sided IE, approximately 40% of whom had a vegetation length of 15 mm or greater, early surgery (i.e., within 7 days of diagnosis) was associated with a significantly lower risk of embolic events compared with conventional treatment in which surgery was deferred until complications occurred (Fig. 25.12).[83]

The reduction in embolic events with early surgical treatment in left-sided IE was confirmed in a small, randomized trial of early surgery versus conventional treatment. Patients with large (>10 mm), left-sided vegetations who underwent surgery within 48 hours of randomization had no embolic events at 6 weeks, compared with 21% of the conventionally treated patients. There was no difference in in-hospital or 6-month mortality rate between the treatment groups.[118] Current American Heart Association (AHA)/American College of Cardiology (ACC) guidelines recognize that surgery for native valve IE may be considered in patients who have mobile vegetations larger 10 mm with or without emboli (class IIb recommendation, level of evidence [LOE] B).[119]

Although vegetation characteristics are clearly important in risk stratification, basing clinical decisions regarding surgery solely on this parameter is problematic because of the considerable interobserver variability on echocardiographic features of vegetations. In a study by Heinle et al., complete observer agreement was achieved on vegetation size in only 73% of cases, mobility in 57%, shape in 37%, and attachment in 40%.[120] These data emphasize the need for careful standardization of examinations. The risk of embolism has been found to decrease rapidly during the first week of antibiotic therapy (Fig. 25.13),[121] a beneficial effect of medical therapy that should be considered when surgery is contemplated for the prevention of IE-related embolic events.

After an embolic event has occurred, the residual vegetation poses a risk for recurrent embolism. However, routine surveillance for embolism in IE has demonstrated that approximately 50% of cases are associated with embolic events (typically to brain, spleen, kidney, or lungs) and that most of these events are clinically silent or asymptomatic. In this situation, the decision of whether to proceed with cardiac surgery is

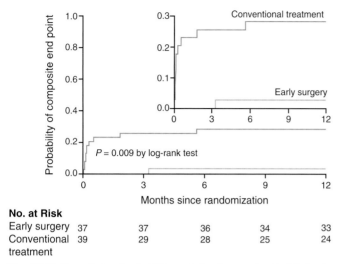

No. at Risk

Early surgery	37	37	36	34	33
Conventional treatment	39	29	28	25	24

Fig. 25.12 Cumulative Probabilities of the Composite End Point in the Randomized Early Surgery Versus Conventional Therapy in Infective Endocarditis (EASE) Trial. Although there was no difference in the mortality rate, the rate of the composite end point of death from any cause, embolic events, recurrence of infective endocarditis, or repeat hospitalization due to the development of congestive heart failure was 3% in the early-surgery group versus 28% in the conventional-treatment group and driven mostly by the reduction in embolic events. (From Kang DH, Kim YJ, Kim SH, et al. Early surgery versus conventional treatment for infective endocarditis. N Engl J Med 2012;366:2466-2473.)

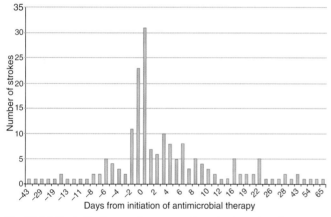

Fig. 25.13 Embolic Events. Frequency of stroke from day of presentation for infective endocarditis (IE), demonstrates a declining number of embolic events during within the first week of antibiotic therapy. (From Dickerman SA, Abrutyn E, Barsic B, et al. The relationship between the initiation of antimicrobial therapy and the incidence of stroke in infective endocarditis: an analysis from the ICE Prospective Cohort Study (ICE-PCS). Am Heart J 2007;154:1086-1094.)

challenged by the subclinical nature of the events and the decreasing risk of embolic events with antibiotic therapy. Conversely, asymptomatic brain infarcts have been associated with a poorer prognosis for IE patents and generally do not increase the risk of cardiac surgery in the absence of cerebral hemorrhage, abscess, or major neurologic impairment.[122]

Neurologic Complications

Neurologic sequelae occur in up to 40% of patients with IE, with most of the events related to septic emboli causing ischemic stroke.[122-124] An even higher percentage of IE patients have radiographic evidence of perfusion abnormalities (especially on MRI with diffusion weighting).[122]

Most of these brain embolic events are not associated with clinical symptoms or signs, but they may still be prognostically important.[124] The most commonly affected brain regions are the middle cerebral artery territory (40%), frontoparietal region (20%), multifocal areas (11%), and thalamus (5%).[125]

In one study, patients who had a stroke in the middle cerebral artery territory had less complete neurologic recovery than those with other infarct areas. In addition to ischemic stroke, IE patients may have other neurologic complications, including intracerebral hemorrhage, subarachnoid hemorrhage, meningoencephalitis, intracerebral abscess, mycotic aneurysm, and enceophalopathy.[126] The relative prevalences of these neurologic complications in IE are shown in Table 25.11.

Mycotic aneurysms result from septic embolization to an arterial intraluminal space or to the vasa vasorum of the cerebral vessels; they most commonly develop at branch-point vessels in the middle cerebral artery territories in the setting of streptococcal IE[71] (Fig. 25.14). They

TABLE 25.11 Neurologic Sequelae of Infective Endocarditis and Estimated Proportions.

Neurologic Complication	Estimated Proportion (%)
Ischemic stroke	70
Intracerebral hemorrhage	10
Subarachnoid hemorrhage	5
Meningoencephalitis	5
Intracerebral abscess	5
Mycotic aneurysm	5
Encephalopathy	—

Modified from Yanagawa B, Pettersson GB, Habib G, et al. Surgical management of infective endocarditis complicated by embolic stroke: practical recommendations for clinicians. Circulation 2016;134:1280-1292.

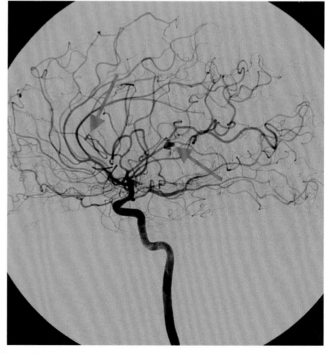

Fig. 25.14 Angiography of a Mycotic Aneurysm. This is same patient as in Fig. 25.11. The cerebral angiogram demonstrates mycotic aneurysms *(arrows)*.

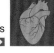

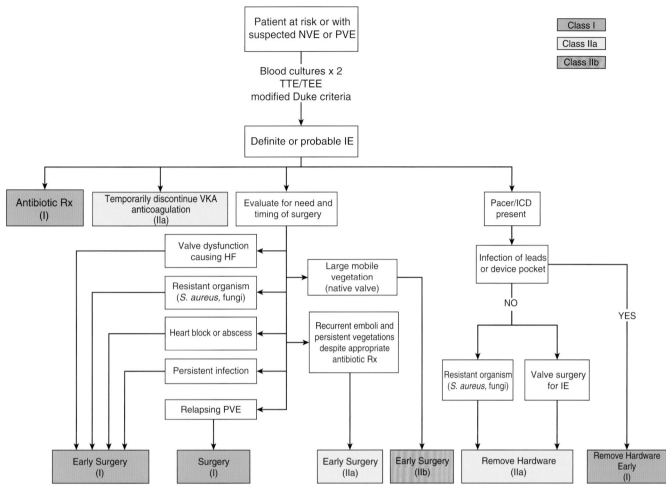

Fig. 25.15 Recommendations for Surgical Treatment of Infective Endocarditis *(IE)*. IE complications that cannot be effectively treated or cured with antibiotic therapy alone are indications for surgery include abscess, recurrent embolic events with residual vegetation, resistant organism, and persistent bacteremia. *HF*, Heart failure; *ICD*, implantable cardioverter-defibrillator; *NVE*, native valve endocarditis; *PVE*, prosthetic valve endocarditis; *Rx*, prescription; *S. aureus*, *Staphylococcus aureus* bacteria; *VKA*, vitamin K antagonist. (From Nishimura RA, Otto CM, Bonow RO, et al. 2014 AHA/ACC guideline for the management of patients with valvular heart disease: executive summary: a report of the American College of Cardiology/American Heart Association Task Force on Practice Guidelines. Circulation 2014;129:2440-2492.)

are infrequent (2%–4% of cases) but very dangerous IE complications with an overall mortality rate greater than 50%.

Brain imaging, including possible CT angiography or magnetic resonance angiography, should be performed for all patients with IE who develop severe, localized headache, neurologic deficits, or meningeal signs. However, the clinical utility of brain imaging for all patients with left-sided IE without symptoms or signs of neurologic complications is not determined.[71]

Surgical Intervention

Guidelines for surgical treatment of IE have been developed by the AHA/ACC and the ESC. They are largely based on observational studies.[71,96,103]

Indications

Surgery is performed during the index hospitalization in about one half of left-sided IE cases,[50] largely for heart failure due to acute, severe valvular regurgitation.[127] In addition to heart failure, other IE complications that would not be effectively treated or cured with antibiotic therapy alone are indications for surgery, including abscess, recurrent embolic events with residual vegetation, resistant organism, or persistent bacteremia (Fig. 25.15).[96,103] These indications are similar for native valve and prosthetic valve IE.

In the absence of large, randomized studies of surgery versus medical therapy alone for IE, multiple observational studies with propensity adjustment for differences in clinical characteristics have been performed to evaluate the outcome of surgery for IE.[128–130] In general, surgery for native or prosthetic valve IE has been associated with lower mortality rates for patients with IE complications. Although the decision to intervene surgically for IE involves consideration of the severity of indication and operative risk, surgery for complicated IE is associated with improved survival even if operative risk is increased compared with medical therapy alone.[131]

In all cases of IE with complications, including highly resistant organisms, multidisciplinary care involving cardiologists, infectious disease specialists, and cardiac surgeons is recommended to assess operative risk and appropriate timing of surgery.[100] Several risk scores

TABLE 25.12 Society of Thoracic Surgeons–Infective Endocarditis (STS-IE) Risk Score for Predicting Operative Mortality and Major Morbidity Associated With Surgery for Active or Healed Endocarditis.	
Risk Factor	Points for Major Morbidity and Operative Mortality
Operative status of emergency, salvage, or with cardiogenic shock	17
Serum creatinine > 2.0 mg/dL or renal failure	12
Intraaortic balloon pump or inotropes used preoperatively	12
Surgery on more than one valve	7
Insulin-dependent diabetes mellitus	7
Active infective endocarditis	7
New York Heart Association functional class IV status	6
Operative status of urgent or emergency without cardiogenic shock	6
History of coronary artery bypass grafting surgery	5
History of valve surgery	5
Female	5
Arrhythmia	5
Age > 60 years	4
Body surface area > 1.9 cm²	1

Modified from Gaca JG, Sheng S, Daneshmand MA, et al. Outcomes for endocarditis surgery in North America: a simplified risk scoring system. J Thorac Cardiovasc Surg 2011;141:98-106.

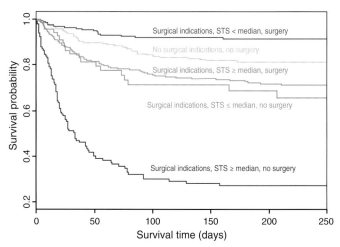

Fig. 25.16 Society of Thoracic Surgeons (STS)–Infective Endocarditis (IE) score and surgical treatment of endocarditis. Probability of 6-month survival according to surgical indications. Although operative risk may be high for some patients with complicated IE, there is evidence of a survival benefit with surgical treatment.

have been developed to predict operative risk of death.[132] Of these risk models, the Society of Thoracic Surgeons–Infective Endocarditis (STS-IE) score is based on the largest cohort of patients who have undergone surgery for active or healed IE; it is internally validated and has shown higher discrimination and calibration than other scores[132,133] (Table 25.12). In this cohort of 19,543 operations for IE, the operative mortality rate was 8%, and death was strongly predicted by operative status (i.e., emergent, urgent, or elective) and active IE with ongoing antibiotic therapy.[133] However, this risk score does not include consideration of the pathogenic organism or other factors associated with worse outcome, such as health care–associated infection.

Although most patients with left-sided IE develop an accepted indication for surgery, about one fourth of them do not undergo surgery during the index hospitalization.[131] Possible reasons for this lack of surgery include high operative risk or, less likely, clinical improvement or resolution of the indication (e.g., mild heart failure symptoms, no additional embolic event, clearance of bacteremia). Although operative risk scores have defined clinical variables associated with worse operative survival, they are not routinely used in clinical practice, and other comorbid conditions have been found to deter surgical intervention when it is otherwise indicated.[131]

Surgery is performed less commonly in patients with S. aureus left-sided IE rather than IE caused by other organisms, even though S. aureus is the most common causative organism and is associated with more IE complications and higher mortality rates.[131] This paradox is related to adverse host factors, including higher rates of sepsis

and health care–associated infection (e.g., hemodialysis) in S. aureus IE.[131,134] Although operative risk may be high for some patients with complicated IE, there is still evidence of a survival benefit with surgical treatment (Fig. 25.16). Left-sided IE caused by S. aureus has been considered a class I indication for surgery before completion of antibiotic therapy in some professional guidelines,[96] but later guidelines from the AHA/ACC and ESC have not recommended surgery in the absence of other IE complications.[71,103]

Optimal Timing

There are inconclusive data to define optimal timing of surgery for complicated IE. Early surgery has been defined as surgery performed at any time before the completion of antibiotic therapy (i.e., 4- to 6-week window),[96] but surgery during this period has been associated with higher mortality rates.[135] ESC guidelines recommend urgent surgery within a few days for most IE complications.[103] A small, randomized study of predominantly streptococcal IE complicated by severe valvular regurgitation and large vegetation found that prompt surgery within 48 hours of randomization was associated with fewer embolic events at 6 months but survival rates similar to those obtained with delayed surgery.[118]

A meta-analysis of 21 observational studies of surgical treatment of IE found that surgery performed at 7 days or less after admission had the lowest risk of all-cause mortality, but no adjustment for operative risk or urgency was performed.[136] Reassuringly, the rate of IE relapse or reinfection of the repaired or replaced valve is low (<5%).[137]

Because valve surgery requires cardiopulmonary bypass and high-dose anticoagulation, there is appropriate concern about conversion of an ischemic to a hemorrhagic stroke, extension of a small hemorrhagic stroke, or neurologic deterioration. A few observational series have evaluated the rate of hemorrhagic conversion and reported incidences of only 1% to 2%.[123,125] Neurologic deterioration after surgery has been reported to be low (6%) and to occur only in patients who had experienced symptomatic ischemic events before surgery.[138] A few observational studies with propensity adjustment for timing of cardiac surgery after ischemic stroke found no statistical increase in mortality rates for patients having surgery less than 2 weeks after the embolic event compared with delayed surgery.[139,140] However, patients who experienced a moderate to severe stroke involving more than 30% of a lobe or multiple emboli had significantly higher operative mortality rates if surgery for IE was performed within 2 weeks rather than later.[108]

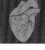

Based on these data, valve surgery may be considered in IE patients with stroke or subclinical cerebral emboli and residual vegetation without delay if intracranial hemorrhage has been excluded by imaging studies and neurologic damage is not severe.[71] However, because the operative mortality rate has been very high (75%) for patients with hemorrhagic stroke undergoing cardiac surgery within 4 weeks of the cerebrovascular event,[108] it is appropriate to delay surgery for at least 4 weeks in these cases.

Surgical Approach

Surgical approaches to valvular endocarditis vary widely. Surgical valve repair rather than replacement has been growing in popularity and is reflected in the STS-IE guideline.[109] For native aortic valve replacement, the selection of a mechanical or biologic valve prosthesis is not dissimilar to that for aortic valve replacement in other valve diseases. If a periannular abscess exists, a mechanical or stented valve is recommended (class IIa, LOE B), or if the destruction is extensive, a homograft is recommended (class IIb, LOE B). For prosthetic valve aortic endocarditis, the same recommendations have been provided. In native mitral IE, mitral valve repair is considered a class I recommendation, with valve replacement class II. For prosthetic mitral IE, the choice for repeat prosthetic valve replacement is not unlike the choice for patients without IE. Patients with active IE who received biologic valve replacements rather than mechanical prostheses had a higher

1-year mortality rate, but this outcome may be related to different host factors (i.e., older patient age, more comorbid medical conditions, and health care–associated infection) and IE complications among patients who received biologic valves rather than to the type of valve itself.[141]

Current guidelines recommend tricuspid valve repair (class I, LOE B) over replacement whenever possible (class IIa, LOE C). However, data from the STS showed that tricuspid valve replacement was more often performed than tricuspid repair or valvulectomy, although all three operations had similar operative mortality rates (7.3% overall, similar to the mortality rate for left-sided IE).[142]

Cardiac Implantable Electronic Device Removal

Eradication of staphylococcal infection from CIEDs is unlikely with antibiotic therapy alone. Complete device and lead removal is recommended for all patients with definite CIED infection as evidenced by valvular or lead IE or sepsis.[143] In the setting of local or pocket infection, complete device and lead removal is recommended. In the setting of CIED without evidence of device infection, the device and leads should be extracted if valvar endocarditis exists. When occult staphylococcal bacteremia occurs, it must be assumed that the CIED is infected and should be removed.[143]

Recommendations for the duration of antibiotic therapy after device removal are shown in Fig. 25.17. For patients who are pacemaker dependent (e.g., underlying severe bradycardia, high-degree heart

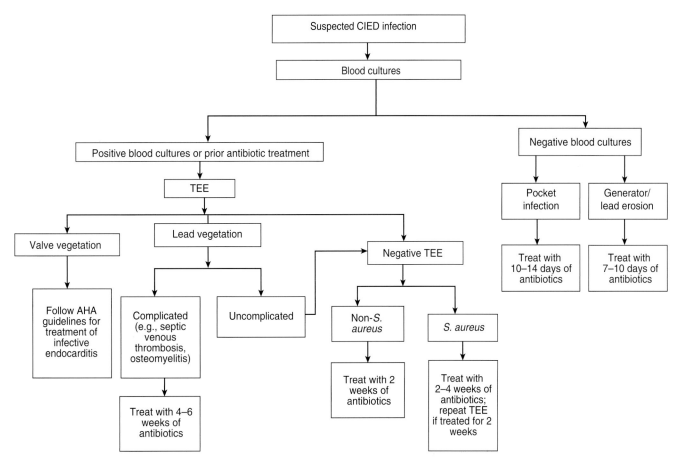

Fig. 25.17 Algorithm for Treatment of a Suspected Cardiac Implantable Electronic Device *(CIED)* Infection. Recommendations are given for the duration of antibiotic therapy after removal of an infected CIED. *AHA,* American Heart Association. (From Baddour LM et al. Update on cardiovascular implantable electronic device infections and their management: a scientific statement from the American Heart Association. Circulation 2010;121:458–477.)

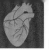

block), temporary or permanent pacemakers may be used without permanent implantation until the infection is eradicated. For patients at high risk for sudden cardiac arrest due to ventricular arrhythmias, a wearable cardioverter-defibrillator vest may provide protection for several months before reimplantation of another permanent device.

The rates of procedural complications and mortality associated with CIED extraction are significantly lower in the current era, although longer-term survival is worse for patients with CIED endocarditis, which is likely related to adverse host factors.[143]

LONG-TERM PROGNOSIS AND FOLLOW-UP

After antibiotic therapy for IE has been completed, the intravenous catheter used for antibiotic administration should be removed promptly to reduce the risk of recurrent bacteremia. Routine blood cultures after antibiotic treatment are no longer recommended in the absence of fever or signs of infection. Patients with a previous history of IE are at higher risk of recurrent infection, and they should be educated regarding symptoms and signs of IE and the need for antibiotic prophylaxis for dental procedures.[71] For IDU patients, referral for addiction treatment should be provided. Reinfection, a recurrence of IE caused by a different microorganism, has been associated with several clinical factors, including IDU, PVE, paravalvular involvement, and chronic dialysis.

Patients with IE who do not undergo valve surgery will likely have chronic valvular regurgitation. Repeat TTE is helpful to establish a new baseline in valve function and ventricular size and function. Patients who survive the first year after IE have an increased mortality rate compared with the general population, particularly younger patients and those with IDU.[144] In a nationwide study of first-time IE in Denmark, the 10-year mortality rate after IE was more than 50%, and cardiovascular disease was the predominant cause.[145] Patients treated with surgery continued to have higher longer-term survival than patients treated with medical therapy alone.[145] For this reason, patients should be serially monitored for symptoms and signs of heart failure due to valvular regurgitation after successful treatment of endocarditis.

REFERENCES

1. Hogevik H, Olaison L, Andersson R, et al. Epidemiologic aspects of infective endocarditis in an urban population. A 5-year prospective study. Medicine (Baltimore) 1995;74:324-339.
2. Berlin JA, Abrutyn E, Strom BL, et al. Incidence of infective endocarditis in the Delaware Valley, 1988-1990. Am J Cardiol 1995;76:933-936.
3. Delahaye F, Goulet V, Lacassin F, et al. Characteristics of infective endocarditis in France 1991: a one year survey. Eur Heart J 1995;16:394-401.
4. Hoen B, Alla F, Selton-Suty C, et al. Changing profile of infective endocarditis: results of a 1-year survey in France. JAMA 2002;288:75-81.
5. Cabell CH, Fowler VG Jr, Engemann JJ, et al. Endocarditis in the elderly: incidence, surgery, and survival in 16,921 patients over 12 years. Circulation 2002;106:547-547.
6. Hill EE, Herijgers P, Claus P, et al. Infective endocarditis: changing epidemiology and predictors of 6-month mortality: a prospective cohort study. Eur Heart J 2007;28:196-203.
7. Lerner PI, Weinstein L. Infective endocarditis in the antibiotic era. N Engl J Med 1966;274:388-393.
8. Tornos P, Iung B, Permanyer-Miralda G, et al. Infective endocarditis in Europe: lessons from the Euro Heart Survey. Heart 2005;91:571-575.
9. Griffin MR, Wilson WR, Edwards WD, et al. Infective endocarditis. Olmsted County, Minnesota, 1950 through 1981. JAMA 1985;254:1199-1202.
10. McKinsey DS, Ratts TE, Bisno AL. Underlying cardiac lesions in adults with infective endocarditis. The changing spectrum. Am J Med 1987;82:681-688.
11. Cherubin CE, Neu HC. Infective endocarditis at the Presbyterian Hospital in New York City from 1938-1967. Am J Med 1971;51:83-96.
12. Duval X, Alla F, Hoen B, et al. Estimated risk of endocarditis in adults with predisposing cardiac conditions undergoing dental procedures with or without antibiotic prophylaxis. Clin Infect Dis 2006;42:e102-e107.
13. Johnson CM, Rhodes KH. Pediatric endocarditis. Mayo Clin Proc 1982;57:86-94.
14. Mathew J, Addai T, Anand A, et al. Clinical features, site of involvement, bacteriologic findings, and outcome of infective endocarditis in intravenous drug users. Arch Intern Med 1995;155:1641-1648.
15. Moreillon P, Que Y. Infective endocarditis. Lancet 2004;363:139-149.
16. Karchmer A. Infective endocarditis. In: Zipes DP, Libby P, Bonow RO, Braunwald E, eds. Heart disease. 7th ed. Philadelphia: Elsevier Saunders; 2005:1633-1656.
17. Grover FL, Cohen DJ, Oprian C, et al. Determinants of the occurece of and survival from prosthetic valve endocarditis. Experience of the VA Cooperative Study on Valve Disease. J Thorac Cardiovasc Surg 1994;108:207-214.
18. Grunkemeier GL, Li HH. Epidemiology and risk factors for prosthetic valve endocarditis. In: Vlessis A, Bolling S, editors. Endocarditis: a multidisciplinary approach to modern treatment. Armonk, NY: Futura Publishing Co.; 1999:85-103.
19. Wang A, Athan E, Pappas PA, et al. Contemporary clinical profile and outcome of prosthetic valve endocarditis. JAMA 2007;297:1354-1361.
20. Regueiro A, Linke A, Latib A, et al. Association between transcatheter aortic valve replacement and subsequent infective endocarditis and in-hospital death. JAMA 2016;316:1083-1092.
21. Greenspon AJ, Patel JD, Lau E, et al. 16-Year trends in the infection burden for pacemakers and implantable cardioverter-defibrillators in the United States 1993 to 2008. J Am Coll Cardiol 2011;58:1001-1006.
22. Polyzos KA, Konstantelias AA, Falagas ME. Risk factors for cardiac implantable electronic device infection: a systematic review and meta-analysis. Europace 2015;17:767-777.
23. Athan E, Chu VH, Tattevin P, et al. Clinical characteristics and outcome of infective endocarditis involving implantable cardiac devices. JAMA 2012;307:1727-1735.
24. Greenspon AJ, Prutkin JM, Sohail MR, et al. Timing of the most recent device procedure influences the clinical outcome of lead-associated endocarditis results of the MEDIC (Multicenter Electrophysiologic Device Infection Cohort). J Am Coll Cardiol 2012;59:681-687.
25. Cabell C, Heidenreich P, Chu V, et al. Increasing rates of cardiac device infections among medicare beneficiaries: 1990-1999. Am Heart J 2004;147:582-586.
26. Klug D, Lacroix D, Savoye C, et al. Systemic infection related to endocarditis on pacemaker leads: clinical presentation and management. Circulation 1997;95:2098-2107.
27. Fernandez-Hidalgo N, Almirante B, Tornos P, et al. Contemporary epidemiology and prognosis of health care-associated infective endocarditis. Clin Infect Dis 2008;47:1287-1297.
28. Fowler VG Jr, Miro JM, Hoen B, et al. Staphylococcus aureus endocarditis: a consequence of medical progress. JAMA 2005;293:3012-3021.
29. Fleischauer AT, Ruhl L, Rhea S, Barnes E. Hospitalizations for endocarditis and associated health care costs among persons with diagnosed drug dependence—North Carolina, 2010-2015. MMWR Morb Mortal Wkly Rep 2017;66:569-573.
30. Chambers HF, Korzeniowski OM, Sande MA. Staphylococcus aureus endocarditis: clinical manifestations in addicts and nonaddicts. Medicine (Baltimore) 1983;62:170-177.
31. Chambers HF, Morris DL, Tauber MG, Modin G. Cocaine use and the risk for endocarditis in intravenous drug users. Ann Intern Med 1987;106:833-836.
32. Frontera JA, Gradon JD. Right-side endocarditis in injection drug users: review of proposed mechanisms of pathogenesis. Clin Infect Dis 2000;30:374-379.
33. Robard S. Blood velocity and endocarditis. Circulation 1963;27:24-30.
34. Foster TJ, McDevitt D. Surface-associated proteins of Staphylococcus aureus: their possible roles in virulence. FEMS Microbiol Lett 1994;118:199-205.
35. Ogawa SK, Yurberg ER, Hatcher VB, et al. Bacterial adherence to human endothelial cells in vitro. Infect Immun 1985;50:218-224.

36. Vuille C, Nidorf M, Weyman AE, Picard MH. Natural history of vegetations during successful medical treatment of endocarditis. Am Heart J 1994;126:1200-1209.

37. Wilson W, Taubert KA, Gewitz M, et al. Prevention of infective endocarditis: guidelines from the American Heart Association: a guideline from the American Heart Association Rheumatic Fever, Endocarditis, and Kawasaki Disease Committee, Council on Cardiovascular Disease in the Young, and the Council on Clinical Cardiology, Council on Cardiovascular Surgery and Anesthesia, and the Quality of Care and Outcomes Research Interdisciplinary Working Group. Circulation 2007;116:1736-1754.

38. Dajani AS, Taubert KA, Wilson W, et al. Prevention of bacterial endocarditis: recommendations by the American Heart Association. J Am Dent Assoc 1997;128:1142-1151.

39. Brooks N. Prophylactic antibiotic treatment to prevent infective endocarditis: new guidance from the National Institute for Health and Clinical Excellence. Heart 2009;95:774-780.

40. Durack DT, Lukes AS, Bright DK. New criteria for diagnosis of infective endocarditis: utilization of specific echocardiographic findings. Duke Endocarditis Service. Am J Med 1994;96:200-209.

41. Ostergaard L, Valeur N, Ihlemann N, et al. Incidence of infective endocarditis among patients considered at high risk. Eur Heart J 2018;39:623-629.

42. DeSimone DC, Tleyjeh IM, Correa de Sa DD, et al. Incidence of infective endocarditis due to viridans group streptococci before and after the 2007 American Heart Association's prevention guidelines: an extended evaluation of the Olmsted County, Minnesota, population and nationwide inpatient sample. Mayo Clin Proc 2015;90:874-881.

43. Desimone DC, Tleyjeh IM, Correa de Sa DD, et al. Incidence of infective endocarditis caused by viridans group streptococci before and after publication of the 2007 American Heart Association's endocarditis prevention guidelines. Circulation 2012;126:60-64.

44. Mackie AS, Liu W, Savu A, et al. Infective endocarditis hospitalizations before and after the 2007 American Heart Association prophylaxis guidelines. Can J Cardiol 2016;32:942-948.

45. Bikdeli B, Wang Y, Kim N, et al. Trends in hospitalization rates and outcomes of endocarditis among Medicare beneficiaries. J Am Coll Cardiol 2013;62:2217-2226.

46. Dayer MJ, Jones S, Prendergast B, et al. Incidence of infective endocarditis in England, 2000-13: a secular trend, interrupted time-series analysis. Lancet 2015;385:1219-1228.

47. Osler W. Gulstonian lectures on malignant endocarditis. Lecture II. Lancet 1885;1:459-464.

48. Osler W. Gulstonian lectures on malignant endocarditis. Lecture I. Lancet 1885;1:415-418.

49. Armstrong WS, Shea M. Clinical diagnosis of infective endocarditis. In: Vlessis A, Bolling S, editors. Endocarditis: a multidisciplinary approach to modern treatment. Armonk, NY: Futura Publishing Co.; 1999:107-134.

50. Murdoch DR, Corey GR, Hoen B, et al. Clinical presentation, etiology, and outcome of infective endocarditis in the 21st century: the International Collaboration on Endocarditis-Prospective Cohort Study. Arch Intern Med 2009;169:463-473.

51. Alpert JS, Krous HF, Dalen JE, et al. Pathogenesis of Osler's nodes. Ann Intern Med 1976;85:471-473.

52. Falcone PM, Larrison WI. Roth spots seen on ophthalmoscopy: diseases with which they may be associated. Conn Med 1995;59:271-273.

53. Pruitt AA. Neurologic complications of infective endocarditis. Curr Treat Options Neurol 2013;15(4):465-476.

54. Masuda J, Yutani C, Waki R, et al. Histopathological analysis of the mechanisms of intracranial hemorrhage complicating infective endocarditis. Stroke 1992;23:843-850.

55. Klein I, Iung B, Wolff M, et al. Silent T2* cerebral microbleeds: a potential new imaging clue in infective endocarditis. Neurology 2007;68:2043.

56. Osler W. Gulstonian lectures on malignant endocarditis: Lectures 1-3. Lancet 1885;1:415-418.

57. Pelletier LL Jr, Petersdorf RG. Infective endocarditis: a review of 125 cases from the University of Washington Hospitals, 1963-72. Medicine (Baltimore) 1977;56:287-313.

58. Von Reyn CF, Levy BS, Arbeit RD, et al. Infective endocarditis: an analysis based on strict case definitions. Ann Intern Med 1981;94:505-518.

59. Andres E, Baudoux C, Noel E, et al. The value of the Von Reyn and the Duke diagnostic criteria for infective endocarditis in internal medicine practice. A study of 38 cases. Eur J Intern Med 2003;14:411-414.

60. Perez-Vazquez A, Farinas MC, Garcia-Palomo JD, et al. Evaluation of the Duke criteria in 93 episodes of prosthetic valve endocarditis: could sensitivity be improved? Arch Intern Med 2000;160:1185-1191.

61. Stockheim JA, Chadwick EG, Kessler S, et al. Are the Duke criteria superior to the Beth Israel criteria for the diagnosis of infective endocarditis in children? Clin Infect Dis 1998;27:1451-1456.

62. Heiro M, Nikoskelainen J, Hartiala JJ, et al. Diagnosis of infective endocarditis. Sensitivity of the Duke vs von Reyn criteria. Arch Intern Med 1998;158:18-24.

63. Sekeres MA, Abrutyn E, Berlin JA, et al. An assessment of the usefulness of the Duke criteria for diagnosing active infective endocarditis. Clin Infect Dis 1997;24:1185-1190.

64. Martos-Perez F, Reguera JM, Colmenero JD. Comparable sensitivity of the Duke criteria and the modified Beth Israel criteria for diagnosing infective endocarditis. Clin Infect Dis 1996;23:410-411.

65. Olaison L, Hogevik H. Comparison of the von Reyn and Duke criteria for the diagnosis of infective endocarditis: a critical analysis of 161 episodes. Scand J Infect Dis 1996;28:399-406.

66. Hoen B, Selton-Suty C, Danchin N, et al. Evaluation of the Duke criteria versus the Beth Israel criteria for the diagnosis of infective endocarditis. Clin Infect Dis 1995;21:905-909.

67. Cecchi E, Parrini I, Chinaglia A, et al. New diagnostic criteria for infective endocarditis. A study of sensitivity and specificity. Eur Heart J 1997; 18:1149-1156.

68. Dodds GA, Sexton DJ, Durack DT, et al. Negative predictive value of the Duke criteria for infective endocarditis. Am J Cardiol 1996;77:403-407.

69. Li JS, Sexton DJ, Mick N, et al. Proposed modifications to the Duke criteria for the diagnosis of infective endocarditis. Clin Infect Dis 2000; 30:633-638.

70. Reference deleted in review.

71. Baddour LM, Wilson WR, Bayer AS, et al. Infective endocarditis in adults: diagnosis, antimicrobial therapy, and management of complications: a scientific statement for healthcare professionals from the American Heart Association. Circulation 2015;132:1435-1486.

72. Fournier PE, Thuny F, Richet H, et al. Comprehensive diagnostic strategy for blood culture-negative endocarditis: a prospective study of 819 new cases. Clin Infect Dis 2010;51:131-140.

73. Heiro M, Helenius H, Sundell J, et al. Utility of serum C-reactive protein in assessing the outcome of infective endocarditis. Eur Heart J 2005;26: 1873-1881.

74. Verhagen DW, Hermanides J, Korevaar JC, et al. Prognostic value of serial C-reactive protein measurements in left-sided native valve endocarditis. Arch Intern Med 2008;168:302-307.

75. Mueller C, Huber P, Laifer G, et al. Procalcitonin and the early diagnosis of infective endocarditis. Circulation 2004;109:1707-1710.

76. Stancoven AB, Shiue AB, Khera A, et al. Association of troponin T, detected with highly sensitive assay, and outcomes in infective endocarditis. Am J Cardiol 2011;108:416-420.

77. Shiue AB, Stancoven AB, Purcell JB, et al. Relation of level of B-type natriuretic peptide with outcomes in patients with infective endocarditis. Am J Cardiol 2010;106:1011-1015.

78. Syed FF, Millar BC, Prendergast BD. Molecular technology in context: a current review of diagnosis and management of infective endocarditis. Prog Cardiovasc Dis 2007;50:181-197.

79. Voldstedlund M, Norum PL, Baandrup U, et al. Broad-range PCR and sequencing in routine diagnosis of infective endocarditis. APMIS 2008; 116:190-198.

80. Harris KA, Yam T, Jalili S, et al. Service evaluation to establish the sensitivity, specificity and additional value of broad-range 16S rDNA PCR for the diagnosis of infective endocarditis from resected endocardial material in patients from eight UK and Ireland hospitals. Eur J Clin Microbiol Infect Dis 2014;33:2061-2066.

81. Kupferwasser LI, Darius H, Muller AM, et al. Diagnosis of culture-negative endocarditis: the role of the Duke criteria and the impact of transesophageal echocardiography. Am Heart J 2001;142:146-152.

82. Greaves K, Mou D, Patel A, Celermajer DS. Clinical criteria and the appropriate use of transthoracic echocardiography for the exclusion of infective endocarditis. Heart 2003;89:273-275.

83. Kim DH, Kang DH, Lee MZ, et al. Impact of early surgery on embolic events in patients with infective endocarditis. Circulation 2010;122:S17-S22.

84. Heidenreich P, Masoudi F, Maini B, et al. Echocardiography in patients with suspected endocarditis: a cost effectiveness analysis. Am J Med 1999;107:198-208.

85. Heidenreich PA, Masoudi FA, Maini B, et al. Echocardiography in patients with suspected endocarditis: a cost-effectiveness analysis. Am J Med 1999;107:198-208.

86. Daniel WG, Mugge A, Martin RP, et al. Improvement in the diagnosis of abscesses associated with endocarditis by transesophageal echocardiography. N Engl J Med 1991;324:795-800.

87. Anguera I, Miro JM, Cabell CH, et al. Clinical characteristics and outcome of aortic endocarditis with periannular abscess in the International Collaboration on Endocarditis Merged Database. Am J Cardiol 2005;96:976-981.

88. Hill EE, Herijgers P, Claus P, et al. Abscess in infective endocarditis: the value of transesophageal echocardiography and outcome: a 5-year study. Am Heart J 2007;154:923-928.

89. Anguera I, Del Rio A, Miro JM, et al. *Staphylococcus lugdunensis* infective endocarditis: description of 10 cases and analysis of native valve, prosthetic valve, and pacemaker lead endocarditis clinical profiles. Heart 2005;91:e10.

90. Kang N, Wan S, Ng CS, Underwood MJ. Periannular extension of infective endocarditis. Ann Thorac Cardiovasc Surg 2009;15:74-81.

91. Victor F, De Place C, Camus C, et al. Pacemaker lead infection: echocardiographic features, management, and outcome. Heart 1999;81:82-87.

92. Baddour LM, Epstein AE, Erickson CC, et al. Update on cardiovascular implantable electronic device infections and their management: a scientific statement from the American Heart Association. Circulation 2010; 121:458-477.

93. Chu VH, Bayer AS. Use of echocardiography in the diagnosis and management of infective endocarditis. Curr Infect Dis Rep 2007;9:283-290.

94. Lo R, D'Anca M, Cohen T, Kerwin T. Incidence and prognosis of pacemaker lead-associated masses: a study of 1,569 transesophageal echocardiograms. J Invasive Cardiol 2006;18:599-601.

95. Feuchtner GM, Stolzmann P, Dichtl W, et al. Multislice computed tomography in infective endocarditis: comparison with transesophageal echocardiography and intraoperative findings. J Am Coll Cardiol 2009;53:436-444.

96. Nishimura RA, Otto CM, Bonow RO, et al. 2014 AHA/ACC guideline for the management of patients with valvular heart disease: executive summary: a report of the American College of Cardiology/American Heart Association Task Force on Practice Guidelines. J Am Coll Cardiol 2014;63:2438-2488.

97. Saby L, Laas O, Habib G, et al. Positron emission tomography/computed tomography for diagnosis of prosthetic valve endocarditis: increased valvular 18F-fluorodeoxyglucose uptake as a novel major criterion. J Am Coll Cardiol 2013;61:2374-2382.

98. Pizzi MN, Roque A, Fernandez-Hidalgo N, et al. Improving the diagnosis of infective endocarditis in prosthetic valves and intracardiac devices with 18F-fluorodeoxyglucose positron emission tomography/computed tomography angiography: initial results at an infective endocarditis referral center. Circulation 2015;132:1113-1126.

99. Chirillo F, Scotton P, Rocco F, et al. Impact of a multidisciplinary management strategy on the outcome of patients with native valve infective endocarditis. Am J Cardiol 2013;112:1171-1176.

100. Botelho-Nevers E, Thuny F, Casalta JP, et al. Dramatic reduction in infective endocarditis-related mortality with a management-based approach. Arch Intern Med 2009;169:1290-1298.

101. Gould FK, Denning DW, Elliott TS, et al. Guidelines for the diagnosis and antibiotic treatment of endocarditis in adults: a report of the Working Party of the British Society for Antimicrobial Chemotherapy. J Antimicrob Chemother 2012;67:269-289.

102. Thuny F, Gaubert JY, Jacquier A, et al. Imaging investigations in infective endocarditis: current approach and perspectives. Arch Cardiovasc Dis 2013;106:52-62.

103. Habib G, Lancellotti P, Antunes MJ, et al. 2015 ESC guidelines for the management of infective endocarditis: the Task Force for the Management of Infective Endocarditis of the European Society of Cardiology (ESC). Endorsed by: European Association for Cardio-Thoracic Surgery (EACTS), the European Association of Nuclear Medicine (EANM). Eur Heart J 2015;36:3075-3128.

104. Iversen K, Ihlemann N, Gill SU, et al. Partial oral versus intravenous antibiotic treatment of endocarditis. N Engl J Med 2019;380(5): 415-424.

105. Chan KL, Dumesnil JG, Cujec B, et al. A randomized trial of aspirin on the risk of embolic events in patients with infective endocarditis. J Am Coll Cardiol 2003;42:775-780.

106. Kiefer T, Park L, Tribouilloy C, et al. Association between valvular surgery and mortality among patients with infective endocarditis complicated by heart failure. JAMA 2011;306:2239-2247.

107. Mills J, Utley J, Abbott J. Heart failure in infective endocarditis: predisposing factors, course and treatment. Chest 1974;66:151-159.

108. Garcia-Cabrera E, Fernandez-Hidalgo N, Almirante B, et al. Neurological complications of infective endocarditis: risk factors, outcome, and impact of cardiac surgery: a multicenter observational study. Circulation 2013;127:2272-2284.

109. Byrne JG, Rezai K, Sanchez JA, et al. Surgical management of endocarditis: the Society of Thoracic Surgeons clinical practice guideline. Ann Thorac Surg 2011;91:2012-2019.

110. Heiro M, Nikoskelainen J, Engblom E, et al. Neurologic manifestations of infective endocarditis: a 17-year experience in a teaching hospital in Finland. Arch Intern Med 2000;160:2781-2787.

111. Dickerman SA, Abrutyn E, Barsic B, et al. The relationship between the initiation of antimicrobial therapy and the incidence of stroke in infective endocarditis: an analysis from the ICE Prospective Cohort Study (ICE-PCS). Am Heart J 2007;154:1086-1094.

112. Lamas C, Boia M, Eykyn SJ. Osteoarticular infections complicating infective endocarditis: a study of 30 cases between 1969 and 2002 in a tertiary referral centre. Scand J Infect Dis 2006;38:433-440.

113. Di Salvo G, Habib G, Pergola V, et al. Echocardiography predicts embolic events in infective endocarditis. J Am Coll Cardiol 2001;37:1069-1076.

114. Tischler MD, Vaitkus PT. The ability of vegetation size on echocardiography to predict clinical complications: a meta-analysis. J Am Soc Echocardiogr 1997;10:562-568.

115. Yang A, Tan C, Daneman N, et al. Clinical and echocardiographic predictors of embolism in infective endocarditis: systematic review and meta-analysis. Clin Microbiol Infect 2019;25(2):178-187.

116. Chu VH, Cabell CH, Benjamin DK Jr, et al. Early predictors of in-hospital death in infective endocarditis. Circulation 2004;109:1745-1749.

117. Thuny F, Di Salvo G, Belliard O, et al. Risk of embolism and death in infective endocarditis: prognostic value of echocardiography: a prospective multicenter study. Circulation 2005;112:69-75.

118. Kang DH, Kim YJ, Kim SH, et al. Early surgery versus conventional treatment for infective endocarditis. N Engl J Med 2012;366:2466-2473.

119. Nishimura RA, Otto CM, Bonow RO, et al. 2014 AHA/ACC guideline for the management of patients with valvular heart disease: a report of the American College of Cardiology/American Heart Association Task Force on Practice Guidelines. Circulation 2014;129:e521-e643.

120. Heinle S, Wilderman N, Harrison JK, et al. Value of transthoracic echocardiography in predicting embolic events in active infective endocarditis. Duke Endocarditis Service. Am J Cardiol 1994;74:799-801.

121. Dickerman SA, Abrutyn E, Barsic B, et al. The relationship between the initiation of antimicrobial therapy and the incidence of stroke in infective endocarditis: an analysis from the ICE Prospective Cohort Study (ICE-PCS). Am Heart J 2007;154:1086-1094.

122. Cooper HA, Thompson EC, Laureno R, et al. Subclinical brain embolization in left-sided infective endocarditis: results from the evaluation by MRI of the brains of patients with left-sided intracardiac solid masses (EMBOLISM) pilot study. Circulation 2009;120:585-591.

123. Yoshioka D, Sakaguchi T, Yamauchi T, et al. Impact of early surgical treatment on postoperative neurologic outcome for active infective endocarditis complicated by cerebral infarction. Ann Thorac Surg 2012;94:489-495; discussion 496.

124. Mirabel M, Sonneville R, Hajage D, et al. Long-term outcomes and cardiac surgery in critically ill patients with infective endocarditis. Eur Heart J 2014;35:1195-1204.

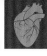

125. Ruttmann E, Willeit J, Ulmer H, et al. Neurological outcome of septic cardioembolic stroke after infective endocarditis. Stroke 2006;37:2094-2099.

126. Yanagawa B, Pettersson GB, Habib G, et al. Surgical management of infective endocarditis complicated by embolic stroke: practical recommendations for clinicians. Circulation 2016;134:1280-1292.

127. Kiefer T, Park L, Tribouilloy C, et al. Association between valvular surgery and mortality among patients with infective endocarditis complicated by heart failure. JAMA 2011;306:2239-2247.

128. Chirouze C, Alla F, Fowler VG Jr, et al. Impact of early valve surgery on outcome of *Staphylococcus aureus* prosthetic valve infective endocarditis: analysis in the International Collaboration of Endocarditis-Prospective Cohort Study. Clin Infect Dis 2015;60:741-749.

129. Lalani T, Cabell CH, Benjamin DK, et al. Analysis of the impact of early surgery on in-hospital mortality of native valve endocarditis: use of propensity score and instrumental variable methods to adjust for treatment-selection bias. Circulation 2010;121:1005-1013.

130. Lalani T, Chu VH, Park LP, et al. In-hospital and 1-year mortality in patients undergoing early surgery for prosthetic valve endocarditis. JAMA Intern Med 2013;173:1495-1504.

131. Chu VH, Park LP, Athan E, et al. Association between surgical indications, operative risk, and clinical outcome in infective endocarditis: a prospective study from the International Collaboration on Endocarditis. Circulation 2015;131:131-140.

132. Varela L, Lopez-Menendez J, Redondo A, et al. Mortality risk prediction in infective endocarditis surgery: reliability analysis of specific scores. Eur J Cardiothorac Surg 2018;53:1049-1054.

133. Gaca JG, Sheng S, Daneshmand MA, et al. Outcomes for endocarditis surgery in North America: a simplified risk scoring system. J Thorac Cardiovasc Surg 2011;141:98-106.

134. Fowler VG, Jr., Miro JM, Hoen B, et al. *Staphylococcus aureus* endocarditis: a consequence of medical progress. JAMA 2005;293:3012-3021.

135. Gaca JG, Sheng S, Daneshmand MA, et al. Outcomes for endocarditis surgery in North America: a simplified risk scoring system. J Thorac Cardiovasc Surg 2011;141:98-106.e1-2.

136. Anantha Narayanan M, Mahfood Haddad T, Kalil AC, et al. Early versus late surgical intervention or medical management for infective endocarditis: a systematic review and meta-analysis. Heart 2016;102:950-957.

137. Chu VH, Sexton DJ, Cabell CH, et al. Repeat infective endocarditis: differentiating relapse from reinfection. Clin Infect Dis 2005;41:406-409.

138. Thuny F, Avierinos JF, Tribouilloy C, et al. Impact of cerebrovascular complications on mortality and neurologic outcome during infective endocarditis: a prospective multicentre study. Eur Heart J 2007;28:1155-1161.

139. Barsic B, Dickerman S, Krajinovic V, et al. Influence of the timing of cardiac surgery on the outcome of patients with infective endocarditis and stroke. Clin Infect Dis 2013;56:209-217.

140. Morita K, Sasabuchi Y, Matsui H, et al. Outcomes after early or late timing of surgery for infective endocarditis with ischaemic stroke: a retrospective cohort study. Interact Cardiovasc Thorac Surg 2015;21:604-609.

141. Delahaye F, Chu VH, Altclas J, et al. One-year outcome following biological or mechanical valve replacement for infective endocarditis. Int J Cardiol 2015;178:117-123.

142. Gaca JG, Sheng S, Daneshmand M, et al. Current outcomes for tricuspid valve infective endocarditis surgery in North America. Ann Thorac Surg 2013;96:1374-1381.

143. Baddour LM, Epstein AE, Erickson CC, et al. Update on cardiovascular implantable electronic device infections and their management: a scientific statement from the American Heart Association. Circulation 2010;121:458-477.

144. Ternhag A, Cederstrom A, Torner A, Westling K. A nationwide cohort study of mortality risk and long-term prognosis in infective endocarditis in Sweden. PLoS One 2013;8:e67519.

145. Ostergaard L, Oestergaard LB, Lauridsen TK, et al. Long-term causes of death in patients with infective endocarditis who undergo medical therapy only or surgical treatment: a nationwide population-based study. Eur J Cardiothorac Surg 2018;54(5):860-866.

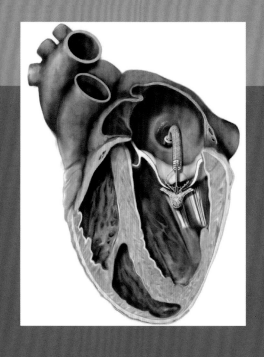

第26章
人工心脏瓣膜

瓣膜置换术是可明确改善瓣膜病患者临床症状和预后的重要治疗方式。人工瓣膜的设计和性能、手术技术等方面的不断完善，使手术治疗的应用范围越来越广。近年来经导管瓣膜介入技术的兴起普及，进一步扩大了手术的适应证及受益人群。因此，熟悉现有人工瓣膜的具体血流动力学特性、耐久性、血栓形成风险等固有局限性，对于临床决策至关重要。同时，瓣膜置换术虽解决了自体瓣膜病变的不良影响，但也带来了需要临床密切关注的人工瓣膜相关并发症，包括栓塞事件、出血、血栓或血管翳引起的瓣膜梗阻、感染性心内膜炎、结构退变（尤其是生物瓣膜）、瓣周反流、溶血性贫血，以及人工瓣膜-患者不匹配等。不同并发症的发生率取决于手术及人工瓣膜的类型、置换瓣膜的位置及其他临床危险因素。

本章对人工瓣膜的类型、机械瓣膜与生物瓣膜之间的比较、置换术后的随访管理、并发症的评估与处理进行了详细阐述。总体而言，瓣膜置换术的终极目标是为瓣膜疾病患者提供有效、持久的解决方案，因此瓣膜的耐久度就成为临床高度关注同时亟须解决的核心问题，无论是手术方式、人工瓣膜的选择或是术后并发症的预防和管理均是服务于该目标。

张 斌

Prosthetic Heart Valves

Philippe Pibarot, Patrick T. O'Gara

CHAPTER OUTLINE

KEY POINTS

- The need for heart valve replacement surgery marks a major milestone in the natural history of valve disease and mandates establishment of a schedule for clinical and echocardiographic surveillance. Surgical repair, especially for primary mitral regurgitation, is preferred whenever anatomically feasible and when supported by the experience of the surgeon.

- Valve replacement surgery substitutes a nonimmunogenic foreign body for the native valve. Hemodynamic performance characteristics vary as a function of valve type and size, and of cardiac output or transvalvular flow. There is some degree of stenosis across any mechanical or stented bioprosthetic valve. A small amount of regurgitation is a normal feature of mechanical valves and of some bioprosthetic valves.

- Mechanical heart valve substitutes are durable but obligate the patient to lifelong anticoagulation with a vitamin K antagonist (VKA), exposing patients to the dual hazards of thromboembolism and bleeding. Bioprosthetic or tissue valves are relatively nonthrombogenic but are susceptible to a predictable rate of structural deterioration over time and the potential need for reoperation. Rates of structural valve deterioration vary as a function of valve type, valve position, and several patient characteristics, such as age at implantation, pregnancy, and altered calcium homeostasis. The durability of an aortic homograft does not exceed that of a bovine pericardial valve.

- Direct oral anticoagulants (i.e., non-VKA) are not approved for use in patients with mechanical heart valves. Management of anticoagulation in pregnant women with mechanical heart valves is very challenging. The choice between warfarin (provided the daily dose does not exceed 5 mg) and low-molecular-weight heparin must be individualized with weekly follow-up during pregnancy.

- The choice of prosthetic heart valve must account for the values and preferences of the informed patient and for the trade-offs regarding durability, anticoagulation, and the aggregate risks of thromboembolism and bleeding. Many patients younger than 60 years of age opt to avoid anticoagulation and accept a bioprosthetic valve with an increased likelihood of reoperation. The introduction of transcatheter aortic valve replacement (TAVR) for the treatment of symptomatic severe aortic stenosis in patients across the entire surgical risk spectrum has changed the dynamic considerably. Shared decision making regarding the type of prosthesis and the manner of implantation (surgical vs. transcatheter) is emphasized. Transcatheter valve-in-valve implantation for aortic or mitral bioprosthetic structural valve deterioration is available for severely symptomatic patients who are considered to be at high or prohibitive risk for reoperation.

- Transthoracic echocardiography (TTE) with color-flow Doppler imaging is an integral feature of patient follow-up after valve replacement surgery. There is good correlation between Doppler and catheterization estimates of mean pressure gradients across prosthetic valves, although in certain instances agreement is less robust. The phenomenon of pressure recovery, which may lead to an overestimate of valve gradient, is particularly problematic for bileaflet mechanical valves in the aortic position. Published tables of normal Doppler echocardiographic parameters for prosthetic valves of various makes and sizes should be consulted to help guide management.

- A baseline postoperative TTE study is obtained during the first 6 to 12 weeks after operation and serves as a reference against which future comparisons can be made as clinically dictated. Transesophageal echocardiography (TEE) is required for the interrogation of prosthetic valves whenever valve dysfunction, paravalvular leak, or endocarditis is suspected. The frequency with which surveillance TTE is performed depends on the valve type. Routine imaging is not required for mechanical prostheses if there are no symptoms or signs of valve dysfunction. Annual TTE examinations may be considered after 5 years and are reasonable after 10 years for bioprosthetic valves. Other imaging modalities (e.g., cardiac computed tomography) may provide corroborative functional information in selected circumstances.
- All patients with prosthetic heart valves should receive antibiotic prophylaxis before dental procedures that involve manipulation of gingival tissue or the periapical region of teeth or the oral mucosa.

Management of prosthetic valve endocarditis requires a multidisciplinary team approach with input from cardiologists, cardiac surgeons, imaging specialists, and infectious disease experts.
- When available, emergency surgery is preferred over fibrinolytic therapy for the management of patients with left-sided prosthetic valve thrombosis (PVT) and shock or New York Heart Association functional class III to IV heart failure. Fibrinolytic therapy is reasonable for patients with small thrombus burden and recent-onset functional class I or II symptoms and for patients with right-sided PVT. There is increasing experience with low-dose, slow-infusion fibrinolytic therapy for mechanical PVT.
- Severe prosthesis–patient mismatch is an important complication for some patients after valve replacement surgery (aortic or mitral). Attempts to implant the largest allowable prosthesis are limited by the anatomic constraints posed by the individual patient. Lesser degrees of mismatch are usually well tolerated.

The past several decades have witnessed extraordinary advancements in patient survival and functional outcomes after heart valve replacement surgery.[1] Continued refinements in prosthetic valve design and performance, operative techniques, myocardial preservation, systemic perfusion, cerebral protection, and anesthetic management have enabled the application of surgical therapy to an increasingly wider spectrum of patients. Minimally invasive surgical approaches and aggressive use of primary valve repair when anatomically appropriate are now routine in most high-volume centers. Heart valve teams have been formed to provide multidisciplinary assessment and treatment in complex cases, including the use of transcatheter aortic and mitral valve interventions when appropriate.[2]

More than 58,000 aortic or mitral valve replacement (MVR) operations (with or without coronary artery bypass) were reported to the Society of Thoracic Surgeons (STS) National Adult Cardiac Database in 2017.[3] Familiarity with the specific hemodynamic attributes, durability, thrombogenicity, and inherent limitations of available heart valve substitutes and their potential for long-term complications is critical for appropriate decision making for patients in whom repair is not appropriate or feasible.

The choice of valve prosthesis is a trade-off between valve durability and the risk of thromboembolism on the one hand and the associated hazards and lifestyle limitations of anticoagulation on the other. The ideal heart valve substitute remains an elusive goal.

TYPES OF PROSTHETIC HEART VALVES

Mechanical Valves

There are three basic types of mechanical prosthetic valves: bileaflet, tilting disk, and ball-cage. The bileaflet SJM Regent Mechanical Heart Valve (Fig. 26.1A) was introduced in 1977 by St. Jude Medical (since acquired by Abbott, Santa Clara, CA) and has become the most frequently implanted mechanical prosthesis worldwide. It consists of two pyrolytic semicircular leaflets or disks with a slit-like central orifice between the two leaflets and two larger semicircular orifices laterally. The opening angle of the leaflets relative to the annulus plane is 75 to 90 degrees. Hemodynamic characteristics compare favorably to those of a tilting disk valve (Tables 26.1 and 26.2). As a performance index, the ratio of effective orifice area (EOA) to the area of the sewing ring ranges from 0.40 to 0.70, depending on valve size. EOAs range from 0.7 cm^2 for a 19-mm valve to 4.2 cm^2 for a 31-mm prosthesis.

Average peak velocities are 3.0 ± 0.8 m/s in the aortic position and 1.6 ± 0.3 m/s in the mitral position.[4,5] Peak instantaneous gradients can be estimated using the Bernoulli equation, but mean gradient calculations are more useful. The phenomenon of pressure recovery across bileaflet and ball-cage aortic valves magnifies the estimate of the difference between left ventricular (LV) and aortic pressures (i.e., the systolic gradient), especially when the latter is derived from measurements obtained close to the valve rather than more distally in the ascending aorta (Fig. 26.2). Additional confounding occurs from the contribution of flow acceleration through the narrow central orifice of a bileaflet valve.

Doppler velocity determinations can overestimate the transvalvular gradient across mechanical bileaflet valves. Published reference tables of expected velocities for the various valve sizes should be consulted, and comparison with baseline postoperative studies should be made to avoid misdiagnosis of prosthetic valve stenosis (see Tables 26.1 and 26.2).[6]

The Carbomedics mechanical heart valve (LivaNova, Arvada, CO) is a variation of the SJM Regent model prosthesis that can be rotated to prevent limitation of leaflet excursion by subvalvular tissue. For a given valve annulus size, the EOAs are generally larger and transprosthetic pressure gradients are lower for the bileaflet mechanical valves compared with the tilting disk valves. Bileaflet valves typically have a small amount of normal regurgitation (i.e., washing jet), designed in part to decrease the risk of thrombus formation. A small central jet and two converging jets emanating from the hinge points of the disks can be visualized on color Doppler flow imaging.[7,8]

Tilting disk or monoleaflet valves use a single circular disk that rotates within a rigid annulus to occlude or open the valve orifice. The disk is secured by lateral or central metal struts. The Medtronic-Hall valve (Medtronic, Inc., Minneapolis, MN) has a thin, circular disk of tungsten-impregnated graphite with pyrolytic coating, secured at its center by a curved, central guide strut within a titanium housing. The sewing ring is made of polytetrafluoroethylene (Teflon). The disk opens to 75 degrees in the aortic model and to 70 degrees in the mitral model.

The disk of the Omniscience valve (Medical CV, Inc., Inner Grove Heights, MN) is made of pyrolytic carbon and has a seamless polyester knit sewing ring. The disk opens to 80 degrees and closes at an angle of 12 degrees to the annular plane.

For both valve types, the major orifice is semicircular in cross section. The non-perpendicular opening angle of the valve occluder tends to slightly increase the resistance to blood flow, particularly in the

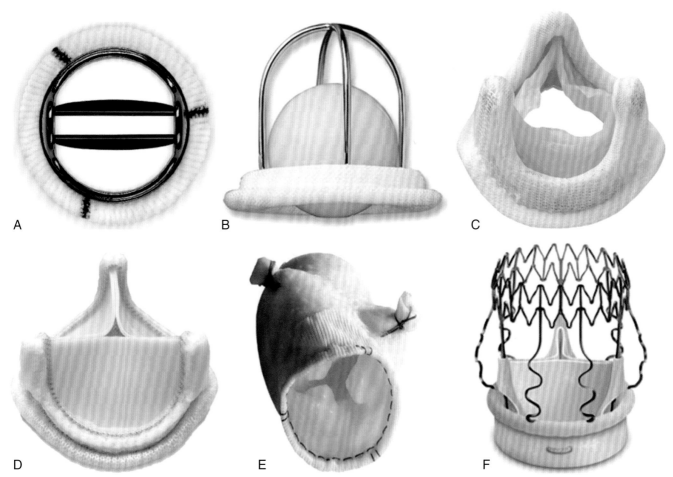

Fig. 26.1 Different Types of Prosthetic Valve Models. (A) SJM Regent Mechanical Heart Valve FlexCuff Sewing Ring (Abbott, Santa Clara, CA). (B) Starr-Edwards ball-cage mechanical valve (Edwards Lifesciences, Irvine, CA). (C) Stented porcine Medtronic Mosaic bioprosthetic valve. (Medtronic Inc., Minneapolis, MN) (D) Stented bovine pericardial Edwards Magna bioprosthetic valve (Edwards Lifesciences). (E) Stentless porcine Medtronic Freestyle bioprosthetic valve (Medtronic Inc.). (F) Sutureless Perceval bioprosthetic valve (Sorin Group USA Inc., a wholly owned subsidiary of LivaNova PLC, Arvada, CO). (A, SJM Regent and FlexCuff are trademarks of Abbott or its related companies. Reproduced with permission of Abbott, © 2019. All rights reserved.)

TABLE 26.1 Normal Doppler Echocardiographic Values for Selected Aortic Valve Prostheses.

Valve	Type	Size	Peak Gradient (mmHg)	Mean Gradient (mmHg)	Peak Velocity (m/s)	Effective Orifice Area (cm²)
Mechanical						
SJM Regent	Bileaflet	19	35.17 ± 11.16	18.96 ± 6.27	2.86 ± 0.48	1.01 ± 0.24
		21	28.34 ± 9.94	15.82 ± 5.67	2.63 ± 0.48	1.33 ± 0.32
		23	25.28 ± 7.89	13.77 ± 5.33	2.57 ± 0.44	1.6 ± 0.43
		25	22.57 ± 7.68	12.65 ± 5.14	2.4 ± 0.45	1.93 ± 0.45
		27	19.85 ± 7.55	11.18 ± 4.82	2.24 ± 0.42	2.35 ± 0.59
		29	17.72 ± 6.42	9.86 ± 2.9	2 ± 0.1	2.81 ± 0.57
		31	16	10 ± 6	2.1 ± 0.6	3.08 ± 1.09
On-X	Bileaflet	19	21.3 ± 10.8	11.8 ± 3.4	—	1.5 ± 0.2
		21	16.4 ± 5.9	9.9 ± 3.6	—	1.7 ± 0.4
		23	15.9 ± 6.4	8.5 ± 3.3	—	2 ± 0.6
		25	16.5 ± 10.2	9 ± 5.3	—	2.4 ± 0.8
		27–29	11.4 ± 4.6	5.6 ± 2.7	—	3.2 ± 0.6

Continued

TABLE 26.1   Normal Doppler Echocardiographic Values for Selected Aortic Valve Prostheses.—cont'd

Valve	Type	Size	Peak Gradient (mmHg)	Mean Gradient (mmHg)	Peak Velocity (m/s)	Effective Orifice Area (cm²)
Medtronic-Hall	Tilting disk	20	34.37 ± 13.06	17.08 ± 5.28	2.9 ± 0.4	1.21 ± 0.45
		21	26.86 ± 10.54	14.1 ± 5.93	2.42 ± 0.36	1.08 ± 0.17
		23	26.85 ± 8.85	13.5 ± 4.79	2.43 ± 0.59	1.36 ± 0.39
		25	17.13 ± 7.04	9.53 ± 4.26	2.29 ± 0.5	1.9 ± 0.47
		27	18.66 ± 9.71	8.66 ± 5.56	2.07 ± 0.53	1.9 ± 0.16
		29	—	—	1.6	—
Omniscience	Tilting disk	19	47.5 ± 3.5	28 ± 1.4	—	0.81 ± 0.01
		21	50.8 ± 2.8	28.2 ± 2.17	—	0.87 ± 0.13
		23	39.8 ± 8.7	20.1 ± 5.1	—	0.98 ± 0.07
Starr-Edwards	Ball-and-cage	21	29		—	1
		22	—	—	4 ± 0	—
		23	32.6 ± 12.79	21.98 ± 8.8	3.5 ± 0.5	1.1
		24	34.13 ± 10.33	22.09 ± 7.54	3.35 ± 0.48	—
		26	31.83 ± 9.01	19.69 ± 6.05	3.18 ± 0.35	—
		27	30.82 ± 6.3	18.5 ± 3.7	—	1.8
		29	29 ± 9.3	16.3 ± 5.5	—	
Bioprosthetic						
Carpentier-Edwards pericardial	Stented bioprosthesis	19	32.13 ± 3.55	24.19 ± 8.6	24.19 ± 8.6	1.21 ± 0.31
		21	25.69 ± 9.9	20.3 ± 9.08	2.59 ± 0.42	1.47 ± 0.36
		23	21.72 ± 8.57	13.01 ± 5.27	2.29 ± 0.45	1.75 ± 0.28
		25	16.46 ± 5.41	9.04 ± 2.27	2.02 ± 0.31	—
		27	19.2 ± 0	5.6	1.6	—
		29	17.6 ± 0	11.6	2.1	—
Carpentier-Edwards	Stented bioprosthesis	19	43.48 ± 12.72	25.6 ± 8.02	—	0.85 ± 0.17
		21	27.73 ± 7.6	17.25 ± 6.24	2.37 ± 0.54	1.48 ± 0.3
		23	28.93 ± 7.49	15.92 ± 6.43	2.76 ± 0.4	1.69 ± 0.45
		25	23.94 ± 7.05	12.76 ± 4.43	2.38 ± 0.47	1.94 ± 0.45
		27	22.14 ± 8.24	12.33 ± 5.59	2.31 ± 0.39	2.25 ± 0.55
		29	22	9.92 ± 2.9	2.44 ± 0.43	2.84 ± 0.51
		31	—		2.41 ± 0.13	—
CryoLife-O'Brien stentless	Stentless bioprosthesis	19	—	12 ± 4.8	—	1.25 ± 0.1
		21	—	10.33 ± 2	—	1.57 ± 0.6
		23	—	8.5	—	2.2
		25	—	7.9	—	2.3
		27	—	7.4	—	2.7
Hancock II	Stented bioprosthesis	21	20 ± 4	14.8 ± 4.1	—	1.23 ± 0.27
		23	24.72 ± 5.73	16.64 ± 6.91	—	1.39 ± 0.23
		25	20 ± 2	10.7 ± 3	—	1.47 ± 0.19
		27	14 ± 3	—	—	1.55 ± 0.18
		29	15 ± 3	—	—	1.6 ± 0.15
Medtronic Mosaic Porcine	Stented bioprosthesis	21	—	12.43 ± 7.3	—	1.6 ± 0.7
		23	—	12.47 ± 7.4	—	2.1 ± 0.8
		25	—	10.08 ± 5.1	—	2.1 ± 1.6
		27	—	9	—	—
		29	—	9	—	—

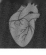

TABLE 26.1   Normal Doppler Echocardiographic Values for Selected Aortic Valve Prostheses.—cont'd

Valve	Type	Size	Peak Gradient (mmHg)	Mean Gradient (mmHg)	Peak Velocity (m/s)	Effective Orifice Area (cm²)
Mitroflow	Stented bioprosthesis	19	18.7 ± 5.1	10.3 ± 3	—	1.13 ± 0.17
		21	20.2	15.4	2.3	—
		23	14.04 ± 4.91	7.56 ± 3.38	1.85 ± 0.34	—
		25	17 ± 11.31	10.8 ± 6.51	2 ± 0.71	—
		27	13 ± 3	6.57 ± 1.7	1.8 ± 0.2	—
Toronto stentless porcine	Stentless bioprosthesis	20	10.9	4.6	—	1.3
		21	18.64 ± 11.8	7.56 ± 4.4	—	1.21 ± 0.7
		22	23	—	—	1.2
		23	13.55 ± 7.28	7.08 ± 4.33	—	1.59 ± 0.84
		25	12.17 ± 5.75	6.2 ± 3.05	—	1.62 ± 0.4
		27	9.96 ± 4.56	4.8 ± 2.33	—	1.95 ± 0.42
		29	7.91 ± 4.17	3.94 ± 2.15	—	2.37 ± 0.67

Modified from Rosenhek R, Binder T, Maurer G, et al. Normal values for Doppler echocardiographic assessment of heart valve prostheses. J Am Soc Echocardiogr 2003;16:1116-1127.

TABLE 26.2   Normal Doppler Echocardiographic Values for Selected Mitral Valve Prostheses.

Valve	Size	Peak Gradient (mmHg)	Mean Gradient (mmHg)	Peak Velocity (m/s)	Pressure Half-Time (ms)	Effective Orifice Area (cm²)
Mechanical						
SJM Regent bileaflet	23	—	4	1.5	160	1
	25	—	2.5 ± 1	1.34 ± 1.12	75 ± 4	1.35 ± 0.17
	27	11 ± 4	5 ± 1.82	1.61 ± 0.29	75 ± 10	1.67 ± 0.17
	29	10 ± 3	4.15 ± 1.8	1.57 ± 0.29	85 ± 0.29	1.75 ± 0.24
	31	12 ± 6	4.46 ± 2.22	1.59 ± 0.33	74 ± 13	2.03 ± 0.32
On-X bileaflet	25	11.5 ± 3.2	5.3 ± 2.1	—	—	1.9 ± 1.1
	27–29	10.3 ± 4.5	4.5 ± 1.6	—	—	2.2 ± 0.5
	31–33	9.8 ± 3.8	4.8 ± 2.4	—	—	2.5 ± 1.1
Medtronic-Hall tilting disk	27	—	—	1.4	78	—
	29	—	—	1.57 ± 0.1	69 ± 15	—
	31	—	—	1.45 ± 0.12	77 ± 17	—
Bioprosthetic						
Carpentier-Edwards stented bioprosthesis	27	—	6 ± 2	1.7 ± 0.3	98 ± 28	—
	29	—	4.7 ± 2	1.76 ± 0.27	92 ± 14	—
	31	—	4.4 ± 2	1.54 ± 0.15	92 ± 19	—
	33	—	6 ± 3		93 ± 12	—
Hancock II stented bioprosthesis	27	—	—	—	—	2.21 ± 0.14
	29	—	—	—	—	2.77 ± 0.11
	31	—	—	—	—	2.84 ± 0.1
	33	—	—	—	—	3.15 ± 0.22
Hancock pericardial stented bioprosthesis	29	—	2.61 ± 1.39	1.42 ± 0.14	105 ± 36	—
	31	—	3.57 ± 1.02	1.51 ± 0.27	81 ± 23	—
Mitroflow stented bioprosthesis	25	—	6.9	2	90	—
	27	—	3.07 ± 0.91	1.5	90 ± 20	—
	29	—	3.5 ± 1.65	1.43 ± 0.29	102 ± 21	—
	31	—	3.85 ± 0.81	1.32 ± 0.26	91 ± 22	—

Modified from Rosenhek R, Binder T, Maurer G, et al. Normal valves for Doppler echocardiographic assessment of heart valve prostheses. J Am Soc Echocardiogr 2003;16:1116-1127.

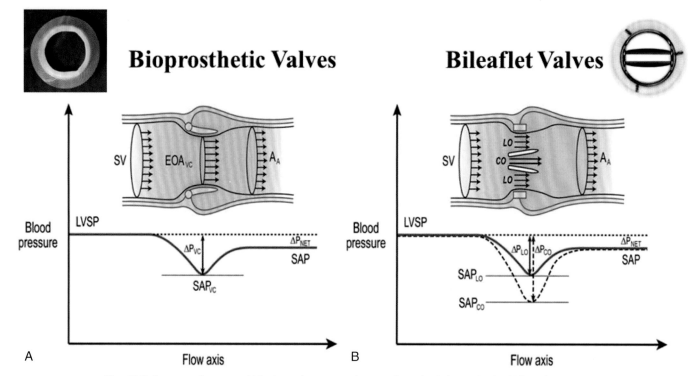

Fig. 26.2 Pressure Recovery. Velocity and pressure changes from the left ventricular (LV) outflow tract to the ascending aorta (A_A) in the setting of a stented bioprosthesis *(left)* and a bileaflet mechanical valve *(right)*. Because of pressure recovery, velocities are lower and systolic aortic pressure *(SAP)* is higher in the distal aorta than at the level of the vena contracta *(VC)*. This phenomenon is more exaggerated in the example of the bileaflet mechanical valve because the velocity is higher in the central orifice *(CO)*, where the pressure drop is higher. Doppler gradients are estimated from the maximal velocity at the level of the VC and represent the maximal pressure drop, whereas catheterization measurements reflect the systolic pressure difference (ΔP) between the LV and the A_A. *EOA,* Effective orifice area; *LO,* lateral orifice; *SP,* systolic pressure; *SV,* stroke volume. (Modified from Zoghbi WA, Chambers JB, Dumesnil JG, et al. Recommendations for evaluation of prosthetic valves with echocardiography and Doppler ultrasound. J Am Soc Echocardiogr 2009;22:975-1014.)

major orifices, resulting in estimated pressure gradients of 5 to 25 mmHg in the aortic position and 5 to 10 mmHg in the mitral position (see Tables 6.1 and 6.2).[9] Tilting disk valves also have a small amount of regurgitation, arising from small gaps at the perimeter of the valve. With the Hall-Medtronic valve, there is a small amount of regurgitation around the central guide strut.[9]

The bulky Starr-Edwards ball-cage valve (Edwards Lifesciences, Irvine, CA) (see Fig. 26.1B), the oldest commercially available prosthetic heart valve, was first used in 1965 and was discontinued in 2007. The ball-cage valve is more thrombogenic and has less favorable hemodynamic performance characteristics than bileaflet or tilting disk valves.

Durability and Long-Term Outcomes
Mechanical valves have excellent long-term durability, up to 50 years for the Starr-Edwards valve and more than 35 years for the SJM Regent valve. Structural valve deterioration (SVD), exemplified by some older-generation Björk-Shiley valves (i.e., strut fracture with disk embolization) and Starr-Edwards prostheses (i.e., ball variance), is now rare. The 10-year rate of freedom from valve-related death exceeds 90% for the SJM Regent and the Carbomedics bilealfet valves.[10] The Medtronic-Hall prosthesis has achieved comparable longevity. Actuarial survival rates, which depend on several patient factors such as age,

gender, ventricular function, coronary artery disease, functional status, and major comorbidities, range from 94% ± 2% at 10 years for SJM Regent valves to 85% ± 3% at 9 years for Omniscience valves and 60% to 70% at 10 years for Starr-Edwards valves (Table 26.3).[11–17]

All patients with mechanical valves require lifelong anticoagulation with a vitamin K antagonist (VKA). Direct-acting oral anticoagulants (DOACs) are not approved for use in this patient subset. In a small phase 2 study, dabigatran was associated with increased rates of thromboembolic and bleeding complications compared with warfarin.[18] Higher-intensity anticoagulation is required for mechanical valves placed in the mitral versus the aortic position, for patients with multiple mechanical prostheses, and often for patients with additional risk factors for thromboembolism (e.g., atrial fibrillation). Even with appropriately targeted anticoagulation, reported rates of thromboembolism range from 0.6 to 3.3 per 100 patient-years for patients with bileaflet or tilting disk valves.[12,13,16,17,19]

Complications related to anticoagulation in this population occur at rates of 0.9 to 2.3 per 100 patient-years.[20] Long-term issues associated with mechanical valves include infective endocarditis, paravalvular leak (PVL), hemolytic anemia, thromboembolism/valve thrombosis, pannus ingrowth, prosthesis–patient mismatch (PPM), and hemorrhagic complications related to anticoagulation (Fig. 26.3).

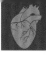

TABLE 26.3 Long-Term Outcome After Mechanical Valve Replacement: Selected Series.

Valve Type	Ref. No.	Years Implanted	N	Mean Age	Survival	COMPLICATIONS (%/PATIENT-YEAR)			
						Thrombo-embolism	Bleeding	Prosthetic Valve Endocarditis	Valve Thrombosis
Bileaflet									
SJM Regent	118	1977–1987	1298	62 ± 13	Event-free: 67% ± 8% at 9 yr	1.5	0.56	0.16	0.09
SJM Regent	25	1978–1991	91	39 (range, 15–50)	Event-free: 94% ± 2% at 10 yr	0.6	0.8	0.4	—
SJM Regent AVR	29	1977–1997	1419	63 ± 14	Actuarial: 82% at 5 yr 51% at 15 yr 45% at 19 yr	—	—	—	—
SJM Regent AVR + CABG	29	1977–1997	971	70 ± 10	Actuarial: 72% at 5 yr 45% at 10 yr 15% at 19 yr	—	—	—	—
Carbomedics	28	1989–1997	1019	61 ± 10	Event-free: 82% at 7 yr Mortality rate: 2.9%/yr	1.0	1.7	0.1	0.1
Tilting Disk									
Medtronic-Hall	24	1977–1987	1104	56	Actuarial: AVR 46% ± 2% at 15 yr	—	1.2	—	—
						1.8			0.05
					MVR 2% ± 4% at 15 yr	1.9			0.19
					DVR 28% ± 5% at 15 yr	1.9			0.13
Ball-Cage									
Starr-Edwards	26	1963–1977	362	40 ± 10 yr	Event-free: AVR 66.4% at 10 yr	1.36	1.06	—	—
					MVR 73.4%	1.25	0.56	—	—
Starr-Edwards	27	1969–1991	1100	57 yr	59.6% at 10 yr 31.2% at 20 yr	1.26	0.18	0.39	0.02

AVR, Aortic valve replacement; *CABG,* coronary artery bypass grafting surgery; *DVR,* double valve replacement; *MVR,* mitral valve replacement; *yr,* year.

Tissue Valves

Tissue or biological valves include porcine and bovine stented and stentless bioprostheses, homografts (or allografts) from human cadaveric sources, and autografts of pericardial or pulmonic valve origin. They provide an alternative, less thrombogenic heart valve substitute for which long-term anticoagulation in the absence of additional risk factors for thromboembolism is not required.

Stented Bioprostheses

The traditional design of a bioprosthetic valve consists of three biological leaflets made from a porcine aortic valve or bovine pericardium and treated with glutaraldehyde to reduce antigenicity. The leaflets are mounted on a metal or polymeric stented ring, and they open to a circular orifice in systole, resembling the anatomy of the native aortic valve (see Fig. 26.1C, D). Most bioprosthetic valves are treated with anticalcifying agents or processes.

Newer-generation bovine pericardial valves (Carpentier-Edwards Magna, Edwards Lifesciences [see Fig. 26.1D] or St. Jude Trifecta, Liva-Nova) offer improved hemodynamic performance compared with earlier-generation porcine bioprostheses (see Tables 26.1 and 26.2). In the aortic position, the antegrade velocity varies as a function of valve size but approximates 2.4 m/s, with a mean gradient of 14 mmHg and an indexed valve area of 1.04 cm²/m². The pericardial aortic valve has a larger EOA at any given valve size between 19 and 29 mm. The average peak gradient in the mitral position is 9 ± 3 mmHg, with an EOA of 2.5 ± 0.6 cm².[21] In a prospective randomized trial of patients with

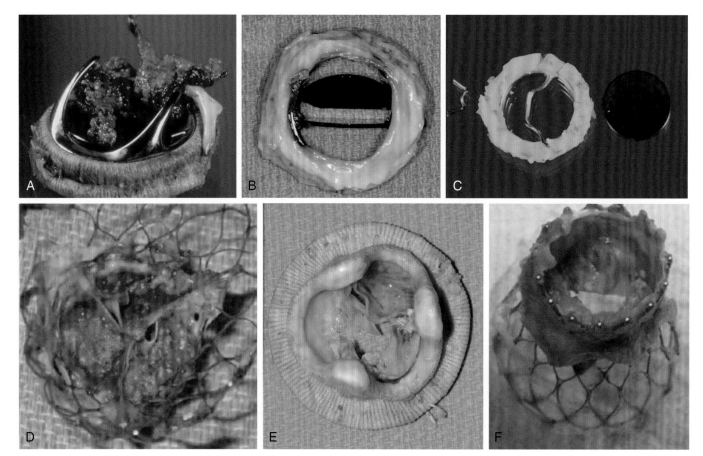

Fig. 26.3 Prosthetic Valve Complications. (A) Obstructing thrombus on a tilting disk prosthetic valve. (B) Pannus ingrowth interacting with leaflet opening in a bileaflet prosthetic valve. (C) Rupture of the outlet strut and leaflet escape in a Björk-Shiley prosthesis. (D) Thrombosis in a self-expanding transcatheter aortic valve. (E) Leaflet calcific degeneration and tear in a porcine bioprosthesis. (F) Leaflet calcific degeneration and stenosis in a self-expanding transcatheter aortic valve. (Courtesy Drs. Siamak Mohammadi, Quebec Heart and Lung Institute [A and C], and Christian Couture [B], Quebec Heart & Lung Institute, Quebec; Gosta Petterson, Cleveland Clinic, Cleveland [E]. D, From Ando T, Briasoulis A, Telila T, et al. Does mild paravalvular regurgitation post transcatheter aortic valve implantation affect survival? A meta-analysis. Catheter Cardiovasc Interv 2018;91:135-147. F, From Seeburger J, Weiss G, Borger MA, et al. Structural valve deterioration of a CoreValve prosthesis 9 months after implantation. Eur Heart J 2013;34:1607.)

aortic valve disease, the Carpentier-Edwards Perimount Magna bovine pericardial valve (Edwards Lifesciences) demonstrated better hemodynamic performance and greater LV mass regression over 5 postoperative years than the newer-generation Medtronic Mosaic porcine valve (Medtronic, Inc.).[22]

A small degree of regurgitation can be detected by color Doppler flow imaging in 10% of normally functioning bioprostheses. One limitation of earlier generations of bioprosthetic valves was their limited durability due to SVD, typically beginning within 5 to 7 years after implantation but varying by position and age at implantation, with tissue changes characterized by calcification, fibrosis, tears, and perforations (see Fig. 26.3).

SVD occurs earlier for mitral than for aortic bioprosthetic valves, perhaps because of exposure of the mitral prosthesis to relatively higher LV closing pressures. The process of SVD is accelerated in younger patients (Fig. 26.4), in those with disordered calcium homeostasis (e.g., end-stage renal disease), and possibly in pregnant women independent of younger age. With most current-generation bioprosthetic pericardial valves, the durability is excellent, with SVD rates of 2% to 10% at 10 years, 10% to 20% at 15 years, and 40% at 20 years[23,24] (Table 26.4; Fig. 26.5). Accelerated SVD and reduced survival have been reported with Mitroflow models 12A/LX.[25]

Stentless Bioprostheses

The rigid sewing ring and stent-based construction of certain bioprostheses allow easier implantation and maintenance of the three-dimensional relationships of the leaflets. However, these features also contribute to impaired hemodynamic performance and accelerated SVD. Stentless porcine valves (see Fig. 26.1E) were developed in part to address these issues. Their use has been restricted to the aortic position. Implantation is technically more challenging, whether they are deployed in a subcoronary position or as part of a mini-root, and they are therefore preferred by only a minority of surgeons.

Early postoperative mean gradients can be less than 15 mmHg (with further improvement in valve performance over time due to aortic root remodeling), leading to lower peak exercise transvalvular gradients and more rapid reduction in LV mass.[26] David et al. reported a rate of freedom from SVD with the stentless Toronto

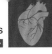

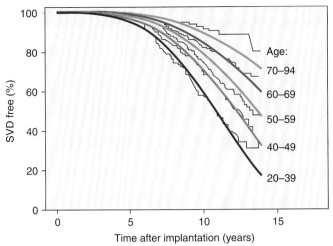

Fig. 26.4 Freedom From Structural Valve Deterioration (SVD). Actuarial Freedom from SVD for 4910 Operative Survivors of Isolated Aortic or Mitral Valve Replacement with a Hancock Porcine Valve (Medtronic, Inc., Minneapolis, MN) or a Carpentier-Edwards porcine valve (Edwards Lifesciences Corporation, Irvine, CA). The curves are stratified by age group and show a significantly lower rate of SVD for older compared with younger patients. A Weibull regression model based on patient age and valve position *(smooth lines)* was used to fit the actuarial Kaplan-Meier curves *(jagged lines)*. (Modified from Grunkemeier GL, Jamieson WRE, Miller DC, et al. Actual vs. actuarial risk of structural valve deterioration. J Thoracic Cardiovasc Surg 1994;108:709-718.)

SPV (St. Jude Medical, St. Paul, MN) at 12 years of 69% ± 4%, 52% ± 8% for patients younger than 65 years, and 85% ± 4% for patients 65 years of age and older.[27] The researchers limited the use of this stentless valve to older patients with small aortic annuli. They also emphasized the marked mortality hazard associated with reoperation for valve failure within 1 year of implantation.[27] Sutureless bioprosthetic valves have been developed to decrease the complexity and duration of implantation of bioprosthetic valves (see Fig. 26.1G).

Homografts

Aortic valve homografts are harvested from human cadavers within 24 hours of death and are treated with antibiotics and cryopreserved at −196°C. They have become most commonly implanted in the form of a total root replacement with reimplantation of the coronary arteries. Homograft valves appear to be resistant to infection and are preferred by many surgeons for management of aortic valve and root endocarditis in the active phase. Neither immune suppression nor routine anticoagulation is required.

Despite earlier expectations, long-term durability beyond 10 years is not superior to that for current-generation pericardial valves,[28] and reoperation may be technically more challenging due to excessive root and leaflet calcification. In an echocardiographic follow-up study of 570 patients with aortic valve homografts, 72% had signs of valve dysfunction at 6.8 ± 4.1 years after implantation, with moderate to severe aortic regurgitation in 15.4%, moderate aortic stenosis in 10%, and severe aortic stenosis in 2.5%.[29] Rates of homograft reoperation at 15 years for SVD, which do not account for all cases of SVD, approximate 20% for patients 41 to 60 years of age and 16% for those older than 60 years at the time of implantation.[30]

Autografts

In the Ross procedure, the patient's own pulmonic valve or autograft is harvested as a small tissue block containing the pulmonic valve, annulus, and proximal pulmonary artery; it is inserted in the aortic position, usually as a complete root replacement with reimplantation of the coronary arteries.[31] The pulmonic valve and right ventricular outflow tract are then replaced with an aortic or a pulmonic homograft. The procedure therefore requires two separate valve operations, a longer time on cardiopulmonary bypass, and a steep learning curve. With appropriate selection of young patients by expert surgeons at experienced centers of excellence, operative mortality rates are less than 1%, and 20-year survival rates are as high as 95% and similar to those of the general population.[31] Advantages of the autograft include its ability to increase in size during childhood growth, excellent hemodynamic performance characteristics, lack of thrombogenicity, and resistance to infection.

The hemodynamic performance characteristics of the pulmonary autograft are similar to those of a normal, native aortic valve. Early homograft stenosis occurs in 10% to 20% of patients and is caused by extrinsic compression from inflammation and adventitial fibrosis.[32,33] The procedure is usually reserved for children and young adults but should be avoided in patients with dilated aortic roots given the unacceptably high incidence of accelerated degeneration, pulmonary autograft dilatation, and significant regurgitation. Significant degrees of aortic regurgitation and the deposition of calcium are additional markers for suboptimal outcomes. In propensity-matched analyses, survival and functional outcomes with the Ross procedure have equaled or exceeded those observed with mechanical or bioprosthetic valve replacement in selected young patients.[31]

Transcatheter Bioprostheses

Transcatheter aortic valve replacement (TAVR) is a valuable alternative to surgical aortic valve replacement (SAVR) in patients with symptomatic severe aortic stenosis across the spectrum of operative risk. The TAVR case volume in the United States surpassed SAVR case volume for treatment of isolated aortic stenosis in 2016, and the gap has continued to widen.[34] Two main types of transcatheter aortic valves are used: balloon-expandable valves and self-expanding valves (see Fig. 12.1 in Chapter 12).

The Edwards Sapien XT and Sapien 3 balloon-expandable valves (Edwards Lifesciences) consist of a three-leaflet pericardial bovine valve mounted in a cobalt-chromium frame. These valves are available in 20-, 23-, 26-, and 29-mm sizes. The most common access routes for TAVR are the transfemoral, transapical, and transaortic routes. Approximately 80% to 90% of TAVR procedures are performed using the transfemoral approach. As catheter sheath sizes decrease (i.e., 14 or 16 Fr for most valves), access is anticipated to shift even more toward the transfemoral approach. The transfemoral approach is associated with lower mortality rates and more rapid recovery compared with alternative access approaches.

The CoreValve Evolut R and Evolut Pro self-expanding valves (Medtronic, Inc.) consist of three leaflets of porcine pericardium seated relatively higher in a nitinol frame to provide true supra-annular positioning of valve leaflets. The valves are available in 23-, 26-, 29-, and 31-mm sizes. The CoreValve Evolut R and Evolut Pro are most frequently implanted using the transfemoral approach.

For a given aortic annulus size, transcatheter valves have larger EOAs and lower transvalvular gradients compared with surgical bioprosthetic valves. Rates of SVD have not been higher with TAVR valves than with SAVR valves.[35,36] Compared with SAVR, transcatheter valve implantation results in higher rates of PVL[37] and heart block

TABLE 26.4 Long-Term Outcome After Tissue Valve Replacement: Selected Series.

Valve Type	Ref. No.	Years Implanted	N	Age (Yr ± SD)	Actuarial Survival	Freedom From (or Annual Rate of) Thrombo-embolism	Freedom From (or Annual Rate of Structural Valve Deterioration
Stented Bioprostheses							
Porcine (Hancock and Carpentier-Edwards)	39	1971–1990	2879	AVR 60 ± 15	77% ± 1% at 5 yr 54% ± 2% at 10 yr 32% ± 3% at 15 yr	92% ± 1% at 10 yr	78% ± 2% at 10 yr 49% ± 4% at 15 yr
				MVR 58 ± 13	70% ± 1% at 5 yr 50% ± 2% at 10 yr 32% ± 3% at 15 yr	86% ± 1% at 10 yr	69% ± 2% at 10 yr 32% ± 4% at 15 yr
Carpentier-Edwards Porcine	40	1975–1986	1195	57.3	57.4% ± 1.5% at 10 yr	(1.6%/pt-yr)	(3.3%/pt-yr)
Carpentier-Edwards Pericardial	42	1984–1995	254	71 (range, 25–87)	80% ± 3% at 5 yr 50% ± 8% at 10 yr 36% ± 9% at 12 yr	67% ± 13% at 12 yr	86% ± 9% at 12 yr
Stentless Bioprostheses							
Toronto SPV	105	1987–1993	123	61 ± 12	91% ± 4% at 6 yr	87% ± 7% at 6 yr	(0%/pt-yr)
Edwards Prima	106	1991–1993	200	68.5 ± 8	95% at 1 yr	(3% at 1 yr)	(AV block requiring pacemaker 7% at 1 yr, mild AR 27% at 1yr)
Homografts							
Cryopreserved	107	1981–1991	18	46	85% at 8 yr		85% at 8 yr
Antibiotic sterilized, subcoronary	108	1973–1983	200	50	81% ± 3% at 10 yr 58% ± 4% at 20 yr	31% ± 5% at 20 yr 81% ± 3% at 10 yr	
Pulmonic Autografts							
Pulmonic autografts	109	1986–1995	195	8 mo–62 yr			95% ± 2% at 2 yr 81% ± 5% at 8 yr
Pulmonary autografts	28	1994–2001	108	38 (range, 19–66)	95% at 5 yr 95% at 10 yr		99% freedom from reoperation at 10 yr

AR, Aortic regurgitation; *AV*, atrioventricular; *AVR*, aortic valve replacement; *MVR*, mitral valve replacement.

necessitating permanent pacemaker insertion. The risks of PVL and heart block have decreased over time with improved case selection and device performance. Moderate to severe PVL is associated with a 2.0- to 2.5-fold increase in mortality rates.[38] Some studies suggest that even mild pulmonary valve regurgitation may have a deleterious impact on outcomes in vulnerable patient subsets (e.g., patients with severe LV concentric hypertrophy and severe diastolic dysfunction without preexisting AR).[39]

Current-generation balloon-expandable valves (Sapien 3) are designed with a skirt at the inflow aspect of the valve stent to reduce the incidence of PVL. Self-expanding valves have slightly larger EOAs and lower gradients but somewhat higher rates of PVL than balloon-expandable valves.[40,41] Self-expanding valves are also associated with a higher incidence of postprocedural PPM.[42,43] Placement of a TAVR valve inside a failed surgically implanted bioprosthesis (valve-in-valve

procedure) is approved for patients who are considered to be at high risk for reoperation.[44]

Comparison of Mechanical and Tissue Valves

Obvious differences between valve types correlate chiefly with durability (i.e., theoretically indefinite for mechanical versus limited for tissue valves) and the need for anticoagulation (i.e., obligatory for mechanical versus none for tissue valves absent other risk factors for thromboembolism). Short- to intermediate-term hemodynamic performance characteristics of low-profile mechanical prostheses (e.g., SJM Regent) are comparable to those of stented tissue valves of similar size. There are no important differences in rates of prosthetic valve endocarditis (PVE), although some series have suggested a higher incidence of early (<1 year) infection with mechanical valves compared with bioprostheses.[45]

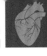

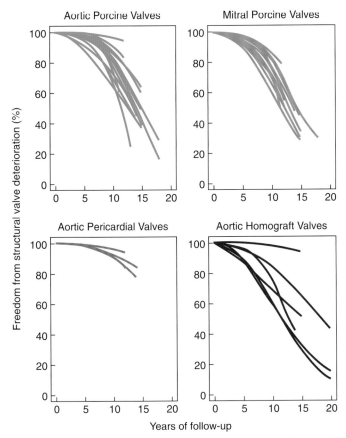

Fig. 26.5 Freedom From Structural Valve Deterioration (SVD). Weibull distribution curves for freedom from SVD for four types of tissue valves. Notice the more gradual rate of SVD for aortic pericardial valves. (Modified from Grunkemeier GL, Li H-H, Naftel DC, et al. Long-term performance of heart valve prostheses. Curr Prob Cardiol 2000;25:73-156.)

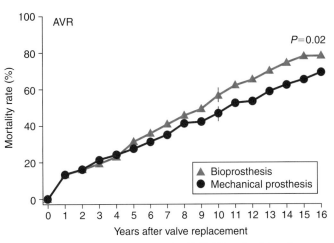

Fig. 26.6 Veterans Affairs Randomized Trial Results. Mortality rates after aortic valve replacement (AVR) with a mechanical prosthesis (Björk-Shiley, Pfizer, Inc., New York, NY) and a stented porcine prosthesis (Hancock, Medtronic, Inc., Minneapolis, MN). At 15 years, the mortality rate was 66% ± 3% for the mechanical valve versus 79% ± 3% for the porcine valve (P = 0.02). (From Hammermeister K, Sethi GK, Henderson WG, et al. Outcomes 15 years after valve replacement with a mechanical versus a bioprosthetic valve: final report of the Veteran Affairs randomized trial. J Am Coll Cardiol 2000;36:1152-1158.)

In the Veterans Affairs randomized trial conducted between 1977 and 1982, patients undergoing aortic valve replacement (AVR) had a better 15-year survival rate with a mechanical valve than with a bioprosthetic valve, whereas there was no difference in survival with mechanical versus biological MVR[46] (Fig. 26.6). With AVR, the increased mortality rate for patients allocated a bioprosthesis was driven largely by the higher rate of SVD. There was an increased risk of bleeding with mechanical valve replacement, but no significant differences were observed for other valve-related complications such as thromboembolism or PVE. A later, smaller randomized trial of patients 55 to 70 years of age with aortic valve disease showed no difference in late survival rates between newer-generation mechanical versus bioprosthetic valves. The rates of SVD and re-operation were higher for patients with bioprostheses, but there were no other differences in secondary end points.[47]

In an analysis of more than 39,000 AVR patients 65 to 80 years of age reported to the STS Adult Cardiac Surgery Database and linked to the Medicare health insurance program, patients receiving a bioprosthesis had a similar adjusted risk of death, higher risks of reoperation and PVE, and lower risks of stroke and bleeding compared with patients receiving a mechanical valve.[48]

Two propensity-matched analyses from New York's Statewide Planning and Research Cooperative System (SPARCS) reported no survival differences for patients 50 to 69 years of age undergoing mechanical versus bioprosthetic aortic or mitral valve replacement.[49,50] Rates of

stroke and bleeding were higher but rates of reoperation were lower among mechanical valve recipients. However, a survival advantage among patients in this age group who underwent mechanical rather than bioprosthetic valve replacement was reported from the Swedish system for the Enhancement and Development of Evidence-based care in Heart disease Evaluated According to Recommended Therapies (SWEDEHEART) register.[51] Stroke risk was similar for the groups, although bleeding rates were higher and the need for reoperation was lower after mechanical valve replacement.

Overall survival and rates of reoperation, stroke, and bleeding after bioprosthetic versus mechanical valve replacement were examined in a 2017 report from the California Office of Statewide Health Planning and Development.[52] Among patients who underwent AVR, receipt of a biological prosthesis was associated with a significantly higher 15-year mortality rate than receipt of a mechanical prosthesis among patients 45 to 54 years of age (hazard ratio = 1.23; P = 0.03), but the same did not hold true for patients 55 to 64 years of age. Among patients 40 to 49 years of age who underwent MVR, receipt of a biological prosthesis was associated with significantly higher mortality rates than receipt of a mechanical prosthesis (hazard ratio = 1.88; P < 0.001); among those 50 to 69 years of age, the mortality rates were 50.0% and 45.3%, respectively (hazard ratio = 1.16; P = 0.01) (Fig. 26.7). There was significant increase in the use of bioprosthetic valves over the 17-year period examined (1996–2013). Rates of reoperation were lower but rates of bleeding and stroke (in some age groups) were higher for those who received a mechanical valve.[52]

CHOICE OF VALVE PROCEDURE AND PROSTHESIS TYPE

Valve Procedure

After the indication for valve intervention is established, the next step is to select the type of procedure (i.e., repair versus replacement) and, if necessary, the type of prosthetic valve preferred by the patient after

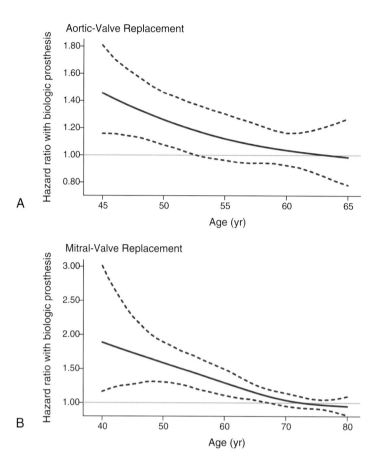

Fig. 26.7 Hazard of Death Associated With a Biologic Prosthesis. Age-dependent hazard of death with a biologic prosthesis compared with a mechanical prosthesis in the aortic (A) or mitral (B) position. These spline analyses suggest that replacement with a biologic valve compared with a mechanical valve is associated with an excess mortality risk for patients undergoing surgical aortic valve replacement who are younger than 55 years of age and for patients undergoing surgical mitral valve replacement who are younger than 70 years of age. (From Goldstone AB, Chiu P, Baiocchi M, et al. Mechanical or biologic prostheses for aortic valve and mitral valve replacement. N Engl J Med 2017;377:1847-1857.)

informed discussion with the implanting surgeon.[44] This choice is based on consideration of several factors, including valve durability, expected hemodynamics for a specific valve type and size, anatomic considerations, surgeon experience, the potential need for long-term anticoagulation, and patient preferences.

Indications for TAVR are evolving, but it is expected that this therapy will soon be available to patients with symptomatic severe aortic stenosis across the entire spectrum of surgical risk.[42,43,53,54] Questions remain about its possible use in patients with bicuspid aortic valve disease (who have been excluded from the randomized, controlled trials of TAVR vs. SAVR)[55] and patients with aortic regurgitation.[56] An additional challenge is to determine the appropriate sequence of procedures in younger patients (e.g., age < 65 years) with aortic stenosis who choose to avoid a mechanical valve and are therefore at risk for repeated surgical and transcatheter interventions for SVD over the following decades.

Practice guideline updates are expected to address recommendations for TAVR versus SAVR as a function of age. It remains difficult in practice to withhold TAVR from patients with a high burden of comorbidities and an expected survival time that is estimated in months, not years. There are several reasons to consider SAVR instead of TAVR, including anatomic concerns (e.g., extent and distribution of calcium), access issues, and the need for concomitant procedures such as root or ascending aortic replacement and coronary bypass grafting.

In patients with chronic severe primary mitral regurgitation who meet an indication for mitral valve surgery, mitral valve repair is recommended instead of MVR when a successful and durable repair can be accomplished.[44] In patients with chronic secondary mitral regurgitation undergoing surgery, MVR may be superior to mitral valve repair in many patients because it is associated with lower rates of recurrent regurgitation and cardiovascular morbidity.[44,57] Transcatheter edge-to-edge repair using a clip device has been approved to treat patients with severe primary mitral regurgitation and prohibitive surgical risk and patients who have heart failure and reduced LV ejection fraction with moderately severe or severe mitral regurgitation after optimization of medical therapy, including cardiac resynchronization when indicated.[58,59] Other transcatheter repair and replacement systems for the treatment of mitral regurgitation are under development.

Tricuspid valve annuloplasty repair is frequently performed at the time of left-sided valve surgery when tricuspid regurgitation is severe or there is significant tricuspid annular dilatation (>40 mm) despite only a mild or moderate degree of tricuspid regurgitation.[24] Tricuspid valve replacement is undertaken for severe valve disease that cannot be repaired, such as advanced rheumatic disease, carcinoid, or destructive endocarditis. Indications for transcatheter tricuspid valve intervention are evolving. Surgical or transcatheter pulmonic valve replacement in adults is rare.

Prosthetic Valve Type

The 2017 international practice guidelines for the management of patients with valvular heart disease (VHD) emphasize the need for shared decision making and recommend a bioprosthesis for patients of any age for whom anticoagulant therapy is contraindicated, cannot be managed appropriately, or is not desired. A mechanical prosthesis is reasonable for AVR or MVR in patients younger than 50 years of age who do not have a contraindication to anticoagulation, whereas a bioprosthesis is reasonable in patients more than 70 years old.[44,60,61] A bioprosthetic or mechanical valve is reasonable in patients between 50 and 70 years of age. A bioprosthesis is reasonable for young women contemplating pregnancy to avoid the hazards of anticoagulation. Whether the age thresholds for improved survival given in the 2017 California report (i.e., mechanical AVR up to age 54 years, mechanical MVR up to age 70 years[52]) will influence patient and surgeon decision making is uncertain.

MEDICAL MANAGEMENT AND SURVEILLANCE AFTER VALVE REPLACEMENT

Anti-Thrombotic Therapy
General Principles

Table 26.5 lists anti-thrombotic regimens recommended in the 2017 American Heart Association (AHA)/American College of Cardiology (ACC) update of the 2014 guideline for the management of patients with VHD for different types of procedures and prosthetic valves.[44,61] All patients with mechanical heart valves require lifelong anticoagulation with a VKA, the intensity of which varies as a function of valve type or thrombogenicity, valve position and number, and additional risk factors for thromboembolism, such as atrial fibrillation, LV systolic dysfunction, a history of thromboembolism, and hypercoagulable state (Fig. 26.8; see Table 26.5).

Anticoagulation should be initiated as soon after surgery as is deemed safe, preferably within the first 2 days, beginning with intravenous unfractionated heparin (UFH) and transitioning to a VKA. The risk of thromboembolism is highest in the first postoperative month. The development of thromboembolism at therapeutic levels of anticoagulation is managed by adding low-dose aspirin or increasing the target International Normalized Ratio (INR) range, or both.

Whether aspirin should be routinely provided to all mechanical heart valve recipients, as recommended by AHA/ACC guidelines, is under reconsideration.[60,61] Anticoagulant therapy with oral direct thrombin inhibitors or anti-Xa agents should not be used in patients with mechanical prostheses.[18,44,61] Although there is no clear consensus, a VKA may be used even in the absence of risk factors for thromboembolism for the first 3 to 6 months after bioprosthetic AVR or MVR,[44,60,61] when the risk of bleeding is low.

TABLE 26.5 Antithrombotic Therapy in Patients With Prosthetic Valves.

	VKA (Target INR)	Aspirin (75–100 mg)	Clopidogrel (75 mg)	Class
MECHANICAL VALVES				
AVR: Bileaflet or current generation single-tilting disc valves and no risk factors for thromboembolism[a]	Yes (INR: 2.5)	Yes[b]	No	I
AVR: Older-generation valves[c] and/or any risk factor for thromboembolism*	Yes (INR: 3.0)	Yes	No	I
MVR: Mechanical valves	Yes (INR: 3.0)	Yes	No	I
AVR: On-X valve and no risk factors for thromboembolism	Yes (INR: 1.5–2.0[b])	Yes	No	IIb
BIOPROSTHETIC VALVES				
AVR or MVR and no risk factors for thromboembolism: first 3–6 months	Yes (INR: 2.5)	Yes	No	IIb
AVR or MVR: after first 3–6 months	No	Yes	No	I
TRANSCATHETER AORTIC VALVES				
First 6 months	No	Yes	Yes	IIb
After first 6 months and no evidence of leaflet thrombosis[e]	No	Yes	No	IIb

[a]Risk factors for thromboembolism: Atrial fibrillation, LV dysfunction (LVEF ≤35%), LA dilation (LA diameter ≥50 mm), previous thromboembolism, and hypercoagulable condition.
[b]If bleeding risk with dual anti-thrombotic therapy is low.
[c]Ball-in-cage valves, older generation of single tilting-disc valves.
[d]INR 2.0–3.0 for first 3 months after AVR.
[e]Leaflet thrombosis is treated with a VKA or DOAC with serial follow-up.
AVR, Aortic valve replacement; *INR*, International Normalized Ratio; *MVR*, mitral valve replacement; *VKA*, vitamin K antagonist.

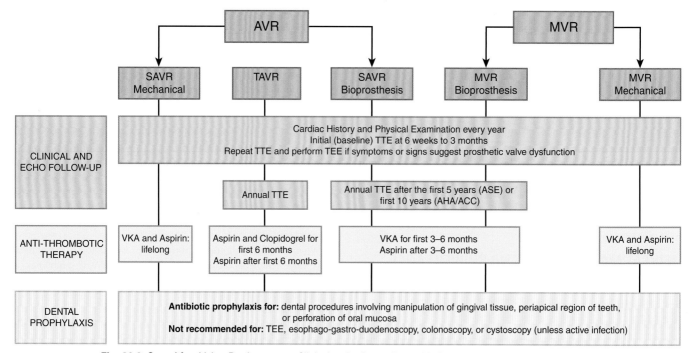

Fig. 26.8 Care After Valve Replacement. Clinical and echocardiographic follow-up, anti-thrombotic therapy, and antibiotic prophylaxis after heart valve replacement. *ACC,* American College of Cardiology; *AHA,* American Heart Association; *ASE,* American Society of Echocardiography; *AVR,* aortic valve replacement; *MVR,* mitral valve replacement; *SAVR,* surgical aortic valve replacement; *TAVR:* transcatheter aortic valve replacement; *TEE,* transesophageal echocardiography; *TTE,* transthoracic echocardiography; *VKA,* vitamin K antagonist. (Data from Nishimura RA, Otto CM, Bonow RO, et al. 2014 AHA/ACC guideline for the management of patients with valvular heart disease: a report of the American College of Cardiology/American Heart Association Task Force on Practice Guidelines. J Am Coll Cardiol 2014;63:e57-e185; Avezum A, Lopes RD, Schulte PJ, et al. Apixaban in comparison with warfarin in patients with atrial fibrillation and valvular heart disease. Findings from the Apixaban for Reduction in Stroke and Other Thromboembolic Events in Atrial Fibrillation (ARISTOTLE) trial. Circulation 2015;132:624-632.)

A report from the Danish National Patient Registry highlighted an association between the discontinuation of warfarin within 6 months after bioprosthetic AVR and an increased risk of cardiovascular death.[62] Longer-term treatment of low-risk bioprosthetic AVR and MVR patients has traditionally consisted of low-dose aspirin, although there are no data to support this practice. There is a growing experience with the use of direct oral anticoagulants (DOACs) in patients after bioprosthetic heart valve replacement or repair who develop a late (nonperioperative) indication for anticoagulation, such as atrial fibrillation. In this context, DOACs demonstrate comparable efficacy and improved safety compared with warfarin.[63]

Protocols for management after TAVR are evolving, but most patients continue to receive dual antiplatelet therapy for several months after the procedure before transitioning to monotherapy (usually aspirin)[44,60,61] (see Fig. 26.8). A small (*N* = 222 patients) randomized, controlled trial of single versus dual antiplatelet therapy after TAVR showed no difference in ischemic outcomes but a significant increase in the risk of major or non–life-threatening bleeding with dual-antiplatelet therapy.[64] These results were confirmed in a small (*N* = 840 patients) meta-analysis comprising three randomized, controlled trials and three observational studies.[65] Additional, larger-scale trials are underway.

There is heightened sensitivity to the development of bioprosthetic valve thrombosis as suggested by an increase of more than 10 mmHg in mean TAVR gradient and computed tomography (CT) evidence of hypoattenuating defects, leaflet thickening, and reduced excursion. This entity is less common among surgical bioprosthetic valve recipients. Treatment with warfarin or a DOAC is recommended.[66]

Interruption of Anti-Thrombotic Therapy

In the planned interruption of oral anticoagulant therapy for noncardiac surgery, the following factors must be taken into account: the nature of the procedure; the magnitude of risk of thromboembolism based on valve type, position, and number; underlying patient risk factors; and the competing risk of periprocedural hemorrhage.[61] Low-risk patients with low-profile bileaflet or tilting disk mechanical valves in the aortic position can usually stop VKA therapy 3 to 5 days before noncardiac surgery and then resume it postoperatively as soon as it is considered safe, without the need for a heparin bridge. In all other mechanical heart valve patients, low-molecular-weight heparin (LMWH) or intravenous UFH should be given before and after surgery, as directed by the surgeon.[44,61]

The use of LMWH avoids the need for preoperative hospitalization. There is a paucity of randomized trial data and tremendous institutional and operator variability in the use of bridging strategies for noncardiac surgery in these patients. A study of patients immediately after mechanical heart valve replacement found the use of LMWH to be a safe and effective bridging strategy until achievement of therapeutic levels of oral anticoagulation.[67]

In bioprosthetic heart valve patients receiving a DOAC, timing of interruption depends on the nature of the procedure, individual drug pharmacokinetics, and renal function. The need for neuraxial anesthesia or intervention demands that the agent be stopped at least 72 hours beforehand.[68] Bridging considerations are similar to those for mechanical heart valve patients and are based on risk-benefit analysis. Familiarity with the use of oral anticoagulant antidotes (e.g., four-factor prothrombin concentrate complex, idarucizumab, andexanet alfa) is beneficial.

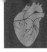

Pregnancy

Pregnant patients with prosthetic heart valves should be followed closely because of the increased hemodynamic burden that can cause or worsen heart failure if there is prosthetic valve dysfunction and because of the hypercoagulable state related to pregnancy that increases the risk of valve thrombosis. All anti-thrombotic regimens carry an increased risk to the fetus and increased risks of miscarriage and maternal bleeding. Patients require appropriate counseling, close monitoring, and adjustment of anticoagulation therapy.

Warfarin therapy appears to be the safest anticoagulant strategy for the mother, although it carries a risk of fetal embryopathy, the aggregate incidence of which has been estimated at 6%.[69,70] Exposure during the 6th to 12th weeks of gestation may be most harmful. However, observational data suggest that the risk of embryopathy may be dose related and that fetal abnormalities are less common (<3%) with maternal doses of warfarin lower than 5 mg/day.[71-73] There is also a small risk of fetal central nervous system abnormalities with first-trimester use of VKAs.

In pregnant patients with mechanical valves, warfarin is reasonable in the first trimester if the dose is 5 mg/day or less, and warfarin is recommended to achieve a therapeutic INR target in the second and third trimesters.[44,61] An alternative is twice-daily, dose-adjusted LMWH throughout pregnancy, aiming for an anti-Xa level between 0.8 and 1.2 IU/mL, assessed 4 hours after a subcutaneous dose. LMWH is not advised if anti-Xa levels cannot be monitored.

Testing should be performed every week, given the pharmacokinetic changes that occur with pregnancy.[44] If UFH is provided, the activated partial thromboplastin time (aPTT) should be twice the control value, or the anti-Xa level should be 0.35 to 0.70 IU/mL. Discontinuation of warfarin with initiation of intravenous UFH is recommended before delivery for pregnant patients with a mechanical valve. Low-dose aspirin can be given safely in the second and third trimesters[44,61] if indicated and if the bleeding risk is low.

Infective Endocarditis Prophylaxis

Patients with prosthetic valves are at increased risk for infective endocarditis because of the foreign valve surface and sewing ring. Antibiotic prophylaxis is recommended for patients with prosthetic valves who undergo dental procedures that involve manipulation of gingival tissue, the periapical region of teeth, or perforation of the oral mucosa. Prophylaxis is not recommended for nondental procedures such as TEE, esophagogastroduodenoscopy, colonoscopy, or cystoscopy (unless there is active infection in these areas)[44,45] (see Fig. 26.8).

Clinical Assessment

Postoperative visits should begin 3 to 6 weeks after valve implantation. The first visit is focused on ensuring a smooth transition from the hospital or rehabilitation facility to home, reconciling medications, and assessing neurocognitive function, wound healing, volume status, heart rhythm, and the auscultatory findings (Fig. 26.9). The history at subsequent visits is tailored to detect symptoms that suggest heart failure or reduced functional capacity, arrhythmia, thromboembolism, or infection. Adherence to the recommended schedule of INR determinations and the relative time spent in the therapeutic range should be assessed for all patients treated with VKAs. Renal function is tracked in patients receiving DOACs.[68] Problems with bleeding should be identified.

A focused cardiovascular examination is repeated at each visit (see Fig. 26.8). Instructions regarding antibiotic prophylaxis are repeated. After the 6-month mark, follow-up visits can be conducted annually unless interim problems arise.

A chest radiograph is obtained by the surgeon at the first visit to assess for residual pleural fluid, pneumothorax, lung aeration, and

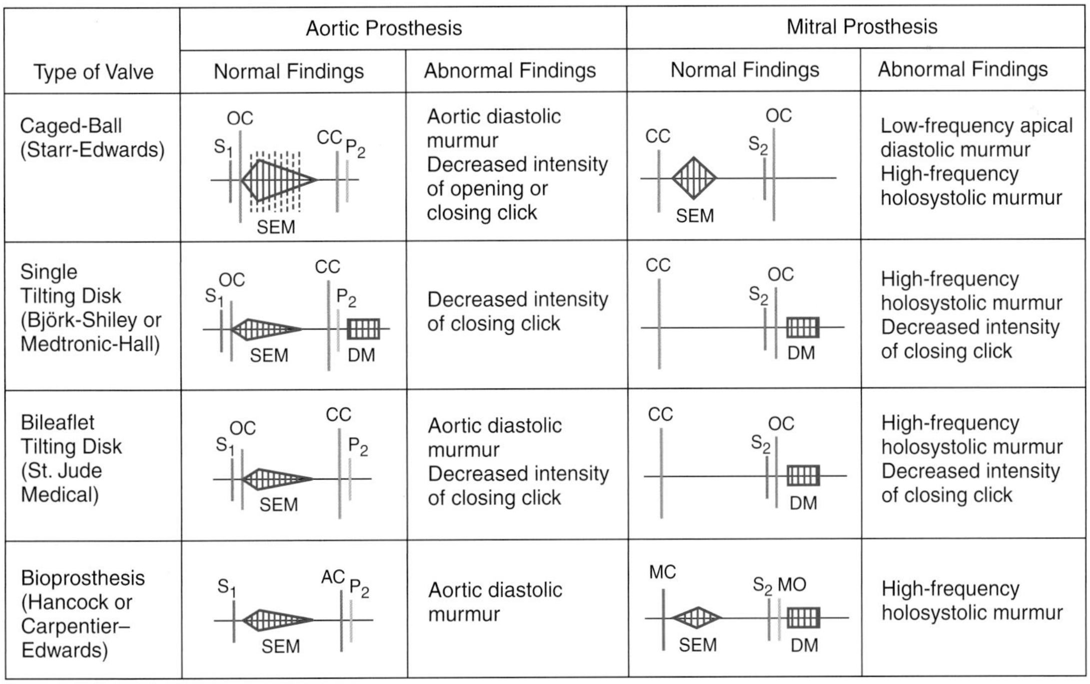

Type of Valve	Aortic Prosthesis		Mitral Prosthesis	
	Normal Findings	Abnormal Findings	Normal Findings	Abnormal Findings
Caged-Ball (Starr-Edwards)	OC, S₁, CC, P₂, SEM	Aortic diastolic murmur. Decreased intensity of opening or closing click	CC, OC, S₂, SEM	Low-frequency apical diastolic murmur. High-frequency holosystolic murmur
Single Tilting Disk (Björk-Shiley or Medtronic-Hall)	OC, S₁, CC, P₂, SEM, DM	Decreased intensity of closing click	CC, OC, S₂, DM	High-frequency holosystolic murmur. Decreased intensity of closing click
Bileaflet Tilting Disk (St. Jude Medical)	OC, S₁, CC, P₂, SEM	Aortic diastolic murmur. Decreased intensity of closing click	CC, OC, S₂, DM	High-frequency holosystolic murmur. Decreased intensity of closing click
Bioprosthesis (Hancock or Carpentier–Edwards)	S₁, AC, P₂, SEM	Aortic diastolic murmur	MC, S₂, MO, SEM, DM	High-frequency holosystolic murmur

Fig. 26.9 Auscultatory Characteristics of Prosthetic Heart Valves. Findings are stratified according to valve type and position. *AC,* Aortic closure; *CC,* closing click; *DM,* diastolic murmur; *MC,* mitral valve closure; *MO,* mitral opening; *OC,* opening click; *P₂,* pulmonary valve closure; *S₁,* first heart sound; *S₂,* second heart sound; *SEM,* systolic ejection murmur. (From Vongpatanasin W, Hillis D, Lange RA. Prosthetic heart valves. N Engl J Med 1996;335:407-416.)

heart size. Electrocardiography is routinely performed and should be reviewed for rhythm, conduction, and dynamic repolarization changes. Postoperative baseline values of hemoglobin, hematocrit, lactate dehydrogenase (LDH), haptoglobin, and bilirubin should be established for patients with mechanical heart valves, allowing future comparisons if hemolysis is suspected. Other laboratory studies are performed as clinically relevant.

Doppler Echocardiography

An initial TTE examination performed 6 weeks to 3 months after prosthetic valve implantation is recommended to assess prosthetic valve and ventricular function and to serve as a baseline for comparison if complications or deterioration occur later[73,74] (see Fig. 26.8). Repeat TTE and TEE are recommended if there is a change in clinical symptoms or signs suggesting valve dysfunction. For patients with a bioprosthetic valve, routine annual TTE follow-up is recommended after year 5 by the American Society of Echocardiography (ASE)[73] but not until year 10 by the 2014 AHA/ACC VHD guideline writing committee[44] (see Fig. 26.8).

Studies based on Doppler-echocardiographic follow-up estimate that 25% to 35% of patients with a bioprosthesis implanted for less than 10 years in the aortic position have some degree of valve degeneration or dysfunction.[75,76] For patients with mechanical valves, routine annual echocardiography is not indicated in the absence of a change in clinical status.[44]

A complete echocardiographic study includes two-dimensional imaging of the prosthetic valve, evaluation of the valve leaflet/occluder morphology and mobility, measurement of the transprosthetic velocity and gradients, valve EOA, Doppler velocity index, estimation of the degree of regurgitation, evaluation of LV size and systolic function, and calculation of systolic pulmonary arterial pressure.[73,74] The fluid dynamics of mechanical valves may differ substantially from those of the native and bioprosthetic valves (see Fig. 26.2). The flow is eccentric in monoleaflet valves and is composed of three separate jets in bileaflet valves. Because the direction of the jets across prosthetic valves may be eccentric, multiwindow continuous-wave (CW) Doppler interrogation is essential to obtain the highest transprosthetic velocity signal. Occasionally, an abnormally high jet gradient corresponding to localized high velocity may be recorded by CW Doppler interrogation through the smaller central orifice of a bileaflet mechanical prosthesis in the aortic or mitral position. This phenomenon may lead to an overestimation of gradient, underestimation of the EOA, and therefore a false impression of prosthesis dysfunction.

Paravalvular regurgitation is more common after TAVR than after SAVR. Moreover, the measurement of valve EOA is more challenging in transcatheter valves than in surgical valves due to the presence of the valve stent in the LV outflow tract. Specific recommendations have been provided by the ASE and the Valve Academic Research Consortium (VARC) for the Doppler-echocardiographic evaluation of TAVR valves.[77]

When needed, echocardiographic data can be supplemented with information obtained from other diagnostic techniques. Fluoroscopy can be very helpful in the evaluation of mechanical leaflet or disk movement, especially in cases of suspected thrombosis. Excessive rocking may indicate dehiscence. Cardiac magnetic resonance (CMR) imaging can provide accurate and quantitative assessment of ventricular volumes and function. CMR or CT angiography can be used to evaluate the size and contour of the aorta, particularly after root or ascending aortic replacement. These modalities also allow assessment of at least the proximal portions of the reimplanted coronary arteries.

Baseline CMR or CT angiography should be performed 3 months after combined aortic valve/ascending aortic surgery, whether valve-sparing in nature or with a valve-graft conduit, and annually thereafter

(Fig. 26.10). Surveillance imaging of this type is especially important for patients with an underlying aortopathy, such as that associated with Marfan syndrome or bicuspid aortic valve disease. Aneurysmal enlargement may occur in other native aortic locations. False aneurysm development along anastomotic suture lines is uncommon but potentially fatal.

EVALUATION AND TREATMENT OF PROSTHETIC VALVE DYSFUNCTION AND COMPLICATIONS

Prosthetic valve dysfunction may be suspected on the basis of a change in clinical status, new auscultatory findings, or the incidental finding of abnormally high flow velocities and gradients detected during routine TTE. Doppler echocardiography is the method of choice to evaluate prosthetic valve function and to identify and quantitate prosthetic valve stenosis or regurgitation and PPM (Figs. 26.11 through 26.14).[73,74] Cinefluoroscopy and multidetector CT can also help in the evaluation of prosthetic valve leaflet structure and mobility[74] (Figs. 26.15 and 26.16).

Prosthetic valve stenosis may be caused by thrombus formation, pannus ingrowth, or a combination of both, by leaflet calcification in the case of bioprosthetic valves, and by vegetations (see Figs. 26.3, 26.15, and 26.16). Prosthetic valve regurgitation may be related to thrombus formation (i.e., mechanical valves), leaflet tearing (i.e., bioprosthetic valves), vegetations, or PVL (see Fig. 26.15G).

Prosthesis–Patient Mismatch

PPM occurs when the size of a normally functioning prosthetic valve is too small in relation to the patient's body size and cardiac output requirements, resulting in abnormally high postoperative gradients. PPM is defined as an indexed EOA of less than 0.85 cm^2/m^2 (severe < 0.65 cm^2/m^2) for aortic prosthetic valves or an indexed EOA of less than 1.2 cm^2/m^2 (severe < 0.9 cm^2/m^2) for mitral prosthetic valves. Given that indexing EOA to body surface area may lead to an overestimation of PPM in obese patients, it is recommended to use lower cutoff values for PPM (i.e., < 0.70 cm^2/m^2 and < 0.55 cm^2/m^2 for overall and severe mismatch in aortic valves; < 1.0 cm^2/m^2 and < 0.75 cm^2/m^2 for overall and severe mismatch in mitral valves) if the body mass index is 30 kg/m^2 or greater.[78]

The prevalence of moderate PPM ranges from 20% to 70% and that of severe PPM from 2% to 20% after aortic or mitral valve replacement.[79–81] Patients with aortic PPM have worse functional class and exercise capacity, reduced regression of LV hypertrophy, more cardiac rehospitalizations, and increased risk of perioperative and late death compared with patients who do not have PPM[81–84] (Fig. 26.17). Patients with mitral PPM have persistent pulmonary hypertension and increased incidence of heart failure and death.[85,86] A greater clinical impact of aortic PPM is also observed in specific groups of patients, such as those with preexisting LV dysfunction or severe LV hypertrophy and/or concomitant mitral regurgitation and those younger than 65 to 70 years of age.

PPM is less frequent with TAVR than with SAVR, particularly in the subset of patients with small aortic annuli.[84] Figs. 26.11 through 26.14 provide algorithms for differentiating between normal prosthetic valve function, PPM, and intrinsic valve dysfunction due to SVD, thrombus, or pannus.

Structural Valve Deterioration

Mechanical prostheses have excellent durability, and SVD is rare with contemporary valves, although mechanical failure (e.g., strut fracture, leaflet escape, occluder dysfunction caused by lipid adsorption) occurred with some models in the past. However, SVD due to leaflet calcification or collagen fiber disruption is the major cause of

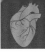

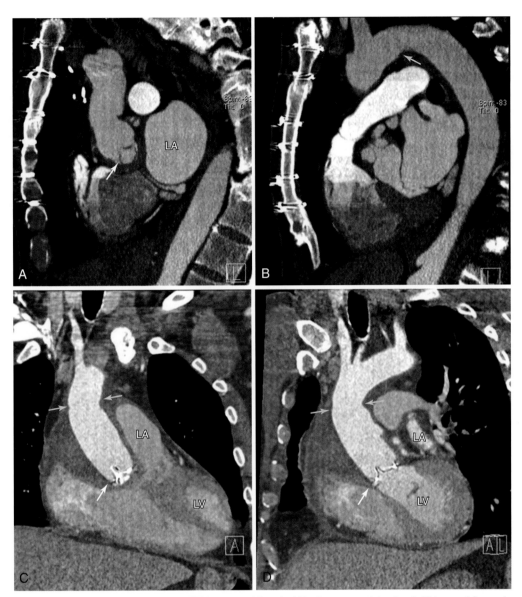

Fig. 26.10 Computed Tomographic (CT) Images of Surgical Replacement of the Aortic Valve and Ascending Aorta. Cardiac CT evaluation of two patients after surgical replacement of the aortic valve and ascending aorta. (A and B) Lateral views of a 58-year-old man with ankylosing spondylitis after aortic valve replacement with a 29-mm St. Jude Toronto Bioroot (St. Jude Medical, Inc., St. Paul, MN) and ascending aortic replacement with hemiarch reconstruction with a 28-mm Vascutek graft (Vascutek Ltd., Renfrewshire, Scotland). (A) Aortic valve prosthesis *(white arrow)* and ascending aorta. (B) Aortic arch *(yellow arrow)*. (C and D) Anterior and anterolateral views of a 41-year-old man with a bicuspid aortic valve and aortic aneurysm after aortic valve replacement with a 27-mm Carpentier Edwards Perimount bovine pericardial valve *(white arrows)* within a 34-mm Dacron graft (Edwards Lifesciences, Irvine, CA). (B–D) *Yellow arrows* indicate the distal anastomoses.

bioprosthetic valve failure. SVD may lead to leaflet stiffening and progressive stenosis or leaflet tear with ensuing transvalvular regurgitation (see Fig. 26.3).

Figs. 26.11 through 26.14 provide algorithms for the quantitation of prosthetic aortic and mitral valve stenosis and regurgitation.[73,74] Although SVD has long been considered a purely passive degenerative process, studies suggest that active and potentially modifiable processes may be involved, including lipid infiltration, inflammation, immune rejection, and active mineralization. Transcatheter valve-in-valve implantation is an alternative to reoperation for patients with prohibitive or high surgical risk and failed bioprosthetic valves.[61,88]

The traditional definition of SVD, which was used in almost all of the AVR series, is based on the composite of valve reintervention or death related to structural valve failure. However, this definition underestimates the true incidence of SVD because it captures only the most severe cases of SVD associated with heart failure symptoms. Moreover, a substantial proportion of patients with severe SVD may not undergo valve reintervention because they are considered to be at high risk for poor outcomes with reoperation or valve-in-valve procedures.

Several deaths may not be appropriately classified as valve related even if SVD has directly or indirectly contributed to the death. A more sensitive and granular definition of SVD based on imaging has been

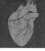

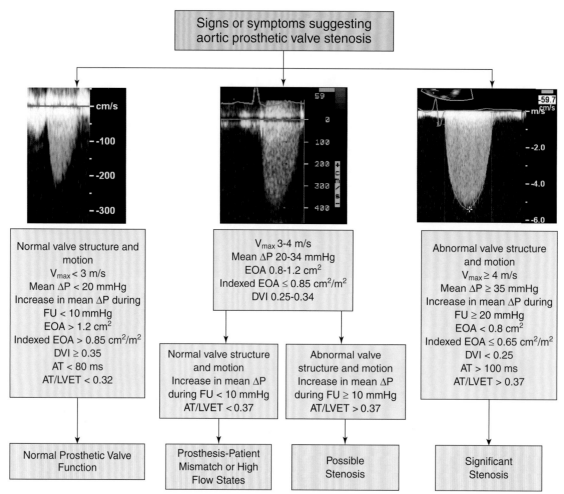

Fig. 26.11 Evaluation of Aortic Prosthetic Valve Stenosis. A practical approach to evaluation of possible prosthetic aortic stenosis begins with standard measures of stenosis severity, including maximal velocity (V_{max}), mean pressure gradient (ΔP), effective orifice area (EOA), and the Doppler velocity index (DVI) (i.e., ratio of left ventricular outflow tract to aortic velocity). Normal values for each valve type and size should be referenced, but simple thresholds of 3 and 4 m/s for V_{max} and 20 and 35 mmHg for mean ΔP are a quick first step. For patients with intermediate measures of stenosis severity, the assessment of valve structure and motion and of the changes in ΔP, EOA, and DVI during follow-up (FU) can help differentiate normal prosthetic valve function with concomitant prosthesis–patient mismatch or high-flow states from prosthetic valve stenosis. The shape of the velocity curve may also be helpful. A triangular short acceleration time (AT; i.e., time to peak velocity) relative to left ventricular ejection time (LVET) suggests normal valve function, whereas a rounded waveform (i.e., increased AT/LVET ratio) suggests significant stenosis. Additional imaging, including transesophageal echocardiography, cinefluoroscopy, or multidetector computed tomography, may be needed to assess valve leaflet structure and motion.

proposed.[89,90] It identifies four stages: stage 0, no SVD; stage 1, morphologic SVD; stage 2, moderate hemodynamic SVD (i.e., occurrence of moderate prosthetic valve stenosis or transvalvular regurgitation during follow-up); and stage 3, severe hemodynamic SVD (i.e., severe stenosis or regurgitation). In a retrospective bioprosthetic surgical AVR series published in 2018,[76] the 10-year incidence of stage 2 or 3 SVD identified by TTE (41%) was much higher than the incidence of aortic valve reintervention for SVD (3.5%). Furthermore, stage 2 or greater SVD was independently associated with a 2.5-fold increase in all-cause mortality, demonstrating the high clinical relevance of this TTE-based definition of SVD.

Paravalvular Leak

PVL occurs external to the prosthetic valve, at the interface between the sewing ring and the native valve annulus (see Fig. 26.15G). It can

occur as a result of inadequate technique, suture dehiscence, compromised native tissue integrity (e.g., dense calcification, extensive myxomatous degeneration), infection, or chronic abrasion of the sewing ring against a calcified or rigid annulus.

The magnitude of the regurgitant volume depends on the size of the orifice. A small and hemodynamically inconsequential PVL is usually discovered incidentally during routine echocardiography with color-flow Doppler imaging; no change in management is indicated. Small PVLs may, however, be associated with significant intravascular hemolysis and anemia as red blood cells are forced through a narrow orifice at high velocities. Despite a high clinical index of suspicion in this circumstance, a new, regurgitant murmur may not be audible. TEE may be necessary to differentiate paravalvular from transvalvular regurgitation and to visualize the defect appropriately, especially with mitral prostheses. Larger PVLs may result in significant volume

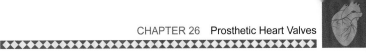

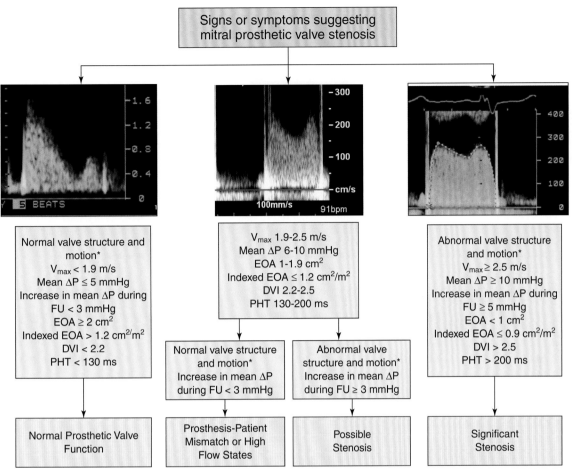

Signs or symptoms suggesting
mitral prosthetic valve stenosis

Normal valve structure and
motion*
V_{max} < 1.9 m/s
Mean ΔP ≤ 5 mmHg
Increase in mean ΔP during
FU < 3 mmHg
EOA ≥ 2 cm²
Indexed EOA > 1.2 cm²/m²
DVI < 2.2
PHT < 130 ms

V_{max} 1.9-2.5 m/s
Mean ΔP 6-10 mmHg
EOA 1-1.9 cm²
Indexed EOA ≤ 1.2 cm²/m²
DVI 2.2-2.5
PHT 130-200 ms

Abnormal valve structure
and motion*
V_{max} ≥ 2.5 m/s
Mean ΔP ≥ 10 mmHg
Increase in mean ΔP during
FU ≥ 5 mmHg
EOA < 1 cm²
Indexed EOA ≤ 0.9 cm²/m²
DVI > 2.5
PHT > 200 ms

Normal valve structure
and motion*
Increase in mean ΔP
during FU < 3 mmHg

Abnormal valve
structure and motion*
Increase in mean ΔP
during FU ≥ 3 mmHg

Normal Prosthetic Valve
Function

Prosthesis-Patient
Mismatch or High
Flow States

Possible
Stenosis

Significant
Stenosis

Fig. 26.12 Evaluation of Mitral Prosthetic Valve Stenosis. The evaluation starts with standard measures of stenosis severity, including maximal velocity *(Vmax)*, mean pressure gradient *(ΔP)*, effective orifice area *(EOA)*, and pressure half-time *(PHT)*. Doppler velocity index *(DVI)* is the ratio of mitral to left ventricular outflow tract to aortic velocity, and an elevated value is abnormal. Normal values for each valve type and size should be referenced, but the thresholds shown are a quick first step. For patients with intermediate measures of stenosis severity, the differential diagnosis includes significant stenosis, prosthesis–patient mismatch, and a high-flow state. Additional imaging *(asterisk)*, including transesophageal echocardiography, cinefluoroscopy, or multidetector computed tomography, may be needed to assess valve leaflet structure and motion. *FU,* Follow-up.

overload and heart failure, to an extent that reoperation or catheter closure might be indicated. Significant PVL may develop during the late postoperative period, often as the result of endocarditis.

PVL is more common after transcatheter than surgical AVR, although its incidence is significantly lower with newer-generation prostheses.[42,43] Because PVL jets after TAVR are often multiple, irregular, and eccentric, imaging and grading can be challenging (see Fig. 26.15H, I). A multiwindow, multiparametric, integrative approach is essential to assess the severity of PVL by Doppler echocardiography (see Figs. 26.13 through 26.15).[37,38,77] Other imaging modalities, such as cine-angiography, cardiac CT, and CMR, and serum biomarkers (e.g., LDH) may be useful to complement or corroborate the echocardiographic findings.[53,74,91] The use of corrective procedures such as repeat balloon dilation, valve-in-valve implantation, or transcatheter leak closure may be considered depending on the severity of the PVL and the risk of procedural complications.[37]

Thromboembolism and Bleeding

Thromboemboli are a major source of morbidity in patients with prosthetic heart valves. The incidence of clinically recognizable events

ranges from 0.6% to 2.3% per patient-year,[20,92] an estimate that does not account for any subclinical episodes that might be detected only with sensitive imaging techniques.[93] Thromboembolic incidence rates are similar for non-anticoagulated patients with bioprostheses and appropriately anticoagulated patients with mechanical valves. Risk factors for thromboembolism include the inherent thrombogenicity of the prosthesis, valve position (mitral > aortic), valve number, time spent out of the therapeutic range of anticoagulation with a VKA, a history of thromboembolism, hypercoagulable state, atrial fibrillation, left atrial enlargement, and LV systolic dysfunction.

Management of a thromboembolic event in patients with mechanical valves usually proceeds along one or more of the following lines:
1. For patients whose INR is subtherapeutic, the dose of the VKA is advanced to achieve the intended INR range.
2. For patients whose INR is in the therapeutic range, the dose of the VKA is advanced to achieve a higher INR range and/or low-dose aspirin is provided if not already used.
3. The patient and family are informed about the increased risks of bleeding.
4. The potential for drug interactions is reviewed.[44]

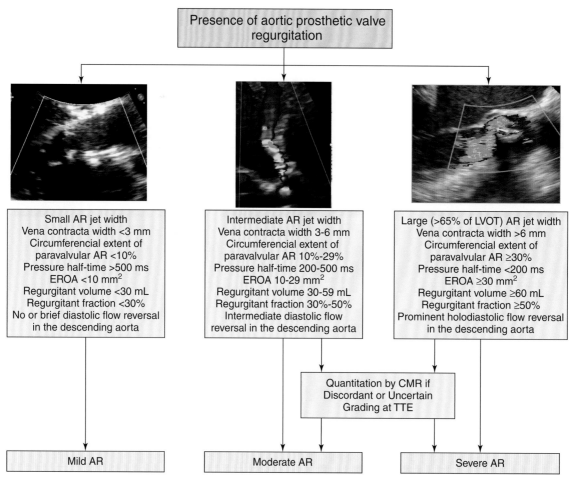

Presence of aortic prosthetic valve
regurgitation

| Small AR jet width
Vena contracta width <3 mm
Circumferencial extent of
paravalvular AR <10%
Pressure half-time >500 ms
EROA <10 mm^2
Regurgitant volume <30 mL
Regurgitant fraction <30%
No or brief diastolic flow reversal
in the descending aorta | Intermediate AR jet width
Vena contracta width 3-6 mm
Circumferencial extent of
paravalvular AR 10%-29%
Pressure half-time 200-500 ms
EROA 10-29 mm^2
Regurgitant volume 30-59 mL
Regurgitant fraction 30%-50%
Intermediate diastolic flow
reversal in the descending aorta | Large (>65% of LVOT) AR jet width
Vena contracta width >6 mm
Circumferencial extent of
paravalvular AR ≥30%
Pressure half-time <200 ms
EROA ≥30 mm^2
Regurgitant volume ≥60 mL
Regurgitant fraction ≥50%
Prominent holodiastolic flow reversal
in the descending aorta |

Quantitation by CMR if
Discordant or Uncertain
Grading at TTE

| Mild AR | Moderate AR | Severe AR |

Fig. 26.13 Evaluation of Aortic Prosthetic Valve Regurgitation. A multiwindow, multiparameter integrative approach is used to identify the type of regurgitation (i.e., transvalvular or paravalvular) and to quantitate its severity by transthoracic echocardiography *(TTE).* The grading of prosthetic aortic regurgitation *(AR)* severity starts with assessment of the semiquantitative parameters of regurgitation. If the grading of AR remains uncertain or discordant with clinical findings by semiquantitative parameters, quantitative parameters (i.e., effective regurgitant orifice area *[EROA]*, regurgitant volume, and regurgitant fraction) should be obtained, if feasible. If quantitation by TTE is not feasible or is discrepant with the patient's symptomatic status (e.g., moderate AR in a patient with severe symptoms), quantitation of regurgitant fraction by cardiac magnetic resonance *(CMR)* should be considered. *LVOT,* Left ventricular outflow tract.

Reoperation to implant a less thrombogenic valve is rarely undertaken for patients with recurrent thromboemboli despite aggressive antithrombotic therapy.

The risk of bleeding, estimated at 1% per patient-year, increases with age and the intensity of anticoagulation. Correction of a supratherapeutic INR should be considered when the INR exceeds 4.5, especially in the presence of active bleeding. Rapid correction of a therapeutic INR may also be necessary because of bleeding or the need for emergency noncardiac surgery. Any INR value higher than 4.0 obtained with a finger-stick device should be verified with a laboratory assay performed on a phlebotomized blood specimen. For patients with minimally elevated INR and no active bleeding, VKA therapy is adjusted or held for one or two doses, after which the INR measurement is repeated.

The 2012 American College of Chest Physicians guideline for antithrombotic therapy recommended against the *routine* use of vitamin K for patients receiving a VKA who have an INR of 4.5 to 10 and no evidence of bleeding. Individual patient circumstances may vary.[94] Oral vitamin K is recommended for patients with an INR higher than

10 and no evidence of bleeding. When oral vitamin K (5 mg) is given in conjunction with temporary discontinuation of a VKA, 1.4 days are required for an INR between 6 and 10 to decline to less than 4.0. Subcutaneous vitamin K is not recommended. For patients with VKA-related bleeding, four-factor prothrombin complex concentrate is preferred over fresh-frozen plasma for more rapid reversal. The additional use of intravenous vitamin K may be considered.

Idarucizumab is a humanized monoclonal antibody that neutralizes the anticoagulant effect of dabigatran and its metabolites.[95] Andexanet alfa is a recombinant modified Xa molecule that targets and sequesters direct and indirect factor Xa inhibitors.[96]

Prosthetic Valve Thrombosis

The incidence of mechanical valve thrombosis is estimated to be 0.3% to 1.3% per patient-year in developed countries but as high as 6% per patient-year in developing countries.[97] Thrombosis of a mechanical heart valve can have devastating consequences (see Figs. 26.3, 26.15, and 26.16). Bioprosthetic (surgical or transcatheter) valve thrombosis is less common, with a reported incidence of 0.03% to 0.5% per

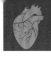

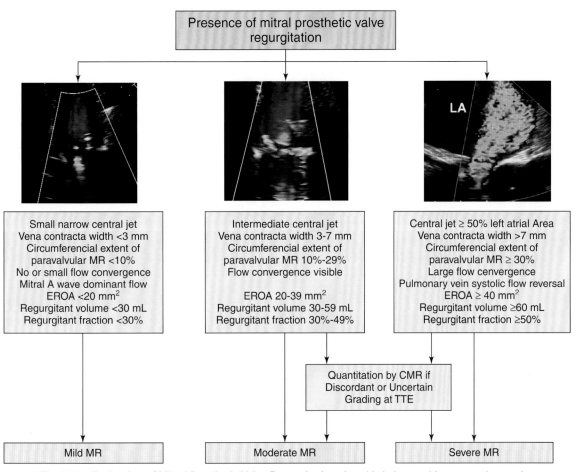

Fig. 26.14 Evaluation of Mitral Prosthetic Valve Regurgitation. A multiwindow, multiparameter integrative approach is used to identify the type of regurgitation (transvalvular vs. paravalvular) and to quantitate its severity. Transesophageal echocardiography *(TEE)* is recommended whenever prosthetic mitral regurgitation *(MR)* is a concern because TTE imaging is limited due to shadowing of the left atrium by the prosthetic valve. Even severe prosthetic MR may not be detected on TTE because of this issue. The grading of MR severity starts with the assessment of the semiquantitative parameters of regurgitation. If the grading of MR remains uncertain or discordant with clinical findings by semiquantitative parameters, quantitative parameters (i.e., effective regurgitant orifice area *[EROA]*, regurgitant volume, and regurgitant fraction) should be obtained, if feasible. If quantitation by TEE is not feasible or is discrepant with the patient's symptoms (e.g., moderate MR in a patient with severe symptoms), quantitation of regurgitant fraction by cardiac magnetic resonance *(CMR)* should be considered.

patient-year.[98] However, studies suggest that subclinical thrombosis may occur in 5% to 15% of patients within the first 2 years after TAVR.[66,99–101]

Clinical suspicion of prosthetic valve thrombosis can be heightened by symptoms of heart failure, thromboembolism, and/or low cardiac output coupled with a decrease in the intensity of the valve closure sounds (i.e., mechanical valves), new and pathologic murmurs, and/or documentation of inadequate anticoagulation. Prosthetic valve thrombosis is more common in the mitral and tricuspid positions than in the aortic position. Although differentiation from pannus formation can be difficult, the clinical context usually allows accurate diagnosis.

Evaluation with TTE/TEE can help guide management decisions.[73,74] In patients with mechanical valves, confirmation of abnormal leaflet or disk excursion in the setting of an occluding thrombus can also be obtained with cine-fluoroscopy or multidetector CT.[74] The latter imaging modality can be useful to identify leaflet thickening and reduced mobility after valve replacement with a bioprosthesis (see Fig. 26.16).[66]

Emergency surgery is reasonable for patients with left-sided prosthetic valve thrombosis and shock or New York Heart Association (NYHA) functional class III–IV symptoms and for patients with a large thrombus burden ($\geq$0.8 cm^2 on TEE).[44] Fibrinolytic therapy is reasonable for patients with recent-onset ($<$2 weeks) NYHA class I–II symptoms and small thrombus burden ($<$0.8 cm^2) or for sicker patients with larger thrombi when surgery is not available or inadvisable. Fibrinolytic therapy is recommended for patients with right-sided prosthetic valve thrombosis.[44] Some patients with no or minimal symptoms and small thrombi can be managed with intravenous UFH alone and then converted to fibrinolytic therapy if unsuccessful. An encouraging report on the efficacy of low-dose, slow-infusion tissue plasminogen activator in pregnant women with prosthetic valve thrombosis should prompt investigation of this approach in other patient subsets.[102]

Any course of fibrinolytic therapy is followed at the appropriate interval by a continuous infusion of UFH during the transition to VKA therapy targeted to a higher INR with or without low-dose aspirin.

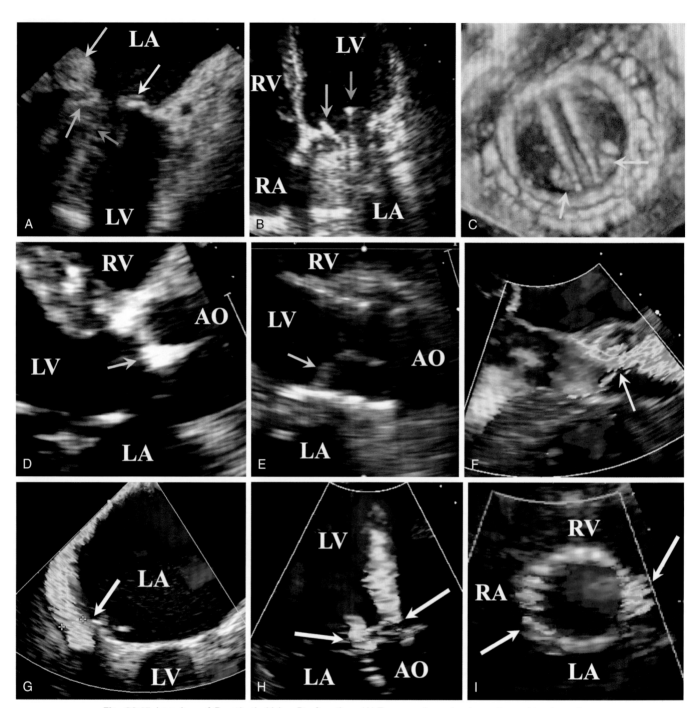

Fig. 26.15 Imaging of Prosthetic Valve Dysfunction. (A) Transesophageal echocardiographic view of an obstructed mitral bileaflet mechanical valve. *Yellow arrow* indicates large thrombus; *white arrow* indicates pannus; *blue arrow* indicates mobile leaflet; *green arrow* indicates immobile leaflet. (B) Transthoracic echocardiographic view of a mitral bileaflet mechanical prosthesis in diastole with a fixed leaflet *(green arrow)*; the other leaflet is still mobile *(blue arrow)*. (C) Mitral bileaflet mechanical valve viewed from the left atrium shows small thrombi *(yellow arrows)* attached to the hinge mechanism of the valve; the motion of the leaflets is not impaired. (D) Transthoracic echocardiographic view of stented bioprosthetic valve with calcific degeneration, thickening, and reduced mobility of the leaflets *(yellow arrow)*. (E and F) Transthoracic echocardiographic views of an obstructive thrombus in a balloon-expandable transcatheter aortic valve. The leaflets are thickened (E) *(yellow arrow)*, and the width of the transprosthetic jet is narrowed (F) *(white arrow)*. (G) Transesophageal color Doppler echocardiographic view of a severe paravalvular leak *(white arrow)* in a mitral mechanical valve. (H and I) Transthoracic color Doppler echocardiographic views (H, apical three-chamber; I, parasternal short-axis) of two paravalvular regurgitant jets *(white arrows)* in a transcatheter aortic valve. *AO,* Aorta. (Courtesy Dr. Steven A Goldstein, Washington Hospital Center [A], and Dr. Arsène Basmadjan, Montreal Heart Institute, Montreal, Canada [G].)

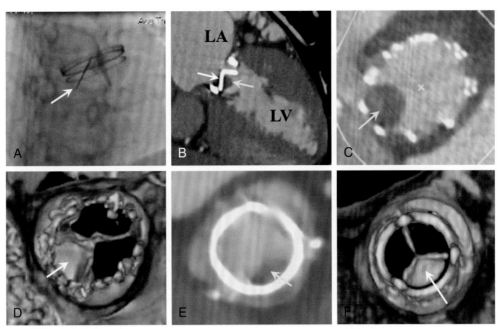

Fig. 26.16 Alternative Imaging Modalities for Detecting Prosthetic Valve Dysfunction. (A) Use of cinefluoroscopy for assessment of mechanical valve leaflet mobility. *White arrow* indicates an immobile leaflet in a mitral bileaflet mechanical valve. (B) Use of multislice computed tomography for assessment of mechanical valve leaflet mobility. *White arrow* indicates an immobile leaflet; *yellow arrow* indicates thrombus. (C–F) Use of four-dimensional multidetector computed tomography to detect subclinical thrombosis in surgical and transcatheter aortic bioprosthetic valves. *Yellow arrows* indicate thrombus; *white arrows* indicate leaflet with restricted mobility. (A, Courtesy Dr. Steven A Goldstein, Washington Hospital Center. C–F, From Mahjoub H, Dahou A, Pibarot P, et al. Prosthetic valve dysfunction, echocardiographic recognition and quantitation of prosthetic valve dysfunction. In: Otto CM, editor. Practice of clinical echocardiography. 5th ed. St. Louis: Elsevier. 2017.)

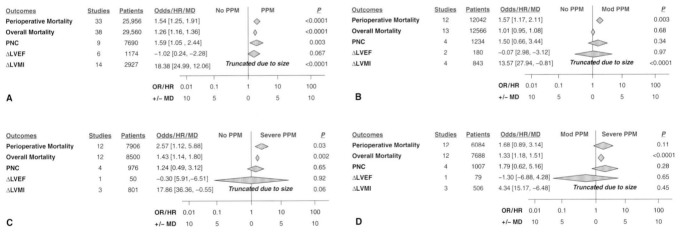

Fig. 26.17 Impact of Prosthesis–Patient Mismatch *(PPM)* on Freedom from Cardiac Events. Summary effects of PPM on outcomes, including the perioperative mortality rate, overall mortality rate, postoperative neurologic complications *(PNC)*, and postoperative change in left ventricular ejection fraction *(LVEF)* and left ventricular mass index (g/m²) *(LVMi)*. (A) Any degree of PPM versus no PPM. (B) Moderate *(Mod)* PPM versus no PPM. (C) Severe PPM versus no PPM. (D) Mod PPM versus severe PPM. *HR*, Hazard ratio; *MD*, mean deviation. (From Dayan V, Vignolo G, Soca G, et al. Predictors and outcomes of prosthesis patient mismatch after aortic valve replacement. JACC Cardiovasc Imaging 2016;9:924-933.)

Serial TTE studies are useful to assess the response to treatment. For patients with suspected or confirmed bioprosthetic valve thrombosis who are hemodynamically stable and have no contraindications to anticoagulation, initial treatment with a VKA is reasonable,[66,99,100] although there is increasing experience with DOACs for this indication.

Infective Endocarditis

PVE, the most severe form of infective endocarditis, occurs in 1% to 6% of patients with valve prostheses, accounting for 10% to 30% of all cases of infective endocarditis.[45] PVE is an extremely serious condition with high mortality rates (30%–50%).

The diagnosis is based on the Modified Duke Criteria and relies predominantly on the combination of positive blood cultures and echocardiographic evidence of prosthetic valve infection, including vegetations, paravalvular abscess, or a new paravalvular regurgitation. TEE is essential for patients with prosthetic valves because of its greater sensitivity in detecting these abnormalities. Studies have suggested that increased uptake of [18]fluorodeoxyglucose measured by positron emission tomography combined with computed tomography (PET-CT) may improve the early diagnosis of prosthetic valve endocarditis,[103] especially when there is a high clinical index of suspicion and echocardiographic data are nondiagnostic.

Despite prompt and appropriate antibiotic treatment, most patients with PVE eventually require surgery. Medical treatment alone is more likely to succeed in late PVE (i.e., occurring > 6 months after surgery) and in nonstaphylococcal infections. Surgery should be considered in the following situations: heart failure; failure of antibiotic treatment; hemodynamically significant prosthetic valve regurgitation, especially if associated with worsening LV function; large vegetations (>10 mm); persistently positive blood cultures despite therapy; recurrent emboli with persistent vegetations; and intracardiac fistula formation.[61]

Even in surgical centers with expertise in the management of these patients, perioperative mortality rates for PVE are as high as 25% to 35%. PVE after TAVR occurs predominantly within the first year; its incidence is low (1% per patient year) but the in-hospital and 2-year mortality rates are high (about 35% and 67%, respectively),[104] likely reflecting patient age and comorbidities. Removal of a previously implanted pacemaker or defibrillator system (including the leads and generator) is recommended for patients with PVE even without definite involvement of the leads or device.

Hemolytic Anemia

The development of a nonimmune hemolytic anemia after valve replacement or repair is usually attributable to PVL with intravascular red blood cell destruction. Diagnosis is based on a high index of suspicion coupled with laboratory evidence of hemolysis, including the characteristic changes in red blood cell morphology (i.e., schistocytes), elevated levels of indirect bilirubin and LDH, a high reticulocyte count, and a depressed serum haptoglobin level.

Reoperation or catheter closure of the defect is indicated when heart failure, a persistent transfusion requirement, or poor quality of life intervenes. Empiric medical measures include iron and folic acid replacement therapy and β-adrenoreceptor blockers. It is important to exclude PVE as a cause.

REFERENCES

1. Søndergaard L, Saraste A, Christersson C, Vahanian A. The year in cardiology 2017: valvular heart disease. Eur Heart J 2018;39(8):650-657.
2. Chambers JB, Prendergast B, Iung B, et al. Standards defining a 'Heart Valve Centre': ESC Working Group on Valvular Heart Disease and European Association for Cardiothoracic Surgery Viewpoint. Eur Heart J 2017;38(28):2177-2183.
3. Society of Thoracic Surgeons. Adult Cardiac Surgery Database. Available at: https://www.sts.org/registries-research-center/sts-national-database/sts-adult-cardiac-surgery-database. Accessed June 21, 2019.
4. Zabalgoitia M. Echocardiographic recognition and quantitation of prosthetic valve dysfunction. In: Otto CM, ed. The Practice of Clinical Echocardiography. Philadelphia: WB Saunders; 2002.
5. Rosenhek R, Binder T, Maurer G, et al. Normal values for Doppler echocardiographic assessment of heart valve prostheses. J Am Soc Echocardiogr 2003;16:1116-1127.
6. Malouf JF, Ballo M, Connolly HM, et al. Doppler echocardiography of 119 normal-functioning St Jude Medical mitral valve prostheses: a comprehensive assessment including time-velocity integral ratio and prosthesis performance index. J Am Soc Echocardiogr 2005;18:252-256.
7. Hixson CS, Smith MD, Mattson MD, et al. Comparison of transesophageal color flow Doppler imaging of normal mitral regurgitant jets in St. Jude Medical and Medtronic Hall cardiac prostheses. J Am Soc Echocardiogr 1992;5:57-62.
8. Lange HW, Olson JD, Pedersen WR, et al. Transesophageal color Doppler echocardiography of the normal St. Jude Medical mitral valve prosthesis. Am Heart J 1991;122:489-494.
9. Yoganathan AP, Heinrich RS, Fontaine AA. Fluid dynamics of prosthetic valves. In: Otto CM, ed. The Practice of Clinical Echocardiography. Philadelphia: W.B. Saunders; 2002.
10. Bryan AJ, Rogers CA, Bayliss K, et al. Prospective randomized comparison of CarboMedics and St. Jude Medical bileaflet mechanical heart valve prostheses: ten-year follow-up. J Thorac Cardiovasc Surg 2007;133:614-622.
11. Thevenet A, Albat B. Long term follow up of 292 patients after valve replacement with the Omnicarbon prosthetic valve. J Heart Valve Dis 1995;4:634-639.
12. Nitter Hauge S, Abdelnoor M, Svennevig JL. Fifteen-year experience with the Medtronic-Hall valve prosthesis: a follow-up study of 1104 consecutive patients. Circulation 1996;94(suppl II):II105-II108.
13. Tatoulis J, Chaiyaroj S, Smith JA. Aortic valve replacement in patients 50 years old or younger with the St. Jude Medical valve: 14-year experience. J Heart Valve Dis 1996;5:491-497.
14. Godje OL, Fischlein T, Adelhard K, et al. Thirty-year results of Starr-Edwards prostheses in the aortic and mitral position. Ann Thorac Surg 1997;63:613-619.
15. Orszulak TA, Schaff HV, Puga FJ, et al. Event status of the Starr-Edwards aortic valve to 20 years: a benchmark for comparison. Ann Thorac Surg 1997;63:620-626.
16. Li HH, Hahn J, Urbanski P, et al. Intermediate-term results with 1,019 Carbomedics aortic valves. Ann Thorac Surg 2001;71:1181-1187.
17. Emery RW, Arom KV, Kshettry VR, et al. Decision-making in the choice of heart valve for replacement in patients aged 60-70 years: twenty-year follow up of the St. Jude Medical aortic valve prosthesis. J Heart Valve Dis 2002;11(suppl 1):S37-S44.
18. Eikelboom JW, Connolly SJ, Brueckmann M, et al. Dabigatran versus warfarin in patients with mechanical heart valves. N Engl J Med 2013;369:1206-1214.
19. Arom KV, Nicoloff DM, Kersten TE, et al. Ten years' experience with the St. Jude Medical valve prosthesis. Ann Thorac Surg 1989;47:831-837.
20. Akins CW. Results with mechanical cardiac valvular prostheses. Ann Thorac Surg 1995;60:1836-1844.
21. Firstenberg MS, Morehead AJ, Thomas JD, et al. Short-term hemodynamic performance of the mitral Carpentier-Edwards PERIMOUNT pericardial valve. Carpentier-Edwards PERIMOUNT Investigators. Ann Thorac Surg 2001;71(suppl 5):S285-S288.
22. Dalmau MJ, González-Santos JM, Blázquez JA, et al. Hemodynamic performance of the Medtronic Mosaic and Perimount Magna aortic bioprostheses: five-year results of a prospectively randomized study. Eur J Cardiothorac Surg 2011;39:844-852.
23. Johnston DR, Soltesz EG, Vakil N, et al. Long-term durability of bioprosthetic aortic valves: implications from 12,569 implants. Ann Thorac Surg 2015;99:1239-1247.
24. Bourguignon T, Bouquiaux-Stablo AL, Candolfi P, et al. Very long-term outcomes of the Carpentier-Edwards Perimount valve in aortic position. Ann Thorac Surg 2015;99:831-837.
25. Senage T, Le Tourneau T, Foucher Y, et al. Early structural valve deterioration of Mitroflow aortic bioprosthesis. Circulation 2014;130:2012-2020.
26. Kunadian B, Vijayalakshmi K, Thornley AR, et al. Meta-analysis of valve hemodynamics and left ventricular mass regression for stentless versus stented aortic valves. Ann Thorac Surg 2007;84:73-78.
27. David TE, Feindel CM, Bos J, Ivanov J, Armstrong S. Aortic valve replacement with Toronto SPV bioprosthesis: optimal patient survival but suboptimal valve durability. J Thorac Cardiovasc Surg 2008;135:19-24.
28. El-Hamamsy I, Eryigit Z, Stevens LM, et al. Long-term outcomes after autograft versus homograft aortic root replacement in adults with aortic valve disease: a randomised controlled trial. Lancet 2010;376:524-531.
29. O'Brien MF, McGiffin DC, Stafford EG, et al. Allograft aortic valve replacement: long-term comparative clinical analysis of the viable cryopreserved and antibiotic 4 degrees C stored valves. J Card Surg 1991;6(suppl 4):534-543.

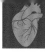

30. O'Brien MF, Hancock S, Stafford EG, et al. The homograft aortic valve: a 29 year, 99.3% follow-up of 1022 valve replacements. J Heart Valve Dis 2001;10:334-344.

31. Mazine A, El-Hamamsy I, Verma S, et al. Ross procedure in adults for cardiologists and cardiac surgeons: JACC State-of-the-Art Review. J Am Coll Cardiol 2018;72:2761-2777.

32. Carr-White GS, Kilner PJ, Hon JK, et al. Incidence, location, pathology, and significance of pulmonary homograft stenosis after the Ross operation. Circulation 2001;104(suppl 1):I16-I20.

33. Briand M, Pibarot P, Dumesnil JG, et al. Midterm echocardiographic follow-up after Ross operation. Circulation 2000;102(suppl 3):III10-III14.

34. Leon MB, Nazif TM, Bapat V. Interpreting national trends in aortic valve replacement: let the buyer beware. J Am Coll Cardiol 2018;71(15):1628-1630.

35. Blackman DJ, Smriti Saraf S, MacCarthy PA, et al. Long-term durability of transcatheter bioprosthetic aortic valves inpatients at lower surgical risk. J Am Coll Cardiol 2019;73:537-545.

36. Sondergaard L, Ihlemann N, Capodanno D, et al. Durability of transcatheter and surgical aortic. J Am Coll Cardiol 2019;73:546-553.

37. Pibarot P, Hahn RT, Weissman NJ, Monaghan MJ. Assessment of paravalvular regurgitation following TAVR: a proposal of unifying grading scheme. JACC Cardiovasc Imaging 2015;8:340-360.

38. Pibarot P, Hahn RT, Weissman NJ, et al. Association of paravalvular regurgitation with 1-year outcomes after transcatheter aortic valve replacement with the SAPIEN 3 valve. JAMA Cardiol 2017;2:1208-1216.

39. Ando T, Briasoulis A, Telila T, et al. Does mild paravalvular regurgitation post transcatheter aortic valve implantation affect survival? A meta-analysis. Catheter Cardiovasc Interv 2017.

40. Abdel-Wahab M, Mehilli J, Frerker C, et al. Comparison of balloon-expandable vs self-expandable valves in patients undergoing transcatheter aortic valve replacement: the CHOICE randomized clinical trial. JAMA 2014;311:1503-1514.

41. Abdelghani M, Mankerious N, Allali A, et al. Bioprosthetic valve performance after transcatheter aortic valve replacement with self-expanding versus balloon-expandable valves in large versus small aortic valve annuli: Insights from the CHOICE trial and the CHOICE-Extend registry. JACC Cardiovasc Interv 2018;11:2507-2518.

42. Mack MJ, Leon MB, Thouran VH, et al. Transcatheter aortic valve replacement with a balloon expandable valve in low risk patients. N Engl J Med 2019;380:1695-1705.

43. Popma JJ, Deeb GM, Yakubov SJ, et al. Transcatheter aortic valve replacement with a self expanding valve in low risk patients. N Engl J Med 2019; 380:1706-1715.

44. Nishimura RA, Otto CM, Bonow RO, et al. 2014 AHA/ACC guideline for the management of patients with valvular heart disease: a report of the American College of Cardiology/American Heart Association Task Force on Practice Guidelines. J Am Coll Cardiol 2014;63:e57-e185.

45. Habib G, Lancellotti P, Antunes MJ, et al. 2015 ESC Guidelines for the management of infective endocarditis: The task force for the management of infective endocarditis of the European Society of Cardiology (ESC) endorsed by: European Association for Cardio-Thoracic Surgery (EACTS), the European Association of Nuclear Medicine (EANM). Eur Heart J 2015;36:3075-3128.

46. Hammermeister K, Sethi GK, Henderson WG, et al. Outcomes 15 years after valve replacement with a mechanical versus a bioprosthetic valve: final report of the Veterans Affairs randomized trial. J Am Coll Cardiol 2000;36:1152-1158.

47. Stassano P, Tommaso LD, Monaco M, et al. Aortic valve replacement: A prospective randomized evaluation of mechanical versus biological valves in patients ages 55 to 70 years. J Am Coll Cardiol 2009;54:1868.

48. Brennan JM, Edwards FH, Zhao Y, et al. Long-term safety and effectiveness of mechanical versus biologic aortic valve prostheses in older patients: results from the Society of Thoracic Surgeons Adult Cardiac Surgery National Database. Circulation 2013;127:1647-1655.

49. Chiang YP, Chikwe J, Moskowitz AJ, et al. Survival and long-term outcomes following bioprosthetic vs mechanical aortic valve replacement in patients aged 50 to 69 years. JAMA 2014;312:1323-1329.

50. Chikwe J, Chiang YP, Egorova NN, et al. Survival and outcomes following bioprosthetic vs mechanical mitral valve replacement in patients aged 50 to 69 years. JAMA 2015;313:1435-1442.

51. Glaser N, Jackson V, Holzmann MJ, et al. Aortic valve replacement with mechanical vs. biological prostheses in patients aged 50-69 years. Eur Heart J 2016;37:2658-2667.

52. Goldstone AB, Chiu P, Baiocchi M, et al. Mechanical or biologic prostheses for aortic valve and mitral valve replacement. N Engl J Med 2017;377: 1847-1857.

53. Adams DH, Popma JJ, Reardon MJ, et al. Transcatheter aortic-valve replacement with a self-expanding prosthesis. N Engl J Med 2014;370:1790-1798.

54. Leon MB, Smith CR, Mack MJ, et al. Transcatheter or surgical aortic-valve replacement in intermediate-risk patients. N Engl J Med 2016;374:1609-1620.

55. Makkar RR, Yoon SH, Leon MB, et al. Association between Transcatheter Aortic Valve Replacement for Bicuspid vs Tricuspid Aortic Stenosis and Mortality or Stroke. JAMA 2019;321(22):2193-2202.

56. Yoon SH, Schmidt T, Bleiziffer S, et al. Transcatheter aortic valve replacement in pure native aortic regurgitation. J Am Coll Cardiol 2017;70:2752-2763.

57. Acker MA, Parides MK, Perrault LP, et al. Mitral-valve repair versus replacement for severe ischemic mitral regurgitation. N Engl J Med 2014;370:23-32.

58. Obadia JF, Messika-Zeitoun D, Leurent G, et al. Percutaneous repair or medical treatment for secondary mitral regurgitation. N Engl J Med 2018; 379:2297-2306.

59. Stone GW, Lindenfeld J, Abraham WT, et al. Transcatheter mitral-valve repair in patients with heart failure. N Engl J Med 2018;379:2307-2318.

60. The Task Force for the Management of Valvular Heart Disease of the European Society of Cardiology (ESC) and the European Association for Cardio-Thoracic Surgery (EACTS). 2017 ESC/EACTS Guidelines for the management of valvular heart disease. Eur Heart J 2017;00:1-53.

61. Nishimura RA, Otto CM, Bonow RO, et al. 2017 AHA/ACC focused update of the 2014 AHA/ACC guideline for the management of patients with valvular heart disease: A report of the American College of Cardiology/American Heart Association Task Force on clinical practice guidelines. J Am Coll Cardiol 2017;70:252-289.

62. Merie C, Køber L, Skov Olsen P, et al. Association of warfarin therapy duration after bioprosthetic aortic valve replacement with risk of mortality, thromboembolic complications, and bleeding. JAMA 2012;308:2118-2125.

63. Avezum A, Lopes RD, Schulte PJ, et al. Apixaban in comparison with warfarin in patients with atrial fibrillation and valvular heart disease. Findings from the Apixaban for Reduction in Stroke and Other Thromboembolic Events in Atrial Fibrillation (ARISTOTLE) Trial. Circulation 2015;132:624-632.

64. Rodes-Cabau J, Masson JB, Welsh RC, et al. Aspirin versus aspirin plus clopidogrel as anti-thrombotic treatment following transcatheter aortic valve replacement with a balloon expandable valve. J Am Coll Cardiol 2017;10:1357-1365.

65. Raheja H, Gatg A, Banerjee K, et al. Comparison of single versus dual anti-platelet therapy after TAVR: a systematic review and meta-analysis (67). Catheter Cardiovasc Interv 2018;92:783-791.

66. Makkar RR, Fontana G, Jilaihawi H, et al. Possible subclinical leaflet thrombosis in bioprosthetic aortic valves. N Engl J Med 2015;373:2015-2024.

67. Dunn AS, Spyropoulos AC, Turpie AG. Bridging therapy in patients on long-term oral anticoagulants who require surgery: the Prospective Perioperative Enoxaparin Cohort Trial (PROSPECT). J Thromb Haemost 2007;5:2211-2218.

68. Steffel J, Verhamme P, Potpara TS, et al. The 2018 European Heart Rhythm Association Practical Guide on the use of non-vitamin K antagonist oral anticoagulants in patients with atrial fibrillation: executive summary. Europace 2018:20:1231-1242.

68. Chan WS, Anand S, Ginsberg JS. Anticoagulation of pregnant women with mechanical heart valves: a systematic review of the literature. Arch Intern Med 2000;160:191-196.

69. Sillesen M, Hjortdal V, Vejlstrup N, et al. Pregnancy with prosthetic heart valves: 30 years' nationwide experience in Denmark. Eur J Cardiothorac Surg 2011;40:448-454.

70. Ansell J, Hirsh J, Hylek E, et al. Pharmacology and management of the vitamin K antagonists: American College of Chest Physicians evidence-based clinical practice guidelines (8th edition). Chest 2008;133(suppl 6):160S-198S.

71. Cotrufo M, De Feo M, De Santo LS, et al. Risk of warfarin during pregnancy with mechanical valve prostheses. Obstet Gynecol 2002;99:35-40.

72. van Driel D, Wesseling J, Sauer PJ, et al. Teratogen update: fetal effects after in utero exposure to coumarins: overview of cases, follow-up findings, and pathogenesis. Teratology 2002;66:127-140.

73. Zoghbi WA, Chambers JB, Dumesnil JG, et al. Recommendations for evaluation of prosthetic valves with echocardiography and Doppler ultrasound: a report from the American Society of Echocardiography's Guidelines and Standards Committee and the Task Force on Prosthetic Valves, developed in conjunction with the American College of Cardiology Cardiovascular Imaging Committee, Cardiac Imaging Committee of the American Heart Association, the European Association of Echocardiography, a registered branch of the European Society of Cardiology, the Japanese Society of Echocardiography and the Canadian Society of Echocardiography, endorsed by the American College of Cardiology Foundation, American Heart Association, European Association of Echocardiography, a registered branch of the European Society of Cardiology, the Japanese Society of Echocardiography, and Canadian Society of Echocardiography. J Am Soc Echocardiogr 2009;22:975-1014.

74. Lancellotti P, Pibarot P, Chambers J, et al. Recommendations for the imaging assessment of prosthetic heart valves: A report from the European Association of Cardiovascular Imaging endorsed by the Chinese Society of Echocardiography, the Interamerican Society of Echocardiography and the Brazilian Department of Cardiovascular Imaging. Eur Heart J Cardiovasc Imaging 2016;17:589-590.

75. Salaun E, Mahjoub H, Dahou A, et al. Hemodynamic deterioration of surgically implanted bioprosthetic aortic valves. J Am Coll Cardiol 2018;72:241-251.

76. Salaun E, Mahjoub H, Girerd N, et al. Rate, timing, correlates, and outcomes of hemodynamic valve deterioration after bioprosthetic surgical aortic valve replacement. Circulation 2018;138:971-985.

77. Kappetein AP, Head SJ, Généreux P, et al. Updated standardized endpoint definitions for transcatheter aortic valve implantation: the Valve Academic Research Consortium-2 consensus document. Eur J Cardiothorac Surg 2012;42:S45-S60.

78. Pibarot P, Dumesnil JG. Valve prosthesis-patient mismatch, 1978 to 2011: from original concept to compelling evidence. J Am Coll Cardiol 2012; 60:1136-1139.

79. Pibarot P, Weissman NJ, Stewart WJ, et al. Incidence and sequelae of prosthesis-patient mismatch in transcatheter versus surgical valve replacement in high-risk patients with severe aortic stenosis- A PARTNER trial cohort A analysis. J Am Coll Cardiol 2014;64:1323-1334.

80. Zorn GL, 3rd, Little SH, Tadros P, et al. Prosthesis-patient mismatch in high-risk patients with severe aortic stenosis: A randomized trial of a self-expanding prosthesis. J Thorac Cardiovasc Surg 2016;151:1014-1023.e3.

81. Herrmann HC, Daneshvar SA, Fonarow GC, et al. Prosthesis-patient mismatch in patients undergoing transcatheter aortic valve replacement: from the STS/ACC TVT registry. J Am Coll Cardiol 2018;72:2701-2711.

82. Fallon JM, DeSimone JP, Brennan JM, et al. The incidence and consequence of prosthesis-patient mismatch after surgical aortic valve replacement. Ann Thorac Surg 2018;106:14-22.

83. Head S, Mokhles M, Osnabrugge R, et al. The impact of prosthesis-patient mismatch on long-term survival after aortic valve replacement: A systematic review and meta-analysis of 34 observational studies comprising 27,186 patients with 133,141 patient-years. Eur Heart J 2012;33:1518-1529.

84. Dayan V, Vignolo G, Soca G, et al. Predictors and outcomes of prosthesis patient mismatch after aortic valve replacement. JACC Cardiovasc Imaging 2016;9:924-933.

85. Unger P, Magne J, Vanden Eynden F, et al. Impact of prosthesis-patient mismatch on mitral regurgitation after aortic valve replacement. Heart 2010;96:1627-1632.

86. Shi WY, Yap CH, Hayward PA, et al. Impact of prosthesis—patient mismatch after mitral valve replacement: a multicentre analysis of early outcomes and mid-term survival. Heart 2011;97:1074-1081.

87. Zoghbi WA, Asch FM, Bruce C, et al. Guidelines for the evaluation of valvular regurgitation after percutaneous valve repair or replacement: a report from the American Society of Echocardiography developed in collaboration with the Society for Cardiovascular Angiography and Interventions, Japanese Society of Echocardiography, and Society for Cardiovascular Magnetic Resonance. J Am Soc Echocardiogr 2019;32(4):431-475.

88. Dvir D, Webb JG, Bleiziffer S, et al. Transcatheter aortic valve implantation in failed bioprosthetic surgical valves. JAMA 2014;312:162-170.

89. Capodanno D, Petronio AS, Prendergast B, et al. Standardized definitions of structural deterioration and valve failure in assessing long-term durability of transcatheter and surgical aortic bioprosthetic valves: a consensus statement from the European Association of Percutaneous Cardiovascular Interventions(EAPCI) endorsed by the European Society of Cardiology (ESC) and the European Association for Cardio-Thoracic Surgery (EACTS). Eur Heart J 2017;38:3382-3390.

90. Dvir D, Bourguignon T, Otto CM, et al. Standardized definition of structural valve degeneration for surgical and transcatheter bioprosthetic aortic valves. Circulation 2018;137:388-399.

91. Van Belle E, Rauch A, Vincent F, et al. Von Willebrand factor multimers during transcatheter aortic-valve replacement. N Engl J Med 2016; 375:335-344.

92. Dellgren G, David TE, Raanani E, et al. Late hemodynamic and clinical outcomes of aortic valve replacement with the Carpentier-Edwards Perimount pericardial bioprosthesis. J Thorac Cardiovasc Surg 2002;124:146-154.

93. Al-Atassi T, Lam K, Forgie M, et al. Cerebral microembolization after bioprosthetic aortic valve replacement: comparison of warfarin plus aspirin versus aspirin only. Circulation 2012;126:S239-S244.

94. Ageno W, Gallus AS, Wittkowsky A, et al. Oral anticoagulant therapy: antithrombotic therapy and prevention of thrombosis, 9th ed. American College of Chest Physicians evidence-based clinical practice guidelines. Chest 2012;141(suppl 2):e44S-e88S.

95. Pollack CV, Reilly PA, van Ryn J, et al. Idarucizumab for Dabigatran Reversal—Full Cohort Analysis. N Engl J Med 2017; 377:431-441.

96. Connolly SJ, Crowther M, Eikelboom JW, et al. Full Study Report of Andexanet Alfa for Bleeding Associated with Factor Xa Inhibitors. N Engl J Med 2019;380:1326-1335.

97. Whitlock RP, Sun JC, Fremes SE, et al. Antithrombotic and thrombolytic therapy for valvular disease: antithrombotic therapy and prevention of thrombosis, 9th ed. American College of Chest Physicians evidence-based clinical practice guidelines. Chest 2012;141(suppl 2):e576S-e600S.

98. Trepels T, Martens S, Doss M, et al. Thromboticx restenosis after minmimally invasive implantation of aortic vakve stent. Circulation 2009; 120(4):e23-e24.

99. Latib A, Naganuma T, Abdel-Wahab M, et al. Treatment and clinical outcomes of transcatheter heart valve thrombosis. Circ Cardiovasc Interv 2015;8:1-8.

100. Kodali SK, Thourani VH, Kirtane AJ. Possible subclinical leaflet thrombosis in bioprosthetic aortic valves. N Engl J Med 2016;374:1591.

101. del Trigo M, Munoz-Garcia AJ, Wijeysundera HC, et al. Incidence, timing and predictors of valve hemodynamic deterioration after transcatheter aortic valve replacement: Multicenter registry. J Am Coll Cardiol 2016;67:644-655.

102. Ozkan A, Cakal B, Karakoyun S, et al. Thrombolytic therapy for the treatment of prosthetic heart valve thrombosis in pregnancy with low-dose, slow infusion of tissue-type plasminogen activator. Circulation 2013;128:532-540.

103. Saby L, Laas O, Habib G, et al. Positron emission tomography/computed tomography for diagnosis of prosthetic valve endocarditis: Increased valvular 18F-fluorodeoxyglucose uptake as a novel major criterion. J Am Coll Cardiol 2013;61:2374-2382.

104. Regueiro A, Linke A, Latib A, et al. Association between transcatheter aortic valve replacement and subsequent infective endocarditis and in-hospital death. JAMA 2016;316:1083-1092.

105. David TE, Feindel CM, Bos J, et al. Aortic valve replacement with a stent-less porcine aortic valve: a six-year experience. J Thorac Cardiovasc Surg 1994;108:1030-1036.

106. Dossche K, Vanermen H, Daenen W, et al. Hemodynamic performance of the PRIMA Edwards stentless aortic xenograft: early results of a multicenter clinical trial. Thorac Cardiovasc Surg 1996;44:11-14.

107. Kirklin JK, Smith D, Novick W, et al. Long-term function of cryopreserved aortic homografts: a ten-year study. J Thorac Cardiovasc Surg 1993;106:154-165.

108. Langley SM, McGuirk SP, Chaudhry MA, et al. Twenty-year follow-up of aortic valve replacement with antibiotic sterilized homografts in 200 patients. Semin Thorac Cardiovasc Surg 1999;11(Suppl 1):28-34.

109. Elkins RC, Lane MM, McCue C. Pulmonary autograft reoperation: incidence and management. Ann Thorac Surg 1996;62:450-455.

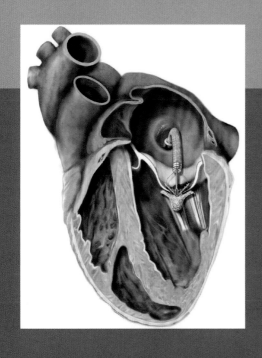

第27章
人工生物瓣膜退化的管理

　　本章由浅入深地阐释人工瓣膜的发展历程，瓣膜毁损的定义、发生机制及其危险因素，以及对于毁损瓣膜再次手术和经导管瓣中瓣植入术的适应证、术前评估、并发症及其应对策略。

　　时至今日，＞90%的瓣膜置换术均使用生物瓣膜。尽管其结构设计和抗钙化处理已经数次改良，但结构性瓣膜衰败仍是限制其长期寿命的重要因素。人工生物瓣膜结构性瓣膜衰败是一个缓慢的过程，其发生发展通常需数年至十余年时间。患者年龄是公认的结构性瓣膜衰败危险因素。除此之外，瓣膜植入位置，肾功能，异常钙磷代谢，高脂血症，妊娠，严重瓣膜-患者不匹配等都与结构性瓣膜衰败密切相关。

　　对于衰败的人工瓣膜，可以选择再次开胸手术或行经导管瓣中瓣植入术进行治疗。尽管再次开胸手术具有更好的血流动力学状态及更少的血管并发症，但其死亡率明显高于首次瓣膜置换术。对于活动性心内膜炎、衰败生物瓣膜尺寸较小、具有冠状动脉梗阻风险和有其他开胸手术指征的患者，建议选择再次开胸手术。随着瓣膜介入技术的发生发展，经导管瓣中瓣植入术的应用日益增加。经导管瓣中瓣植入术与首次经导管主动脉瓣置换术相比，其死亡率、瓣环损伤、主动脉夹层和传导阻滞的发生率均明显更低。但在经导管瓣中瓣植入术中，残余狭窄、瓣膜血栓和瓣膜异位的发生率较高。通过术前充分评估及术中合理决策，可以显著降低上述不良事件的发生率。

郭　帅

Management of Bioprosthetic Valve Degeneration

Danny Dvir

CHAPTER OUTLINE

KEY POINTS

- The choice of surgical valve replacement or transcatheter valve-in-valve (VIV) implantation for bioprosthetic valve failure depends on careful consideration of patient characteristics and surgical valve and anatomic parameters by a multidisciplinary heart valve team.
- Clinical outcomes after a transcatheter VIV procedure differ from those after a native valve transcatheter aortic valve implantation; with VIV, there are fewer mechanical complications and lower rates of mortality, conduction defects, and paravalvular regurgitation.
- Adverse effects after VIV transcatheter aortic valve replacement (TAVR) for a failed surgical bioprosthesis include residual stenosis, clinical thrombosis, malpositioning, and coronary obstruction.

- Approaches to reduce the risk of stenosis after transcatheter aortic valve implantation include supra-annular positioning of the transcatheter valve, avoidance of underexpansion of the valve, and intentional fracturing of the bioprosthetic valve ring.
- Clinical thrombosis after VIV TAVR occurs in about 8% of patients, necessitating careful postimplantation monitoring and appropriate anticoagulation.
- A novel approach to prevention of coronary ostial obstruction with a VIV procedure is the bioprosthetic or native aortic scallop intentional laceration to prevent iatrogenic coronary artery obstruction (BASILICA) procedure.

HISTORY OF PROSTHETIC HEART VALVES

The evolution of prosthetic heart valves begins with the work of innovative physicians backed by industry support. The first implantation of a homograft in the descending aorta was performed by Murray in 1956.[1] In 1961, Albert Starr and Lowell Edwards introduced clinical orthotopic valve replacement therapy using mechanical valve models.[2] A few years later, Donald Ross and Barratt Boyes introduced aortic homografts and pulmonary autografts into clinical practice, and the work of Carlos Duran and others led to the implantation of porcine aortic and mitral valves.[3–5] Significant growth of porcine bioprosthetic aortic valve replacements was mainly led by Hancock Laboratory, Edwards Lifesciences (Irvine, CA), Medtronic (Minneapolis, MN), and Shiley.

In 1969, Alain Carpentier introduced the use of glutaraldehyde for prevention of degeneration of porcine aortic valves.[6] In 1971, Marian Ionescu designed the first-generation bovine pericardial valves.[7] In the early 1980s, several types of second-generation bioprosthetic valves were clinically available. Later, transcatheter pulmonary valves were implanted, and in 2002, the first transcatheter aortic valve replacement

(TAVR) was performed by Alian Cribier, marking the start of the transcatheter valve replacement era.[8,9]

Tissue bioprosthetic valves are used in almost all surgical implantations and in all clinical transcatheter valve implantations.[10–13] Bioprosthetic valves are favored over mechanical valves because of lower thrombogenicity and lack of obligatory long-term anticoagulation. Novel anticoagulants do not reduce the risk of thrombogenicity effectively enough in these cases, and the use of mechanical valves is rapidly decreasing.[14] In 1997, more than 50% of valve replacements in the United States used mechanical valves; a decade later, their use had decreased to less than 25%.[15] Currently, bioprosthetic tissue valves are used in more than 90% of valve replacements, with TAVR procedures accounting for a large portion of that group in the aortic position.

Although bioprostheses are much less prone to clinical thrombosis than mechanical valves, tissue valves are associated with structural valve degeneration (SVD), potentially limiting long-term durability.[16] The updated American Heart Association (AHA)/American College of Cardiology (ACC) guidelines recommend that selection of the type of prosthetic heart valve to be implanted should be based on a shared decision-making process that accounts for the patient's values and

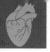

preferences.[17,18] It should include a discussion about the risks of anticoagulant therapy and the potential risk of associated reintervention.

The age cutoff for considering mechanical valve implantation is defined as less than 50 years in the AHA/ACC guidelines. In the European Society of Cardiology (ESC) guidelines, the cutoffs are less than 60 years for aortic valves and less than 65 years for mitral valves.[19]

CHARACTERISTICS OF BIOPROSTHETIC HEART VALVES

Numerous prosthetic heart valve designs and a large variety of proprietary anticalcification treatments are available (see Chapter 26). These devices differ in their tissue characteristics, frame designs, and implantation methods.[20] They commonly have unique fluoroscopic appearances, which is essential for optimal VIV deployment. This chapter focuses on the more common heart valve subgroup: bioprosthetic tissue valves (see Fig. 26.1 in Chapter 26).

Bioprosthetic valves can be classified according to their method of implantation (i.e., transcatheter vs. surgical). Surgical bioprosthetic valves are commonly stratified according to type of tissue (porcine vs. bovine pericardial) or according to frame design (i.e., stented, stentless, or sutureless). Transcatheter valves are commonly categorized as balloon-expandable versus mechanically expandable or self-expandable devices.

Initially, most surgical bioprosthetic aortic valves were implanted in the plane of the annulus (i.e., intra-annular position); today, many are implanted above the annulus (i.e., supra-annular position), allowing for a larger orifice and possibly decreasing the risk of prosthesis–patient mismatch (PPM).

Bioprosthesis leaflets are conventionally attached to the internal aspect of the stent posts, although several surgical bioprosthetic valves are designed with externally mounted leaflets, including the Mitroflow (Livanova, London, England) and Trifecta (St. Jude Medical, now Abbott Cardiovascular, Santa Clara, CA) valves. This design may enable a better hemodynamic profile and reduce the risk of PPM, but the risk of coronary obstruction after VIV is higher in certain anatomic conditions.

Valve leaflets are commonly fashioned from animal tissue (i.e., xenografts) and sometimes from human valves (i.e., homografts and autografts). Most bioprostheses are made of porcine valve tissue or bovine pericardium, whereas transcatheter valves are occasionally made of porcine pericardial tissue. The tissue is commonly preserved in glutaraldehyde; cross-linking of collagen fibers reduces antigenicity, enzymatic degradation, and remodeling of the extracellular matrix.[21,22]

Stented surgical bioprosthetic valves include a support structure made of Elgiloy, a cobalt-chromium-nickel-molybdenum alloy (Elgiloy Specialty Metals, Sycamore, IL); titanium; or Delrin, an acetal homopolymer (DuPont de Nemours, Inc., Wilmington, DE). The frame is attached to a circular or scallop-shaped basal ring. The semirigid materials of the frame absorb some of the forces acting on the leaflets, with the aim of prolonging leaflet durability. The basal ring is frequently covered by a sewing cuff, which facilitates suturing to the native tissue during cardiac surgery. The sewing ring determines the position of the valve in relation to the patient's tissue annulus. A supra-annular sewing ring is designed to secure the surgical heart valve fully above the patient's tissue annulus, whereas an intra-annular ring secures it fully or mostly within the patient's tissue annulus.[23]

Stentless bioprostheses lack a firm support structure. These valves include homografts and porcine (e.g., Freestyle [Medtronic]) and bovine (e.g., Freedom Solo [Livanova]) pericardial tissue valves, and they offer more natural flow in the aortic root.[24] Homografts can be explanted from recipients of heart transplants or from organ donors. They can be implanted as a full root or with the use of a subcoronary

technique or occasionally a modified subcoronary technique. Novel surgical bioprostheses (e.g., rapid-deployment valves) include the Intuity valve (Edwards Lifesciences) and the sutureless Perceval valve (Livanova).[25] They enable reduction in aortic cross-clamp and cardiopulmonary bypass times.

Prosthetic valves are defined in several dimensions. The most common feature is the label size, which traditionally represents the external diameter of the inflow portion.[26,27] Inconsistencies and controversies exist regarding the sizing and labeling of bioprosthetic valves.[27] Non-uniform or incomplete reporting of bioprosthesis materials and physical dimensions by the industry was described in a 2019 position statement.[28]

For VIV sizing, it is the inner diameter of the valve that is most relevant.[29] These measures include the manufacturer-defined inner diameter (ID) and the inner diameter of the valve as measured by sizing tools (true ID); the latter takes into consideration the valve leaflets inside the frame. There is significant discrepancy between the manufacturer ID and the true ID.[28] The true ID is commonly 1 to 3 mm smaller than the reported ID. Several applications are used for decision making based on these characteristics.

Other relevant prosthetic valve measures include the height of the frame and leaflets when deflected. Occasionally, the length of the leaflet corresponds to the length of the frame, but not always. Leaflet length and the degree to which the leaflets can be deflected are important measures that can influence the risk for coronary obstruction after VIV.[30]

MECHANISMS OF FAILURE OF BIOPROSTHETIC HEART VALVES

There are numerous causes of prosthetic heart valve failure (Box 27.1). Mechanical valves are prone to thrombosis, whereas bioprosthetic valves are prone to valve degeneration (Fig. 27.1). SVD is an acquired intrinsic bioprosthetic valve abnormality. It is deterioration of the leaflets or supporting structures that results in thickening, calcification, tearing, or disruption of the prosthetic valve material with eventual associated valve hemodynamic dysfunction, manifested as stenosis and/or regurgitation.[31,32]

There are two main pathways for SVD: the biochemical pathway, which is mostly related to the interaction between the leaflets and the blood and leads to intrinsic cusp calcification, and the biomechanical pathway, which is related to the stress on the leaflets and can result in leaflet tear.[33] Commonly, the process of SVD is a result of the combined effect of the biochemical and biomechanical pathways manifested by progressive degeneration with periods of accelerated hemodynamic deterioration.

The literature on SVD is extensive and includes numerous definitions for this abnormal condition.[34–37] Freedom from reoperation,

---

BOX 27.1   Main Causes for Failure of Prosthetic Heart Valves

Structural valve degeneration
Thrombosis
Endocarditis
Prosthesis–patient mismatch
Pannus formation
Paravalvular leakage
Malposition
Underexpansion or stent creep

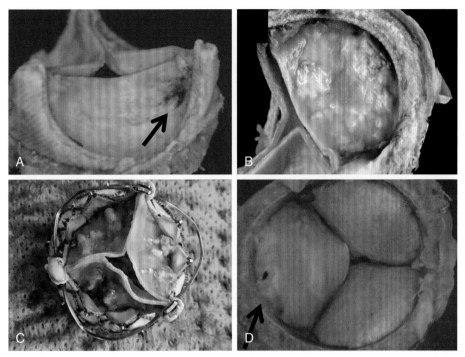

Fig. 27.1 Examples of Degenerated Bioprostheses. (A) Carpentier-Edwards Perimount valve (Edwards Lifesciences) leaflet tear *(arrow)*. (B) Carpentier-Edwards Magna Ease valve (Edwards Lifesciences) leaflet calcification. (C) Engager THV (Medtronic) leaflet restriction and calcification. (D) Carpentier-Edwards Perimount valve (Edwards Lifesciences) leaflet tear, ventricular side *(arrow)*. (From Dvir D, Bourguignon T, Otto CM, et al. Standardized definition of structural valve degeneration for surgical and transcatheter bioprosthetic aortic valves. Circulation 2018;137:388-399.)

which was considered the primary end point in many studies, is a poor surrogate for SVD because reintervention (surgical or transcatheter) may be performed for causes other than SVD. Conversely, reintervention may not be performed if SVD goes undetected because of a lack of echocardiographic follow-up.

In 2018, a standard definition of SVD of bioprosthetic valves was published, specifying stages according to the hemodynamic severity of the failed valve (Fig. 27.2).[38] The process of valve degeneration typically is gradual, taking place over years. The stages of SVD are based on the state of the implanted valve and not on the patient's clinical status. Stage 1 includes early morphologic leaflet changes without hemodynamic sequelae. Stage 2 SVD refers to morphologic abnormalities of valve leaflets associated with hemodynamic dysfunction and is divided according to the type of dysfunction (i.e., stenosis and/or regurgitation of moderate degree) after exclusion of PPM, paravalvular leak (PVL), and other non-SVD conditions. Some patients with stage 2 SVD, especially those with mixed failure, may have symptoms and may be considered for reintervention. Stage 3 includes the development of severe stenosis or severe regurgitation, or both.

There are many risk factors for early SVD. Patient age is widely considered to be associated with the risk of SVD: young age at implantation is associated with early valve degeneration.[31] Other correlates for early SVD include the position of the device (i.e., mitral and tricuspid valves degenerate more rapidly than aortic valves), renal dysfunction (e.g., end-stage kidney disease, dialysis therapy), abnormal calcium/phosphate metabolism, very severe dyslipidemia (e.g., patients with homozygous familial hypercholesterolemia), pregnancy, severe PPM, and others.

The type of the device also is related to the risk of SVD. Some devices that were associated with early failures were taken off the market.[39,40]

Certain valves are more prone to a specific type of failure than others. Bovine pericardial valves tend to fail more often by stenosis, whereas porcine leaflets tend to fail more commonly by regurgitation.

In the current TAVR era, patients with failed bioprosthetic valves can be treated with this less invasive approach, providing a strong argument in favor of a more meticulous echocardiographic surveillance regimen. Consensus documents support yearly echocardiographic surveillance in all patients,[38] but there is a discrepancy about when to begin: from the first year in the ESC guidelines or 10 years after implantation in the AHA/ACC guidelines.[18,19]

OPEN HEART SURGERY FOR BIOPROSTHETIC HEART VALVE FAILURE

Reoperation is a procedure widely considered to carry increased risk: the mortality rate is higher than for those undergoing first surgery, although some registries have found conflicting evidence.[41,42] Data from the Society of Thoracic Surgeons (STS) database show an in-hospital mortality rate of 4.6% among 3380 patients (mean age, 68 years; average STS Predicted Risk of Mortality [PROM] score, 5.4%) who underwent repeat aortic valve replacement.[43] This record represents the largest reported population and is an important reference for clinical outcomes of repeat surgery in the VIV era.

The group with bioprosthetic valves who underwent repeat open heart surgery included 2213 patients. The operative mortality rate was 4.7%, and the composite rate of operative mortality and major morbidity was 21.9%. Stroke was reported for 1.8% of patients, and a pacemaker was required in 11.5%. Selected high-volume centers achieved lower 30-day mortality rates of 2% to 3% after repeat surgery.[44–46] Surgical reoperation was the main therapeutic modality

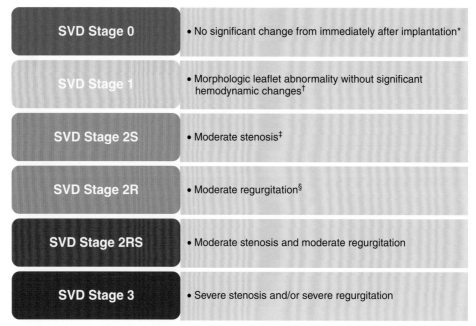

Fig. 27.2 Definitions of Structural Valve Deterioration (SVD). The SVD definition excludes infective endocarditis, valve thrombosis, isolated prosthesis–patient mismatch without deterioration in valve function, isolated paravalvular regurgitation, and frame distortion without abnormal leaflet function. Nevertheless, these conditions may account for stage 1 SVD because the bioprosthesis may be prone to early SVD. *No significant new hemodynamic abnormality (mean gradient < 20 mmHg and intravalvular regurgitation less than moderate) and no morphologic leaflet abnormality (e.g., leaflet thickening). †Leaflet calcification, sclerosis, thickening, or new leaflet motion disorder. ‡Must include > 10 mmHg increase from baseline status with concomitant decrease in effective orifice area (EOA) and Doppler velocity index (DVI). Thrombotic leaflet thickening should be clinically excluded. If it is reversible with anticoagulation, it should be considered as valve thrombosis. §If the main component is paravalvular, it should not be considered as SVD. (From Dvir D, Bourguignon T, Otto CM, et al. Standardized definition of structural valve degeneration for surgical and transcatheter bioprosthetic aortic valves. Circulation 2018;137:388-399.)

for patients with prosthetic valve stenosis and/or regurgitation before the era of transcatheter therapies. Repeat open heart surgery is becoming less common when the less invasive transcatheter VIV procedure is available.[47]

It is challenging to compare results of repeat open heart surgery with those of transcatheter VIV because the patient populations are significantly different. VIV is commonly performed in high-risk patients 70 to 85 years of age, whereas open heart surgery is commonly performed in patients who are younger than 70 years of age and have many fewer comorbidities. Nevertheless, several studies have been published.[48–50] The small cohort comparisons showed similar short-term and 1-year survival rates for patients undergoing open heart reoperation compared with VIV; hospital stay was shorter in the VIV group, and there was less need for a pacemaker or for conversion to open heart surgery. Those having repeat open heart surgery had better hemodynamics and fewer vascular complications.

Table 27.1 is a list of patient characteristics, surgical valve features, and anatomic parameters that may favor a repeat open heart surgical approach or a transcatheter VIV approach. The evidence indicates that selected patients with failed bioprosthetic heart valves can benefit from open heart surgery. These include patients with active endocarditis, those with small surgical valves who may benefit from root enlargement, those at risk for coronary obstruction with aortic VIV, those at risk for left ventricular outflow tract obstruction with mitral VIV, and those who are candidates for open heart surgery for other conditions. In rare cases, patients with failed bioprosthetic valves have occult infective endocarditis that may damage the newly implanted valve after

VIV; they may be better treated with open heart surgery that includes surgical debridement of the previously implanted valve, especially because endocarditis after TAVR is associated with very poor prognosis.[51]

The role of advanced imaging modalities, including positron emission tomography/computed tomography (PET-CT), in the pre-VIV evaluation needs to be determined.[52,53] It is conceivable that an implanted valve after repeat open heart surgery can serve as a better platform for a future VIV than a transcatheter valve that will eventually require a second VIV procedure. In such cases, open heart surgical valve replacement may allow better, less invasive therapeutic options years later.[54]

TRANSCATHETER AORTIC VALVE-IN-VALVE IMPLANTATION

Before the TAVR era, patients with failed bioprostheses who were considered to be at high surgical risk had limited options for minimally invasive treatment. Some of these patients were treated by supportive medical therapy, but the associated prognosis was poor.

Although balloon valvuloplasty alone could potentially improve valve function in selected patients with predominant stenosis as the mechanism of failure of their bioprosthesis, the limited efficacy of balloon dilation and the fact that degenerated bioprosthetic leaflets are at high risk for tearing did not support this clinical use. Anecdotally, attempts at balloon dilatation were occasionally futile, and some cases resulted in severe regurgitation or were followed by emergent surgical procedures.[55,56] As a result, isolated balloon interventions

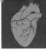

TABLE 27.1   Clinical Characteristics That May Favor Repeat Open Heart Surgery or Transcatheter Valve-in-Valve Implantation in Patients With Failed Bioprosthetic Valves.

Favors Open Heart Surgery	Favors Transcatheter Valve-in-Valve Procedure
Patient Characteristics	
Low risk for open heart surgery	At high risk for open heart surgery
Patient age < 60 yr	Patient age > 70 yr
Prolonged expected longevity	Poor candidate for general anesthesia
Candidate for open heart surgery for other reasons	Renal failure
Patient choice	Patient choice
Surgical Valve/Ring Characteristics	
Small surgical valve	Large surgical valve
Severe prosthesis-patient mismatch	—
Noncircular and/or rigid mitral or tricuspid ring	Circular semirigid or flexible mitral or tricuspid ring
Mixed paravalvular and intravalvular leakage	Good fluoroscopic markers for positioning
Possible active endocarditis	Expandable surgical valve ring
Anatomic Parameters	
Poor transfemoral artery access for aortic VIV	Favorable transcatheter access
Poor transseptal access for mitral VIV	Calcified aortic root
High risk for malposition with VIV	Porcelain aorta
Risk for coronary obstruction with aortic VIV	
Risk for LVOT obstruction with mitral VIV or valve-in-ring procedure	

LVOT, Left ventricular outflow tract; *VIV*, valve-in-valve procedure.

for the treatment of degenerated bioprosthetic valves were widely avoided. Nevertheless, improvement may be achieved with balloon dilation alone in selected cases of recently implanted bioprosthetic valves without leaflet calcification or in some cases of transcatheter heart valves (THVs) with underexpansion.[57]

Preclinical and Early Clinical Studies

VIV implantation was a minimally invasive method suggested to treat failed bioprostheses. In a sheep model, six animals were implanted with a Mosaic (Medtronic) bioprosthesis, followed by implantation of bovine jugular valves mounted onto a stent and inserted off-pump.[58]

Later, the feasibility of implanting an early-generation transcatheter balloon-expandable valve was evaluated in seven pigs.[59] Carpentier-Edwards valves (Edwards Lifesciences) were implanted in the aortic and mitral positions, followed in each case by transapical VIV implantation of a 23-mm Cribier-Edwards valve. Good hemodynamic function was observed and confirmed by autopsy.

In several of these bench testing studies,[60–62] the hemodynamics after implantation of a 23-mm Edwards-SAPIEN transcatheter valve (derived from the original Cribier-Edwards design) within various sizes of Carpentier-Edwards Perimount valves were extensively examined. Postprocedural aortic valve gradients negatively correlated with surgical valve device size, and transcatheter valves with a supravalvular design resulted in better hemodynamic gains. Initial reports of aortic VIV feasibility appeared in 2007 from research groups in Canada and Germany. A Canadian registry (N = 24) was soon followed by an Italian registry (N = 25), two German registries (N = 20, N = 47), and numerous other case reports and small case series documenting mainly favorable outcomes.[63–82]

TAVR practice in the United States was captured in the STS/ACC Transcatheter Valve Therapy (TVT) Registry, which describes the trends of VIV procedures across the years.[83] The proportion of VIV procedures increased from 2.5% in 2012 to 6.1% in 2017. With the dramatic

increase in the use of bioprosthetic valves over the past 2 decades, in addition to increased patient longevity and extension of TAVR to patients with previous cardiac surgery, it is conceivable that the proportion of VIV procedures may grow to 10% or more of all TAVR cases.

VIV using several different devices is an approved and indicated therapy in the United States, Canada, and Europe. It is indicated in published guidelines for the treatment of failed bioprosthetic valves. The 2017 AHA/ACC focused guideline update indicated VIV therapy for severely symptomatic patients who have bioprosthetic valve failure with stenosis or regurgitation, for whom reoperation carries high or prohibitive risk and in whom improvement in hemodynamics is anticipated (class IIa indication).[18]

This indication was based solely on registry data without any randomized trial comparing this transcatheter approach with that of open heart surgery. After the expansion of TAVR to include lower-risk patient populations, it became very challenging to design a study that could randomly assign patients with previous open heart surgery, who are commonly considered to be at increased surgical risk, to repeat open heart surgery.

Several large studies have evaluated patients undergoing aortic VIV procedures (Table 27.2). The Valve-in-Valve International Data (VIVID) Registry was introduced in 2010 to collate this increasing but widely distributed experience.[84,85] The registry now includes the largest cohort of VIV procedures, with more than 4100 VIV cases collected from 127 centers worldwide. Other registries include a VIV registry in the PARTNER study, the CoreValve U.S. registry, the VIVA registry, and a VIV cohort from the TVT Registry.[83,86–89]

Patients undergoing aortic VIV therapy are commonly between the ages of 70 and 85 years and have a failed bioprosthetic valve that was implanted 7 to 12 years earlier. The median time to VIV is 9 years (interquartile range, 6–12 years), and it is significantly shorter for patients who have predominant valve stenosis rather than regurgitation (8 vs. 10 years, P = 0.04). In approximately 80% of cases, the failed

TABLE 27.2 Large, Multicenter Studies of Aortic Valve-in-Valve TAVR in High-Risk Patients.

	VIVID Aortic	PARTNER 2	CoreValve US	VIVA	TVT
Patient Characteristics					
Study population (N)	2318	365	227	202	1150
Age (yr)	78	79	77	80	79
STS PROM (mean %)	8.8	9.1	9.0	6.6	6.9
Implantation Rate by Valve Type (% of Patients)					
CoreValve	39.1	0	100	9.4	19
Evolut	14.2	0	0	90.6	42
SAPIEN XT	26.9	100	0	0	25
SAPIEN 3	13.9	0	0	0	14
Outcomes at 30 Days					
Mortality rate (%)	4.4	2.7	2.2	2.5	2.9
Stroke (%)	1.4	2.7	0.9	3.0	1.7
Coronary obstruction (%)	2.3	0.8	0.9	2.5	0.6
Annular rupture (%)	0	0	0	0	0
PVL ≥ moderate (%)	5.2	3.2	3.5	2.8	3.3
Conversion to open surgery (%)	0.7	0.6	0.5	0.5	0.2
New pacemaker (%)	6.7	1.9	8.1	8.0	3.0
Mean gradient (mmHg)	16.2	17.7	17.0	17.5	16.0
Valve area (cm^2)	1.2	1.1	1.4	1.3	1.3
Length of stay (days)	7	5	—	7	3
Mortality rate at 1 yr (%)	13.3	12.4	14.6	8.8	11.7

PROM, Predicted Risk of Mortality score; PVL, paravalvular leakage; STS, Society of Thoracic Surgeons; TAVR, transcatheter aortic valve replacement; VIV, valve-in-valve procedure.

bioprosthesis is a stented surgical valve, and the most common label sizes are 21, 23, and 25 mm.[84] Small surgical valves (≤21 mm) account for almost one third of the candidates for aortic VIV. The mechanism of failure may include predominant stenosis, predominant regurgitation, or a mixture of the two.

Until several years ago, most aortic VIV experience had been obtained with the Medtronic CoreValve or the Edwards SAPIEN XT device. Numerous other transcatheter devices have been used, and the clear majority of aortic VIV procedures are performed with Evolut (Medtronic) or SAPIEN 3 (Edwards) devices.[83]

Clinical Outcomes After Transcatheter Aortic Valve-in-Valve Implantation

Clinical outcomes for aortic VIV are different from those for conventional TAVR in several respects (Table 27.3). Matched comparisons between conventional TAVR and aortic VIV cases showed lower mortality rates for the VIV group, even after adjusting for differences in baseline characteristics.[83] The frame and ring of stented bioprosthetic valves enable protection of surrounding structures when a valve is implanted inside. As a result, the risk of rare mechanical complications such as annular injury or aortic dissection is lower for VIV procedures. Conduction defects are also much less common.

The rate of pacemaker implantation after VIV is consistently less than 10%. Even with devices, such as the Lotus valve (Boston Scientific Corporation, Marlborough, MA), that are commonly associated with a greater need for pacemaker implantation during conventional TAVR, the rate of pacemaker implantation is low after VIV (5% risk in the VIVID Registry). The frame of the failed bioprosthetic valve enables good support for sealing after VIV, and as a result, the risk of PVL is very low if the previously implanted valve did not have a PVL.

Some adverse events are more common in VIV procedures. They include residual stenosis (especially in small and stenotic surgical

TABLE 27.3 Main Complications After Valve-in-Valve TAVR or Native Valve TAVR.

Complication	Stented Valve TAVR	Stentless VIV	THV VIV	Conventional TAVR
Valve stenosis	+++	+	+	+
Clinical thrombosis	++	+	++	+
Coronary obstruction	++	+++	+++	+
Malpositioning	+	++	+	+
Paravalvular leakage	−	++	+	++
Annular rupture	−	+	−	+

TAVR, Transcatheter aortic valve replacement; THV, transcatheter heart valve; VIV, valve-in-valve procedure; −, no cases; +, uncommon; ++, common; +++, very common.

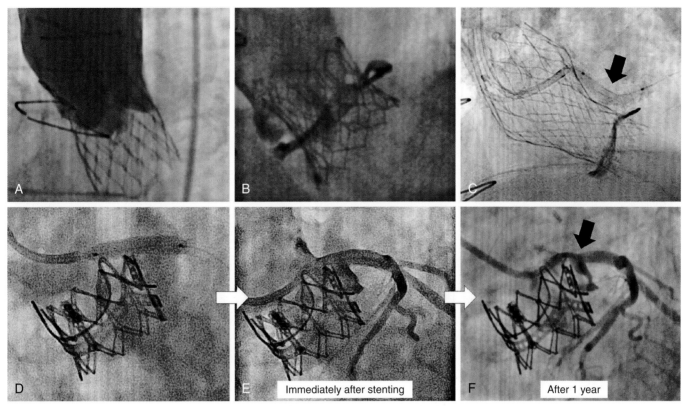

Fig. 27.3 Case Examples of Coronary Obstruction After Transcatheter Aortic Valve Replacement (TAVR) and Prevention by Stent Implantation. (A) Coronary obstruction after TAVR using a CoreValve (Medtronic) in a Toronto stentless porcine valve (SPV) (St. Jude Medical). (B) Coronary obstruction after TAVR using a SAPIEN 3 valve (Edwards Lifesciences) in a Mitroflow valve (Livanova). (C) Prevention of coronary obstruction using the chimney/snorkel technique, in which a stent is prepositioned, undeployed, in the coronary tree during TAVR and then deployed after valve deployment in the coronary inflow to deflect the aortic valve leaflet *(arrow)*. (D–F) Delayed coronary obstruction *(arrow)* after the chimney/snorkel technique for left coronary obstruction after aortic valve-in-valve implantation of a SAPIEN XT valve in a Magna valve (both Edwards Lifesciences). (From Komatsu I, Mackensen GB, Aldea GS, et al. Bioprosthetic or native aortic scallop intentional laceration to prevent iatrogenic coronary artery obstruction. Part 1: how to evaluate patients for BASILICA. Eurointervention 2019;15:47-54.)

valves), clinical thrombosis, malpositioning (especially in regurgitant stentless valves and those with poor fluoroscopic markers), and coronary obstruction (Fig. 27.3).

Patients display significant clinical improvement after aortic VIV. Approximately 90% are in New York Heart Association (NYHA) functional class I/II 30 days after the procedure.[85] These patients show a significant increase in day-to-day capabilities, with an average absolute increase of more than 30 points in Kansas City Cardiomyopathy Questionnaire (KCCQ) score and a significant 66-m average increase in 6-minute walk distance early after the procedure[86,87] (Fig. 27.4). In one study of aortic VIV, the average left ventricular (LV) mass index decreased from 136.4 ± 37.4 g/m^2 at baseline to 125.0 ± 34.0 g/m^2 at 30 days and 109.1 ± 28.2 g/m^2 at 3 years ($P < 0.0001$).[87] Significant LV mass regression is considered a very favorable prognostic signal.

Clinical outcomes after aortic VIV procedures are significantly related to the characteristics of the surgical valve. Small and stenotic surgical valves are associated with inferior clinical outcomes. Data from the VIVID Registry stratifying patients according the size of the surgical valve showed that those with small surgical valves (label size ≤ 21 mm) had a worse 1-year mortality rate after VIV than those with intermediate or large surgical valves (25.2% vs. 18.2% and 6.7%, respectively).[85] Later, smaller analyses with lower-risk patient populations failed to

show differences in 1-year mortality rates.[89] The mechanism of failure is consistently linked to clinical outcomes after the procedure and especially to the risk of elevated postprocedural gradients.

Clinical outcomes may differ according to the type of transcatheter device implanted during aortic VIV. Several studies have compared different devices in this scenario. The VIVID Registry data revealed differences in hemodynamics between intra-anular transcatheter devices and those with potential supra-anular function.[84,85] Two studies compared transcatheter devices. A comparison between the CoreValve/Evolut platform and the Portico device (Abbott, Abbott Park, IL) used for aortic VIV showed similar early mortality and stroke rates but a higher 1-year mortality rate and more cases with residual PVL in the Portico arm.[90] A matched comparison between SAPIEN XT and SAPIEN 3 devices showed similar hemodynamic profiles and risks for residual stenosis with VIV implantation in small bioprosthetic valves.[91,92] Patients receiving a SAPIEN 3 VIV had a greater requirement for pacemaker implantation and fewer vascular complications than those receiving a SAPIEN XT valve.

There is no dedicated calculated risk score for aortic VIV candidates. Operative risk scores for open heart surgery are commonly used as surrogates. In an analysis comparing several common risk score calculators, the Logistic EuroSCORE, EuroSCORE II, and STS scores

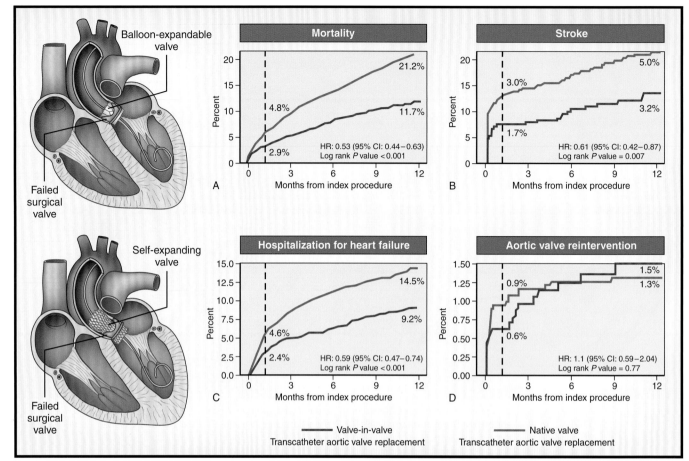

Fig. 27.4 Valve-in-Valve (VIV) Transcatheter Aortic Valve Replacement (TAVR) Versus TAVR for Native Aortic Stenosis. Outcomes are shown for patients in the STS/ACC Registry who underwent VIV TAVR ($n = 1150$) compared in a 1:2 fashion with patients undergoing native valve TAVR ($n = 2259$) between November 9, 2011, and June 30, 2016, with matching based on sex, inoperable or extreme risk designation, hostile chest or porcelain aorta, 5-m walk time, and STS PROM score for reoperation. *ACC*, American College of Cardiology; *CI*, confidence interval; *HR*, heart rate; *PROM*, Predicted Risk of Mortality assessment tool; *STS*, Society of Thoracic Surgeons. (From Tuzcu EM, Kapadia SR, Vemulapalli S, et al. Transcatheter aortic valve replacement of failed surgically implanted bioprostheses: the STS/ACC Registry. J Am Coll Cardiol 2018;72:370-382.)

all overestimated 30-day mortality rates, but the highest predictability occurred with the EuroSCORE II.[93]

Malpositioning after aortic VIV in stented bioprosthetic valves is uncommon. However, the risk of misplacement and need for implantation of a second transcatheter valve is much higher with specific bioprosthetic valves. Data from the VIVID Registry show that malpositioning occurred in 5.3% of stented bioprosthetic valves with adequate fluoroscopic visibility; the rate was higher for patients who had stented valves and poor fluoroscopic markers (11.6%) and for those with stentless surgical valves (13.2%). Malpositioning is associated with acute kidney injury and higher early mortality rates. Independent correlates for device malpositioning include isolated regurgitation as the mechanism of failure, a self-expanding transcatheter valve, and lack of fluoroscopic markers.

Valve-in-Valve Procedure for Severe Prosthesis–Patient Mismatch

PPM is a condition in which an implanted prosthetic valve is too small for the patient's body size.[94] Severe PPM is defined as a postimplantation effective orifice area (EOA) index of less than 0.65 cm²/m² in nonobese patients (body mass index [BMI] < 30 kg/m²) and less than

0.6 cm²/m² in obese patients (BMI ≥ 30 kg/m²). Severe PPM occurs in approximately 5% to 10% of TAVR procedures with supra-anular device function and in 10% to 25% of surgical aortic valve replacement (SAVR) procedures.[95,96] Compared with patients with up to moderate PPM, patients with severe PPM after TAVR or SAVR have higher long-term mortality rates, inferior postprocedure clinical improvement, worse device durability, and higher rates of reintervention.[97,98]

Data from the VIVID Registry show that patients with severe PPM (7.6% of the registry) who underwent aortic VIV procedures had significantly worse clinical outcomes[99] (Fig. 27.5). After adjusting for surgical valve label size, the finding of preexisting severe PPM was associated with an increased risk of death at 1 year (odds ratio = 1.88). It seems that at least part of the previously confirmed association between small surgical valves and worse clinical outcomes after VIV is related to severe PPM and not directly to the small size of the surgical valve.[85] Patients with severe PPM more frequently had elevated postprocedural transvalvular gradients.[99] Attempts to decrease the risk of stenosis in aortic VIV procedures performed for patients with severe PPM may include bioprosthetic valve ring fracture (BVF) (discussed later).[100]

Worse clinical outcomes for patients with severe PPM of their implanted valve are a strong argument for preventing severe PPM in the

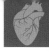

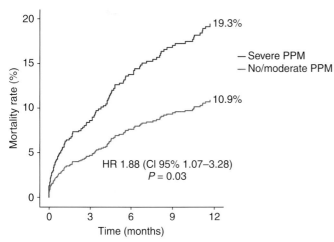

Fig. 27.5 Clinical Outcomes After Aortic Valve-in-Valve (VIV) Procedures. Adjusted 1-year mortality rate after VIV aortic TAVR according to severe prosthesis–patient mismatch (PPM). Data from the transcatheter Valve-in-Valve International Data (VIVID) Registry included 1168 patients, of whom 89 (7.6%) had preexisting severe PPM. (From Pibarot P, Simonato M, Barbanti M, et al. Impact of pre-existing prosthesis-patient mismatch on survival following aortic valve-in-valve procedures. JACC Cardiocasc Interv 2018;11:133-141.)

> **BOX 27.2 Correlates For Stenosis After Aortic Valve-in-Valve Procedures**
>
> Preprocedural characteristics
> - Stenosis as the baseline mechanism of failure
> - Preprocedural severe prosthesis–patient mismatch
> - Stented surgical valve
> - Small surgical valve (internal diameter ≤ 20 mm)
>
> Procedural characteristics
> - Intra-annular transcatheter heart valve
> - Deep transcatheter heart valve position
> - Lack of bioprosthetic valve ring fracture
>
> Postprocedural characteristics
> - Leaflet thrombosis
> - Postprocedural prosthesis–patient mismatch
> - Structural valve degeneration

index procedure. Safety concerns related to these surgical strategies have been raised, but favorable results in selected cohorts have been shown.[101] Preventive measures may include root enlargement and preferential use of a device with a larger EOA and therefore lower risk for PPM. Several studies have reported better hemodynamic results using surgical bioprostheses with supra-annular position rather than intra-annular devices.[102,103] Sutureless rapid-deployment valves and stentless devices have been proposed as an alternative to root enlargement; they have an acceptable safety profile while allowing for a better EOA.[104,105] Since the start of the VIV era, the size of implanted surgical valves has increased, and the rate of severe PPM has decreased.[106]

Persistent Stenosis After Aortic Valve-in-Valve Procedures

With greater operator experience and improved devices compared with those used a decade ago, the rates of most adverse events after VIV procedures are decreasing. Nevertheless, stenosis after aortic VIV remains a significant issue.[107] Elevated aortic valve gradients are relatively common after VIV and are considered the Achilles' heel of these procedures.[85] In contrast to open heart surgery, in TAVR procedures, a device is added without decalcification or any tissue removal. Adding a transcatheter valve to a previously implanted bioprosthesis creates a Russian-doll phenomenon in which the newly implanted valve is smaller than the previous device. If the newly implanted valve is similar in size to the previous one, it will commonly be extremely underexpanded. Residual stenosis after aortic VIV can be at least partially explained by the nondistensible nature of stented bioprosthetic valve rings.[26] Underexpansion has been shown in vitro to create localized regions of high stress that may result in accelerated degeneration.[108]

The average mean aortic valve gradient after VIV (12–20 mmHg) is significantly higher than the average mean gradient in conventional TAVR procedures (6–14 mmHg), creating unique challenges for VIV procedures.[109] Correlates for stenosis after aortic VIV can be divided into preprocedural, procedural, and postprocedural characteristics (Box 27.2). Preprocedural correlates for stenosis include baseline

severe PPM involving a small, a predominantly stenotic, or a stented surgical valve. Postprocedural correlates include clinical thrombosis and SVD of the newly implanted valve.

There are several procedural correlates for elevated gradients after the procedure. They are modifiable and selected at operator discretion. The type, size, and deployment position of the THV are important considerations in optimizing hemodynamic outcomes. In a simplified view, there are two main valve designs: intra-annular valves, in which the leaflets are positioned at the level of the annulus, and supra-annular valves, in which the leaflets function above the annulus. Among the commercially available THVs, the SAPIEN XT and SAPIEN 3 valves (Edwards Lifesciences) are intra-annular, and the CoreValve and Evolut valves (Medtronic) are potentially supra-annular (when implanted high). Because supra-annular devices have their functional section operating in a more elevated position, it is natural that a more complete expansion of the valve can be attained, with better hemodynamic results. This conclusion has been supported by multiple in vitro studies.[110,111]

In one bench study, the gradient across an intra-annular THV greatly depended on surgical valve size, with mean gradients of 9.1 mmHg in a 23-mm Perimount surgical valve, 19.5 mmHg in a 21-mm bioprosthesis, and 46.5 mmHg in a 19-mm bioprosthesis.[60] Other bench studies found the supra annular position to be superior to the annular position in producing lower gradients after implantation of a CoreValve in a Trifecta surgical valve.[112] The importance of supra-annularity has also been supported by clinical data: for small surgical valves with internal diameters less than 20 mm; elevated gradients were found in 59% of SAPIEN procedures.

The relation of elevated gradients to surgical valve size is not as significant in supra-annular implants. These devices allow for a larger orifice and less restriction caused by the surgical valve if implanted high.[60] In a clinical study, implantation depth was shown to be an important independent factor for elevated mean gradient in addition to the THV valve type and the surgical valve mechanism of failure.[113]

Bench testing and clinical data show that for each THV device, there is an ideal high position that may safely decrease the risk of elevated postprocedural gradients[112–114] (Fig. 27.6). Implantation up to a depth of 4 mm (for Evolut devices) or implantation of up to 20% of the device frame below the surgical valve ring (for SAPIEN 3) is considered to represent the optimal cutoff point. SAPIEN 3 positioning in aortic VIV is optimally performed by positioning the central marker bottom up to 6 mm above the surgical valve ring to gain the high implantation

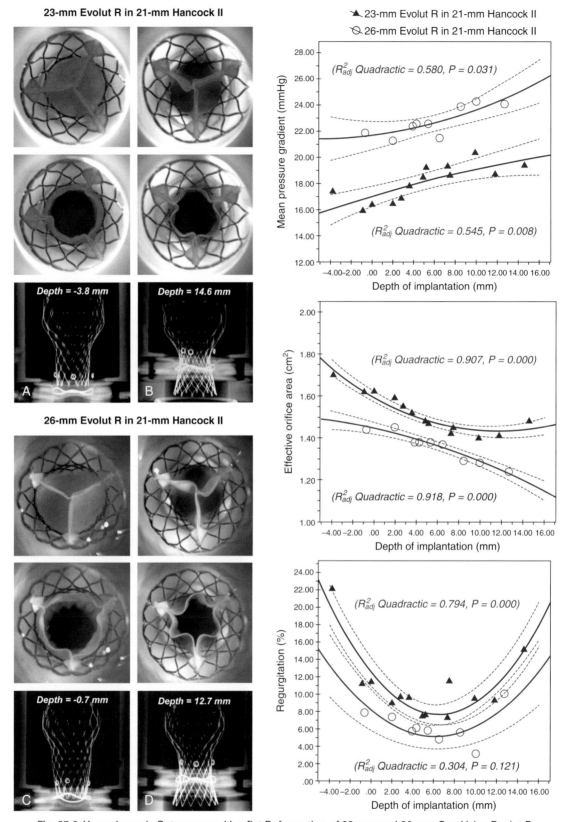

Fig. 27.6 Hemodynamic Outcomes and Leaflet Deformation of 23-mm and 26-mm CoreValve Evolut R Devices Within 21-mm Hancock II Bioprostheses at Different Implantation Depths. (A) 23-mm Evolut R at 3.8 mm. (B) 23-mm Evolut R at 14.6 mm. (C) 26-mm Evolut R at 0.7-mm. (D) 26-mm Evolut R at 12.7 mm. *Dashed lines* represent 95% confidence intervals. A *P* value less than .05 was regarded as statistically significant. R^2_{adj}, Adjusted R squared. (From Azadani AN, Reardon M, Simonato M, et al. Effect of transcatheter aortic valve size and position on valve-in-valve hemodynamics: an in vitro study. J Thorac Cardiovasc Surg 2017;153:1303-1315.)

target.[92] One study suggested that focusing during deployment on the central marker for positioning and not on the top of the SAPIEN 3 frame could be helpful.[92] Although higher device positioning may allow for better hemodynamics, an excessively high position can lead to malpositioning, embolism, challenges in coronary access, and in rare cases, coronary obstruction.[115,116]

In selecting a device during the procedure, operators should consider the importance of using a large THV device in borderline conditions to improve postoperative hemodynamics.[114] If significant oversizing is attempted in VIV conditions with a relatively large THV device, it is essential to position it high to avoid an underexpansion effect on the implanted valve and severe pin-wheeling of the leaflets in diastole.

The small THV devices (e.g., 20-mm SAPIEN 3) allow for less THV deformation when implanted in smaller surgical valves. However, a smaller THV may naturally create severe PPM by its small EOA, and careful preprocedural calculations should be conducted to avoid suboptimal results. Many reports of success with intentional cracking of the ring of the bioprosthesis with ultra-high-pressure inflation of relatively noncompliant balloons to facilitate the expansion of THV have been published[100,115,117–122] (Fig. 27.7).

The aim of BVF is to allow further expansion of the implanted (or about to be implanted) THV; this increases the valve area that can be achieved with VIV and reduces the likelihood of PPM.[100] Patients with small surgical valves, who are at risk for elevated residual gradients after VIV, seem to benefit most from this technique. Clinical data show that a variety of surgical valve rings can be effectively fractured with high-pressure inflations.[118]

Bioprostheses differ in the pressure that results in ring fracture.[123] Several surgical valves, such as the Epic (St. Jude Medical) and Mosaic (Medtronic) valves, fracture at relatively low pressure. Other surgical valves, such as the Hancock II (Medtronic), Trifecta, older-generation Carpentier-Edwards, and Avalus (Medtronic) valves, cannot be fractured using available balloons, although their sewing rings and frames can occasionally be stretched. Other bioprostheses, such as the Inspiris valve (Edwards Lifesciences), have rings that allow dilation under low pressure; this may facilitate a more effective VIV procedure without the potential risks associated with high-pressure balloon inflation.

The safety of BVF, the target population, and optimal candidates for this approach still must be determined. Observed and theoretical risks posed by BVF, including major complications, are uncommon but can be serious. Whether BVF is best performed before or after implantation of the THV is unknown. Performing BVF before VIV may result hemodynamic instability, whereas high-pressure inflation after the VIV procedure may damage the newly implanted transcatheter valve, with possible durability issues and, in rare cases, acute valvular regurgitation. Long-term follow-up data are needed to understand whether BVF improves clinical outcomes except for the acute hemodynamic benefit observed.

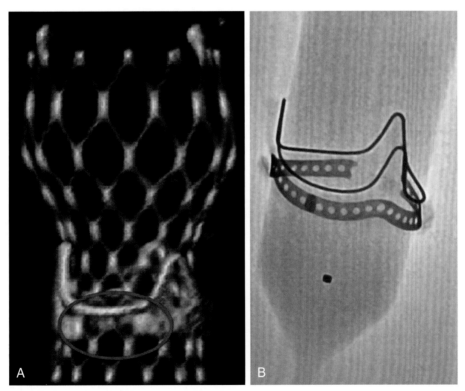

Fig. 27.7 Cracking the Bioprosthesis Ring Can Facilitate Expansion of the Transcatheter Heart Valve. (A) Postoperative computed tomographic image demonstrates the single fracture point *(red circle)* in a 21-mm Edwards Magna tissue valve in a patient who underwent valve-in-valve transcatheter aortic valve replacement using a 23-mm Medtronic Evolut R valve followed by bioprosthetic valve fracture using a 22-mm True Dilation Balloon (CR Bard, Murray Hill, NJ) and high-pressure inflation. (B) Fluoroscopic image obtained during previous bench testing of a 21-mm Edwards Magna tissue valve fractured with the use of a 22-mm True Dilation balloon shows similarities. (From Allen KB, Chhatriwalla AK, Saxon JT, et al. Bioprosthetic valve fracture: technical insights from a multicenter study. J Thorac Cardiovasc Surg 2019;158:1317-1328.)

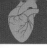

Clinical Thrombosis of Aortic Valve-in-Valve Prostheses

Clinical valve thrombosis is an underrecognized adverse event in TAVR in general and especially in the VIV population. It is possible that some of the residual stenosis seen at follow-up after aortic VIV can be reduced with effective anticoagulation. Hypoattenuated leaflet thickening occurs in approximately 10% to 20% of conventional TAVR procedures.[124–126] This relatively common manifestation is prevented by anticoagulation but is not often associated with elevated transvalvular gradients, and almost all of these patients are asymptomatic. Clinical valve thrombosis with hemodynamic significance is rare after conventional TAVR.[127] However, bench testing and clinical data suggest that clinical thrombosis after aortic VIV is significantly more common.[128–132]

In an analysis from the VIVID Registry, the incidence of clinical thrombosis after VIV was 7.6%.[133] These cases were typically diagnosed 3 to 6 months after the procedure. Most patients presented with worsening symptoms, and almost all had an increase in transvalvular gradients that significantly decreased after anticoagulation therapy. Clinical thrombosis was less common among patients who were discharged on oral anticoagulation and much more common among those with Mosaic or Hancock II stented porcine bioprostheses. It was calculated that approximately 20% of patients with Mosaic or Hancock II bioprostheses who are treated with aortic VIV and not anticoagulated could have clinical thrombosis later.[133]

These findings have many clinical implications. Severe increase in mean gradient early after VIV is a signal for possible thrombotic complications and the need for careful monitoring. After VIV, it is essential for patients to have a good baseline assessment of the hemodynamic result and meticulous follow-up, including a 30-day echocardiographic assessment to allow early identification of thrombotic complications. In the meantime, selected patients undergoing aortic VIV procedures, especially those who have specific surgical valves that are prone to clinical thrombosis after VIV and are not amenable to meticulous echocardiographic follow-up, may benefit from a 3- to 6-month period of anticoagulation therapy unless they are at increased risk for bleeding complications. Anticoagulation trials in specific subsets of TAVR populations would help guide future postoperative protocols to prevent thrombotic complications.

Coronary Obstruction After Aortic Valve Implantation

Reduction in coronary blood flow after TAVR is a serious complication.[30,134] It commonly manifests clinically with abrupt severe hypotension or electrocardiographic changes immediately or shortly after valve implantation.[135] Echocardiographic regional left ventricular dyskinesia should also prompt immediate assessment for aortography. The in-hospital mortality rate after coronary obstruction is approximately 50%. The risk of coronary obstruction is approximately 10 times higher for aortic VIV (2%–3%) than for conventional TAVR procedures (0.2%–0.5%).[136,137] Likewise, delayed coronary obstruction, occurring hours or even days after the procedure, is significantly more common after VIV than after conventional TAVR.

Displacement of a bioprosthetic valve leaflet by the newly implanted THV often is the main cause of the obstruction.[30,138] Aortic valve leaflets are in a closed position during diastole, and the widely open sinus of Valsalva enables a large pool of blood to be delivered to the coronary arteries. After TAVR, an abnormal condition exists in which a deflected bioprosthetic leaflet does not close in diastole, and the flow to the sinus of Valsalva is diminished. This is clinically relevant for cases in which the deflected leaflet can rise above the plane of the coronary artery while the gap between that deflected leaflet and the sinus wall or sinotubular junction (STJ) is narrow.[30,138] Patients with a low coronary ostia origin and narrow sinuses of Valsalva are prone to coronary obstruction (Box 27.3).

VIVID classification defines the anatomic relationships of the coronary ostia and divides them into three main types according to the location of the ostia and the size of the sinuses or STJ that will determine the risk of coronary obstruction[138] (Fig. 27.8). In type I, a coronary ostium lies above the top of the deflected leaflet, and the deflected leaflet is unable to cover the flow to the coronary artery, even if the sinuses are narrow. In type II, the deflected leaflet may go beyond the level of the coronary ostium, and in these cases, the risk of coronary obstruction depends on the capacity of the sinuses to accommodate the deflected leaflet (type IIA, wide sinuses; type IIB, effaced sinuses). Occasionally, implanted valves have leaflets that can extend above the level of the STJ when deflected. These conditions may not carry a risk of coronary obstruction after TAVR as long as the sinuses and STJ are wide (type IIIA). However, coronary obstruction by the deflected leaflet may occur if the sinuses (type IIIB) or the STJ alone (type IIIC) is narrow.

In an analysis from the VIVID Registry that included 1612 aortic VIV procedures, coronary obstruction was more common in stentless bioprostheses or stented bioprostheses with externally mounted leaflets than in the more commonly encountered stented bioprostheses with internally mounted leaflets.[139] No association has been shown between the type of THV and the risk of immediate coronary obstruction. However, there is a higher risk of delayed coronary obstruction with self-expandable devices. Identification of patients at risk for coronary obstruction is crucial to avoid this rare but potentially fatal complication.[138] Although CT is the gold standard in assessing the risk for coronary obstruction, conventional coronary angiography and aortography in the catheterization laboratory can convey important basic screening information for that risk.

Poor contrast opacification of the aortic root is relatively common in patients with a regurgitant bioprosthetic surgical valve undergoing aortography. Semiselective injection of contrast into a coronary ostium or solely into the coronary sinus base may improve assessment of the geometric relationship between the failed surgical valve and the coronary ostia with minimal use of contrast. Injection performed in the left anterior oblique (LAO)–cranial projection, in which the posts of a stented bioprosthesis are aligned in 1-2 fashion (i.e., obtaining a leaflet side view projection) can delineate the relationship between the left main ostium and the potential deflected leaflet. It can easily show whether the ostium originates above the post of the surgical valve (type I), in which case no risk for obstruction exists. Another

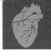

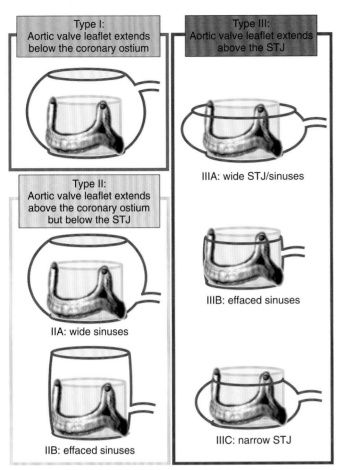

Fig. 27.8 Risk of Coronary Obstruction and Valve-in-Valve International Data (VIVID) Registry Classification. VIVID classification of coronary ostia and aortic root morphologies influences the risk of coronary obstruction after transcatheter aortic valve replacement (TAVR). *STJ*, Sinotubular junction. (From Komatsu I, Mackensen GB, Aldea GS, et al. Bioprosthetic or native aortic scallop intentional laceration to prevent iatrogenic coronary artery obstruction. Part 1: how to evaluate patients for BASILICA. Eurointervention 2019;15:47-54.)

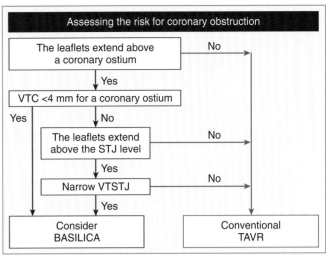

Fig. 27.9 Assessment of the Risk for Coronary Obstruction and BASILICA Procedure Consideration. Assessment starts with observing the relationship between the coronary ostia and leaflet commissures. If the coronary ostia originate above the commissures, the leaflet will not reach far enough to cover the coronary artery. If the commissure comes above, the distance between the virtual transcatheter heart valve (THV) and the coronary ostium *(VTC)* is measured. If it is less than 4 mm, a BASILICA procedure should be considered. If the VTC is greater than 4 mm, the risk for sinotubular junction *(STJ)* inflow obstruction should be checked by evaluating the relationship between the STJ and the leaflet commissures. If the virtual THV-to-STJ distance *(VTSTJ)* is small, BASILICA may be considered. However, there are insufficient data to suggest a high risk of obstruction in cases with a small VTSTJ. The operator also needs to assess leaflet bulkiness and the position of stent posts in case they are in front of a coronary ostium. *TAVR*, Transcatheter aortic valve replacement. (From Komatsu I, Mackensen GB, Aldea GS, et al. Bioprosthetic or native aortic scallop intentional laceration to prevent iatrogenic coronary artery obstruction. Part 1: how to evaluate patients for BASILICA. Eurointervention 2019;15:47-54.)

important aspect of coronary angiography is that it can identify the size of the territory at risk if occlusion occurs. Patency of bypass grafts, significant collateral flow, and coronary dominancy may alter the clinical significance of coronary occlusion.

CT allows three-dimensional assessment of the aortic root's anatomy, including the coronary ostia height, the width and height of the sinus of Valsalva, and the STJ. CT delineates valve tissue characteristics, bulkiness, and calcification. The virtual THV-to–coronary ostium distance (VTC) is a CT-obtained parameter that combines the risk factors of coronary height, sinus width, and THV size and accounts for bioprosthetic valve root canting.[30,140] This is optimally performed by superimposition of a virtual ring simulating the diameter of the anticipated expanded THV, positioned on the geometric center of the surgical prosthesis, followed by a caliper measurement from the ring toward each coronary ostium (Fig. 27.9).

A short VTC distance predicts coronary obstruction: an optimal cutoff level of 4 mm best identifies patients at risk with high sensitivity and high specificity (85% and 89%, respectively), albeit with a low positive predictive value related to the low incidence of coronary obstruction in clinical practice.[139] When the top of the deflected leaflets can cover the STJ, the distance between the deflected leaflet and the

STJ wall (VTSTJ) should also be measured. There are still uncertainties related to actual postimplantation THV diameter, position, shape, and canting, all of which are influenced by numerous factors that are challenging to predict before TAVR.[138]

Bailout coronary stenting is feasible with coronary obstruction.[141,142] Because coronary access after obstruction by the leaflet is challenging, it is reasonable to perform coronary protection before TAVR by positioning a guidewire (with or without an undeployed stent) in the coronary artery that can be brought back to stent the coronary ostium if necessary. The stent is deployed alongside the THV toward the ostium of the coronary artery to keep the bioprosthetic leaflet away from the ostium (chimney or snorkel stenting; see Fig. 27.3). However, this technique of stent protection is associated with a risk of stent jailing if there is no need to deploy the stent.

The long-term outcomes of the bailout techniques are suboptimal. Concerns include stent thrombosis, restenosis, and extremely challenging reaccess to the coronary artery.[30,143] Emergent coronary artery bypass surgery is another option if bailout stenting or other transcatheter techniques are impossible, but it is commonly a high-risk procedure.

To avoid coronary obstruction, a procedure to maintain coronary flow has been proposed. The bioprosthetic or native aortic scallop intentional laceration to prevent iatrogenic coronary artery obstruction (BASILICA) procedure directly addresses the pathophysiology of coronary artery obstruction by lacerating the leaflet in front of the threatened coronary artery[144–147] (Fig. 27.10). The concept of BASILICA is

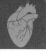

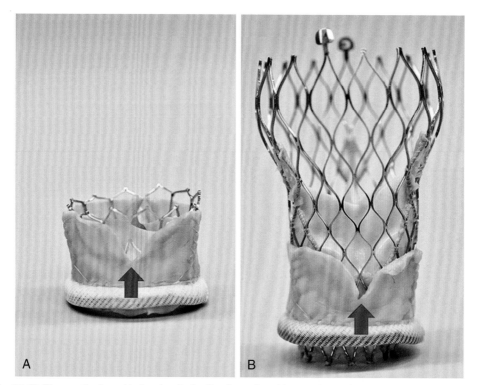

Fig. 27.10 Bioprosthetic or Native Aortic Scallop Intentional Laceration to Prevent Iatrogenic Coronary Artery Obstruction (BASILICA). Through the gap (*red arrows*) in the lacerated leaflet, flow to the coronary sinus can be maintained (i.e., triangle of flow). Results of BASILICA are shown with a SAPIEN 3 valve (Edwards Lifesciences) (A) and an Evolut R valve (Medtronic) (B) implanted in a Mitroflow (Livanova) valve. (From Komatsu I, Mackensen GB, Aldea GS, et al. Bioprosthetic or native aortic scallop intentional laceration to prevent iatrogenic coronary artery obstruction. Part 1: how to evaluate patients for BASILICA. Eurointervention 2019;15:47-54.)

that the intentionally sliced leaflet splays after transcatheter aortic valve implantation, creating a triangular space that allows blood flow toward the sinus and from it to the coronary artery that otherwise would be occluded.

The steps in the BASILICA procedure include leaflet traversal and later laceration, both by an electrified wire. Accurate traversal is guided by fluoroscopy, using front and side views of the bioprosthetic valve leaflet and transesophageal echocardiography (TEE).[148] Clinical data are limited, although procedural and short-term outcomes have shown favorable results, with ability to prevent coronary obstruction in almost all cases without the need to deploy a stent.[149] There may be additional aortic root hydrodynamic benefits of BASILICA, with the potential to reduce the risk for thrombosis and improve valve durability.[150,151]

BASILICA requires a deeper anatomic understanding of coronary cusps and leaflets to achieve precise traversal and laceration. Two perpendicular fluoroscopic angles that can be derived by CT are used. These are the front and side projection angles, which are unique for each coronary cusp.[148] The eccentric location of each coronary ostium in relation to each coronary cusp is especially important when BASILICA is performed in very narrow sinuses and can be identified by CT.

After surgical implantation, left main ostia conventionally originate in front of the center of the left cusp, whereas right coronary ostia commonly deviate mildly toward the commissure between the right and noncoronary cusps. After TAVR, the location of the coronary ostia in relation to the leaflets is random. The suboptimal ability to assess the neosinus size after TAVR and the risk for obstruction should be viewed in relation to the procedural risk of BASILICA. The BASILICA technique may continue to evolve and include dedicated tools that may enable a safe and effective approach for the prevention of coronary obstruction.

Aortic Valve-in-Valve Implantation in Uncommon Bioprostheses

Approximately 15% to 20% of aortic VIV procedures are performed in nonstented surgical bioprostheses. They include stentless surgical valves, those used for rapid deployment (i.e., sutureless valves), and THVs. Clinical outcomes for these diverse subgroups vary.

Stentless bioprosthetic valves lack a metallic frame and have no fluoroscopic markers. They include homografts, autografts, and a variety of bioprostheses such as Freestyle, Freedom, Toronto SPV, and Prima (Edwards Lifesciences).[20] These valves more commonly fail with regurgitation rather than stenosis, and their clinical use has decreased in recent years. VIV procedures in failed stentless valves are associated with higher rates of procedural complications.

Data from the VIVID Registry were used to compare stentless and stented valves in 1598 VIV procedures (18% stentless).[152] Patients with failing stentless bioprostheses were younger than patients with failing stented devices; the mechanism of bioprosthetic failure was predominantly aortic regurgitation in 56.0% of stentless and 20.0% of stented devices. Stentless VIV procedures were more commonly performed with the patient under general anesthesia and with TEE guidance, and self-expandable devices were more commonly used in these procedures. Compared with stented VIV TAVR, stentless VIV TAVR more frequently involved initial device malposition (10.3% vs.

6.2%; $P = 0.014$), a second transcatheter device (7.9% vs. 3.4%; $P < 0.001$), coronary obstruction (6.0% vs. 1.5%; $P < 0.001$), and more than mild PVL ($P < 0.001$). However, the rates of post-VIV severe PPM and elevated postprocedural gradients were lower with stentless than with stented valves. There were nonsignificant trends toward increased mortality rates at 30 days (6.6% vs. 4.4%; $P = 0.12$) and 1 year (15.8% vs. 12.6%; $P = 0.15$) in stentless versus stented VIV TAVR.

Several surgical valves are designed for rapid deployment. The Perceval (Livanova) and Intuity (Edwards Lifesciences) valves are being increasingly implanted. Because of their potential benefits with regard to length of operation and improved hemodynamics, these prostheses are often implanted in patients who are already at relatively high risk and prone to PPM and for whom reoperation is a high-risk procedure. VIV intervention may play a major role in treating suitable patients with failed rapid-deployment valves.

Data on VIV covering 30 failed sutureless valves (including 24 Perceval valves) from the VIVID Registry have been published.[153] Sutureless VIV procedures were mainly performed in patients with relatively small body size, a characteristic associated with a greater risk of PPM. Postprocedural gradients were lower in sutureless VIV than in matched stented VIV procedures, and there were no documented cases of coronary obstruction. Sutureless VIV procedures need to be studied further.

VIV procedures inside THV devices are not rare. They are classified as acute VIV procedures, prompted mainly by device malposition, and VIV procedures performed for THV degeneration. There are many more data on acute VIV procedures than on VIV for THV degeneration,[154] mainly because TAVR is a relatively new procedure that in the early years was associated with some risk of device malposition related to operator inexperience and device characteristics (e.g., short frame, inability to reposition) that made them more prone to malposition. With the large increase in TAVR procedures worldwide and better operator skills and device characteristics, one may expect many fewer aortic VIV procedures in THV devices caused by malposition and more necessitated by device degeneration. Data on clinical outcomes of aortic VIV in failed THV devices are limited.[155,156] The main challenges in these procedures are related more to the risks of coronary obstruction, valve thrombosis, and coronary access and much less to the risks associated with other aortic VIV procedures, such as elevated postprocedural gradients and device malposition. Novel techniques to prevent coronary obstruction in these cases (e.g., BASILICA) are being developed.

FUTURE PERSPECTIVES

Bioprosthetic valves have been increasingly implanted in the past 2 decades instead of mechanical valves. These devices are prone to SVD and ultimately to valve failure. Of concern is the potential for an upcoming pandemic of bioprosthesis failures, particularly as younger patients are treated. These valves may require a less invasive approach when they fail, and the practice of VIV is expected to grow significantly. Current devices and techniques facilitate successful treatment of most degenerated surgical valves.

The main limitations of aortic VIV are directly related to the lack of space in the aortic root (i.e., residual stenosis) and to mechanical complications associated with deflection of failed device tissue (i.e., coronary obstruction). Emerging tools and techniques enable operators to manipulate existing devices and implant new ones inside them safely. Optimal bioprosthetic valves may have a superb durability record in addition to ease of treatment when they fail, but durability should not be viewed as the only consideration in the long-term

management of these cases. Some bioprosthetic valves are not amenable to safe and effective VIV.

The ability to treat failed bioprosthetic valves with VIV with good efficacy and minimal risk (i.e., optimal valve treatability) is an important concept. Considering the available evidence, it seems that advanced transcatheter techniques, such as BVF and BASILICA, may help prevent adverse events after VIV, but continued research is needed.

Other issues are related to the growing need to treat failed THV devices. Novel strategies to remove or displace the failed leaflets of current THVs, thereby facilitating THV-in-THV implantation and enabling coronary access, are in development. Careful preprocedural screening and better operator understanding and techniques will result in further improvements in clinical outcomes for patients undergoing VIV. As long as prosthetic valves have limited durability, we can expect that the techniques and tools to treat them will continue to evolve.

REFERENCES

1. Murray G. Homologous aortic-valve-segment transplants as surgical treatment for aortic and mitral insufficiency. Angiology 1956;7(5): 466-471.
2. Starr A, Edwards ML. Mitral replacement: clinical experience with a ball-valve prostheses. Ann Surg 1961;154:726-740.
3. Ross DN. Homograft replacement of the aortic valve. Lancet 1962;2:487.
4. Ross DN. Replacement of mitral and aortic valves with a pulmonary autograft. Lancet 1967;2:956.
5. Duran CG, Gunning AJ. Heterologous aortic valve transplantation in the dog. Lancet 1965;2:114.
6. Carpentier A, Lemaigre G, Robert L, et al. Biological factors affecting long-term results of valvular heterografts. J Thorac Cardiovasc Surg 1969;38:467.
7. Ionescu MI, Pakrashi BC, Holden MP, et al. Results of aortic valve replacement with fascia lata and pericardial grafts. J Thorac Cardiovasc Surg 1972;64:340.
8. Bonhoeffer P, Boudjemline Y, Saliba Z, et al. Percutaneous replacement of pulmonary valve in a right ventricle to pulmonary artery prosthetic conduit with valve dysfunction. Lancet 2000;356:1403-1405.
9. Cribier A, Eltchaninoff H, Bash A, et al. Percutaneous transcatheter implantation of an aortic valve prosthesis for calcific aortic stenosis: first human case description. Circulation 2002;106(24):3006-3008.
10. Dunning J, Gao H, Chambers J, et al. Aortic valve surgery: marked increases in volume and significant decreases in mechanical valve use—an analysis of 41,227 patients over 5 years from the Society for Cardiothoracic Surgery in Great Britain and Ireland National database. J Thorac Cardiovasc Surg 2011;142(4):776-782.e3. doi: 10.1016/j.jtcvs.2011.04.048.
11. van Geldorp MWA, Eric Jamieson WR, Kappetein AP, et al. Patient outcome after aortic valve replacement with a mechanical or biological pros-thesis: weighing lifetime anticoagulant-related eventrisk against reoperation risk. J Thorac Cardiovasc Surg 2009;137:881-886, 886e1-5.
12. Glaser N, Jackson V, Holzmann MJ, et al. Aortic valve replacement with mechanical vs. biological prostheses in patients aged 50-69 years. Eur Heart J 2016;37(34):2658-2667. doi: 10.1093/eurheartj/ehv580.
13. Eikelboom JW, Connolly SJ, Brueckmann M, et al. Dabigatran versus warfarin in patients with mechanical heart valves. N Engl J Med 2013;369(13):1206-1214.
14. Isaacs AJ, Shuhaiber J, Salemi A, et al. National trends in utilization and in-hospital outcomes of mechanical versus bioprosthetic aortic valve replacements. J Thorac Cardiovasc Surg 2015;149:1262-1263.
15. Brown JM st al. J Thorac Cardiovasc Surg. 2009;137(1):82-90.
16. Côté N, Pibarot P, Clavel MA. Incidence, risk factors, clinical impact, and management of bioprosthesis structural valve degeneration. Curr Opin Cardiol 2017;32:123-129.

17. Repack A, Ziganshin BA, Elefteriades JA, Mukherjee SK. Comparison of quality of life perceivedby patients with bioprosthetic versus mechanicalvalves after composite aortic root replacement. Cardiology 2016;133:3-9.

18. Nishimura RA, Otto CM, Bonow RO, et al. 2017 AHA/ACC Focused Update of the 2014 AHA/ACC Guideline for the Management of PatientsWith Valvular Heart Disease: A Report of the American College of Cardiology/American HeartAssociation Task Force on Clinical Practice Guidelines. J Am Coll Cardiol 2017;70(2):252-289.

19. Baumgartner H, Falk V, Bax JJ, et al. 2017 ESC/EACTS Guidelines for the management of valvular heart disease. Eur Heart J 2017;38(36): 2739-2791. doi: 10.1093/eurheartj/ehx391.

20. Bapat V, Mydin I, Chadalavada S, et al. A guide to fluoroscopic identification and design of bioprosthetic valves: a reference for valve-in-valve procedure. Catheter Cardiovasc Interv 2013;81(5):853-861.

21. Schoen FJ, Levy RJ. Calcification of tissue heart valve substitutes: Progress toward understanding and prevention. Ann Thorac Surg 2005;79:1072-1080.

22. Hilbert SL, Ferrans VJ. Porcine aortic valve bioprostheses: morphologic and functional considerations. J Long Term Eff Med Implants 1992;2: 99-112.

23. ISO. International Standard, ISO 5840:2015. Cardiovascular Implants— Cardiac Valve Prostheses. International Organization for Standardization (ISO), 2015. www.iso.org.

24. Kon ND, Westaby S, Amarasena N, et al. Comparison of implantation techniques using freestyle stentless porcine aortic valve. Ann Thorac Surg 1995;59(4):857-862.

25. Pfeiffer S, Fischlein T, Santarpino G. Sutureless sorin perceval aortic valve implantation. Semin Thorac Cardiovasc Surg 2017;29(1):1-7. doi: 10.1053/j.semtcvs.2016.02.013.

26. Webb JG, Dvir D. Transcatheter aortic valve replacement for bioprosthetic aortic valve failure: the valve-in-valve procedure. Circulation 2013; 127(25):2542-2550.

27. Christakis GT, Buth KJ, Goldman BS, et al. Inaccurate and misleading valve sizing: a proposed standard for valve size nomenclature. Ann Thorac Surg 1998;66:1198-1203.

28. Durko AP, Head SJ, Pibarot P, et al. Characteristics of surgical prosthetic heart valves and problems around labelling: a document from the European Association for Cardio-Thoracic Surgery (EACTS)-The Society of Thoracic Surgeons (STS)-American Association for Thoracic Surgery (AATS) Valve Labelling Task Force. Ann Thorac Surg 2019; 108(1):292-303.

29. Bapat VN, Attia R, Thomas M. Effect of valve design on the stent internal diameter of a bioprosthetic valve: a concept of true internal diameter and its implications for the valve-in-valve procedure. JACC Cardiovasc Interv 2014;7(2):115-127.

30. Dvir D, Leipsic J, Blanke P, et al. Coronary obstruction in transcatheter aortic valve-in-valve implantation: preprocedural evaluation, device selection, protection, and treatment. Circ Cardiovasc Interv 2015;8(1).

31. Côté N, Pibarot P, Clavel MA. Incidence, risk factors, clinical impact, and management of bioprosthesis structural valve degeneration. Curr Opin Cardiol 2017;32:123-129.

32. Fatima B, Mohananey D, Khan FW, et al. Durability data for bioprosthetic surgical aortic valve: a systematic review. JAMA Cardiol 2019;4(1):71-80.

33. Schoen F, Levy R. Tissue heart valves: current challenges and future research perspectives. J Biomed Mater Res 1999;47:439-465.

34. Capodanno D, Petronio AS, Prendergast B, et al. Standardized definitions of structural deterioration and valve failure in assessing long-term durability of transcatheter and surgical aortic bioprosthetic valves: a consensus statement from the European Association of Percutaneous Cardiovascular Interventions endorsed by the European Society of Cardiology and the European Association for Cardiothoracic Surgery. Eur Heart J 2017;0:1-10. doi: 10.1093/eurheartj/ehx303.

35. Zoghbi WA, Chambers JB, Dumesnil JG, et al. Recommendations for evaluation of prosthetic valves with echocardiography and doppler ultrasound: a report From the American Society of Echocardiography's Guidelines and Standards Committee and the Task Force on Prosthetic Valves, developed in conjunction with the American College of Cardiology Cardiovascular Imaging Committee, Cardiac Imaging Committee of the American Heart Association, the European Association of Echocardiography, a registered branch of the European Society of Cardiology, the Japanese Society of Echocardiography and the Canadian Society of Echocardiography, endorsed by the American College of Cardiology Foundation, American Heart Association, European Association of Echocardiography, a registered branch of the European Society of Cardiology, the Japanese Society of Echocardiography, and Canadian Society of Echocardiography. J Am Soc Echocardiogr 2009;22:975-1014.

36. Akins CW, Miller DC, Turina MI, et al. Guidelines for reporting mortality and morbidity after cardiac valve interventions. J Thorac Cardiovasc Surg 2008;135:732-738.

37. Edmunds LH, Clark RE, Cohn LH, et al. Guidelines for reporting morbidity and mortality after cardiac valvular operations. J Thorac Cardiovasc Surg 1996;112:708-711.

38. Dvir D, Bourguignon T, Otto CM, et al. Standardized definition of structural valve degeneration for surgical and transcatheter bioprosthetic aortic valves. Circulation 2018;137(4):388-399.

39. Masters RG, Walley VM, Pipe AL, Keon WJ. Long-term experience with the Ionescu-Shiley pericardial valve. Ann Thorac Surg 1995;60: 288-291.

40. David TE, Feindel CM, Bos J, et al. Aortic valve replacement with Toronto SPV bioprosthesis: optimal patient survival but suboptimal valve durability. J Thorac Cardiovasc Surg 2008;135(1):19-24.

41. Onorati F, Biancari F, De Feo M, et al. Outcome of redo surgical aortic valve replacement in patients 80 years and older: results from the Multicenter RECORD Initiative. Ann Thorac Surg 2014;97: 537-543.

42. Dalrymple-Hay MJ, Crook T, Bannon PG, et al. Risk of reoperation for structural failure of aortic and mitral tissue valves. J Heart Valve Dis 2002;11:419-423.

43. Kaneko T, Vassileva CM, Englum B, et al. Contemporary outcomes of repeat aortic valve replacement: a benchmark for transcatheter valve-in-valve procedures. Ann Thorac Surg 2015;100(4):1298-1304; discussion 1304. doi: 10.1016/j.athoracsur.2015.04.062.

44. Potter DD, Sundt TM, Zehr KJ, et al. Operative risk of reoperative aortic valve surgery. J Thorac Cardiovasc Surg 2005;129:94-103.

45. Naji P, Griffin BP, Sabik JF, et al. Characteristics and outcomes of patients with severe bioprosthetic aortic valve stenosis undergoing redo surgical aortic valve replacement. Circulation 2015;132(21):1953-1960.

46. Leontyev S, Borger MA, Davierwala P, et al. Redo aortic valve surgery: early and late outcomes. Ann Thorac Surg 2011;91(4):1120-1126.

47. Attias D, Nejjari M, Nappi F, et al. How to treat severe symptomatic structural valve deterioration of aortic surgical bioprosthesis: transcatheter valve-in-valve implantation or redo valve surgery? Eur J Cardiothorac Surg 2018;54(6):977-985.

48. Erlebach M, Wottke M, Deutsch MA, et al. Redo aortic valve surgery versus transcatheter valve-in-valve implantation for failing surgical bioprosthetic valves: consecutive patients in a single-center setting. J Thorac Dis 2015;7:1494-1500.

49. Silaschi M, Wendler O, Seiffert M, et al. Transcatheter valve-in-valve implantation versus redo surgical aortic valve replacement in patients with failed aortic bioprostheses. Interact Cardiovasc Thorac Surg 2016.

50. Spaziano M, Mylotte D, Thériault-Lauzier P, et al. Transcatheter aortic valve implantation versus redo surgery for failing surgical aortic bioprostheses: a multicentre propensity score analysis. EuroIntervention 2017;13(10):1149-1156.

51. Amat-Santos IJ, Messika-Zeitoun D, Eltchaninoff H, et al. Infective endocarditis after transcatheter aortic valve implantation: Results from a large multicenter registry. Circulation 2015;131:1566-1574.

52. Saby L, Laas O, Habib G, et al. Positron emission tomography/computed tomography for diagnosis of prosthetic valve endocarditis: Increased valvular 18F-fluorodeoxyglucose uptake as a novel major criterion. J Am Coll Cardiol 2013;61:2374-2382.

53. Lam DH, Itani M, Dvir D. Evaluation of failed prosthetic valves in the valve-in-valve era: Potential for utilizing positron emission tomography/

computed tomography to recognize infective endocarditis. Catheter Cardiovasc Interv 2019. doi: 10.1002/ccd.28185.

54. Aldea GS, Dvir D. Exuberance meets harsh realities in the bioprosthetic tissue valve era. J Thorac Cardiovasc Surg 2018;155(5):e145-e146.

55. McKay CR, Waller BF, Hong R, et al. Problems encountered with catheter balloon valvuloplasty of bioprosthetic aortic valves. Am Heart J 1988; 115:463-465.

56. Orbe LC, Sobrino N, Mate I, et al. Effectiveness of balloon percutaneous valvuloplasty for stenotic bioprosthetic valves in different positions. Am J Cardiol 1991;68:1719-1721.

57. Vahanian A, Alfieri O, Andreotti F, et al. Guidelines on the management of valvular heart disease (version 2012): the Joint Task Force on the Management of Valvular Heart Disease of the European Society of Cardiology (ESC) and the European Association for Cardio-Thoracic Surgery (EACTS). Eur J Cardiothorac Surg 2012;42(4):S1-S44.

58. Boudjemline Y, Pineau E, Borenstein N, et al. New insights in minimally invasive valve replacement: description of a cooperative approach for the off-pump replacement of mitral valves. Eur Heart J 2005;26(19): 2013-2017.

59. Walther T, Falk V, Dewey T, et al. Valve-in-a-valve concept for transcatheter minimally invasive repeat xenograft implantation. J Am Coll Cardiol 2007;50(1):56-60.

60. Azadani AN, Jaussaud N, Matthews PB, et al. Transcatheter aortic valves inadequately relieve stenosis in small degenerated bioprostheses. Interact Cardiovasc Thorac Surg 2010;11(1):70-77.

61. Azadani AN, Jaussaud N, Ge L, et al. Valve-in-valve hemodynamics of 20-mm transcatheter aortic valves in small bioprostheses. Ann Thorac Surg 2011;92(2):548-555.

62. Azadani AN, Tseng EE. Transcatheter valve-in-valve implantation for failing bioprosthetic valves. Future Cardiol 2010;6(6):811-831.

63. Webb JG. Transcatheter valve in valve implants for failed prosthetic valves. Catheter Cardiovasc Interv 2007;70:765-766.

64. Wenaweser P, Buellesfeld L, Gerckens U, Grube E. Percutaneous aortic valve replacement for severe aortic regurgitation in degenerated bioprosthesis: The first valve in valve procedure using the corevalve revalving system. Catheter Cardiovasc Interv 2007;70:760-764.

65. Bedogni F, Laudisa ML, Pizzocri S, et al. Transcatheter valve-in-valve implantation using Corevalve Revalving System for failed surgical aortic bioprostheses. JACC Cardiovasc Interv 2011;4(11):1228-1234.

66. Eggebrecht H, Schäfer U, Treede H, et al. Valve-in-valve transcatheter aortic valve implantation for degenerated bioprosthetic heart valves. JACC Cardiovasc Interv 2011;4(11):1218-1227.

67. Dvir D, Assali A, Vaknin-Assa H, et al. Transcatheter aortic and mitral valve implantations for failed bioprosthetic heart valves. J Invasive Cardiol 2011;23(9):377-381.

68. Sharp AS, Michev I, Colombo A. First trans-axillary implantation of Edwards Sapien valve to treat an incompetent aortic bioprosthesis. Catheter Cardiovasc Interv 2010;75:507 510.

69. Khawaja MZ, Haworth P, Ghuran A, et al. Transcatheter aortic valve implantation for stenosed and regurgitant aortic valve bioprostheses corevalve for failed bioprosthetic aortic valve replacements. J Am Coll Cardiol 2010;55:97-101.

70. Rodés-Cabau J, Dumont E, Doyle D, Lemieux J. Transcatheter valve-in-valve implantation for the treatment of stentless aortic valve dysfunction. J Thorac Cardiovasc Surg 2010;140(1):246-248.

71. Kempfert J, Van Linden A, Linke A, et al. Transapical off-pump valve-in-valve implantation in patients with degenerated aortic xenografts. Ann Thorac Surg 2010;89:1934-1941.

72. Gotzmann M, Mugge A, Bojara W. Transcatheter aortic valve implantation for treatment of patients with degenerated aortic bioprostheses—valve-in-valve technique. Catheter Cardiovasc Interv 2010;76:1000-1006.

73. Pasic M, Unbehaun A, Dreysse S, et al. Transapical aortic valve implantation after previous aortic valve replacement: Clinical proof of the "valve-in-valve" concept. J Thorac Cardiovasc Surg 2011;142:270-277.

74. Seiffert M, Franzen O, Conradi L, et al. Series of transcatheter valve-in-valve implantations in high-risk patients with degenerated bioprostheses in aortic and mitral position. Catheter Cardiovasc Interv. 2010;76:608-615.

75. Wilbring M, Alexiou K, Tugtekin SM, et al. Transcatheter valve-in-valve therapies: Patient selection, prosthesis assessment and selection, results, and future directions. Curr Cardiol Rep 2013;15:341.

76. Webb JG, Wood DA, Ye J, et al. Transcatheter valve-in-valve implantation for failed bioprosthetic heart valves. Circulation 2010;121:1848-1857.

77. Conradi L, Silaschi M, Seiffert M, et al. Transcatheter valve-in-valve therapy using 6 different devices in 4 anatomic positions: Clinical outcomes and technical considerations. J Thorac Cardiovasc Surg 2015; 150(6):1557-1565, 1567.e1-3; discussion 1565-1567. doi: 10.1016/j. jtcvs.2015.08.065.

78. Ihlberg L, Nissen H, Nielsen NE, et al. Early clinical outcome of aortic transcatheter valve-in-valve implantation in the Nordic countries. J Thorac Cardiovasc Surg 2013;146(5):1047-1054; discussion 1054. doi: 10.1016/j.jtcvs.2013.06.045.

79. Latib A, Ielasi A, Montorfano M, et al. Transcatheter valve-in-valve implantation with the Edwards SAPIEN in patients with bioprosthetic heart valve failure: the Milan experience. EuroIntervention 2012; 7(11):1275-1284. doi: 10.4244/EIJV7I11A202.

80. Scholtz S, Piper C, Horstkotte D, et al. Valve-in-valve transcatheter aortic valve implantation with CoreValve/Evolut R© for degenerated small versus bigger bioprostheses. J Interv Cardiol 2018;31(3):384-390. doi: 10.1111/joic.12498.

81. Ussia GP, Barbanti M, Ramondo A, et al. The valve-in-valve technique for treatment of aortic bioprosthesis malposition an analysis of incidence and 1-year clinical outcomes from the italian CoreValve registry. J Am Coll Cardiol 2011;57(9):1062-1068. doi: 10.1016/j. jacc.2010.11.019.

82. Diemert P, Seiffert M, Frerker C, et al. Valve-in-valve implantation of a novel and small self-expandable transcatheter heart valve in degenerated small surgical bioprostheses: the Hamburg experience. Catheter Cardiovasc Interv 2014;84(3):486-493. doi: 10.1002/ccd.25234.

83. Tuzcu EM, Kapadia SR, Vemulapalli S, et al. Transcatheter Aortic Valve Replacement of Failed Surgically Implanted Bioprostheses: The STS/ACC Registry. J Am Coll Cardiol 2018;72(4):370-382.

84. Dvir D, Webb J, Brecker S, et al. Transcatheter aortic valve replacement for degenerative bioprosthetic surgical valves: results from the global valve-in-valve registry. Circulation 2012;126(19):2335-2344. doi: 10.1161/ CIRCULATIONAHA.112.104505.

85. Dvir D, Webb JG, Bleiziffer S, et al. Transcatheter aortic valve implantation in failed bioprosthetic surgical valves. JAMA 2014;312(2):162-170. Available at: http://www.ncbi.nlm.nih.gov/pubmed/25005653.

86. Webb JG, Mack MJ, White JM, et al. Transcatheter aortic valve implantation within degenerated aortic surgical bioprostheses: PARTNER 2 valve-in-valve registry. J Am Coll Cardiol 2017;69(18):2253-2262. doi: 10.1016/j.jacc.2017.02.057.

87. Webb JG, Murdoch DJ, Alu MC, et al. 3-year outcomes after valve-in-valve transcatheter aortic valve replacement for degenerated bioprostheses: The PARTNER 2 registry. J Am Coll Cardiol 2019;73(21):2647-2655.

88. Deeb GM, Chetcuti SJ, Reardon MJ, et al. 1-year results in patients undergoing transcatheter aortic valve replacement with failed surgical bioprostheses. JACC Cardiovasc Interv 2017;10(10):1034-1044.

89. Tchétché D, Chevalier B, Holzhey D, et al. TAVR for failed surgical aortic bioprostheses using a self-expanding device: 1-year results from the prospective VIVA postmarket study. JACC Cardiovasc Interv 2019;12(10):923-932.

90. Alnasser S, Cheema AN, Simonato M, et al. Matched comparison of self-expanding transcatheter heart valves for the treatment of failed aortic surgical bioprosthesis: insights from the Valve-in-Valve International Data Registry (VIVID). Circ Cardiovasc Interv 2017;10(4):e004392. doi: 10.1161/CIRCINTERVENTIONS.116.004392.

91. Seiffert M, Treede H, Schofer J, et al. Matched comparison of next- and early-generation balloon-expandable transcatheter heart valve implantations in failed surgical aortic bioprostheses. EuroIntervention 2018;14(4):e397-e404.

92. Simonato M, Webb J, Bleiziffer S, et al. Current generation balloon-expandable transcatheter valve positioning strategies during aortic valve-in-valve procedures and clinical outcomes. JACC Cardiovasc Interv 2019;12(16):1606-1617.

93. Aziz M, Simonato M, Webb JG, et al. Mortality prediction after transcatheter treatment of failed bioprosthetic aortic valves utilizing various international scoring systems: Insights from the Valve-in-Valve International Data (VIVID). Catheter Cardiovasc Interv 2018;92(6):1163-1170.

94. Pibarot P, Dumesnil JG. Prosthesis-patient mismatch: definition, clinical impact, and prevention. Heart 2006;92:1022-1029.

95. Pibarot P, Weissman NJ, Stewart WJ, et al. Incidence and sequelae of prosthesis-patient mismatch in transcatheter versus surgical valve replacement in high-risk patients with severe aortic stenosis: a PARTNER trial cohort—a analysis. J Am Coll Cardiol 2014;64(13):1323-1334.

96. Zorn GL III, Little SH, Tadros P, et al. Prosthesis-patient mismatch in high-risk patients with severe aortic stenosis: a randomized trial of a self-expanding prosthesis. J Thorac Cardiovasc Surg 2016;151(4):1014-1022, 1023.e1-3.

97. Head SJ, Mokhles MM, Osnabrugge RLJ, et al. The impact of prosthesis-patient mismatch on long-term survival after aortic valve replacement: a systematic review and meta-analysis of 34 observational studies comprising 27 186 patients with 133 141 patient-years. Eur Heart J 2012;33:1518-1529.

98. Herrmann HC, Daneshvar SA, Fonarow GC, et al. Prosthesis-patient mismatch in patients undergoing transcatheter aortic valve replacement: from the STS/ACC TVT registry. J Am Coll Cardiol 2018;72(22):2701-2711.

99. Pibarot P, Simonato M, Barbanti M, et al. Impact of pre-existing prosthesis-patient mismatch on survival following aortic valve-in-valve procedures. JACC Cardiovasc Interv 2018;11(2):133-141.

100. Sathananthan J, Sellers S, Barlow AM, et al. Valve-in-Valve Transcatheter Aortic Valve Replacement and Bioprosthetic Valve Fracture Comparing Different Transcatheter Heart Valve Designs: An Ex Vivo Bench Study. JACC Cardiovasc Interv 2019;12(1):65-75.

101. Peterson MD, Borger MA, Feindel CM, David TE. Aortic annular enlargement during aortic valve replacement: improving results with time. Ann Thorac Surg 2007;83(6):2044-2049.

102. Botzenhardt F, Eichinger WB, Bleiziffer S, et al. Hemodynamic comparison of bioprostheses for complete supra-annular position in patients with small aortic annulus. J Am Coll Cardiol 2005;45(12):2054-2060.

103. Badano LP, Pavoni D, Musumeci S, et al. Stented bioprosthetic valve hemodynamics: is the supra-annular implant better than the intra-annular? J Heart Valve Dis 2006;15(2):238-246.

104. Beckmann E, Martens A, Alhadi F, et al. Aortic valve replacement with sutureless prosthesis: better than root enlargement to avoid patient-prosthesis mismatch? Interact Cardiovasc Thorac Surg 2016;22:744-749. Available at: http://www.ncbi.nlm.nih.gov/pubmed/26920726.

105. Kunadian B, Vijayalakshmi K, Thornley AR, et al. Meta-analysis of valve hemodynamics and left ventricular mass regression for stentless versus stented aortic valves. Ann Thorac Surg 2007;84(1):73-78.

106. Silaschi M, Conradi L, Treede H, et al. Trends in surgical aortic valve replacement in more than 3,000 consecutive cases in the era of transcatheter aortic valve implantations. Thorac Cardiovasc Surg 2016;64(5):382-389.

107. Yao RJ, Simonato M, Dvir D. Optimising the haemodynamics of aortic valve-in-valve procedures. Interv Cardiol 2017;12(1):40-43.

108. Abbasi M, Azadani AN. Leaflet stress and strain distributions following incomplete transcatheter aortic valve expansion. J Biomech 2015;48(13):3663-3671. Available at: http://dx.doi.org/10.1016/j.jbiomech.2015.08.01

109. Bleiziffer S, Erlebach M, Simonato M, et al. Incidence, predictors and clinical outcomes of residual stenosis after aortic valve-in-valve. Heart 2018;104(10):828-834.

110. Zenses AS, Mitchell J, Evin M, et al. In vitro study of valve-in-valve performance with the CoreValve self-expandable prosthesis implanted in different positions and sizes within the Trifecta surgical heart valve. Comput Methods Biomech Biomed Engin 2015;18:2086-2087. Available at: http://www.tandfonline.com/doi/full/10.1080/10255842.2015.1069634.

111. Midha PA, Raghav V, Condado JF, et al. How can we help a patient with a small failing bioprosthesis? An in vitro case study. JACC Cardiovasc Interv 2015;8(15):2026-2033.

112. Simonato M, Azadani AN, Webb J, et al. In vitro evaluation of implantation depth in valve-in-valve using different transcatheter heart valves. EuroIntervention 2016;12:909-917.

113. Simonato M, Webb J, Kornowski R, et al. Transcatheter replacement of failed bioprosthetic valves: large multicenter assessment of the effect of implantation depth on hemodynamics after aortic valve-in-valve. Circ Cardiovasc Interv 2016;9(6):e003651. doi: 10.1161/CIRCINTERVENTIONS.115.003651.

114. Azadani AN, Reardon M, Simonato M, et al. Effect of transcatheter aortic valve size and position on valve-in-valve hemodynamics: an in vitro study. J Thorac Cardiovasc Surg 2017;153(6):1303-1315.

115. Chhatriwalla AK, Allen KB, Saxon JT, et al. Bioprosthetic valve fracture improves the hemodynamic results of valve-in-valve transcatheter aortic valve replacement. Circ Cardiovasc Interv 2017;10(7):e005216. doi: 10.1161/CIRCINTERVENTIONS.117.005216.

116. Bapat VN, Attia RQ, Condemi F, et al. Fluoroscopic guide to an ideal implant position for SAPIEN XT and CoreValve during a Valve-in-Valve procedure. JACC Cardiovasc Interv 2013;6(11):1186-1194.

117. Nielsen-Kudsk JE, Andersen A, Therkelsen CJ, et al. High-pressure balloon fracturing of small dysfunctional Mitroflow bioprostheses facilitates transcatheter aortic valve-in-valve implantation. EuroIntervention 2017;13(9):e1020-e1025. Available at: http://www.pcronline.com/eurointervention/124th_issue/156.

118. Allen KB, Chhatriwalla AK, Saxon JT, et al. Bioprosthetic valve fracture: technical insights from a multicenter study. J Thorac Cardiovasc Surg 2019;158(5):1317-1328.e1. doi: 10.1016/j.jtcvs.2019.01.073.

119. Saxon JT, Allen KB, Cohen DJ, Chhatriwalla AK. Bioprosthetic valve fracture during valve-in-valve TAVR: bench to bedside. Interv Cardiol 2018;13(1):20-26.

120. Johansen P, Engholt H, Tang M, et al. Fracturing mechanics before valve-in-valve therapy of small aortic bioprosthetic heart valves. EuroIntervention 2017;13(9):e1026-e1031.

121. Nielsen-Kudsk JE, Andersen A, Therkelsen CJ, et al. High-pressure balloon fracturing of small dysfunctional Mitroflow bioprostheses facilitates transcatheter aortic valve-in-valve implantation. EuroIntervention 2017;13(9):e1020-e1025.

122. Tanase D, Grohmann J, Schubert S, et al. Cracking the ring of Edwards Perimount bioprosthesis with ultrahigh pressure balloons prior to transcatheter valve in valve implantation. Int J Cardiol 2014;176:1048-1049.

123. Allen KB, Chhatriwalla AK, Cohen DJ, et al. Bioprosthetic valve fracture to facilitate transcatheter valve-in-valve implantation. Ann Thorac Surg 2017;104:1501-1508.

124. Chakravarty T, Sondergaard L, Friedman J, et al. Subclinical leaflet thrombosis in surgical and transcatheter bioprosthetic aortic valves: an observational study. Lancet 2017;389(10087):2383-2392.

125. Makkar RR, Fontana G, Jilaihawi H, et al. Possible subclinical leaflet thrombosis in bioprosthetic aortic valves. N Engl J Med 2015;373(21):2015-2024.

126. Sondergaard L, De Backer O, Kofoed KF, et al. Natural history of subclinical leaflet thrombosis affecting motion in bioprosthetic aortic valves. Eur Heart J 2017;38(28):2201-2207.

127. Jose J, Sulimov DS, El-Mawardy M, et al. Clinical bioprosthetic heart valve thrombosis after transcatheter aortic valve replacement: incidence, characteristics, and treatment outcomes. JACC Cardiovasc Interv 2017;10(7):686-697.

128. Vahidkhah K, Javani S, Abbasi M, et al. Blood stasis on transcatheter valve leaflets and implications for valve-in-valve leaflet thrombosis. Ann Thorac Surg 2017;104(3):751-759. doi: 10.1016/j.athoracsur.2017.02.052.

129. Hatoum H, Moore BL, Maureira P, et al. Aortic sinus flow stasis likely in valve-in-valve transcatheter aortic valve implantation. J Thorac Cardiovasc Surg 2017;154(1):32-43.e1.

130. Vahidkhah K, Azadani AN. Supra-annular Valve-in-Valve implantation reduces blood stasis on the transcatheter aortic valve leaflets. J Biomech 2017;58:114-122.

131. Midha PA, Raghav V, Okafor I, Yoganathan AP. The effect of valve-in-valve implantation height on sinus flow. Ann Biomed Eng 2017;45(2):405-412.

132. Midha PA, Raghav V, Sharma R, et al. The fluid mechanics of transcatheter heart valve leaflet thrombosis in the neosinus. Circulation 2017;136(17):1598-1609.

133. Abdel-Wahab M, Simonato M, Latib A, et al. Clinical valve thrombosis after transcatheter aortic valve-in-valve implantation. Circ Cardiovasc Interv 2018;11(11):e006730. doi: 10.1161/CIRCINTERVENTIONS.118.006730.

134. Flecher EM, Curry JW, Joudinaud TM, et al. Coronary flow obstruction in percutaneous aortic valve replacement. An in vitro study. Eur J Cardiothorac Surg 2007;32:291-294.

135. Ribeiro HB, Nombela-Franco L, Urena M, et al. Coronary obstruction following transcatheter aortic valve implantation: a systematic review. JACC Cardiovasc Interv 2013;6(5):452-461. Available at: http://www.ncbi.nlm.nih.gov/pubmed/23602458.

136. Ribeiro HB, Nombela-Franco L, Urena M, et al. Coronary obstruction following transcatheter aortic valve implantation: a systematic review. JACC Cardiovasc Interv 2013;6:452-461.

137. Ribeiro HB, Webb JG, Makkar RR, et al. Predictive factors, management, and clinical outcomes of coronary obstruction following transcatheter aortic valve implantation: insights from a large multicenter registry. J Am Coll Cardiol 2013;62:1552-1562.

138. Komatsu I, Mackensen GB, Aldea GS, et al. Bioprosthetic or native aortic scallop intentional laceration to prevent iatrogenic coronary artery obstruction. Part 1: how to evaluate patients for BASILICA. EuroIntervention. 2019;15(1):47-54.

139. Ribeiro HB, Rodés Cabau J, Blanke P, et al. Incidence, predictors, and clinical outcomes of coronary obstruction following transcatheter aortic valve replacement for degenerative bioprosthetic surgical valves: insights from the VIVID registry. Eur Heart J 2018;39:687-695.

140. Blanke P, Soon J, Dvir D, et al. Computed tomography assessment for transcatheter aortic valve in valve implantation: the vancouver approach to predict anatomical risk for coronary obstruction and other considerations. J Cardiovasc Comput Tomogr 2016;10(6):491-499.

141. Abramowitz Y, Chakravarty T, Jilaihawi H, et al. Clinical impact of coronary protection during transcatheter aortic valve implantation: first reported series of patients. EuroIntervention 2015;11(5):572-581.

142. Chakravarty T, Jilaihawi H, Nakamura M, et al. Pre-emptive positioning of a coronary stent in the left anterior descending artery for left main protection: a prerequisite for transcatheter aortic valve-in-valve implantation for failing stentless bioprostheses? Catheter Cardiovasc Interv 2013. doi: 10.1002/ccd.25037.

143. Jabbour RJ, Tanaka A, Finkelstein A, et al. Delayed coronary obstruction after transcatheter aortic valve replacement. J Am Coll Cardiol 2018;71(14):1513-1524.

144. Komatsu I, Mackensen GB, Aldea GS, et al. Bioprosthetic or native aortic scallop intentional laceration to prevent iatrogenic coronary artery obstruction. Part 2: how to perform BASILICA. EuroIntervention 2019;15(1):55-66.

145. Lederman RJ, Babaliaros VC, Rogers T, et al. Preventing coronary obstruction during transcatheter aortic valve replacement: from computed tomography to BASILICA. JACC Cardiovasc Interv 2019;12(13):1197-1216.

146. Dvir D, Khan J, Kornowski R, et al. Novel strategies in aortic valve-in-valve therapy including bioprosthetic valve fracture and BASILICA. EuroIntervention 2018;14:AB74-AB82.

147. Khan JM, Dvir D, Greenbaum AB, et al. Transcatheter laceration of aortic leaflets to prevent coronary obstruction during transcatheter aortic valve replacement: concept to first-in-human. JACC Cardiovasc Interv 2018;11:677-689.

148. Komatsu I, Leipsic J, Webb JB, et al. Imaging of aortic valve cusps using commissural alignment: guidance for transcatheter leaflet laceration with BASILICA. JACC Cardiovasc Imaging 2019;12(11 Pt 1):2262-2265. doi: 10.1016/j.jcmg.2019.04.019.

149. Khan JM, Greenbaum AB, Babaliaros VC, et al. The BASILICA trial: prospective multicenter investigation of intentional leaflet laceration to prevent TAVR coronary obstruction. JACC Cardiovasc Interv 2019;12(13):1240-1252.

150. Khodaee F, Qiu D, Dvir D, Azadani AN. Reducing the risk of leaflet thrombosis in transcatheter aortic valve-in-valve implantation by BASILICA: a computational simulation study. EuroIntervention 2019;15(1):67-70.

151. Hatoum H, Maureira P, Lilly S, Dasi LP. Impact of leaflet laceration on transcatheter aortic valve-in-valve washout: BASILICA to solve neosinus and sinus stasis. JACC Cardiovasc Interv 2019;12(13):1229-1237.

152. Duncan A, Moat N, Simonato M, et al. Outcomes following transcatheter aortic valve replacement for degenerative stentless versus stented bioprostheses. JACC Cardiovasc Interv 2019;12(13):1256-1263.

153. Landes U, Dvir D, Schoels W, et al. Transcatheter aortic valve-in-valve implantation in degenerative rapid deployment bioprostheses. EuroIntervention 2019;15(1):37-43.

154. Makkar RR, Jilaihawi H, Chakravarty T, et al. Determinants and outcomes of acute transcatheter valve-in-valve therapy or embolization: a study of multiple valve implants in the U.S. PARTNER trial (Placement of AoRTic TraNscathetER Valve Trial Edwards SAPIEN Transcatheter Heart Valve). J Am Coll Cardiol 2013;62(5):418-430.

155. Barbanti M, Webb JG, Tamburino C, et al. Outcomes of redo transcatheter aortic valve replacement for the treatment of postprocedural and late occurrence of paravalvular regurgitation and transcatheter valve failure. Circ Cardiovasc Interv 2016;9(9):e003930.

156. Schmidt T, Frerker C, Alessandrini H, et al. Redo TAVI: initial experience at two German centres. EuroIntervention 2016;12(7):875-882.

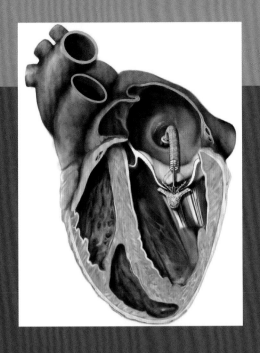

第28章
妊娠期心脏瓣膜疾病

妊娠期心脏瓣膜疾病的相关情况包括已知有心脏瓣膜疾病而来评估潜在母胎风险的怀孕前妇女，已知有心脏瓣膜疾病但未接受孕前咨询的处于怀孕期的妇女，以及在怀孕期间被诊断出患有心脏瓣膜疾病的妇女。无论何种情况，妊娠期间正常的生理变化，如心输出量增加，可能加重瓣膜病变引起的症状及体征。同样，在非妊娠状态下，无症状的合并心脏瓣膜疾病的妇女也可能在妊娠期间出现失代偿表现。虽然在发达国家，怀孕通常是安全的，但患有心脏病的妇女在怀孕期间死亡的风险是无心脏病妇女的100倍，尤其是表现为纽约心功能分级 Ⅲ～Ⅳ级、二尖瓣重度狭窄、主动脉瓣重度狭窄、肺动脉高压及存在机械心脏瓣膜的孕产妇，上述情况是其发生不良事件及结局的高危因素。而且，在妊娠期间，由于自身心脏病带来的药物、辐射或手术等因素，对胎儿亦存在潜在影响。因此，准确的风险评估、孕前咨询及在怀孕期间和围产期采用多学科综合管理至关重要。尽管心脏瓣膜疾病增加了孕产妇和胎儿的风险，但在有经验的中心，在其多学科团队的精心管理下，大多数患有心脏瓣膜疾病的妇女可成功完成妊娠。

周 政

Valvular Heart Disease in Pregnancy

Karen K. Stout, Eric V. Krieger

KEY POINTS

- Pregnancy increases cardiac output and intravascular volume, which increases gradients across stenotic lesions and can exacerbate heart failure in patients with severe valvular stenosis.
- Intravascular volume increases in the immediate postpartum period, and high-risk patients require 48 to 72 hours of close monitoring after delivery.
- The risk of cardiovascular events ranges between 5% and 70% for women with heart disease. Women with higher New York Heart Association class, mitral or aortic stenosis, mechanical valves, pulmonary hypertension, or multiple lesions are at highest risk.

- Women at increased risk for adverse maternal or fetal outcomes should be referred to experienced centers.
- Vaginal delivery is safe for most patients with cardiac lesions. In most cases, cesarean section should be reserved for obstetric indications.
- For women with mechanical valves, meticulous uninterrupted anticoagulation is essential, but morbidity rates remain elevated for this population. Warfarin is recommended for most women in the second and third trimesters despite higher fetal risk. However, the anticoagulation strategy needs to be individualized for each patient.

Although pregnancy is typically safe in developed countries, women with cardiac disease have 100 times greater risk of dying during pregnancy than women without heart disease. Accurate risk assessment, prenatal counseling, and a multidisciplinary approach during pregnancy and in the peripartum period are therefore critical.[1]

Valvular heart disease in pregnant women includes those with known valve disease who come in before pregnancy for evaluation of potential maternal and fetal risk; women with known valve disease who come in during pregnancy without preconception counseling; and women without known cardiac disease who are diagnosed during pregnancy. In each situation, the normal physiologic changes of pregnancy may exacerbate the hemodynamics of the valve lesion, and women who are asymptomatic in the nongravid state may decompensate during pregnancy.

Management is complicated by the potential effects of medication, irradiation, or surgery on the fetus. Despite increased maternal and fetal risks, most women with valvular heart disease can successfully complete pregnancy with careful management by a multidisciplinary team at an experienced center.

PHYSIOLOGIC CHANGES OF PREGNANCY

Normal Hemodynamic Changes

Pregnancy

During pregnancy, there are substantial increases in plasma volume, erythrocyte volume, and cardiac output (Fig. 28.1).[2–6] Cardiac output increases by up to 45%, mostly due to a 20% to 30% increase in heart rate. There is a smaller increase in stroke volume.[7–10] The increase in

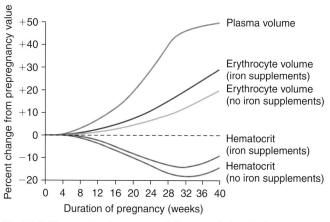

Fig. 28.1 Plasma, Erythrocyte, and Hematocrit Levels During Pregnancy. During pregnancy, there are substantial increases in the plasma and erythrocyte volumes. (From Pitkin RM. Nutritional support in obstetrics and gynecology. Clin Obstet Gynecol 1976:19:489-513.)

cardiac output begins as early as 10 weeks of gestation, with the maximal cardiac output achieved in most by 24 weeks (Fig. 28.2).[9,11,12] Pulmonary pressures should remain normal during pregnancy because there is a decrease in pulmonary vascular resistance through vascular recruitment in the high-capacitance pulmonary circulation.[13] Left ventricular (LV) filling pressures also should remain normal.[14]

During pregnancy, an increase in venous tone augments preload[15] while a decrease in aortic stiffness and alterations in the microcirculation reduce afterload.[7] The decrease in systemic vascular resistance offsets the increase in cardiac output so that blood pressure decreases slightly during pregnancy. LV wall stress decreases by about 30%, reducing the oxygen demand of the myocardium.[5,16] Several studies have suggested that LV contractility may be mildly depressed, although the magnitude of this change is unlikely to be clinically significant.[5,16,17] Stroke volume is maintained in the setting of decreased contractility by the altered loading conditions of pregnancy. At term, the relationship between LV filling pressure and stroke-work index is comparable to that in the nonpregnant state.[18]

Positional Changes

The effects of positional change on hemodynamics may be more prominent in women with valve disease. In the supine position, the gravid uterus can compress the inferior vena cava, resulting in decreased preload, stroke volume, and cardiac output. This can be avoided by use of the left lateral decubitus position.[19] Some patients may also need to labor in the left lateral decubitus position to maintain cardiac output.

Peripartum and Postpartum Changes

Peripartum hemodynamics is affected by uterine contractions, the pain of labor and delivery, and blood loss. Pain increases heart rate, blood pressure, and stroke volume. Uterine contractions reintroduce blood into the circulating blood pool. The increase in intravascular volume with each contraction is accompanied by an increase in heart rate, and cardiac output is augmented by about 20% during each contraction (Fig. 28.3). In the setting of valvular disease, these hemodynamic alterations may result in clinical deterioration.[20,21] Labor and delivery are associated with mild increases in LV diastolic pressure, which may lead to pulmonary edema in a patient with decreased LV compliance. The increase in intravascular volume that occurs with uterine contraction can increase LV end-diastolic pressure and pulmonary edema.

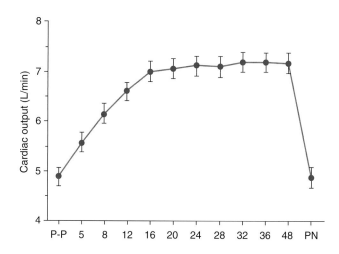
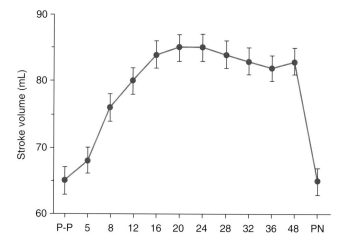
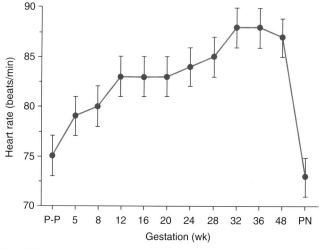

Fig. 28.2 Increases in cardiac output, stroke volume, and heart rate from the nonpregnant state by week of gestation. *P-P,* Prepregnancy; *PN,* postnatal. (From Hunter S, Robson SC. Adaptation of the maternal heart in pregnancy. Br Heart J 1992;68:540-543.)

Blood loss from vaginal delivery partially compensates for the increased blood volume of pregnancy, but acute changes may not be well tolerated by women with valvular heart disease. This is particularly true when the LV diastolic pressure-volume relationship is very steep, as in women with severe aortic stenosis (AS): a small loss of volume

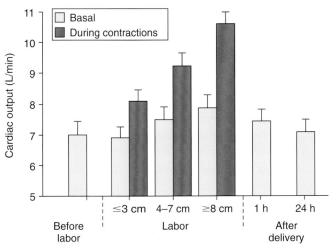

Fig. 28.3 Changes in Cardiac Output During Normal Labor. The increase in intravascular volume with each contraction is accompanied by an increase in the heart rate. (From Hunter S, Robson SC. Adaptation of the maternal heart in pregnancy. Br Heart J 1992;68:540-543.)

and preload may result in a large fall in cardiac output. However, the volume changes with cesarean section are even greater than with vaginal delivery.[6,22] Cesarean section is rarely indicated for cardiac reasons.

After delivery of the placenta, stroke volume and cardiac output rise by about 10% and remain elevated for approximately 24 hours. Over the next 2 weeks, cardiac output declines by 25% to 30%, related to decreases in heart rate and intravascular volume[23,24] (Fig. 28.4). In some patients, symptoms occur after delivery because of intravascular and extravascular volume shifts that result in spontaneous volume loading.[18,25] Although hemodynamics return toward baseline by 6 to 12 weeks after delivery, the new postpartum baseline may be different from the prepregnancy state. For example, LV and aortic dimensions may remain slightly larger than at baseline.[8,24]

Evaluation by Echocardiography
Normal Anatomic Changes
Echocardiographic findings reflect the normal physiologic changes of pregnancy. LV end-diastolic diameter increases by 2 to 3 mm, with no change in the end-systolic dimension, and fractional shortening and ejection fraction are increased compared with baseline values.[26–32] The aortic root and LV outflow tract diameters increase by 1 to 2 mm, and this increase often persists after pregnancy.[33,34] Left atrial area increases by about 2 cm²,[29] in association with an increase in serum atrial natriuretic peptide levels.[35,36] There is a small increase in mitral annulus diameter and a larger increase in tricuspid annulus diameter.[29] A small pericardial effusion is seen in 25% of healthy women during pregnancy.[36]

Doppler Changes
The increased cardiac output of pregnancy leads to increased transvalvular flow velocities. Aortic and LV outflow velocities increase by about 0.3 m/s. The peak transmitral early ventricular filling (E) velocity increases by up to 0.1 m/s, and the late diastolic filling (A) velocity, which reflects atrial contraction, increases by 0.1 to 0.2 m/s.[9,29] The greater increase in A velocity compared with E velocity results in a shift from the normal E/A ratio seen in young adults to an equalized or reversed E/A ratio. The pulmonary venous flow pattern shows an increase in velocity, but not in duration, of the pulmonary venous A wave.[7] For these reasons, pregnant women can appear to have diastolic dysfunction on echocardiography.

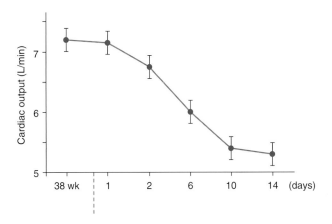

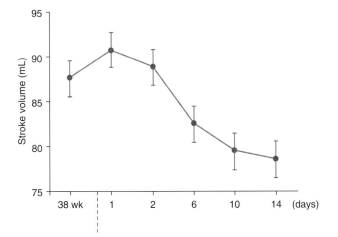

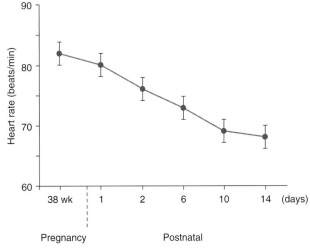

Fig. 28.4 Changes in Cardiac Output, Stroke Volume, and Heart Rate After Normal Delivery. After delivery of the placenta, the stroke volume rises and remains elevated for approximately 24 hours. Over the next 2 weeks, cardiac output declines by 25% to 30%, related to decreases in heart rate and intravascular volume. (From Hunter S, Robson SC. Adaptation of the maternal heart in pregnancy. Br Heart J 1992;68:540-543.)

Mild tricuspid and pulmonic regurgitation are common during pregnancy, as is physiologic mitral regurgitation (MR), which is most likely to be caused by annular dilation.[37] Gradients across native and prosthetic valves increase in pregnancy due to increased flow and increased heart rate. Changes seen with specific cardiac lesions are discussed later.

EPIDEMIOLOGY

The incidence of rheumatic heart disease has declined in industrialized nations over the past 40 years.[38,39] During that same period, there has been an increase in the number of adults with congenital heart disease. Other causes of valve disease, including connective tissue disorders such as Marfan syndrome, are increasingly recognized in pregnancy. Although rheumatic heart disease remains common among pregnant women in economically developing countries, congenital and genetic valvulopathies are more common in industrialized nations.

Patients with congenital or genetic valve disease frequently have additional associated cardiovascular abnormalities. Some patients have a systemic right ventricle or aortic pathology that introduces additive risk. The spectrum of valve disease in pregnancy makes risk assessment somewhat difficult, but general risk factors and risks based on specific valvular lesions can be identified.

RISK FACTORS FOR ADVERSE OUTCOMES

The European Society of Cardiology (ESC) has created the Registry on Pregnancy and Cardiac Disease (ROPAC) and prospectively enrolled more than 1300 pregnant women with heart disease. Among the enrollees with valvular heart disease, the maternal mortality rate was 2.1%, and the hospitalization rate was 38%. This may be an overestimate for North American and European centers because the majority of deaths occurred among women in low-resource countries.[1] Risk is not increased uniformly for all pregnant women with valve disease. Accurate identification of risk factors for adverse outcomes allows preconception counseling and decisions about appropriate monitoring during pregnancy.[40]

A multicenter Canadian study of Cardiac Disease in Pregnancy (CARPREG) prospectively enrolled consecutive pregnant women with all types of heart disease.[41] Predictors of adverse maternal events were a history of cardiac events before pregnancy, New York Heart Association (NYHA) functional class greater than II, cyanosis, left heart obstruction, and systemic ventricular dysfunction. These factors allowed prediction of the risk of maternal events (Table 28.1; Fig. 28.5).[42,43] In this series, the live birth rate was 98%. Maternal risk factors for fetal or neonatal death are listed in Box 28.1.[44] Adverse neonatal events occurred in 20% of pregnancies, including premature birth in 18% and small-for-gestational-age birth weight in 4% of pregnancies. Among the infants of women who had a congenital heart disease but not a recognized genetic syndrome, 7% had congenital heart disease.

In this same study population, 302 pregnancies of women with heart disease were compared with 575 pregnancies of women without heart disease. The rate of maternal cardiac complications was 17% among women with heart disease and 0% in the control group. Heart failure and arrhythmias accounted for most of the cardiac complications (94%). There were two postpartum maternal deaths due to heart failure or pulmonary hypertension. The risk of neonatal complications was 2.3 times normal (Fig. 28.6). The additive effects of maternal cardiac and obstetric risk factors support referral of patients with these conditions to high-risk obstetric clinics (see Fig. 28.5).[45]

The CARPREG study was updated in 2018 in CARPREG II, a prospective study of 1938 pregnancies in women with cardiovascular disease, approximately two thirds of whom had congenital heart disease.[43] On multivariable analysis, 10 clinical predictors of adverse maternal events were identified. Each score was weighted, and a new CAPREG score was developed (see Table 28.1). The strongest predictors of adverse events were prior cardiac events, baseline NHYA class III or higher, cyanosis, and presence of a mechanical heart valve. Other multivariable predictors of adverse outcomes included ventricular

TABLE 28.1 Predictors of Maternal Cardiovascular Events in Pregnancy: Risks for Adverse Maternal Outcomes.

Predictors of Adverse Maternal Events in CARPREG[41]
- Prior cardiac event (heart failure, transient ischemic attack, stroke before pregnancy, or arrhythmia)
- Baseline NYHA functional class > II or cyanosis
- Left heart obstruction (mitral valve area < 2 cm², aortic valve area < 1.5 cm², peak LV outflow tract gradient > 30 mmHg by echocardiography)
- Reduced systemic ventricular systolic function (ejection fraction < 40%)

CARPREG risk score: for each CARPREG predictor that is found, a point is assigned. Risk estimation of maternal cardiovascular complications: 0 points, 5%; 1 point, 27%; >1 point, 75%.

Predictors of Adverse Maternal Events in CARPREG II[43]

• Prior cardiac events or arrhythmia	3 points
• Baseline NYHA functional class III–IV or cyanosis	3 points
• Mechanical valve	3 points
• At least mild systemic ventricular systolic dysfunction	2 points
• High-risk left-sided valve disease/LVOT obstruction	2 points
• Pulmonary hypertension	2 points
• Coronary artery disease	2 points
• High-risk aortopathy	2 points
• No prior cardiac intervention	1 point
• Late pregnancy assessment	1 point

CARPREG II risk score: risk estimation of maternal cardiovascular complications: 0–1 points, 5%; 2 points, 10%; 3 points, 15%; 4 points, 22%; >4 points, 41%.

Predictors of Adverse Maternal Events in ZAHARA[42]
- History of arrhythmia event
- Baseline NYHA functional class > II
- Left heart obstruction (aortic valve peak gradient > 50 mmHg)
- Mechanical valve prosthesis
- Moderate to severe systemic atrioventricular valve regurgitation
- Moderate to severe subpulmonary atrioventricular valve regurgitation
- Use of cardiac medication before pregnancy
- Repaired or unrepaired cyanotic heart disease

CARPREG, Cardiac Disease in Pregnancy study; *LV*, left ventricular; *LVOT*, left ventricular outflow tract; *NYHA*, New York Heart Association; *ZAHARA*, Zwangerschap bij vrouwen met een Aangeboren HARtAfwijking (Pregnancy in Women with Congenital Heart Disease [Dutch study]).
Modified from Regitz-Zagrosek V, Blomstrom Lundqvist C, Borghi C, et al. ESC guidelines on the management of cardiovascular diseases during pregnancy: the Task Force on the Management of Cardiovascular Diseases during Pregnancy of the European Society of Cardiology (ESC). Eur Heart J 2011;32:3147-3197, with the addition of the CARPREG II risk score.

dysfunction, left-sided obstructive lesions, pulmonary hypertension, coronary artery disease, aortopathy, no prior cardiac intervention, and late pregnancy assessment (Fig. 28.7).

In another study of 1302 pregnancies of women with congenital heart disease (ZAHARA), the overall rate of maternal complications

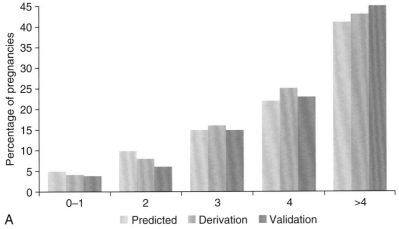

PREDICTOR	POINTS
Prior cardiac events or arrhythmias	3
Baseline NYHA III-IV or cyanosis	3
Mechanical valve	3
Ventricular dysfunction	2
High-risk left-sided valve disease/ left ventricular outflow tract obstruction	2
Pulmonary hypertension	2
Coronary artery disease	2
High-risk aortopathy	2
No prior cardiac intervention	1
Late pregnancy assessment	1

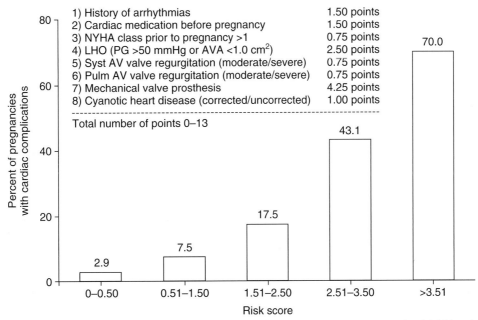

Fig. 28.5 Frequency of Maternal Primary Cardiac Events. Expected maternal cardiovascular risk (%) and observed cardiovascular events (%) for the CARPREG II (A) and ZAHARA (B) cardiovascular risk scores. *AV*, Atrioventricular; *AVA*, aortic valve area; *LHO*, left heart obstruction; *NYHA*, New York Heart Association; *PG*, pressure gradient; *Pulm AV*, subpulmonic atrioventricular; *Syst AV*, systemic atrioventricular. (Data from Drenthen W, Boersma E, Balci A, et al. Predictors of pregnancy complications in women with congenital heart disease. Eur Heart J 2010;31:2124-2132; Silversides CK, Grewal J, Mason J, et al. Pregnancy outcomes in women with heart disease: the CARPREG II study. J Am Coll Cardiol 2018;71:2419-2430.)

was 7.6%. The strongest predictors of adverse maternal events were presence of a mechanical valve, mitral stenosis (MS) or AS, NYHA class greater than II, a history of arrhythmia, and need for cardiac medications before pregnancy. Risk factors were additive, and women with more than one risk factor had a greater than 18% risk of a maternal complication during pregnancy (see Table 28.1).[42]

Using results from published risk models and expert opinion, the World Health Organization (WHO) developed a consensus-based document to risk-stratify women with cardiovascular disease into four categories (Box 28.2).[48] The WHO risk I category designates women with no perceived increased risk, such as those with mitral valve prolapse or repaired ventricular septal defect. Pregnancy is

contraindicated in women with WHO risk IV lesions, such as those with severe symptomatic AS or MS and women with pulmonary arterial hypertension. Although the WHO criteria are derived from expert consensus, they have outperformed CARPREG and ZAHARA in their ability to predict risk[49-51] (Fig. 28.8). The ESC recommends that maternal risk assessment be performed with regard to the WHO risk classification.[52]

Aortic dilation occurs in women with bicuspid aortic valve, tetralogy of Fallot, transposition of the great vessels, or truncus arteriosus and in those who have undergone Ross repair for AS. The risk of aortic rupture or dissection during pregnancy is up to four times greater than at baseline.[53]

BOX 28.1 Maternal Risk Factors for Fetal Complications

Predictors of adverse fetal events
- Cyanosis[41,44,158]
- NYHA functional class > II[41]
- Left heart obstruction[41,158]
- Smoking[41,44,158]
- Anticoagulation[41]
- Multiple gestations[41,44]
- Arrhythmia[158]
- Cardiac medications before pregnancy[44]
- Mechanical heart valve[44]

NYHA, New York Heart Association.

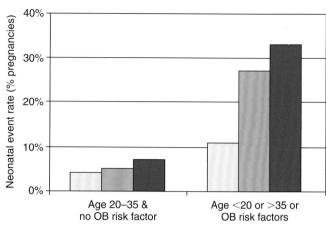

Fig. 28.7 Effect of Age and Maternal Risk Factors on Neonatal Complication Rates. Frequency of neonatal complications when patients are divided into two groups by the presence or absence of maternal noncardiac risk factors. Obstetric *(OB)* high-risk characteristics include smoking, use of anticoagulation, multiple gestations, and younger or older maternal age. *Light blue bars* represent the control group. *Medium blue bars* represent the group of patients with heart disease without left heart obstruction (LHO) or poor functional class/cyanosis. *Dark blue bars* represent high-risk cardiac patients with LHO or poor functional class/cyanosis. (From Siu SC, Colman JM, Sorensen S, et al. Adverse neonatal and cardiac outcomes are more common in pregnant women with cardiac disease. Circulation 2002;105:2179-2184.)

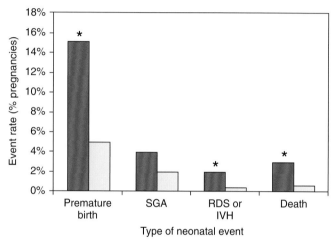

Fig. 28.6 Neonatal Complications in Women With and Without Heart Disease. Specific types of neonatal complications in 302 pregnancies of women with heart disease *(purple bars)* compared with 572 pregnancies in women without heart disease *(light blue bars)*. The asterisk indicates $P < 0.005$ for heart disease versus controls. *Premature birth* indicates delivery before 37 weeks of gestation; *Death* includes fetal and neonatal deaths. *IVH*, Intraventricular hemorrhage; *RDS*, respiratory distress syndrome; *SGA*, small-for-gestational-age birth weight; (From Siu SC, Colman JM, Sorensen S, et al. Adverse neonatal and cardiac outcomes are more common in pregnant women with cardiac disease. Circulation 2002;105:2179-2184.)

BOX 28.2 Pregnancy Risk According to the Modified World Health Organization Classification

WHO risk I: No detectable increased risk of maternal mortality and no or only mild increase in morbidity
- Uncomplicated, small or mild pulmonary stenosis, patent ductus arteriosus, or mitral valve prolapse
- Successfully repaired simple lesions (atrial or ventricular septal defect, patent ductus arteriosus, anomalous pulmonary venous drainage)
- Isolated atrial or ventricular ectopic beats

WHO risk II: Small increased risk of maternal mortality or moderate increase in morbidity
- Unrepaired atrial or ventricular septal defect
- Repaired tetralogy of Fallot

WHO risk II or III (depending on the individual)
- Mild LV impairment
- Native or tissue valvular heart disease not considered WHO I or IV
- Marfan syndrome without aortic dilation
- Aorta < 45 mm associated with bicuspid aortic valve
- Repaired aortic coarctation

WHO risk III: Significantly increased risk of maternal mortality or severe morbidity; expert counseling is required. If pregnancy is decided on, intensive specialist cardiac and obstetric monitoring is needed throughout pregnancy, childbirth, and the puerperium.
- Mechanical heart valve
- Systemic right ventricle
- Fontan circulation
- Unrepaired cyanotic heart disease
- Other complex congenital heart disease
- Aortic dilation of 40–45 mm in Marfan syndrome
- Aortic dilation of 45–50 mm in bicuspid aortic valve

Pregnancy increases the risk of dissection through several mechanisms: estrogen interferes with collagen deposition, elastase accelerates destruction of the elastic lamellae, and relaxin decreases collagen synthesis.[54,55] The risk of dissection in congenital abnormalities does not appear to be as high as the risk in genetic connective tissue disorders. The risk of dissection in women with bicuspid aortic valve appears to be greatest during the third trimester of gestation and at larger diameters, particularly larger than 45 mm (WHO risk III).[54,56,57] Among patients with Marfan syndrome, the risk appears to be highest for those with aortic diameters larger than 40 mm.[58–60]

These studies emphasize the importance of placing the valvular disease in the context of a patient's other cardiac lesions because risk factors for adverse outcomes may be additive. Functional class is important in risk assessment, independent of the underlying hemodynamic abnormality.

Continued

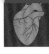

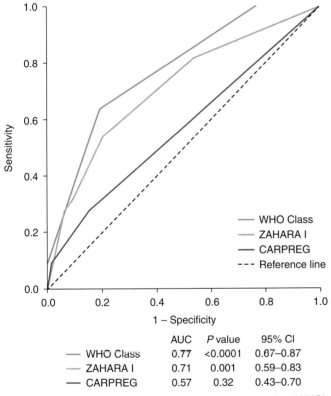

	AUC	P value	95% CI
WHO Class	0.77	<0.0001	0.67–0.87
ZAHARA I	0.71	0.001	0.59–0.83
CARPREG	0.57	0.32	0.43–0.70

Fig. 28.8 Predictive Accuracy of World Health Organization (WHO), CARPREG, and ZAHARA Findings for Maternal Cardiac Events. Receiver operating characteristics demonstrate that the modified WHO classification outperforms the ZAHARA and CARPREG models in predicting maternal cardiovascular events. *AUC,* Area under the curve; *CI,* confidence interval. (From Balci A, Sollie-Szarynska KM, van der Bijl AG, et al. Prospective validation and assessment of cardiovascular and offspring risk models for pregnant women with congenital heart disease. Heart (British Cardiac Society) 2014;100:1373-1381.)

BASIC CLINICAL APPROACH

Evaluation of Disease Severity

The first step in evaluation of the pregnant woman with possible valve disease is to establish a specific diagnosis and determine the severity of disease. The history and physical examination are important to identify cardiac symptoms or abnormal findings on cardiac examination.

Healthy pregnant women frequently have symptoms or examination findings that may suggest heart disease (Box 28.3). A systolic murmur is detected in 80% of pregnant women and typically represents a benign flow murmur.[61] A diastolic murmur or a murmur inconsistent with a flow murmur indicates pathology.

Echocardiography is warranted for pregnant women with a murmur if there is a previous history of cardiac disease, cardiac symptoms, arterial oxygen desaturation, a grade 3/6 or louder systolic murmur, or any diastolic murmur. For these patients, echocardiography allows accurate diagnosis of the location and severity of valve disease, identification of associated hemodynamic abnormalities (e.g., pulmonary hypertension), and assessment of left and right ventricular systolic and diastolic dysfunction.

Transthoracic echocardiography (TTE) is usually adequate to characterize valvular and ventricular function, but in patients with poor acoustic windows or complex anatomy, it may not be sufficient. Transesophageal echocardiography (TEE) may be an adequate surrogate, depending on the information needed. Cardiac magnetic resonance imaging (CMR) appears to be safe in pregnant women, particularly after the first trimester, and it can accurately quantify valvular regurgitation, ventricular dimensions, and ventricular function.[62] Gadolinium contrast is not required for the evaluation of ventricular and valvular function. The safety of gadolinium is controversial in pregnancy, and because it crosses the placenta, it is usually avoided.

Functional status plays an important role in risk stratification. Poor functional class is a risk factor for maternal and fetal complications. In addition to a careful symptom history, exercise testing may have a role in preconception counseling. If there is a significant valvular lesion and impaired functional status, valve surgery before pregnancy may be considered.

Management During Pregnancy
Clinical Monitoring

After the diagnosis of valve disease has been established, the cardiologist should work with a specialist in high-risk obstetrics to determine the optimal intervals for evaluation, assess the potential need for medical therapy, discuss issues related to labor and delivery, and determine and document contingency plans if the patient's condition deteriorates during pregnancy.

Patients with moderate or greater valve disease benefit from close monitoring during pregnancy in a high-risk obstetrics clinic to prevent maternal and fetal complications. Disease severity and the clinical course determine the frequency of evaluation. At each visit, a provider should elicit early evidence of orthopnea, paroxysmal nocturnal dyspnea, decreased exercise tolerance, chest pain, dyspnea, or palpitations. Any change in exercise tolerance or subtle symptoms should prompt reevaluation and repeat imaging. The patient and providers should discuss postpartum interventions and plans for future pregnancies early in the pregnancy.

Medical Therapy

Medications should be carefully reviewed before pregnancy to avoid those that have adverse fetal effects. If a medical therapy is not essential and may not be safe in pregnancy, it should be discontinued. For example, a woman taking an angiotensin-converting enzyme inhibitor for asymptomatic aortic regurgitation should discontinue it during pregnancy. Medications that are critical to maintaining clinical stability may need to be continued or changed before pregnancy. If the patient is receiving teratogenic medications that are essential to maintain stability, pregnancy is likely ill advised.

Occasionally, nonpharmacologic measures such as bed rest, oxygen supplementation, avoiding the supine position, and patient education can be effective at reducing symptoms. Diuretics and β-blockers are used extensively during pregnancy, particularly for patients with MS, to counter the tachycardia of pregnancy. Because metoprolol undergoes accelerated metabolism during pregnancy, the dose should be titrated to heart rate effect in consultation with the obstetrics team.[63] Other β-blockers have similarly accelerated metabolism, and many programs have found atenolol to be most effective; however, atenolol has a class D pregnancy rating from the U.S. Food and Drug Administration because it causes intrauterine growth restriction. Loop diuretics are appropriate to treat pulmonary congestion, but diuretics can precipitate oligohydramnios and therefore should be used with caution.[64]

Effects of Intercurrent Illness

Women with valve disease who are initially well may abruptly decompensate with superimposition of another hemodynamic stress such as an intercurrent febrile illness.[65] Infection may lead to symptoms of angina or heart failure due to the increased metabolic demands from fever and tachycardia. Vaccination against influenza and pneumococcus is appropriate.

Heritability

Women with congenital heart disease, including congenital valve disease, are more likely to have children with congenital heart disease.[66] Bicuspid aortic valve is autosomal dominant in many families, although penetrance is incomplete.[67,68] Children of patients with bicuspid aortic valve are more likely to have associated conditions such as coarctation of the aorta, aortopathy, or hypoplastic left heart syndrome.[67,69]

Fetal echocardiography allows diagnosis of fetal congenital heart disease.[70] However, some congenital heart diseases, such as coarctation of the aorta or patent ductus arteriosus, are difficult or impossible to diagnosis by fetal echocardiography. For women with congenital heart disease, fetal echocardiography is appropriate and provides the opportunity to identify significant cardiac defects and plan appropriately for care of the infant after delivery. If a significant cardiac abnormality is identified, pediatric cardiologists, perinatologists, and cardiac surgeons can be consulted to discuss management. For patients considering termination of pregnancy, the timing of fetal echocardiography should take into account the laws regarding elective termination.

Management in the Peripartum Period

Guidelines do not recommend antibiotic prophylaxis for vaginal delivery in women by valvular heart disease.[52,71,72]

Peripartum Hemodynamic Monitoring

In patients with severe valvular disease, particularly clinically tenuous patients with severe symptomatic left-sided obstructive lesions, a planned delivery with invasive hemodynamic monitoring should be considered. Placement of a pulmonary artery catheter and arterial line allows continuous monitoring of hemodynamics and optimization of preload and afterload during labor and delivery and in the early postpartum period. For high-risk patients, monitoring may be continued for 24 to 48 hours after delivery to avoid deterioration caused by the intravascular fluid shifts that occur during this period.

Type of Delivery

Most women with heart disease should undergo vaginal delivery. Cesarean delivery is reserved for obstetric indications.[52] There is no difference in peripartum complication rates between vaginal delivery and cesarean delivery for women with heart disease.[45] Among 599 consecutive pregnant women with heart disease, 27% were delivered by cesarean section, 96% of them for obstetric indications. Maternal cardiac status was the indication for cesarean section in only 4% of these patients.

Many high-risk obstetrics centers recommend induction of labor to ensure the availability of an experienced cardiac and obstetrics team for patient management. The optimal timing of induction is near term, with a favorable cervix. Prolonged induction is discouraged. Pain control is especially important in women with heart disease to minimize catecholamine surges and changes in heart rate and systemic vascular resistance. Epidural analgesia can cause hypotension, which usually responds to volume infusion. If the fetus has a cardiac abnormality, a planned delivery allows prompt care of the newborn infant. Many centers avoid the Valsalva maneuver to minimize maternal hemodynamic stress. However, this practice is not evidence based and may increase the risk of severe lacerations and postpartum hemorrhage.[73] Cesarean delivery is sometimes performed for women with aortic dimensions greater than 45 mm, chronic aortic dissection, or anticoagulation.[52]

Timing of Surgical Intervention

For women with valvular heart disease who are evaluated before pregnancy, risk assessment can assist in deciding whether surgical intervention before pregnancy is necessary. Most women with mild to moderate valve disease tolerate pregnancy well, and valve surgery can be safely deferred. In cases of severe valve dysfunction, decision making is more difficult. If valve repair is likely, such as mitral valve repair for MR or balloon valvuloplasty for MS, intervention before pregnancy is often appropriate.

If correction requires valve replacement, the advantages of correcting the hemodynamic abnormality must be weighed against the risks of having a prosthetic valve during pregnancy. Mechanical valves require anticoagulation and are associated with high rates of maternal complications (discussed later). Tissue valves have limited durability, and they may exhibit accelerated deterioration in young patients. Some studies suggest that pregnancy hastens valve degeneration, whereas others suggest that the rate of degeneration is related to the young age of the patients, not to pregnancy.

Individualized recommendations are needed, balancing the risk of anticoagulation against the risk of reoperation.[74–76] For all young women undergoing valve replacement surgery, the possibility of a subsequent pregnancy should be taken into account in deciding on the type of valve prosthesis. We rarely recommend placement of a mechanical heart valve in a woman planning pregnancy because of the high incidence of complications with mechanical valves that can occur during pregnancy.

In women with valvular heart disease who are first seen during pregnancy, surgical intervention usually can be deferred until the postpartum period, even if valve disease is severe. However, surgical intervention may be performed during pregnancy in women with valvular heart disease and hemodynamic compromise that does not respond to medical management. Valve surgery during pregnancy has an estimated maternal mortality rate of 3%, similar to the incidence in nonpregnant women, but there is also a fetal loss rate of between 12% and 50%.[77–81]

Risk factors for adverse maternal or fetal outcomes include NYHA class greater than III, LV dysfunction, and emergent procedures, particularly in aortic dissection. To minimize cardiopulmonary bypass time, the most adept surgeon available should perform these surgical procedures because risks to the fetus increase with increasing bypass time.[82] Fetal outcomes appear best when the cardiopulmonary flow rate is greater than 2.4 L/min/m^2, mean arterial pressure is greater than 70 mmHg, and body temperature is near normal.[81] Percutaneous mitral or aortic valvuloplasty can be performed during pregnancy with abdominal shielding to limit fetal radiation exposure. However, complications at the time of valvuloplasty that require urgent surgical intervention would likely have adverse fetal outcomes.

Women with severe valve disease that is medically managed during pregnancy should be referred for surgical intervention after delivery using the same criteria as for valve disease in nonpregnant patients. However, a postpartum improvement in well-being combined with the responsibilities of caring for an infant may result in poor compliance with follow-up visits. A reasonable approach is to evaluate the valve disease carefully during pregnancy, discuss the options with the patient, and if intervention is indicated, proceed with valve surgery or balloon valvuloplasty early in the postpartum period, possibly during the same hospital admission.

SPECIFIC VALVULAR LESIONS AND OUTCOMES

Aortic Stenosis

Severe AS is a high-risk lesion in pregnancy and was found to be a predictor of adverse outcomes in the ZAHARA and CAPREG studies and the WHO classification. The cause of AS in pregnant women usually is congenital, and AS often affects a unicuspid or bicuspid valve.[41,83] Many of these patients have undergone surgical valvuloplasty or commissurotomy in childhood. In 20% of patients with unicuspid aortic valve who received commissurotomy, restenosis requires reoperation at a mean of 13 years after the initial surgery—an age when pregnancy is most likely.[84]

In women with AS, the increased stroke volume of pregnancy is associated with an increase in transvalvular velocity and pressure gradient. Valve area calculations and the dimensionless valve index are reliable and are unlikely to change substantially during pregnancy. Many previously asymptomatic women with AS have symptom onset during pregnancy because of the increased systemic metabolic demands and a limited ability to increase stroke volume.[83,85] Congestive heart failure symptoms also may be caused by decreased LV compliance. The relative tachycardia of pregnancy limits the time for diastolic coronary blood flow, sometimes leading to angina. Superimposed hemodynamic stress, such as infection or anemia, can lead to clinical deterioration in women who were previously tolerating pregnancy.

AS is associated with increased maternal and fetal risk, and the level of risk is related to the severity of LV outflow obstruction.[83,85–87] Symptoms typically increase by one NYHA functional class in about one half of patients. Congestive heart failure is the most common complication, occurring in up to 40% of cases.[41,85,88]

The largest prospective study of pregnancy outcomes for women with AS is the ROPAC, which included 96 women with moderate or severe AS. There were no maternal deaths, but 21% of the patients had a cardiovascular hospitalization during pregnancy, most commonly for heart failure. The hospitalization rate was highest (42%) among women with preexisting severe symptomatic AS.[88] The risk of neonatal complications was also high, affecting as many as 25% of pregnancies in women with AS.[41,88] The most common neonatal complications

were prematurity and small for gestational age birth weight, which may be caused by reduced placental perfusion.[1,89,90]

Most women with mild or moderate stenosis had no cardiac events during pregnancy. Conversely, approximately 40% of those with severe stenosis had events, even if they were asymptomatic before pregnancy.[89,91] Clinical deterioration during pregnancy may persist after delivery and may increase the probability of late interventions in this population.[92]

Echocardiography allows quantification of AS and identification of any associated abnormalities such as aortic aneurysms. Peak and mean aortic gradients rise by approximately 50% between the first and second trimesters because of increased stroke volume before plateauing for the third trimester.[93] The aortic valve area and dimensionless valve index, however, should remain unchanged.

Although AS increases maternal risk, most cases are successfully managed medically. Even when stenosis is severe, maternal death is rare.[85,88,94] If symptoms occur, conservative treatment options include bedrest, diuretics, and rarely, oxygen supplementation. Intercurrent febrile events can be managed with fever reduction and bed rest. With refractory symptoms or hemodynamic compromise, monitoring in the intensive care unit with optimization of preload and afterload may be needed. Balloon aortic valvuloplasty and aortic valve replacement have been performed in patients with severe AS after failure of medical therapy.[88,95–97] Transcatheter aortic valve replacement (TAVR) has been performed during pregnancy as an alternative to surgical aortic valve replacement.[98]

Mitral Stenosis

MS is most often caused by rheumatic valve disease, although congenital MS is encountered.[39] The murmur of MS is difficult to appreciate in the pregnant patient. Echocardiography allows evaluation of stenosis severity and associated regurgitation and the estimation of pulmonary systolic pressure. During pregnancy, increased cardiac output and tachycardia lead to an increase in the mean diastolic inflow gradient of approximately 30%.[93]

Previously asymptomatic patients with MS may first experience symptoms during pregnancy because of the associated hemodynamic changes.[41] A mild decrease in functional status is experienced by 43% of patients, and 30% experience a more severe reduction, although even women without cardiovascular disease have a decrease in functional status with pregnancy.[64] The increased transmitral flow rate and shortened diastolic filling time lead to an increase in left atrial pressure, which may result in pulmonary edema and an obligatory rise in pulmonary artery pressure.

Symptoms most often begin during the second trimester; 30% to 43% of patients with MS develop heart failure, 10% to 20% develop tachyarrhythmias, 50% have a change in medication, and 43% require hospitalization during pregnancy.[64,99] In a large, prospective cohort study published in 2018, 23% of woman with MS were hospitalized during their pregnancy, and 48% of those with severe MS developed heart failure.[100]

β-Blockers may help pregnant women with MS by increasing the diastolic filling time, which results in a decrease in left atrial pressure and an increase in forward stroke volume.[101] Diuretics may be used judiciously to treat volume overload. Because diuresis can impair uteroplacental blood flow, caution must be exercised in their use. For women with rheumatic mitral valve disease, it also is important to continue antibiotic prophylaxis to prevent recurrent rheumatic fever during pregnancy (Fig. 28.9).

Admission to the intensive care unit with placement of a pulmonary artery catheter may be needed to guide medical therapy in severely symptomatic patients. In cases unresponsive to medical therapy,

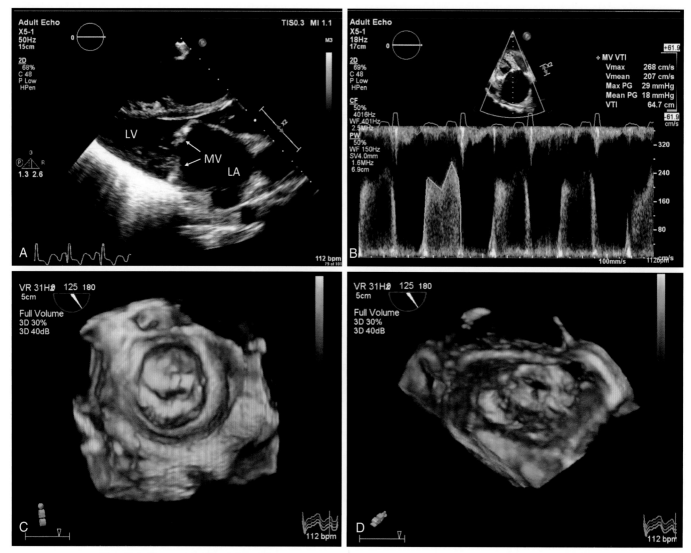

Fig. 28.9 Rheumatic Mitral Stenosis. A 39-year-old woman was seen during the second trimester of her fifth pregnancy. Examination revealed dyspnea and crackles, and she was found to be in atrial fibrillation with a rapid ventricular response. (A) Transthoracic echocardiography shows rheumatic mitral stenosis with characteristic thickening and doming of the mitral leaflets in diastole in a parasternal long-axis view and evidence of a dilated right heart due to pulmonary hypertension. (B) The mean diastolic mitral valve gradient was 18 mmHg at a heart rate of 125 beats/min, indicating severe mitral stenosis. Despite diuresis and rate control, the patient remained very symptomatic. Transesophageal echocardiography was performed to facilitate balloon mitral valvuloplasty. (C) The mitral valve from the left atrial side shows leaflet tip thickening, commissural fusion, and a small effective orifice area (see Video 28.9C ▶). (D) The mitral valve from the left ventricular side shows a slit orifice, commissural fusion, and doming of the valve (see Video 28.9D ▶). After valvuloplasty, the diastolic gradient was 7 mmHg, valve regurgitation remained mild, and the patient improved. *LA,* Left atrium; *LV,* left ventricle; *MV,* mitral valve.

balloon mitral valvuloplasty can be performed during pregnancy. Abdominal shielding limits radiation exposure. Alternatively, TEE guidance can be used to minimize exposure.[102–107] If radiation exposure is kept below 5 rads, the risk of teratogenicity is very low. If exposure is greater than 10 rads, the risks of teratogenicity, central nervous system abnormalities, and childhood cancers increase, and consideration should be given to pregnancy termination.

Immediate and long-term results of balloon valvuloplasty are good even when it is performed during pregnancy. In a study of 71 NYHA class III–IV patients who underwent valvuloplasty, 98% were NYHA class I–II at the end of pregnancy. Event-free survival at 44 months was 54%. Most of the events were initiation of medical therapy, with some

patients undergoing repeat valvuloplasty or mitral valve surgery. The neonates born after maternal valvuloplasty had no clinical abnormalities and normal growth and development.

A 2010 Cochrane review of 68 publications described 1289 women who underwent percutaneous balloon valvuloplasty or surgery for MS during pregnancy. There was a 3% incidence of minor adverse events and a 0.7% rate of major complications.[108] These and other data suggest that if medical therapy fails, percutaneous valvuloplasty is an acceptable option.[109,110]

Patients at highest risk for significant decompensation are those with moderate or severe MS and cardiac symptoms before pregnancy.[64,99,111,112]

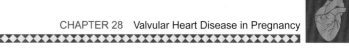

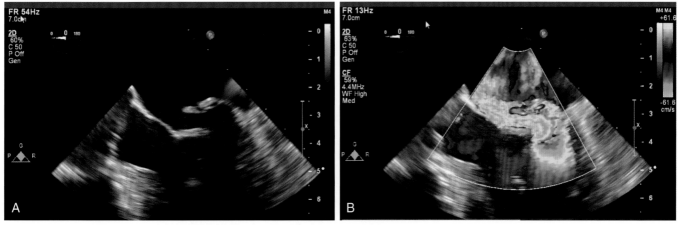

Fig. 28.10 Aortic Regurgitation. A 26-year-old woman with a history of intravenous drug use was seen at 24 weeks' gestation with acute heart failure. She had a wide pulse pressure and a diastolic murmur. (A) The parasternal long-axis view shows a vegetation on the aortic valve with normal left ventricular size. (B) Color Doppler image shows a broad jet of aortic regurgitation. (C) Pulse-wave Doppler of the descending aorta shows holodiastolic flow reversal consistent with severe regurgitation.

Fig. 28.11 Mitral Regurgitation. A 33-year-old woman with a history of a murmur was seen at 20 weeks' gestation with worsening dyspnea. Transthoracic echocardiography suggested significant mitral regurgitation, but acoustic windows were poor. (A) The transesophageal echocardiogram shows flail posterior leaflet. (B) Color Doppler image shows severe eccentric mitral regurgitation (see Video 28.11B ▶).

Aortic Regurgitation

Aortic regurgitation (Fig. 28.10) is uncommon in pregnant women. Causes include a bicuspid aortic valve, previous valvotomy, endocarditis, rheumatic valve disease, and aortic root dilation. In cases of aortic disease, as in Marfan syndrome, the risk of pregnancy is more closely linked to the risk of the aortic dissection than to the aortic regurgitation. In theory, the decrease in systemic vascular resistance and shortened diastole of pregnancy might decrease aortic regurgitant severity. In reality, aortic regurgitation severity is unchanged because the decrease in systemic vascular resistance is counterbalanced by the increased intravascular volume and slight increase in aortic root dimension associated with pregnancy. Typically, patients with aortic regurgitation tolerate pregnancy well. If symptoms occur, a careful evaluation to distinguish worsening of valve disease from other causes of symptoms is warranted.

Mitral Regurgitation

MR in pregnancy (Fig. 28.11) may be caused by mitral valve prolapse, endocarditis, or rheumatic disease. Mild to moderate MR is well tolerated. Mitral valve prolapse is not associated with increased maternal

risk unless severe MR exists.[112,113] Even severe MR may be well tolerated unless atrial fibrillation or pulmonary hypertension complicates the presentation. There have been case reports of clinical deterioration during pregnancy due to acute severe MR due to chordal rupture caused by endocarditis or myxomatous mitral valve disease.

Management of MR includes careful monitoring during pregnancy and at the time of labor and delivery. There are no data to support the use of vasodilators for MR in pregnancy, and pregnancy itself is a powerful afterload reducer.

Right-Sided Valve Disease

Pulmonic stenosis in pregnancy is congenital or postoperative in origin; if severe, it is likely to have been treated in infancy or childhood. Severe native pulmonic stenosis is rare in adults because milder forms of pulmonic stenosis rarely progress to severe stenosis during adulthood. Severe pulmonic stenosis during pregnancy usually is caused by restenosis or prosthetic valve dysfunction in patients with congenital heart disease. Mild to moderate pulmonic stenosis is well tolerated in pregnancy.[64,113] If Doppler tricuspid regurgitant jet velocity is used to estimate right ventricular systolic pressure, the transpulmonic gradient must be subtracted to obtain pulmonary pressure when pulmonic stenosis exists.

Pulmonic stenosis accounted for about 10% of all patients in a series of 599 pregnancies in women with heart disease.[41] There were no adverse cardiac events in these 58 pregnancies, and only 1 patient had worsening cardiac symptoms. However, neonatal complications occurred in 17% of the pregnancies.[41] In a systematic review, there were no maternal cardiovalvular events among 123 women with pulmonic stenosis of a total of 2491 pregnancies.[114] However, noncardiac complications were common, with a higher than expected rate of pregnancy-induced hypertension and fetal complications such as prematurity, small for gestational age, and intrauterine growth retardation.[115] However, these findings have not been confirmed in other studies, and the mechanism for increased pregnancy-induced hypertension is not evident. Tricuspid stenosis in pregnancy is rare, but treatment with percutaneous balloon valvuloplasty has been reported.

Right-sided valve regurgitation is generally well tolerated in pregnancy. Pulmonic regurgitation is caused by congenital heart disease and is most often a sequela of a previous surgical procedure, such as repair of tetralogy of Fallot (Fig. 28.12). Among patients with repaired tetralogy of Fallot, maternal and fetal complication rates are usually low, but severe pulmonic regurgitation with impaired right ventricular function, LV dysfunction, and severe pulmonary hypertension are risk factors for maternal cardiac events.[116,117] Severe pulmonic regurgitation combined with another risk factor (e.g., twin pregnancy, right ventricular dysfunction, a concomitant right-sided obstructive lesion) may increase the risk of adverse outcomes.[118]

Because of the low rate of maternal and fetal complications associated with pulmonic regurgitation, prophylactic pulmonic valve replacement is not necessarily indicated before pregnancy in asymptomatic women.[118] Tricuspid regurgitation may be caused by Ebstein anomaly or previous endocarditis.[41,119]

Prosthetic Valves

In patients with heart valve prostheses, the hemodynamic changes of pregnancy result in increased transvalvular velocities, even with no change in valve function. Prosthetic aortic valves demonstrate a 50% increase in peak and mean gradients by the end of the second trimester, and prosthetic mitral valve mean gradients increase by approximately 35%.[93] Valve area should remain stable during pregnancy. A baseline echocardiographic study early in pregnancy is useful in case symptoms occur later in pregnancy.

Outcomes

The major management issues in women with heart valve prostheses are anticoagulation for mechanical valves and the risk of valve degeneration with tissue valves. Women with tissue or mechanical heart valves have significantly worse outcomes with pregnancy than women without valvular disease; the maternal mortality rate is greater than 1% in most series.[119–123] Older-generation mechanical valves, such as ball-in-cage valves, appear to have higher complication rates but are unlikely to be encountered in pregnant women in the modern era.[121–124]

Women with bioprosthetic valves have fewer thromboembolic or bleeding complications, although they may have adverse outcomes due to bioprosthetic valve dysfunction or myocardial dysfunction.[124] Data regarding the effect of pregnancy on bioprosthetic valves are conflicting. Some series suggest a rapid deterioration during or after pregnancy,[74,122,123,125,126] perhaps because high flow or high calcium turnover during pregnancy can precipitate valve degradation.[75,121] Others have suggested that newer-generation bioprosthetic valves fare better and have found no impact of pregnancy on valve durability.[74–76,126–130]

It remains controversial whether pregnancy accelerates valve degeneration or the degeneration seen in pregnant women reflects the relatively rapid valve degeneration seen in younger patients generally.

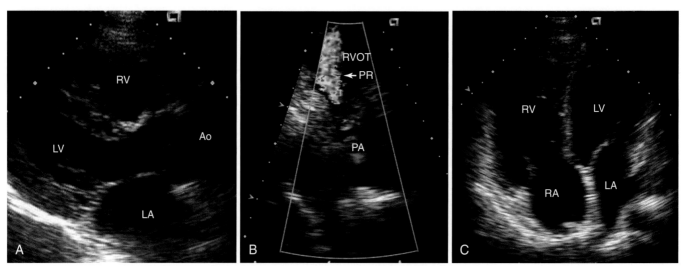

Fig. 28.12 Tetralogy of Fallot. A 28-year-old asymptomatic woman with tetralogy of Fallot was seen in the clinic at 15 weeks' gestation. At 3 years of age, she had had surgical repair with closure of the ventricular septal defect (VSD) and a transannular right ventricular outflow patch for relief of pulmonic stenosis. She had undergone long-term follow-up for pulmonic regurgitation and RV enlargement. (A) The parasternal long-axis view shows an overriding aorta *(Ao)*, VSD patch, and RV enlargement. (B) Color Doppler image of the pulmonic valve and main pulmonary artery *(PA)* demonstrates pulmonic regurgitation *(PR)*. (C) The apical four-chamber view shows RV enlargement with normal systolic function. *LA*, Left atrium; *LV*, left ventricle; *RVOT*, right ventricular outflow tract.

Pregnancy in women with a pulmonic autograft (Ross procedure) has been reported, but the experience with pregnancy after this procedure is limited.[131,132]

Anticoagulation

The importance of effective anticoagulation during pregnancy in women with mechanical prosthetic valves is clear;[126,134] finding an effective regimen that is safe for mother and fetus is difficult.[122,133,134] Each option for anticoagulation during pregnancy carries risks for the mother and fetus. Overall, the maternal complication rate is high among women with mechanical valves; the rate of thromboembolism ranges from 2.5% to 11%, depending on the strategy of anticoagulation used and the types of valves included.[123,135,136] The recommended anticoagulation strategy from the 2014 American Heart Association (AHA)/American College of Cardiology (ACC) valvular heart disease guidelines is shown in Fig. 28.13.[75]

Because warfarin is the most effective form of anticoagulation for mechanical heart valves, there has been a shift toward encouraging the use of warfarin in pregnancy. The 2014 AHA/ACC valve guidelines and the 2011 ESC guidelines for the management of cardiovascular disease in pregnancy recommend continuation of oral anticoagulation throughout the first trimester if the warfarin dose is less than 5 mg/day. Both guidelines favor warfarin during the second and third trimesters regardless of dose.[52,72]

Warfarin provides the lowest risk of thromboembolic complications during pregnancy.[137] The major risks are miscarriage, embryopathy, and fetal bleeding. The risks of warfarin therapy during pregnancy include first-trimester teratogenicity, particularly between the 6th and 12th weeks of gestation. There also may be an increased risk of central nervous system abnormalities with exposure to warfarin at any time during pregnancy.[138] There is a substantial risk of bleeding in the anticoagulated fetus, especially at the time of delivery, and it is necessary to make a transition to unfractionated heparin at approximately 35 weeks' gestation.[52,139]

The incidence of warfarin embryopathy is less than 5% to well over 10%.[65,121,136,139–142] In an attempt to consolidate disparate data, literature reviews are available. One review found a rate of warfarin embryopathy of 6.4%,[136] whereas another found a rate of 7.4% of live births.[76] A reasonable estimate is 4% to 10%. Miscarriage rates may be as high as 29%.[123,137]

Warfarin embryopathy appears to be dose dependent. Women taking more than 5 mg/day had a fetal complication rate of 88%, and embryopathy was seen in 8%. Conversely, in women taking 5 mg or less per day, the fetal complication rate was 15% with no embryopathy. A subsequent study found that adverse fetal events were reduced by 90% for women who took less than 5 mg/day compared with women who took higher doses. Use of low-dose warfarin (>5 mg/day, targeting an international normalized ratio (INR) of 1.5 to 2.0 for patients with mechanical aortic valves has been attempted but was associated with high rates of valve thrombosis.[143] Because of the risk of teratogenicity with warfarin, shared decision making with the patient is critical when choosing an anticoagulation strategy.

Women taking oral anticoagulation should switch to unfractionated heparin or low-molecular-weight heparin (LMWH) at 36 weeks' gestation. Those taking LMWH should switch to unfractionated heparin at least 36 hours before delivery to reduce the risk of maternal hemorrhage. If a woman on oral anticoagulation requires emergent delivery, the risk of maternal hemorrhage is high. Anticoagulation should be reversed, and cesarean delivery is preferred to prevent intracranial hemorrhage in the anticoagulated fetus.[52]

LMWH is safe for the fetus, does not cross the placenta, and can provide effective anticoagulation when used in therapeutic doses and meticulously monitored.[144,145] LMWH is dosed according to peak anti-Xa levels. However, even with therapeutic peak levels (0.7–1.2 U/mL), subtherapeutic trough levels are found in many cases. Periodic monitoring of trough levels is useful, and dose adjustment should be performed by a team with expertise in LMWH dosing.[146] Weight-based fixed dosing of LMWH is absolutely contraindicated.[147] Valve thrombosis occurs in 4% to 9% among pregnant women taking LMWH and occurs most commonly when LMWH is incorrectly prescribed or taken. The vast majority of valve thromboses in women on LMWH occurs in women with therapeutic Xa levels.[148–150]

A disadvantage of heparin therapy is development of osteoporosis, with a small risk (<2%) of symptomatic fractures but a higher risk (33%) of a detectable decrease in bone density.[150–153] Unfractionated heparin offers significant challenges in administration and monitoring of the anticoagulation effect, and there is frequent need for dose adjustment. Indwelling catheters increase the risk of prosthetic valve endocarditis, and it can be difficult to obtain stable therapeutic anticoagulation with subcutaneous bolus dosing.[126,154] In general, the use of unfractionated heparin during pregnancy is associated with a higher risk of thromboembolic complications compared with warfarin.[135]

There are no randomized, controlled trials comparing options for anticoagulation of mechanical heart valves in pregnancy. A Danish nationwide registry found similar levels of maternal complications across 30 years with various strategies of anticoagulation.[155] A large meta-analysis demonstrated lowest maternal risk with warfarin and highest maternal risk with unfractionated heparin.[136] Other available data are include cohort studies, small case series, or case reports. The literature provides reviews and opinions but few quality data on which to base recommendations. Major cardiac societies emphasize the importance of continuous effective anticoagulation with frequent monitoring throughout pregnancy. The guidelines discuss several options for achieving continuous effective anticoagulation, favoring oral anticoagulation in most situations (Fig. 28.14).

With any approach, close monitoring is essential to maintain therapeutic anticoagulation and to avoid bleeding or thrombotic complications. Without meticulous management, the complication rate is high.[121] Many of the hemorrhagic and thromboembolic complications associated with anticoagulation and prosthetic valves during pregnancy can be avoided by a rigorous approach to management and monitoring of anticoagulation.

Acute valve thrombosis during pregnancy is a potentially catastrophic event. Recombinant tissue plasminogen activator does not cross the placenta and is not known to cause teratogenicity in animals.[156] Thrombolytics can cause placental bleeding, however, and may result in premature labor or placental abruption.[157] In a prospective series of 28 prosthetic valve thrombosis episodes in pregnancy, low-dose, slow infusion of tissue plasminogen activator under TEE guidance provided complete lysis in all cases. There was one instance of placental hemorrhage managed with delivery.[158] Considering the high rates of fetal loss associated with emergent valve replacement in pregnancy, low-dose slow-infusion thrombolysis is an appealing option for hemodynamically stable pregnant patients with valve thrombosis.

New anticoagulants such as oral direct thrombin inhibitors or oral Xa inhibitors should not be used in patients with mechanical heart valves.

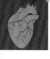

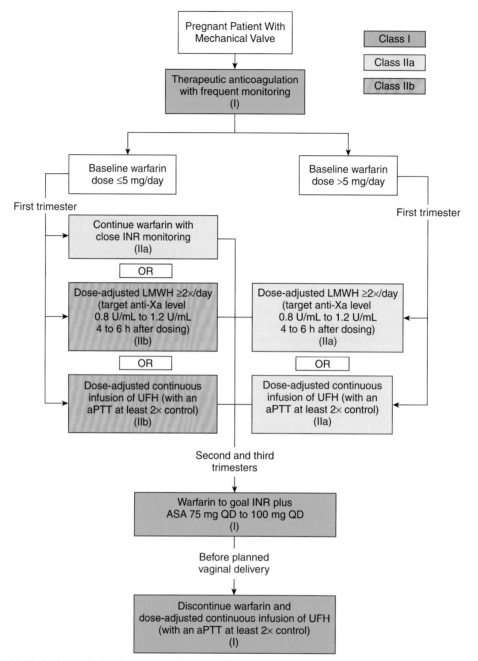

Fig. 28.13 **Anticoagulation in Pregnant Patients With Mechanical Heart Valves.** American Heart Association (AHA)/American College of Cardiology (ACC) guidelines for anticoagulation in pregnant women with mechanical heart valves. *aPTT,* Activated partial thromboplastin time; *anti-Xa,* anti–factor X assay; *ASA,* aspirin; *INR,* international normalized ratio; *LMWH,* low-molecular-weight heparin; *QD,* once daily; *UFH,* unfractionated heparin. (From 2014 AHA/ACC guideline for the management of patients with valvular heart disease. Circulation.2014;129:2440-2492. ©2014 American Heart Association, Inc.)

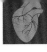

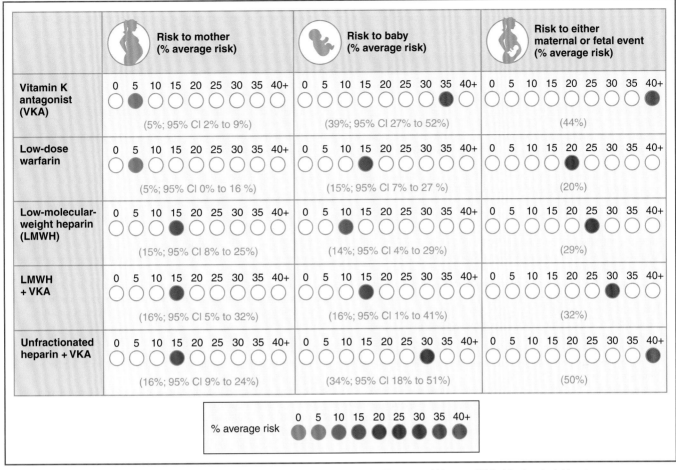

Fig. 28.14 Risks of Various Anticoagulation Strategies in Pregnant Women With Mechanical Heart Valves. Maternal and fetal risks with different anticoagulation regimens were determined from a meta-analysis. Maternal risk is lowest on a vitamin K antagonist *(VKA)* regimen, and fetal risk is lowest on a low-molecular-weight heparin *(LMWH)* regimen. The risk of a maternal or fetal complication during pregnancy is lowest with a low-dose warfarin regimen, although even low-dose warfarin carries a substantial risk of a poor outcome. *CI,* Confidence interval. (Redrawn from Steinberg ZL, Dominguez-Islas CP, Otto CM, et al. Maternal and fetal outcomes of anticoagulation in pregnant women with mechanical heart valves. J Am Coll Cardiol 2017;69:2681-2691.)

REFERENCES

1. Roos-Hesselink JW, Ruys TP, Stein JI, et al. Outcome of pregnancy in patients with structural or ischaemic heart disease: results of a registry of the European Society of Cardiology. Eur Heart J 2012.
2. Cole P, St. John Sutton M. Cardiovascular physiology in pregnancy. In: Douglas PS, ed. Cardiovascular health and disease in women. Philadelphia: W.B. Saunders; 1993:305-328.
3. Katz VL. Physiologic changes during normal pregnancy. Curr Opin Obstet Gynecol 1991;3:750-758.
4. Capeless EL, Clapp JF. Cardiovascular changes in early phase of pregnancy. Am J Obstet Gynecol 1989;161:1449-1453.
5. Gilson GJ, Samaan S, Crawford MH, et al. Changes in hemodynamics, ventricular remodeling, and ventricular contractility during normal pregnancy: a longitudinal study. Obstet Gynecol 1997;89:957-962.
6. Tihtonen K, Koobi T, Yli-Hankala A, Uotila J. Maternal hemodynamics during cesarean delivery assessed by whole-body impedance cardiography. Acta Obstet Gynecol Scand 2005;84:355-361.
7. Mesa A, Jessurun C, Hernandez A, et al. Left ventricular diastolic function in normal human pregnancy. Circulation 1999;99:511-517.
8. Robson SC, Dunlop W. When do cardiovascular parameters return to their preconception values? Am J Obstet Gynecol 1992;167:1479.
9. Mabie WC, DiSessa TG, Crocker LG, et al. A longitudinal study of cardiac output in normal human pregnancy. Am J Obstet Gynecol 1994;170:849-856.
10. Easterling TR, Benedetti TJ. Measurement of cardiac output by impedance technique. Am J Obstet Gynecol 1990;163:1104-1106.
11. Easterling TR, Benedetti TJ, Schmucker BC, Millard SP. Maternal hemodynamics in normal and preeclamptic pregnancies: a longitudinal study. Obstet Gynecol 1990;76:1061-1069.
12. Hunter S, Robson SC. Adaptation of the maternal heart in pregnancy. Br Heart J 1992;68:540-543.
13. Robson SC, Hunter S, Boys RJ, Dunlop W. Serial changes in pulmonary haemodynamics during human pregnancy: a non-invasive study using Doppler echocardiography. Clin Sci (Lond) 1991;80:113-117.
14. Clark SL, Cotton DB, Lee W, et al. Central hemodynamic assessment of normal term pregnancy. Am J Obstet Gynecol 1989;161:1439-1442.
15. Edouard DA, Pannier BM, London GM, et al. Venous and arterial behavior during normal pregnancy. Am J Physiol 1998;274:H1605-H1612.
16. Geva T, Mauer MB, Striker L, et al. Effects of physiologic load of pregnancy on left ventricular contractility and remodeling. Am Heart J 1997;133:53-59.
17. Mone SM, Sanders SP, Colan SD. Control mechanisms for physiological hypertrophy of pregnancy. Circulation 1996;94:667-672.

18. Clark SL. Cardiac disease in pregnancy. Crit Care Clin 1991;7:777-797.

19. McLennan FM, Haites NE, Rawles JM. Stroke and minute distance in pregnancy: a longitudinal study using Doppler ultrasound. Br J Obstet Gynaecol 1987;94:499-506.

20. Robson SC, Dunlop W, Boys RJ, Hunter S. Cardiac output during labour. Br Med J (Clin Res Ed) 1987;295:1169-1172.

21. Lee W, Rokey R, Miller J, Cotton DB. Maternal hemodynamic effects of uterine contractions by M-mode and pulsed-Doppler echocardiography. Am J Obstet Gynecol 1989;161:974-977.

22. Strickland RA, Oliver WC, Jr., Chantigian RC, et al. Anesthesia, cardiopulmonary bypass, and the pregnant patient. Mayo Clin Proc 1991;66:411-429.

23. Robson SC, Dunlop W, Hunter S. Haemodynamic changes during the early puerperium. Br Med J (Clin Res Ed) 1987;294:1065.

24. Robson SC, Hunter S, Boys RJ, Dunlop W. Hemodynamic changes during twin pregnancy. A Doppler and M-mode echocardiographic study. Am J Obstet Gynecol 1989;161:1273-1278.

25. Clark SL, Horenstein JM, Phelan JP, et al. Experience with the pulmonary artery catheter in obstetrics and gynecology. Am J Obstet Gynecol 1985;152:374-378.

26. Easterling TR, Schmucker BC, Benedetti TJ. The hemodynamic effects of orthostatic stress during pregnancy. Obstet Gynecol 1988;72:550-552.

27. Robson SC, Hunter S, Moore M, Dunlop W. Haemodynamic changes during the puerperium: a Doppler and M-mode echocardiographic study. Br J Obstet Gynaecol 1987;94:1028-1039.

28. Robson SC, Hunter S, Boys RJ, Dunlop W. Serial study of factors influencing changes in cardiac output during human pregnancy. Am J Physiol 1989;256:H1060-H1065.

29. Sadaniantz A, Kocheril AG, Emaus SP, et al. Cardiovascular changes in pregnancy evaluated by two-dimensional and Doppler echocardiography. J Am Soc Echocardiogr 1992;5:253-258.

30. Rubler S, Damani PM, Pinto ER. Cardiac size and performance during pregnancy estimated with echocardiography. Am J Cardiol 1977;40:534-540.

31. Vered Z, Poler SM, Gibson P, etal. Noninvasive detection of the morphologic and hemodynamic changes during normal pregnancy. Clin Cardiol 1991;14:327-334.

32. Laird-Meeter K, van de Ley G, Bom TH, et al. Cardiocirculatory adjustments during pregnancy — an echocardiographic study. Clin Cardiol 1979;2:328-332.

33. Easterling TR, Benedetti TJ, Schmucker BC, et al. Maternal hemodynamics and aortic diameter in normal and hypertensive pregnancies. Obstet Gynecol 1991;78:1073-1077.

34. Hart MV, Morton MJ, Hosenpud JD, Metcalfe J. Aortic function during normal human pregnancy. Am J Obstet Gynecol 1986;154:887-891.

35. Bradley TD, Logan AG, Kimoff RJ, et al. Continuous positive airway pressure for central sleep apnea and heart failure. N Engl J Med 2005;353:2025-2033.

36. Pouta AM, Rasanen JP, Airaksinen KE, et al. Changes in maternal heart dimensions and plasma atrial natriuretic peptide levels in the early puerperium of normal and pre-eclamptic pregnancies. Br J Obstet Gynaecol 1996; 103:988-992.

37. Campos O, Andrade JL, Bocanegra J, et al. Physiologic multivalvular regurgitation during pregnancy: a longitudinal Doppler echocardiographic study. Int J Cardiol 1993;40:265-272.

38. Boudoulas H. Etiology of valvular heart disease. Expert Rev Cardiovasc Ther 2003;1:523-532.

39. Soler-Soler J, Galve E. Worldwide perspective of valve disease. Heart 2000; 83:721-725.

40. Stout KK, Daniels CJ, Aboulhosn JA, et al. 2018 AHA/ACC guideline for the management of adults with congenital heart disease: a report of the American College of Cardiology/American Heart Association Task Force on Clinical Practice Guidelines. J Am Coll Cardiol 2019;73(12):1494-1563.

41. Siu SC, Sermer M, Colman JM, et al. Prospective multicenter study of pregnancy outcomes in women with heart disease. Circulation 2001;104: 515-521.

42. Drenthen W, Boersma E, Balci A, et al. Predictors of pregnancy complications in women with congenital heart disease. Eur Heart J 2010;31: 2124-2132.

43. Silversides CK, Grewal J, Mason J, et al. Pregnancy outcomes in women with heart disease: the CARPREG II study. J Am Coll Cardiol 2018;71(21): 2419-2430.

44. Khairy P, Ouyang DW, Fernandes SM, et al. Pregnancy outcomes in women with congenital heart disease. Circulation 2006;113:517-524.

45. Siu SC, Colman JM, Sorensen S, et al. Adverse neonatal and cardiac outcomes are more common in pregnant women with cardiac disease. Circulation 2002;105:2179-2184.

46. Reference deleted in review.

47. Reference deleted in review.

48. Thorne S, MacGregor A, Nelson-Piercy C. Risks of contraception and pregnancy in heart disease. Heart 2006;92:1520-1525.

49. Lu CW, Shih JC, Chen SY, et al. Comparison of 3 risk estimation methods for predicting cardiac outcomes in pregnant women with congenital heart disease. Circ J 2015;79:1609-1617.

50. Pijuan-Domenech A, Galian L, Goya M, et al. Cardiac complications during pregnancy are better predicted with the modified WHO risk score. Int J Cardiol 2015;195:149-154.

51. Balci A, Sollie-Szarynska KM, van der Bijl AG, et al. Prospective validation and assessment of cardiovascular and offspring risk models for pregnant women with congenital heart disease. Heart 2014;100:1373-1381.

52. Regitz-Zagrosek V, Blomstrom Lundqvist C, Borghi C, et al. ESC Guidelines on the management of cardiovascular diseases during pregnancy: the Task Force on the Management of Cardiovascular Diseases during Pregnancy of the European Society of Cardiology (ESC). Eur Heart J 2011;32:3147-3197.

53. Kamel H, Roman MJ, Pitcher A, Devereux RB. Pregnancy and the risk of aortic dissection or rupture: a cohort-crossover analysis. Circulation 2016;134:527-533.

54. Immer FF, Bansi AG, Immer-Bansi AS, et al. Aortic dissection in pregnancy: analysis of risk factors and outcome. Ann Thorac Surg 2003;76:309-314.

55. Bryant-Greenwood GD, Schwabe C. Human relaxins: chemistry and biology. Endocr Rev 1994;15:5-26.

56. Nienaber CA, Fattori R, Mehta RH, et al. Gender-related differences in acute aortic dissection. Circulation 2004;109:3014-3021.

57. McKellar SH, MacDonald RJ, Michelena HI, et al. Frequency of cardiovascular events in women with a congenitally bicuspid aortic valve in a single community and effect of pregnancy on events. Am J Cardiol 2011;107:96-99.

58. Milewicz DM, Dietz HC, Miller DC. Treatment of aortic disease in patients with marfan syndrome. Circulation 2005;111:e150-e157. doi:10.1161/01.CIR.0000155243.70456.F4.

59. Lind J, Wallenburg HCS. The Marfan syndrome and pregnancy: a retrospective study in a Dutch population. Eur J Obstet Gynecol Reprod Biol 2001;98:28-35.

60. Meijboom LJ, Vos FE, Timmermans J, et al. Pregnancy and aortic root growth in the Marfan syndrome: a prospective study. Eur Heart J 2005;26:914-920.

61. Mishra M, Chambers JB, Jackson G. Murmurs in pregnancy: an audit of echocardiography. BMJ 1992;304:1413-1414.

62. De Wilde JP, Rivers AW, Price DL. A review of the current use of magnetic resonance imaging in pregnancy and safety implications for the fetus. Prog Biophys Mol Biol 2005;87:335-353.

63. Wadelius M, Darj E, Frenne G, Rane A. Induction of CYP2D6 in pregnancy. Clin Pharmacol Ther 1997;62:400-407.

64. Hameed A, Karaalp IS, Tummala PP, et al. The effect of valvular heart disease on maternal and fetal outcome of pregnancy. J Am Coll Cardiol 2001; 37:893-899.

65. Elkayam U, Gleicher N. Cardiac problems in pregnancy: diagnosis and management of maternal and fetal disease. 3rd ed. New York: Wiley-Liss; 1998.

66. Siu SC, Colman JM. Heart disease and pregnancy. Heart 2001;85:710-715.

67. Cripe L, Andelfinger G, Martin LJ, et al. Bicuspid aortic valve is heritable. J Am Coll Cardiol 2004;44:138-143.

68. Huntington K, Hunter AG, Chan KL. A prospective study to assess the frequency of familial clustering of congenital bicuspid aortic valve. J Am Coll Cardiol 1997;30:1809-1812.

69. Biner S, Rafique AM, Ray I, et al. Aortopathy is prevalent in relatives of bicuspid aortic valve patients. J Am Coll Cardiol 2009;53:2288-2295.

70. Gardiner HM. Fetal echocardiography: 20 years of progress. Heart 2001;86(Suppl 2):II12-II22.

71. Wilson W, Taubert KA, Gewitz M, et al. Prevention of infective endocarditis: guidelines from the American Heart Association: a guideline from the American Heart Association Rheumatic Fever, Endocarditis, and Kawaski

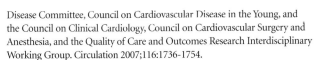

Disease Committee, Council on Cardiovascular Disease in the Young, and the Council on Clinical Cardiology, Council on Cardiovascular Surgery and Anesthesia, and the Quality of Care and Outcomes Research Interdisciplinary Working Group. Circulation 2007;116:1736-1754.

72. Nishimura RA, Otto CM, Bonow RO, et al. 2014 AHA/ACC Guideline for the Management of Patients With Valvular Heart Disease: a report of the American College of Cardiology/American Heart Association Task Force on Practice Guidelines. Circulation 2014;129:e521-e643.

73. Ouyang DW, Khairy P, Fernandes SM, et al. Obstetric outcomes in pregnant women with congenital heart disease. Int J Cardiol 2010;144:195-199.

74. Badduke BR, Jamieson WR, Miyagishima RT, et al. Pregnancy and childbearing in a population with biologic valvular prostheses. J Thorac Cardiovasc Surg 1991;102:179-186.

75. Jamieson WR, Miller DC, Akins CW, et al. Pregnancy and bioprostheses: influence on structural valve deterioration. Ann Thorac Surg 1995; 60:S282-S286; discussion S287.

76. Hung L, Rahimtoola SH. Prosthetic heart valves and pregnancy. Circulation 2003;107:1240-1246.

77. Mahli A, Izdes S, Coskun D. Cardiac operations during pregnancy: review of factors influencing fetal outcome. Ann Thorac Surg 2000;69:1622-1626.

78. Pomini F, Mercogliano D, Cavalletti C, et al. Cardiopulmonary bypass in pregnancy. Ann Thorac Surg 1996;61:259-268.

79. Parry AJ, Westaby S. Cardiopulmonary bypass during pregnancy. Ann Thorac Surg 1996;61:1865-1869.

80. Avila WS, Gouveia AM, Pomerantzeff P, et al. Maternal-fetal outcome and prognosis of cardiac surgery during pregnancy. Arq Bras Cardiol 2009;93:9-14.

81. John AS, Gurley F, Schaff HV, et al. Cardiopulmonary bypass during pregnancy. Ann Thorac Surg 2011;91:1191-1196.

82. Arnoni RT, Arnoni AS, Bonini RC, et al. Risk factors associated with cardiac surgery during pregnancy. Ann Thorac Surg 2003;76:1605-1608.

83. Lao TT, Sermer M, MaGee L, et al. Congenital aortic stenosis and pregnancy—a reappraisal. Am J Obstet Gynecol 1993;169:540-545.

84. Horstkotte D, Loogen F. The natural history of aortic valve stenosis. Eur Heart J 1988;9(Suppl E):57-64.

85. Easterling TR, Chadwick HS, Otto CM, Benedetti TJ. Aortic stenosis in pregnancy. Obstet Gynecol 1988;72:113-118.

86. Arias F, Pineda J. Aortic stenosis and pregnancy. J Reprod Med 1978;20: 229-232.

87. Shime J, Mocarski EJ, Hastings D, et al. Congenital heart disease in pregnancy: short- and long-term implications. Am J Obstet Gynecol 1987;156:313-322.

88. Orwat S, Diller GP, van Hagen IM, et al. Risk of pregnancy in moderate and severe aortic stenosis: from the Multinational ROPAC Registry. J Am Coll Cardiol 2016;68:1727-1737.

89. Yap SC, Drenthen W, Pieper PG, et al. Risk of complications during pregnancy in women with congenital aortic stenosis. Int J Cardiol 2008;126: 240-246.

90. Roberts JM, Gammill HS. Preeclampsia: recent insights. Hypertension 2005;46:1243-1249.

91. Silversides CK, Colman JM, Sermer M, et al. Early and intermediate-term outcomes of pregnancy with congenital aortic stenosis. Am J Cardiol 2003;91:1386-1389.

92. Tzemos N, Silversides CK, Colman JM, et al. Late cardiac outcomes after pregnancy in women with congenital aortic stenosis. Am Heart J 2009;157: 474-480.

93. Samiei N, Amirsardari M, Rezaei Y, et al. Echocardiographic evaluation of hemodynamic changes in left-sided heart valves in pregnant women with valvular heart disease. Am J Cardiol 2016;118:1046-1052.

94. Brian JE, Jr., Seifen AB, Clark RB, et al. Aortic stenosis, cesarean delivery, and epidural anesthesia. J Clin Anesth 1993;5:154-157.

95. Lao TT, Adelman AG, Sermer M, Colman JM. Balloon valvuloplasty for congenital aortic stenosis in pregnancy. Br J Obstet Gynaecol 1993;100:1141-1142.

96. Sreeram N, Kitchiner D, Williams D, Jackson M. Balloon dilatation of the aortic valve after previous surgical valvotomy: immediate and follow up results. Br Heart J 1994;71:558-560.

97. Banning AP, Pearson JF, Hall RJ. Role of balloon dilatation of the aortic valve in pregnant patients with severe aortic stenosis. Br Heart J 1993; 70:544-545.

98. Hodson R, Kirker E, Swanson J, et al. Transcatheter aortic valve replacement during pregnancy. Circ Cardiovasc Interv 2016;9:e004006.

99. Silversides CK, Colman JM, Sermer M, Siu SC. Cardiac risk in pregnant women with rheumatic mitral stenosis. Am J Cardiol 2003;91:1382-1385.

100. van Hagen IM, Thorne SA, Taha N, et al. Pregnancy outcomes in women with rheumatic mitral valve disease: results from the registry of pregnancy and cardiac disease. Circulation 2018;137:806-816.

101. al Kasab SM, Sabag T, al Zaibag M, et al. Beta-adrenergic receptor blockade in the management of pregnant women with mitral stenosis. Am J Obstet Gynecol 1990;163:37-40.

102. Ben Farhat M, Gamra H, Betbout F, et al. Percutaneous balloon mitral commissurotomy during pregnancy. Heart 1997;77:564-567.

103. Gupta A, Lokhandwala YY, Satoskar PR, Salvi VS. Balloon mitral valvotomy in pregnancy: maternal and fetal outcomes. J Am Coll Surg 1998;187:409-415.

104. Patel JJ, Mitha AS, Hassen F, et al. Percutaneous balloon mitral valvotomy in pregnant patients with tight pliable mitral stenosis. Am Heart J 1993;125:1106-1109.

105. Ribeiro PA, Fawzy ME, Awad M, et al. Balloon valvotomy for pregnant patients with severe pliable mitral stenosis using the Inoue technique with total abdominal and pelvic shielding. Am Heart J 1992;124:1558-1562.

106. Ruzyllo W, Dabrowski M, Woroszylska M, et al. Percutaneous mitral commissurotomy with the Inoue balloon for severe mitral stenosis during pregnancy. J Heart Valve Dis 1992;1:209-212.

107. Stoddard MF, Longaker RA, Vuocolo LM, Dawkins PR. Transesophageal echocardiography in the pregnant patient. Am Heart J 1992;124:785-787.

108. Henriquez DD, Roos-Hesselink JW, Schalij MJ, et al. Treatment of valvular heart disease during pregnancy for improving maternal and neonatal outcome. Cochrane Database Syst Rev 2011;(5):CD008128.

109. Esteves CA, Munoz JS, Braga S, et al. Immediate and long-term follow-up of percutaneous balloon mitral valvuloplasty in pregnant patients with rheumatic mitral stenosis. Am J Cardiol 2006;98:812-816.

110. Mangione JA, Lourenco RM, dos Santos ES, et al. Long-term follow-up of pregnant women after percutaneous mitral valvuloplasty. Catheter Cardiovasc Interv 2000;50:413-417.

111. Reimold SC, Rutherford JD. Clinical practice. Valvular heart disease in pregnancy. N Engl J Med 2003;349:52-59.

112. Tang LC, Chan SY, Wong VC, Ma HK. Pregnancy in patients with mitral valve prolapse. Int J Gynaecol Obstet 1985;23:217-221.

113. Jana N, Vasishta K, Khunnu B, et al. Pregnancy in association with mitral valve prolapse. Asia Oceania J Obstet Gynaecol 1993;19:61-65.

114. Drenthen W, Pieper PG, Roos-Hesselink JW, et al. Outcome of pregnancy in women with congenital heart disease: a literature review. J Am Coll Cardiol 2007;49:2303-2311.

115. Drenthen W, Pieper PG, Roos-Hesselink JW, et al. Non-cardiac complications during pregnancy in women with isolated congenital pulmonary valvar stenosis. Heart (British Cardiac Society) 2006;92:1838-1843.

116. Veldtman GR, Connolly HM, Grogan M, et al. Outcomes of pregnancy in women with tetralogy of fallot. J Am Coll Cardiol 2004;44:174-180.

117. Meijer JM, Pieper PG, Drenthen W, et al. Pregnancy, fertility, and recurrence risk in corrected tetralogy of Fallot. Heart 2005;91:801-805. doi:10.1136/hrt.2004.034108.

118. Greutmann M, Von Klemperer K, Brooks R, et al. Pregnancy outcome in women with congenital heart disease and residual haemodynamic lesions of the right ventricular outflow tract. Eur Heart J 2010;31: 1764-1770.

119. Connolly HM, Warnes CA. Ebstein's anomaly: outcome of pregnancy. J Am Coll Cardiol 1994;23:1194-1198.

120. Pavankumar P, Venugopal P, Kaul U, et al. Pregnancy in patients with prosthetic cardiac valve. A 10-year experience. Scand J Thorac Cardiovasc Surg 1988;22:19-22.

121. Sbarouni E, Oakley CM. Outcome of pregnancy in women with valve prostheses. Br Heart J 1994;71:196-201.

122. Born D, Martinez EE, Almeida PA, et al. Pregnancy in patients with prosthetic heart valves: the effects of anticoagulation on mother, fetus, and neonate. Am Heart J 1992;124:413-417.

123. van Hagen IM, Roos-Hesselink JW, Ruys TP, et al. Pregnancy in women with a mechanical heart valve: data of the European Society of Cardiol-

ogy Registry of Pregnancy and Cardiac Disease (ROPAC). Circulation 2015;132:132-142.

124. Lawley CM, Lain SJ, Algert CS, et al. Prosthetic heart valves in pregnancy, outcomes for women and their babies: a systematic review and meta-analysis. BJOG 2015;122:1446-1455.

125. Hanania G, Thomas D, Michel PL, et al. Pregnancy and prosthetic heart valves: a French cooperative retrospective study of 155 cases. Eur Heart J 1994;15:1651-1658.

126. Salazar E, Izaguirre R, Verdejo J, Mutchinick O. Failure of adjusted doses of subcutaneous heparin to prevent thromboembolic phenomena in pregnant patients with mechanical cardiac valve prostheses. J Am Coll Cardiol 1996;27:1698-1703.

127. El SF, Hassan W, Latroche B, et al. Pregnancy has no effect on the rate of structural deterioration of bioprosthetic valves: long-term 18-year follow up results. J Heart Valve Dis 2005;14:481-485.

128. Avila WS, Rossi EG, Grinberg M, Ramires JA. Influence of pregnancy after bioprosthetic valve replacement in young women: a prospective five-year study. J Heart Valve Dis 2002;11:864-869.

129. Cleuziou J, Horer J, Kaemmerer H, et al. Pregnancy does not accelerate biological valve degeneration. Int J Cardiol 2010;145:418-421.

130. Salazar E, Espinola N, Roman L, Casanova JM. Effect of pregnancy on the duration of bovine pericardial bioprostheses. Am Heart J 1999;137: 714-720.

131. Dore A, Somerville J. Pregnancy in patients with pulmonary autograft valve replacement. Eur Heart J 1997;18:1659-1662.

132. Yap SC, Drenthen W, Pieper PG, et al. Outcome of pregnancy in women after pulmonary autograft valve replacement for congenital aortic valve disease. J Heart Valve Dis 2007;16:398-403.

133. Sareli P, England MJ, Berk MR, et al. Maternal and fetal sequelae of anticoagulation during pregnancy in patients with mechanical heart valve prostheses. Am J Cardiol 1989;63:1462-1465.

134. Vongpatanasin W, Hillis LD, Lange RA. Prosthetic heart valves. N Engl J Med 1996;335:407-416.

135. North RA, Sadler L, Stewart AW, et al. Long-term survival and valve-related complications in young women with cardiac valve replacements. Circulation 1999;99:2669-2676.

136. Chan WS, Anand S, Ginsberg JS. Anticoagulation of pregnant women with mechanical heart valves: a systematic review of the literature. Arch Intern Med 2000;160:191-196.

137. Steinberg ZL, Dominguez-Islas CP, Otto CM, et al. Maternal and fetal outcomes of anticoagulation in pregnant women with mechanical heart valves. J Am Coll Cardiol 2017;69:2681-2691.

138. Hall JG, Pauli RM, Wilson KM. Maternal and fetal sequelae of anticoagulation during pregnancy. Am J Med 1980;68:122-140.

139. Ville Y, Jenkins E, Shearer MJ, et al. Fetal intraventricular haemorrhage and maternal warfarin. Lancet 1993;341:1211.

140. Vitale N, De Feo M, De Santo LS, et al. Dose-dependent fetal complications of warfarin in pregnant women with mechanical heart valves. J Am Coll Cardiol 1999;33:1637-1641.

141. Cotrufo M, De Feo M, De Santo LS, et al. Risk of warfarin during pregnancy with mechanical valve prostheses. Obstet Gynecol 2002;99:35-40.

142. Khamooshi AJ, Kashfi F, Hoseini S, et al. Anticoagulation for prosthetic heart valves in pregnancy. Is there an answer? Asian Cardiovasc Thorac Ann 2007;15:493-496.

143. Bian C, Wei Q, Liu X. Influence of heart-valve replacement of warfarin anticoagulant therapy on perinatal outcomes. Arch Gynecol Obstet 2012;285:347-351.

144. Ginsberg JS, Hirsh J, Turner DC, et al. Risks to the fetus of anticoagulant therapy during pregnancy. Thromb Haemost 1989;61:197-203.

145. Ginsberg JS, Kowalchuk G, Hirsh J, et al. Heparin therapy during pregnancy. Risks to the fetus and mother. Arch Intern Med 1989;149: 2233-2236.

146. Goland S, Schwartzenberg S, Fan J, et al. Monitoring of anti-Xa in pregnant patients with mechanical prosthetic valves receiving low-molecular-weight heparin: peak or trough levels? J Cardiovasc Pharmacol Ther 2014;19:451-456.

147. Oran B, Lee-Parritz A, Ansell J. Low molecular weight heparin for the prophylaxis of thromboembolism in women with prosthetic mechanical heart valves during pregnancy. Thromb Haemost 2004; 92:747-751.

148. Rowan JA, McCowan LM, Raudkivi PJ, North RA. Enoxaparin treatment in women with mechanical heart valves during pregnancy. Am J Obstet Gynecol 2001;185:633-637.

149. Yinon Y, Siu SC, Warshafsky C, et al. Use of low molecular weight heparin in pregnant women with mechanical heart valves. Am J Cardiol 2009;104:1259-1263.

150. Ginsberg JS, Kowalchuk G, Hirsh J, et al. Heparin effect on bone density. Thromb Haemost 1990;64:286-289.

151. Dahlman T, Lindvall N, Hellgren M. Osteopenia in pregnancy during long-term heparin treatment: a radiological study post partum. Br J Obstet Gynaecol 1990;97:221-228.

152. Barbour LA, Kick SD, Steiner JF, et al. A prospective study of heparin-induced osteoporosis in pregnancy using bone densitometry. Am J Obstet Gynecol 1994;170:862-869.

153. Dahlman TC. Osteoporotic fractures and the recurrence of thromboembolism during pregnancy and the puerperium in 184 women undergoing thromboprophylaxis with heparin. Am J Obstet Gynecol 1993;168: 1265-1270.

154. Shapiro NL, Kominiarek MA, Nutescu EA, et al. Dosing and monitoring of low-molecular-weight heparin in high-risk pregnancy: single-center experience. Pharmacotherapy 2011;31:678-685.

155. Sillesen M, Hjortdal V, Vejlstrup N, Sorensen K. Pregnancy with prosthetic heart valves - 30 years' nationwide experience in Denmark. Eur J Cardiothorac Surg 2011;40:448-454.

156. Leonhardt G, Gaul C, Nietsch HH, et al. Thrombolytic therapy in pregnancy. J Thromb Thrombolysis 2006;21:271-276.

157. Keyser DL, Biller J, Coffman TT, Adams HP, Jr. Neurologic complications of late prosthetic valve endocarditis. Stroke 1990;21:472-475.

158. Ozkan M, Cakal B, Karakoyun S, et al. Thrombolytic therapy for the treatment of prosthetic heart valve thrombosis in pregnancy with low-dose, slow infusion of tissue-type plasminogen activator. Circulation 2013;128:532-540.